Musculoskeletal Disorders
in the Workplace:
Principles and Practice

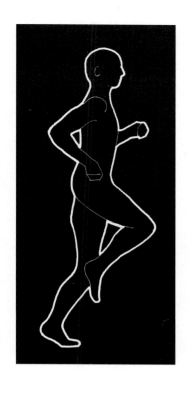

Musculoskeletal Disorders in the Workplace: Principles and Practice

Margareta Nordin, Dr.Med.Sci.
Director Occupational & Industrial Orthopaedic Center,
Hospital for Joint Diseases, New York University Medical Center, New York,
New York

Gunnar B.J. Andersson, M.D., Ph.D.
Professor and Chairman, Department of Orthopaedic Surgery,
Rush-Presbyterian-St. Luke's Medical Center, Chicago, Illinois

Malcolm H. Pope, Dr.Med.Sci., Ph.D.
Professor and Director, Iowa Spine Research Center, University of Iowa,
Iowa City, Iowa

Project Editor: Dawn Leger, Ph.D.
Illustrator: Cristina Mickley Burwell, M.A.
Foreword by Victor H. Frankel, M.D., Ph.D.

with 368 illustrations

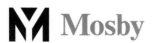 Mosby

St. Louis Baltimore Boston Carlsbad Chicago Naples New York Philadelphia Portland
London Madrid Mexico City Singapore Sydney Tokyo Toronto Wiesbaden

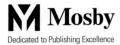

Mosby

Dedicated to Publishing Excellence

A Times Mirror Company

Vice President and Publisher: Anne S. Patterson
Editor: Robert Hurley
Associate Developmental Editor: Christine Pluta
Project Manager: Linda Clarke
Production Editor: Veda King
Design Manager: Nancy J. McDonald
Manufacturing Manager: William A. Winneberger, Jr.

Printed in the United States of America
Composition by Carlisle Communications
Printing/binding by Maple-Vail Book Manufacturing Group

Mosby–Year Book, Inc.
11830 Westline Industrial Drive
St. Louis, Missouri 63146

Library of Congress Cataloging in Publication Data

Musculoskeletal disorders in the workplace: principles and practice /
  [edited by] Margareta Nordin, Gunnar B.J. Andersson, Malcolm H.
  Pope.
      p.   cm.
    Includes bibliographical references and index.
    ISBN 0-8016-7984-2
    1. Musculoskeletal system—Wounds and injuries. 2. Occupational
diseases. 3. Industrial accidents. I. Nordin, Margareta.
II. Pope, M.H. (Malcolm Henry), 1941- . III. Andersson, Gunnar,
1942- .
    [DNLM: 1. Musculoskeletal Diseases—therapy. 2. Musculoskeletal
Diseases—prevention & control. 3. Human Engineering.
4. Occupational Diseases—etiology. WE 140 M9854 1997]
RD732.M875   1997
617.5' 8044—dc20
DNLM/DLC
for Library of Congress   96-24116
                                                                        CIP

97 98 99 00 01 / 9 8 7 6 5 4 3 2 1

Contributors

Kai-Nan An, Ph.D.
Director
Orthopaedics Biomechanics Laboratory
Mayo Clinic
Rochester, Minnesota

Gunnar B.J. Andersson, M.D., Ph.D.
Professor and Chairman
Department of Orthopaedic Surgery
Rush-Presbyterian-St. Luke's Medical Center
Chicago, Illinois

Thomas P. Andriacchi, Ph.D.
Director, Section of Biomechanics
Associate Chairman for Research
Department of Orthopaedic Surgery
Rush-Presbyterian-St. Luke's Medical Center
Chicago, Illinois

James A. Antinnes, B.S.
Graduate Research Assistant
School of Medicine
Pennsylvania State University
Milton S. Hershey Medical Center
Hershey, Pennsylvania

Thomas J. Armstrong, Ph.D.
Professor
Center for Ergonomics
University of Michigan
Ann Arbor, Michigan

Michele Crites Battié, Ph.D., P.T.
Chair
Department of Physical Therapy
Faculty of Rehabilitation Medicine
University of Alberta
Edmonton, Alberta, Canada

Jane Bear-Lehman, M.S., O.T.R.
Assistant Professor
Program in Occupational Therapy
College of Physicians and Surgeons
Columbia University
New York, New York

Michael S. Bednar, M.D.
Assistant Professor for Hand Surgery
Department of Orthopaedic Surgery
Loyola University Medical Center
Maywood, Illinois

Stanley J. Bigos, M.D.
Professor
Department of Orthopaedic Surgery
University of Washington School of Medicine
Seattle, Washington

Donald S. Bloswick, Ph.D., P.E., C.P.E.
Associate Professor
Department of Mechanical Engineering
University of Utah
Salt Lake City, Utah

Paul J. Bonzani, OTR/L, CHT
Occupational Therapist
New England Baptist Hospital
Boston, Massachusetts

Christopher Carlson-Dakes, M.S.
Graduate Research Assistant
Department of Industrial Engineering
University of Wisconsin-Madison
Madison, Wisconsin

Don B. Chaffin, Ph.D.
Professor and Director
Center for Ergonomics
University of Michigan
Ann Arbor, Michigan

Paul S. Cooper, M.D.
Assistant Professor
Department of Orthopaedic Surgery
School of Medicine
University of Connecticut
Farmington, Connecticut

Frances Cuomo, M.D.
Associate Chief, Shoulder and Elbow Service
Department of Orthopaedic Surgery
Hospital for Joint Diseases
New York University Medical Center
New York, New York

Jiri Dvorak, M.D.
Chair, Spine Unit
Department of Neurology
Schulthess Hospital
Zurich, Switzerland

Ulf Eklund, M.D.
Orthopaedic Surgeon
Department of Orthopaedics
Molndal Hospital
Molndal, Sweden

Lawrence J. Fine, M.D., Dr.P.H.
Director
Division of Surveillance, Hazard Evaluations, and Field
Studies
National Institute for Occupational Safety and Health
Cincinnati, Ohio

David Keith Fram, J.D.
Attorney Advisor
Office of Legal Council
United States Equal Employment Opportunity
Commission
Washington, District of Columbia

John D. Frymoyer, M.D.
Dean
College of Medicine
University of Vermont
Burlington, Vermont

Freddie H. Fu, M.D.
Professor of Orthopaedic Surgery
Vice Chairman
Clinical Department of Orthopaedic Surgery
Center for Sports Medicine and Rehabilitation
Pittsburgh, Pennsylvania

Arun Garg, Ph.D.
Professor
Department of Industrial and Systems Engineering
University of Wisconsin
Milwaukee, Wisconsin

Judith Goodwin Greenwood, Ph.D., M.P.H.
Director of Research and Information
West Virginia Worker's Compensation Division
Charleston, West Virginia

Nortin M. Hadler, M.D., F.A.C.P.
Professor of Medicine and Microbiology/Immunology
Division of Rheumatology
School of Medicine
University of North Carolina
Chapel Hill, North Carolina

Scott Haldeman, D.C., M.D., Ph.D.
Associate Clinical Professor
Department of Neurology
University of California, Irvine
Santa Ana, California

Michael R. Hawes, Ph.D.
Associate Dean of Research and Graduate Studies
Human Performance Laboratory
Facilities of Kinesiology and Medicine
University of Calgary
Calgary, Alberta, Canada

Jay Himmelstein, M.D., M.P.H.
Assistant Chancellor for Health Policy
Director, Occupational and Environmental
Health Program
Department of Family and Community Medicine
University of Massachusetts Medical Center
Worcester, Massachusetts

Beat Hintermann, M.D.
Orthopaedic Surgeon
Department of Orthopaedic Surgery
Kantonsspital
University of Basel
Basel, Switzerland

Debra E. Hurwitz, Ph.D.
Assistant Professor
Department of Orthopaedic Surgery
Rush-Presbyterian-St. Luke's Medical Center
Chicago, Illinois

Beth D. Keelan, OTR/L, CHT
Occupational Therapist
New England Baptist Hospital
Boston, Massachusetts

John D. Kemp
President
Very Special Arts
Washington, District of Columbia

Stephan Konz, Ph.D., P.E.
Professor
Department of Industrial Engineering
Kansas State University
Manhattan, Kansas

Karl H.E. Kroemer, Dr.Ing.
Director
Industrial Ergonomics Laboratory
Virginia Polytechnic Institure and State University
Blacksburg, Virginia

Shrawan Kumar, Ph.D., D.Sc.
Professor
Department of Physical Therapy
Faculty of Rehabilitation Medicine
University of Alberta
Edmonton, Alberta, Canada

Steve A. Lavender, Ph.D.
Assistant Professor
Department of Orthopaedic Surgery
Rush-Presbyterian-St. Luke's Medical Center
Chicago, Illinois

Dawn Leger, Ph.D.
Research Associate
Occupational and Industrial Orthopaedic Center
Hospital for Joint Diseases
New York University Medical Center
Associate Research Scientist
School of Education
New York University
New York, New York

William C. Lennen, M.D.
Staff Physician
Naval Medical Center
Portsmouth, Virginia

Jess H. Lonner, M.D.
Chief Resident
Department of Orthopaedic Surgery
Hospital for Joint Diseases
New York University Medical Center
New York, New York

Marianne Magnusson, Dr.Med.Sci.
Associate Faculty
Associate Research Fellow
Iowa Spine Research Center
College of Medicine
University of Iowa
Iowa City, Iowa

Marjorie G. Mangieri, M.S., OTR/L
Occupational Therapist
Occupational Health and Rehabilitation, Inc.
Boston, Massachusetts

Paul H. Marks, M.D., FRCSC
Staff Orthopaedic Surgeon
Division of Orthopaedics
Department of Surgery
Orthopaedic and Arthritic Hospital
University of Toronto
Toronto, Ontario, Canada

William S. Marras, Ph.D.
Professor and Director
Biodynamics Laboratory
Industrial and Systems Engineering Department
Ohio State University
Columbus, Ohio

Bernard J. Martin, Ph.D., Dr.Sci.
Assistant Professor
Center for Ergonomics
University of Michigan
Ann Arbor, Michigan

Tom G. Mayer, M.D.
Executive Medical Director
Productive Rehabilitation Institute of Dallas for
Ergonomics (PRIDE) Research Foundation
Dallas, Texas

Lewis H. Millender, M.D.
Chief
Occupational Medical Center
New England Baptist Hospital
Boston, Massachusetts

Benno M. Nigg, Dr.sc.nat.
Professor and Director
Human Performance Laboratory
Faculties of Kinesiology, Medicine and Engineering
University of Calgary
Calgary, Alberta, Canada

Margareta Nordin, Dr.Med.Sci.
Director
Occupational and Industrial Orthopaedic Center
Hospital for Joint Diseases
New York University Medical Center
Research Associate Professor
Department of Environmental Medicine
New York University School of Medicine
New York, New York

Seoungyeon Oh, M.S.
Graduate Research Assistant
Department of Industrial Engineering
University of Wisconsin
Madison, Wisconsin

Malcolm H. Pope, Dr.Med.Sci., Ph.D.
Professor and Director
Iowa Spine Research Center
Department of Biomedical Engineering
University of Iowa
Iowa City, Iowa

Glenn Pransky, M.D., M.Occ.H.
Associate Director and Associatae Professor
Occupational and Environmental Health Program
Department of Family and Community Medicine
University of Massachusetts Medical Center
Worcester, Massachusetts

Laura Punnett, Sc.D.
Associate Professor
Department of Work Environment
University of Massachusetts
Lowell, Massachusetts

Robert G. Radwin, Ph.D.
Professor
Department of Industrial Engineering
University of Wisconsin
Madison, Wisconsin

Jane A. Rajan, Ph.D., M.Erg.S., C.P.E.
Director
ErgonomiQ Limited
St. Albans, Hertfordshire, United Kingdom

Mark S. Redfern, Ph.D., C.P.E.
Associate Professor
Departments of Otolaryngology and Industrial Engineering
University of Pittsburgh
Pittsburgh, Pennsylvania

David M. Rempel, M.D.
Assistant Professor of Medicine
Ergonomics Program, Richmond Field Station
School of Medicine
University of California, San Francisco
Richmond, California

Per A.F.H. Renström, M.D., Ph.D.
Professor
Department of Orthopaedics and Rehabilitation
McClure Musculoskeletal Research Center
College of Medicine
University of Vermont
Burlington, Vermont

G. James Sammarco, M.D., F.A.C.S.
Volunteer Professor of Orthopaedic Surgery
Department of Orthopaedic Surgery
University of Cincinnati Medical Center
Center for Orthopaedic Care, Inc.
Cincinnati, Ohio

Aaron Sandler, B.S.
Graduate Research Assistant
Department of Biomechanics
Yale University
New Haven, Connecticut

Craig D. Silverton, D.O.
Assistant Professor
Department of Orthopaedics
Rush-Presbyterian-St. Luke's Medical Center
Chicago, Illinois

Mary Louise Skovron, Dr.P.H.
Director, Musculoskeletal Epidemiology Unit
Hospital for Joint Diseases
New York University Medical Center
Assistant Professor
Department of Environmental Medicine
New York University School of Medicine
New York, New York

Dan M. Spengler, M.D.
Professor and Chairman
Department of Orthopaedics and Rehabilitation
Vanderbilt University Medical Center
Nashville, Tennessee

Jeffrey M. Spivak, M.D.
Associate Chief, Spine Service
Department of Orthopaedic Surgery
Hospital for Joint Diseases
New York University Medical Center
New York, New York

K. Tapio Videman, M.D., Dr. Med. Sci.
Professor in Sports Medicine
Department of Health Sciences
University of Jyväskylä
Jyväskylä, Finland

James N. Weinstein, D.O.
Professor
Department of Orthopaedic Surgery
University of Iowa
Director, Spine Diagnostic and Treatment Center
Iowa City, Iowa

Sherri Weiser, Ph.D.
Coordinator, Psychological Services
Occupational and Industrial Orthopaedic Center
Hospital for Joint Diseases
New York University Medical Center
New York, New York

Sam W. Wiesel, M.D.
Chair
Department of Orthopaedic Surgery
Georgetown University Medical Center
Washington, District of Columbia

David G. Wilder, Ph.D., P.E.
Senior Scientist
Iowa Spine Research Center
Visiting Associate Professor
Department of Biomedical Engineering
University of Iowa
Iowa City, Iowa

John R. Wilson, Ph.D.
Professor
Institute for Occupational Ergonomics
Department of Manufacturing Engineering and
Operations Management
University of Nottingham
Nottingham, United Kingdom

Edwin T. Wyman, M.D.
Assistant Clinical Professor
Department of Orthopaedic Surgery
Harvard Medical Center
Visiting Orthopaedic Surgeon
Massachusetts General Hospital
Boston, Massachusetts

Carl H. Zetterberg, M.D., Ph.D.
Professor
Occupational Unit, Orthopaedic Division
Sahlgren Hospital
Göteborg, Sweden

Joseph D. Zuckerman, M.D.
Chair, Department of Orthopaedic Surgery
Chief, Shoulder Surgery
Hospital for Joint Diseases
New York University Medical Center
New York, New York

Foreword

Medical professionals work in an increasingly specialized world brought on by an explosion of knowledge, the demand from society for "the very best" in services, and the need for expertise to keep pace with technological change and innovation. Modern medical history, in particular, is replete with examples of sudden bursts of information that challenged the growth of new domains and abilities. The period of World War II saw an explosion of medical knowledge, rapidly dividing General Surgery into numerous subspecialties. Similarly, the 1970s was a critical period in orthopaedic surgical practice as many subspecialties developed that allowed greater expert use of modern technology.

Occupational orthopaedics is a relatively young specialty that is still evolving rapidly. As in sports medicine, we have learned that it is not sufficient to examine and treat injuries alone. After recovery, an injured football player is expected to return to the game and perform at his previous level of athletic ability. The injured industrial worker is also expected to return to his or her previous level of performance, accomplishing a particular task within a reasonable time frame. Although the average orthopaedic surgeon may be well-versed with the conditions of the gridiron, he or she may not be familiar with the requirements and limitations of the industrial playing field. In industrial medicine, it is not only necessary to "fix" the worker; one must have an idea about how to fix the workplace to prevent further injury. Like sports medicine, the management and prevention of industrial injury demands a dedicated and knowledgeable cadre of physicians, surgeons, and therapists who are able to apply modern knowledge and expertise to a successful medical program.

This volume brings together chapters authored by the most knowledgeable group of surgeons, physicians, scientists, ergonomists, and therapists currently addressing the prevention and management of workplace injury. The editors, Drs. Nordin, Andersson, and Pope, are world leaders in their respective fields of ergonomics/therapy, orthopaedic surgery, and engineering, and have created a most versatile and practical tool for the many allied-health professionals involved with work-related injuries. I am certain that this treatise will have a strong impact within the industry and on the management of patients well into the 21st century.

Victor H. Frankel, M.D., Ph.D.
President
Hospital for Joint Diseases
New York University Medical Center
New York, New York

Contents

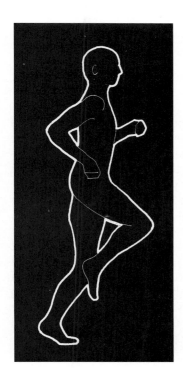

Introduction

There have been great advances in the prevention, treatment, and rehabilitation of work-related musculoskeletal disorders throughout the industrialized world. Because every sector of the economy is undergoing changes and adjustments and the healthcare delivery system itself is under scrutiny, a comprehensive analysis of the nature of work-related musculoskeletal disorders is needed. Provided in this text is the latest information about ergonomics and a segmental evaluation of recommended approaches for clinical evaluation and patient care for a broad spectrum of healthcare providers working in the area of occupational medicine. Work-related musculoskeletal disorders are very costly to the economy. Good ergonomics and prevention strategies of other kinds will save money in the long run.

Each chapter of the book provides insight into the implications of work-related musculoskeletal disorders for the patient and the healthcare team of physicians, therapists, and ergonomists. The information presented herein complements the broad-spectrum textbooks by focusing exclusively on the work-related aspects of musculoskeletal disorders. The clinical evaluation and treatment information looks at disorders identified as common-site injuries from epidemiologic studies and discusses treatment options in terms of return to work and workplace adaptation. Experts in each area have written about the latest advances in their specialties with specific reference to the workplace, and each chapter draws on ground-breaking research studies at universities and medical centers across the United States and Europe.

BASIC CONCEPTS

The chapters in this section cover the "basic concepts" that underlie the information provided in the remainder of the text. The reader should be familiar with the concepts of epidemiology and biomechanics. Each segmental chapter discusses the epidemiologic research related to that body segment and the types of injuries that occur in different industries. This information is collected by using a variety of research tools, including surveillance systems that describe the latest methods for collecting information about injury prevention and reporting in the workplace.

Readers will also encounter an explanation of the biomechanics of the skeletal system: how it works in a purely mechanical manner. Each group of chapters about specific body segments includes more detailed information about biomechanics. Additionally, there is a brief introduction to the muscular system that may be a useful reference for the more detailed discussions of diagnosis and treatment of work-related disorders that follow.

Researchers in every specialty are recognizing the importance of pain control and psychosocial factors that influence the prevention, treatment, and outcome of work-related musculoskeletal disorders. The control of pain is an important component in any treatment program, especially when the goal is a return to work and a reduction in chronicity for certain disorders such as low back pain. The biopsychosocial model looks at the relationship of lifestyle, work stress and job satisfaction, and psychological criteria that have an impact on the outcome for patients injured at the workplace. Throughout the text, examples of the importance of recognizing and addressing psychosocial concerns abound. Recognition of these issues is growing, and all healthcare providers should be cognizant of these findings.

Section 2 concludes with an overview of the magnitude of the problem. The cost of work-related musculoskeletal disorders has skyrocketed in the last decade, and control of the cost—economic, social, and personal—has become a priority in the workplace. Containment and even reduction of the cost of these injuries are discussed throughout the text in terms of better diagnosis and treatment, as well as prevention of future injuries by proper job design and workplace adaptation, all of which are dealt with in depth in Section 3, ergonomics.

ERGONOMICS

The section on ergonomics focuses on how the workplace can be adapted to the worker, which is the very definition of ergonomics. For too many years, workers have been asked to adapt themselves to unfriendly and even harmful workplaces, spaces that were too tight or too hot, vibrating, or mentally stressful, dangerous, or tedious. Over

time, workers may experience increasing levels of pain, or they may be subject to falls, slips, or strains that cause acute injury. Although workers can sometimes be taught safe posture and lifting techniques, for example, it is often necessary to change the workplace to eliminate a hazardous working condition. The chapters in the section on ergonomics discuss the research and guidelines for workplace adaptation and worker education that can contribute to a decline in the numbers of work-related musculoskeletal injuries. The field of ergonomics is constantly changing and growing to accommodate new laws and demands, and the important tools—job analysis, task analysis, and workplace design—are presented in detail.

PREVENTION

All the data collected about work-related injury and the efforts of ergonomists are geared toward the prevention of injury in the workplace. There are many levels of prevention, and each embodies the best hopes of the healthcare profession to prevent injury, avoid chronicity, and reduce work-related disability. This section emphasizes the importance of the physician working in concert with the ergonomist to deal with each individual case and modify the workplace for an injured worker and all others who might follow. Physicians working in the field of occupational health must understand the nature of the workplace and the cause of the injury, as well as the biopsychosocial treatment of the patient, in order to recommend the course of treatment that will have the best outcome for each individual worker.

CLINICAL EVALUATION AND PATIENT CARE

Section 5 has been arranged according to body segment: low back area; neck, shoulder, and elbow; wrist and hand; hip and knee; and foot and ankle. Within each segment there are chapters dealing with the epidemiology of the problem for that body segment: where and why injuries are likely to occur and how they can be identified and prevented. There are also chapters on the biomechanics of the body segment and chapters that discuss clinical examination of patients with a complaint. Treatment is discussed for each type of injury, including the indications and prognoses for surgical intervention. Finally, each section includes a discussion of workplace adaptation for each particular body segment and types of injuries, drawing upon epidemiologic data and research in ergonomics, biomechanics, and engineering.

LEGAL ISSUES

This final section looks at the legal issues that have a direct impact on the healthcare delivery system in the United States, with a brief comparison to the European experience. If an injured worker is involved in worker's compensation or another type of litigation, diagnosis and treatment of the injury are greatly compromised. Harking back to the importance of psychosocial issues in the treatment of work-related musculoskeletal disorders, the presence of an attorney in the treatment picture is a very important consideration for the physician, more so if a disability evaluation is called for. Passage of the Americans with Disabilities Act presents new challenges for employers as well as occupational healthcare providers, and the last two chapters discuss the implications of the law for physicians as well as workers.

New advances in the field represent a challenge to healthcare providers as knowledge about the biomechanics of work and the importance of ergonomics increases. In the United States, passage of the Americans with Disabilities Act challenges workers, employers, and healthcare professionals to take a new look at the workplace and find ways to improve its ergonomics. This effort, combined with a new understanding of the diagnosis and treatment of musculoskeletal disorders, fosters a sense of optimism about the health of the American workplace. The U.S. Agency for Health Care Policy and Research (AHCPR) recently completed a comprehensive review of the treatment of acute low back problems. The ACHPR issued a clinical practice guideline that sets the standard for the diagnosis and treatment of acute low back injuries, based on years of clinical research reported in the literature, and those findings set the tone for this document and are presented herein. These new laws draw the employer and the worker into a closer alliance against injury and disability, and it is the role of the healthcare provider to facilitate that relationship. If we all work together to apply these principles, the workplace can only improve and, with it, the lives of all workers.

Margareta Nordin
Gunnar B. J. Andersson
Malcolm H. Pope

PART I

Basic Concepts

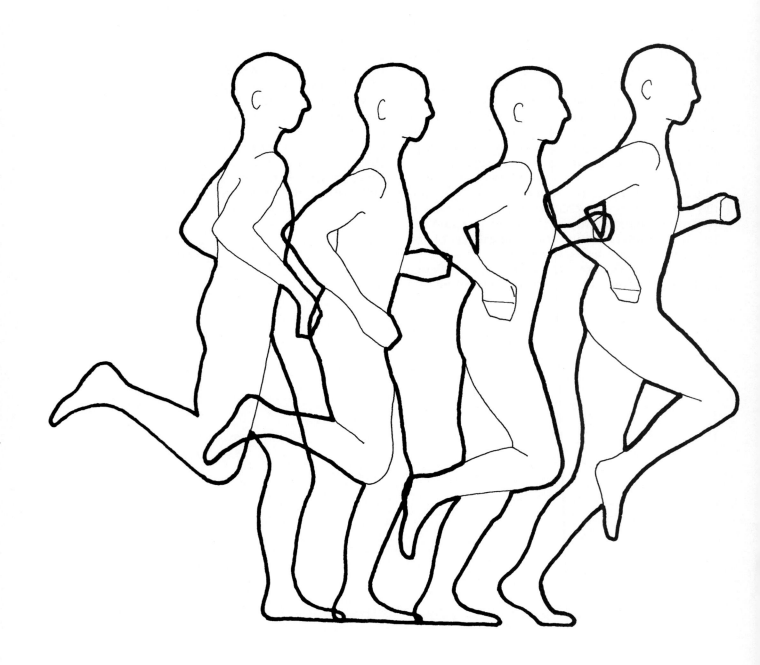

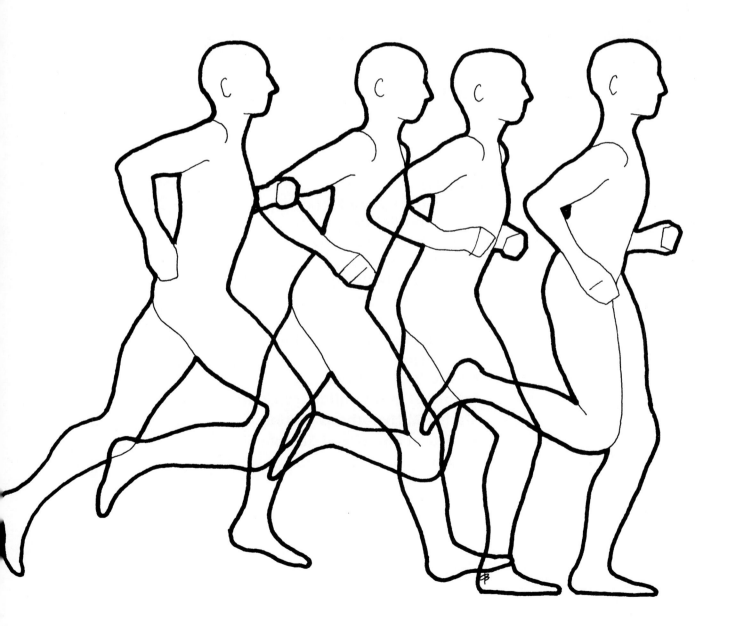

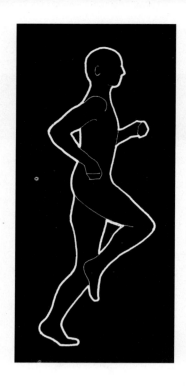

Chapter 1

Epidemiology

Mary Louise Skovron

CONTENTS

The literature on the epidemiology of occupational musculoskeletal disorders is often confusing because of conflicting evidence on the importance of various potential risk or causal factors. This chapter describes basic epidemiologic methods so that the reader may be able to evaluate critically the published literature on occupational musculoskeletal disorders. Most examples will be drawn from the literature on occupational low back pain, but the reader should be aware that similar methodologic standards must be applied to the literature on upper extremity disorders.

Epidemiology is the study of the distribution and determinants of diseases and injuries in human populations.[8] It consists of a developed methodology for testing scientific hypotheses in groups of individuals rather than in a laboratory setting. With knowledge of the intrinsic strengths and limitations of the design and execution of studies reported in the literature, it is possible to evaluate the strength of the evidence derived from these studies and even to make sense of conflicting results from different studies on the same topic. In this chapter we present an overview of the basic terminology used in epidemiology and the characteristics and generic strengths and limitations of analytic (hypothesis testing) study designs, with an emphasis on observational study designs.

There are several types of epidemiologic studies. Descriptive epidemiology is a means of monitoring the health of a population, identifying health problems, and compiling information that can be used for the development of causal hypotheses. Analytic epidemiology, which is the second major division of epidemiologic methods, is a set of epidemiologic study methods that is used to test specific hypotheses.

MEASURES OF DISEASE FREQUENCY

The fundamental strategy of epidemiology is the analysis of relative and absolute measures of disease frequency and a comparison of the characteristics of individuals with and without disease. The most obvious measures of disease frequency are case counts and their variations, which are often referred to as *numerator data*. They describe the frequency of the disorder without reference to the underlying population at risk. Examples of sources of case count data include back injury reports to the Occupational Safety and Health Administration (OSHA) by employers, worker's compensation records, records of visits to the workplace health facility, and surveys of the workforce. In clinical practice, the simple case count is usually derived by chart review (retrospec-

tively) or by enrollment of patients seen during a given period (prospectively). Disease frequency can also be expressed as a proportionate ratio, a ratio of cases of a particular disorder to cases of all disorders in the population of interest. In 1985, for example, occupational back injuries accounted for 26% of all closed compensation cases in a sample of nine states.[9]

Without being related to the underlying population at risk, however, numerator data cannot provide useful information regarding the risk or probability of acquiring the disorder. Without information about the characteristics of the underlying population or at least a comparison to the characteristics of people without the disorder, descriptions of the characteristics of cases also fail to provide sufficient information to test hypotheses about disease causality. For instance, approximately 400,000 disabling occupational back injuries were reported in 1990 in 23 states.[9] Without reference to the number of people at risk it is not possible to estimate the risk of back injury in the population or to test hypotheses regarding risk factors for back injury. For this reason, rates are used to express disease frequency when the objective is to assess the risk of disease or determinants of diseases or their outcomes.

Rates and Ratios

Rates describe the frequency of a disease or disorder per unit size of the population per unit time of observation. The rates commonly used in epidemiology are morbidity and mortality rates. The general form of a morbidity or mortality rate is

$$\frac{Number\ of\ cases}{\substack{Number\ of\ persons \\ at\ risk}} \times 100\ (1000,\ etc.)\ per\ unit\ time$$

The most frequently used morbidity rates in epidemiologic research are the *incidence rate* and the *prevalence rate*. The incidence rate is based on new cases of a disease or disorder (or new disease events), whereas the prevalence rate is based on existing cases. Because they are based on new versus existing cases, incidence and prevalence rates have different uses and different limitations.

In a sense, the incidence rate is a rate of change, the frequency with which people change from the nondiseased to the diseased state. Therefore the appropriate denominator is the population at risk of acquiring the disease (that is, those who are nondiseased at the start of the time interval). The incidence rate may be quantified in a number of ways—for example, as the number of new events per 1000 persons per year—when the population is stable and the number of new events is counted each year. Alternatively, it may be quantified as the number of new events per 1000 person-years, as is done in prospective studies where a fixed population is followed until either disease, the end of the study, or loss to follow-up occurs. In practice, although the best denominator for incidence rates is the number of people disease-free at the start of the time interval, surveillance incidence rates (and prevalence rates) that are based on case reports often use the total population derived from census data or from workforce estimates. Data from the United States, Canada, and the United Kingdom suggest that the average annual incidence is approximately 1 to 2 per 100 workers per year.[9,14,18]

The prevalence rate is the number of existing cases of disease in a given population in a given time period. For example, the 1-year prevalence of disabling back pain is as high as 25%.[4,5] *Point prevalence* is the number of cases per unit population at one moment of counting, for example, all persons receiving disability because of back pain in the workforce of a metropolitan electrical utility company on January 1, 1994, expressed per 1000 population. For point prevalence, the unit of time is often not expressed because the period of time is effectively instantaneous. Period prevalence is the number of cases existing at one time or another during a definable time interval such as 1-year, 5-year, or lifetime prevalence. Some epidemiologists do not express prevalence as a rate because in practice it is often derived from surveys that are difficult to assign to a specific time interval.

There are a number of factors other than the risk factor under study that may affect the incidence and prevalence rates. These include demographic characteristics of the underlying population, most obviously age distribution,[4] since age is known to be associated with the onset of almost all diseases. Gender and ethnicity distributions must also be taken into account when incidence rates are interpreted. Other influences can distort the apparent incidence rate, including certain company policies, worker's compensation claims, and health care system influences that affect the likelihood of seeking medical attention, of being diagnosed with a given disease or disorder, or of having the disorder reported. These factors should be considered when measures of disease frequency are evaluated, particularly when changes are assessed over time or different populations are compared.

To eliminate the effects of differences in these factors, the rates may be adjusted or standardized algebraically. The adjusted rates express the risk of acquiring the disease in the populations being compared as if they had the same age, sex, and ethnicity distributions. Alternatively, if it is not necessary to have a single summary index of disease risk, the morbidity rates within population strata defined by age, sex, and ethnicity may be compared.

The number of existing cases of a disease or disorder at any time is a function of both the rate of new cases (incidence) and the duration of that disorder. Therefore, when a population is stable and the duration of a disorder is also stable, it is possible to estimate prevalence from incidence and vice versa according to the following approximation:

$$Prevalence \approx Incidence \times Duration$$

Thus a change in prevalence may reflect changes in the incidence rate, duration, or both. For example, the prevalence of low back pain in a population may change because of alterations in individual, work-related, or other environmental risk factors affecting incidence rate, or because treatment changes alter the duration of back pain episodes and risk of chronicity. It is occasionally the case that improved treatment will extend the duration of a disorder with the result that the prevalence increases in the face of a decreasing incidence, as occurred some decades ago with Down syndrome. The survival of infants with Down syndrome had improved because of improved medical and surgical management of their associated disorders. The prevalence of Down syndrome increased, although the incidence declined as a result of prenatal screening programs.

DESCRIPTIVE EPIDEMIOLOGY

The first step often undertaken in epidemiology is development of the descriptive epidemiology of a disease or disorder. Descriptive epidemiology supports the development of causal hypotheses but does not in itself support conclusions about disease causality or about any hypotheses. In descriptive epidemiology the frequency of a disorder in the population is characterized in terms of person (e.g., age, sex, ethnicity-specific incidence rates, economic, behavioral, occupational, and other factors), place (rural versus urban, type of housing, national variations, type of industry, job requirements), and time (long-term trend, seasonality, occasionally day of the week or time of day). In classic epidemiology, causal hypotheses are developed by inductive reasoning from the descriptive epidemiology and available information regarding anatomy, pathology, physiology, and so forth. Specific hypotheses are formulated and tested by means of analytic studies. As the results of hypothesis-testing (analytic) studies are accrued, they are added to the basis for causal inference, depending on their strengths and generalizability, and hypotheses are supported, modified, or negated. In interpreting the evidence from all scientific sources, the rules of causal inference are applied.[6] Briefly, the hypothesized cause must be demonstrated to have preceded the disease by a length of time sufficient to allow disease development and expression (time sequence of events). The disease should be more common in those with the hypothesized cause than in those without it (increased risk in those exposed to the hypothesized cause), and as the intensity or duration of exposure to the hypothesized cause increases, the frequency of the disorder should increase (dose-response relationship). The association between the hypothesized causal factor and the disease should be consistently demonstrated in methodologically sound studies and should be biologically plausible. In addition, the specificity of an association (i.e., the extent to which the hypothesized causal factor is associated with only one disease or disorder) adds weight to a causal hypothesis, but it is not necessary for causal inference; for example, cigarette smoking is accepted as a cause of lung cancer, although the association is not specific. Cigarette smoking is also associated with a number of other cancers, obstructive pulmonary disease, heart disease, and a variety of disorders, including osteoporosis, low back pain, and in particular, herniated intervertebral disks.

ANALYTIC EPIDEMIOLOGY

Analytic, or hypothesis-testing, epidemiology relies on two types of study designs. These are observational and interventional study designs. In observational studies, exposure to the hypothesized causal factor and development of the disease in the population under study occur in the natural course of events; the investigator does not cause them to occur. The study is designed and executed to maximize the extent to which it can be seen as a natural experiment, that is, the extent to which all extraneous sources of variation are eliminated and only the exposure to the putative cause and the frequency of disease vary between populations being compared. It is often the case that once substantial observational evidence has accrued, causality is widely accepted. However, it is desirable in etiologic epidemiology and almost universally required in evaluations of treatment that the final test of the hypothesis be in interventional or experimental studies.

In experimental studies the investigator causes individuals or groups of individuals in the population to receive the treatment in question. To demonstrate ethically the causal role of a risk factor for which there is only observational evidence, the investigator would prevent exposure to the risk factor for a group of people. In both types of interventional design strategies a comparison group that does not receive the intervention is necessary. All other factors that might influence the outcome of the study (potential confounding factors) can be eliminated or controlled by the investigator. Because the conditions of the study are much more under control of the investigator, interventional studies can more closely approximate true experiments than can observational studies. When such studies are well designed and executed, they provide very strong support (or negation) for a hypothesis.

All the analytic study designs have potential problems of internal and external validity that must be solved by the investigator either in the study design or in the data analysis. Internal validity is the extent to which a study is a true test of the specific hypothesis, that is, the extent to which all possible biases of measurement or information and all possible confounding variables are eliminated as explaining the observed study result. External validity is the extent to which the study results are generalizable to the population of interest, namely, whether the study subjects are representative of the population at risk. If the potential validity problems have been solved in either the design or analysis of the study, the study evidence is strengthened.

Because it is not possible to study the entire universe of potentially eligible subjects, epidemiologic studies are conducted on samples of the population of interest. Even a study of an entire city or the workforce of a company constitutes a sample. The method of sampling should not introduce selection biases. For example, a volunteer study is potentially susceptible to selection bias because the health behavior and health status of people who volunteer for research are well documented to be better than those of refusers. No characteristics of the individuals should affect the likelihood of selection for the study, including their knowledge of the question at issue, their beliefs about the risk factors or about the cause of the disease being studied, or any characteristic such as age, sex, or education that could be independently associated with both the disease and the hypothesized causal factor.

It is important for the internal validity of the study results that the information collected be accurate and complete. If there is inaccuracy (measurement error) in the information collected, the ability to detect the association of interest will be reduced. If the accuracy of the information is worse for one exposure group than for another, the effect on the study results may not be predictable. For this reason, an evaluation of the accuracy (or validity) of measurements is necessary for any study. Research reports should describe the validity of the sources of information. Questionnaires or reporting methods that have been validated in the study population or in similar populations or circumstances should be used. The problem of validity of information is particularly important in research on occupational musculoskeletal disorders because the methods of both case diagnosis[15] and measurement of work exposure[17] have substantial limitations.

Before specific study designs can be discussed, the term *confounding* must be defined. Confounding occurs when the study results can be explained by a factor extraneous to the hypothesis being tested. A potential confounding factor must be associated with both the disease in question and the hypothesized causal factor. That is, the proportion of diseased persons who have the confounding exposure must be different from the proportion of nondiseased persons with the confounding exposure. It is also necessary that the proportion of those with the hypothesized causal factor who have the confounding exposure be different from the proportion of those not exposed to the hypothesized causal factor who have the confounding factor. For example, a study that found an association between job satisfaction and the risk of occupational back injury could be confounded by the physical requirements of work if heavy work was a risk factor for back injury and was also associated with lack of job satisfaction in the studied population. Potential confounding factors can be eliminated in the design of the study by restricted or matched sampling or, in the data analysis phase, by stratified or multivariate analysis, for example. If in the study just described the statistical analyses controlled for physical requirements of work or if the researchers conducted an exploratory analysis and found no association between job satisfaction and the physical requirements of work, the potential for confounding would be eliminated. In experimental studies, potential confounding should be successfully eliminated by truly random, blind assignment of subjects to the different treatments under study. Comparability of the treatment groups should be confirmed by presentation of the baseline characteristics of each group on entry to the study.

Confounding invalidates a study as a test of the hypothesis. The study's results cannot be taken as evidence of causality or efficacy of treatment. Lack of generalizability, as opposed to confounding, does not invalidate a study's results, but merely restricts inference to populations similar to those under study.

Observational study designs are applicable in both clinical and etiologic epidemiology. In etiologic epidemiology the researcher tests whether a hypothesized factor is a determinant or cause of disease in previously healthy people, whereas in clinical epidemiology one tests whether particular characteristics, risk factors, or clinical interventionsare determinants of the prognosis or outcome in diseased individuals. The classic observational analytic study designs are the cohort study, the case-control study, and the cross-sectional study.

Cohort Study (Prognostic Study)

The cohort study (sometimes also called a prospective study) is the observational design that when well designed and executed, produces the soundest results in terms of incidence rates and disease etiology or prognostic determinants of all the observational study designs.

The hallmark of a cohort study is that a nondiseased population is identified and characterized with respect to the hypothesized risk factor, important covariates, and potential confounders. The population is observed for a period of time adequate for development of the disorder, and the new cases of disease (incident cases) are recorded.

The Boeing study of aircraft workers is an example of a cohort study. Approximately 3000 volunteers were enrolled. The potential risk factors examined included demographic characteristics, body habitus, aerobic capacity, and strength; physical requirements of work; and prior medical, surgical, and back pain history. Additional assessments included questions about psychological characteristics and job satisfaction, which approximately half the participants agreed to complete. The workers were then followed for 3 years with the outcome of interest being an episode of low back pain that caused work loss.[1,2]

Because it may take decades for disease to develop, cohort studies are often undertaken by identifying subjects from existing records documenting their health status and exposure to the causal factor in the past and by ascertaining subsequent exposure and development of disease in the more recent past or in the near future. This type of cohort study is called a historical, or

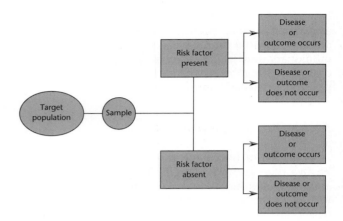

Figure 1-1 Cohort study.

retrospective, cohort study because at least the exposure and possibly the disease events happened before the study was conducted. When the subjects are enrolled at the time of exposure onset and followed forward in time, the cohort study may be referred to as a follow-up, or prospective, cohort study (**Fig. 1-1**).

Loss to follow-up is a potential problem in cohort studies. If a substantial proportion of subjects are lost to the study for any reason, for example, having moved out of the region, it would be expected that fewer cases of the disease in question would arise in the study than originally planned. The number of study cases may ultimately be too small to yield stable estimates of the incidence rates and, consequently, estimates of the relative risk. In this case, the observed relative risk would have to be very large to be accepted as supporting the causal hypothesis. For example, consider a cohort study examining the causal role of occupational repetitive motion in carpal tunnel syndrome. New workers hired in 1965 through 1970 are enrolled and followed forward for 10 years, with information on new cases of carpal tunnel syndrome coming from the company medical department records. If 30% of the workers retire, take disability pensions, die, get another job, or leave the company for other reasons, there is a substantial loss to follow-up. A bias in loss to follow-up occurs if the workers who leave the company are those with the highest exposure to repetitive work movements and those who leave because upper extremity problems consistent with preclinical carpal tunnel syndrome are making it more difficult for them to do the job. The observed relative risk is an underestimate of the true relative risk because the detected incidence of carpal tunnel syndrome among those with repetitive-motion jobs is lower than the true incidence and the detected incidence among those not exposed is not affected. Biased loss to follow-up leading to underestimates of incidence in the unexposed would produce an inflated observed relative risk. High proportions lost to follow-up, or higher proportions lost in one exposure category than another (selective loss to follow-up), leave open the possibility of biased loss to follow-up with consequent distortion of the study findings.

Another form of selection bias can occur. This bias, called selective survival or selective attrition, occurs when people who have both the exposure and the disease have a different probability of dropping out of the population available to be included in the study than do people who are not exposed and get the disease. This type of bias can easily occur in cross-sectional and case-control studies. It can also occur in a particular variant of the cohort study called the prevalent cohort study. For example, a prevalent cohort study examining occupational repetitive motion as a risk factor for carpal tunnel syndrome that enrolled workers who were first employed between 1965 and 1970 and were still actively employed in 1995 could be affected by selective attrition if carpal tunnel syndrome by and large developed within 15 years of employment and workers tended to leave the company when carpal tunnel syndrome developed.

Because most diseases or conditions are relatively uncommon or take a long time to develop, cohort studies require the enrollment of a large number of subjects who may need years of follow-up. Outcome studies in which the outcome of interest is rare or develops long after the intervention present similar requirements. It can be more efficient in terms of time and the number of subjects studied to address the hypothesis by means of a case-control study, as described in the next section.

Case-Control Study

The essential feature of the case-control study that differentiates it from the other observational study types is that individuals are selected for the study on the basis of the presence of the disease or disorder in question (cases) and compared with individuals selected for the study on the basis of the absence of the disease under study (controls). The presence or absence of the hypothesized causal factor is then ascertained in both case and control subjects. Although this appears on its face to be a simple undertaking, case-control studies present a number of methodologic challenges that must be solved for the study results to be valid (**Fig. 1-2**).

The study by Punnett, Fine, and Keyserling[10] in which frequency, quantity, and position of lifting were examined as risk factors for occupational back injury among auto workers is a case-control study. Cases of back pain were identified from workers' self-reports and confirmed by medical evaluation, and controls were sampled from workers who reported themselves free of back pain for the previous year, again confirmed by medical evaluation. The positional and lifting requirements of the work of the two groups were then compared.

Case-control studies frequently suffer from information biases. For example, if information on exposure to the risk factor of interest comes from a different source for case and control subjects, biased exposure informa-

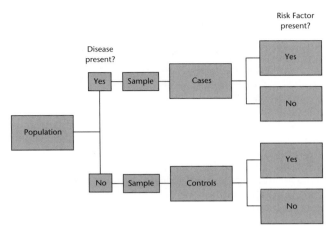

Figure 1-2 Case-control study.

tion is possible. Recall bias, in which a case subject is more or less likely to recall an event in the past than is a control subject, is also possible. There is also the problem of unbiased recall failure, in which subjects are asked to recall events or conditions that took place so long ago that they cannot be remembered. Establishing that exposure to the factor of interest took place long enough before the outcome to be a biologically plausible determinant is difficult for certain types of hypotheses; for example, a case-control study examining preexisting degenerative disk disease as a determinant of chronicity (symptom duration greater than 6 months) in workers with chronic back pain could not establish that the disk problem predated chronicity based on clinical or imaging examinations at the time of study. These problems are avoided if the case-control study uses exposure or prognostic information that was recorded, for example, in medical or prescription records, long enough before the disease condition being studied to be a biologically plausible cause and to obviate recall problems.

Well-designed and well-conducted case-control studies may provide evidence as robust as that of cohort studies at considerably less cost and in considerably less time. However, because of the difficulty in avoiding the problems just described, case-control studies often produce weaker causal evidence than do cohort studies.

Cross-Sectional Study

Cross-sectional studies simultaneously ascertain exposure to risk factors (or the presence of prognostic factors) and the presence of the disease or disorder or outcome in question in a population sampled without regard to the presence of either. This type of sampling is sometimes called naturalistic sampling. In contrast to a cohort study, which follows subjects over time and ascertains incidence, a cross-sectional study ascertains conditions present at the moment of study, that is, the prevalence of the disorder or outcome in question at the time of the study. The estimates of relative risk derived from cross-sectional studies are therefore estimates of prevalence relative risk.

Population-based cross-sectional studies of low back pain often address, among other factors, the association of the type of work (occupation, physical requirements, and so forth) with low back pain (**Fig. 1-3**).[13,15]

Cross-sectional or survey studies are often undertaken because unlike case-control studies, they require few *a priori* decisions with regard to the selection of subjects and, unlike cohort studies, it is not necessary to wait for the study outcome. These advantages are offset by their susceptibility to some of the problems of both cohort and case-control studies. When uncommon diseases or exposures are being studied, a large number of people must be included, as in cohort studies. If information on exposures or on determinants of interest is collected at the time of the study rather than from previously existing records, there can be recall biases, recall failure, and problems in establishing the time sequence of events, just as in case-control studies. Nevertheless, for relatively common disorders (outcomes) and risk factors (determinants), cross-sectional studies may be a useful first step in exploring a hypothesis. Because of their many limitations, however, cross-sectional studies rarely produce robust results for evaluating the importance of causal or prognostic factors.

When the literature on a problem consists predominantly of cross-sectional studies, it is often the case that the analytic epidemiology of that problem is in its infancy. Until recently, much of the epidemiologic information on occupational low back pain was derived from descriptive and cross-sectional studies.[12] In the past 5 or 6 years there has been a substantial advance in the quantity and quality of observational analytic studies of work-related back pain. The epidemiologic investigation of upper extremity disorders began later than that of low back pain. Consequently, knowledge of the risk factors for work-related upper extremity disorders is less developed.

The intrinsic strengths and limitations of the basic observational study designs are summarized in **Table 1-1**.

Experimental Study Designs: Clinical Trials

The distinction between observational and interventional study designs is that in observational designs the investigator does not cause the exposure to the causal factor or treatment for the purposes of the study, whereas in interventional designs the investigator does cause subjects to be exposed to different factors or treatments. Observational study designs are susceptible to treatment assignment biases in which the treatment the patients receive is influenced by certain patient characteristics, for example, lifestyle or clinical severity, that can confound the results. Clinical trials, in which the treating physicians or the investigators control which treatment patients receive, are also susceptible to such biases. For this reason, randomized controlled trials (RCTs), where only chance influences which treatment eligible patients receive, are the preferred method of evaluating therapeutic interventions.

The validity of RCTs depends on all the methodologic features described for the observational study designs and more. The study must be confined to those patients who have agreed to participate. Comparisons of treatment outcomes in patients who agree to participate with those in patients who refuse to participate are not valid. Assignment of patients to treatments must be

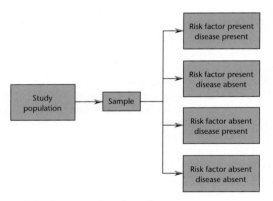

Figure 1-3 Cross-sectional study.

Table 1-1	Strengths (+) and limitations (−) of the observational study designs		
Feature	**Cohort Study**	**Case-Control Study**	**Cross-Sectional Study**
Selective survival	+	+	−
Recall bias	+	−	−
Loss to follow-up	−	+	+
Time sequence of events	+	−	−
Time to complete	−	+	+
Expense	−	+	+/−

done by using accepted methods of randomization, which are described in the report, and the resulting comparability of the treatment groups on important covariates should be described, usually in a table summarizing the baseline characteristics of the treatment groups. On the occasions when, by chance, randomization does not result in comparable groups, potential confounding must be controlled in the statistical analysis. **Figure 1-4** is a schematic representation of appropriate design in an RCT.

Ordinarily in randomized trials, the treating physician and the patient should be blind to which treatment group the patient has been assigned. If this is not possible, assessment of the study outcome should be done by an independent evaluator to avoid observer and participant biases in assessing the outcome. This is particularly important when the outcome being assessed is subjective. Information should be collected in the same way and with the same frequency in all treatment groups. Eligibility and exclusion criteria should be described and be appropriate to the question being addressed. Treatments should be clearly described, and patient compliance, dropouts from the study, and complications should be described and equivalent in both groups. Finally, the outcomes studied should be appropriate to the treatment or condition in question. There are a number of general health status assessment measures that are used, including, for example, the SF-36,[16] a standardized multidimensional assessment instrument that includes functional capacity, pain, locomotion, mental status, and affect. In addition, there are a number of assessment instruments for back pain disability that have been extensively used in research, such as the Oswestry[3] and the Roland.[11] Recently the reliability and validity of the newly developed Quebec Back Pain Disability Scale have been reported.[7]

STATISTICAL ISSUES

Methods of Analysis

The statistical analysis of any study result should be appropriate to the hypothesis and to the structure of the data collected. When, for instance, the study examines the difference in Oswestry scores associated with a conditioning program as compared with usual care for subacute low back pain, comparisons of the mean scores in the treatment groups may be appropriate. If it is necessary to control for pretreatment differences between the groups, the analysis will use multivariate methods such as analysis of covariance or multiple regression. Occasionally, because of the statistical characteristics of the outcome being assessed it may be necessary to transform it (e.g., log transformation, square root transformation) and analyze the transformed variable. It is often the case that the outcome variable distribution or the conditions of the study do not conform to the requirements of the usual statistical hypothesis tests such as *t*-tests, analysis of covariance, and regression analysis. In these cases, a nonparametric method of statistical analysis such as the Wilcoxon method is appropriate.

When the hypothesis addresses the relative frequency of an event such as a back injury rate, the relative incidence of back injury in the subjects exposed to the risk factor and those not exposed is evaluated. A ratio of the incidence rates, called the *relative risk,* is used to express the association. The larger the relative risk, the stronger the observed association and the stronger the evidence in favor of the research hypothesis. A relative risk of 1 indicates no effect of the hypothesized causal factor on the risk of disease. The relative risk may be adjusted for important covariates or to eliminate potential confounding. There are also other statistics that estimate the relative risk. The *odds ratio,* the ratio of the odds of the disease in those exposed to the odds of disease in those unexposed, provides a good estimate of the relative risk in cohort studies. It also has valuable statistical properties because it can be estimated by using logistic regression. The effects of confounding variables can be controlled or the simultaneous effects of several causal variables or covariates can be estimated by using multiple logistic regression.

Another way of estimating the risk of disease in cohort studies is failure-time, or survival, analysis. The cumulative probability of acquiring the disease is often displayed as a failure-time curve and expressed as the cumulative hazard. The cumulative probability of acquiring disease in those exposed and those unexposed can be similarly displayed; the *hazard ratio* is an estimate of the relative risk of acquiring the disease. In prognostic or outcome studies the failure-time curve may be interpreted as a survival curve, in which case the hazard ratio is an estimate of the relative risk of recovery associated with the prognostic factor in question. Cox proportional hazards regression, which can be used when there are several predictor variables of interest or when potential confounders must be controlled, is a method of estimating the simultaneous effects of multiple variables.

An advantage of survival analysis is that all study subjects contribute information for as long as they remain in the study. The reader should be aware, however, that if the number of dropouts during the course

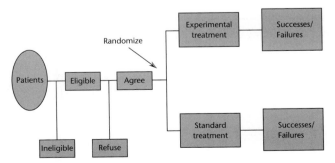

Figure 1-4 Randomized control trial.

of the study is substantial, estimates of the hazard ratio toward the end of the follow-up period are based on relatively small numbers and are consequently unstable.

Estimates and Confidence Limits

Research is conducted on a sample of persons or other units of observation drawn from a target population. The results of any given study are estimates of the true means, proportions, relative risks, and so forth in the population from which the samples were drawn. The precision of a study estimate of the population value, or parameter, of a measurement is described by the standard error of estimate. The standard error (*SE*) is the square root of the ratio of the variance (s^2), or variability of the measurement in the sample, to the number of subjects (*N*) in the study. For example,

$$SE_{Mean} = \sqrt{\frac{s^2}{N}}$$

Variance is affected by a number of factors, including interindividual variability, intraindividual variability (such as diurnal variations), and instrument variability. Designing or executing a study to reduce any of these components will reduce the variance of the measurement, thus reducing the standard error and increasing the stability of the estimate of the population parameter. The larger the number of subjects on whom the estimate is based, the smaller the standard error and the more confident we can be in its representation of the population parameter.

Because sample results are estimates of population parameters, it is increasingly becoming the standard of reporting to describe the precision of the estimates as a range within which the population parameter probably lies. This is the *confidence limit* around the estimate and is by convention expressed as the 95% confidence limit. For example, the 95% confidence limit for a mean is approximated by

$$95\% \text{ Confidence interval} = Mean \pm 2\,SE_{Mean}$$

Statistical Hypothesis Testing

Because there is always sampling error, estimates may be expected to vary from sample to sample. Consequently, study results must be subjected to statistical hypothesis testing; that is, study results must be tested to determine the probability that the observed results from a specific study could have occurred by chance alone.

The statistical hypothesis test evaluates the null hypothesis that the observed study results occurred because of sampling error when there was no true association in the population from which the study subjects were sampled. The probability of making this type of error is designated as *Alpha*. If the observed association is large enough that this kind of error is improbable, the null hypothesis is rejected. The investigators then accept the alternative hypothesis, that the observed estimates of relative risk or differences between treatments reflect the true situation in the population from which the samples were drawn. By convention, the cutoff of *Alpha* for rejecting the null hypothesis is usually set at .05. Then if the probability (*p* value) that the observed results are due to sampling error is less than .05, that is, less than alpha, the null hypothesis is rejected and the results are declared statistically significant. Thus, statistically significant results are simply results that we have decided, within an acceptable margin of error, probably did not occur by chance. Further, the larger the observed association relative to the underlying variability of the outcome being measured, the more likely that it will be declared statistically significant.

Statistical Power and Sample Size

Statistical hypothesis tests actually involve two probabilities. The probability of making a type I error by incorrectly rejecting the null hypothesis, that is, by declaring an observed association to be statistically significant when in fact it is the result of sampling error, is referred to as *Alpha*, as described in the preceding paragraph. There is also the probability of incorrectly accepting the null hypothesis, that is, declaring that the study results are due to sampling error (not statistically significant) when in fact they reflect a true association in the population from which the study subjects were drawn. This is the type II error and its probability is *Beta*. The complementary probability that a study will be able to correctly reject the null hypothesis when it is false, that is, correctly detect an association when there is one in the population at large, is referred to as statistical

Table 1-2 Population conditions, statistical hypothesis test results, error types and designations		
Hypothesis Test Result	**Population Condition**	
	NULL HYPOTHESIS TRUE **NO ASSOCIATION**	**NULL HYPOTHESIS FALSE** **ASSOCIATION EXISTS**
Accept null hypothesis No association	*Correct*	*Type II error (beta)*
Reject null hypothesis Association exists	*Type I error (alpha)*	*Correct*

power (1–*Beta*). **Table 1-2** illustrates the different conditions and possible results of a statistical hypothesis test.

In the planning phase of research the investigators should make a determination of how strong an association would be clinically significant, i.e., how large an estimated relative risk or how big a difference between treatments. Because the validity of the study requires that it be a true test of the research hypothesis, it is important to design the study so that a clinically significant association will have a good chance of being declared statistically significant, that is, so that the study has sufficient power to detect a clinically significant association. The larger the sample size, the more power the statistical test has to detect associations; in other words, as expected differences or relative risks get smaller, the number of subjects studied must increase to have adequate power to test the hypothesis. Conversely, with very large numbers of study subjects it is possible to declare trivial associations statistically significant. When studies with small sample sizes report results that are not statistically significant, they should also report how an association would have been required for there to have good power to detect it. The reader should also evaluate whether the observed difference and its upper confidence limit, although not statistically significant, are clinically significant. When studies with huge numbers of subjects report statistically significant results, the reader should decide whether the differences are trivial in clinical terms, even though they are statistically significant.

SUMMARY

The validity of clinical research depends on a number of factors. The hypothesis must be formulated specifically enough to be testable. The appropriate study subjects should be eligible, and there should not be differential participation. The information collected should be appropriate to the hypothesis and accurate. The study design and information sources should avoid potential information biases. Potential confounders should be eliminated in the study design or controlled in the statistical analysis. At the time the study is designed, a clinically significant hypothesized result should be specified, the plan of statistical analysis determined, and the necessary number of study subjects defined. Study management should avoid the introduction of differential loss to follow-up, unblinding, and other potential problems. The statistical analysis should be appropriate to the structure of the data and to the hypothesis. Finally, although the discussion should place the study in the context of other work and what is already known about the question, the specific conclusions should not go beyond what was actually tested in the study.

References

1. Battie MC et al: A prospective study of the role of cardiovascular risk factors and fitness in industrial back pain, *Spine* 14:851, 1989.

2. Bigos SJ et al: A prospective study of work perceptions and psychosocial factors affecting the report of back injury, *Spine* 16:1-6, 1991.

3. Fairbank JCT et al: The Oswestry low back pain disability questionnaire, *Physiotherapy* 66:271, 1980.

4. Gyntelberg F: One-year incidence of low back pain among male residents of Copenhagen aged 40-59, *Danish Med Bull* 21:30-36, 1974.

5. Haber LD: Disabling effects of chronic disease and impairment, *J Chronic Dis* 24:469-487, 1971.

6. Kelsey JL, Thompson D, Evans AS: *Methods in observational epidemiology,* New York, Oxford University Press, 1986.

7. Kopec JA: The Quebec back pain disability index. Measurement properties, *Spine* 20:341-352, 1995.

8. Mausner JS, Kramer S: *Mausner and Bahn epidemiology: an introductory text,* ed 2, Philadelphia, WB Saunders, 1985; p. 1.

9. National Safety Council: *Accident facts 1991,* Chicago, NSC, 1991, pp 38, 40.

10. Punnett L, Fine LJ, Keyserling WM: Back disorders and non-neutral trunk positions of automobile assembly workers, *Scand J Work Environ Health* 17:337-346, 1991.

11. Roland M, Morris R: A study of the natural history of back pain. I. Development of a reliable and sensitive measure of disability in low back pain, *Spine* 8:141-144, 1983.

12. Skovron ML: Epidemiology of low back pain, *Baillieres Clin Rheumat* 76:559-573, 1992.

13. Skovron ML et al: Sociocultural factors and back pain, *Spine* 19:129-137, 1994.

14. Svensson H-O, Andersson GBJ: Low back pain in 40-47 year old men: Work history and work environment, *Spine* 8:272-276, 1983.

15. On the accuracy of history, physical examination, and erythrocyte sedimentation rate in diagnosing low back pain in general practice, *Spine* 20:318-327, 1995.

16. Ware JE Jr, Sherbourne CD: The MOS 36-item short form health survey (SF-36), *Med Care* 30:473-483, 1992.

17. Winkel J, Mathiassen SE: Assessment of physical work load in epidemiologic studies: concepts, issues and operational considerations, *Ergonomics* 37:979-988, 1994.

18. Wood PHN, Baddeley EM: Epidemiology of back pain. In Jayson M, editor: *The lumbar spine and back pain,* ed 2, London, Churchill Livingstone, 1980; pp. 1-15.

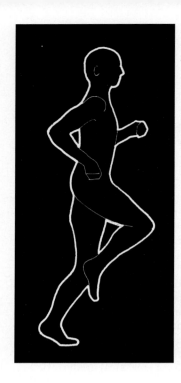

Chapter 2

Surveillance Systems

Lawrence J. Fine

CONTENTS

The use of surveillance systems at both the national and local level is critical to the prevention of work-related musculoskeletal disorders (WMDs) because surveillance should be used to determine where to focus the prevention efforts and whether these efforts are effective.[3] Occupational surveillance is the ongoing and systematic collection, analysis, and interpretation of data related to either occupational exposures (hazard surveillance) or adverse health outcomes (injuries, disorders, or diseases).[3,23] Surveillance data are often derived from information collected for some administrative purpose or as the result of a regulatory demand; therefore, the data are generally not as accurate as data collected during a planned research study. However, surveillance data can be collected much more efficiently and less expensively than research data. An effective surveillance system conducts each of the aforementioned steps effectively and results in the initiation of preventive actions.[22]

GOALS

The goals of surveillance are intimately linked to the use of surveillance data in prevention activities. The first goal of surveillance systems for WMDs is the identification of new or previously unrecognized problems. Identification will occur when a musculoskeletal disorder has been associated with a specific work process or occupation.[10] This generally happens through two types of surveillance data: either the identification of

cases without definite information about the size of the population from which the cases are drawn (Sentinel Health Event) or from a surveillance source of cases that include some information on both the number of cases and the size of the population at risk. An example of the first type is a recent report of carpal tunnel syndrome (CTS) in cardiologists and cardiovascular technicians that is linked to the performance of intraaortic balloon pump and sheath removal for cardiac catheterization and percutaneous transluminal coronary angioplasty.[20] An example of the second type is the increase in worker's compensation claims for knee joint inflammation in carpet installers and tile setters (**Table 2-1**).[21] This example also illustrates the differences between surveillance and research data sources. The worker's compensation claims for knee joint inflammation from states all over the United States are most likely a heterogeneous set of clinical entities, whereas cases in a research study would usually be established to have a disease status with a more homogeneous and validated definition. The level of resources required to study a representative population of each of the occupational groups in **Table 2-1** would be quite large. The research study would require a few years to complete. Despite the limitations characteristic of many surveillance systems, large excessive risks often correctly identify serious problems as in this example.[23]

The second goal of surveillance is to determine the magnitude of the WMD problem at either the national, state, or local level. This is the most important goal of surveillance from the perspective of prevention. Surveillance data can be used to determine where to focus prevention efforts.

At the national level, surveillance data can be used to identify which industries are at high risk. One of the few national representative sources of data for WMDs is collected by the Bureau of Labor Statistics (BLS) in the Department of Labor, which surveys a representative sample of private sector employers with more than 11 employees each year. The number of occupational illnesses and injuries is collected from each surveyed employer. This system has a number of limitations because of the limited amount of data collected and the

| Table 2-1 | Worker's compensation claims in 1979 for knee-joint inflammation from kneeling, leaning, repetition of pressure, or striking against a stationary object |

Occupation	Number of Claims	Percentage of Claims	Percentage of Workforce	Occupational Knee Morbidity Rate*
Carpet installers	46	6.2	0.06	108.0
Tile setters	16	2.2	0.04	53.0
Brick/stone masons	9	1.2	0.20	6.0
Millwrights	3	0.4	0.15	2.7

Percentage of claims/percentage of workforce.

Table 2-2	Industries with high and low rates of disorders associated with repeated trauma—1990 (Bureau of Labor Statistics, U.S. Department of Labor, November 1991)	
Industry	**Standard Industrial Classification**	**Incidence Rate**
Meat-packing plants	2011	1336
Poultry slaughtering	2015	696
Refrigerator manufacturing	3632	473
Grocery stores	5411-9	2
Electronic component manufacturing	3671-9	2

methods used to classify specific injuries or illnesses. Despite its limitations, the system has been used to identify some industries with a high risk of suspected WMDs of the upper extremity (**Table 2-2**).[6] Disorders such as CTS are classified in the BLS as disorders associated with repeated trauma.

Data in **Table 2-2** illustrate some of the limitations of surveillance data. Some of the differences between the low- and high-risk industries in **Table 2-2** could be due to the lower ratio of high-risk jobs to low-risk jobs in the broader Standard Industrial Classifications reported for the lower-risk industries. For example, the job of checker, which is a common job within the grocery-store three-digit 541 Standard Industrial Classification, has been identified as a risk job for several WMDs of the upper extremity.[4,17] Despite the fact that it includes some high-risk jobs, the grocery store industry is evidently characterized mostly by lower-risk jobs or less effective reporting of cases than is the manufacturing sector. Variation in the accuracy of the classification of health outcomes or the type and level of occupational exposures can be expected in most surveillance systems.

Despite the limitations of this surveillance system, it has identified some industries with substantial WMD problems. This type of surveillance analysis should trigger activities to evaluate whether the probable elevated rates of WMD are related to occupational causes and suggest preventive programs to reduce the magnitude of the problem.[8,9]

Analysis of surveillance data collected at the local level in a manufacturing or service sector firm can also identify areas of the firm with an elevated rate of WMDs that deserve further investigation. These local surveillance systems are typically based on one or more of the following data sources: (1) OSHA 200 log, an important source of data for the BLS surveillance system; (2) in-plant medical records or logs; or (3) worker's compensation records. By analyzing the *magnitude* of the WMD problem it is often possible to find job categories or departments with elevated rates (**Table 2-3**). In this example, a mail order facility was investigated, and 1 year of the dispensary log for an in-plant medical department was reviewed. The employees were considered possible cases if they reported appropriate symptoms or requested/reported medical treatment by a healthcare provider. On the basis of these data, it may be concluded in this facility, further data and ergonomic job analyses should be directed at the likely high-risk job categories of stocking inventory and order filling. Because resources for reducing exposure are almost always limited, whether at a national, state, or local level, surveillance data can be used to allocate resources for further investigation and preventive activities.

A surveillance system can not only determine the magnitude of the WMD problem in terms of the number of cases but can also be useful in suggesting some of the causes of the problem, for example, analysis of nature and cause of back injuries in databases of approximately 200,000 workers and compensation claims from 15 states during 1981 through 1990.[4] The most common type of injury was strain/sprain (93%), and the most common cause of these strains/sprains was lifting, or slips and falls (**Tables 2-4 and 2-5**).[15] Two occupational activities, lifting and the pushing or pulling of objects at work, should be the focus of substantial further investigation and preventive actions. Optimally, greater use of surveillance data in resource allocation decisions will lead to a more rational allocation of resources. For example, given the magnitude of the low back pain problem, the amount of preventive resources directed at this problem by society is modest.

The third goal of surveillance systems is to track trends in the number of workers exposed to occupational hazards or in the number of workers with injuries, disorders, and diseases over time. This can lead to the detection of new WMD problems or to the evaluation of prevention programs and the determination of some of the costs associated with WMDs. Increases or decreases in the number of cases or changes in the rate of disorders may be due to changing levels of exposure or changes in the reporting of disorders independent of their level of occurrence. Trends can be tracked at either the national or local level. This increase in the number of cases of disorders associated with repeated trauma in

Table 2-3	Possible cases of work-related musculoskeletal disorder for 1990 in a mail order facility	
Job Category (Number of Cases/ Number of Workers)	**Percentage of Hand Cases (Number of Cases/Number of Workers)**	**Percentage of Back Cases (Number of Cases/Number of Workers)**
Mail opening	2 (3/128)	6 (8/128)
Keyboard—lower repetition rate	3 (15/459)	2 (11/459)
Keyboard—higher repetition rate	5 (9/164)	5 (8/164)
Stocking inventory	13 (13/104)	13 (13/104)
Order filling	14 (26/183)	16 (30/183)

Table 2-4	Worker's compensation back cases by injury description
Injury Description	**Percentage of All Back Claims**
Strain	83.0
Sprain	10.1
Contusion	2.3
Herniated disk	0.4
Others	4.2

From National Council on Compensation Insurance, "Worker's Compensation Back Pain Claim Study," Chapter IX, Exhibit IX-A, B, page 68, 1992. Copyright 1992 NCCI. All rights reserved. Reprinted with permission.

Table 2-5	Worker's compensation back strains/sprains by causes of injury description
Cause of Back Strains/Sprains	**Percentage of Claims**
Lifting, holding, or carrying an object	56.8
Slips and falls	19.4
Pushing and/or pulling	11.7
Using a tool/machine	3.3
Motor vehicle	3.0
Others	5.8

Modified from National Council on Compensation Insurance, "Workers Compensation Back Pain Claim Study," Chapter IX, Exhibit IX-A, B, p. 68. Copyright 1992 NCCI. All rights reserved. Reprinted with permission.

Table 2-6	Occupational skin disorders and disorders associated with repeated trauma, from 1982 to 1992 in the United States private sector	
Year	**Number of Skin Disorders**	**Number of Repeated Trauma Disorders**
1982	41,900	22,600
1983	39,500	26,700
1984	42,500	34,700
1985	41,800	37,000
1986	41,900	45,500
1987	54,200	72,900
1988	58,000	115,300
1989	62,100	146,900
1990	60,900	185,400
1991	58,201	223,000
1992	62,900	281,800

Bureau of Labor Statistics, U.S. Department of Labor: Annual Report, 1993, The Bureau.

the BLS national surveillance system has led to efforts by both the Occupational Safety and Health Administration (OSHA) and the American National Standard Institute (ANSI) to initiate efforts to develop standards that address the problem of WMDs (**Table 2-6**).[6,12,16]

The trend of increases in disorders associated with repeated trauma could be explained by an increase in the number of WMDs or by an increase in both the reporting of these disorders by workers and the recording of these disorders by their employers. The relative role of these three factors in explaining this apparent epidemic is unclear. There is some evidence for increas-

Table 2-7	Evaluation of a job redesign with OSHA 200 log and job risk factor data		
Variable		**Before Redesign**	**After Redesign**
Number of possible work-related musculoskeletal disorders (20 employees at risk)		14	0
Lost time days		321	0
Score on job risk factor—ANSI checklist		15	9

Based on Narayan M, Rudolph L: Ergonomic improvements in a medical device assembly plant: a field study. Paper presented at the Human Factors Society, 1993. Estimates of the ANSI checklist scores were based on our reading of the job description of the redesigned job and as a result are only approximate.

ing employer reporting since skin disorders increased by approximately 50% and other illness categories increased by more than twofold, although none of the illness categories increased at the rate of the repeated-trauma category. Given the widespread media coverage for some WMD disorders such as CTS and the attention that CTS has received by the medical profession, there has probably been increased reporting by workers.[20] The most difficult factor to ascertain is whether there has been an actual increase in the incidence of WMDs. Changes in technology and labor practices in some industries, such as the meat packing industry, also likely contributed to the increased repeated-trauma cases by causing an increase in the incident rate in the 1980s.

The goal of tracking trends in the number of WMD cases can be effective in evaluating the success of an intervention program to reduce the number of WMD cases. The use of surveillance data is particularly important for this type of evaluation because although feasible, large-scale research evaluations of intervention programs are very difficult and costly to conduct. Surveillance evaluations may involve both the levels of occupational exposures (hazard) and health outcome data (**Table 2-7**).[14] In the example in **Table 2-7**, surveillance information on both exposure and health was assessed for a manufacturing job that was redesigned. This redesign was conducted after an initial analysis of the OSHA 200 log and discussions with management and workers had identified the job as having an elevated rate of possible WMDs.[14] Hazard surveillance was performed by a walk-through inspection using an ergonomic checklist to identify possible high-risk jobs. As a result of the analysis of both types of surveillance data, a high-risk job was selected for more detailed job analysis and redesign to reduce the risk of WMD from that job. The job had several risk factors, including forceful pinch grips and awkward neck, forearm, wrist, and trunk postures, as well as contact points between areas of the upper extremity and the machinery.

This example illustrates how surveillance data can be used to evaluate intervention activities. However, a dramatic reduction in the rate of WMDs from job redesign does not always occur. In summary, the other goals of surveillance are to identify new problems, determine the magnitude of problems, and evaluate trends over time. Included cluded in these goals is the ability to identify when existing control (prevention) has failed and the possibility to target limited prevention resources to areas of highest disease risk or hazard exposure. Accomplishing these goals requires systematic collection of data in an efficient manner, analysis of the collected data, and dissemination of results of the surveillance analysis.

SITE-SPECIFIC OR ORGANIZATION-SPECIFIC SURVEILLANCE

Surveillance activities conducted at specific workplaces or within a single organization are more important and common than surveillance activities at the national or state level. The identification of either cases of WMD or occupational exposure (hazard surveillance or exposure assessment) before cases of WMD have developed should trigger further evaluation of the workplace. If high levels of exposure are found, the exposure can be reduced by the implementation of either administrative or engineering controls. Recently, ANSI initiated a standard development project (ANSI Z-365: Control of Cumulative Trauma Disorders). This project has described the components of an effective surveillance system.[1,2] A surveillance system should have a health component that can identify possible or definite cases of WMD and a hazard component to examine jobs and work tasks to determine whether there is ongoing exposure to known or suspected causes of WMD. Examples of such exposure are repetitive lifting of objects weighing more than 50 lbs or repetitive and forceful movements of the wrist occurring every few seconds. The most effective workplace surveillance system will have both a medical or health and a hazard or exposure component.

HAZARD SURVEILLANCE

Although hazard surveillance components are less common in current surveillance activities, they are vital. They provide the opportunity to identify and intervene in cases of hazardous exposure before an injury or disorder develops. When the hazardous exposure involves only small groups (fewer than 25 workers), there may be only one or two cases of WMD per year. With so few cases occurring it will be hard to identify a job as one with a possible problem by use of health surveillance alone. This is particularly true if many years of health surveillance data are not available for analysis or if all the jobs within an organization have the same level of exposure so that an analysis that compares workers with low and high exposure cannot be conducted. With an effective hazard surveillance system, hazards may be readily identified regardless of the number of exposed workers. The ability of a hazard surveillance system to identify hazardous exposures is less dependent on the number of exposed workers but rather depends on the overall accuracy of the methods used to identify the nature and intensity of the exposure.

Hazard surveillance can be conducted in at least three ways: (1) ergonomic experts can conduct regular inspections of workplaces followed by detailed job analyses; (2) trained workers, supervisors, or occupational health personnel can analyze jobs with checklists or other simple methods that provide a systematic approach to identifying possible risk factors present on a job; and (3) interviews with workers are also a useful way to identify potential hazardous exposure, particularly because workers have the most detailed information on how their jobs are performed. For example, a checklist for WMDs of the upper extremity might evaluate the repetitive nature of a job, the presence or absence of awkward postures such as reaching overhead, or the use of power tools. Several checklists have been proposed and at least one has been partially validated.[12,18] The most hazardous jobs will often entail exposure to multiple risk factors; it is often possible to combine these methods into a comprehensive approach. The first step would involve both interviews with workers and checklist evaluations of all jobs in an organization. From this hazard surveillance and other health surveillance information, jobs could be prioritized for more sophisticated or intensive evaluation to identify hazardous exposure. The purpose of the more sophisticated evaluation is to precisely assess the nature of the exposures and evaluate possible methods to reduce exposure.[2] Such evaluations are often done by either ergonomists or engineers and require substantial training. In these evaluations each movement of the worker on the job is carefully characterized and the forces on each part of the body are estimated. Some methods compare the forces on the body with some estimate of the body's ability to withstand these forces without injury, based not only on characteristics of the job but also on characteristics of the individual. Although there is no single widely accepted and validated method for sophisticated job analyses, many methods are similar in their overall approach. Commonly, some of the hazardous exposures identified by the hazard surveillance activities

will be so clearly hazardous and ways to reduce the level of exposure will be so obvious that the more sophisticated evaluation will be unnecessary.

Training of employees and supervisors is critical to conducting hazard surveillance activities. However, the initial training can be limited to approximately 1 week. Involvement of employees in hazard surveillance and the development of possible ways to reduce exposure are extremely useful because of their detailed knowledge of work processes. The success of hazard surveillance activities conducted by workers hinges on ensuring that those workers are regularly provided with time on the job to conduct these activities.

With regard to precision in estimating the level of exposure, hazard surveillance activities occupy one pole of a spectrum, with sophisticated job analyses at the other end of the spectrum. Hazard surveillance assessments should be completed quickly and with modest accuracy by nonprofessionals, whereas sophisticated job analyses will require considerably more time to be completed but will be more accurate in the identification of risk factors. Either approach can be used to assess changes in the level of job exposure after a job has been changed for any reason. Although there is little controversy about the general approach of using a checklist and worker interviews for hazard surveillance, there is some disagreement about the accuracy of hazard surveillance checklists when used by nonexperts. Most likely, future guidelines and standards for surveillance activities will incorporate recommendations for hazard surveillance of existing and new work processes.

HEALTH AND MEDICAL SURVEILLANCE

There are two major approaches to conducting health surveillance for WMDs. The first relies on *existing data sources* such as the OSHA 200 log data, whereas the second actively seeks to collect current health information by using *health or symptom questionnaires and interviews or physical examinations*. In addition to the OSHA 200 log data, these other existing sources include worker's compensation and occupational health service records. Some types of nonhealth records may also be useful, such as job bidding or transfer requests and absentee records. Each type of surveillance has its advantages and disadvantages (**Table 2-8**).

One weakness of the existing data sources is the lack of uniformity in how cases are routinely classified or coded. The result is inhomogeneous disease or disorder categories. An example would be the category in the OSHA 200 log in which most CTS cases would be classified. Cases of noise-induced hearing loss should also be classified as repetitive trauma. In the new system for classifying data collected in the annual BLS survey, some of the problems have been addressed. The worker's compensation system has similar problems. One of the reasons for the lack of precision in coding WMDs in both the OSHA and the worker's compensation systems

Table 2-8	Two types of health surveillance for work-related musculoskeletal disorders
Existing Data Sources Such as Worker's Compensation Records	**Questionnaires, Interviews, and Physical Examinations**
System usually designed for other administrative purposes	System designed specifically for surveillance
Relatively inexpensive	Moderate to high cost
Usually requires addition of coding of surrogate of exposure such as job title	Often contains at least job title information, can be linked to risk factor analysis
Examples: OSHA 200 log, occupational health service log, early retirement, medical insurance, absentee and transfer records, accident reports, product quality productivity	Examples: confidential questionnaires without personal identifiers, questionnaire interviews, physical examinations, workplace walk-throughs, job checklist, job analyses

From American National Standards Institute: ANSI Z-365: two types of health surveillance for work-related musculoskeletal disorders (draft), ANSI, 1994; p. 5-4.

is that individual cases are generally coded by the employer or medical provider, who identifies the case rather than by trained coders. Unlike most other medical data systems, worker's compensation systems often rely not on the International Classification of Disease (ICD) system but rather on the ANSI coding scheme for the nature of the injury or illness and the affected body part.[2] Several worker's compensation systems, including that of Massachusetts, have added a special code for CTS to the ANSI coding scheme. One study of the validity of CTS diagnoses in the Massachusetts worker's compensation system found that the majority of claims for CTS classified under the special code for CTS had a physician's diagnosis of CTS in the medical record and most of these had confirmatory nerve conduction studies.[11] However, within the much more numerous claims under the ANSI codes for inflammation, sprain, or neurologic disorders of the upper extremities, as many as 10% to 20% may have been CTS cases.[11] The impact of these limitations in coding the functioning of the surveillance system to accurately identify high-risk jobs or industries is variable. Training of the individuals who will be coding surveillance data can substantially increase the reliability of these data. Validation studies should also be performed for other common conditions. The impact of these limitations in coding is to reduce the utility of surveillance systems to identify all of the moderate- and high-risk jobs or industries. However, industries or occupations that are identified as high risk will generally be truly high risk. This lack of consistency in coding also limits our ability to compare data between two surveillance systems.

The principal advantage of using existing data sources is their low cost. Because questionnaires, interviews, and physical examinations may require additional resources, many organizations have relied on existing data sources to conduct surveillance activities.

A review of hazard surveillance and existing health surveillance data will often be helpful in determining when to add periodic questionnaires or physical examinations to a health surveillance system.

It would be necessary to seek additional information in two situations. The first situation occurs when observation of the workplace suggests that there is common or frequent exposure to known risk factors but the existing surveillance data suggest that there are no problems; in this case one might want to confirm the absence of problems by more actively seeking to identify possible cases of WMD. The absence of problems will commonly be due to one of two reasons: a small number of exposed workers or underreporting of the correct number. A possible solution to the problem of a small number of exposed workers in some situations is to use hazard surveillance data to group jobs with similar exposure into homogeneous groups for the purpose of analysis. This depends on having both an adequate exposure assessment and a record system with detailed information on which job a worker is performing. Another reason there may be no reports of WMD is that there may be obstacles or disincentives to the reporting of a possible disorder to supervisors or health professionals. For example, if an organization gives awards to departments without lost-time injuries or work-related disorders, either supervisors or co-workers may discourage reporting. Confidential interviews with workers can be used to determine whether underreporting is occurring. The second situation when more active collection of surveillance data is indicated is when there is simply no existing surveillance information to determine whether there is a problem. For example, in many sectors of the economy OSHA logs are not required, and in some states, CTS is not recognized by the worker's compensation system as a compensable disorder.

Individuals who report pain or discomfort on a

questionnaire constitute a heterogeneous group. Some will have mild or intermittent symptoms that have not been severe enough for the individual to have sought medical care, whereas others will have had severe symptoms that have led them to seek medical attention from their private or company physician. Others with symptoms will have decided to either accept their symptoms or seek nonphysician providers such as chiropractic practitioners.

The most common method to actively seek information on the presence of symptoms is the use of a questionnaire. Symptom questionnaires may be administered in a number of ways. They may be simply distributed to workers and self-administered; they may be administered in a group with a trained person available to answer questions about the questionnaire and ensure that they are filled out completely; and finally, they may be filled out by an interviewer either separately or as part of a physical examination. The latter method will generally provide the most uniform data, provided that the interviewers have been trained; however, the group-administered method can also provide uniform data in many situations. If workers are fearful of providing health information, the use of self-administered questionnaires without any personal identifying information is an option to be considered.

Analysis of questionnaire data requires some training. Generally, one must decide what will constitute a case. A typical definition used by the National Institute for Occupational Safety and Health (NIOSH) in health hazard evaluations, for example, is based on symptom-meeting criteria such as frequency (more than once a month) and severity (more than 2 on a 5-point scale). The purpose of these definitions is to improve the uniformity or consistency of the data collected, thereby improving the quality of the surveillance data. The goal is to ensure that cases have a common set of characteristics. Clearly, this is more feasible with clinical syndromes that have distinct physical findings and less so with WMDs such as low back pain that are commonly defined by pain in a specific body region.

The prevalence of symptoms will generally be higher than the prevalence of possible cases of WMD in the OSHA log or worker's compensation records. Symptom questionnaires are not used to establish a clinical diagnosis unless accomplished by physical examination.

Despite the limitations of symptom questionnaires, they can be used to identify and prioritize jobs for job analysis, ongoing surveillance monitoring using existing health data, and possible job redesign. If employees feel free to report all types of possible work-related complaints to occupational health care providers and those health records are incorporated into a health surveillance system, the routine use of symptom questionnaires may not be necessary. However, the combination of symptom questionnaires and use of existing health data will most effectively identify and monitor problem areas.

One of the most interesting additional uses of questionnaire data is the evaluation of job modifications.[7] Brief symptom questionnaires (postural discomfort surveys) are used immediately before a change in a job and then several weeks after the change. The discomfort scores by body region are compared for two reasons: to see whether there is improvement in the expected body areas and to then evaluate whether some unexpected problem area has developed.

Because symptoms are subjective and physical examination may be more objective, physical examination has been discussed as an additional component of a surveillance system. The examination consists of inspection, palpation, and active range-of-motion and muscle testing. An additional simple neurologic examination is performed, and several special tests of function such as Phalen's sign may be conducted. The principal advantage of the physical examination is that in some cases it can provide a more specific and uniform classification of the patient's symptoms and the severity of the disorder. However, some common WMDs such as low back pain often have no specific physical findings. In the absence of symptoms, physical examination contributes little useful surveillance information. The role of physical examination is critical in the clinical evaluation of employees with musculoskeletal complaints; however, if barriers to reporting do not exist, periodic physical examinations as a routine surveillance activity are probably not essential for surveillance purposes.

Analysis of health surveillance data is conceptually similar to the analysis of epidemiologic research data. Common epidemiologic concepts such as incidence and prevalence rates are often used. Statistical methods to estimate the random variability of the data are common. In the analysis of surveillance and epidemiologic data, issues of misclassification and random or systematic errors in assessing either exposure or health outcomes should be considered. Errors caused by misclassification are likely to be more common in surveillance data than in epidemiologic research data. When the goal of the analysis is to determine whether a specific group of workers or jobs is associated with an elevated risk, the use of an internal-comparison reference group from the same organization rather than some external comparison is very useful because the identification of cases within an organization and their reporting are likely to be similar. National symptom rates for a limited number of WMD symptoms may also be used for comparison.[5] Efforts to make surveillance data more accurate by standardization of the collection and coding of data are useful, as is the training of personnel involved in the surveillance system.

Whereas random and systematic errors in surveillance data limit the conclusions that can be drawn, these limitations are less important because the goals of surveillance analysis are less rigorous than in epidemiologic research, where the goal is to test a specific hypothesis. Surveillance analyses should be interpreted less quantitatively and more qualitatively. Frequently in the analysis of surveillance data, the variation in risk between jobs, departments, or industries is so large that real differences in risk can be characterized by simple statistical analyses and are unlikely to be explained principally by errors in the classification of disease, confounding factors, or random errors. Nevertheless, surveillance data should always be interpreted cautiously, given their limitations. The goal of the analysis of surveillance data is to trigger further investigation if a problem is detected, not to definitively establish its presence or absence.

The primary goals of surveillance are distinct from those of screening programs. The classic purpose of screening from the patient's perspective is to identify patients who have asymptomatic disease in order to initiate therapy early in the natural course of the disease. The expected benefit is that earlier treatment will be less invasive and more successful. This classic rationale for screening makes little sense for most WMDs because they do not have a detectible asymptomatic period. Carpal tunnel syndrome may be considered an exception to this generalization by some because it may be possible to detect asymptomatic declines in median nerve function, but there is little evidence that most of these asymptomatic cases will progress to symptomatic CTS.[19]

For some WMDs there is a period of definite symptoms and even physical findings during which most workers will continue to work. There is some limited evidence and a reasonable theoretical basis for the hypothesis that intervention as soon as possible in the symptomatic period will reduce the time for recovery to occur once exposure has been reduced or has ceased. Surveillance programs that include the use of questionnaires will identify some individuals with symptoms of short duration that should be further evaluated.

SUMMARY

The most common surveillance systems used to evaluate WMD problems are based on OSHA 200 log data, the occupational health service (in-plant medical records), or worker's compensation records. These records are often analyzed for each facility or department within an organization and have been used to achieve many surveillance goals.

There are three principal surveillance goals. The first goal of surveillance for WMD is the identification of new or previously unrecognized problems. The second goal is to determine the magnitude of the WMD problem at either the national, state, or local level. The third goal is to track trends in the number of workers exposed to occupational hazards, or the number of workers with injuries, disorders, and diseases over time. Evaluation of preventive activities is often feasible with surveillance data. The identification of possible hazardous exposure and elevated rates of WMDs should trigger further evaluation and preventive efforts. Surveillance of WMDs is feasible at both the national and local level. At the local level this should include hazard surveillance. If there are no barriers to reporting the symptoms of WMDs, if the workforce has been educated about the causes of WMDs, and if there is prompt evaluation of workers with possible complaints, then health surveillance based on existing sources of data may be sufficient. The usual sources of existing data are worker's compensation data and the OSHA 200 log. Symptom questionnaires are very useful in cases where there have been barriers to reporting or where there are no existing data sources, such as in the many sectors of the economy where OSHA 200 logs are not required. Although surveillance data need to be interpreted cautiously given their inherent limitations, surveillance data often correctly identify hazardous working conditions and can be used to monitor their elimination.

References

1. American National Standards Institute: *ANSI Z-365: control of cumulative trauma disorders* (draft), ANSI, 1994.

2. American National Standards Institute: *ANSI Z-365: two types of health surveillance for work-related musculoskeletal disorders* (draft), ANSI, 1994; P 4-5.

3. Baker LB, Hanker PA, Fine LJ: Surveillance in occupational illness and injury: concepts and content, *Am J Public Health* 79(suppl): 9-11, 1989.

4. Baron S et al.: *Health hazard evaluation 88-344-2092: Shoprite Supermarkets*, NJ and NY, NIOSH Report No HHE 88-344-2092, NTIS Report No PB91-212431, U.S. Department of Health & Human Services, Public Health Service, Centers for Disease Control and Prevention, National Institute for Occupational Safety and Health, 1990.

5. Behrens V et al: The prevalence of back pain, hand discomfort, and dermatitis in the U.S. working population. 84: 1780-1785, 1994.

6. Bureau of Labor Statistics, U.S. Department of Labor: *Annual report*, 1993, The Bureau.

7. Corlett EN, Bishop RP: A technique for assessing postural discomfort, *Ergonomics* 19: 175-182, 1976.

8. Hales T et al.: *Health hazard evaluation 88-180-1958: John Morrell & Co*, Sioux Falls, SD, NIOSH Report No HHE 88-180-1958, NTIS Report No PB80-128992, U.S. Department of Health & Human Services, Public Health Service, Centers for Disease Control and Prevention, National Institute for Occupational Safety and Health, 1989.

9. Hales T et al.: *Health hazard evaluation 89-251-1997: Cargill Poultry Division*, Buena Vista, GA, NIOSH Report No HHE 89-251-1997, NTIS Report No PB901-183989, U.S. Department of Health & Human Services, Public Health Service, Centers for Disease Control and Prevention, National Institute for Occupational Safety and Health, 1990.

10. Halperin W: Occupational health surveillance, *Health Environ Dig* 8:3-5, 1993.

11. Karrick SA et al.: Use of state workers' compensation data for occupational carpal tunnel syndrome surveillance: A feasibility study in Massachusetts, *Am J Ind Med* 25: 837-850, 1994.

12. Keyserling WM: Analysis of manual lifting tasks: a qualitative alternative of the NIOSH work practices guide, *Am Ind Hyg Assoc J* 50:165-173, 1989.

13. Keyserling WM et al.: A checklist for evaluating ergonomic risk factors associated with upper extremity cumulative trauma disorders, *Ergonomics* 36: 807-831, 1993.

14. Narayan M, Rudolph L: *Ergonomic improvements in a medical device assembly plant: a field study.* Paper presented at the Human Factors Society, Seattle, Wash., 1993.

15. National Council on Compensation Insurance: *Workers' compensation back pain claim study*, New York, 1992, The Council.

16. Occupational Safety and Health Administration: *Record keeping guidelines for occupational injuries and illnesses*, O.M.B. No 1220-0029, U.S. Department of Labor, Bureau of Labor Statistics, September 1986.

17. Osorio AM, Ames R, Jones J: *Carpal tunnel syndrome among grocery store workers*, FI-86-005, Berkeley, Calif, California Occupational Health Program, California Department of Health Services, 1989, p 61.

18. Putz-Anderson V: *Cumulative trauma disorders: a manual for musculoskeletal diseases of the upper limbs*, New York, 1988, Taylor & Francis.

19. Median sensory distal amplitude and latency: comparisons between nonexposed managerial/professional employees and industrial workers, *Am J Ind Med*, 24: 175-189, 1993.

20. Stevens K: The carpal tunnel syndrome in cardiologists, *Ann Intern Med* 112:796, 1990 (letter).

21. Tanaka S et al: Morbidity from repetitive knee trauma in carpet and floor layers, *Br J Ind Med* 44:611-620, 1987.

22. Thacker SB, Berkelman RL: History of public health surveillance. In Halperin W, Baker EL, Monson RR, editors: *Public health surveillance*, New York, 1992, Van Nostrand Reinhold.

23. Thun M et al: Morbidity from repetitive knee trauma in carpet and floor layers, *Br J Ind Med* 44:611-620, 1987.

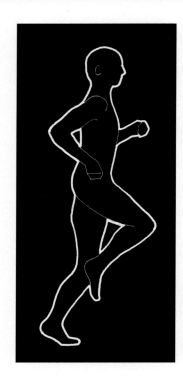

Chapter 3

Biomechanics of Skeletal Systems

Malcolm H. Pope

CONTENTS

The musculoskeletal system can be understood through the application of some basic concepts of biomechanics. Biomechanics applies the principles of physical science (mechanics) to the materials making up the structures and systems of the human body.

JOINT MECHANICS

The links of the human body facilitate our movements. The links pivot at the joints, are guided by the ligaments, and are powered by the muscles. The body links, when rotating relative to each other, rotate around an axis. This is not usually an unchanging axis but one that moves. The location at any point in time is called the *instant center* (**Figure 3-1**). Kinematically, most joint motion is a combination of rolling and sliding. **Figure 3-2** shows how, with rolling, the instant center is at the intersection of the surfaces.

The forces in the joints are usually estimated by the principles of force and moment balance. Simply stated, the principle is that at equilibrium the forces up must equal the forces down and the clockwise moments must equal the counterclockwise moments. In **Figure 3-3**, an example is given of pelvis equilibrium. Forces of 2000 N can be reached in the joint. If we assume that one limb weighs one-sixth of body weight, then $W = \frac{5}{6}$ body weight. For a 60-kg person, $W = 500$ N. If $d_1 = 0.05$ m and $d_2 = 0.15$ m, the moment equilibrium is

$$d_1 M = d_2 W$$

$$\therefore M = \frac{0.15}{0.05} \times 500 = 1500 \text{ N}$$

For force equilibrium,

The joint reaction force (*J*)
$$= M + W = 1500 + 500 = 2000 \text{N}$$

(this assumes that *M* and *W* are parallel forces).

In activities typical of industry, we must take into account the dynamic forces. The torque around a joint is given by *T*:

$$T = \text{mass moment of inertia} \times \text{angular acceleration}$$
$$= I\Theta$$
$$= Md$$

Because the inertia of a body segment is a constant and the muscle moment arm is a constant, this equation shows that an increase in joint acceleration means greater forces on the joint and in the muscles. Occupationally, this can lead to muscle fatigue, increased joint forces, and eventually osteoarthritis.

MATERIALS OF THE BODY

Bone

Bone is the major structural material of the human body. It is essentially a composite material made up of osteons (the Haversian System) embedded in a matrix of ground substance. **Figure 3-4** reveals that bone has a different response at different strain rates.[11] At higher rates, it is stronger but exhibits less plastic behavior. Bone is also anisotropic, which means that it has different properties in different directions.[11]

In mature humans there are two types of bone, compact (or haversian) and cancellous. Cortical bone is stiffer and stronger than cancellous bone. Cancellous bone fractures at strains of 75%, but cortical bone

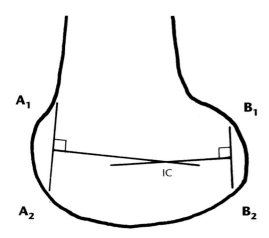

Figure 3-1 The instant center (*IC*) calculation. The perpendicular bisector of $B_1\,B_2$ intersects with the perpendicular bisector of $A_1\,A_2$ to form the IC.

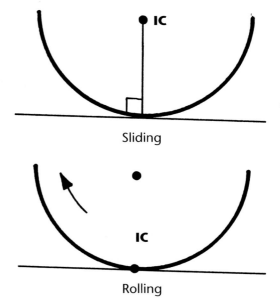

Figure 3-2 Sliding versus rolling.

fractures when the strain exceeds 2%.[3] Typical stress-strain curves for cortical bone, metal, and glass are given in **Figure 3-5**. The variations in material stiffness are reflected in the slopes of the curves in the elastic region. Metal is the stiffest material.

Bone has different strengths in compression, shear, and tension. Because it is stronger in compression, a bone under bending tends to break on the tensile side. Bone fractures fall into three general categories: low-energy, high-energy, and very high-energy fractures. A low-energy fracture is exemplified by a fall leading to a fracture, a high-energy fracture is sustained during automobile accidents, and a very high-energy fracture is produced by a gunshot. Because of the strain rate dependency of bone (**Fig. 3-6**), these fractures have differ-

ent characteristics with higher-energy fractures characterized by a greater number of fracture fragments.[5]

A fracture can also be caused by repeated applications of a lower load. This type is termed a *fatigue fracture* and is produced either by few repetitions of a high load or by many repetitions of a relatively normal load. These fractures can occur in industry under repetitive loading (continuous strenuous physical activity), which causes the muscles to become fatigued and reduces their ability to contract. As a result, they are less

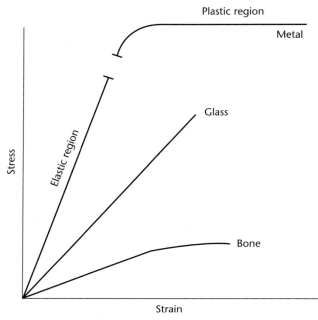

Figure 3-5 Stress-strain curves for three materials. Metal is the stiffest material. Glass is termed brittle; it has elastic behavior but fails with little deformation. Cortical bone, which has both ductile and brittle regions, exhibits nonlinear elastic behavior.

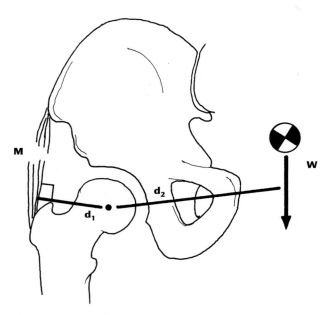

Figure 3-3 Equilibrium of the hip.

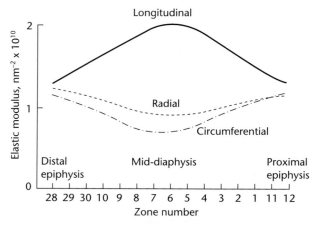

Figure 3-4 Variation of elastic moduli as a function of distance from epiphyses. (*From Pope MH and Outwater JO: J Biomech 7:61-66, 1974*).

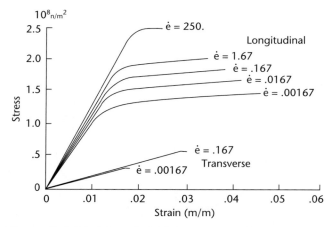

Figure 3-6 Modulus of elasticity versus strain rate, compact bovine bone. (*From Crowningshield RD and Pope MH: Ann Biomed Eng 2:217-225, 1974*).

able to store energy and thus neutralize stresses on the bone.

A progressive loss of bone density, which is part of the normal aging process, is far more dramatic in post-menopausal females. The result is a marked reduction in the amount of cancellous bone and thinning of cortical bone. The longitudinal trabeculae become thinner, and some of the transverse trabeculae are even reabsorbed.[13] This decrease in total bone tissue and the slight decrease in bone size reduce bone strength and stiffness. Patients with osteoporosis will be more likely to suffer femoral neck and vertebral fractures, but all of the bones are weaker.

Soft Tissues

Tendons and ligaments are made up of mostly collagen and some ground substance. These tissues derive their strength and flexibility from collagen. The ligamentum flavum of the spine is unusual in having a substantial proportion of elastin, which gives these structures great elasticity. The collagen fibers are nearly parallel in tendons, which equips them to withstand high unidirectional loads. The collagen fibers in ligaments are less oriented, usually because ligaments have multiple attachment sites.

When a tendon or ligament is mechanically loaded, the resulting load-elongation curve has several regions that characterize the tissue's behavior (**Fig. 3-7**). The initial region of the load-elongation curve is usually called the toe region. The behavior is due to a change in the wavy pattern of the relaxed collagen fibers, which become straighter as loading progresses.[7,16]

Like most biologic materials, the behavior of ligaments and tendons is viscoelastic, or rate dependent, so these structures increase in strength and stiffness with an increased loading rate. An additional viscoelastic effect is the slow deformation, or creep, that occurs when tendons and ligaments are subjected to a constant low load over an extended period such as a workday. Injury mechanisms in a tendon are influenced by the amount of force produced by the contraction of the muscle to which the tendon is attached and the cross-sectional area of the tendon in relation to that of its muscle. Aging results in a decline in the strength, stiffness, and ability to withstand deformation.[17] Therefore, this should be taken into account in aging workers.

Few in vivo studies of strain of tendons or ligaments have been performed. Kear and Smith[9] found that strain in the lateral digital extensor tendons of sheep reached 2.6% while the sheep were trotting rapidly. This suggests that during normal activity, a tendon in vivo is subjected to less than one fourth of its ultimate stress. Beynnon et al[2] have measured the strain in the anterior cruciate ligament in vivo. Strain was found to vary as a function of flexion angle (**Fig. 3-8**) and as a function of activity.

Cartilage

As noted earlier, very high loads occur across the diarthrodial joints. Although the geometry of joints

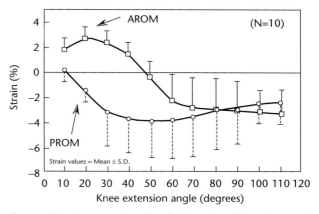

Figure 3-8 Average data for all 10 study subjects for active and passive motion of the knee joint in a graph of anteromedial band strain (%) versus knee angle. (*From Beynnon B et al:* Int Orthop *16:1-12, 1992*).

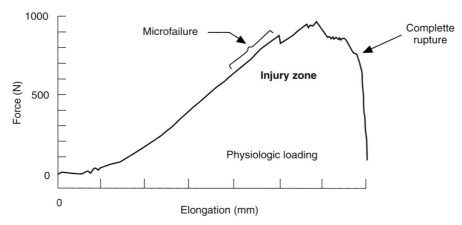

Figure 3-7 Progressive failure of the anterior cruciate ligament in tension at a physiologic strain rate. (*Courtesy Noyes, 1976.*) The joint was displaced 7 mm before the ligament failed completely.

varies, it is axiomatic that the function of articular cartilage in diarthrodial joints is to increase the area of load distribution and provide a smooth, wear-resistant bearing surface.

Like other biologic materials, articular cartilage is a mixture of materials. Articular cartilage is a biphasic (solid-fluid) material: a collagen-proteoglycan solid matrix (25% by weight) surrounded by freely movable interstitial fluid (75% by weight). The biomechanical properties of articular cartilage that are vital to function are the intrinsic material properties of the solid matrix and the frictional resistance to the flow of interstitial fluid through the porous permeable solid matrix. The other property that is important is the mechanism to maintain the lubricating fluid film between the opposing articulating surfaces and maintain a constant nutrient flow to the chondrocytes within the matrix. Walker et al[18,19] coined the term "boosted lubrication" in which the solvent component of the synovial fluid passes into the articular cartilage during squeeze film action and a concentrated pool of proteins is left to lubricate the surfaces. It becomes more difficult, as the two articular surfaces approach each other, for the macromolecules in the synovial fluid to escape from the gap between the surfaces because they are physically large. The water and small molecules can still escape into the articular cartilage through the cartilage surface and into the joint space at the joint periphery.

Although it is clear that articular cartilage has the ability to provide for the diarthrodial joint a self-lubrication feature that operates under normal physiologic joint-loading conditions, it is unlikely that the varied demands during normal function can be satisfied by a single mode of lubrication. A schematic view of mixed-mode lubrication is given in **Figure 3-9.**[1]

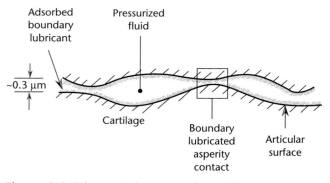

Figure 3-9 Schematic depiction of mixed lubrication operating in articular cartilage. Boundary lubrication occurs at places where the thickness of the fluid film is on the same order as the roughness of the bearing surfaces. Fluid film lubrication takes place in areas with more widely separated surfaces. (*Modified from Armstrong CG and Mow VC: Friction, lubrication and wear of synovial joints. In Owen R, Goodfellow J, and Bullough P, editors:* Scientific foundations of orthopaedics and traumatology, *London, 1980, Heinemann: pp 223-232.*)

Nerve Tissue

The peripheral nerves can be considered complex structures composed of nerve fibers, layers of connective tissue, and blood vessels. Many industrial medical problems are related to acute or chronic trauma to the nerves (e.g., sciatica, carpal tunnel syndrome, and Raynaud's disease).

Nerve fibers appear to be extremely susceptible to trauma, but because they are surrounded by the epineurium and perineurium, they are protected. Only when these layers are compromised will injury occur. External trauma can result in deterioration in nerve function. Common types of nerve injury are stretching by rapid extension and compression inflicted by crushing. Stretching induces changes in intraneural blood flow before the nerve fibers rupture, whereas compression of a nerve can cause injury to both nerve fibers and blood vessels in the nerve, mainly at the edges of the nerve.

When tension is applied to a nerve, initial elongation of the nerve under a very small load is followed by a region in which stress and elongation show a linear elastic relationship (**Fig. 3-10**). As the limit of the linear region is approached, the nerve fibers start to rupture inside the endoneurial tubes and inside the intact perineurium.[8] Finally, the epineurium and perineurium rupture, and the nerve behaves like plastic material.

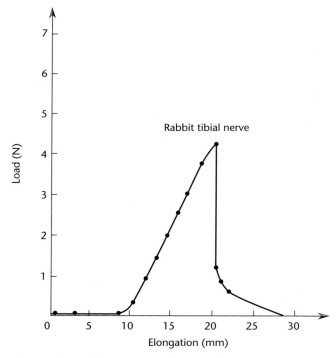

Figure 3-10 The initial portion of the curve indicates elongation without any measurable load. After the load begins to increase, the curve shows a region in which the nerve behaves like elastic material. This linear portion extends nearly to the point of peak load. Beyond peak load, the mechanical capacity of the nerve deteriorates sharply.

Maximal elongation at the elastic limit is about 20%, and complete structural failure occurs at a maximum elongation of 30%.[15] The maximal load that can be sustained by the median and ulnar nerves is in the range of 70 to 220 N and 60 to 150 N, respectively.[14]

Tensile injuries of peripheral nerves are usually associated with severe trauma because nerve fibers in a nerve under tension rupture before the endoneurial tubes and perineurium do. The regenerating axons may have intact pathways to follow during their growth. Compression of a nerve can induce symptoms such as numbness, pain, and muscle weakness.[14] Compression at about 30 mm Hg may also lead to depletion of axonally transported proteins distal to the compression site.[6] Pressure above 80 mm Hg causes the nerve in the compressed segment to become completely ischemic.

Regeneration following transection of a peripheral nerve is dependent on both biologic and biomechanical factors. Nerve fibers grow at about 1 mm/day. Aging of peripheral nerves can be manifested as alterations in vibratory perception, ankle jerks, and nerve conduction velocity.

Muscle

The main structural unit of skeletal muscle is the muscle fiber organized into fascicles encased in the perimysium. The fibers are composed of myofibrils, which in turn are composed of (thin) filaments of the protein actin and (thick) filaments of the protein myosin.

Shortening of the muscle results from the relative movement of the actin and myosin filaments past one another. The force of contraction is developed by movement of the myosin cross-bridges in contact with the actin filaments. Troponin and tropomyosin regulate the making and breaking of the contacts between filaments; the calcium ion turns the contractile activity on and off. Each repeat of this pattern is a sarcomere, the functional unit of the contractile system. The tendons and the endomysium, perimysium, and epimysium represent parallel and series elastic components that stretch with active contraction or passive muscle extension.

Muscles may contract concentrically, isometrically, or eccentrically, depending on the relationship between muscle tension and resistance. The types of muscle work

are given in **Table 3-1**. Concentric and eccentric contractions involve dynamic work in which the muscle moves a joint or controls its movement. Isometric contractions involve static work in which the joint position is unchanged. These contractions rarely occur in occupational work. Isometric contractions produce greater tension than do concentric contractions. The tension developed in an eccentric contraction may even exceed that developed during an isometric contraction.[10] Isokinetic contraction is dynamic muscle work in which movement of the joint is kept at a constant velocity, and the velocity of shortening or lengthening of the muscle is constant. Isoinertial contraction is also dy-

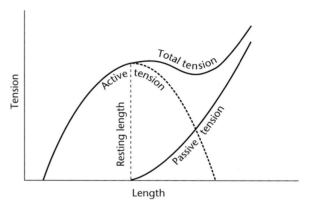

Figure 3-11 The active and passive tension exerted by an entire muscle contracting isometrically and tetanically is plotted against the muscle's length. Active tension is produced by the contractile muscle components and passive tension by the series and parallel elastic components, which become stressed when the muscle is stretched beyond its resting length. The greater the amount of stretching, the larger the contribution of the elastic component to the total tension. The shape of the active curve is generally the same in different muscles, but the passive curve and hence the total curve varies depending on how much connective tissue (elastic component) the muscle contains. (*Modified from Crawford GNC and James NT: The design of muscles. In Owen R, Goodfellow J, and Bullough P, editors:* Scientific foundations of orthopaedics and traumatology, *London, 1980, Heinemann: pp 67-74.*)

Table 3-1	Definitions of muscle contractions
Type	**Definition**
Isometric	The external length of the muscle does not change. Same as *static.*
Isotonic	The internal force of the muscle does not change but the muscle shortens. Same as *concentric.*
Eccentric	The external force is greater than the internal force of the muscles, so the muscle lengthens.
Isokinetic	A dynamic exercise in which the speed of motion is constant.
Isoinertial	Contraction against a constant load. The torque generated by the muscle causes acceleration.

namic muscle work in which the resistance against which the muscle must contract remains constant. If the moment produced by the muscle is equal to or less than the resistance to be overcome, the muscle length remains unchanged and the muscle contracts isometrically. If the moment is greater than the resistance, the muscle shortens and causes acceleration of the body part.

An isotonic contraction is a muscle contraction in which the tension is constant throughout a joint's range of motion. Because the muscle force moment arm changes throughout the range of joint motion, the muscle tension must also change. Therefore, isotonic muscle contraction does not usually occur in physiologic joint motion.

Force production in muscle is influenced by the length-tension, load-velocity, and force-time relationships of the muscle. The length-tension relationship in a whole muscle is influenced by both active (contractile) and passive (series and parallel elastic) components.

Two other factors that increase force production are prestretching of the muscle and a rise in muscle temperature caused by stretching activity. Active tension in **Figure 3-11** shows the tension developed by the contractile elements of the muscle.[4] Passive tension reflects the tension developed when the muscle exceeds its resting length and the noncontractile elements are stretched. This passive tension is mainly developed in the parallel and series elastic components. Under contraction, the combined active and passive tensions produce the total tension. As a muscle is progressively stretched beyond its resting length, passive tension rises and active tension decreases.

SUMMARY

Biomechanical factors can help explain injuries to the musculoskeletal system. Loads in the joints are extremely high because of the lever arm and the high muscle forces. Materials of the human body are usually viscoelastic and anisotropic. Cartilage is a biphasic material with its properties guaranteed by mixed-mode lubrication. Nerve function is affected by tension and compression overload. Muscle contractions can be divided into isometric (static), concentric, eccentric, isokinetic, isoinertial, and isotonic.

References

1. Armstrong CG, Mow VC: Friction, lubrication and wear of synovial joints. In Owen R, Goodfellow J and Bullough P, editors: *Scientific foundations of orthopaedics and traumatology,* London, 1980, Heinemann: pp 223-232.

2. Beynnon B et al: The measurement of anterior cruciate ligament strain in-vivo, *Int Orthop* 16:1-12, 1992.

3. Carter DR, Hayes WC: Compact bone fatigue damage. A microscopic examination, *Clin Orthop* 127:265-274, 1977.

4. Crawford GNC, James NT: The design of muscles. In Owen R, Goodfellow J, and Bullough P, editors: *Scientific foundations of orthopaedics and traumatology,* London, 1980, Heinemann: pp 67-74.

5. Crowningshield RD, Pope MH: The response of compact bone in tension at various strain rates, *Ann Biomed Eng* 2:217-225, 1974.

6. Dahlin LB et al: Changes in fast axonal transport during experimental nerve compression at low pressures, *Exp Neurol* 84:29, 1984.

7. Elliott DH: Structure and function of mammalian tendon, *Biol Rev* 40:392, 1965.

8. Haftek J: Stretch injury of peripheral nerves. Acute effects of stretching on rabbit nerve, *J Bone Joint Surg Br* 52:354, 1970.

9. Kear M, Smith RN: A method for recording tendon strain in sheep during locomotion, *Acta Orthop Scand* 46:896, 1975.

10. Norkin C, Levange P: *Joint structure and function: a comprehensive analysis,* Philadelphia, 1983, FA Davis Co.

11. Pope MH, Outwater JO: Mechanical properties of bone as a function of position and orientation, *J Biomech* 7:61-66, 1974.

12. Siffert RS, Levy RN: Trabecular patterns and the internal architecture of bone, *Mt Sinai J Med* 48:221, 1981.

13. Sunderland S: *Nerves and nerve injuries,* ed 2, Edinburgh, 1978, Churchill Livingstone International.

14. Sunderland S, Bradley KC: Stress-strain phenomena in human peripheral nerve trunks, *Brain* 84:102, 1961.

15. Viidik A: Biomechanics and functional adaptation of tendons and joint ligaments. In Evans FG, editor: *Studies on the anatomy and function of bones and joints,* Berlin, 1966, Springer-Verlag: pp 17-39.

16. Viidik A, Danielsen CC, Oxlund H: Fourth International Congress of Biorheology Symposium on Mechanical Properties of Living Tissues: on fundamental and phenomenological models, structure and mechanical properties of collagen, elastic and glycosaminoglycan complexes, *Biorheology* 19:437, 1982.

17. Walker PS et al: "Boosted lubrication" in synovial joints by fluid entrapment and enrichment, *Ann Rheum Dis* 27:512, 1968.

18. Walker PS et al: Mode of aggregation of hyaluronic acid protein complex on the surface of articular cartilage, *Ann Rheum Dis* 29:591, 1970.

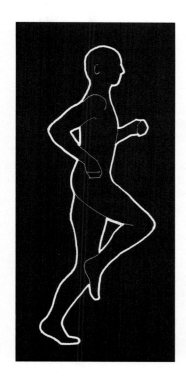

Chapter 4

The Skeletal Muscle

Margareta Nordin

CONTENTS

The human body system contains three muscle types: cardiac muscle, which composes the heart; smooth (nonstriated or involuntary) muscle, which lines the hollow internal organs; and skeletal (striated or voluntary) muscle, which attaches the skeleton via the tendons and causes it to move. Skeletal muscles provide strength and protection to the skeleton by distributing loads and absorbing shocks. They enable the linkage of bones in the skeleton to move.[40]

Movement or maintenance of posture usually represents the action of muscle groups rather than individual muscles. There are about 430 skeletal muscles in the human body. They are found in pairs on the right and left sides of the body and constitute approximately 40% to 45% of the total body weight. Skeletal muscle mass decreases with age, disuse, and immobilization.

Skeletal muscle is a highly dynamic tissue. The role of skeletal muscle is to perform both dynamic and static work. Dynamic work permits motion and positions the body segments in space; static work maintains body posture. During direct or indirect trauma to the body, skeletal muscle also acts as a shock absorbent.

A brief overview of the structure of skeletal muscle will be presented, with a focus on muscle strain and pain, by far the most common diagnosis in patients seeking care in an occupational setting. The chapter will describe types of muscle work, muscle remodeling (overuse, disuse, immobilization), and the effects of physical training.

BASIC STRUCTURE OF SKELETAL MUSCLE

Skeletal muscle is surrounded by a fibrous connective tissue fascia called the *epimysium* (**Fig. 4-1**). The muscle itself is composed of many bundles, or fascicles, each of which is encased in a dense connective tissue or tissue sheath (the *perimysium*). Each fascicle is composed of muscle fiber, that is, long cylindrical multinucleated cells. Skeletal muscle is well vascularized with capillary blood vessels between the muscle fibers. The muscle fibers are surrounded by the *endomysium,* a loose connective tissue. The *sarcolemma*—a thin elastic sheet—lies beneath the endomysium. Each muscle fiber consists of numerous delicate strands, *myofibrils,* which are the contractile elements of muscles. The myofibril is a series of smaller filaments in a repeated pattern called a *sarcomere.* The sarcomere is the functional unit of the contractile system of the muscle and has a banding pattern that is formed by thick and thin filaments, myosin and actin proteins. Each actin filament is a double helix appearing

as two strands of beads spiraling around each other. The *cross-bridges* between myosin filaments and actin filaments are the essential elements in the mechanism of muscle contraction. Tropomyosin and troponin proteins regulate interdigitation of the actin and myosin filaments. For a more extensive review, interested readers are recommended to read Garrett and Best[19] and Caplan et al.[9]

In general, each end of the skeletal muscle is attached to the bone by tendons, which have no active contractile properties. The epimysium of skeletal muscle is continuous with that of the tendons, and together these fibers act as a structural framework for the attachment of bones and muscle fibers. The force produced by the contracting muscle is transmitted to skeletal bone through these connective tissues and tendons.

INSERTIONS

The insertion points and connection of tendon to bone and tendon to muscle are particularly vulnerable to load as a change in material characteristics occurs. The structure of the insertion of a tendon to bone is similar to that of a ligament. The insertion consists of four zones: a parallel collagen fiber zone, unmineralized fibrocartilage, mineralized fibrocartilage, and cortical bone.[11] The change from a more tendinous material to more bony material produces a gradual change in mechanical properties, such as increased stiffness. The larger the cross-sectional area of the muscle, the greater the tensile load transmitted to the tendon and the insertion area. In the insertion of muscle tissue into a tendon, the collagen fibers extend well into the muscle and the muscle fibers insert with an oblique angle. When a muscle-tendon unit is stretched in laboratory conditions, a healthy tendon seldom fails. Failure usually occurs at the bone-tendon unit, at the myotendinousjunction, or within the muscle tissue itself.[39,49] These injuries are commonly called *strain* but can also be labeled muscle pull, muscle tear, or various other names.[19] *Sprain* refers to collagenous tissues such as ligaments or tendons. Sprain and strain are frequently used together in clinical settings, and this pairing implies injury to both muscle and ligament.

THE MOTOR UNIT

The motor unit forms the functional unit of the skeletal muscle. It includes a single motor neuron and all the muscle fibers innervated by it. The motor unit is the smallest part of a muscle that can contract independently. If a motor unit is excited, all muscle fibers respond as one. This is called the all-or-none response to stimulation, that is, they either contract maximally or not at all.

The number of muscle fibers forming a motor unit is closely related to the degree of control required of the muscle. For example, in large muscles that perform

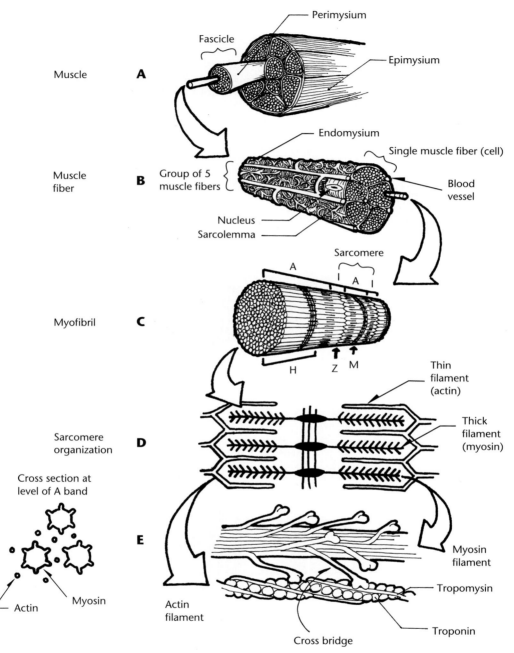

Figure 4-1 Basic structure of the skeletal muscle. From Pittman MI, Peterson L: Biomechanics of skeletal muscle. (*In Nordin M, Frankel VH, editors:* Basic biomechanics of the musculoskeletal system, *ed 2, Philadelphia, 1989, Lea & Febiger: pp 89-111.*)

coarse movements such as the gastrocnemius, the motor unit contains 1000 to 2000 muscle fibers. In the extraocular muscles, each motor unit may contain fewer than a dozen muscle fibers. The higher the control required for fine movements, the smaller the number of muscle fibers per motor unit.

The fibers of each motor unit are dispersed throughout the muscle along with fibers of other units. Muscle recruitment therefore implies that the more motor units that are stimulated, the higher the contraction of the muscles and consequently the higher the force production.

MUSCLE CONTRACTION

A brief description of the events during excitation, contraction, and relaxation of a skeletal muscle fiber is essential. The motor neuron is composed of an axon originating from the body cell in the anterior horn of the spinal cord. The axon branches near its end to innervate several skeletal muscle fibers and thereby form a neuromuscular junction with each fiber (see **Fig. 4-2**). The muscle membrane—the sarcolemma—lies directly under the terminal branches of the axon. The sarcolemma is known as the motor end plate or the motor end-plate membrane.[45] The final branches of the axon form the terminal through which acetylcholine is stored in synaptic vesicles. When an action potential is initiated and propagated in a motor axon, it causes the release of acetylcholine from the axon terminal at the neuromuscular junction and the contraction begins.[19,34,44] The box on p. 37 summarizes the events during excitation, contraction, and relaxation of skeletal muscle fiber.[40]

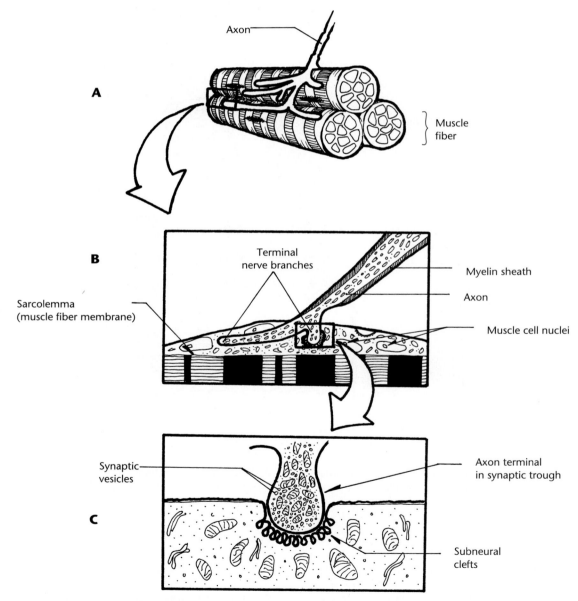

Figure 4-2 Schematic representation of the innervation of muscle fibers. (*From Pittman MI, Peterson L: Biomechanics of skeletal muscle. In Nordin M, Frankel VH, editors: Basic biomechanics of the musculoskeletal system, ed 2, Philadelphia, 1989, Lea & Febiger: pp 89-111.*)

MUSCLE FIBER TYPE

The fiber composition of a skeletal muscle depends on the function of that muscle. For example, the function of the soleus muscle in the calf is primarily to maintain posture, that is, an endurance characteristic. Most skeletal muscles, however, perform both endurance-type activity and high-intensity strength activities. Therefore these muscles generally contain a mixture of different muscle fiber types. As a result of histologic and histochemical observations, the fiber types in skeletal muscles are classified on the basis of their different contractile and metabolic properties.[14,16] **Table 4-1** identifies the properties of the three most common types of skeletal muscle fibers: type I, type IIA, and type IIB. The classification system takes into consideration the speed of contraction, myosin adenosine triphosphate (ATP) activity, the primary source of ATP production, glycolytic enzyme activity, the number of mitochondria, capillaries, myoglobin content, muscle color, glycogen content, fiber diameter, and the rate of fatigue.[34]

Type I fibers (slow-twitch, oxidative) are functionally characterized by a relatively slow contraction time,

---

Events during excitation, contraction, and relaxation of muscle fiber.

1. An action potential is initiated and propagated in a motor axon.

2. This action potential causes the release of acetylcholine from the axon terminals at the neuromuscular junction.

3. Acetylcholine is bound to receptor sites on the motor end-plate membrane.

4. Acetylcholine increases the permeability of the motor end plate to sodium and potassium ions and thereby produces an end-plate potential.

5. The end-plate potential depolarizes the muscle membrane (sarcolemma) and generates a muscle action potential that is propagated over the membrane surface.

6. Acetylcholine is rapidly destroyed by acetylcholinesterase on the end-plate membrane.

7. The muscle action potential depolarizes the transverse tubules.

8. Depolarization of the transverse tubules leads to the release of calcium ions from the terminal cisternae of the sarcoplasmic reticulum surrounding the myofibrils. These ions are released into the sarcoplasm in the direct vicinity of the regulatory proteins tropomyosin and troponin.

9. Calcium ions bind to troponin, which allows movement of the tropomyosin molecule away from the myosin receptor sites on the actin filament that it had been blocking and releases the inhibition that had prevented actin from combining with myosin.

10. Actin combines with myosin ATP (receptor sites on the myosin cross-bridges bind to receptor sites on the actin chain):

$$A + M \times ATP \rightarrow A \times M \times ATP$$

11. Actin activates the myosin ATPase found on the myosin cross-bridge, thereby enabling ATP to be split (hydrolyzed). This process releases energy used to produce movement of the myosin cross-bridges:

$$A \times M \times ATP \rightarrow A \times M + ATP + P_1$$

12. Oarlike movements of the cross-bridges produce relative sliding of the thick and thin filaments past each other.

13. Fresh ATP binds to the myosin cross-bridge, the actin-myosin bond breaks, and the cross-bridge dissociates from actin:

$$A \times M + ATP \rightarrow A + M \times ATP$$

14. Cycles of binding and unbinding of actin with the myosin cross-bridges at successive sites along the actin filament (steps 11, 12, and 13) continue as long as the concentration of calcium remains high enough to inhibit action of the troponin-tropomyosin system.

15. The concentration of calcium ions falls as they are pumped into the terminal cisternae of the sarcoplasmic reticulum by an energy-requiring process that splits ATP.

16. Calcium dissociates from troponin, and the inhibitory action of troponin-tropomyosin is restored. The actin filament slides back and the muscle lengthens. In the presence of ATP, actin and myosin remain in the dissociated, relaxed state.

Data from Pittman MI, Peterson L: In Nordin M, Frankel VH, editors: Basic biomechanics of the musculoskeletal system, ed 2, Philadelphia, 1989, Lea & Febiger.

Table 4-1	Properties of three types of skeletal muscle fibers		
Feature	**Type I:** **Slow-twitch,** **Oxidative**	**Type IIA:** **Fast-twitch,** **Oxidative-Glycolytic**	**Type IIB:** **Fast-twitch,** **Glycolytic**
Speed of contraction	Slow	Fast	Fast
Myosin-ATPase activity	Low	High	High
Primary source of ATP production	Oxidative phosphorylation	Oxidative phosphorylation	Anaerobic glycolysis
Glycolytic enzyme activity	Low	Intermediate	High
Number of mitochondria	Many	Many	Few
Capillaries	Many	Many	Few
Myoglobin content	High	High	Low
Muscle color	Red	Red	White
Glycogen content	Low	Intermediate	High
Fiber diameter	Small	Intermediate	Large
Rate of fatigue	Slow	Intermediate	Fast

Data from Pittman MI, Peterson L: In Nordin M, Frankel VH, editors: Basic biomechanics of the musculoskeletal system, *ed 2, Philadelphia, 1989, Lea & Febiger.*

their anaerobic glycolytic activity is slow, and they have a high potential for aerobic activity because of the high content of mitochondria. Type I fibers are difficult to fatigue because many capillaries deliver oxygen and nutrients to the fiber and a relatively slow rate of ATP breakdown occurs. Well suited for prolonged low-intensity work, type I fibers are smaller in diameter and each fiber produces relatively little tension. The popular name of type I fibers—"red fibers"—is derived from the color given by the high content of myoglobin.

Type II muscle fibers are classified as A, B, and C. Type IIC fibers are rare and are considered to be undifferentiated fibers that may be transitory. These fibers will not be described in this text. Functionally, type IIA and IIB fibers are characterized by relatively fast contraction. Type IIA fast-twitch oxidative-glycolytic fibers are also red because of their high myoglobin content. The fast contraction time is combined with a well-developed capacity for both aerobic (oxidative) and anaerobic (glycolytic) activity. Type IIA fibers have a well-developed capillary system and can maintain contractile activity for relatively long periods and at a high rate of activity. They do, however, fatigue quicker because the rate of ATP splitting is high.

Type IIB fast-twitch glycolytic fibers are primarily suited for anaerobic activity. These fibers have few capillaries and contain little myoglobin, and thus their color is often referred to as white. Type IIB fibers fatigue easily because the rate of ATP splitting quickly depletes the glycogen in the muscle fiber. These fibers are of larger diameter and can therefore produce high tension for only short spurts before they fatigue.

In the average population, about 50% to 55% of skeletal muscle fibers are type I, 30% to 35% are type IIA, and about 15% are type IIB. It should be pointed out that these percentages vary greatly among individuals. For example, as large as a 90% variation has been observed in the type I fibers predominantly found in erector spinae muscles. It is generally believed that fiber types are genetically determined.[12,20,25]

Elite athletes may have a different fiber-type distribution than the average population. Essen[18] and Saltin et al[46] reported that endurance athletes can exhibit up to 80% type I fibers whereas sprinters may have as few as 30%.

TYPES OF MUSCLE WORK

Muscle work is usually divided into *static* and *dynamic* work. Static work implies that no mechanical work is performed and the posture or joint position is maintained. The muscle has produced an isometric contraction, that is, muscle tension equals the external load and the muscle length is virtually constant.

Dynamic work implies that mechanical work is performed and joint motion is produced. Dynamic work is divided into *concentric* and *eccentric* contractions. Dur-

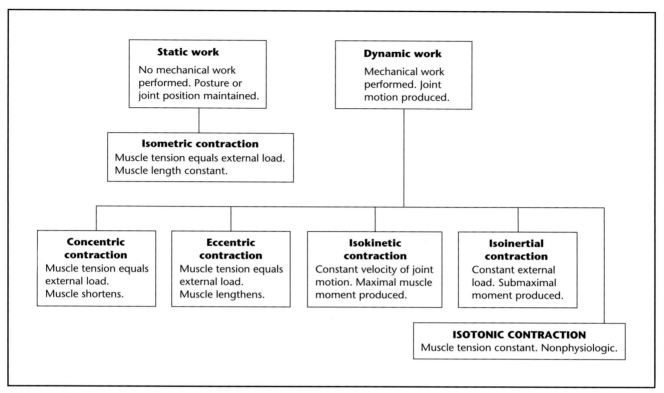

Figure 4-3 Types of muscle work and contraction.

ing concentric contractions, muscle tension overcomes the external load and the muscle shortens. Eccentric contractions occur when the muscle tension does not overcome the external load and the muscle lengthens. Greater muscle tension is produced in eccentric contraction than in either isometric contraction or concentric contraction.[28,29,31,41] A particular type of contraction seldom occurs in isolation but rather in combination.[28] For example, during a lift bending forward to pick up an object, the erector spinae first undergoes an eccentric contraction. During the lift of the object, the back muscles perform a concentric contraction. Finally, while holding the object and maintaining the posture, the contraction becomes isometric.

Dynamic work can furthermore be divided into *isokinetic, isoinertial,* and *isotonic* contractions (see **Fig. 4-3**).[30,44] Isokinetic contraction is defined as a contraction made under a constant velocity of joint motion when a subject is asked to produce a maximal voluntary contraction. Isoinertial contraction is a constant external load on the limb where a submaximal contraction is produced to overcome the external load. Finally, during an isotonic contraction, the muscle tension remains constant when it is monitored by electromyography or other means. This type of contraction is nonphysiologic and is usually only produced in a laboratory setting.

MUSCLE PERFORMANCE MEASUREMENTS

Muscle performance is commonly measured to describe the strength, endurance, and coordination abilities of an individual. These measurements are helpful for documenting progress in patient treatment. Protocols and standardized progress measurements are part of a good rehabilitation program, but there is weak evidence that these measurements are helpful in predicting an individual's work capacity.[2,5,10] A host of different devices are available on the market to measure strength and endurance capabilities. There are also systems to measure function through functional capacity evaluation.[24] Such specialized measurements are discussed in the latter part of this book under each body part.

More important as a global view, the question arises as to whether measurements of muscle function are important. The question deserves some attention and can be answered with a firm yes.[3] If the goal is to document the specific deficits of a muscle function, we need to measure the function to the best of our ability to design an appropriate training program. We can measure progress and determine the success or failure of the treatment, which is an important measure of the outcome of any prescribed treatment.

The next question is how to measure muscle function. This deserves much attention by the clinical and/or research team. Kroemer et al have reviewed the taxonomy for human strength measurements.[30] They point out that since muscle performance or strength cannot currently be measured directly at the muscle level, it is usually performed outside the body at the interface with some kind of a dynamometer. This poses difficulty for experimental controls or in a clinical setting. The more restricted the test, the less functional will be the practical application for an occupational healthcare provider, who must decide whether a patient can resume work or not.

For example, in isometric muscle testing, displacement, velocity, acceleration, and jerk are assumed to be nonexistent. The exposure to the muscle or muscle group can be constant or controlled in terms of the force exerted, external mass imposed, and repetition involved. In a dynamic job or task, only the external mass (object) and the repetitions can be more easily controlled. Therefore the measurement method chosen to document any improvement in the outcome of exercise or training is entirely dependent on the question posed.

There is little evidence that good correlation exists between strength and endurance in the performance of functional tasks in a normal population. Parnianpour et al[43] studied back muscle performance in 131 healthy women. They investigated the isometric and isokinetic strength and isometric endurance of trunk muscles. A number of significant correlations were found, but they were too weak to have any predictive power. These results were in agreement with other studies.[35,38,42,52] In clinical work this means that a strength test of a muscle group may not predict the endurance or functional ability of that limb. Mital and Karwoski[38] showed that the use of a static strength test to develop a human performance limit for a dynamic task is fundamentally incorrect because the inertia forces are ignored. In work-related muscle impairment, this information is helpful to clinicians. For example, improvement in a simple static-force handgrip test by a patient with a hand injury may not elucidate the patient's ability to maneuver a paced machine. The determination of functional ability and working capacity related to a specific muscle impairment is still in need of much research because the relationship between the two is confounded by several factors such as pain, joint stiffness, and fear avoidance behavior.

MUSCLE REMODELING

Muscle tissue remodels in the same way as any other skeletal tissue such as bone, cartilage, and ligament. Muscle tissue atrophies in response to disuse and immobilization and hypertrophies in response to greater than usual demands.

Immobilization and Disuse

Disuse and immobilization of a muscle have many similar effects. When a muscle is immobilized for a long time, changes occur in muscle size and structure and its physiologic and metabolic properties. Clinical and laboratory studies suggest that early or even immediate motion may prevent atrophy after injury or surgery. If a muscle is not subjected to its normal loading condition, that is, force production and length changes, it may lead to motion limitation and increased pain. Motion itself acts as a pain reliever. Although the mechanism for pain relief induced by motion is not entirely understood, the clinical observation is frequently reported. Among the first changes occurring with immobilization is the loss of muscle weight. More muscle weight is lost in the initial days after injury or disuse than in subsequent days. Prolonged bed rest leads to 1.0% to 1.5% loss of muscle mass per day.[13] All muscle fibers exhibit some atrophy on a microscopic level; however, type I fibers are most affected. Their cross-sectional area decreases and the potential for oxidative enzyme activity is reduced.[17,21,26,47]

Parallel with muscle mass loss during disuse is a loss of force production and endurance in the muscle. The ability to do prolonged work is negatively affected, which may harm the work capacity and perhaps increase the risk for reinjury. Biochemical changes occurring during immobilization or disuse include lower energy supplies and increased levels of lactic acid.[7,36] Other changes such as decreased protein synthesis and insulin sensitivity have also been reported.[19] Immobilization should therefore be kept to a minimum and motion promoted if the goal is to prevent the secondary effects of disuse of the skeletal muscles.[23]

Physical Training

Skeletal muscle is strikingly able to adapt to exercise and training. Most training and exercise programs for unspecific pain symptomatology involve strength training, endurance (aerobic) training, stretching, and sometimes power (anaerobic) training.

Strength training involves high force and low repetition. It results in increased muscle bulk through the increased cross-sectional area of the muscle fibers,[37] but it is unclear whether an increase in the number of fibers occurs.[50] Studies have shown that the best results for increased strength are obtained if the resistance is high and the motion is performed only a few times through the entire range of motion. Several sets of training are recommended, and different muscle groups are trained sequentially. The initial improvement from strength training is better motor unit recruitment. Subsequently there will be an effect of hypertrophy of the fibers.[25,51] An increased muscle mass results in decreased stress on each muscle fiber for the same load.

Endurance (aerobic) training involves medium to low loads and a high amount of repetition. The effects of endurance training on the cardiovascular system are an increased stroke volume of the heart and improved oxidative metabolism of the muscle fibers by an improved blood flow to the muscles through the development of more capillaries. Endurance training affects mainly type II fibers and their oxidative capacity but has little effect on muscle strength and bulk.

Finally, anaerobic training—so-called power spurts—consists of exercises with a duration of a few minutes to seconds. This type of training effects metabolic changes leading to an increased level of stored phosphagens and an increased ability for anaerobic glycolysis. These changes have mostly been documented in type II fibers. A well-designed muscle training program must therefore contain a variety of exercises to "impress" all muscle fiber types.

Stretching is commonly used in occupational rehabilitation. It implies specific exercises to stretch out the muscle-tendon-bone complex. The effect of stretching is to increase range of motion by increasing the length of the musculotendinous unit. When the unit is stretched or elongated passively, a certain tension develops. The tension decreases with time if the muscle and tendon remain stretched. This phenomena is called *stress relaxation* and is used clinically. Once stress relaxation has occurred (about 20 to 30 seconds), we can slowly stretch some more. Other viscoelastic properties such as the *strain rate,* that is, the velocity at which the stretching is performed, also affect the musculotendinous unit. A quick stretch results in increased muscle stiffness, whereas slow stretching allows for more elongation. Additionally, a cold muscle is stiffer than a warm muscle that has been subjected to a "warm-up routine."

Overuse

Overuse or sports-induced inflammation may also occur in an occupational setting. The mechanism is not completely understood but is currently the subject of intensive research.[32] The theory behind overuse is the occurrence of either macrotrauma by impact/contact or microtrauma by repeated cyclic loading.[32] **Figure 4-4** schematically demonstrates the different theoretical pathways of incurred inflammation. In the context of this chapter, the question is whether to immobilize or exercise patients diagnosed with overuse symptomatology in an occupational setting. If we accept the model of tissue inflammation caused by tissue injury, the inflammatory phase will alter function mainly through pain inhibition and changes in proprioceptive feedback. Muscle strength will decrease secondary to neurologic deconditioning.[27] Commonly, a reduction in flexibility occurs as a result of scar tissue formation.

Most working people are not Olympic athletes; however, we can still learn from this model that activity alterations seem to be the most successful and that injured workers should not stop being active but change their activity constellation during the healing process. The key to the right treatment is, of course, the correct diagnosis; that is, differentiation between overuse and

disuse in a working patient. The other key to successful rehabilitation is the willingness of the employer to change the working environment inasmuch as patients with overuse inflammation do not heal with intensive exercises or by returning to a highly repetitive job. Once the acute symptomatology has subsided, activity should gradually be resumed and prevention exercises instituted.

A conceptual model for work-related neck and upper extremity musculoskeletal impairment has been suggested by Armstrong et al.[1] The model describes a progressive association between exposure, dose, capacity, and response to mechanical load and is intended to enhance understanding of the development of painful conditions in the muscles and tendons. Many questions must still be answered concerning the suggested model inasmuch as outcome studies have yet to prove the efficacy of interventions such as job alteration and exercise programs as a primary prevention intervention; in addition basic research is needed on muscle and tendon strain and so forth. Nevertheless, the importance of this model is that it emphasizes the complexity of the problem of exposure and impairment.

EFFICACY OF EXERCISE PROGRAMS IN OCCUPATIONAL SETTINGS

Exercises are frequently prescribed for the prevention and treatment of nonspecific musculoskeletal ailments. Exercises are a popular intervention because they are relatively inexpensive and noninvasive, provide an active rather than passive approach, and have several positive secondary effects. Exercise has been shown to be a mood elevator, reduce pain, and give the participant a sense of control.[8] The effect of exercises in acute nonspecific pain symptomatology in work-related ailments is poorly documented. In a recent literature review, the Agency for Health Care Policy and Research[6] (AHCPR) for patients with acute nonspecific low back pain screened 92 studies as regards to exercises and training. Few of the reviewed studies were from occupational health-care providers. The results showed that exercises for low back pain (nonspecific or mechanical) were most efficacious in the prevention of chronicity if started as low-stress aerobic exercises. The exercises should be geared toward endurance training, at first set by quota and designed to cause minimal stress (load) on the back.[33] No evidence supports stretching as effective in this patient category. In another large review related to whiplash-associated disorders by the Quebec Task Force[48] it was concluded that the independent effect of exercises has not been evaluated. However, the cumulative evidence again suggests that exercises in combination with other interventions are beneficial in both the short and long term after sustained injury. Both reviews are in agreement that inactivity and immobilizing types of treatment are detrimental for patients with a

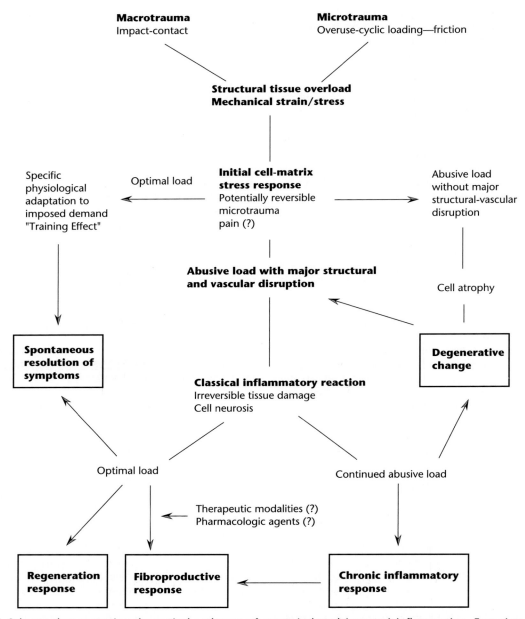

Figure 4-4 Schema demonstrating theoretical pathways of sports-induced (overuse) inflammation. From Leadbetter WB: An introduction to sports-induced soft-tissue inflammation. (*In Leadbetter WB, Buckwalter JA, Gordon SL, editors: Sports-induced inflammation: clinical and basic science concepts, Park Ridge, Ill, 1990, American Academy of Orthopedic Surgeons: pp 3-23.*)

"benign" strain in the spine. Patients must be carefully screened before such a recommendation (see Chapter 21).

One study looked at strength training for the neck musculature and its effect on pain and function of the neck. Middle-aged working women exercised twice weekly for 8 weeks.[4] Each session (12 minutes) consisted of three sets of 12 repetitions of resisted rotation and flexion, with the work performed and measured by using a neck ergometer built in-house. The results were amazingly good, including an average of a 25% increase in muscle strength and complete abolition of pain. Although the study lacked a blinded evaluator, the concept that strength training functions as a "pain killer" is interesting. Although it is attractive to attribute the results to the improved neuromuscular function, a causal relationship has not been proven. However, two previous studies support these findings.[15,22] There is a lack of well-designed studies that look at what type of training and exercises provide the greatest benefits to patients in the healing process. There is also a lack of studies in which exercise has been used as the sole intervention for patients with nonspecific work-related musculoskeletal pain.

SUMMARY

The structural unit of skeletal muscle is the fiber. Three main types of fibers are identified: type I slow twitch oxidative and types IIA and IIB fast twitch, oxidative-glycolytic fibers. The fibers are composed of myofibrils, thin filaments of the protein actin and thick filaments of the protein myosin. The force of the contraction is caused by the interaction between actin and myosin.

A particularly vulnerable area of skeletal muscle is the myotendinous and the bone-tendon insertions, areas in which strain most commonly occurs. Muscle tissue remodels and is very receptive to a change in activity. Decreased activity can lead to a painful disuse condition, whereas too much activity may lead to an overuse condition. The theory behind the two is entirely different. The role, type, duration, and intensity of exercises need to be studied more in relation to strain and cumulative repetitive exposure to nonspecific, work-related painful conditions of the musculoskeletal system.

ACKNOWLEDGMENT
This chapter was partially funded by NIOSH CDC GRANT No. U60/CCU 206153.

References

1. Armstrong T et al: A conceptual model for work-related neck and upper limb musculoskeletal disorders, *Scand J Work Environ Health* 19:73-84, 1993.

2. Battie M: *The reliability of physical factors as predictors of the occurrence of back pain reporters: a prospective study within industry*, thesis, Gothenburg, Sweden, 1989, Gothenburg University.

3. Bellamy N: *Musculoskeletal clinical metrology*, Boston, 1993, Kluwer Academic Publishers.

4. Berg HE, Berggren G, Tesch PA: Dynamic neck strength training effect on pain and function, *Arch Phys Med Rehabil* 75:661-665, 1994.

5. Biering-Sorensen F: Physical measurements as risk indicators for low back trouble over a one-year period, *Spine* 9:106-119, 1984.

6. Bigos SJ et al: *Acute low back problems in adults*. Clinical practice guideline No 14, AHCPR Pub No 95-0642, Rockville, Md, 1994, Agency for Health Care Policy and Research, Public Health Service, US Department of Health and Human Services.

7. Booth FW: Physiologic and biochemical effects of immobilization on muscle, *Clin Orthop* 219:15-20, 1987.

8. Campello M, Nordin M, Weiser S: Physical exercise and low back pain: a review, *Scand J Med Sci Sports* (in press).

9. Caplan A, et al: Skeletal muscle. In Woo SL-Y and Buckwalter J, editors: *Injury and repair of the musculoskeletal soft tissues*, Park Ridge, Ill, 1987, American Academy of Orthopaedic Surgeons; pp 213-291.

10. Chaffin DB, Park KS: A longitudinal study of low-back pain as associated with occupational weight lifting factors, *Am Ind Hyg Assoc J* 32:513-525, 1973.

11. Cooper RR, Misol S: Tendon and ligament insertion: a light and electron microscopic study, *J Bone Joint Surg Am* 52:1-20, 1970.

12. Costill PL, et al: Adaptations in skeletal muscles following strength training, *J Appl Physiol* 46:96-99, 1976.

13. Deyo RA: Non-operative treatment of low back disorders. Differentiating useful from useless therapy. In Frymoyer JW, editor: *The adult spine: principles and practice*, New York, 1991, Raven Press: pp 1567-1580.

14. Dubowitz V: Cross-innervated mammalian skeletal muscle, *J Physiol* 193:481, 1967.

15. Dyrssen T, Svedenkrans M, Paasikivi J: Muskelträning vid besvär i nacke och skuldror effektiv behandling för att minska smärtan, *Lakartidningen* 86:2116-2120, (in Swedish).

16. Engel WK: The essentiality of histo- and cystochemical studies of skeletal muscle in investigation of neuromuscular disease, *Neurology* 12:778, 1962.

17. Eriksson E: Rehabilitation of muscle function after sport injury. Major problems in sports medicine, *Int J Sports Med* 2:1-5, 1981.

18. Essen B: Intramuscular substrate utilization during prolonged exercise, *Ann N Y Acad Sci* 301:30, 1977.

19. Garrett WE, Best TM: Anatomy, physiology, and mechanics of skeletal muscle. In Simon SR, editor: *Orthopaedic basic science*, Park Ridge, Ill, 1994, American Academy of Orthopaedic Surgeons; pp 89-125.

20. Gollnick PD: Relationship of strength and endurance with skeletal muscle structure and metabolic potential, *Int J Sports Med* 3(suppl):26-32, 1982.

21. Haggmark T, Eriksson E: Cylinder or mobile cast brace after knee ligament surgery: a clinical analysis and morphologic and enzymatic study of changes in the quadriceps muscle, *Am J Sports Med* 7:48-56, 1979.

22. Highland TR et al: Changes in isometric strength and range of motion of the isolated cervical spine after eight weeks of clinical rehabilitation, *Spine* 17(suppl):77-82, 1992.

23. Hultman G, et al: Body composition, endurance, strength, cross-sectional area, and density of mm erector spinae in men with and without low back pain, *J Spinal Disord* 6:114-123, 1993.

24. Isernhagen SJ: *The comprehensive guide to work injury management,* Gaithersburg, Md, 1995, Aspen Publishers, Inc.

25. Jansson E, Sjodin B, Tesch P: Changes in muscle fibre type distribution in man after physical training. A sign of fibre type transformation, *Acta Physiol Scand* 104:235-237, 1978.

26. Jansson E et al: Increase in myoglobin content and decrease in oxidative enzyme activities by leg muscles immobilization in man, *Acta Physiol Scand* 132:515-517, 1988.

27. Kibler BW: Concepts in exercise rehabilitation of athletic injury. In Leadbetter WB et al, editors: *Sports-induced inflammation: clinical and basic science concepts,* Park Ridge, Ill, 1990, American Academy of Orthopaedic Surgeons; pp 759-769.

28. Komi PV: Neuromuscular performance: factors influencing force and speed production, *Scand J Sports Sci* 1:2-15, 1979.

29. Komi PV, and Buskirk ER: Effect of eccentric and concentric muscle conditioning on tension and electrical activity of human muscle, *Ergonomics* 15:417-434, 1972.

30. Kroemer KHE et al: On the measurement of human strength, *Int J Ind Ergonom* 6:199-210, 1990.

31. Kroll PG: *The effect of previous contraction condition on subsequent eccentric power production in elbow flexor muscles,* unpublished doctoral dissertation, New York, 1987, New York University.

32. Leadbetter WB: An introduction to sports-induced soft-tissue inflammation. In Leadbetter WB et al, editors: *Sports-induced inflammation: clinical and basic science concepts,* Park Ridge, Ill, 1990, American Academy of Orthopaedic Surgeons; pp 3-23.

33. Lindstrom I et al: The effect of graded activity on patients with subacute low back pain: a randomized prospective clinical study with an operant-conditioning behavioral approach, *Phys Ther* 72:279-293, 1992.

34. Luciano DS, Vander AJ, Sherman JH: *Human function and structure,* New York, 1978, McGraw Hill; pp 113-136.

35. Marras WS, King AI, Joynt RL: Measurements of the loads on the lumbar spine under isometric and isokinetic conditions, *Spine* 9:176-187, 1984.

36. Max SR: Disuse atrophy of skeletal muscle: loss of functional activity of mitochondria, *Biochem Biophys Res Commun* 46:1394-1398, 1972.

37. McDonaugh MJ, Davies CTM: Adapted response of mammalian skeletal muscle to exercise with high loads, *Eur J Appl Physiol* 52:139-155, 1984.

38. Mital A, Karwoski W: *Use of simulated job dynamic strength (SJDS) in screening workers for manual lifting task.* Proceedings of the twenty-ninth annual meeting of the Human Factors Society, Baltimore, Md., 1985, p 513.

39. Nikolaou PK et al: Biomechanical and histological evaluation of muscle after controlled sprain injury, *Am J Sports Med* 15:9-14, 1987.

40. Nordin M, Frankel VH: *Basic biomechanics of the musculoskeletal system,* ed 2, Philadelphia, 1989, Lea & Febiger.

41. Norkin C, Levange P: *Joint structure and function: a comprehensive analysis,* Philadelphia, 1983, F A Davis Co.

42. Ostering R, Bates B, James S: Isokinetic and isometric torque relationship, *Arch Phys Med Rehabil* 58:254-259, 1977.

43. Parnianpour M et al: Correlation between different tests of trunk strength. In Buckle P, editor: *Musculoskeletal disorders at work,* New York, 1987, Taylor & Francis Publishers, Inc.

44. Pittman MI, Peterson L: Biomechanics of skeletal muscle. In Nordin M, Frankel VH, editors: *Basic biomechanics of the musculoskeletal system,* ed 2, Philadelphia, 1989, Lea & Febiger; pp 80-111.

45. Prichard JW: Nerve. In Albright JA, Brand RA, editors: *The scientific basis of orthopaedics,* E Norwalk, Conn, 1979, Appleton & Lange Books; pp 385-414.

46. Saltin B et al: Fiber types and metabolic potentials of skeletal muscles in sedentary man and endurance runners, *Ann N Y Acad Sci* 301:3-29, 1977.

47. Sargeant AJ et al: Functional and structural changes after disuse of human muscle, *Clin Sci* 52:337-342, 1977.

48. Spitzer WO et al: Scientific monograph of the Quebec Task Force on Whiplash-Associated Disorders: redefining "whiplash" and its management, *Spine* 20(suppl 8):1-73, 1995.

49. Taylor DC et al: Viscoelastic properties of muscle-tendon units: the biomechanical effects of stretching, *Am J Sports Med* 18:300-309, 1990.

50. Taylor NA, Wilkinson JG: Exercise-induced skeletal muscle growth: hypertrophy or hyperplasia? *Sports Med* 3:190-200, 1986.

51. Tesch PA: Acute and long-term metabolic changes consequent to heavy-resistance training, *Med Sport Sci* 26:67-68, 1987.

52. Thorstensson A, Nilsson J: Trunk muscle strength during constant velocity movements, *Scand J Rehabil Med* 14:61-68, 1982.

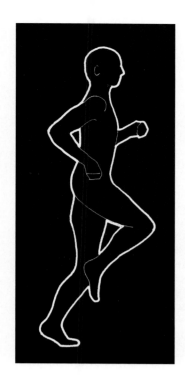

Chapter 5

Basic Pain Mechanism and Its Control

James N. Weinstein

CONTENTS

Despite the enormity of the problem of low back pain, its causes remain largely obscure. In the last 50 years much of the focus has been on ruptured or herniated intervertebral disks. Other suspected sources of low back pain include the nerve roots, the lumbar facet joints, the paraspinal muscles, and the posterior longitudinal ligament (PLL).

Occupational factors contributing to the prevalence of low back pain are difficult to research because of the uncertainty of cause and exposure. Healthy workers are more difficult to assess than "unhealthy workers," and injury mechanisms remain unclear. Disability may be related to work factors, individual factors, and medical, legal, and social factors. Known work factors, including heavy lifting, static work postures, bending and twisting, and exposure to vibration, are all associated with an increased risk of back pain. Psychosocial and psychological factors in the workplace include satisfaction with work as an important risk factor in low back pain disability. Gender appears to be of little importance with respect to low back symptoms, although women seem to have an increased prevalence after menopause.

According to the Arthritis Foundation, 40% of all visits to neurosurgeons and orthopaedists are for complaints of back pain. It is estimated that more than 70% of the population experiences low back pain at some time during adulthood; by inference, the longer one lives, the greater one's chances for the development of low back pain. Despite the frequency of this complaint, back pain is notoriously difficult to diagnose and treat, partly because of the complex structure of the spine. Only 10% to 15% of patients with low back pain complaints have a known cause.[13] Symptoms do not always correspond with the severity of this disorder. Relatively minor, self-limiting injuries can produce incapacitating pain, whereas extensive pathology may initially cause mild symptoms. Therefore, the only rule that can be stated with confidence is that clinical manifestations do not necessarily reflect the cause or severity of disease. In this chapter, anatomy and neurophysiology will be examined as they relate to low back pain.

SOURCES OF LOW BACK PAIN

Just what are the sources involved in the generation of low back pain in sciatica? Over the past decade, Kuslich et al[27] reported nearly 200 consecutive patients studied prospectively. The authors used progressive regional anesthesia in 193 consecutive patients undergoing decompression for a herniated disk or lumbar spinal stenosis. Interestingly, when touched or even cut, the lumbar fascia was anesthetic. The supraspinous ligament produced some level of back pain, but the muscles never produced pain in response to general pressure. On the other hand, when the base of the muscles was touched, especially at the site of blood vessels or nerves at the attachment to bone, localized low back pain often resulted. It is hypothesized that the pain is probably derived from local vessels and nerves rather than from the muscle bundles themselves. A normal nerve root is generally insensitive to pain. However, with retraction over a long period of time, mild paresthesias did result but did not cause significant pain. Stimulation of a compressed or stretched nerve root consistently produced pain in the same sciatic distribution the patient had before surgical intervention. Therefore, it appears that sciatica can only be reproduced when a previously stretched, compressed, or swollen nerve root is stimulated. In the case of stretched, compressed, or swollen nerve roots, sciatica was reproduced with either pressure or stretch on the caudal dura, the nerve root sleeve, the ganglion, or the nerve distal to the ganglion. The ganglion, a very mechanosensitive structure, was more tender than other parts of the nerve root. Pain was almost eliminated in each case by injection of 0.5 cc of 1% lidocaine (Zylocaine) beneath the nerve root sheath proximal to the site of compression.

In Dr. Kuslich's population of patients, two thirds experienced similar preoperative pain when the outer part of the annulus was stimulated. Again, local anesthetic would obliterate this pain. Buttock pain was only produced by simultaneous stimulation or pressure on the nerve root and the outer surface of the annulus.

Referred pain is interesting, and it is clear from Kuslich and his colleagues[27] that the central part of the annulus and the PLL produce central back pain. Stimulation to the right or left of center of the PLL was associated with pain on the side of the stimulus.

The vertebral end plates appear to be pressure sensitive, and curettage results in deep rather than superficial low back pain. In many cases the pain was more severe than the preoperative pain. The facet joints did produce sharp and localized pain in the region of dissection. Interestingly, the findings around the facet joints were inconsistent and the pain often perceived as deep and dull. In the case of the facet joints, intraarticular injections were not necessary for relieving the pain, but periarticular injections always blocked the pain around the facet joint. In this series, neither the facet synovium nor its articular cartilage produced symptoms. The ligamentum flavum, epidural fat, nucleus pulposus, bony lamina, posterior dura, and spinous processes caused pain during mechanical stimulation.

Perineural fibrosis or scarring is sometimes thought to be responsible for pain. The scar itself, however, is never tender, whereas the nerve root itself is frequently very sensitive. It is hypothesized that the sensitivity or pain of a scar may be secondary to repair of the nerve now sensitive to compression and/or tension.

THE INTERVERTEBRAL DISK AND NERVE ROOTS

Hirsch et al[19] reported that hypertonic saline injected into the disk produces severe pain, "identical to a real lumbago," that could not be localized but was described as deep aching across the back. Mooney,[36] in a review of the current literature, concluded that the disk may be the primary source of the production of low back pain. However, mechanisms of pain production remain uncertain.

FACET JOINTS

The facet joint capsules are richly innervated[19,22,39,44] and can undergo extensive stretch during physiologic loading.[9] Whether the facet joint pain is due to capsular deformation, bony impingement, or a combination thereof remains unanswered. Through injections of hypertonic saline into the facet joint capsules, Lewis and Kellgren were able to produce typical low back symptoms, including radiation of pain into the posterior of the thigh.[29] Similar studies reported by Ghormley,[14] Mooney,[35] and Shealy[40] have suggested that facet joint pathology plays an important role in low back pain.

A literature review of facet block success rates and facet rhizolysis has been reported by Helbig and Casey.[18] They demonstrated a 50% to 60% success rate. A definitive set of diagnostic criteria regarding what part the facet syndrome plays in the mixed success rates of these treatment modalities is needed. Lilius et al[30] found no statistical difference in the treatment outcomes of those who receive facet injections with a cortical steroid and analgesic as compared with those injected with saline. Jackson et al[23] performed facet injections on 454 patients but were unable to select patients responsive to the injections.

MUSCULAR PAIN

The most common diagnosis for low back pain is an acute sprain or strain. However, scientific evidence for low back pain of muscle origin is lacking.[1] Some patients are known to have palpable findings in their back muscles during physical examination with associated increased myeloelectric activity, whereas others have suggested no increased activity.[8,24]

LUMBAR NERVE ROOTS

Smyth and Wright[41] placed nylon threads into various lumbar tissue sites during operations on the spine. These threads exited the surgical wound and were pulled upon in the postoperative period to determine pain and sensitivity in the affected spinal tissues. The most common pain site was the annulus fibrosus. Nerve roots compressed by disks or bony impingement were thought to be the cause of sciatica and were painful and sensitive. Normal or uninvolved nerve roots were not associated with pain. Greenbarg et al also reported that compressed and inflamed nerve roots were very sensitive to mechanical manipulation.[15] As previously pointed out, Kuslich et al[27] demonstrated that stimulation of stretched, compressed, or swollen nerve roots caused significant pain in 90% of their patients and the nerve root was the only tissue site that upon stimulation reproduced the patient's sciatica. In fewer than 10% of their cases, the uninvolved normal nerves, when stimulated, produced significant pain.

NEUROPHYSIOLOGY

Sensory nerve fibers are often assigned to one of four groups (I to IV) based on conduction velocity.[17] Group IV consists of unmyelinated C fibers and group III includes the thinly myelinated A delta fibers. In general, pain fibers belong to either group III or IV, but not all group III and IV fibers are associated with muscle pain. Mense and Meyer[34] reported on the activity of group III and IV muscle units from anesthetized cats. Group III fibers were low-threshold pressure-sensitive units. Nociceptive and contraction-sensitive units were also seen. Group IV units included nociceptive, low-threshold pressure-sensitive, contraction-sensitive, and thermosensitive units. In these small-diameter afferents, nonnociceptive units outnumbered nociceptive units 62% to 38%.

Nonneurogenic pain mediators like bradykinin are known to excite muscle units. This has been shown to be an excitement of afferent fibers from muscle groups III and IV. Prostaglandin E(PGE_2) is known to enhance this action.[33] Inflammation-induced myositis is known to increase the neurophysiologic background activity of group III and IV units and is associated with lowering of the threshold of group IV units.[3]

Several neurophysiologic investigators have demonstrated inflammation to be a provocateur of nerves and joints, making them more sensitive to movement than normal joints. Cavanaugh et al have studied the lumbar facet joint,[6] and the ankle joint has been studied with inflammation models.[7,16,21] Some of these models have demonstrated that group III and IV units are more sensitive to stretch and have higher resting discharge rates than do controls. Grigg et al[16] found that group IV units were much more readily activated by normal joint movements in inflamed joints than in normal joints.

Over the years there has been a great deal of interest in the lumbar facet joints, but limited work regarding the neurophysiology and the possible sources of pain. To that end, Cavanaugh et al,[5,6] Yamashita et al,[45,46] and Avramov et al[2] have undertaken a series of neurophysiologic studies in rabbits. These studies have indicated that the facet joint capsule or pericapsular area in the adjacent musculotendinous junctions contains both low- and high-threshold mechanoreceptors, low-threshold receptors or proprioceptors, and high-threshold pain receptors. It is interesting that these tissues are not only mechanosensitive but also chemosensitive and that localized injections of inflammatory agents such as carrageenan and kaolin produce ongoing neuronal discharge. Likewise, localized injection with synthetic substance P, a neuromodulator of pain, also activates nociceptors and proprioceptors in the facet joints and deep back muscles. Bradykinin and serotonin chemical mediators of inflammation also activate nociceptive units in and around the facet joint.

Loading of the spine can also activate high- threshold units and phasic units but cannot be maintained. On the other hand, chemical mediators do maintain the discharge. Mechanosensitive units in the rabbits were found in the multifidus, rotatory, and intermaxillary muscles, as well as in and around the facet joint capsule and border regions at the junction of the capsule and musculotendinous insertions. Inflamed units often showed vigorous multiunit response to stretch and demonstrated a decrease in discharge rate from the inflamed tissue when lidocaine or hydrocortisone were applied.

Preliminary work on neural activity within the spinal canal has been reported by Cavanaugh et al.[4] They have seen activation of mechanosensitive units from dorsal roots after various mechanical manipulations and application of algesic substances to the lumbar spinal canal. However, only occasionally did probing into the disk or PLL evoke a neural discharge. Pulling of the ventral dura was accompanied by multiunit activation. It is hard to know whether these dural units themselves are responsible or adjacent tissues that receive traction when the dura is pulled.

CHEMICAL MEDIATORS OF NOCICEPTION

Chemical inflammation is often mediated by amines (histamine, 5-hydroxytryptamine), kinins (including bradykinin), arachidonic acid derivatives (prostaglandins and leukotrienes), kinin- forming enzymes (killikrein), plasmin, products of the complement system, and components of polymophonuclear leukocytes. The major pain-producing substances involved in inflammation, however, appear to be related to reactions of bradykinin, 5-hydroxytryptamine (serotonin), and PGE_1. In a study on human volunteers, interdermal injection of histamine and bradykinin producedshort-lasting pain but prolonged edema and erythema.[10] Bradykinin has been shown to excite group III and IV muscle afferent fibers,[12,32] and subdermal injections of prostaglandins and histamine or bradykinin are associated with intense pain that is considerably greater than

when these agents are injected alone. Aspirin, known to block the synthesis of prostaglandins, may produce its analgesic effect by preventing the sensitization of pain receptors to prostaglandins. Leukotrienes are chemotactic for polymorphonuclear leukocytes that accumulate in areas of inflammation and, when injected interdermally, are known to sensitize c-nociceptors to mechanically stimulate and cause hyperalgesia.[25] These substances are not affected by nonsteroidal antiinflammatory drugs, which normally block the cyclooxygenation of arachidonic acid.[28]

NEUROGENIC MEDIATORS

Substance P is an 11–amino acid polypeptide identified immunohistochemically in various regions of the peripheral and central nervous system, as well as the functional spinal unit. Substance P is thought to play a major role in the transmission and modulation of pain signals.[20] Release of substance P to and from the dorsal horn is reported to increase during acute noxious mechanical stimuli[26] and in the polyarthritic state.[38]

Sensitization as a result of substance P on peripheral nerve endings has not been resolved. Fitzgerald and Lynn[11] report only weak excitation of cutaneous receptors in cats and rabbits by synthetic substance P. On the other hand, Nakamura-Craig and Smith[37] reported that multiple injections of subthreshold doses of substance P in the rat paw caused long-lasting hyperalgesia. Synthetic substance P applied to receptive fields in and around the facet joint was accompanied by an increase in spontaneous discharge rates. Therefore, substance P may contribute to the transmission of both nociceptive and, in some cases, proprioceptive sensations in the primary afferent units of the lumbar facet and adjacent soft tissue.

Casual links between environmental factors (such as vibration) and functional spinal unit degeneration mediated by biologic events are currently being explored.[43] In this model it is proposed that neuropeptides released from the dorsal root ganglion induced by environmental and structural factors mediate a progressive degeneration of the functional spinal unit by stimulating the synthesis of inflammatory agents (PGE_2) and various degradative enzymes (such as proteases). This now weakened functional spinal unit is increasingly susceptible to environmental factors, which in turn lower the threshold necessary to stimulate neuropeptide activity, thereby perpetuating the degenerative spiral.

In the work by Levine et al[28] and Lotz et al,[31] arthritis was induced by an infusion of substance P and was decreased or inhibited by substance P antagonists. If substance P is released in and around the functional spinal unit, it is therefore in theory capable of stimulating or activating various proteases that in effect degrade collagen and negatively affect the mechanics of the functional spinal unit.

The interrelationships between these neurogenic

and nonneurogenic mediators described in the injury and repair process are obviously important when the degenerative spiral or aging associated with osteoarthritis is considered. Paradigms have recently been proposed that suggest that cytokines leaking from degenerative facet joints may, in and of themselves, be injurious to nerve tissue per se.[42] The interaction and reactions of these systems must be better understood if treatment algorithms are to be efficacious and lead to positive outcomes.

SUMMARY

In the classic model of disease, patients often have symptoms and significant pathology. However, more often than not, patients have many symptoms and little pathology or a great deal of pathology and no symptoms. In occupational low back pain it is more challenging to also consider the psychosocial aspects and their effects on the perception of pain. These issues have been poorly understood, but clearly, injured tissues are capable of being a source of chronic pain. On the other hand, psychological factors can create a pain spiral unrelated to the routine, or explained, injury and repair processes. The lack of understanding of the perception of pain and how our perceptions interact in the development and manifestations of pain itself remains unknown. In the United States, one family in three includes someone suffering from pain. Pain is not necessarily related to an injury; in some cases pain is related to an emotional response that may be more painful.

With proper education, appropriate expectations, and a comprehensive approach to diseases and pain management, the majority of our patients can expect successful outcomes. Still, in many cases residual pain must be expected and dealt with. Through a better understanding of pain itself—the pathophysiology, neurochemistry, anatomy, and psychology of pain—we must continue to seek more efficacious and responsible therapies for our patients.

References

1. Andersson G: The epidemiology of spinal disorders. In Frymoyer JW, editor: *The adult spine: principles and practice,* New York, 1991, Raven Press; pp. 107-146.

2. Avramov A et al: Effects of controlled mechanical loading on group II, III, and IV afferents from the lumbar facet joint and surrounding muscle: an *in vitro* study, *J Bone Joint Surg Am* (in press).

3. Berberich P, Hoheisel U, Mense S: Effects of carrageenan-induced myositis on the discharge properties of group III and IV muscle receptors in the cat, *J Neurophysiol* 59: 1395-1409, 1988.

4. Cavanaugh JM et al: *Initial electrophysiological studies of neurons of the lumbar spinal canal.* Proceedings of the International Society for the Study of the Lumbar Spine, Chicago, May 20-24, 1992.

5. Cavanaugh JM et al: Sensory innervation of soft tissues of lumbar spine in the rat, *J Orthop Res* 7:389-397, 1989.

6. Cavanaugh JN et al: *An inflammation model of low back pain.* Proceedings of the International Society for the Study of the Lumbar Spine, Boston, 1990, p 46.

7. Coggeshall RE et al: Discharge characteristics of fine medial articular afferents at rest and during passive movements of inflamed knee and joints, *Brain Res* 272:185-188, 1983.

8. Denslow JS, Clough GH: Reflex activity in the spinal extensors, *J Neurophysiol* 1:430-437, 1941.

9. El-Bohy AA, Goldberg SJ, King AI: *Measurement of facet capsular stretch.* 1987 Biomechanics symposium, Applied Mechanics Division, 84:161-164, 1987 Conference of the American Society of Mechanical Engineers, Cincinnati, 1987.

10. Ferreria SH: Prostaglandins, aspirin-like drugs and analgesia, *Nature* 240:200-203, 1972.

11. Fitzgerald M, Lynn B: The weak excitation of some cutaneous receptors in cats and rabbits by synthetic substance P, *J Physiol* (Lond) 66P-67P, 1976.

12. Franz M, Mense S: Muscle receptors with group IV afferent fibers responding to application of bradykinin, *Brain Res* 92:369-383, 1975.

13. Frymoyer JW et al: Posterior support structures, part A: clinical perspective. In Frymoyer JW and Gordon SL, editors: *New perspectives in low back pain,* Park Ridge, Ill, 1989, American Academy of Orthopaedic Surgeons; pp 217-248.

14. Ghormley RK: Low back pain with special reference to the articular facets, with presentation of an operative procedure, *JAMA* 17:73, 1933.

15. Greenbarg PE er al: Epidural anesthesia for lumbar spine surgery, *J Spinal Disord* 1:139-143, 1988.

16. Grigg P, Schaible HG, Schmidt RF: Mechanical sensitivity of group III and IV afferents from posterior articular nerve in normal and inflamed cat knee, *J Neurophysiol* 55:635-643, 1986.

17. Guyton AC: Sensory receptors and their basic mechanisms of action. In *Textbook of medical physiology,* Philadelphia, 1981, WB Saunders; pp 588-596.

18. Helbig T, Casey CK: The lumbar facet syndrome, *Spine* 13:61-64, 1988.

19. Hirsch C, Ingelmark BE, Miller M: The anatomical basis for low back pain, *Acta Orthop Scand* 33:1-17, 1963.

20. Hokefelt T et al: Experimental immunohistochemical studies on the localization and distribution of substance

P in cat primary sensory neurons, *Brain Res* 100:235-252, 1975.

21. Iggo A: Sensory receptors in inflamed tissues, *Adv Inflammation Res* 10:352-355, 1985.

22. Jackson HC, Winkelmann RK, Bickel WH: Nerve endings in the human spinal column and related structures, *J Bone Joint Surg Am* 48:1272-1281, 1966.

23. Jackson RP, Jacobs RR, Montesano PX: Facet joint injection in low back pain: a prospective statistical study, *Spine* 13:966-971, 1988.

24. Kraft GH, Johnson EW, Laban MM: The fibrositis syndrome, *Arch Phys Med Rehabil* 49:155-162, 1968.

25. Kumazawa T, Mizumura K: The polymodal receptors in the testes of dogs, *Brain Res* 136:553-558, 1977.

26. Kurahashi Y et al: Evidence that substance P and somatostatin transmit separate information related to pain in the spinal dorsal horn, *Brain Res* 325:294-298, 1985.

27. Kuslich SD, Ulstrom CL, Michael CJ: The tissue origin of low back pain and sciatica: a report of pain response to tissue stimulation during operation on the lumbar spine using local anesthesia, *Orthop Clin North Am* 22:181-187, 1991.

28. Levine JD et al: The role of polymorphonuclear leukocytes in hyperalgesia, *J Neurosci* 5:3025-3029, 1985.

29. Lewis T, Kellgren JH: Observations relating to referred pain, visceromotor reflexes and other associated phenomena, *Clin Sci* 4:47-71, 1939.

30. Lilius G et al: Lumbar facet syndrome: a randomized clinical trial, *J Bone Joint Surg Br* 71:681-684, 1989.

31. Lotz M, Carson DA, Vaughan JH: Substance P activation of rheumatoid synoviocytes: neural pathway in the pathogenesis of arthritis, *Science* 235:893-895, 1987.

32. Mense S: Nervous outflow from skeletal muscle following chemical noxious stimulation, *J Physiol* (Lond) 267:75-88, 1977.

33. Mense S: Sensitization of group IV muscle receptors to bradykinin by 5-hydroxytryptamine and prostaglandin E$_2$, *Brain Res* 225:95-105, 1981.

34. Mense S, Meyer H: Different types of slowly-conducting afferent units in cat skeletal muscle and tendon, *J Physiol* (Lond) 363:404-417, 1985.

35. Mooney V: The facet syndrome, *Clin Orthop* 115:149-156, 1976.

36. Mooney V: Where is the pain coming from? *Spine* 12:754-759, 1987.

37. Nakamura-Craig M, Smith TW: Substance P and peripheral inflammatory hyperalgesia, *Pain* 38:91-98, 1989.

38. Oku R, Satoh M, Takagi H: Release of substance P from the spinal dorsal horn is enhanced in polyarthritic rats, *Neurosci Lett* 74:315-319, 1987.

39. Ozaktay AC et al: *Fine nerve fibers and endings in the fibrous capsule of the lumbar facet joint.* Proceedings of the thirty-seventh annual meeting of the Orthopaedic Research Society, vol 16, Anaheim, Calif, 1991, p 353.

40. Shealy CN: Facet denervation in the management of back pain and sciatic pain, *Clin Orthop* 115:157-164, 1976.

41. Smyth MJ, Wright V: Sciatica and the intervertebral disc: an experimental study, *J Bone Joint Surg* 40:1401-1418, 1958.

42. Wehling P, Bandara G, Evans CH: Synovial cytokines impair the function of the sciatic nerve in rats: a possible element in the pathophysiology of radicular syndromes, *Neuro-Orthop* 7:55-59, 1989.

43. Weinstein JN: The role of neurogenic and non neurogenic mediators as they relate to pain in the development of osteoarthritis (a clinical review), *Spine* 17(suppl 10) (special edition of the Cervical Spine Research Society), 1992.

44. Wyke B: The neurology of low back pain. In Jayson MIV, editor: *The lumbar spine and back pain,* ed 2, London, 1980, Pitman Publishing: pp 265-339.

45. Yamashita T et al: Mechanosensitive afferent units in the lumbar facet joint, *Bone Joint Surg Am* 72:865-870, 1990.

46. Yamashita T et al: Effects of substance P on the mechanosensitive units in the lumbar facet joint and adjacent tissue, *J Orthop Res* (in press).

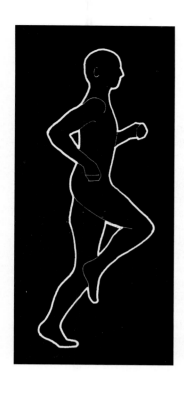

Chapter 6

Psychosocial Aspects of Occupational Musculoskeletal Disorders

Sherri Weiser

CONTENTS

The spectrum and impact of occupational and musculoskeletal disorders have been described in Chapters 1 and 7. Until recently, attempts to unravel the mystery of these disorders concentrated on the physical demands of the job and the physical vulnerabilities of the worker. It was soon clear that this problem did not easily lend itself to reductionistic approaches. Although certain physical loads and tasks have been associated with the development of musculoskeletal problems, the strength of these associations has been disappointingly weak.[55] Furthermore, a determination of physical vulnerability before injury is nearly impossible. Even when a physical defect has been established (e.g., disk herniation), the correspondence with actual disability is often low.

Like all human conditions, occupational musculoskeletal disorders can be infinitely complex. A thorough understanding of these disorders requires a consideration of influences beyond the physical. The worker's psychological attributes and social reality may have significant bearing on the onset, progression, and outcome of occupational musculoskeletal disorders. A biopsychosocial perspective offers much in the way of understanding these disorders.

The biopsychosocial model and its relevance to occupational musculoskeletal disorders will be described in this chapter, as well as current research derived from this model. This review will be limited to studies in which injuries are considered to be either a result of working or exacerbated by working. Also, intervention strategies will be discussed from a biopsychosocial perspective.

THE BIOPSYCHOSOCIAL MODEL

The notion of a link between the mind and body has existed throughout history. It was Walter Canon,[5] however, who substantiated this idea with his scientific explanation of the "fight or flight" response. His research identified the organism's physical reactions to psychological stress. Selye[48] later showed how these responses, if left unchecked, can over time cause severe damage to vulnerable organs and body systems and may even cause death.[48] Today, the relationship between the mind and the body is studied extensively. Psychological factors have been shown to have an impact on a spectrum of diseases involving virtually all bodily organs and systems.[18]

The biopsychosocial model, first described by Engel in 1977, extends beyond mind and body to include the impact of social factors on illness. Influenced by models of stress and illness, Engel concluded that any illness must be viewed from a multidimensional perspective that takes biologic, psychological, and social factors into consideration. Furthermore, these factors are not independent, as a medical model would suggest, but interrelated. It was by understanding this perspective, Engel believed, that physicians would be prepared to take on the complexities of health and illness.[7]

The biopsychosocial model soon became the prevailing view among those involved in pain research. In 1965 the gate control theory outlined the channels of pain transmission through neurologic pathways.[39] It further asserted that pain transmission may be modulated by cognitive and affective states. This model was fundamental in explaining the disparities between physical findings and the phenomenologic experience of pain. The gate control theory laid the groundwork for modern approaches to treating chronic pain.

In 1992, Waddell[56] presented a detailed analysis of low back pain with the use of a biopsychosocial model (see **Fig. 6-1**). In it, the many levels on which pain is experienced are defined. The physical injury is interpreted cognitively, resulting in a corresponding emotion. For example, a man who believes that he has a herniated disk is more apt to be anxious and depressed than a man who believes that he has a sprain. The man with the "herniated disk" may also display more avoidance behavior initially than the man who thinks he sprained his back. This process takes place within a

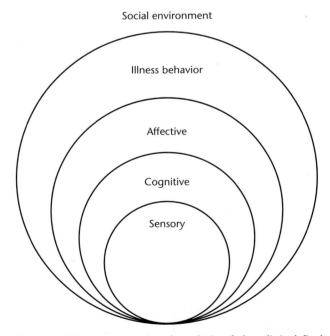

Figure 6-1 A cross-sectional analysis of the clinical findings and assessment of low back pain and disability at one point in time. (*Waddell G: Biopsychosocial analysis of low back pain. In Nordin M, Vischer TL, editors:* Common low back pain: prevention of chronicity, *London, 1992, Bailliere Tindall.*)

social context that is constantly providing feedback and modifying the individual's response.

Waddell also points out that feedback loops exist among all levels in the model and that a change in one component affects the others. If the man with the supposed herniation sees a physician and is assured that the problem is only a sprain, his belief has changed. As a result, his affect and pain behavior will change, and nociception may be experienced as less severe. These feedback loops are particularly important in chronic low back pain, wherein the original injury is often resolved. In these cases, psychological and social variables are even greater determinants of functional status than in cases of acute back pain when nociception is responsible for much of the illness behavior.

Occupational musculoskeletal injuries are clearly amenable to biopsychosocial analysis. They either occur at work or are believed to be the result of work. Therefore, the cognitive, affective, behavioral, and social elements of such an injury are inextricably related to the workplace. Recently, a number of studies have demonstrated the impact of psychological and social factors on occupational musculoskeletal injuries. What has emerged is evidence that these factors have as much and, in some cases, more predictive value than physical and environmental factors.

The following is a review of recent studies. Most have concentrated on low back pain because it is the most prevalent musculoskeletal complaint. However, disorders of the upper extremities have been investigated as well. The studies refer to a wide range of occupations with great variation in physical and psychological demands. It should be noted that most studies apply a multicausal model and analyze a number of variables simultaneously. Each component of Waddell's model will be discussed in turn.

PSYCHOSOCIAL FACTORS

Cognitive Factors

Cognitive factors include beliefs about illness as well as mental coping strategies. Cognitive factors are important because, as previously explained, they play a role in determining affect. It is also generally thought that it is easier to change false or maladaptive beliefs than maladaptive emotions. As such, they provide a window for intervention. The literature on low back pain has shown these factors to have value in predicting outcome and guiding treatment.[61] The few studies on occupational musculoskeletal disorders (mostly low back pain) and cognitive factors bear this out.

Sandstrom and Esbjornsson[47] investigated the beliefs of patients with low back pain about whether they would return to work following a rehabilitation program. They found that the patient's projection predicted work status 4 years hence. These results may indicate a motivational state on the part of the patient or may merely show that patients are the best judge of their condition. However, they lend support to the notion that beliefs have prognostic value.

Lacroix et al[27] found that patients who claimed to understand their low back pain had a better outcome than patients who did not understand what was wrong with them. They conclude that understanding facilitated compliance. An alternative explanation may be that understanding reduces the distress associated with uncertainty. Also, patients who do not understand their problem may be more likely to seek other opinions and engage in more healthcare utilization than others. This type of behavior may be associated with delayed recovery.

Fear of pain has been shown to be a motivating factor in the patient's avoidance of normal activities. Waddell[56] has developed a questionnaire to assess the extent to which patients believe that normal activities affect their back pain. The scale has been used to determine to what extent the patient's behavior is guided by the fear of engaging in work and leisure activities. Preliminary results have found these beliefs to be predictive of work loss caused by low back pain. Modifying these beliefs can be the determining factor in the patient's rehabilitation.

More recently, Sivik and Delimar[49] found psychological differences between injured workers who attributed the injury to a work accident and those who did not. It should be noted that most of the former group had disability claims outstanding. Nonetheless, the accident group appeared to be more psychologically healthy than the nonaccident group on most variables including hypochondriasis, anxiety, and muscular tension. These findings may suggest that patients with back pain of no identifiable origin are more psychologically distressed than those who can attribute the pain to a specific incident. However, the direction of the relationship between these variables is unclear.

Linton et al[36] compared three groups of female nurses from the same workplace: those off work because of back pain, those with back pain but not off work, and those working without pain. Several factors were found to distinguish between the three groups: differences in coping strategies in general, catastrophizing (imagining the worst), physical health, and perceived health. Their findings support previous studies that showed a relationship between coping and the outcome of low back pain.[46,54]

Cognitive factors seem to be important in the understanding of occupational musculoskeletal disorders. More prospective studies need to be done, however. Also, the mechanisms by which cognition has an impact on an injury are poorly understood. For example, is the belief that one can overcome an injury motivational, or does it result in a salutary emotional state that buffers the effects of stress on the musculoskeletal system? These relationships require clarification.

Affective States

Numerous studies have attempted to link personality to the onset, progression, or outcome of musculoskeletal disorders. The assumption here is that certain patients are predisposed to chronicity and that these patients can be identified early. Longitudinal studies of this nature are few, and retrospective studies have been disappointing. It may be concluded from these studies that it is not possible to predict whose pain will become chronic by personality type. The prevailing belief appears to be that certain personality traits may be magnified by or are a result of chronic illness. It is more common now to focus on specific reactions to injury. These reactions fall under the categories of psychological distress.

Psychological distress refers to negative affective states. The Minnesota Multiphasic Personality Inventory (MMPI) is the most popular and controversial tool for studying these states. A critique of its use in patients with low back pain can be found elsewhere.[61] To date, the MMPI has been used predominantly in patients with low back pain and has yielded conflicting results.

Two studies of recently injured workers found no relationship between the three scales most often associated with chronic low back pain—hypochondriasis, hysteria, and depression—and return-to-work status.[6,27] However, a prospective study of healthy workers found four MMPI scales (hysteria, psychopathic deviance, schizophrenia, and low back pain) that distinguished those who reported back injury from those who did not.[2] Further analysis of these data showed that several items on the hysteria scale were particularly predictive of back injury report: lassitude/malaise, denial of social anxiety, and to a lesser extent, the need for affection.[15]

Two additional studies found that specific MMPI scales determined tertiary risk factors for low back pain. Barnes et al[1] found that hypochondriasis was related to poor outcome in a functional restoration program. Later, Gallagher et al[16] studied 150 patients with chronic pain and showed that the hysteria scale was inversely related to return-to-work status for patients with low back pain 6 months posttreatment. Finally, as part of a multivariate study, Feuerstein and Thebarge[9] found that the depression and the psychasthenia (anxiety) scales of the MMPI differentiated between patients with chronic back, neck, or shoulder problems who were working and patients with chronic pain who were not.

Feyer et al[10] compared 257 nurses, 256 postal workers, and 45 pain clinic patients on patterns of psychosocial symptoms and work-related low back complaints. Using a general measure of psychological distress, the correlational study found more symptoms in the patient population. This was true despite the fact that pain complaints were similar between patients and working subjects. Of equal interest was that working patients and workers without pain did not differ on the measure of distress. Additionally, psychological distress was unrelated to the decision to take sick leave. However, it was related to the decision to leave work completely.

Several studies have looked at the association between personality or psychological distress and a variety of musculoskeletal complaints. Flodmark and Aase[12] identified aspects of the type A behavior pattern, specifically speed and hard-driving competitiveness, as correlates of neck, shoulder, and low back pain in 58 factory workers. Patients who endorsed these items, particularly speed, for the previous week had more physical complaints than others. In a study of upper limb disorders, Helliwell et al[20] found that anxiety, depression, and related somatic complaints were associated with a history of pain and current pain. Pain was also related to workload, indicating an interaction between load and psychological status.

In a prospective study of 697 employees at three metal industry plants, Leino and Magni[31] found that depression and symptoms of stress at baseline predicted reports of musculoskeletal pain in the back, neck, and shoulders 3 years later. In men, these factors also predicted clinical findings. Musculoskeletal symptoms predicted symptoms of stress at time 2 as well, showing a reciprocal relationship between the two variables. Musculoskeletal symptoms at time 1, however, did not predict future depression. This may indicate that depression is a risk factor for the development of physical problems.

Other measures of psychological distress have been used to predict the outcome of tertiary prevention programs for workers with low back pain. Factors associated with poor outcome include high levels of pain, depression, high scores on the premorbid pessimism scale of the Millon Behavioral Health Inventory (MBHI), and external locus of control.[1,16,43] A good outcome in one study was predicted by high scores on the cooperative scale of the MBHI.[1] This finding underscores the need to look for the adaptive attributes of patients as well as the maladaptive traits.

Lustman et al[38] studied 56 patients in a work-hardening program retrospectively. All suffered from musculoskeletal pain, although the affected region was not specified. Histories of alcohol abuse or depression were found in 64.3% of these patients. Within this subgroup, most had psychiatric histories. The authors conclude that these factors may predispose workers to injury. They caution healthcare providers against assuming that distress is merely the result of injury. Only speculative results can be drawn from correlational studies, however.

The evidence shows that the psychological status of the individual is an important component in a work-related injury. Specifically, measures of distress (i.e., depression, anxiety) seem to show some consistent relationships to musculoskeletal complaints despite wide variation in methods of assessment. An argument may be made for the causal relationship between distress and musculoskeletal disorders at various stages. The relationship between distress and early symptom reporting suggests that multidisciplinary attempts to prevent the progression of occupational musculoskeletal injuries should start early. Future studies that include the adaptive traits of the patient may give a more complete picture of the sequelae of disability.

Pain Behavior

Behavior is a way of communicating beliefs and emotional states to the outside world. Because pain behavior is often nonverbal and manifest, it can be measured unobtrusively. Pain behavior includes grimacing, bracing, guarding, groaning, limping, overreacting, and being inactive.[26,57] In patients with chronic pain, pain behavior is sometimes considered to be a sign of symptom magnification or an indication of a psychological overlay to illness. This behavior has been called illness or pain behavior.

Using Waddell's signs and pain drawings, Greenough, Taylor, and Fraser[19] could predict the outcome of surgery in 151 spinal fusion patients at 2 years postsurgery. Patients with few signs and anatomically consistent drawings were functioning better and were more satisfied than those whose scores were inconsistent with physical findings. The significance of pain behavior in the acute and subacute stages of injury is a topic for future investigation.

PERCEPTIONS OF THE SOCIAL ENVIRONMENT

Work Perceptions

Attributes of the work environment are by definition extrinsic to the worker. They include aspects of the job itself as well as the social and corporate culture. These factors, however, are rarely measured objectively. Instead, researchers rely heavily on workers' self-reports. Self-reports ensure that individuals' subjective opinions are reflected in the responses. Therefore, in reality, they are perceptions of the work environment and not clearly separate from intrinsic factors. Individuals who tend to endorse questionnaire items that indicate negative affective states may also endorse items that indicate high levels of work stress. The tendency to respond negatively has been called negative affectivity.[59] It can bias results by making relationships spuriously high whenever self-report measures are used. This notwithstanding, perceptions of the work environment are studied to shed light on the etiology and treatment of occupational musculoskeletal disorders.

Work satisfaction and work stress are distinct constructs; an individual can certainly be satisfied with and even choose a highly stressful job. However, they are clearly related and many of the same variables are used to explain satisfaction and work stress. For example, the support of coworkers can increase satisfaction and reduce stress. Reducing stress may also increase satisfaction. Despite this, these terms are sometimes used interchangeably in the literature. Therefore it is important to be aware of how variables are defined and measured when any research on this topic is reviewed.

In a cross-sectional study, Linton and Warg[35] investigated the relationships between attributions of back injury, work satisfaction, and low back pain in 145 employees. Work satisfaction was measured by one item assessing general satisfaction. Using the hypothetical case of an injured worker, they found that white-collar employees were more likely to attribute the cause of an injury to the worker. Blue-collar workers, on the other hand, attributed the injury to the workplace. This attribution was also related to a history of back pain. Work dissatisfaction was also associated with the belief that the injury was caused by the work environment, and it was associated with reports of previous back pain.

A recent study conceptualized work satisfaction as consisting of work content, work-related social support, work-related hygienic factors, and perception of healthiness of the work environment.[32] They also found a positive relationship between the multidimensional measure of work satisfaction and neck and shoulder symptoms in 232 Finnish female office employees.

In a well-known prospective investigation of factory employees, work satisfaction, assessed by a single item, was the best predictor of back injury reporting among all psychological variables.[2] More recently, using a prospective design, Ready et al[44] found that work satisfaction (also assessed univariately) and other lifestyle factors could discriminate between nurses who reported back pain and those who did not.

At least one study found no relationship between work dissatisfaction and disability from occupational low back pain.[10] Here, work dissatisfaction was computed as the difference between the ideal work environment and the perceived actual environment. However, these results do not necessarily contradict previous findings. It is possible to conceive of satisfaction and dissatisfaction as unipolar constructs. That is, a person may be satisfied and dissatisfied simultaneously. These factors may have different effects on occupational musculoskeletal complaints. This is an area for future investigation.

Work stress is a common concept associated with occupational musculoskeletal disorders. Like job satisfaction, work stress has been defined in a variety of ways. It can be measured univariately or as the product of several underlying dimensions. The scale chosen reveals the investigators' understanding of the construct. A number of models have been proposed to explain the relationship between work stress and health. Two in particular, the models of Karasek et al[25] and Smith and Sanfort,[51] seem to have attracted the most attention.

Karasek and colleagues identify the psychosocial variables of greatest importance. According to these authors, they are the demands placed on the worker and the amount of control the worker has over the job. These factors are said to interact to determine perceptions of work stress.[25] Typically, these factors are measured by self-report. Smith and Sainfort's balance theory of job design[51] proposes that psychological and physical factors interact to affect health. Evidence for this model requires objective measures of physical stressors, which are often difficult to obtain. These models complement each other and can be tested simultaneously.

One study with direct bearing on both models is that of Houtman et al.[22] In a cross-sectional analysis of 5865 workers, high work pace, low decision latitude, and high physical demands were associated with back, joint, and muscle pain and reports of chronic pain as well as psychosomatic complaints. Similar findings have been shown elsewhere. In a recent study of 131 dentists, 41% complained of neck-shoulder problems and 37% complained of low back problems.[29] Dentists who reported their work to be too physically or mentally demanding had greater reports of muscle problems in the past year than others. Eskelinen et al[8] conceptualized work stress similarly and added the variable of "control." In a sample of 1799 males and 2456 females in 40 different municipal occupations, work stress was related to musculoskeletal symptoms as well as other physical complaints.

Pickett and Lees[42] also found psychological demands to be associated with problems. They assessed work stress as the portion of time the worker reported being under emotional or mental stress. Seventy-eight female data entry clerks reported high levels of stress and physical complaints. Complaints of pain in the neck, shoulders, back, hand, wrist, legs, and muscles in general were significantly more frequent in subjects who perceived their work stress level as high. Lancourt and Kettlehut[28] prospectively studied 134 patients with low back pain and found that patients with fewer problems, whether work-related or personal, were more likely to return to work than those with many problems. These factors showed greater predictive value than did the physical findings. Their results also suggest that different factors are associated with returning to work for patients with acute and chronic pains.

Leino and Lyyra[30] measured work stress with a 10-item scale. Here, social support was measured independently by six items referring to work, friends, and family. Stress was associated with musculoskeletal complaints and predicted clinical findings at a 10-year follow-up of blue-collar but not white-collar workers. Social support was negatively related to morbidity, but this finding was not significant. Feuerstein and Thebarge[9] found similar but significant findings. They used a work perception scale with three dimensions as part of a multivariate study: relationship, personal growth, and system maintenance and change. In a sample of 165 patients they found that reported job stress could discriminate between patients with chronic pain disorders who work and those who do not. Specifically, supervisor support and work pressure were the best discriminators.

From these and other studies, social support has emerged as a variable of interest. Social support may be defined as the perception of having someone to rely on for emotional or instrumental sustenance. The perception of support is thought to buffer the impact of stress on an individual's health. However, findings regarding social support have provided an ambiguous picture. One study found coworker support to be positively associated with back pain in a sample of 787 nurses.[50] Although the idea of social support may be compelling, the reader should be aware that support can have variable effects. For instance, in the case of an injured worker, coworker support—if offered in terms of encouragement to return to work—can have a positive impact on recovery. It is equally plausible that support from coworkers can have deleterious effects on recovery if it is of the kind that encourages the worker to remain on disability in order to be compensated for the injury. It is important that the exact nature of social support be specified before conclusions can be drawn.

Cumulative evidence suggests that perceptions about work dramatically affect occupational musculoskeletal disorders. The exact mechanisms by which this works remain unknown. For example, work stress has been implicated in the development of repetitive strain injuries (RSIs), particularly hand and arm disorders, in visual display terminal (VDT) operators.[40] However, the relationship is believed to be indirect. The introduction of VDTs into the work environment has altered work practices and has generated boring work, repetitive gestures, increased demand for output, lack of control, and few rest breaks. All these factors are believed to be associated with increased risk for injuries. It is also possible that work perceptions have a direct effect on musculoskeletal disorders by influencing the meaning of the injury and the associated distress or by causing physical strain that leaves the worker more vulnerable to injury. In a recent review, Bongers et al[4] attempts to shed light on these relationships. They conclude that high correlations between psychosocial factors and physical demands on the job make it difficult to assess the impact of these factors. More studies using subjective and objective measures of the work environment are needed to provide causal models and address these issues.

Other Social Factors

In the United States, a worker who sustains an injury on the job may file a claim for worker's compensation. The purpose of compensation is to provide the worker with a normal income while the worker is undergoing rehabilitation. Compensation status has been linked to rehabilitation outcome in contrary ways. Patients with pending compensation claims have been shown to have poorer outcomes than those not receiving compensation.[6,13] It has been suggested that compensation payments reinforce the worker for not working. However, Barnes et al[1] found that patients with chronic pain who are receiving high levels of compensation were more likely to be working 1 year after rehabilitation than those with lower levels of compensation. They reasoned that patients receiving more money had more satisfying jobs and in turn were more motivated to return to work. Clearly, however, the relationship between compensation and health status is complex and deserves comment.

Implicit in the compensation agreement is the notion that the injured worker is actively "working" at getting better.[11] Anecdotally, it is often heard that remuneration serves as a disincentive to return to work. In the author's experience, it is never the compensation payments that deter patients from getting well if they are determined to do so. Instead, compensation makes it easier for those disinclined to be rehabilitated to remain disabled. However, this is almost never a case of true malingering and more often the result of a mismanaged disability claim and the patient's reaction to a paradoxical process.

Frequently, the injured worker places the blame for the accident on the workplace, whereas the employer is more likely to blame the worker.[35] This situation ultimately leads to adversarial relationships between the worker and employer. The worker is perceived to be manipulating the system to derive undeserved benefits (in other words, "he's not really sick"). The employer is perceived to be a merciless slave driver thinking only of financial loss and not of the employee's suffering.

Rarely is either scenario entirely true. Most often, the worker and the employer fall victim to the roles assigned to them in the extremely powerful social influence of the compensation system. Walker[58] has described how the compensation system engenders a sense of helplessness in the injured worker. Employees trying to negotiate their way out of compensation are confronted with obstacles at every turn: from suspicious employers to attorneys who discourage returning to work for short-term gains. After a series of discouraging encounters, patients give up and give in to the role of "disabled" worker. According to Holloway,[21] this is an adaptive response to a deleterious system and is the only way the patient can receive validation.

Indeed, Reid, Ewan, and Lowy[45] found the quest for validation to be a powerful motivator in 52 patients with repetitive strain injury (RSI) in Australia. Because RSI is poorly understood, these patients were often viewed as neurotic by physicians. This contributed to the patient's emphasis on physical symptoms, doctor shopping, and a tendency to deny any psychological problem. These authors point out that because so little is known about the course of these problems, patients are in a no-win situation. They truly want to get better but fear that if they try to minimize symptoms, they may reinjure themselves and will not get the compensation they deserve.

The family system is another powerful social structure that influences workers with a musculoskeletal complaint. Stutts and Kasdan[53] studied 83 worker's compensation patients who were being seen for independent medical examinations. Fifty-two percent of these patients had a family member who was disabled. The authors postulate that a "disabled support system," where norms of disability and an acceptance of this status are cultivated in the family, encourage the adoption of disability status on the part of the patient. Because no control group was used and the study was correlational, this conclusion, although interesting, is speculative.

It may be surmised that the worker, once injured, enters a new realm of the disabled. This new realm has a social reality that can dramatically direct the course of recovery. The worker's compensation system may foster the precise behavior and attitudes it was designed to protect the worker from, disability and distress. Family systems are also influential in the patient's progress. In the worst case, these forces can challenge the individual's self-determination to recover from an injury. It is therefore prudent to consider these factors whenever an occupational musculoskeletal disorder is managed.

DEVELOPING INTERVENTIONS

The Role of the Healthcare Professional

Clinicians inclined to adhere to a biopsychosocial model are advised to do so from the first visit. Beliefs about disability may be rooted in past experience but are certainly solidified when a worker becomes injured. In one study, Hyytiainen[23] found that metal industry workers had positive attitudes in general about preventing back pain. However, these attitudes declined with age and with the report of a low back pain episode. This speaks to the need for active management at the first sign of a musculoskeletal problem.

Every encounter with healthcare professionals and medical management systems provides an opportunity for intervention. Waddell[56] has astutely observed the powerful effects a physician can have on the patient. Information that is vague, incomplete, or incomprehensible to a layperson can render the patient confused, helpless, and afraid. For example, the diagnosis of a herniated disk can be a disability sentence in the mind of a patient. Diagnostic film results are often held up as proof. It is the healthcare provider's responsibility to explain the implications of any diagnosis in terms the patient can understand. In the case of disk herniation, the patient needs to know that pain and disability are often self-limiting and that many patients with this condition maintain their usual lifestyles.

Making sure that the patient has a realistic picture of the diagnosis and the prognosis is the first step. Patients who seem overly distressed can be questioned about other life circumstances. Questions about work are particularly important when the injury is work related. There is often residual anger toward the employer. Patients sometimes believe that it is the employer's responsibility to make sure they get well. If patients understand the normal course of low back pain and are encouraged to take responsibility for their recovery from the onset (even if they are not responsible for the injury), they may be spared the ordeal of becoming a compensation failure.

Primary healthcare professionals also have a responsibility to make appropriate referrals for their patients. Information given by the physician can be reinforced or contradicted by secondary caregivers. Contradictory information is one of the major causes of distress and can lead to endless doctor shopping and prolongation of recovery. At the very least, the physician should be aware of the treatment philosophy of any facility to which they are referring patients. Ideally, the patient should be referred to a facility that adheres to current guidelines for the treatment of acute low back pain.[3] In this case, patients who exceed the expected recovery time can be assessed in a timely fashion. If warranted, they can begin a multidisciplinary program that addresses psychosocial issues. **Figure 6-2** illustrates an optimal framework for psychosocial interventions.

There are a great many studies that testify to the efficacy of the multidisciplinary approach in treating patients with chronic pain.[61] However, the application of a biopsychosocial model in the acute and subacute phases of treatment is a relatively new concept. In a recent investigation, Main found that psychological distress measured at the onset of injury predicts future disability (Main, personal communication, June 15, 1994). This study supports the need for early intervention. Indeed, programs that have applied a multidisciplinary approach early have had positive outcomes.

A behavioral approach pioneered by Fordyce is the easiest to implement early in treatment. This program consists of time-contingent care in which medication levels, exercise goals, and duration of treatment are preset and not determined by the patient. The idea is to provide environmental contingencies that reinforce "well" behavior and ignore "pain" behavior. In a benchmark study, Fordyce et al.[14] compared this approach

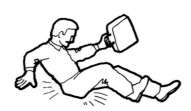

Onset of pain

- Explain the biopsychosocial model
- Address concerns about pain, including the course, diagnosis, and prognosis
- Emphasize the patient's role in recovery
- Make appropriate referral if indicated

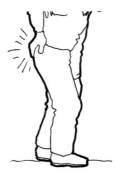

Two weeks after

- Address concerns again, old and new
- Address social factors including attitudes about work, as well as family and friend's responses to pain
- Reinforce patient's role in recovery again
- Make appropriate referral if indicated

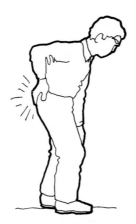

Four weeks after

- Address concerns again, old and new
- Address social factors again
- Reinforce patient's role in recovery again
- Refer for multidisciplinary evaluation and possible treatment

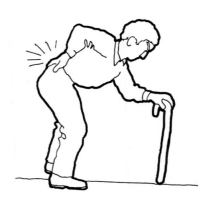

Seven weeks after

- Address concerns again
- Address social factors again
- Reinforce patient's role in recovery
- Refer for multidisciplinary evaluation and treatment

Figure 6-2 Application of the biopsychosocial model: general guidelines for primary healthcare providers.

with traditional care in which patients were told to "let pain be your guide." Subjects with back pain for less than 10 days were randomly assigned to one of the two conditions and were followed at 6 weeks and then 9 to 12 months after treatment. Although no differences were noted at 6 weeks, long-term follow-up showed significantly greater improvement in functioning for the treatment group.

Other studies have shown the benefits of multidisciplinary care for an acute population. The psychosocial component of these programs often includes relaxation training and cognitive coping strategies as well as time-contingent care. Gill et al[17] described significant decreases in pain and improvement in function and work status among 50 acute patients entering a 4-week program for low back pain. Linton and Bradley[33] found similar results in an 18-month follow-up study of 36 subjects with recent-onset back pain. They also projected from baseline data the costs that would have been incurred if the subjects had not attended the program and showed significant financial benefits of an early-care multidisciplinary program.

These findings suggest that primary healthcare physicians would do well to start patients on the road to recovery by following a biopsychosocial approach at the onset. Establishing a good rapport with the patient, giving clear and intelligible information, encouraging an active approach to treatment, and making appropriate referrals at the first sign of delayed recovery can go a long way toward reducing occupational musculoskeletal disorders.

The Role of the Workplace

A comprehensive model of prevention and treatment must include the cooperation of management at all levels. Steffy et al[52] demonstrated the importance of involving high level management in efforts to reduce accidents at work. They implemented a stress management program at two hospitals and one industrial plant that included organizational changes as well as individual techniques. The reductions in accident-related costs following this program were staggering at all three sites. Stress management programs aimed at employees alone have yet to demonstrate such effects.[41]

Once injured, the employee enters a medical system that all too often offers inappropriate or delayed care and contradictory advice. Wiesel Boden, and Feffer[60] have demonstrated the impact of a quality-based management system in reducing disability and associated costs. At a power company employing over 5300 workers, the authors implemented a protocol that included early reporting of injury, early examination at a centralized facility, and a computerized database.

Feedback gleaned over the 10-year period was used to modify and improve care. As a result, the authors developed algorithms for treating back and neck pain. This program resulted in a myriad of improvements, including a decrease in workdays lost, surgeries performed, and medical expenses incurred.

The argument for managed care of injured workers fits well within the biopsychosocial model. For one thing, it addresses the fears and concerns of patients early and gets them well on their way to recovery. The message to patients is that they can get better quickly with proper care. When this is implemented at the workplace, it also conveys the sense that management cares enough to make sure that the worker receives appropriate treatment in a timely manner.

It has already been shown that negative attitudes about work can have adverse effects on the course of musculoskeletal complaints. However, the attitudes of supervisors and coworkers can influence attempts to resume work activities. Linton and Bradley[33] note that simple ergonomic changes and encouragement from coworkers can make the difference between an easy adjustment period or a difficult one. The attitudes of supervisors are generally a reflection of the organizational climate. Managers must be vigilant of the message they send to subordinates when it comes to accommodating an injured employee who is newly returned to work.

Many employees suffer from sporadic musculoskeletal complaints that do not require lost workdays. Management can engage in secondary prevention by providing programs on-site and supporting their use. Linton and his colleagues[24,34] have demonstrated the efficacy of mind/body techniques in preventing an increase in occupational injuries in the workplace. In one study, subjects were instructed to take relaxation breaks every half hour. Despite problems with adherence, this technique reduced the development of neck and shoulder pain over the course of the day. In a more recent controlled study, Linton et al[37] demonstrated the advantage of a behaviorally based treatment program at the workplace in preventing chronic disability in nurses and nurses aides. At 6 months after the intervention, the treatment group showed superior results in regard to pain intensity, distress, life satisfaction, pain behavior, and sicklisting.

The Role of Society

Any discussion of the biopsychosocial model in treating occupational musculoskeletal diseases would be remiss if it did not look at the contribution of society. Much of the problem from this standpoint was already covered in the previous, albeit brief discussion of the compensation system. A society that reinforces injured workers for staying out of work holds some responsibility for the suffering and related costs of musculoskeletal disorders. Those in power would do well to consider a biopsychosocial model when policies are created. Given what we now know about the course of low back pain, it is reasonable to expect the injured worker to return to work within 2 months. Exceptions occur when other medical or psychological problems exist. Fordyce suggests that patients who languish beyond this time should receive appropriate medical referrals or forego compensation status. In any case, their primary diagnosis should no longer be "low back pain" (Fordyce, personal communication, October 5, 1994). Just as rehabilitation programs now seek to not reward pain behavior, so may society do the same by modifying a failing compensation system.

SUMMARY

Traditional treatments for occupational musculoskeletal disorders have fallen short of expectations. The biopsychosocial model goes beyond physical factors to include psychological and social elements that affect the worker before and after an injury. Investigations into the practical application of this model are most convincing. Studies have shown that psychosocial factors are at least as important and often more important than physical factors in determining disability. Programs that have attempted to prevent injury or the chronicity associated with occupational musculoskeletal disorders have flourished when they include a biopsychosocial framework. It is suggested that this model be implemented by primary healthcare providers, employers, and society at large. Because we all share the burden of disability, we must all share in the solution. Much can be done by the physician, the workplace, and society to make this process easier and more successful for everyone.

References

1. Barnes D et al: Psychosocioeconomic predictors of treatment success/failure in chronic low-back pain patients, *Spine* 14:427-430, 1988.

2. Bigos S, Battie M, Spengler D: A prospective study of work perceptions and psychosocial factors affecting the report of back injury, *Spine* 16:1-6, 1991.

3. Bigos S et al: *Acute low back pain problems in adults.* Clinical practice guideline No 14, AHCPR Pub No 95-0642, Rockville, Md, 1994, Agency for Health Care Policy and Research, Public Health Service, US Department of Health and Human Services.

4. Bongers PM et al: Psychosocial factors at work and musculoskeletal disease, *Scand J Work Environ Health* 19:297-312, 1993.

5. Canon W: *Bodily changes in pain, hunger, fear and rage,* ed 2. New York, 1936, Appleton-Century-Crofts.

6. Cats-Baril W, Frymoyer J: Identifying patients at risk of becoming disabled because of low back pain. The Vermont Rehabilitation Engineering Center Predictive Model, *Spine* 16:1168-1172, 1991.

7. Engel GL: The need for a new medical model, *Science* 196:129-136, 1977.

8. Eskelinen L et al: Work-related stress symptoms of aging employees in municipal occupations, *Scand J Work Environ Health* 17(suppl):87-93. 1991.

9. Feuerstein M, Thebarge RW: Perceptions of disability and occupational stress as discriminators of work disability in patients with chronic pain, *J Occup Rehabil* 1:185-195, 1991.

10. Feyer AM et al: Role of psychosocial factors in work-related low back pain, *Scand J Work Environ Health* 18:368-375, 1992.

11. Fleeson W: *Going on comp,* Duluth, Minn, 1991, Med-Ed Books & Publishers.

12. Flodmark B, Aase G: Musculoskeletal symptoms and type A behaviour in blue collar workers, *Br J Ind Med* 49:683-687, 1992.

13. Fordyce WE: *Behavioral methods for chronic pain and illness,* St. Louis, 1976, Mosby–Year Book.

14. Fordyce WE: Acute back pain: a control group comparison of behavioral vs. traditional management methods, *J Behav Med* 9:127-140, 1986.

15. Fordyce WE et al: MMPI scale 3 as a predictor of back injury report: what does it tell us? *Clin J Pain* 8:222-226, 1992.

16. Gallagher RM et al: Determinants of return-to-work among low back pain patients, *Pain* 39:55-67, 1989.

17. Gill C et al: Low back pain: program description and outcome in a case series, *J Orthop Sports Phys Ther* 20:11-16, 1994.

18. Goleman D, Gurin D, editors: *Mind body medicine: how to use your mind for better health,* New York, 1993, Consumer Reports Books.

19. Greenough CG, Taylor LJ, and Fraser RD: Anterior lumbar fusion: a comparison of noncompensation patients with compensation patients, *Clin Orthop* 300:30-37, 1994.

20. Helliwell PS et al: Work related upper limb disorder: the relationship between pain, cumulative load, disability and psychological factors, *Ann Rheum Dis* 51:1325-1329, 1992.

21. Holloway G: Susto and the career path of the victim of an industrial accident: a sociological case study, *Soc Sci Med* 38:989-997, 1994.

22. Houtman IL et al: Psychosocial stressors at work and musculoskeletal problems, *Scand J Work Environ Health* 20:139-145, 1994.

23. Hyytiainen K: Attitudes towards prevention of low back disorders in industry, *Occup Med* 44:83-86, 1994.

24. Kamwendo K, Linton S: Can pause-gymnastics prevent neck and shoulder pain? *Sjukgymnasten* 7:12-14, 1986.

25. Karasek R et al: Job decision latitude, job demands, and cardiovascular disease. In Salvendy G and Smith M, editors: *Machine pacing and occupational stress,* London, 1981, Taylor & Francis Publishers, Inc; pp 694-705.

26. Keefe F, Block A: Development of an observation method for assessing pain behavior in chronic low back pain patients, *Behav Ther* 13:363-375, 1982.

27. Lacroix JM et al: Low back pain. Factors of value in predicting outcome, *Spine* 15:495-499, 1990.

28. Lancourt J, Kettelhut M: Predicting RTW for lower back pain patients receiving worker's compensation, *Spine* 17:629-640, 1992.

29. Lehto TU, Helenius HY, Alaranta HT: Musculoskeletal symptoms of dentists assessed by a multidisciplinary approach, *Community Dent Oral Epidemiol* 19:38-44, 1991.

30. Leino P, Lyyra A: The effects of mental stress and social support on the development of musculoskeletal morbidity in the engineering industry. In Sakurai H et al, editors: *Occupational epidemiology,* Amsterdam, 1990, Elsevier Science, Inc: pp 267-272.

31. Leino P, Magni G: Depressive and distress symptoms as predictors of low back pain, neck-shoulder pain and other musculoskeletal morbidity: a 10-year follow-up of metal industry employees, *Pain* 53:89-94, 1993.

32. Levoska S, Keinanen-Kiukaanniemi S: Psychosocial stress and job satisfaction in female office employees with and without neck-shoulder symptoms, *Work Stress* 8:255-262, 1994.

33. Linton SJ, Bradley LA: An 18 month follow-up of a secondary prevention program for back pain: help and hindrance factors related to outcome maintenance, *Clin J Pain* 8:227-236, 1992.

34. Linton SJ, Kamwendo J: Low back schools. A critical review, Phys Ther 67:1375-1383, 1987.

35. Linton SJ, Warg LE: Attributions (beliefs) and job satisfaction associated with back pain in an industrial setting, *Percept Mot Skills* 76:51-62, 1993.

36. Linton SJ et al: Psychological factors related to health, back pain and dysfunction, *J Occup Rehabil* 4:3-10, 1994.

37. Linton SJ et al: The secondary prevention of low back pain: a controlled study with follow-up, *Pain* 36:197-207, 1989.

38. Lustman PJ et al: Prior psychiatric problems in rehabilitation clients with work-related injuries, *J Occup Rehabil* 1: 227-233, 1991.

39. Melzack R, Wall P: Pain mechanisms: a new theory, *Science* 150:971-979, 1965.

40. Ong CN: Musculoskeletal disorders in operators of VDTs, *World Health Forum* 15:161-64, 1994.

41. Pelletier K, Lutz R: Mindbody goes to work: a critical review of stress management programs in the workplace, *Advances* 6:28-34, 1989.

42. Pickett CW, Lees RE: A cross-sectional study of health complaints among 79 data entry operators using video display terminals, *J Soc Occup Med* 41: 113-116, 1991.

43. Polatin P et al: A psychosociomedical prediction model of response to treatment by chronically disabled workers with low back pain, *Spine* 14:956-961, 1988.

44. Ready AE et al: Fitness and lifestyle parameters fail to predict back injury in nurses, *Can J Appl Physiol* 18:80-90, 1993.

45. Reid J, Ewan C, Lowy E: Pilgrimage of pain: the illness experiences of women with repetition strain injury and the search for credibility, *Soc Sci Med* 32:601-612, 1991.

46. Rosenstiel A, Keefe F: The use of coping strategies in chronic low back pain patients: relationship to patient characteristics and current adjustment, *Pain* 17:33-44, 1983.

47. Sandstrom J, Esbjornsson E: Return to work after rehabilitation. The significance of the patient's own prediction, *Scand J Rehabil Med* 18:29, 1986.

48. Selye H: *The stress of life,* New York, 1956, McGraw Hill.

49. Sivik TM, Delimar D: Characteristics of patients who attribute chronic pain to minor injury, *Scand J Rehabil Med* 26:27-31, 1994.

50. Skovron ML et al: Work organization and low back pain in nursing personnel, *Ergonomics* 30:359-366, 1987.

51. Smith M, Sainfort P: A balance theory of job design for stress reduction, *Int J Ind Ergonom* 4:67-79, 1989.

52. Steffy BD et al: A demonstration of the impact of stress abatement programs on reducing employees accidents and their costs, *Am J Health Promot* Fall: 25-32, 1986.

53. Stutts JT, Kasdan M: Disability: a new psychosocial perspective, *J Occup Med* 35:825-827, 1993.

54. Turner J, Clancy S: Strategies for coping with chronic low back pain: relationship to pain and disability, *Pain* 24:355-364, 1986.

55. Ursin H et al: Muscle pain and coping with working life in Norway: a review, *Work Stress* 7:247-258, 1993.

56. Waddell G: Biopsychosocial analysis of low back pain. In Nordin M and Vischer TL, editors: *Common low back pain: prevention of chronicity,* London, 1992 Bailliere Tindall.

57. Waddell G: Understanding the patient with back pain. In Jayson M editor: *The lumbar spine and back pain,* ed 3, Edinburgh, 1987, Churchill Livingstone, International.

58. Walker JM: Injured worker helplessness: critical relationships and systems level approach for intervention, *J Occup Rehabil* 2:201-209, 1992.

59. Watson D, Clark C: Negative affectivity: the disposition to experience aversive emotional states, *Psychol Bull* 96:465-490, 1984.

60. Wiesel SW, Boden SD, Feffer HL: A quality based protocol for management of musculoskeletal injuries, *Clin Orthop* 301:164-176, 1994.

61. Weiser S, Cedraschi C: Psychosocial issues in the prevention of chronic low back pain: a literature review. In Nordin M and Vischer TL, editors: *Common low back pain: prevention of chronicity,* London, 1992, Bailliere Tindall.

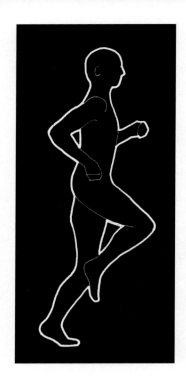

Chapter 7

Cost and Control of Industrial Musculoskeletal Injuries

John D. Frymoyer

CONTENTS

Work-related musculoskeletal disorders cost a great deal of money. To paraphrase one of America's most colorful senators, Everett Dirkson, "A billion here and a billion there, pretty soon it adds up to real money." Today the costs of health care in general, or work-related musculoskeletal disorders in specific, are the source of great debate. Although the debate is most public in the United States, the issues are affecting all industrialized nations. In response to the rising costs, this country is moving toward greater government regulation, whereas many European countries are moving away from their more socialized systems, as seen in the "privatization" of the English Health Service.

The rising costs of health care and the associated public debate are occurring in the context of three major societal forces affecting all industrialized nations: a growing and competitive international marketplace, international healthcare reform, and a significant downturn in the economies of many countries. Although the outcome of the debates is not yet certain, industry, insurers, health professions, and government anticipate that there will be significant and perhaps profound changes in how individual patients with work-related musculoskeletal disorders will be managed in the future.

Work-related low back pain and its cost in the United States are the focus of this chapter. The issues and the societal response to them are generalizable. Three broad issues will be discussed: what is driving the escalating costs of work-related musculoskeletal disorders, what the magnitude of the problem is, and what strategies can be employed to gain better control of these costs.

WHAT IS DRIVING THE ESCALATING COST OF WORK-RELATED MUSCULOSKELETAL DISORDERS?

The economics of work-related musculoskeletal disorders are rooted in multiple complex medical, legal, and social phenomena. There is strong evidence that the rise in healthcare costs, in general, is related to the growth in medical technology, particularly during the past two decades. The dramatic increase in costs specific to musculoskeletal disorders has resulted from enactment and continuing implementation of the worker's compensation law, the complex psychosocial and legal issues surrounding "disability behavior," and probably the widespread acceptance of the concept of "cumulative trauma." The Americans with Disabilities Act (ADA)

may also drive up societal costs, but the overall impact is as yet unknown.

The Impact of Medical Technology

The single most important driving force in the rise in healthcare costs has been the continuous growth of sophisticated medical technology. Aaron and Schwartz[1] have analyzed the costs of medical care and determined that inflation, improved pay for healthcare providers, and in some instances, the changing demographics of the population to a more aged society have had some impact on increasing medical costs. However, they concluded that the increase in cost and use of medical technology has been the single most important factor.

The low back paradigm demonstrates this point. Before 1934, low back pain was considered a benign ailment, usually part of the general and accepted aches and pains termed "rheumatism." Physicians and surgeons focused primarily on infectious diseases and major trauma as the identifiable causes of more serious spinal disorders. Tuberculosis, not low back pain, served as the major impetus for the development of spinal fusion in 1914. An occupational causation was only attributed in cases in which a worker suffered major trauma resulting in a spinal fracture.

By 1930 the medical profession was considering other potential causes and diagnoses, largely because of the radiologic identification of structural aberrations such as facet arthritis and narrowed disks. These investigators surmised but did not prove that these abnormalities caused back pain. Mixter and Barr[19] gave further credence to a structural rather than rheumatic causation of back pain when they described herniated nucleus pulposus as a cause of sciatica. In addition, they surmised that this condition was most likely traumatic in etiology and resulted in basic structural weakening of the spine. Based on this theory, they proposed that surgical management of nerve compression should be accompanied by lumbar spinal fusion.[19]

Frymoyer and Donaghy[12] reported on the first patient in whom Mixter and Barr made the diagnosis of herniated lumbar disk. In a refreshing display of candor, Mixter was later to comment, "Newton is of historic significance because he was the first person in whom we recognized the herniated lumbar disk as such. He is the man who started all the damn trouble." It is also noteworthy that Barr et al[2] many years later concluded that spinal fusion had no additive benefits in the management of these patients.

Following Mixter and Barr's clinical discovery, the number of patients identified with herniated nucleus pulposus grew, but the number requiring surgery remained small. To consider a patient for surgery required painful tests such as lipoidal myelography. Anesthetics were risky and complications common, thereby giving the practitioner ample reason to be cautious. Technical advances in spinal imaging, anesthesia, and operating instruments have removed these obstacles, and today lumbar spinal surgery is considered "routine." Not surprisingly, the number of diagnostic tests for low back disorders has grown rapidly, as has the number of surgical interventions. The precise costs of computed tomography (CT) and magnetic resonance imaging (MRI) have not been reported, but there is little doubt that the proliferation of these tests for musculoskeletal disorders has been significant. Today it is common for a patient with a short history of back pain and questionable sciatica to have an MRI and undergo lumbar percutaneous diskectomy. Despite the growing popularity of this approach, a recent prospective, randomized, controlled study showed that only 36% of the patients treated by lumbar percutaneous diskectomy had a satisfactory outcome 1 year after the intervention.[23] By comparison, 66% of the patients treated by chymopapain had a favorable outcome for the duration of the surveillance.

The past decade has also seen the proliferation of internal fixation devices thought, but not proved, to enhance spinal fusion. Perhaps because of this technology, lumbar spinal fusions are again popular for low back pain. Dependent on the outcome criterion used, the success of these operations in populations of "compensable low back pain" ranges from 20% to 60%. Despite the absence of clearly established benefit, it is estimated that the rate of lumbar spine surgery may have doubled in the United States during the past decade.

This low back paradigm could easily apply to a variety of common musculoskeletal disorders, including carpal tunnel syndrome, one of the more costly causes of work-related musculoskeletal disorders. Like low back pain, carpal tunnel syndrome was hardly recognized until after World War II and was rarely the source of medical attention, yet today it is a major source of work-related musculoskeletal disability. As with low back disorders, the practitioner has many new diagnostic and therapeutic modalities available such as percutaneous techniques to decompress the median nerve. Again, the proliferation of technology is not necessarily associated with improved results. A recent study showed that percutaneous median nerve decompression has significant complications. The investigators recommend that the technique be considered experimental.[5]

Based on such evidence, technology has been found to be one of the driving forces in the escalating costs of health care and occupational injuries. However, it remains unclear whether these diagnostic and therapeutic approaches are affecting outcomes, particularly approaches that measure return to work.

The Impact of Social Reform

Before World War II, the cost of work-related musculoskeletal disorders was hardly worthy of public concern, much less debate, but the stage had been set by the enactment of worker's compensation programs in Europe and later the United States. Hadler[17] traced the history of worker's compensation and noted that it grew out of Bismark's social reforms in Germany in the latter part of the nineteenth century. By the turn of the century, England had enacted similar social legislation. As Hadler[17] notes, the new law was based on two critical precedents: "the continuing need for identifying the unworthy by means of 'disability determination,' and the new need to single out those whose work incapacity is a consequence of accidental workplace injury for special treatment under worker's compensation programs." Unlike Germany and England, which established national programs, the United States evolved a patchwork of state-enacted programs. In fact, some states did not have worker's compensation until 1934. These laws set the basic social framework in which disability costs could soar. However, it is unlikely that this social framework alone would have caused the profound changes in work-related musculoskeletal disorders had it not been for the major growth in medical technology.

Cumulative Trauma

Elsewhere in this volume (Chapter 12), the issues of cumulative trauma are addressed. The conceptual model is simple. The tissues of the human body undergo mechanical and biologic changes as a result of the repetitive stresses to which these tissues are subjected. Over time, this leads to tissue failure manifested in disorders such as lumbar disk herniation, carpal tunnel syndrome, and tendinitis. Widespread acceptance of this "injury" mechanism has resulted in many musculoskeletal conditions having greater legitimacy as a source of impairment and disability. Hadler[17] believes that "cumulative trauma" has had a major impact on the number and type of patients whose benign health conditions result in chronic disability.

"Disability Behavior"

Many patients with work-related musculoskeletal conditions improve with simple, conventional, nonoperative therapy. Failure of treatment can result from many factors, but when it occurs, the final common pathway is chronic disability. This small but growing subset of disabled patients has been shown to account for 70% to 90% of the costs of work-related musculoskeletal conditions.[3,13]

Consider again the low back paradigm. It is known that the majority of patients with low back pain improve rapidly, regardless of the inciting cause, as shown in **Figure 7-1**.[11] Even if the patient has sciatica proven to be secondary to a herniated lumbar disk, the majority will improve without surgical intervention. When a patient with low back pain does not improve over a period of 4 to 7 weeks, a small subset of 1% to 3% will be found to have a serious disorder usually related to a specific rheumatic disorder, tumor, or major structural defect. The remainder have no significant demonstrable structural causation, and nonspecific diagnoses such as "fibromyalgia," "chronic lumbosacral sprain," and "degenerative disk disease" are considered.

As the duration of disability continues, this population can be characterized by multiple medical and psychosocial phenomena.

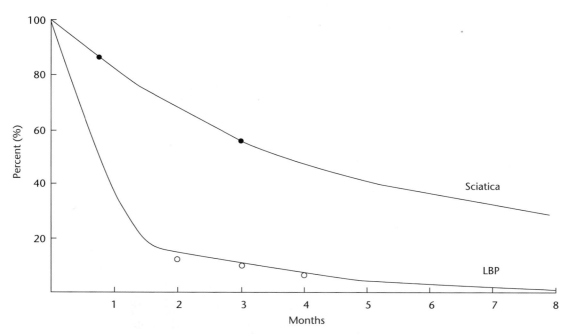

Figure 7-1 Recovery from low back pain and sciatica as a function of time. (*Modified from Frymoyer JW:* N Engl J Med *318:291-300, 1988, by permission.*)

1. **Demographics**

   Cats-Baril and Frymoyer[7] analyzed the demographic attributes of the United States population studied in the Second National Health and Nutrition Examination Survey (NHANES II) survey of noninstitutionalized adults. Disability was defined as being out of work for any cause (not exclusively musculoskeletal) for a period of 3 weeks. In comparison to the nondisabled cohorts, the disabled had a lower educational level and lower incomes and their jobs required heavier work.

2. **Occupational factors**

   There is ample evidence that the physical demands of a job relate to specific occupational disabilities. Repetitive movements and jobs requiring specific postures of the hand and wrist are associated with an increased risk of carpal tunnel syndrome. Similarly, low back disability is associated with requirements for heavy, repetitive lifting, particularly when twisted postures are required. However, a more potent set of predictors is the job environment. The characteristics of these environments entail repetitive boring activities and promote diminished job satisfaction. Poor relationships with supervisors and co-workers can antedate disability, as shown in the Boeing study.[3]

3. **Social factors**

   The attribution of causation to an occupational event is predictively associated with a greater risk for continued disability.[8]
   When the legal profession is involved, the chances for a return to work are significantly limited.[16]

4. **Psychological factors**

   Chronic disability is associated with a variety of psychological complaints measurable by a number of psychological testing instruments. These include anxiety, depression, and somatization (a morbid concern with symptoms). Not unexpectedly, there is a "chicken-egg" debate. Does psychological disturbance antedate the "injury" or is it a result of the disability? The Boeing study[3] would suggest that psychological disturbances may in fact antedate an "injury" and its resultant disability. Not all studies confirm this point.

5. **Medical factors**

   As disability continues, the probability of elucidating a verifiable structural disorder diminishes. Undaunted, the medical profession seeks to study and restudy these patients with powerful imaging techniques. Not surprisingly, the occupationally disabled cohort has undergone many more tests. Furthermore, this population often undergoes surgery with predictably poorer results. Virtually all analyses of outcome failure in low back surgery show that the most potent predictor of failure is an uncertain preoperative diagnosis. This was particularly well shown in a study by Norton,[21] who found in his cohort of worker's compensation patients with low back pain that over 50% did not meet the accepted criteria for lumbar disk herniation yet underwent surgical treatment with poor results and resultant high costs.

   Unfortunately, the results of medical intervention are also worse for patients receiving compensation, even when there is a medically verifiable indication for the selected treatment. For example, Hanley and Levy[18] analyzed the outcomes of spinal fusion for ischemic spondylolisthesis. Patients without compensation had an 86% satisfactory outcome rate, whereas those with compensation had only a 36% rate of satisfactory results.

Finally, the probability that such surgical intervention will occur is significantly influenced by the geographic region. Throughout the industrialized world, wide variations are identified in many forms of surgery and low back surgery in particular.[10] **Figure 7-2** shows the international distribution. Significant variations are identified even within the same state (**Figure 7-3**).[24] This type of difference is characteristic of medical deci-

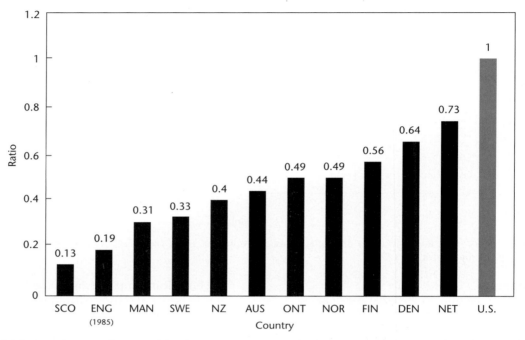

Figure 7-2 Variations in annual rates of lumbar spine surgery between nations. Note the almost tenfold differences between Scotland and the United States. (*From Graig L:* Health of nations: an international perspective on US health care reform, *ed 2, Chicago, 1991, The Wyatt Co.*)

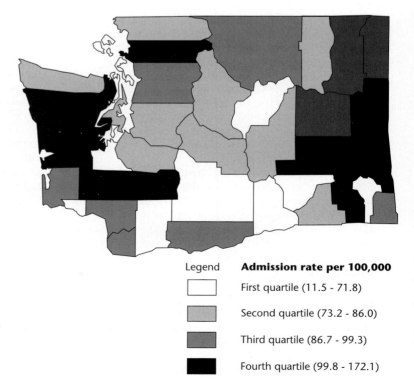

Figure 7-3 Variations in the annual rates of lumbar spine surgery within the state of Washington show highly significant differences. (*From Volinn E et al:* Spine *17:575-579, 1992.*)

Legend   **Admission rate per 100,000**

First quartile (11.5 - 71.8)

Second quartile (73.2 - 86.0)

Third quartile (86.7 - 99.3)

Fourth quartile (99.8 - 172.1)

sion making when the preferred treatment is debatable. There is no evidence that these variations can be explained by inherent differences in the occupational requirements or epidemiology of disease.

WHAT IS THE MAGNITUDE OF THE PROBLEM?

Throughout the industrialized world, the costs of health care have risen, but the greatest growth has been in the United States, as shown in **Figure 7-4**.[14] These

differences are even more striking when the per capita costs are analyzed, as in **Figure 7-5**. As already noted, the most important factors driving costs for work-related musculoskeletaldisorders are the growth in technology and the impact of chronic disability. The growth in chronic disability has been striking, particularly in low back disorders. From 1957 to 1976, Social Security disability claims grew at a rate slightly greater than population growth, but low back claims exceed population growth by a multiple of 14 (**Figure 7-6**).[9] In other nations a similar growth was observed. For example, Waddell[25] reports that the days of sick certification

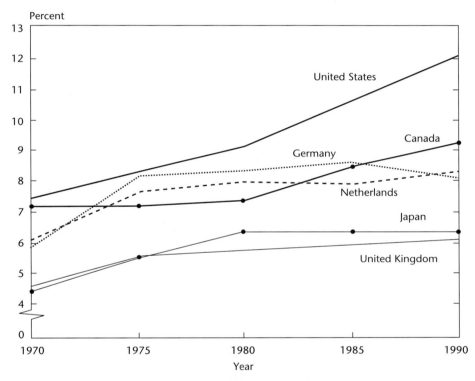

Figure 7-4 The costs of health care as a percentage of gross domestic product illustrate the dramatic increase in U.S. health care costs as compared with other industrialized nations. (*From Graig L:* Health of nations: an international perspective on US health care reform, *ed 2, Chicago, 1991, The Wyatt Co.*)

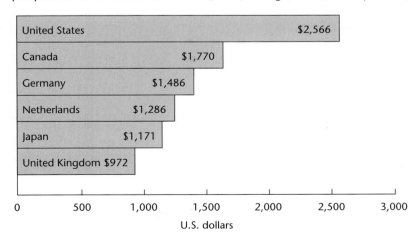

Figure 7-5 The cost of health care per capita again shows the major differences in U.S. costs versus other industrialized nations. (*From Graig L:* Health of nations: an international perspective on US health care reform, *ed 2, Chicago, 1991, The Wyatt Co.*)

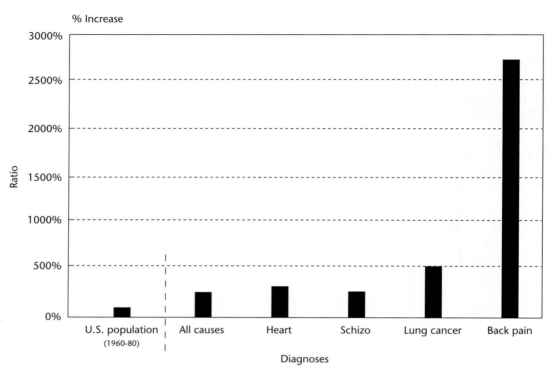

Figure 7-6 The rate of increase for Social Security disability claims for spinal disorders is compared with other chronic and often disabling disease processes as well as population growth. Note the dramatic difference between low back pain and these other conditions during the period 1957 to 1976. (*From Cats-Baril WL, Frymoyer JW: The economics of spinal disorders. In Frymoyer JW, editor:* The adult spine, *New York, 1991, Raven Press: pp 55-105.*)

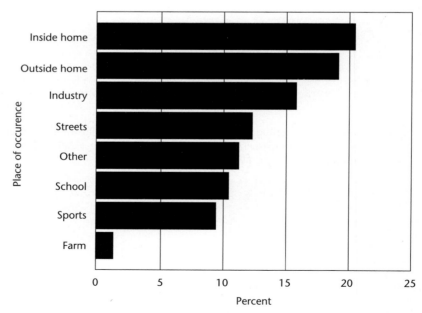

Figure 7-7 The place of occurrence for musculoskeletal injuries in the United States is shown for the interval 1985 to 1988. **Note:** These figures include injuries that are either medically attended or result in at least one-half day of restricted activity. (*From Praemer A, Furner S, and Rice DP, editors:* Musculoskeletal conditions in the United States, *Chicago, 1992, American Academy of Orthopaedic Surgeons.*)

remained fairly constant from 1950 to 1980 whereas low back sickness certification doubled. In Sweden, the number of individuals suffering permanent disability increased 3800% during the same time interval.[20]

Grazier et al[15] calculated the impact and cost of musculoskeletal injuries, and in 1991 these data were recalculated and updated to 1988.[22] This analysis showed that the annual rate of musculoskeletal impairments per annum was approximately 124 per 1000 for both work-related and non–work-related causes. Back and spinal disorders represented 51.7% of all musculoskeletal impairments. The resultant activity limitation resulted in over 382.2 million days in which activity was restricted. Again, back and spinal impairments accounted for almost half of the total.

To place this information in an occupational context, it is important to realize the place of occurrence of all injuries in the United States. These data are shown in **Figure 7-7**. It is estimated that there were 1.8 million disabling work injuries in the United States in 1990, 60,000 of which resulted in permanent impairment. Musculoskeletal injuries accounted for the majority of occupational injuries and illnesses that resulted in work loss. The type of injuries included sprains and strains, which accounted for 43%; fractures, 9.6%; dislocations, 2%; and tendinitis, 1.1%. The back was the most frequently reported anatomic site and accounted for almost one quarter of the total musculoskeletal injuries.

The financial consequences of musculoskeletal disease were estimated to be $126 billion: $61 billion for direct medical costs and $65 billion for indirect costs. The indirect costs included lost work days and lowered productivity. The direct costs of musculoskeletal conditions accounted for 12.7% of all healthcare costs in this nation. Injuries accounted for $26.1 billion. However, the contribution of work-related musculoskeletal injuries was not calculated.

The specific costs of low back pain were calculated in the earlier study of Grazier et al,[15] and in 1990 we attempted to update this information.[9] Although this extrapolation contains a number of debatable assumptions, these data give a picture of the potential range of costs. In making this analysis we had considerably greater comfort in estimating the direct cost estimates but were less certain about the indirect cost calculation.

Within the worker's compensation system it is common for one third of the costs to be direct medical expenses, whereas the remaining two thirds are related to indemnification costs. We calculated that the total cost for low back pain might range from $25 billion to an astronomic $100 billion, depending on the range of assumptions, but the most realistic assumptions placed the figure at $35 billion.

Because spinal disorders account for 50% of all musculoskeletal impairments and 50% of the lost work days, this cost figure is well within the range of expenditure that might be expected for spinal disorders. How much of this cost is attributable to surgery was also unclear, but it is known that 250,000 lumbar disk operations and 90,000 fusions were performed in 1988.

Back pain represents 25% to 40% of worker's compensation claims and is the most common and costly cause of such claims. The next most common disorders relate to finger injuries, which represent 11% of the total. Again, the chronicity of the condition and the intervention required are highly significant.

For example, it is estimated that a worker's musculoskeletal injury that is uncomplicated and not serious carries with it a cost of $500. When surgery is performed, the costs rise to $30,000 per case. When the worker has a chronic disabling condition, the costs further increase to $80,000.[6]

We can derive the following points from these data: (1) musculoskeletal disorders are very common and costly, (2) work-related musculoskeletal disorders are an extremely common and costly subset, (3) the costs have continued to rise at rates disproportionate to population growth, and (4) the major driver of cost is chronic disability.

WHAT CAN BE DONE?

The social, political, legal, and medical complexity of work-related musculoskeletal injuries has created a major dilemma for all industrialized nations as they attempt to control the escalating costs. Not surprisingly, a variety of social, engineering, and legal approaches have been considered. From a medical perspective, the key element would seem to be control of chronic disability and perhaps the more judicious application of technology.

Preventive strategies can be divided into primary, secondary, and tertiary techniques. Primary methods attempt to prevent the condition's occurrence in the first place. The usual methods are education, job redesign, and preemployment screening. There has been little evidence that preemployment screening has much impact on later work-related musculoskeletal disorders. The effects of education have been debated but seem more effective in preventing acute, major injuries than in preventing more subtle conditions such as typical occupational back pain. Job redesign has been advocated and is particularly effective when the job requirements involve repetitive stereotyped activity. Thus job and tool redesign is of particular utility in the prevention of carpal tunnel syndrome and similar upper extremity musculoskeletal conditions. When the jobs are less stereotypic, the costs and effectiveness of job redesign are somewhat less certain.

Secondary prevention is an attempt to improve the rate of recovery in a worker who has acquired a condition such as a job-related musculoskeletal injury. These interventions are particularly well suited to the prevention of work-related musculoskeletal injuries, especially those in which a major injury mechanism such as a fracture is not present. Not all experts will agree.

Weisel, Feffer, and Rothman[26] described a method for the prevention of back-related disability. In the initial study, all patients with low back pain were examined by an unbiased expert in musculoskeletal disease present at the work site within a few days of the injury. The injured workers were permitted to use their routine medical care, but their progress in recovery was measured against an algorithm. With this simple expedient, all of the following measures showed improvement: days lost from work, cost, and the number of surgical interventions. Over the ensuing decade, they have streamlined the process such that the care can now be monitored against algorithms. Computer technology has allowed this monitoring to progress without experts at the work site. The approach has been broadened to other work-related musculoskeletal conditions such as knee and shoulder pain. As a result of these interventions, the industries where these techniques have been employed have sustained a significant reduction in lost work days and costs.[4] Similar effects have been demonstrated for other work-related musculoskeletal conditions by these investigators.

The other approach that remains unproven is an attempt to identify early in the course of an occupational injury those people who are at risk for chronic disability. The hypothesis has been that for this group, more aggressive, early rehabilitative interventions might be cost effective. Our analysis of patients with low back pain has indicated that the "at risk" population can be identified with a fairly high level of confidence.[8] The key factors are perception of others being at fault, worker's compensation, and legal intervention. However, the single most important predictor is the duration of time lost from work. From a medical perspective, the key should be careful monitoring of care with the use of time-dependent points when further interventions should be considered. This general principle is very similar to the methods described previously whereby a patient's progress is monitored against an algorithm.

Finally, tertiary prevention include those techniques that attempt to optimize function in a person who has an impairment and disability. Clearly the goal should be to prevent a person from reaching that status. Tertiary prevention is discussed in Chapter 18. What the most cost-effective strategies are has not been subjected to rigorous analysis. However, intensive rehabilitation seems to offer the best potential for returning a person to work, particularly when low back pain is the cause of the disability.

References

1. Aaron H, Schwartz WB: Rationing health care: the choice before us, *Science* 274:418-422, 1990.

2. Barr JS et al: Evaluation of end results in treatment of ruptured lumbar intervertebral discs with protrusion of nucleus pulposus, *Surg Gynecol Obstet* 25:250-256, 1967.

3. Bigos SJ, Battie MC: The impact of spinal disorders in industry. In Frymoyer JW, editor: *The adult spine*, New York, 1991, Raven Press; pp 147-153.

4. Boden SD, Wiesel SW, Feffer HL: *A quality-based protocol for the management of low back pain and sciatica: a ten-year prospective outcome study.* Presented to the International Society for the Study of the Lumbar Spine Scientific Program, Marseilles, France, June 19, 1993.

5. Brown RA et al: Carpal tunnel release. A prospective, randomized assessment of open and endoscopic methods, *J Bone Joint Surg Am* 75:1265-1275, 1993.

6. Bureau of National Affairs: Back injuries: costs, causes, cases, and prevention, Washington, DC, 1988, Bureau of National Affairs.

7. Cats-Baril WL, Frymoyer JW: Demographic features associated with the prevalence of disability in the general population: analysis of the NHANES I database, *Spine* 16:671-674, 1991.

8. Cats-Baril WL, Frymoyer JW: Identifying patients at risk of becoming disabled due to low back pain: the Vermont Rehabilitation Engineering Center predictive model, *Spine* 16:605-607, 1991.

9. Cats-Baril WL, Frymoyer JW: The economics of spinal disorders. In Frymoyer JW, editor: *The adult spine*, New York, 1991, Raven Press; pp 95-105.

10. Deyo RA: Practice variations, treatment fads, rising disability: do we need a new clinical research paradigm? *Spine* 18:2152-2161, 1993.

11. Frymoyer JW: Low back pain and sciatica, *N Engl J Med* 318:291-300, 1988.

12. Frymoyer JW, Donaghy RM: The ruptured intervertebral disc with involvement of the spinal canal, *N Engl J Med* 211:210-215, 1985.

13. Frymoyer JW et al: Risk factors in low back pain: an epidemiological study in men, *J Bone Joint Surg Am* 66:1048-1055, 1983.

14. Graig L: *Health of nations: an international perspective on U.S. health care reform*, ed 2, Chicago, 1991, Wyatt Co.

15. Grazier KL et al, editors: *The frequency of occurrence, impact, and cost of musculoskeletal conditions in the United States*, Chicago, 1984, American Academy of Orthopaedic Surgeons.

16. Haddad GH: Analysis of 2932 workers' compensation back injury cases, *Spine* 12:765-769, 1987.

17. Hadler NM: Backache and humanism. In Frymoyer JW, editor: *The adult spine*, New York, 1991, Raven Press; pp 55-60.

18. Hanley EN, Levy JA: Surgical treatment of isthmic lumbosacral spondylolisthesis: analysis of variables influencing results, *Spine* 14:48-50, 1989.

19. Mixter WJ, Barr JS: Rupture of the intervertebral disc with involvement of the spinal canal, *N Engl J Med* 211:210-215, 1934.

20. Netteelbladt E: *Opuscula Med* (Sweden) 30:54, 1985.

21. Norton WL: Chemonucleolysis versus surgical discectomy: comparison of costs and results in workers' compensation claimants, *Spine* 11:440-443, 1986.

22. Praemer A, Furner S, Rice DP, editors: *Musculoskeletal conditions in the United States,* Chicago, 1992, American Academy of Orthopaedic Surgeons.

23. Revel M et al: Percutaneous lumbar discectomy versus chemonucleolysis in the treatment of sciatica: a randomized multicenter trial, *Spine* 18:1-7, 1993.

24. Volinn E et al: Small area analysis of surgery for low back pain, *Spine* 17:575-579, 1992.

25. Waddell G: 1987 Volvo Award in Clinical Sciences: a new clinical model for the treatment of low back pain, *Spine* 12:632-644, 1987.

26. Wiesel SW, Feffer HL, Rothman RH: Industrial low back pain: a prospective evaluation of a standardized diagnostic and treatment protocol, *Spine* 9:199-203, 1984.

PART II

Ergonomics

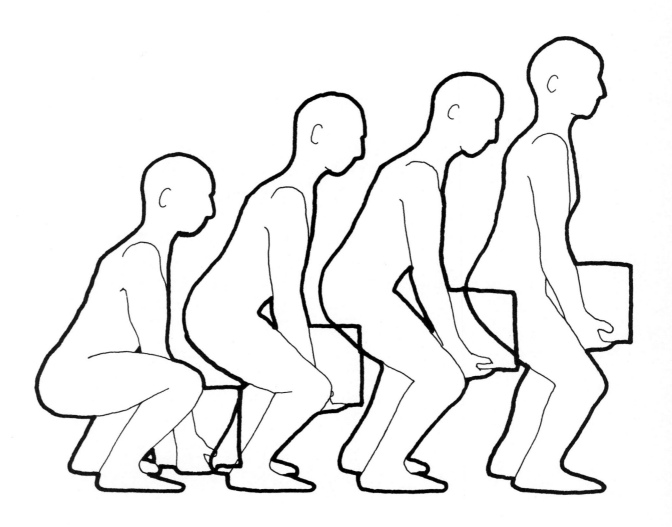

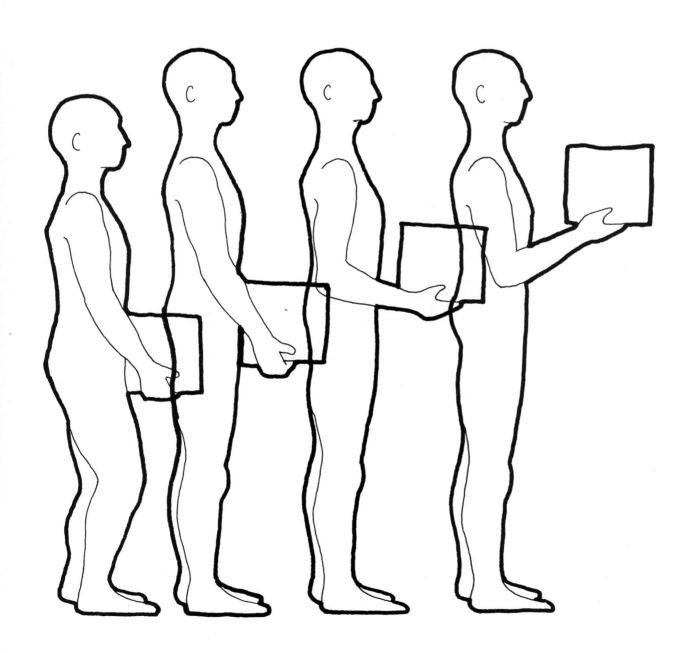

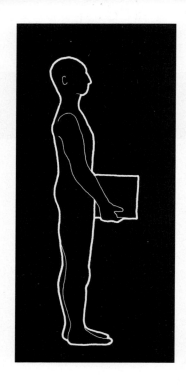

Chapter 8

Posture

Marianne Magnusson

CONTENTS

No posture is good enough to be comfortably maintained for long periods of time. Any prolonged posture will lead to static loading of the muscles and joint tissues and, consequently, cause discomfort. The human being's natural behavior is to change posture often. Even during sleep, posture adjustments are necessary.

At the workplace, standing and sitting are the two basic postures. These two postures have their specific advantages and disadvantages for mobility, exertion of force, energy consumption, circulatory demands, coordination, and motion control.

EPIDEMIOLOGY

The Lumbar Spine

Magora[67] found in his studies that both too much and too little sitting or standing were related to high incidences of low back pain (LBP). An increased risk of prolapsed lumbar disk has been reported among persons who have had sedentary occupations for several years.[55] Some studies on the epidemiology of LBP, not specific for diagnoses, have found that both sedentary occupations and occupations with very heavy loading increase the risk for LBP.[35,68] This paradox may be explained by prolapsed disks being related to sedentary occupations, whereas other disorders such as muscle strain and ligamentous injury are associated with heavy work. In fact, jobs involving manual materials handling have been reported to not be associated with an increased risk for a prolapsed disk. This may be due to the fact that lumbar disks are very resistant to compressive loads and that such loads can fracture the vertebral end plate before causing damage to the disk.[29]

Several studies, most of which are retrospective, have indicated an increased risk for back pain in people with predominantly seated working postures.[49,58,59,67,76] They also show that prolonged sitting aggravates back pain in people with ongoing symptoms. The risk of low back problems seems to be increased from prolonged sitting in a vibrational environment such as the professional driving of vehicles.[62,64] Kelsey and Hardy,[56] in an epidemiologic survey, stated the evidence for the fact that driving motor vehicles increases the risk of prolapsed lumbar disks. They suggest the combination of vibration and prolonged sitting, with little freedom to change posture, as plausible causative factors. Bent-over postures seem to carry an increased risk for LBP.[59,77] Frymoyer et al[32] found both bending and twisting to be significantly related to LBP, and Troup, Roantree, and Archibald[94] found frequent bending and twisting in combination with lifting to be the most frequent cause of back injuries in England.

The Neck, Shoulder, and Arm

In most epidemiologic studies on neck and shoulder pain, the exposure is defined by job title rather than job characteristics such as an objectively quantified load or a detailed description of working postures, arm and head movements, materials handled, and work organization. This makes epidemiologic studies slightly difficult to interpret. The multifactorial etiology, the poorly defined syndromes, and the age factor contribute to the lack of well-identifed cause-effect relationships.

In the only study that specifically addressed the relationship between musculoskeletal pain in the upper extremities and working posture, nontraumatic musculoskeletal disorders were diagnosed in nearly 40% of the patients visiting the occupational health clinic.[14] Almost 70% of the patients with shoulder pain stated that they worked with their hands at or above shoulder level.

Hagberg and Wegman[42] in a metaanalysis found significant odds ratios (ORs) above 1.0 for cervical spondylosis in meat carriers, dentists, miners, and heavy workers, thereby suggesting high loading on the cervical spine as the causal exposure. Extreme forward flexion of the cervical spine was suggested as the causative factor for cervical syndrome in civil servants.[45] The assumed causative factor for tension neck syndrome is static contraction of the neck and shoulder muscles to counteract the weight of the head.[39,98] Therefore, the greater the angle of neck flexion, the greater the load in the muscles and joints. A high OR was found in keyboard operators, which may reflect the exposure of a static load on the upper trapezius muscle as measured by electromyography (EMG).[41]

In a study that included machine operators, carpenters, and office workers it was found that working in twisted or bent postures increased the occurrence of neck and shoulder symptoms, an association that was most evident for machine operators.[92]

Many studies suggest shoulder muscle "overload" as being the major cause for the increasing incidence of "occupational" shoulder pain.[36,40,47,99,100] A clear relationship between exposure groups and chronic tendinitis has been demonstrated in three studies.[14,47,48] One of the common exposure factors was long periods of time with the arm in an abducted or flexed position. Herberts et al[48] found a significantly higher prevalence of tendinitis in shipyard welders and plate workers when compared with a control group. In those with diagnosed tendinitis, the welders were younger and had worked a much shorter time than the plate workers. Both jobs were rated high in physical workload, but the plateworkers' jobs were dynamic whereas welding was classified as a static task. Burt, Hornung, and Fine[17] found an 11% prevalence of shoulder symptoms in newspaper employees, and the symptoms were associated with the amount of time spent typing at computer terminals, which was thought of as time spent in a static sitting posture with the arms unsupported. Hagberg and Wegman[42] demonstrated an association between elevated work heights and the prevalence of rotator cuff tendinitis and found an OR of 11 for work at shoulder height as compared with work below that level.

Awkward postures of the wrist, for example, working with the wrist not straight, repetitive forceful work, and vibration, are risk factors for cumulative trauma disorders affecting the wrist.[89]

Hip and Knee

Törner[93] found that subjective musculoskeletal symptoms were common mainly from the lower part of the back, neck/shoulders, and knees among fishermen. The occurrence of physical signs, particularly in the shoulders and knees, was similar among fishermen and welders, whereas welders experienced more subjective symptoms from the shoulders and knees. Sick reporting and medical consultations for these symptoms were not frequent, however, among fishermen.

Work that involves much loaded knee bending carries an increased risk for osteoarthritis of the knee (OR, 2.2,[30]), and the risk is two to three times greater for male shipyard workers, farmers, construction workers, and firemen.[60,74,77,96]

There seems to be a clearly increased risk for the development of osteoarthrosis of the hip in farmers, the relative risk ranging from 9.7 to 12.4 in different studies.[12,23,51,91] Severe disease is associated with prolonged standing at work and heavy lifting. The relative risk for disability pensions because of osteoarthritis of the hip in men over 59 years was 12.4 (6.7 to 23.0) for those with high exposure to physical load as compared with those with low exposure.[97] Professional ballet dancers have been shown to have a high prevalence of osteoarthritis of both the hips and knees.[11]

STANDING POSTURES

Effects on the Musculoskeletal System

Postural muscles are always active in the standing posture, although their activity is small when the trunk is unloaded and in erect standing.[4-7, 18,69,70,87] The center of gravity of the upper part of the body is anterior to the spine. Muscle forces are required to counterbalance this forward-bending moment of the motion segments to maintain equilibrium.[6,57] Muscle activity is further increased and changed to counterbalance the larger moment created by a forward-bending posture, an outstretched arm, or any other external weight.[8,85] When a person bends forward, muscle activity increases with increased trunk flexion, but the activity ceases almost completely when full flexion is reached.[6] Okada[75] studied forward-bending postures at different angles, with and without extra external loads, and found increased muscle activity until 45 to 60 degrees of flexion was reached, after which the activity decreased. An explanation for the "EMG silence" in full flexion is a

reflex-induced inhibition of the muscle activity.[31] Carr et al[20] suggested that passive tissues—ligaments and capsules—counteract the forward-bending moment. Others have proposed that the thoracolumbar fascia is important in resisting the forward-bending moment.[33] Electromyographic activity has also been established during static forward-bent postures. The EMG activity increased with both increased bending (up to the zone of EMG silence) and increased external weight.[6,86] When the trunk is hyperextended, back muscle activity occurs during the initial phase and in full extension.[31,69,78] The activity of the abdominal muscles increases while being stretched throughout the whole range of motion. In lateral flexion, increased muscle activity is found on both sides of the spine, but mainly on the contralateral side to balance the flexed posture[79] (Fig. 8-1).

When the trunk is rotated, the back muscles are active on both sides of the spine. Some studies have shown similar levels of activity on both sides,[19,82]

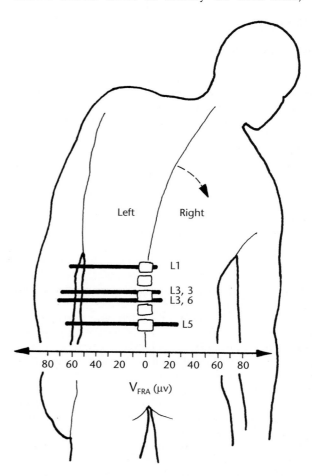

Figure 8-1 During bending to the side, substantial muscle activity is required on the contralateral side of the trunk to maintain equilibrium. (*Modified from Andersson GBJ, Örtengren R, and Herberts P:* Orthop Clin North Am *18:85-96, 1977.*)

whereas others have observed differences.[24,52,69] In their study, Andersson, Örtengren, and Herberts[6] showed that with the combination of lateral flexion and rotation with an external load, high levels of activity on the contralateral side of the lumbar region and on the ipsilateral side of the thoracic region were recorded. This asymmetric muscle contraction can lead to unequal stress concentrations on the different components of the spine, with an increased risk of injury.

Disk pressure measurements obtained in vivo in the standing posture indicate that the load roughly corresponds to the mass above the level of measurement, about 40% of the body mass at the L3 level.[4,9,73] When one leans forward, the intradiscal pressure increases parallel to the increased load moment.[7,72,86] Sideways bending and twisting increase the disk pressure by only 20% to 25% (**Fig. 8-2**).

Changes in stature—stadiometry—have been used as a measure of spinal loading.[22,65,95] The effect of the hyperextension adopted in overhead working tasks showed that lordosis was significantly associated with a relative gain in stature, thus suggesting that increased lumbar extension reduces the load on the disks. Studies of overhead work are more concerned with loads on the neck and shoulders rather than the lower part of the back,[38,100] although sustained hyperextension is considered a possible cause of lumbar symptoms caused by ligamentous or facet joint capsule strain.[28,102] In the hyperextended posture, the facet joints become load bearing and can be damaged by compressive loads as low as 500 N.[1]

Standing work in a vibrating or moving environment (as with fishermen) may result in the worker adopting a bent-knee stance to reduce shock loading to the spine. Standing unloaded in ship motions caused a 70% increase in L4/L5 compression in comparison with standing unloaded in still conditions. Ship motions also increased the moment in L4/L5, the knees, and the ankles when standing unloaded.[93] The pathomechanisms behind the development of osteoarthrosis of the hip and knee are suggested to possibly be dynamic forces from stress on the joint that result in microfractures of the cartilage and subchondral bone when shock-absorbing capacity is exceeded. Static compression impedes movement of the joint; this may impair nutrient transportation and metabolic elimination in the cartilage, which has neither blood vessels nor lymphatic drainage.[96]

Very little muscle activity is demanded to keep the head in a normal upright position. The forward-bending moment that is created by balancing the head requires only low activity of the cervical erector spinae musculature. In the forward-flexed position of the head, the major load will be carried by the C7-T1 joint. When compared with the normal upright position, the forward-flexed position creates a 3.6 times greater load at this level[27] (**Fig. 8-3**).

The load on the cervical spine increases by wearing a helmet, especially if the helmet is equipped with a lamp that increases the forward-bending moment.[37,90]

When the neck is in a hyperextended position, it is balanced by the muscles and ligaments anterior to the cervical spine. The very low muscle activity in both flexed and extended postures indicates that the load moment is mainly counterbalanced by passive connective tissues such as joint capsules and ligaments.[45]

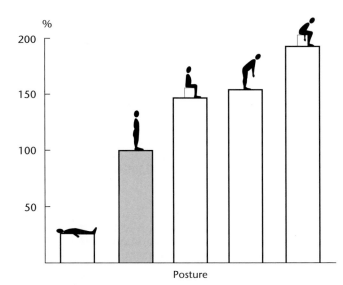

Figure 8-2 The relative loads on the third lumbar disk for various body positions in living subjects in relation to the upright standing posture, depicted as 100%. (*Modified from Nachemson AL:* Spine *1:59-71, 1976.*)

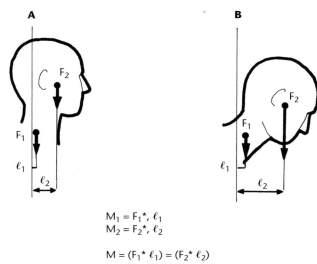

$$M_1 = F_1{}^* , \ell_1$$
$$M_2 = F_2{}^* , \ell_2$$

$$M = (F_1{}^* \ \ell_1) = (F_2{}^* \ \ell_2)$$

Figure 8-3 Forces acting on the cervical spine in upright and flexed positions of the neck and head. (*From Hagberg M:* Arbetsmiljöns betydelse för besvär i skuldra och halsrygg, *Arbetsmiljöfonden, No 1, 1988.*)

The complex function of the shoulder joint, which consists of four separate joints and 15 muscles requiring synchronized activity, makes the shoulder a very complicated biomechanical unit.[50,62,81] The calculation of joint reaction forces at the glenohumeral joint when the arm is elevated is a great problem because of the large number of muscles involved, the various force contributions of the different muscles, and so forth. Poppen and Walker[80] as well as Inman, Saunders, and Abbott[50] found the glenohumeral joint forces at 90 degrees of abduction to be close to body weight. Great muscle forces are thus necessary to keep the arm elevated, in particular in working postures where the hand is positioned at or above shoulder level and even more if a hand tool is held.

From an ergonomic point of view, it has become more important to detect the development of muscular fatigue rather than focus on muscular force to prevent pain and injury. Local muscle fatigue is considered a limiting factor for monotonous and long-lasting static work, although the work can be regarded as light. Muscle fatigue has been defined as failure to maintain constant force[25] because of a complex metabolic process. Chaffin[21] and Basmajian and DeLuca[13] have defined localized muscular fatigue. Localized muscle fatigue can arise from sustained muscular work and is accompanied by motor decrement and pain confined to the muscle.[21] The main factor in local muscular fatigue is reduced blood flow in the contracting muscle because of increased intramuscular pressure (IMP)[26] and a consequent accumulation of metabolites. This vascular shortfall can appear when the relative force exceeds 15% to 20% of the maximum voluntary contraction (MVC).[61]

Electromyographic studies have shown localized muscle fatigue in several of the shoulder muscles in work situations with the hand at or above shoulder level.[38,53] Sigholm et al[88] found that the degree of upper arm elevation was the most important factor determining shoulder load whereas upper arm rotation was of little importance and a hand weight was of less importance. Hand weight was an important factor for the load on the supraspinatus and infraspinatus muscles.[48] In overhead work with the neck extended and the arms elevated, sometimes with a hand tool as an extra load, the shoulder muscles must engage in considerable muscular activity to keep the arm in this position; at the same time, the load moment on the neck is increased, particularly at the C7-T1 level (**Fig. 8-4**).

Kadefors, Petersen, and Herberts[53] measured localized muscle fatigue of the shoulder muscles in three typical working situations and found localized muscle fatigue in both experienced and unexperienced welders in overhead work only. In experienced welders, fatigue was confined to the supraspinatus muscle, whereas fatigue in inexperienced welders was abundant in several other muscles, thereby suggesting a higher risk than normal to acquire tendinitis at the supraspinatus tendon insertion in overhead work.[46]

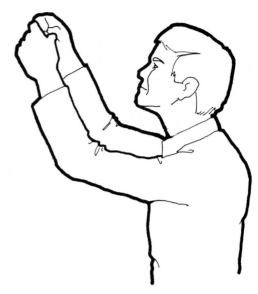

Figure 8-4 In overhead work, considerable stress is placed on the cervical facet joints as a result of the hyperextended position of the neck at the same time that the elevated arm position requires large static muscle forces.

The advantages with the standing working posture are the close accessibility, the mobility, and the possibility for using more strength. The disadvantages are that the standing posture is more energy consuming and loads the lower extremity joints more than the seated posture.

THE SEATED POSTURE

Effects on the Musculoskeletal System

The seated posture is determined by both the design of the chair and the task to be performed. The height and inclination of the seat, the position and shape of the backrest, and the presence of armrests influence the seated posture. Because all postures become uncomfortable and may be a risk factor for LBP if maintained too long, the chair should permit alterations in posture.[101] A "semisitting" posture is often desirable to facilitate changes between standing and sitting when different tasks are performed. A forwardly bent position is a common seated working position adopted when desk work is being performed and in light mechanical work that demands high precision such as dentistry, jewelry, and watchmaking. Backward-leaning positions are preferred at rest, but also in such tasks as car driving and computer programming.

When sitting, the pelvis rotates backward and the lumbar lordosis decreases.[2,10,16,54,84] The disk pressure in a seated unsupported upright posture measured at the L3 level is 40% in excess of the value obtained in upright standing.[71] This pressure corresponds to an

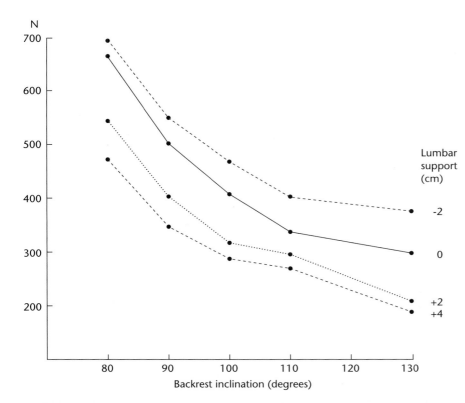

Figure 8-5 The disk pressure decreases when the backrest inclination is increased and when a lumbar support is used. (*Modified from Andersson GBJ et al:* Scand J Rehabil Med *6:104-114, 1974*).

approximate load of 700 N. The reduced lumbar lordosis, which creates an increased load moment, and the disk deformation itself caused by the lumbar spine flattening are most likely strong contributing factors for the increased disk pressure in unsupported sitting. Andersson and Örtengren performed an extensive series of experiments to establish the spinal load while sitting in different chairs and with different back supports.[3-5,9] These studies confirm that the disk pressure is significantly higher in unsupported sitting than in standing (**Fig. 8-5**). The lowest pressure was found in the upright straight position. The disk pressure was influenced by several different factors of support. Inclination of the backrest, as well as a lumbar support, resulted in decreased disk pressure. The disk pressure decreased with the amount of backrest inclination. The larger the inclination, however, the less the decrease. The effect of a lumbar support was more pronounced when the backrest inclination was small. The use of armrests also resulted in decreased disk pressure (**Fig. 8-6**).

Electromyographic studies of the erector spinae musculature have shown similar activity levels during standing as during unsupported sitting.[4,5,18,31] It is generally agreed that myoelectric activity decreases in sitting when the back is slumped forward, when the arms are supported, when a backrest is used, and when leaning backwards.* The parameter that has the majr influence on myoelectric activity is the backrest inclination. In one of the studies by Andersson et al[10] it was

*References 2, 4, 9, 18, 31, 52, 63, 83, 84.

shown that when the backrest-seat angle was increased, muscle activity at all levels of the back decreased.

When the backrest inclination was greater than 110 degrees, the effect of further inclination decreased, however. A lumbar support had only minor influence on muscle activity, whereas it was of great importance on disk pressure. The muscular activity of the spinal musculature increases when the knees are bent more than 90 degrees, whereas extension of the knees reduces the activity. This is probably due to the combined actions of various muscles that rotate the pelvis and thus influence the lumbar curve.[54]

Forklift drivers and farmers are exposed to long periods of twisted posture. The twisted posture in a vibrational environment has been shown to cause increased energy consumption as compared with twisted posture or vibration as single exposure variables.[66] Seated whole body vibration in a position that ensures muscular activity of the erectorspinae muscles caused faster and more pronounced muscular fatigue in the lumbar erector spinae muscles when compared with the absence of vibration.[43] Whole body vibration caused increased spinal height loss in seated subjects, thus suggesting increased spinal load as compared with a seated posture without vibration[65] (**Fig. 8-7**).

The load on the neck is correlated to the trunk and head position. The load moment is balanced by muscle forces and tension of the passive connective tissues. Thus flexion of the entire spine in the sitting posture increases EMG activity in the cervical spinae, trapezius, and thoracic erector spinae muscles. For even a 30-

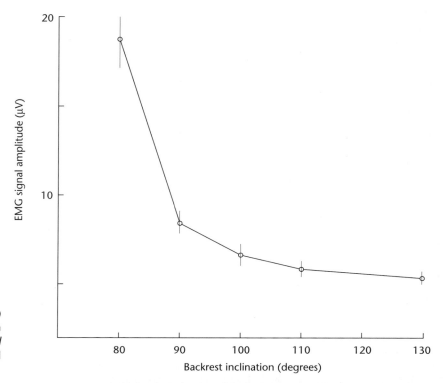

Figure 8-6 Myoelectric activity (EMG) decreases when the backrest inclination is increased. (*From Andersson GBJ and Örtengren R:* Scand J Rehabil Med Suppl *3:73-90, 1974.*)

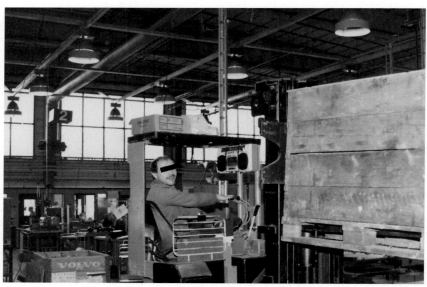

Figure 8-7 The twisted posture in a vibrational environment stresses the entire spine by the extreme posture and the vibrational effect on the muscles and circulatory demands.

degree inclination angle from the vertical, the moment and corresponding muscle force values are 50% higher than the values achieved at 0 degrees. The lowest activity is obtained when the trunk is leaning slightly backward and the neck is vertical. It appears that the cervical extensor muscles may produce muscle fatigue symptoms quite quickly when head inclination angles become significant. Chaffin,[21] using EMG frequency shifts, found that the endurance time of young healthy females was considerably decreased when the neck inclination angle exceeded 30 degrees. In extreme head

positions with the neck fully flexed, the extensor muscles of the cervical spine are not increased in comparison to the neutral upright head position, although the load moment of the C7-T1 motion segment is increased three to four times.[45] The stress on the ligaments and joint capsules is considerable during extreme flexed positions of the cervical spine (**Fig. 8-8**).

Work tasks that demand continuous arm movement generate load patterns with a static component of the shoulder joint.[99] In an optimal seated work posture, the upper trapezius static load level is 2% to 3% MVC.[41]

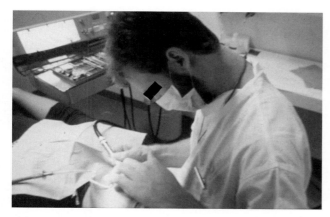

Figure 8-8 In extreme neck flexion, the load moment of the C7-T1 motion segment is increased three to four times.

Optimal posture was defined as a vertical position or slightly backward inclination of the spine, an approximately vertical positon of the upper part of the arm, and a work task at about elbow height without material handling (i.e., data entry work). In this position, intramuscular pressure was close to zero in the upper trapezius, supraspinatus, and infraspinatus muscles, thus suggesting normal blood flow in these muscles. Elevation of the shoulders without raising the arms may increase the load level on the upper trapezius to about 20% MVC.[40] Any deviation of the arm from the vertical position increases the load on the upper trapezius and the rotator cuff muscles, and both EMG amplitude and IMP increase linearly with increased shoulder torque.[38] The IMP and the EMG amplitude are markedly reduced if a given shoulder torque is obtained during flexion instead of abduction. At an abduction of 30 degrees (in a plane 45 degrees to the frontal plane) without a hand load, the IMP in the upper trapezius is only 15 mm Hg whereas the corresponding value in the supraspinatus muscle is about 80 mm Hg. Blood flow in the supraspinatus muscle is significantly impeded at an IMP of about 40 mm Hg. Therefore, the supraspinatus muscle is very vulnerable in work situations with elevated arms.

Leg support is important for distribution and reduction of the load on the buttocks and the back of the thighs. The feet should therefore be permitted to rest firmly on the floor or foot support to avoid lower leg weight being supported by the thighs resting on the seat. If there is pressure against the thighs close to the knees, this may create clinical problems in terms of swelling of the legs and pressure on the sciatic nerve. It has been shown that the volume of the legs increases by 4% during prolonged sitting. When a chair is too high, the feet do not reach the floor and pressure on the thighs becomes uncomfortable.[2,84] When a chair is too low, the small knee and hip angles soon become uncomfortable, and the pelvis rotates backward and flexes the spine.[54,58]

The seated posture leads to an inactivity that may itself be injurious. Lack of motion leads to an accumulation of metabolites, which probably accelerates degeneration of the disks. Experimental studies have shown a close relationship between bone mineral content (BMC) and static compressive strength in lumbar vertebral segments.[15,34,44]

The advantages of the seated working posture are that it provides the stability required for tasks with high visual and motor control, it is less energy consuming than standing, it is less loading on lower extremity joints, and it reduces the hydrostatic pressure on the lower extremity circulation. The disadvantages are the increased load on the back and neck, the risk for decalcification, and the low demands on the circulation.

SUMMARY

The following considerations about the workplace and work performance should be taken into account in all kinds of work as a measure of preventing musculoskeletal disorders or reducing the risk of impairment following an injury.

1. Provide the possibility for variation between standing and sitting.
2. Avoid flexed, twisted, and hyperextended standing postures.
3. Avoid extreme postures of the head.
4. Avoid work at or above shoulder level.
5. Provide a chair with good back support.
6. Avoid lifting in flexed or twisted postures.

References

1. Adams MA et al: Posture and the compressive strength of the lumbar spine, *Clin Biomech* 9:5-14, 1994.

2. Åkerblom B: *Standing and sitting posture,* thesis, Univ. Stockholm, Sweden, 1948.

3. Andersson GBJ, Jonsson B, Örtengren R: Myoelectric activity in individual lumbar erector spinae muscles in sitting. A study with surface and wire electrodes, *Scand J Rehabil Med Suppl* 3:91-108, 1974.

4. Andersson GBJ, Örtengren R: Lumbar disk pressure and myoelectric back muscle activity during sitting II. Studies on an office chair, *Scand J Rehabil Med* 6:115-121, 1974.

5. Andersson GBJ, Örtengren R: Myoelectric back muscle activity during sitting, *Scand J Rehabil Med Suppl* 3:73-90, 1974.

6. Andersson GBJ, Örtengren R, Herberts P: Quantitative electromyographic studies of back muscle activity related

to posture and loading, *Orthop Clin North Am* 8:85-96, 1977.

7. Andersson GBJ, Örtengren R, Nachemson A: Intradiscal pressure, intraabdominal pressure and myoelectric back muscle activity related to posture and loading, *Clin Orthop* 129:156-164, 1977.

8. Andersson GBJ, Örtengren R, Schultz A: Analysis and measurement of the loads on the lumbar spine during work at a table, *J Biomech* 13:513-520, 1980.

9. Andersson GBJ, et al: Lumbar disk pressure and myoelectric back muscle activity during sitting. I. Studies on an experimental chair, *Scand J Rehabil Med*, 6:104-114, 1974.

10. Andersson GBJ et al: The influence of backrest inclination and lumbar support on lumbar lordosis, *Spine* 4:52-58, 1979.

11. Andersson S et al: Degenerative joint disease in ballet dancers, *Clin Orthop* 238:233-236, 1989.

12. Axmacher B, Lindberg H: Coxarthrosis in farmers, *Clin Orthop* 287:82-86, 1993.

13. Basmajian JV, DeLuca CJ: *Muscles alive. Their functions revealed by electromyography,* Baltimore, 1985, Williams & Wilkins; pp 83-91.

14. Bjelle A, Hagberg M, Michaelsson G: Clinical and ergonomic factors in prolonged shoulder pain among industrial workers, *Scand J Work Environ Health* 5:205, 1979.

15. Brinkmann P et al: Fatigue fracture of human lumbar vertebrae, *Clin Biomech* 2:94-96, 1987.

16. Burandt U: Röntgenuntersuchung über die Stellung von Becken und Wirbelsäule beim Sitzen auf vorgeneigten Flachen, *Ergonomics* 12:356-364, 1969.

17. Burt S, Hornung R, Fine LJ: *NIOSH Health Hazard Evaluation Report* HETA 89-250-2046, Cincinnati, 1990, National Institute for Occupational Health and Safety.

18. Carlsöö S: *Writing desk, chair and posture of work,* Stockholm, 1963, Anatomiska Institute Stockholm Univ.

19. Carlsöö S: The static muscle load in different work positions: an electromyographic study, *Ergonomics* 4:193-198, 1961.

20. Carr D et al: The lumbodorsal fascial compartment, *Trans Orthop Res Soc* 9:252, 1984.

21. Chaffin DB: Localized muscle fatigue: definition and measurement, *J Occup Med* 15:346-354, 1973.

22. Corlett EN, Eklund JAE: Change of stature as an indication of load on the spine. In Corlett EN, Wilson J, and Manenica I, editors: *The ergonomics of working postures,* London, 1986, Taylor & Francis Publishers, Inc: pp 232-242.

23. Croft P et al: Osteoarthritis of the hip: an occupational disease in farmers, *BMJ* 304:1269-1272, 1992.

24. Donish ER, Basmajian JV: Electromyography of deep muscles in man, *Am J Anat* 133:25-31, 1972.

25. Edwards RTH: Human muscle function and fatigue, *Ciba Found Symp* 82:1-18, 1981.

26. Edwards RTH, Hill DK, McDonell M: Myothermal and intramuscular pressure measurements during isometric contractions of the human quadriceps muscle, *J Physiol (Lond)* 224:58-59, 1972.

27. Ekholm J et al: *Effekt på rörelseorganen av belastningsreducerande åtgärder vid medeltungt stående materialhanteringsarbete och sittande monteringsarbete med små komponenter, forskningsrapport,* Stockholm, 1983, Karolinska Institutet, Stockholm Univ.

28. Evans DP: Extended-heel shoes, *Rheum Rehabil* 19:103-108, 1980.

29. Farfan HF, Huberdeau RM, Dubow HI: Lumbar intervertebral disk degeneration, *J Bone Joint Surg Am* 54:492-510, 1972.

30. Felson D et al: Occupational physical demands, knee bending and knee osteoarthritis; results from the Framingham study, *J Rheumatol* 18:1587-1592, 1991.

31. Floyd WF, Silver PHS: The function of the erector spinae muscles in certain movements and postures in man, *J Physiol* (Lond) 129:184, 1955.

32. Frymoyer JW et al: Epidemiologic studies of low back pain, *Spine* 5:419-423, 1980.

33. Gracovetsky S, Farfan HF, Lamy C: The mechanism of the lumbar spine, *Spine* 6:249-262, 1981.

34. Granhed H, Hansson T, Jonson R: The bone mineral content and ultimate compressive strength of lumbar vertebra of a cadaver study, *Acta Orthop Scand* 60:105-109, 1989.

35. Gyntelberg F: One year incidence of low back pain among male residents of Copenhagen aged 40-59, *Dan Med Bull* 21:30-36, 1974.

36. Hagberg M: Arbetsmiljöns betydelse för besvär i skuldra och halsrygg, *Arbetsmiljöfonden rapport No 1,* 1988.

37. Hagberg M: Arbetsrelaterade besvär i halsrygg och skuldra, *Arbetarskyddsfonden rapport No 2,* 1982.

38. Hagberg M: Electromyographic signs of shoulder muscle fatigue in two elevated arm positions, *Am J Phys Med* 60:111-121, 1981.

39. Hagberg M: Occupational musculoskeletal stress and disorders of the neck and shoulder: a review of possible pathophysiology, *Int Arch Occup Environ Health* 53:269-278, 1984.

40. Hagberg M: Shoulder pain—pathogenesis. In Hadler NM, editor: *Clinical concepts in regional musculoskeletal illness,* New York, 1987, Grune & Stratton, Inc: pp 191-200.

41. Hagberg M, Sundelin G: Discomfort and load on the upper trapezius muscle when operating a wordprocessor, *Ergonomics* 29:1637-1645, 1986.

42. Hagberg M, Wegman DH: Prevalence rates and odds ratios of shoulder-neck disease in different occupational groups, *Br J Ind Med* 44:602-610, 1987.

43. Hansson T, Magnusson M, Broman H: Back muscle fatigue and seated whole body vibrations: an experimental study in man, *Clin Biomech* 6:173-178, 1991.

44. Hansson T, Roos B, Nachemson A: The bone mineral content and ultimate compressive strength in lumbar vertebrae, *Spine* 1:46-55, 1980.

45. Harms-Ringdahl K et al: Load moments and myoelectric activity when the cervical spine is held in full flexion and extension, *Ergonomics* 29:1539-1552, 1986.

46. Herberts P, Kadefors R: A study of painful shoulder in welders, *Acta Orthop Scand* 47:381-387, 1976.

47. Herberts P, Kadefors R, Andersson GP: Shoulder pain in industry: an epidemiological study on welders, *Acta Orthop Scand* 52:299-306, 1981.

48. Herberts P et al: Shoulder pain and heavy manual labor, *Clin Orthop* 191:166-178, 1984.

49. Hult L: The Munkfors investigation, *Acta Orthop Scand Suppl* 16, 1954.

50. Inman VT, Saunders JB, Abbott LC: Observations on the function of the shoulder joint, *J Bone Joint Surg* 26:1-30, 1944.

51. Jacobsson B, Dalen N, Tjörnstrand B: Coxarthrosis and labour, *Int Orthop* 11:311-313, 1987.

52. Jonsson B: *The lumbar part of the erector spinae muscle: a technique for electromyographic studies of the function of its individual muscles,* thesis, Univ. of Göteborg, Sweden, 1976.

53. Kadefors R, Petersen I, Herberts P: Muscular reaction to welding work: an electromyographic investigation, *Ergonomics* 19:543-558, 1976.

54. Keegan JJ: Alterations of the lumbar curve related to posture and seating, *J Bone Joint Surg Am* 35:589-603, 1953.

55. Kelsey JL: An epidemiological study of the relationship between occupations and acute herniated lumbar intervertebral disks, *Int J Epidemiol* 4:197-205, 1975.

56. Kelsey JL, Hardy RJ: Driving motor vehicles as risk factor for acute herniated lumbar intervertebral disc, *Am J Epidemiol* 102:63-73, 1975.

57. Klausen K: The form and function of the loaded human spine, *Acta Physiol Scand* 65:176-182, 1965.

58. Kroemer KHE, Robinette JC: Ergonomics in the design of office furniture, *Ind Med Surg* 38:115-125, 1969.

59. Lawrence JS: Rheumatism in coal miners. Part III, occupational factors, *Br J Ind Med Surg* 12:249-261, 1955.

60. Lindberg H, Montgomery F: Heavy labor and the occurrence of gonarthrosis, *Clin Orthop* 214:235-236, 1987.

61. Lindström L, Kadefors R, Petersen I: An electromyographic index for localized muscle fatigue, *J Appl Physiol,* 43:750-754, 1977.

62. Lucas DB: Biomechanics of the shoulder joint, *Arch Surg* 107:425-432, 1973.

63. Lundervold AJS: Electromyographic investigations of position and manner of working in typewriting, *Acta Physiol Scand Suppl* 84:1-171, 1951.

64. Magnusson M et al: Measurement of height loss during whole body vibrations, *J Spinal Disord* 5:198-203, 1992.

65. Magnusson M et al: Measurement of time-dependent height loss during sitting, *Clin Biomech* 5:137-142, 1990.

66. Magnusson M et al: The metabolic cost of various occupational exposures, *Ergonomics* 30:55-60, 1987.

67. Magora A: Investigation of the relation between low back pain and occupation. 3. Physical requirements: sitting, standing and weight lifting, *Ind Med Surg* 41:5-9, 1972.

68. Magora A: Investigation of the relation between low back pain and occupation. Six medical histories and symptoms, *Scand J Rehabil Med* 6:81-88, 1974.

69. Morris JM, Benneer G, Lucas DB: An electromyographic study of the intrisic muscles of the back in man, *J Anat* 96:509-520, 1962.

70. Morris JM, Lucas DB, Bresler B: Role of the trunk in stability of the spine, *J Bone Joint Surg Am* 43:327-351, 1961.

71. Nachemson AL: Disk pressure measurements, *Spine* 6:93-97, 1981.

72. Nachemson AL: The effect of forward leaning on lumbar intradiscal pressure, *Acta Orthop Scand* 35:314-328, 1965.

73. Nachemson AL, Elfström G: Intravital dynamic pressure measurements in lumbar disks. A study of common movements, manoeuvers and exercises, *Scand J Rehabil Med* 2(suppl 1):1-40, 1970.

74. Nilsson BE: The Tore Nilson Sy on the etiology of degenerative joint disesase, *Acta Orthop Scand Suppl* 2653, 1993.

75. Okada M: Electromyographic assessment of muscular load in forward bending postures, *J Fac Sci Univ Tokyo* 8:311, 1970.

76. Patridge RE, Anderson JA: *Back pain in industrial workers.* Proceedings of the Twelfth International Rheumatism Congress, 1969, p 284 (abstract).

77. Patridge RE, Duthie JJR: Rheumatism in dockers and civil servants. A comparison of heavy manual and sedentary workers, *Ann Rheum Dis* 27:559-568, 1968.

78. Pauly JE: An electromyographic analysis of certain movements and exercises. I. Some deep muscles of the back, *Anat Rec* 155:223-234, 1966.

79. Pope MH et al: The role of the prerotation of the trunk in axial twisting efforts, *Spine* 10:1041-1045, 1987.

80. Poppen NK, Walker PS: Forces at the glenohumeral joint in abduction, *Clin Orthop* 135:165-170, 1978.

81. Poppen NK, Walker PS: Normal and abnormal motion of the shoulder, *J Bone Joint Surg Am* 58:1-4, 1976.

82. Portnoy H, Morin F: Electromyographic study of the postural muscles in various positions and movements, *Am J Physiol* 186:122-126, 1956.

83. Rosemeyer B: Eine Methode zur Bechenfixierung im Arbeitssitz, *Z Orthop* 110:514, 1972.

84. Schobert H: *Sitzhaltung, Sitzschaden, Sitzmöbel,* Berlin, 1962, Springer-Verlag.

85. Schultz AB et al: Analysis and quantitative myoelectric measurements of loads on the lumbar spine when holding weights in standing postures, *Spine* 7:390-397, 1982.

86. Schultz AB et al: Loads on the lumbar spine, *J Bone Joint Surg Am* 64:713-720, 1982.

87. Schultz AB et al: Lumbar trunk muscle use in standing isometric heavy exertions, *J Orthop Res* 5:320-329, 1987.

88. Sigholm G et al: Electromyographic analysis of shoulder muscle load, *J Orthop Res* 1:379-386, 1984.

89. Silverstein B: *The prevalence of upper extremity cumulative trauma disorders in industry,* dissertation, Ann Arbor, 1985, University of Michigan.

90. Tamminen S: Biomekanisk analys av gruvhjälmens belastning på nacke, Examensarbete vid Arbetarskyddsstyrelsens kurs för företagsgymnaster, 1980, Stockholm Univ.

91. Thelin A: Hip joint arthrosis: an occupational disorder among farmers, *Am J Ind Med* 18:339-343, 1990.

92. Tola S et al: Neck and shoulder symptoms among men in machine operating, dynamic work and sedentary work, *Scand J Environ Health* 14:299-305, 1988.

93. Törner M: *Musculoskeletal stress in fishery causes, effects and preventive measures,* thesis, ISBN 91-628-0232-1, Göteborg, Sweden, 1991, University of Göteborg.

94. Troup JDG, Roantree WB, Archibald RM: *Survey of cases of lumbar spinal disability.* A methodological study, Med Officer's Broadsheet, London, 1970, National Coal Board.

95. Tyrrell AR, Reilly T, Troup JDG: Circadian variation in stature and the effects of spinal loading, *Spine* 10:161-164, 1985.

96. Vingård E: Work, sports, overweight and osteoarthrosis of the hip, thesis, Karolinska Institutet, 1995, Arbete & Hälsa.

97. Vingård E et al: Disability pensions due to musculoskeletal disorders among men in heavy occupations, *Scand J Soc Med* 20:31-36, 1992.

98. Waris P: Occupational cervico-brachial syndromes, *Scand J Work Environ Health* 6(suppl 3):3-13, 1979.

99. Westgaard RH, Aarås A: Postural muscle strain as a causal factor in the development of musculoskeletal illnesses, *Appl Ergonom* 15:162-174, 1984.

100. Wiker S, Chaffin DB, Langolf GD: Shoulder posture and localized muscle fatigue and discomfort, *Ergonomics* 32:211-237, 1989.

101. Wilder DG, Pope MH, Frymoyer JW: The biomechanics of lumbar disk herniation and the effect of overload and instability, *J Spinal Disord* 1:16-32, 1988.

102. Yang KH, King AI: Mechanism of facet load transmission as a hypothesis for low back pain, *Spine* 99:557-565, 1984.

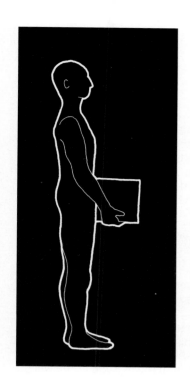

Chapter 9

Manual Material Handling: The Science

Arun Garg

CONTENTS

Overexertion injuries account for about 25% of all reported occupational injuries.[89] Lifting, pushing, or pulling of loads is involved in 87% of overexertion injury claims.[89] A significantly higher incidence of low back pain (LBP) has been reported among workers with heavy industry jobs than among workers with less strenuous jobs.* Others have reported either a moderate difference or no significant difference in the frequency of LBP between workers on light and heavy jobs.† Worker's compensation claims and insurance data show that LBP is much more prevalent in heavy physical jobs.[18,40,88,89]

MANUAL MATERIAL HANDLING

Workers with heavy manual jobs are more likely to develop compensable back injuries than other workers.[88,89,147,148,172] The severity of back pain is also significantly greater in manual workers than in those with light jobs.[18,27,138,173] Wickström[172] reported that those with heavy jobs had a four times greater lifetime prevalence of lumbar insufficiency, a three times greater prevalence of recurrent attacks of lumbago, and a two times greater prevalence of pronounced sciatica than those with light jobs. A higher prevalence of disk degeneration has also been reported among those who perform heavy physical work.[83,92,96,106]

It is widely recognized that an increased load on an already afflicted back produces more pain.[18,83,113,131,148] Also, it is reasonable to assume that back symptoms are much more likely to interfere with work when it is heavy; for example, a worker with a backache would have more difficulty performing a heavy job than a light one.[146,148] Hult[83] reported that 43.5% of those in heavy work versus 25.5% of those in light work had been off work because of LBP. Individuals with severe LBP try to find a job without much manual material handling.[89]

A musculoskeletal injury can be triggered by direct trauma, a single overexertion, repetitive loading, or frequent and sustained loading (static muscular work). Repetitive loading may cause fatigue failure, and this may not become obvious until ultimate failure occurs. In this regard, the final event may be trivial and could occur outside the workplace. For example, Bergquist-Ullman and Larson[18] noted that 44% of their patients reported a sudden onset of LBP whereas the remaining 56% had a more insidious onset. It is also important to note that tissue heals if given sufficient time.

*References 19, 20, 28, 92, 99, 106, 111-114, 159, 166-168, 172.
†References 36, 83, 93, 138, 148, 149.

It is believed that an overexertion injury occurs because physical stresses from manual material handling exceed tissue tolerance. In other words, job physical demands exceed the worker's physical capability. There are four different ergonomic criteria for overexertion injuries:

1. Biomechanical criteria
2. Psychophysical criteria
3. Physiological criteria
4. Static muscular work (postural stresses) criteria

It is believed that an overexertion injury can occur if any of the four criteria is exceeded.

Biomechanical Criteria

Biomechanical criteria deal with forces and moments on body joints and soft tissues. The human body acts as a lever system. External forces, such as the weight of a load and body segment weights, create rotational moments (torques) at various body joints. The skeletal muscles counteract these moments. Because the moment arms of the muscles are much smaller than the moment arms of the external forces and body segment weights, small external forces produce large muscle, ligament, and joint forces. For example, consider the task of holding a weight of 20 lb in both hands, as shown in **Figure 9-1**.[161] Under static equilibrium condi-

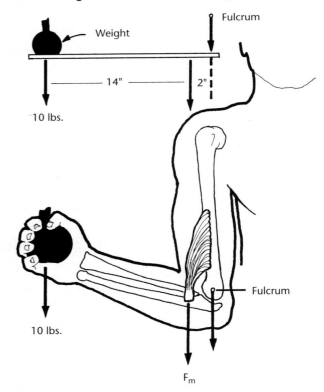

Figure 9-1 Person holding a 10-lb object. The fulcrum is in the center of rotation for elbow flexion and extension. In the posture shown, the primary elbow flexor is the brachialis muscle. *(Modified from Tichauer ER: The biomechanical basis of ergonomics, New York, 1978, John Wiley & Sons.)*

tions, the sum of the clockwise moments is equal to the sum of the counterclockwise moments:

$$(-10 \text{ lb}) (14 \text{ in}) + (F_m) (2 \text{ in}) = 0$$
$$F_m = 70 \text{ lb} \tag{1}$$

Therefore, holding a 10-lb load in each hand creates a muscle force (F_m) about seven times greater than the weight. The elbow joint reactive force, R_e, is obtained by balancing the forces along the vertical axis:

$$(-10 \text{ lb}) + (70 \text{ lb}) + R_e = 0$$
$$R_e = -60 \text{ lb (downward)} \tag{2}$$

In the preceding example the effect of body weight (weight of the lower part of the arm) was ignored. Let us assume that the body weight above the L5/S1 disk (BW) is 100 lb and consider the ask of holding a weight of 20 lb in both hands, as shown in **Figure 9-2**.[164] Under static equilibrium conditions,

$$-(w)(x) - (BW)(z) + (F_m)(y) = 0$$
$$F_m = \frac{(w)(x) + (BW)(z)}{y} \tag{3}$$
$$F_m = \frac{(20 \times 12) + (100 \times 6)}{2}$$
$$= 420 \text{ lb}$$

The compressive (F_c) and shear (F_s) forces on the L5/S1 disk, as shown in **Figure 9-3**, are computed by balancing the forces along and perpendicular to the spine:

$$-(W)(\sin\theta) - (BW)(\sin\theta) - F_m + F_c = 0$$
$$F_c = (W)(\sin\theta) + (BW)(\sin\theta) + F_m \tag{4}$$
$$= (20 \times 0.94) + (100 \times 0.94) + 420$$
$$= 533 \text{ lb}$$

$$(-W)(\cos\theta) - (BW)(\cos\theta) + F_s = 0$$
$$F_s = (W)(\cos\theta) + (BW)(\cos\theta) \tag{5}$$
$$= (20 \times 0.34) + (100 \times 0.34)$$
$$= 41 \text{ lb}$$

Simple biomechanical analyses show the following:

1. Relatively small forces applied with the during activities such as lifting, holding, lowering, carrying, pushing, and pulling produce large internal muscle forces because of the small moment arms of the muscles involved. This can produce high stresses (tension) in muscles in certain body postures, even when relatively light loads are lifted.
2. High internal muscle forces during a voluntary exertion produce equally large forces on adjoining skeletal structures. This concept of muscles loading skeletal structures is extremely important in the biomechanics of the lower part of the back. The handling of light loads in certain postures produces large compressive loads on the spine—a downward force perpendicular to the surface of the upper vertebra that compresses the intervertebral disk.
3. Often, several muscles contribute to the moment requirement at a joint, and a unique mathematical solution is not possible without the assumption

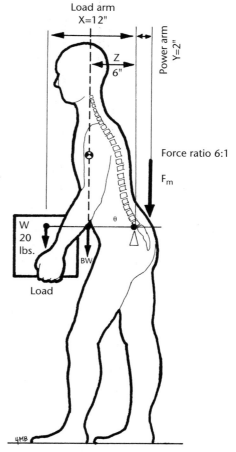

Figure 9-2 Lever system for the lower part of the back. *(Modified from Troup JDG and Edwards FC: Manual handling and lifting, London, 1985, Her Majesty's Stationery Office.)*

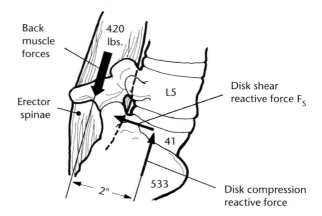

Figure 9-3 Forces on the low back area from the example in Figure 9-2. *(Adapted from Pope MH et al: Occupational low back pain: assessment, treatment and prevention, St Louis, 1991, Mosby–Year Book.)*

that the system is statically indeterminate. It is not clear which particular biomechanical objective is dominant during the performance of a manual task.

4. Several studies have shown the presence of antagonistic muscle activity, especially when the trunk is laterally bent and/or axially rotated. Biomechanically, antagonistic muscle activity results in greater compressive and shear forces on the spine.

5. Under certain load-lifting conditions, the ligamentous tissues of the lumbar spine may provide significant passive resistance, called restorative moment, to external moments. At present it is not clear under what conditions antagonistic muscles and ligaments play an important role.

COMPRESSIVE STRENGTH OF THE LUMBAR SPINAL COLUMN

The maximum amount of compression that can be tolerated by the lumbar spinal motion segments has been estimated from axial compression loading tests on cadaver specimens. Ultimate compressive strength is defined as the magnitude of the load at failure in a single test. In general, the ultimate compressive strength varies between approximately 2 and 12 kN (**Fig. 9-4**). Jäger and Luttmann[86] found that the mean value of the lumbar compressive strength from 477 experiments was 4.9 ± 2.2 kN. Recently, Brinckmann, Biggemann, and Hilweg[24] showed ultimate compressive strength ranging from 2.1 to 8.8 kN, with the exception of one cadaver column. Approximately 30% of the motion segments fractured at loads below 4 kN, and approximately 63% had ultimate compressive strengths of 6 kN or less. The large variability in measured compressive strengths within a study and between different studies makes it difficult to provide a single value of spinal compressive strength that would be valid for all persons.

The disk is strongest in young adults and weakens slowly with age. Sonada[158] estimates that female spinal compression tolerance is approximately 17% less than that of males. This would be consistent with the smaller force-bearing area of the vertebral bodies in a female spine.

The vertebrae are also subject to fatigue failure from repeated loading. Under repeated loading by a compressive force, the height of the motion segment decreases slowly because of viscoelastic deformation and creep. A sudden irreversible loss of height is interpreted as *fatigue failure*. Brinckmann, Biggemann, and Hilweg[24] showed that the probability of a fatigue fracture increases with both the number of load cycles and the magnitude of relative cycle load (percentage of the ultimate compressive strength). They postulated that fatigue fractures of the lumbar vertebrae might occur in vivo; however, several issues, such as the time interval for load cycles, periods of rest, strain rate, and maximum load in consecutive load cycles, need to be addressed before these results can be applied in vivo.

EPIDEMIOLOGIC SUPPORT FOR THE IMPORTANCE OF DISK COMPRESSION

In 1973, Chaffin and Park[32] reported that incidence rates for LBP are related to compressive forces on the L5/S1 disk (**Fig. 9-5**). Further, LBP incidence rates are nine times higher when the predicted compressive forces are greater than 650 kg (6.5 kN) than when they are below 250 kg (2.5 kN). Brigham and Garg[23] analyzed 109 cases of overexertion injuries over a period of 3 years in one company. There were 10 back injuries—8 muscular strains and 2 disk injuries. Among the muscular strains, the average estimated compressive force was 5.34 kN. For the 2 disk injuries, the average compressive force was 7.97 kN.

Anderson[4] reported a 40% increase in incidence rates among jobs requiring compressive forces above 3.4 kN as compared with forces below that level. In a study of 6912 incumbent workers in 55 industrial jobs in five industries, Herrin, Jariedi, and Anderson[80] concluded that "the biomechanical criterion of maximal back compression appears to be a good predictor of the risk of

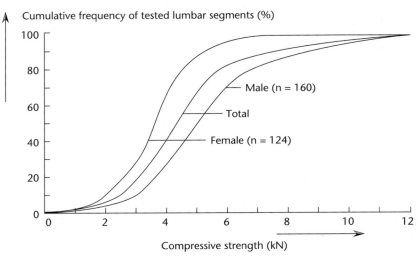

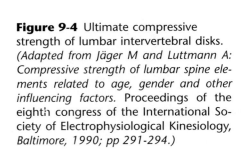

Figure 9-4 Ultimate compressive strength of lumbar intervertebral disks. *(Adapted from Jäger M and Luttmann A: Compressive strength of lumbar spine elements related to age, gender and other influencing factors. Proceedings of the eighth congress of the International Society of Electrophysiological Kinesiology, Baltimore, 1990; pp 291-294.)*

not only back incidents but also overexertion injuries in general.''

Ultimate strength under a given compressive load may be lower when the spine is subjected to additional shearing and rotational forces. However, it is difficult to support a lower limit for ultimate compressive strength at this time based on current knowledge of spinal compressive strength; in vitro observations may not be applicable in vivo, and several low-back injury mechanisms, independent of disk compression, have been proposed.

CREEP

Body stature undergoes normal diurnal shrinkage, on the order of 1.1%, that is attributed to loss of disk height secondary to the cumulative effects of compressive loading during the day.[100] Losses in overall stature were demonstrated among healthy young adult males bearing a shoulder load of 88 N for 20 minutes in an erect posture. Recovery took approximately 10 minutes. Shrinkage rates are closely related to the calculated levels of spinal compression at L3.[47]

Whenever a compressive load produces intradiscal pressure that is greater than the disk's osmotic pressure, fluid is expelled from the disk. This is called *creep*.[91] As fluid is expelled from the disk, the height of the disk decreases (narrows). This narrowing affects the dynamics of the three-joint complex. In particular, the areas of contact between the load-bearing surfaces of the facet joints change as they are compressed and strained. In addition, the intervertebral joint becomes stiffer. Thus motion segments with disks affected by creep exhibit a

decreased capacity to dissipate energy and decreased ultimate strength when placed under a compressive load.[61]

DISK SHEAR FORCE

The disk shear forces experienced in flexion, extension, lateral flexion, and axial rotation are also important. These shear forces are resisted primarily by the posterior facet joints in the lumbar spine and the annulus fibrosus of the disk. Under normal physiological conditions, the facets can resist shear forces.[49] However, the limit to such forces is not well documented.[154] Cyron and Hutton,[35] Troup,[163] Lamy et al,[104] and Farfan, Osteria, and Lamy[48] reported about 2000 to 3000 N of shear forces as the failure limit for the articular facets. If a disk space is narrowed by degeneration, abnormally high stresses on the facet joints may result.[49] These authors also suggest that interarticular facets, being unstable, are more vulnerable to injury and, with their rich blood supply and nerve endings (in synovial membrane), are likely to cause considerable pain. Further, facet joints may be injured simultaneously whenever there is a disk injury or may be injured exclusively without a disk injury.

Psychophysical Criteria

The basic premise for psychophysical criteria is that most of the musculoskeletal and back injuries are caused by overexertion as a result of a mismatch between a worker's strength and job strength requirements. In other words, the job's physical requirements exceed the physical strength of the worker. These criteria

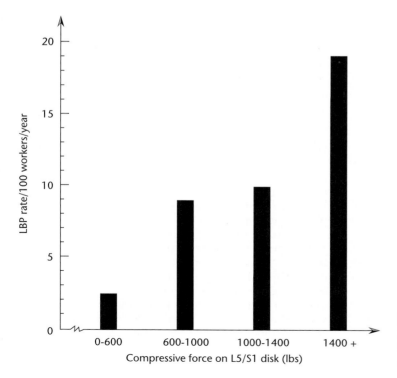

Figure 9-5 Relationship between low back incidence rate and predicted compressive force on the L5/S1 disk. *(Adapted from Chaffin DB and Park KS: Am Ind Hyg Assoc J 32:513-525, 1973.)*

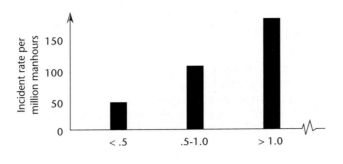

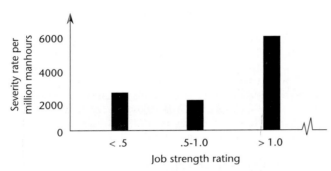

Figure 9-6 The incidence and severity of low back disorders according to job strength rating. *(From Chaffin DB, Park KS:* Am Ind Hyg Assoc J *32:513-525, 1973.)*

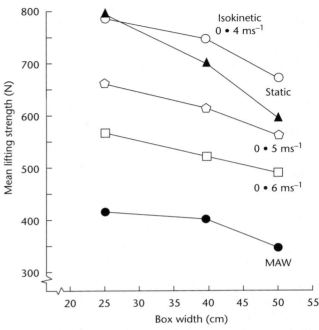

Figure 9-7 A comparison of static strength, isokinetic strength, and maximum acceptable weight. *(From Garg A, Beller D:* Int J Ind Erg *6:231-240, 1990.)*

are called psychophysical because the measurement of human strength is influenced by the worker's motivation and willingness to tolerate some discomfort and/or pain.

Chaffin and Park,[32] from data involving 103 jobs in five manufacturing plants, reported that a job with even one highly back-stressing lifting task could appreciably increase the risk of back pain complaints (**Fig. 9-6**). Similarly, Herrin, Jariedi, and Anderson[80] concluded that overexertion injuries can be related to job physical stress and, in addition to compressive force, the percentage of the population capable of performing the most stressful element of the job is perhaps the best single index. This index can be based on either static strength or psychophysically determined maximum acceptable weights and forces.

Liles et al[109] reported that the disabling back injury rate increased with an increase in the percentage of overstressed workers. Ayoub, Selan, and Liles[11] also reported a relationship between the job severity index and the frequency and severity of back injuries. Other studies have also found that an inability to demonstrate a lifting strength equal to that required on the job is a significant risk factor.*

When strength data are used for job design and evaluation or for administering a preemployment strength test for worker selection, the data and the test

*References 5, 32, 97, 98, 113, 142.

must be job specific, that is, they should be exactly related to job physical requirements. Standardized pre-employment strength testing (including strength tests that do not relate to job physical demands) is not effective.[15]

Regarding practical applications, a question often asked is which strength should be used for job design and physical ability testing. In this regard, there are four types of strengths:

1. Static strength
2. Maximum acceptable weight and force
3. Isokinetic strength
4. Isoinertial strength

Data on job-specific isoinertial strength and its effectiveness in preventing overexertion injuries in the workplace are lacking. Further, based on the author's experience, there is concern that the commercially available isoinertial testing equipment may not simulate job physical requirements.

According to Garg and Beller,[59] there are major differences between static strength, maximum acceptable weight, and isokinetic strength, which is highly dependent on the speed of lifting (**Fig. 9-7**). At slow speed, mean isokinetic strength appears to be equal to mean static strength, and at high speed, mean isokinetic strength appears to be equal to the maximum acceptable weight. The moderate correlations between the three types of strengths (.65 to .82) suggest that it is highly questionable whether one type of strength can be estimated from another type of strength for a given individual.[59]

From a practical standpoint, the type of strength selected will have a major impact on recommended weight limits for job design and on an individual's performance in a physical ability test (**Fig. 9-7**). For the present it is recommended that ergonomists use maximum acceptable weights and static strengths for job design with the understanding that using static strength will result in higher allowable limits. Extensive data on maximum acceptable weights and forces are available in the literature.* For physical ability testing, the effectiveness of maximum acceptable weights is not well documented.

The complexities associated with isokinetic strength and its relationship to a person's "safe" maximum dynamic lifting capability are not fully understood. It is recommended that for the present, the use of isokinetic strength measurements be avoided for both job design and physical ability testing.

Physiological Criteria

The physiological basis for manual material handling is summarized in the schematic on p. 92. Muscle fatigue results from the accumulation of incompletely oxidized metabolic breakdown products of glycogen. Lactic acid is the primary fatigue product formed from pyruvic acid if there is not enough oxygen in the cell for oxidative metabolism. Muscles cannot use the lactic acid as a substrate for further energy generation. The lactic acid is returned to the liver by the blood supply to be converted to blood glucose or stored as glycogen. This takes time.

It is generally believed that both the intensity of effort and endurance time at a given intensity level are related to a person's aerobic capacity for dynamic muscular work involving large muscle groups. Kamon and Ramanathan[90] estimated the maximum aerobic capacity for an average 35-year-old male worker to be less than 15 kcal/min. Aerobic capacities for men and women, based on data from the American Heart Association, are summarized in **Table 9-1**.[3] However, several factors affect aerobic capacity:

1. Age: aerobic capacity decreases with age and is 30% lower at age 65 that at age 25.
2. Gender: females, on average, have 30% lower aerobic capacity than men.
3. Physical fitness: aerobic capacity increases with physical fitness.
4. Whole-body versus upper-body work: on average, aerobic capacity is 30% lower for arm work.
5. Nature of work: each task has its own maximum aerobic capacity. Aerobic capacities for lifting are significantly lower than those based on a bicycle ergometer (**Table 9-2**).[140]

*References 11, 57, 58, 60, 127, 128, 157.

Table 9-1	Aerobic capacities (kcal/min) for American men and women.	
Fitness Class	**Men**	**Women**
Low	<8.6	<6.2
Fair	8.6-11.3	6.2-8.4
Average	11.7-14.3	8.7-10.3
Good	14.7-18.1	10.6-13.7
High	>18.5	>14.0

From American Heart Association: Exercise testing and training of apparently healthy individuals: a handbook for physicians, *Dallas, 1972, American Heart Association.*

Table 9-2	Comparison of maximum O_2 uptake and heart rate for lifting with a bicycle ergometer.	
Weight Lifted (lb)	**Percentage of Vo_2 Max for Bicycle**	**Maximum Heart Rate**
2	54	144
15	64	160
50	75	164
80	80	182
Bicycle ergometer	100	187

From Petrofsky JS, Lind AR: J Appl Physiol Respir Environ Exerc Physiol *45:64-68, 1978.*

Past studies recommended 33% of the maximum aerobic power of a normal healthy person as the maximum energy expenditure rate that should be expended for an 8-hour workday (or 5 kcal/min for men and 3.5 kcal/min for women).[64,68,145] However, most data now suggest that the range should be between 25% and 30% of bicycle ergometer Vo_2 max for an 8-hour shift.[64,145] From a literature review it is clear that there are three major components for determining acceptable levels of energy expenditure[64]: (1) design limit versus maximum permissible limit, (2) lift location (above or below 76 cm or 30 inches), and (3) an adjustment for the continuous duration of lifting (1, 1 to 2, or 2 to 8 hours). At the design limit, at least half of the women and most of the men will find the tasks acceptable. At the maximum permissible limit (MPL), about 25% of the men and a few women will find the tasks acceptable. The recommendations from the National Institute For Occupational Health and Safety (NIOSH) to accommodate 75% of female workers (design limit) and 25% of male workers (MPL) are summarized in **Tables 9-3** and **9-4**.[145]

Table 9-3	Energy expenditure limits to accommodate 75% of female workers.		
Lift Location, Inches (cm)	**Duration of Lifting**		
	1 hr	1-2 hr	2-8 hr
V < 30 (75)	4.72	3.78	3.12
V ≥ 30 (75)	3.30	2.65	2.18

V, *vertical height.*
From Garg A, Rodgers SH, Yates JW: The physiological basis for manual lifting. In Kumar S, editor: Advances in industrial ergonomics and safety IV, *London, 1992, Taylor & Francis: pp 867-874.*

Table 9-4	Energy expenditure limits to accommodate top 25% of male workers.		
Lift Location, Inches (cm)	**Duration of Lifting**		
	1 hr	1-2 hr	2-8 hr
V < 30 (75)	6.75	5.40	4.45
V ≥ 30 (75)	5.40	4.05	3.12

From Garg A, Rodgers SH, Yates JW: The physiological basis for manual lifting. In Kumar S, editor: Advances in industrial ergonomics and safety IV, *London, 1992, Taylor & Francis: pp 867-874.*

Repetitive lifting
↓
Accumulation of fatigue
↓
Overexertion injury

- Pain/discomfort experienced in muscles can be due to fatigue
- Chronic exhaustion: most frequent contributing factor to back pain

Although a relationship between energy expenditure and the incidence of musculoskeletal injuries from manual material handling has not been established, there is considerable indirect evidence that frequent manual material handling, especially repetitive lifting, is an important risk factor associated with the frequency, severity, and resultant disability of LBP.* Jensen[87] and Marras et al[118] found a direct relationship between the incidence of LBP and the frequency of lifting. Garg, Haggland, and Mericle[64] showed that a combination of moderate to heavy loads and frequent lifting, walking, and carrying can result in physical fatigue as demonstrated by energy expenditure, heart rate, and subjective fatigue. Similarly, the introduction

*References 7, 18, 33, 52, 82, 83, 96, 111, 112, 168.

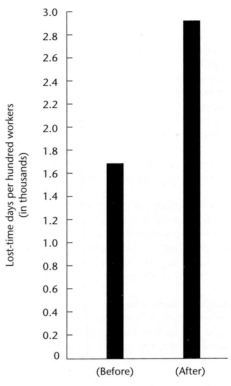

Figure 9-8 Effect of production standards on severity of injuries. *(Severity rates for musculoskeletal injuries before and after introduction of production standards from Garg A, Hagglund G, and Mericle K:* AIIE Trans *18(3):235-245, 1986.)*

of unreasonable production standards results in high energy expenditure and a significant increase in job-related injuries.[64] For example, Garg, Haggland, and Mericle[64] reported that the severity rate increased from 1700 lost workdays to 2900 lost workdays per 100 workers per year after the introduction of production standards (**Fig. 9-8**). In addition to fatigue, repetitive manual material handling can result in uncoordinated muscle action and could accelerate the wear and tear of connective tissues.

Static Muscular Work Criteria

Static muscular work (postural stresses) leads to reduced blood flow to the affected muscles in proportion to the intensity of exertion (percentage of maximum voluntary contraction [MVC]). Reduced blood flow results in the accumulation of lactic acid, which causes localized muscle fatigue.[44,145]

JOB RISK FACTORS

Several studies have shown an association between heavy physical work and the incidence of LBP, the prevalence of disk degeneration, and the risk of compensable back injury.[55] Similarly, the severity of LBP is significantly higher in heavy physical work, most likely

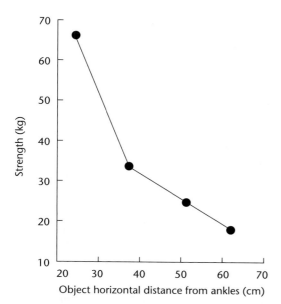

Figure 9-9 Strength decreases sharply with an increase in horizontal distance of the hands from the ankles. *(Modified from Garg A et al: Hum Factors 25:527-539, 1983.)*

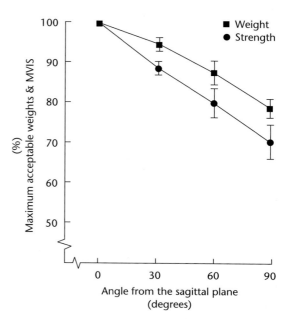

Figure 9-10 Effects of twisting on maximum acceptable weight and static strength. Data are expressed as percentages of values in the sagittal plane. *(Adapted from Garg A, Badger D: Ergonomics, 29:879-892, 1986; and Garg A, Banaag J: Ergonomics 31(1):77-96, 1988.)*

because back symptoms interfere with work much more and, as a result, there is a greater need to report LBP.[55] Other job risk factors include sudden or unexpected maximal effort; haste; speed and inattention; bending, stretching, and reaching; a combination of lifting, bending, and twisting; lowering, carrying, and holding; pushing and pulling; and the maintenance of a flexed posture.[55]

Risk factors associated with the lifting and lowering of loads are described in the list that follows. A discussion of these risk factors can be found in work by Garg.[55] Among all these factors, the product of the weight of the load and the horizontal distance of the hands from the spinal axis appears to be the most important risk factor.[33,54,118,150] The following is a brief summary of the effects of task variables on the four criteria:

1. Weight of the load: compressive force, required strength, energy expenditure, and postural stresses increase with an increase in weight of the load. Keep the weight as low as possible.
2. Horizontal location of hands: compressive force increases and strength decreases (**Fig. 9-9**) with an increase in horizontal distance. The horizontal distance should be minimized as much as possible through job design and worker education and training.
3. Vertical location of hands: workers are strongest when lifting loads near floor level. However, this results in high compressive and shear forces on the lower part of the back. Lifting above the shoulder results in reduced strength, and hyperextension of the back causes the concentration of compressive

force on the posterior third of the disks. Ideal lifting height is between knuckle and chest height.
4. Distance of lift: increased distance of lifting results in reduced strength and higher energy expenditure. The ideal distance of a lift is 10 inches or less.
5. Asymmetric lifting: asymmetric lifting occurs under the following conditions: twisting, lateral bending, asymmetric placement of hands, asymmetric center of mass, or lifting with one hand. Asymmetric lifting results in high compressive and shear forces, reduced strength (**Fig. 9-10**), and a high circulatory load (heart rate).
6. Frequency of lifting: an increase in frequency causes an increase in energy expenditure and physical fatigue.
7. Couplings: lack of good handles or handhold cutouts reduces strength by 5% to 10%.
8. Nature of the object: sagging objects, unstable contents, or hot surfaces make lifting much more difficult and result in increased stress on the worker.
9. Temperature: heat and/or humidity adds to the circulatory load and results in a higher heart rate, heat stress, and early fatigue. Cold makes muscles less efficient and increases energy expenditure, and extra clothing may impede efforts.
10. Organizational stressors: time pressures, incentive rates, negative attitudes toward injury, and so forth can produce muscle tension and contribute to injury rates. Anxiety may cause muscle tension that can lead to pain, and pain leads to more anxiety

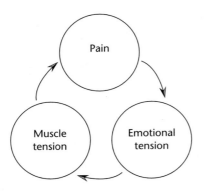

- Anxiety causes muscle tension, which leads to pain.

- Pain leads to more anxiety, more muscle tension, etc.

- A vicious cycle...

Figure 9-11 Possible relationship between anxiety, muscle tension, and pain.

and more muscle tension; this becomes a vicious cycle (**Fig. 9-11**).

PREVENTION OF OVEREXERTION INJURIES

Several different approaches have been used in industry to reduce overexertion injuries and, in particular, low back injuries. These include selection of workers (radiologic screening, medical history, anthropometry, and preemployment strength testing), physical fitness, lifting technique, back belts, and ergonomic job design. The pros and cons of some of these are reviewed in the following section.

Lifting Technique

As discussed in greater detail in Chapter 10, several different lifting techniques have been recommended over the past several years. The most common recommendation is to bend the knees, keep the back straight, and then lift with the leg muscles. It has been assumed that this posture would allow the worker to keep the load close to the body, thereby resulting in smaller and more uniformly distributed compressive force and lower shear force on the back. However, if the worker cannot keep the load between the knees, which is most often true in industry, the moment arm of the load is much greater with the squat lifting posture than with the freestyle lifting posture (**Fig. 9-12**). Observations of workers in industry show that they typically use a combination of trunk and knee flexion when lifting an object from the floor. The degree of trunk flexion versus knee flexion varies from worker to worker and from object to object. Garg and Saxena,[71] observing workers

in three different warehouses who were required to lift loads frequently, found that practically no workers bent their knees and kept their backs straight when lifting objects near the floor level. Other investigators have also observed that the stoop lifting technique is frequently used. Davis, Troup, and Burnhard[39] reported that young adult untrained males, when asked to lift a heavy weight by using their legs and not their backs, tend to convert the bent-knee lift into a straight-knee lift. As summarized in the box on p. 95, no significant evidence exists that one lifting technique is superior to another technique. Whereas a few studies have reported a significant reduction in reported LBP disability, others have found that the lifting technique has little or no effect. As a result, it is recommended that instructions on lifting technique be avoided. On the other hand, workers should be advised to observe the following:

1. Do not overexert yourself. Test the load. If the load is too heavy for you, get help.
2. Do not jerk or speed up. Lift in a smooth and controlled manner.
3. Keep the load as close to the body as possible. Walk as close as possible to the load. Pull the load and/or tilt the load toward you before lifting.
4. Do not twist while lifting (especially with a heavy load). Turn and take a step.
5. Follow the above rules for lowering the load.
6. Take frequent microbreaks if you feel tired.

Physical Fitness

It is widely believed that improved physical fitness among workers would be associated with a reduction in overexertion and low back injuries. However, it is not clear how to define physical fitness and how it relates to job physical requirements. Further, it is not clear exactly what training is appropriate and how it can be provided without risk of injury to the targeted population (5% of all injuries suffered by firefighters occur during physical fitness training). Physical fitness is often expressed in terms of spinal flexibility, strength, isometric endurance time, and/or aerobic capacity. Some investigators have reported that physical fitness and conditioning have a significant preventive effect on back injuries.[8,25,119,120,125,126] Others have found that physical fitness and training have little or no effect in preventing back injuries.* The majority of studies suggest that flexibility, strength, and aerobic capacity without relating to job physical requirements are poor predictors of future overexertion and low back injuries. Further, in normal as opposed to deconditioned individuals, the expected gains in strength and aerobic capacity from physical fitness are not very large.[9] In summary, the importance of physical fitness and training in reducing musculoskeletal injuries is generally accepted, but the epidemiologic literature at present does not support the efficacy of physical fitness and training as a primary

*References 14-16, 18, 34, 41, 42, 53, 93, 94.

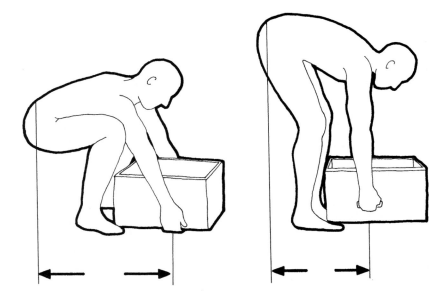

Figure 9-12 Horizontal distance (H) between the spine and the center of grasp is greater with the squat posture than with a freestyle posture if the load cannot be brought between the knees. *(Based on data from Garg A et al:* Hum Factors *25(5):527-539, 1983.)*

Pros and cons of specific lifting techniques

1. The squat lifting posture places the quadriceps muscles at severe mechanical disadvantage, and an average worker cannot develop sufficient force to raise a heavy load.

2. Detailed biomechanical analyses show that the squat lifting method may indeed produce higher compressive forces on the lower part of the back (see **Fig. 9-13**).

3. No significant difference is found in intradiscal pressure for the two methods of lifting (straight back/bent knee and bent back/straight knee).[141]

4. Lifting strength with the squat lifting posture is lower than lifting strength with the freestyle posture (**Table 9-5**).[76] Also, both static and isokinetic trunk extensor strength increases with an increase in trunk flexion angle.[29,121]

5. Energy expenditure with the squat lifting posture is higher than energy expenditures for the stoop and freestyle lifting postures (see **Fig. 9-14**).[71]

6. Ratings of perceived exertion for the squat and freestyle lifting postures are about the same (**Table 9-5**).

7. Productivity decreases and energy expenditure and the heart rate increase when workers are forced to adopt a squat lifting posture (**Fig. 9-15**).

8. Most workers use a combination of trunk and knee flexion. The degree of trunk versus knee flexion varies from worker to worker and from object to object.

9. Some flexion of the spine appears to be advantageous because it transfers some force to the posterior ligaments, provides nutrition to the disk, and gives greater compressive strength to the disk.[1]

---

intervention for preventing musculoskeletal injuries. Injuries from training and physical fitness programs are frequent, and the benefits and risks from these programs are not clear.

Back Belts, Braces, and Corsets

Spinal supports may have the following possible effects:

1. Limitation of movement
2. Increase in intraabdominal pressure (IAP)
3. Reduction in abdominal and back muscle activity
4. Warming of the skin

The primary reason for recommending spinal supports for healthy workers is the belief that a tight-fitting belt can increase IAP, which helps relieve compressive force

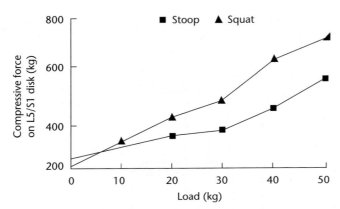

Figure 9-13 Estimated compressive force on the L5/S1 disk for squat and stoop postures when the load cannot be brought between the knees. *(Adapted from Garg A and Herrin GD:* AIIE Trans *11(4):293-302, 1979.)*

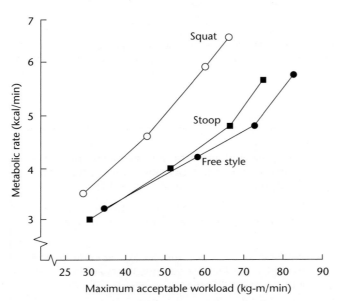

Figure 9-14 Energy expenditures for three different lifting postures. The Squat lifting posture is more fatiguing than the stoop or freestyle lifting postures. *(Adapted from Garg A, Saxena U:* Am Ind Hyg Assoc J *40(10):894-902, 1979.)*

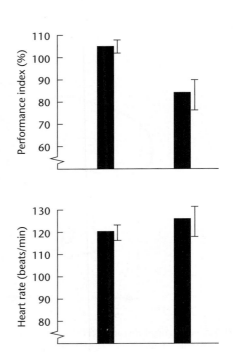

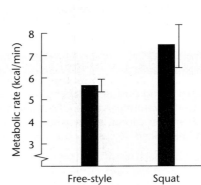

Figure 9-15 Performance standards (productivity), heart rates, and energy expenditures for warehouse workers when using the squat and freestyle lifting postures. Productivity decreases while heart rate and energy expenditures increase when the squat lifting posture is used. *(Adapted from Garg A and Saxena U:* Am Ind Hyg Assoc J *46(2):53-59, 1985.)*

Table 9-5 Lifting technique, maximum acceptable weights, and ratings of perceived exertion.

Box Size (in)	Maximum Acceptable Weights			Ratings of Perceived Exertion (RPE)	
	FREESTYLE (LB)	SQUAT (LBS)	DECREASE (%)	FREESTYLE RPE	SQUAT RPE
10	85	69	29	15.7	15.4
15	75	63	19	16.0	15.1
20	64	59	8	15.8	15.3
25	59	53	10	16.0	15.6

From Garg A et al: Hum Factors *25:527-539, 1983.*

on the spine as well as tension in the back muscles. It is common at the start of a manual handling activity to hold the breath and close the glottis. The muscles of the abdominal wall and pelvic floor contract and pressure increases in both the thoracic and abdominal cavities. The increased pressure in the thorax stiffens the rib cage, provides a stable base for the activity of the upper limbs, and supplements the thoracic erector spinae musculature.[13,38,130] A pressure increase in the abdominal cavity appears to supplement the lumbar extensor mechanism and reduces compressive force on the spine, particularly when the spine is flexed.[162] It was estimated that increased IAP reduces the load on the spine by as much as 40%.*

Recent studies show that IAP does not play any significant role in relieving intradiscal pressure or tension in back extensors.† Reasons include the following: (1) abdominal muscle forces produce a flexion moment and counterbalance the action of IAP[76,124,132,141,162]; (2) an increase in IAP does not decrease the activity of dorsal musculature in a flexed or axially rotated position[75]; (3) there is no relationship between IAP and abdominal musculature[79,118]; (4) there is little correlation between IAP and electromyographic (EMG) findings, measured intradiscal pressure, and estimated compressive force[123,151,152]; (5) there is a delay in onset of the production of IAP and muscle moment, and this lag increases with an increase in velocity[115]; and (6) fatigue or training has not been shown to have an effect on IAP.[108]

Some studies have shown that corsets, although increasing the resting IAP by about 10 to 15 mm Hg, do not raise the peak pressure during a controlled lift.[77,102,130] Other studies have shown that peak IAP is 8% to 20% (about 15 to 20 mm Hg) greater with belts than without belts.[78,105,125] The weights lifted in these studies were 160 to 200 lb, 280 lb, and 300 to 350 lb, and most differences were observed with the heaviest weights.[105] These are certainly much greater loads than the typical weights lifted in most manual material handling activities in industry. Whereas Lander, Simonton, and Giacobbe[105] and Hilgen and Smith[81] reported somewhat lower EMG values with a belt than without a belt, McGill, Norman, and Sharratt[125] found no change in erector spinae EMG findings. Further, EMG amplitude increased with a belt in the rectus abdominus, external oblique, andintercostal muscles.[125] Waters and Morris[170] found that spinal braces produced little or no change in muscle activity in the abdominal wall. Lander, Simonton, and Giacobbe[105] reported that L5/S1 moments were 11% to 16% greater (raw data) and the estimated compressive forces were 4% to 10% higher with a belt than without a belt. McGill et al[125] reported that the use of a belt did not affect estimated compressive force on the lower part of back. Also, lifts were performed a little faster with a belt and there was a greater emphasis on hip extension than knee exten-

sion.[78,81,105] Circuit weight training caused stature losses of 3.6 mm without a belt and 2.9 mm with a belt, but the difference was not significant ($p > .05$).[22]

Regarding the effects of belts on lifting strength, McCoy et al reported that belts increased the maximum acceptable weight of lifts by 13% to 19% with respect to controls (no belts).[121] Woodhouse et al,[174] using isokinetic measurements, found that belts had no significant effects on peak lifting force, total muscular work, or average muscular power. Amendola[2] found no significant differences in maximum acceptable weights when lifting with and without external supports.

Several different studies have concluded that lumbar spinal supports reduce the range of motion of the lumbar spine in both normal and patient groups.[77,102,139] In this regard, rigid supports restrict spinal movement much more than fabric-based supports.[77] However, Seguin and McGill[155] reported that although wearing a belt significantly increased the passive stiffness of the trunk about the axial rotation and lateral-bending axes, it made no difference in trunk flexion and extension. Similarly, Milton et al[126] reported that the use of spinal supports by patients did not improve performance in either spinal motion or straight-leg raising.

Thicker or padded lumbar support can raise the skin temperature in the lumbar area by 2°C.[77] Others have reported continued complaints from workers that the brace was too hot.[121,143,169]

Subjectively, some workers feel more secure, stable, and comfortable with spinal support than without it.[22,102,105] Similarly, among patients with LBP, wearing a lumbar support results in significant relief of symptoms.[110,126,139]

Walsh and Schwartz[169] and Reddell et al[143] studied the effects of lumbar support on low back injuries in the workplace. Walsh and Schwartz[169] studied 81 male warehouse workers in a grocery distribution center divided into three groups: true controls, back school only, and back school plus wearing custom-molded lumbosacral orthoses. Pretesting and 6-month follow-up posttesting data were compared for each group. There were no significant changes in abdominal strength, productivity, and accident rate in all three groups. The group with back school plus orthoses had significantly less lost time (2.9 versus 0.5 lost workdays). However, a further analysis of the data shows that the most improvement was in the high-risk group (those patients with previous injury). The low-risk group (those patients without a previous history of back injury) showed no significant differences (**Table 9-6**).

Reddell et al[143] studied 642 baggage handlers over an 8-month period. There were four treatment groups: belt only, 1-hour training class, belt and 1-hour training class, and control group. The study found no significant differences in the low back injury incident rate, restricted workday injury incident rate, lost workday and restricted workday rate, and worker's compensation cost rate among the four groups. About 58% of the participants in the belt groups discontinued use of the belt

---

*References 29, 38, 45, 46, 65, 130, 151, 160.
†References 75, 76, 108, 115, 123, 132, 141, 151.

before the end of 8 months. Some of the reasons for discontinuation of belt use included the belt being too hot; the belt rubbing, pinching, and bruising ribs; and the belt making the back sore. Participants who wore a belt for a while and then discontinued its use had significantly higher lost workday injury incident rates than did either the group receiving training only or the control group (**Fig. 9-16**). The study concluded that the use of belts may in fact increase the risk of injury when a belt is not worn after a period of wearing one.

Grew and Deane[77] concluded that despite exercises, wearing a corset over a long term can cause a loss of tone in the abdominal muscles. Similarly, Harman et al[78] warned that "someone who lifts regularly with a belt should be extremely cautious about lifting without one." Strengthening of abdominal and back muscles for those who lift while wearing a belt has been recom-

mended.[78,105,139] Perry[139] suggested that belts should never be prescribed without a plan to eliminate them. However, Walsh and Schwartz[169] did not find a loss in abdominal muscle strength from wearing back braces. Similarly, McGill, Norman, and Sharratt[125] concluded that wearing a belt during lifting activities should not result in a loss of abdominal muscle strength because EMG values never exceeded 15% of the EMG values produced by an isometric MVC.

Finally, there is concern that use of a belt can put an added strain on the cardiovascular system. In this regard, Hunter et al[84] reported an 8-mm to 20-mm Hg increase in systolic blood pressure and a 5-beat to 10-beat/min increase in heart rate as a result of wearing a back belt for dead lifting and bicycling exercises. The study concluded that individuals with a compromised cardiovascular system are probably at greater risk when exercising with back supports. Also, it has been shown that large IAP and intrathoracic pressure impede blood flow back to the heart.

In summary, it does not appear that back belts assist in relieving stresses either to the spine or to the back muscles. Epidemiologic studies show that back belts do not reduce the incidence or severity of work-related injuries among healthy workers. There is concern that they may lead to a false feeling of security. Based on the current data, the prescription of back belts to workers is not justified.

Ergonomic Job Design

Job design is an ergonomic approach that attempts to fit the job to the worker. (A detailed discussion of job analysis is contained in Chapter 15.) It is widely believed that the most effective control for musculoskeletal injuries and low back injuries in particular is ergo-

Table 9-6	The effect of prophylactic orthoses on low back injury in the workplace.			
	Lost Workdays			
	LOW RISK		**HIGH RISK**	
Group	Before	After	Before	After
Controls	0	0.3	1.1	1.6
Back school	0	0.9	6.1	4.1
Back school + orthosis	0	0.1	6.8	0.9

From Walsh NE, Schwartz RK: Am J Phys Med Rehabil 69:246-250, 1990.

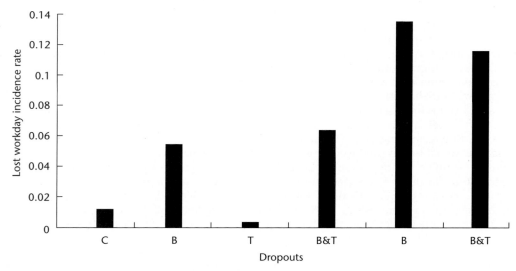

Figure 9-16 Lost workday incidence rate for back injuries among the four groups: *C*, controls; *B*, belt only; *T*, training only; *B & T*, belt and training; *dropouts*, workers who discontinued wearing the belt before the end of 8 months. *(Adapted from Reddel CR et al: Appl Erg 23(5):319-329, 1992.)*

nomic job design. Several studies have demonstrated that musculoskeletal injuries are related to job physical stress (or resulting strain) and that such injuries can be significantly reduced by designing the job so that it is within the physical capability of a large percentage of the working population. Stress or resulting strain from the job can be defined as follows:

$$\text{Strain} = \frac{\text{Job physical demands}}{\text{Worker physical capacity}} \qquad (6)$$

Whereas the previously mentioned and other approaches focus on the denominator, that is, they attempt to improve the worker's physical capacity, ergonomic job design focuses on the numerator, that is, it attempts to reduce the job's physical demands. In this regard, several different criteria need to be satisfied to ensure that workers are not exposed to unreasonable stresses. The different criteria, acceptable level for each criterion, and some of the available tools for job design and evaluation are listed in **Tables 9-7** and **9-8**.

The benefits of ergonomic job design may include the following:

1. Reduction in the incidence of injuries
2. Reduction in the severity of injuries (lost and restricted workdays)
3. Increase in productivity and improvement in quality
4. Reduction in cost
5. Decrease in the risk of litigation (Occupational Health and Safety Administration, Equal Employment Opportunity Commission, and so forth)

Snook, Campanelli, and Hart[156] reported that a worker was three times more susceptible to low back injury if the worker were performing a job that fewer than 75% of the working population could perform without overexertion. The authors suggested that the ergonomic approach would be more effective if jobs were designed so that they were within the physical capability of 90% of the working population. Other investigators have drawn more or less similar conclusions[11,32,80,109,118] and have shown that work-related injuries are related to job physical demands (**Fig. 9-17**).

Rowe believes that the real objective is to minimize disability rather than the incidence of injuries.[147, 148]

Table 9-8	Tools for ergonomic job evaluation.
Tool	**Criteria Evaluated**
Biomechanical models 2-D 3-D	Compressive and shear forces on LB Static strength
Psychophysical tables	Maximum acceptable weights and forces
Energy expenditure model	Energy expenditure
Revised NIOSH guide	Compressive force Strength Energy expenditure Epidemiology
Borg scales	Perceived stresses

2-D, *two-dimensional;* 3-D, *three-dimensional;* LB, *lower part of back;* NIOSH, *National Institute for Occupational Safety and Health.*

Table 9-7	Recommended ergonomic design criteria.
Criteria	**Acceptable Limit**
Compressive force	≤770 lb
Strength	≥75% capable
Energy expenditure	3.1 kcal/min (whole body) 2.2 kcal/min (arm work)
Heart rate	100-105 beats/min (whole body) 90-95 beats/min (arm work)
Postural stress	Avoid as much as possible Acceptable level depends on percent MVC, exertion time, and recovery time
Perceived stress	Light

MVC, *maximum voluntary contraction.*

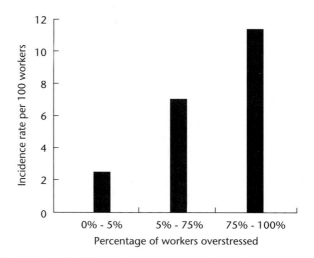

Figure 9-17 Effect of percentage of employees overstressed on incidence rates of back complaints per 100 workers. *(Adapted from Jensen RC:* Top Acute Care Trauma Rehabil *2(3):1-15, 1988, which is based on data from Liles et al.[115])*

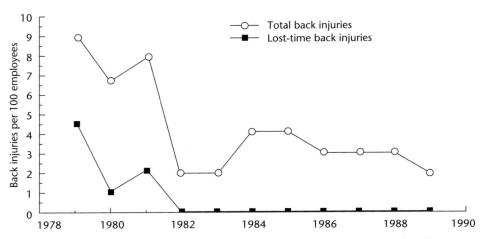

Figure 9-18 Ergonomic intervention (1982) has much greater impact on disability (lost-time back injuries) than on the incidence rate (total back injuries). *(Adapted from Ridyard DT: A successful applied ergonomics program for preventing occupational back injuries. In Das B, editor:* Advances in industrial ergonomics and safety II, *London, 1990, Taylor & Francis: pp 25-142.)*

Studies have shown that ergonomic job design has a much greater impact on disability than on the incidence of injuries (**Fig. 9-18**). Since ergonomic job design reduces job physical demands to accommodate a large percentage of workers, generally 75% to 90%, it may have the same effect as placing the workers on light-duty work.

TOOLS FOR JOB EVALUATION AND DESIGN

Motion and Time Study and Predetermined Motion-Time Data

The most common approach to establish production standards or expected work output from workers is a stopwatch time study or predetermined motion-time data systems.[12] Unfortunately, the primary emphasis from this approach is on time, that is, how long it takes to perform the job once working at normal speed. This approach does not address stress and strain on the body. Several different studies have shown that production standards based on a traditional approach (1) can result in very high energy expenditure and heart rates (**Fig. 9-19**)[6,64,129,195]; (2) are inconsistent with the physiological demands of work (**Fig. 9-19**)[6,64]; and (3) can produce unacceptable levels of biomechanical, psychophysical, and postural stress on the workers.[56] Work measurement gives the time required to perform a job; the time should be modified by some physiologic response of the body. Additionally, biomechanical, psychophysical, and ergonomic evaluations should be made to determine that these stresses do not exceed acceptable levels.

Worker Feedback

An alternative to a stopwatch time study is to obtain subjective feedback from the workers on (1) how stress-ful the job is and (2) which body part is most affected. Borg scales[21] (**Table 9-9**) can be used to quantify stresses perceived by workers. The advantage of this approach is that the analyst can have an integrated response of the body from all different types of stress on the worker. The disadvantage of this approach is that it is subjective and feedback from the worker can be affected by personal biases. Job dissatisfaction, pressure from co-workers, and disputes between management and unions can result in artificially high ratings. Similarly, the fear of loss of a job or the fear of an unfavorable reaction from management can cause artificially low ratings.

In spite of these limitations, obtaining subjective feedback from workers is often worthwhile because it is sometimes not possible to simulate all the different physical requirements of a job. Also, workers may perform some tasks that are not observed by the analyst. Regarding an acceptable level of perceived stress, under controlled laboratory conditions studies have shown that during maximum voluntary exertion for static strength, isokinetic strength, and maximum acceptable weights and work loads, subjects generally give ratings of perceived exertion (RPE) between 13 and 15 on the Borg RPE scale.[58] Similarly, Owen and Garg[58] reported RPE scores of 13 to 15 for manually lifting and transferring of patients in a long-term healthcare facility. Garg, Hagglund, and Mericle[64] reported RPE scores between 13 and 16.5 from order selectors in three different grocery warehouses. Based on these studies it appears that for safe job design, the RPE should be less than 13. In the absence of epidemiologic studies relating RPE scores to the incidence of injuries, a value of about 11 (light) seems to be more reasonable.

Biomechanical Models

Simple two-dimensional static-strength models are available to simulate the physical requirements and

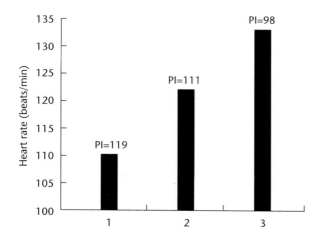

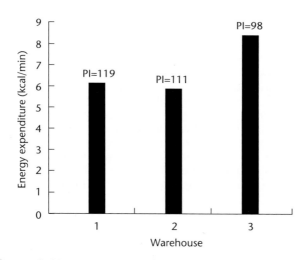

Figure 9-19 Heart rates and energy expenditures from three different warehouses. Mean performance standards (*PI*) based on a traditional approach are also listed. *(Adapted from Garg A, Hagglund G, Mericle K: AIIE Trans 18:235-245, 1986.)*

Table 9-9	Borg scales for subjective feedback.
Borg's RPE Scale	**Borg's CR-10 Scale**
6 No exertion at all	0 Nothing at all
7	0.5 Extremely weak (just
8 Extremely light	noticeable)
9 Very light	1 Very weak
10	2 Weak (light)
11 Light	3 Moderate
12	4
13 Somewhat hard	5 Strong (heavy)
14	6
15 Hard	7 Very strong
16	8
17 Very hard	9
18	10 Extremely strong (almost
19 Extremely hard	maximal)
20 Maximal	• Maximal

RPE, *rating of perceived exertion*
From Borg G: Scand J Work Environ Health 16*(suppl):55-58, 1990.*

The estimated compressive force can be compared with the acceptable limit of 770 lb to determine how hazardous the job is. Regarding strength, the lowest percentile value from the six different body joints (elbow, shoulder, L5/S1, hip, knee, and ankle) is used.

In **Figure 9-20**, a value of 72% for the hip joint for females shows that the simulated lifting task would produce the maximum stress on the hip joint. Further, it estimates that about 72% of female workers have sufficient strength to lift the 54-lb load in the posture shown without overexertion. The remaining female workers would be overexerting themselves when attempting to lift this load. The estimated compressive forces of 960 and 862 lb on male and female spines exceed the 770-lb value recommended by NIOSH.[133,171]

Detailed three-dimensional biomechanical models of the trunk are also available.* However, major assumptions are made in the estimation of internal muscle forces because of the statically indeterminate system. At present it is not clear under what conditions antagonistic muscles and ligaments play an important role and the biomechanical objective function that the body attempts to minimize. It is also difficult to obtain postural data in three dimensions in an industrial setting, and small errors in postural data can lead to large errors in model prediction. Therefore the user should be well trained and very careful when these models are used.

One criticism of static models is that lifting is a dynamic activity. Static models tend to underestimate forces and moments because the inertial loads are ignored.[†] Some of these models are EMG driven.[103,116,117,122,123] However, muscle recruitment

resulting compressive force on the L5/S1 disk. One such model is available from the Center for Ergonomics, University of Michigan (**Fig. 9-20**). Use of the model requires data on posture (body link angles), nature of the task involved (the lifting, pushing, pulling, and so forth), number of hands used (one or two), and magnitude of force (the weight lifted). Postural data are usually obtained from a photograph showing a side view of the worker (sagittal-plane photograph). The model also allows the option of selecting different heights and body weights to represent different-sized workers. Output from the model includes (1) the estimated compressive force on the L5/S1 disk for male and female subjects and (2) the percentage of capable males and females based on static-strength simulation of the job.

*References 17, 85, 103, 123, 151, 152.
†References 25, 51, 61, 85, 116, 117, 165.

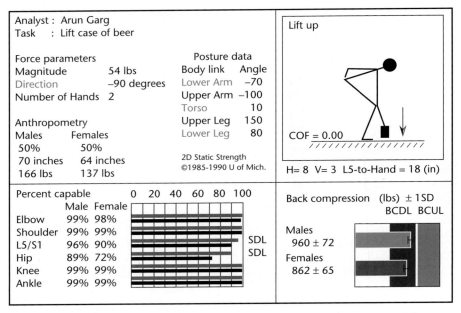

Figure 9-20 Printout from the University of Michigan's two-dimensional static-strength model.

patterns may vary from person to person and from time to time in any one person.[43,134,151,153] Task variables can affect the relationship between force and EMG values.[135] At present, the dynamic biomechanical models are of limited practical use in analyzing the stress from manual handling jobs in an industrial setting:

1. Ultimate compressive strengths of lumbar vertebral bodies are not available under different dynamic loading conditions.
2. Volitional muscle strengths and tissue limits for various body joints have not been systematically studied as a function of angular velocity and acceleration.
3. The human body has viscoelastic properties and may tolerate much higher forces for a very short duration.
4. It is difficult to obtain postural data in three dimensions as a function of time.
5. A large number of assumptions are made to determine internal forces, especially under asymmetric lifting conditions. Inclusion of dynamic factors may compound these errors.

It is concluded that for the present, one has to rely on static biomechanical models to determine compressive and shear forces on the spine from manual material handling jobs in an industrial setting.

Energy Expenditure Model

The most comprehensive and widely used model for estimating energy expenditure for manual material handling jobs is from Garg, Chaffin, and Herrin.[62] The model is based on the assumption that a job can be divided into simple tasks and the average energy expenditure for the job can be predicted by estimating the energy expenditure of the simple tasks and the time duration of the job. Energy expenditure for simple tasks is estimated from regression equations based on experimental data. Energy expenditure for each task is a function of task variables (such as weight of the object, frequency, technique, distance, and height) and individual variables (such as body weight and gender). The average energy expenditure is simply equal to the sum of the energy demands of the tasks and maintenance of body postures averaged over time. Mathematically,

$$\dot{E}_{job} = \frac{\sum_{i=1}^{n} \dot{E}_p \times t_i + \sum_{j=1}^{m} \Delta E_{T_j}}{T} \tag{7}$$

where

$\dot{E}_{job}$ = Average energy expenditure for the job (kcal/min)
$\dot{E}_p$ = Energy expenditure for the ith posture (kcal/min)
t_i = Time spent in the ith posture (min)
n = Total number of body postures used in the job
ΔE_{T_j} = Net energy cost (over and above the maintenance of body posture) for the jth task in the job (kcal)
m = Total number of tasks in the job
T = Time duration of the job (min)

Model validation on 48 jobs resulted in a correlation of .95 and a coefficient of variation of 10%. The model accounted for 91% of the variation in measured energy expenditure. The model gives a structure to most factors, except training and environment, that affect energy expenditure in manual material handling jobs.

Task Number	Task	Task Description	Energy Expenditure (kcal/min)
	Table 9-10 Example of energy expenditure for various tasks using Garg's model.		
1	Lifting	25 lb, 4 times, stoop, floor to 30-in height	1.19
2	Turning 180 degrees	4 times with 25-lb load	0.33
3	Carrying	4 times, 25 lb, against thighs, 10 ft at 2.5 mph	1.22
4	Setting the object on the conveyor	6 times, 25 lb	0.43
5	Turning back	6 times, 0 lb	0.28
6	Walking back	6 times, 10 ft at 3 mph	0.71
7	Posture	Standing	1.53
TOTAL			5.69

From Garg A, Beller D: A comparison of isokinetic lifting strength with static strength and maximum acceptable weight with special reference to speed of lifting, Ergonomics *37: 1363-1374, 1994.*

Furthermore, partitioning of a job into task factors also shows which particular tasks are most stress producing and is thus useful for job design.

As an example, consider the following job. A worker lifts a 25-lb compact box from the floor, turns 180 degrees, carries the object against the thighs 10 feet at 2.5 mph, sets the object on a conveyor belt, turns back (180 degrees), and walks back to the machine at 3 mph. The job is performed four times per minute. The energy expenditures for the different tasks are shown in **Table 9-10**.

The compressive force and the strength requirement of the aforementioned job are well within the acceptable criteria. However, **Table 9-10** shows that the energy expenditure requirements are excessive. Only a few selected male and female workers can be expected to maintain 5.69 kcal/min for an 8-hour workday. If the machine can be placed close to the conveyor, thus eliminating carrying and walking, the energy expenditure will be reduced to 3.76 kcal/min. Raising the machine so that the worker does not have to lift from the floor will further reduce the energy expenditure.

REVISED NIOSH LIFTING EQUATION

The principal products of the revised NIOSH lifting equation[171] are the recommended weight limit (RWL) and the lifting index (LI). The RWL is defined as the weight of the load that nearly all healthy workers could lift and/or lower for a specific set of task conditions and over a period of time (up to 8 hours) without an increased risk of lifting-related overexertion or low back injury developing. The LI provides a relative estimate of the level of physical stress associated with a particular manual lifting task.

Assumptions and Limitations

The lifting equation is limited to the following conditions for which it was designed:

- A two-handed, smooth, continuous lifting motion is used. The equation is not applicable to one-handed lifting or if the lifting task is performed at high speed.
- The lifting posture is unrestricted. The lifting equation is not applicable if the task is performed in a constrained or restricted work space.
- Foot traction is adequate. Worker/floor surface coupling provides at least a 0.4 (preferably 0.5) coefficient of static friction.
- The ambient environment is moderate. Extremes of temperature, humidity, or vibration add additional stress to the worker. Independent heart rate assessments would be needed to account for the added effects of temperature and/or humidity.
- Other manual handling activities (such as holding, walking, carrying, climbing, pushing, and pulling) are minimal. Independent measures of energy expenditure[62] are required if other nonlifting activities are common.
- A smooth, continuous lowering motion can be treated as lifting.
- Object length (frontal-plane dimension) is less than or equal to 25 inches (65 cm). To be more exact, separation between the hands should be less than 25 inches.

Criteria for the Revised Lifting Equation

The revised NIOSH lifting equation is based on four criteria, which are summarized in **Table 9-11**. If the weight of the object is less than or equal to the RWL, the lifting task will satisfy the criteria listed in **Table 9-11**.

Table 9-11	Criteria for recommended weight limit.
Criteria	**Limit**
Compressive force	770 lb (350 kg)
Strength	≥ 75% for females 99% for males
Energy expenditure Near floor level Bench height	≤3.12 kcal/min ≤2.18 kcal/min
Epidemiologic	Nominal risk

From Garg A, Chaffin DB, Herrin GD: Am Ind Hyg Assoc J 39:661-674, 1978.

DEFINITIONS

1. Recommended Weight Limit

$$RWL = LC \times HM \times VM \times DM \times AM \times CM \times FM \quad (8)$$

where

LC = Load constant
HM = Horizontal multiplier
VM = Vertical multiplier
DM = Distance multiplier
AM = Asymmetric multiplier
CM = Coupling multiplier
FM = Frequency multiplier

The six multipliers are the penalties for deviating from the ideal lifting situation. The ideal lifting situation is defined as lifting at a 30-inch (75 cm) height, with hands close to the body (up to 10 inches [25 cm] from the ankles), to a distance of up to 10 inches (25 cm), with no twisting, with good grasp, with a lifting frequency of once every 5 minutes or less, and with the lifting duration not to exceed 1 hour.

Because the six multipliers are penalties, none of them can be more than 1. In other words, under ideal conditions when all six multipliers are 1, RWL = LC. Therefore, the load constant is the maximum weight allowed to be lifted to satisfy the four criteria in **Table 9-11**.

2. Lifting Index

$$LI = \frac{\text{Load weight (lb)}}{\text{Recommended weight limit (lb)}} \quad (9)$$

The job is considered "safe" if the LI is less than or equal to 1. As the LI increases, the risk of overexertion injury increases. However, the relationship between the risk of injury and LI is not linear. An LI of 2.0 is worse than an LI of 1.5.

3. Load Constant

The load constant is 51 lb (23 kg).

4. Horizontal Multiplier

$$HM = (10/H) \quad (10)$$

a. Ten inches ≤ H ≤ 25 inches.
b. If $H < 10$ inches, $HM = 1.0$.
c. If $H > 25$ inches, $HM = 0$.
d. H is defined as the horizontal location (inches) of the hands forward of the midpoint between the ankles at the origin (beginning) of the lift (**Fig. 9-21**), or the horizontal distance from the ankles (malleolus) to the center of the grasp (middle knuckle). If the two hands and/or feet are not symmetric, H can be determined as

$$H = \frac{(H \text{ for right hand} + H \text{ for left hand})}{2} \quad (11)$$

It is strongly recommended that H be measured. In those situations where H cannot be measured and a rough estimate is desired, H can be estimated as follows:

$$H = 8 + W/2 \quad (\text{for } V \geq 10 \text{ inches}) \quad (12)$$
$$H = 10 + W/2 \quad (\text{for } V < 10 \text{ inches}) \quad (13)$$

where V = vertical height of the hands from the floor.

5. Vertical Multiplier

$$VM = (1 - .0075 \,|\, V - 30|) \quad (14)$$

a. $0 \leq V \leq 70$ inches.
b. If $V < 0$ inches, $VM = 0$
c. If $V > 70$ inches, $VM = 0$
d. V is the vertical location of the hands (inches) above the floor at the origin (beginning) of the lift (**Fig. 9-22**).

6. Distance Multiplier

$$DM = (0.82 + 1.8/D) \quad (15)$$

a. 10 inches ≤ D ≤ 70 inches.
b. If $D < 10$ inches, $DM = 1.0$.
c. If $D > 70$ inches, $DM = 0$.
d. D is the vertical travel distance of the hands (inches) between the destination (end point) or the highest point during the lift and origin of the lift (**Fig. 9-23**). D can be estimated as follows:

$$D = V \text{ at destination} - V \text{ at origin} \quad (16)$$

7. Asymmetric Multiplier

$$AM = (1 - .0032 \times A) \quad (17)$$

a. Zero ≤ A ≤ 135 degrees
b. If $A > 135$ degrees, $AM = 0$
c. A is the asymmetric angle. It is defined as the angle that the asymmetry line makes from the midsagittal plane in degrees (**Fig. 9-23**). The asymmetry line is defined as the line joining the midpoint between the ankles with the midpoint of the hands projected on the floor. When the hands are in front of the feet (in the sagittal plane), $A = 0$. When the hands are oriented at 90 degrees as compared with the feet, $A = 90$ degrees. The asymmetric angle (A)

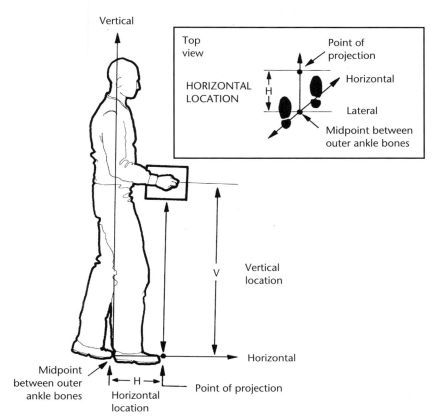

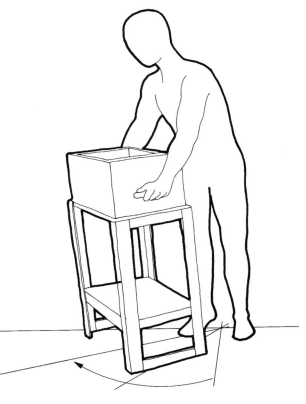

Figure 9-21 Definition of horizontal distance (*H*) used in the revised NIOSH lifting equation. *(Adapted from Waters TR et al: Ergonomics 36:749-776, 1993; personal communications with T Waters.)*

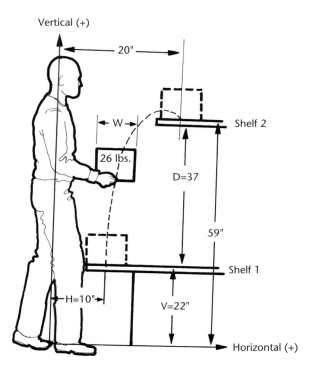

Figure 9-22 Definitions of vertical location (*V*) and travel distance (*D*) used in the revised NIOSH lifting equation. *(Adapted from Waters TR et al: Ergonomics 36(7):749-776, 1993; personal communications with T. Waters.)*

Figure 9-23 Definition of the asymmetric angle (*A*) used in the revised NIOSH lifting equation.

Table 9-12	Coupling multiplier.	
Coupling	V < 30 in (< 75 cm)	V ≥ 30 in (≥ 75 cm)
Good	1.0	1.0
Fair	0.95	1.0
Poor	0.90	0.90

V, *vertical height.*

includes twisting at different body joints such as the ankles, knees, hips, pelvis, trunk, and shoulders.

8. Coupling Multiplier

The coupling multiplier, given in **Table 9-12**, depends on the type of coupling (good, fair, or poor) and the vertical height of the hands at the beginning of the lift.

The following are the definitions of good, fair, and poor couplings:

Good
- $L \leq 16$ inches (40 cm), $H \leq 12$ inches (30 cm), and good handles (or hand-hold cutouts)
- Easy to handle loose parts and objects with wrap-around grasp and without excessive wrist deviation

Fair
- $L \leq 16$ inches (40 cm), $H \leq 12$ inches (30 cm), and poor handles (or hand-hold cutouts)
- $L \leq 16$ inches (40 cm), $H \leq 12$ inches (30 cm), and 90-degree fingers can be flexed 90 degrees (for example, when lifting a box without handles)
- Easy-to-handle loose parts and objects with 90-degree finger flexion and without excessive wrist deviation

Poor
- $L > 16$ inches (40 cm) or
- $H > 12$ inches (30 cm) or
- Difficult-to-handle parts or
- Sagging objects or
- Asymmetric center of mass or
- Unstable contents or
- Hard-to-grasp object or
- Use of gloves

Good handles
- Length ≥ 4.5 inches (11.5 cm)
- Diameter = 0.75 to 1.5 inches (1.9 to 3.8 cm)
- Clearance between the handle and the object ≥ 2 inches (5 cm)
- Cylindrical shape
- Smooth, nonslip surface

Good hand-hold cutouts
- Length ≥ 4.5 inches (11.5 cm)
- Height ≥ 1.5 inches (3.8 cm)

- Clearance ≥ 2 inches (5 cm)
- Thickness ≥ 0.43 inches (1.1 cm)
- Semioval shape
- Smooth, nonslip surface

9. Frequency Multiplier

The frequency multiplier, given in **Table 9-13**, is a function of the frequency of lifting (lifts per minute), the vertical height of the hands at the beginning of the lift (V), and the duration of continuous lifting. Frequency (*F*) is defined as the number of lifts per minute. The following recommendations are made regarding the frequency multiplier:

- If *F* is less than 0.2 lifts per minute (once every 5 minutes), $F = 0.2$.
- Use frequency averaged over 15 minutes.
- Add all the periods of lifting in one shift to determine duration.
- Separate high-frequency and low-frequency durations and analyze them separately.

10. Rest Allowances

The revised NIOSH lifting equation requires mandatory rest allowances (RT) depending on the job's physical demands. Work time (WT) is the period spent doing work on the job. The following guidelines are recommended to determine the amount of RT if needed (see guidelines for RT, item 11):

- **If continuous lifting duration ≤ 1 hour,**

$$\text{Rest time (min)} = 1.2 \times \text{Work time (min)} \tag{18}$$

- **If continuous lifting duration ≤ 2 hours,**

$$\text{Rest time (min)} = 0.3 \times \text{Work time (min)} \tag{19}$$

- **If continuous lifting duration ≤ 8 hours,**

No additional fatigue allowances other than normal allowances (midmorning break, lunch break, midafternoon break) (20)

11. Guidelines for Allowances

a. If object weight $\leq$ RWL for 8 hours, *no* additional allowance is required.
b. RWL for 8 hours < object weight $\leq$ RWL for 2 hours, RT = 0.3 × WT, provided WT $\leq$ 2 hours
c. RWL for 2 hours < object weight $\leq$ RWL for 1 hour, RT = 1.20 × WT, provided WT $\leq$ 1 hour
d. If object weight > RWL for 1 hour, Not recommended without administrative and/or engineering controls
e. Light work can be performed during RT.

12. Origin and Destination Analysis

- Compute the RWL at the origin of the lifting/lowering task.
- For tasks requiring significant control at the destination of lifting/lowering

Table 9-13	Frequency multiplier.					
			Work Duration			
Frequency	**≤ 8 hr**		**≤ 2 hr**		**≤ 1 hr**	
(Lifts/min)	**V < 30 in**	**V ≥ 30 in**	**V < 30 in**	**V ≥ 30 in**	**V < 30 in**	**V ≥ 30 in**
0.2	0.85	0.85	0.95	0.95	1.00	1.00
0.5	0.81	0.81	0.92	0.92	0.97	0.97
1	0.75	0.75	0.88	0.88	0.94	0.94
2	0.65	0.65	0.84	0.84	0.91	0.91
3	0.55	0.55	0.79	0.79	0.88	0.88
4	0.45	0.45	0.72	0.72	0.84	0.84
5	0.35	0.35	0.60	0.60	0.80	0.80
6	0.27	0.27	0.50	0.50	0.75	0.75
7	0.22	0.22	0.42	0.42	0.70	0.70
8	0.18	0.18	0.35	0.35	0.60	0.60
9	0.00	0.15	0.30	0.30	0.52	0.52
10	0.00	0.13	0.26	0.26	0.45	0.45
11	0.00	0.00	0.00	0.23	0.41	0.41
12	0.00	0.00	0.00	0.21	0.37	0.37
13	0.00	0.00	0.00	0.00	0.00	0.34
14	0.00	0.00	0.00	0.00	0.00	0.31
15	0.00	0.00	0.00	0.00	0.00	0.28
>15	0.00	0.00	0.00	0.00	0.00	0.00

V, *vertical height.*
Note: 30 inches = 75 cm.

—Compute the RWLs at both the origin and destination.
—Take the lower of the RWLs at the origin and destination.
• Both origin and destination analyses are *required* if the
—Worker has to regrasp the load near the destination.
—Worker has to momentarily hold the object at the destination.
—Worker has to position or guide the load at the destination.

13. Simple-Task (Single-Task) versus Multiple-Task Analysis

Before data collection, the analyst must determine whether the job should be analyzed as a single-task or multiple-manual lifting task.

• A *single-task* job is defined as a lifting job in which the task variables (H, V, D, A, C, or F) do not significantly change from task to task. This analysis can also be used if only one task is of interest (e.g., worst-case task). Obviously, the latter analysis will ignore the cumulative effect of other tasks.
• *Multiple-task manual lifting jobs* are jobs in which there are significant differences in one or more task variables. A specialized procedure is used to analyze multitask manual lifting jobs. (A computer program entitled "Revised NIOSH Guide Program for Manual Lifting" is available from the author.)

14. Procedure for Analyzing Lifting/Lowering Jobs (Single-Task Analysis)

a. Determine whether the job needs to be analyzed only at the origin (beginning) of the lift or at both the origin and destination of the lift.

Table 9-14 The six multipliers for the revised NIOSH equation.

HORIZONTAL MULTIPLIER (HM)			
H (in)	HM	H (in)	HM
< 10	1.00	18	0.56
10	1.00	19	0.53
11	0.91	20	0.50
12	0.83	21	0.48
13	0.77	22	0.45
14	0.71	23	0.43
15	0.67	24	0.42
16	0.63	25	0.40
17	0.59	>25	0

DISTANCE MULTIPLIER (DM)			
D (in)	DM	D (in)	DM
< 10	1.00	22	0.90
10	1.00	24	0.90
11	0.98	25	0.89
12	0.97	30	0.88
13	0.96	35	0.87
14	0.95	40	0.87
15	0.94	50	0.86
16	0.93	60	0.85
18	0.92	70	0.85
20	0.91	>70	0

VERTICAL MULTIPLIER (VM)			
V (in)	VM	V (in)	VM
0	0.78	38	.94
2	0.79	40	0.93
4	0.81	42	0.91
6	0.82	44	4.90
8	0.84	46	0.88
10	0.85	48	0.87
12	0.87	50	0.85
14	0.88	52	0.84
16	0.90	54	0.82
18	0.91	56	0.81
20	0.93	58	0.79
22	0.94	60	0.78
24	0.96	62	0.76
26	0.97	64	0.75
28	0.99	66	0.73
30	1.00	68	0.72
32	0.99	70	0.70
34	0.97	>70	0
36	0.96		

ASYMMETRIC MULTIPLIER (AM)			
A (degrees)	AM	A (degrees)	AM
0	1.00	75	0.76
5	0.98	80	0.74
10	0.97	85	0.73
15	0.95	90	0.71
20	0.94	95	0.70
25	0.92	100	0.68
30	0.90	105	0.66
35	0.89	110	0.65
40	0.87	115	0.63
45	0.86	120	0.62
50	0.84	125	0.60
55	0.82	130	0.58
60	0.81	135	0.57
65	0.79	>135	0
70	0.78		

From Waters TR et al: Ergonomics 36:749-776, 1993.

| Table 9-14 | The six multipliers for the revised NIOSH equation—continued. |

COUPLING MULTIPLIER (CM)

Coupling	V < 30 in	V ≥ 30 in
Good	1.0	1.0
Fair	0.95	1.0
Poor	0.90	0.90

FREQUENCY MULTIPLIER TABLE

Frequency	Work duration					
	≤8 hr		≤2 hr		≤1 hr	
(Lifts/mi)	V < 30 in	V ≥ 30 in	V < 30 in	V ≥ 30 in	V < 30 in	V ≥ 30 in
0.2	0.85	0.85	0.95	0.95	1.00	1.00
0.5	0.81	0.81	0.92	0.92	0.97	0.97
1	0.75	0.75	0.88	0.88	0.94	0.94
2	0.65	0.65	0.84	0.84	0.91	0.91
3	0.55	0.55	0.79	0.79	0.88	0.88
4	0.45	0.45	0.72	0.72	0.84	0.84
5	0.35	0.35	0.60	0.60	0.80	0.80
6	0.27	0.27	0.50	0.50	0.75	0.75
7	0.22	0.22	0.42	0.42	0.70	0.70
8	0.18	0.18	0.35	0.35	0.60	0.60
9	0.00	0.15	0.30	0.30	0.52	0.52
10	0.00	0.13	0.26	0.26	0.45	0.45
11	0.00	0.00	0.00	0.23	0.41	0.41
12	0.00	0.00	0.00	0.21	0.37	0.37
13	0.00	0.00	0.00	0.00	0.00	0.34
14	0.00	0.00	0.00	0.00	0.00	0.31
15	0.00	0.00	0.00	0.00	0.00	0.28
>15	0.00	0.00	0.00	0.00	0.00	0.00

b. Collect data on the average and maximum weight of the object—H, V, D, A, C, F, and duration of lifting in hours, either at the origin or at both the origin and destination of the lift.

c. Determine the six multipliers by using either the formulas or **Table 9-14**.

d. Compute RWL by multiplying 51 lb and the six multipliers (see Equation 8).

e. Compute LI by dividing the weight of the object by the RWL (see Equation 9).

f. Determine whether the job is "safe" or needs improvement.

15. Example (Single-Task Analysis)

Consider a job called "loading punch press stock." The job requires lifting a supply reel and loading it into

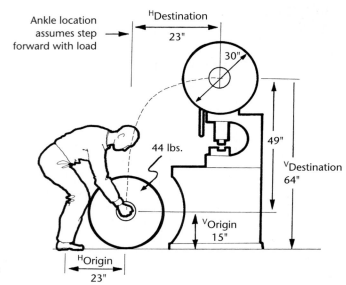

Figure 9-24 Loading punch press stock; example discussed in the text.

a punch press (**Fig. 9-24**). Because the worker has to hold the supply reel to guide it into the punch press, the job is analyzed at both the origin and destination of the lift. The job is performed once per shift, and it takes 1 minute to load the supply reel. Therefore the duration of continuous lifting is less than 1 hour and frequency of lifting is less than once every 5 minutes. The supply reel weighs 44 lb. Assume that the following measurements were made on the six task variables:

Variable	Origin	Destination
H	23 in	23 in
V	15 in	64 in
D	49 in	49 in
A	0	0
C	Fair	Fair
F	<0.2	<0.2

Next, the multipliers corresponding to the six task variables are obtained from **Table 9-14**, and the RWLs are computed at both the origin and destination of the lift by multiplying the six multipliers and the load constant of 51 lb:

	LC	HM	VM	DM	AM	CM	FM	RWL
Origin	51	0.43	0.89	0.86	1	0.95	1	15.9
Destination	51	0.43	0.75	0.86	1	1	1	14.1

The smaller of the RWLs at the origin and destination is 14.1 lb. Therefore the RWL for this job is 14.1 lb. The

Lifting Index is computed as follows:

$$LI = \frac{44}{14.1} = 3.12$$

The analysis shows that the greatest penalty or hazard from performing this job is the horizontal multiplier, which has a value of 0.43, or a 57% (1 − 0.43) penalty for reaching and lifting at a horizontal distance of 23 inches. Therefore efforts should be directed to reduce *H*. There is no penalty for the frequency of lifting and the asymmetric angle. The other three variables (vertical location, travel distance, and coupling) have relatively much smaller penalties.

The LI of 3.12 suggests that the job is unsafe for most female and male workers. The job can be made safer by using engineering controls such as a mechanical device (hoist, small crane) to load the supply reel. Although engineering controls are the most desired solution to manual material handling problems, they may be expensive. An alternate solution is administrative controls such as using two workers to lift and load the supply reels. The disadvantage is that this would require education and training of workers and some kind of enforcement that always requires two workers to load the supply reel. The data were collected again with two workers lifting the supply reel, and RWLs were computed as follows. Note that in this case the supply reel is placed flat on the floor and there is 30-degree asymmetry at the destination. Further, the couplings are assumed to be poor at the destination.

	H	V	D	A	C	F
Origin	10	0	64	0	Fair	<0.2
Destination	10	64	64	30	Poor	<0.2

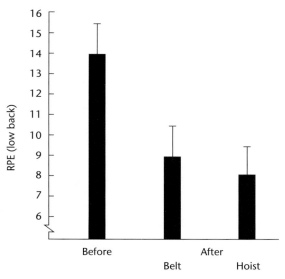

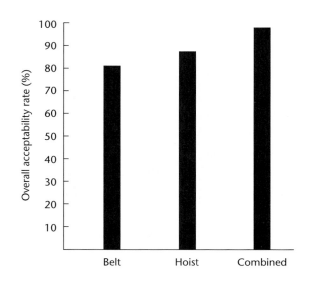

Figure 9-25 Acceptability rates and ratings for perceived exertion before and after ergonomic intervention. *(Based on data from Garg A, Owen B:* Ergonomics *35:1353-1375, 1992.)*

	LC	HM	VM	DM	AM	CM	FM	RWL
Origin	51	1.0	0.78	0.85	1.0	0.95	1.0	32.1
Destination	51	1.0	0.75	0.85	0.90	0.90	1.0	26.3

$$RWL = 26.3 \text{ lb}$$
$$WT = \frac{44}{2} = 22 \text{ lb}$$
$$LI = \frac{22}{26.3} = 0.84$$

Now, the LI of 0.84 is less than 1. Therefore the job is much safer than before. According to the revised NIOSH guide, more than 75% of females and practically all male workers can perform this job without a significant risk of overexertion injury or back injury.

In the analysis just presented, the weight of the supply reel per worker was assumed to be 22 lb; that is, it was assumed that the weight was equally divided between the two workers. Even with 40% and 60% weight distribution—with 18 lb of weight supported by one worker and 26 lb by the other—the job will be safe. The highest LI will be 26/26, or 1.0.

A CASE STUDY USING ERGONOMICS

Simple ergonomic interventions can have a powerful impact on work-related overexertion injuries, even in occupations that are known to have very high incident and severity rates for back injuries. Nursing personnel have both high injury and disability rates, which appear to be rising; rates are higher than the published statistics, and nurses perceive back pain as an inevitable part of the job. The problem appears to be greater in nursing homes than in hospitals.[66]

Attempts to lower the injury rates in hospitals and nursing homes have focused on the worker (nurses and nursing aides). These include education and training on lifting techniques, body mechanics, back care, and physical fitness. However, this type of approach has had little impact. The problem of lifting a patient is more difficult than lifting a heavy weight. A patient's weight, shape, size, unpredictability, and combativeness, space limitations, and unadjustable furniture make the job very hazardous.[66]

Garg and Owen[66] concentrated on reducing job physical demands. A prospective epidemiologic study was performed in two units (140 beds and 57 nursing assistants [NAs]) of a nursing home. These two units were selected because the residents were the most difficult to handle. The study involved the following phases:

1. A determination of patient-handling tasks perceived to be most stressful by the NAs[137]
2. An ergonomic evaluation of the work performed by NAs before the introduction of change[67]
3. A pilot study to identify and locate assistive devices, to establish criteria for their selection, and to perform preliminary trials of these devices[136]
4. A laboratory study to select patient-handling devices that were less stressful than existing methods in the nursing home[72,73]
5. The introduction of selected devices in the nursing home and training of NAs in their use with patients (intervention)
6. Postintervention measurement of back injury incidence and severity rates, acceptability rates, biomechanical task demands, and perceived level of physical stress[66]

Selected devices and interventions included shower chairs, walking belts using a gentle rocking and pulling technique, carefully selected hoists, ramp-type weighing

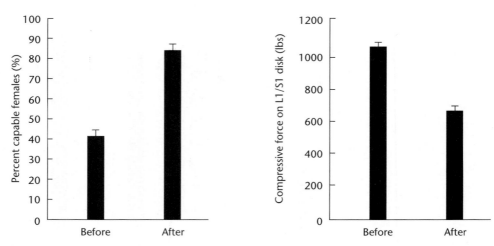

Figure 9-26 Effects of ergonomic intervention on estimated force and strength requirements of the job. *(Based on data from Garg A, Owen B:* Ergonomics *35:1353-1375, 1992.)*

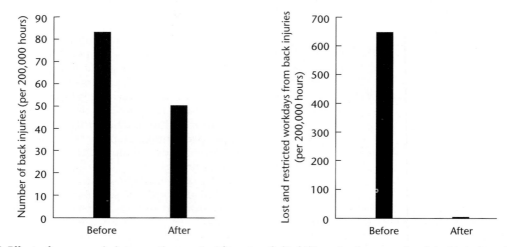

Figure 9-27 Effect of ergonomic intervention on incidence and disability rates from work-related injuries. *(Based on data from Garg A, Owen B:* Ergonomics *35:1353-1375, 1992.)*

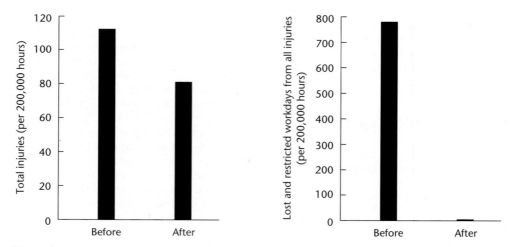

Figure 9-28 Effect of ergonomic intervention on incidence and disability rates from all work related injuries. *(Based on data from Garg A, Owen B:* Ergonomics *35:1353-1375, 1992.)*

scales, raising of commodes, adjustment of toilet hand rails, adaptive clothing for some residents, modification of shower rooms, and so forth. Postintervention data were collected for 9 months in unit 1 and for 4 months in unit 2.

The study found very high acceptability of these recommendations (**Fig. 9-25**). Regarding stress on the spine, compression was reduced from an average of 1067 lb before intervention to 440 lb after intervention (**Fig. 9-26**). The strength requirements of the job decreased considerably after intervention (**Fig. 9-26**). Subjectively, the mean rating of perceived exertion on the Borg RPE scale dropped from "somewhat hard" and "hard" to less than "very light" (**Fig. 9-27**).

The incidence rate for back injuries dropped by almost 50% (**Fig. 9-27**). Most importantly, not a single day was lost or restricted because of back injuries after the intervention (**Fig. 9-27**). Injuries to other parts of the body showed similar patterns (**Fig. 9-28**).

The use of resident transferring equipment resulted in an elimination or a reduction in certain resident-handling transfers. This has an important implication, inasmuch as it is believed that each stressful patient-handling event involves some risk of back and overexertion injury and this risk can be minimized by reducing the number of stressful patient-handling transfers.[87]

The study shows that ergonomic interventions need not be complicated or expensive to be effective, but they must be developed thoughtfully. Management commitment, worker participation, and consultation with both management and workers are essential for ergonomic intervention to be effective.

PUSHING AND PULLING

Pushing and pulling objects account for 9% of all back strains and sprains[99] and 18% of all back injuries.[156] Patients with LBP are more likely to engage in more pushing and pulling than patients without LBP.[36,52] The primary concerns with pushing and pulling objects include

1. High forces on the spine
2. High strength requirements
3. Risk of slipping and falling
4. Body posture

Lee[107] estimated that compressive forces on the L5/S1 disk were lower for pushing than for pulling. In pushing, the external force moments were often found to act in extension and the stabilizing muscles were the rectus abdominus rather than the erector spinae. For pushing, there was no significant effect of grip height on compressive force. For pulling, the compressive force increased significantly with a decrease in grip height from 43 inches (109 cm) to 26 inches (66 cm). In addition, there was a slight increase in compressive force when the grip height was raised from 43 inches to 60 inches. Thus based on compressive force, the ideal grip height

appears to be about 43 inches. The observation that pushing is less stressful than pulling is also supported by IAP measurements. Davis and Stubbs[37] showed that tensing of the anterior abdominal muscles creates higher gastric pressure when pushing than when pulling. The increased pressures during pushing may provide additional spinal stabilization. Finally, body weight is used more effectively in pushing than in pulling because subjects tend to incline the torso more in pushing than in pulling. This assists in counterbalancing the push force on the hands.

Static pushing and pulling strengths decrease with an increase in handle height (**Table 9-15**).[30,60] Thus there appears to be a trade-off between compressive force on the spine and pushing/pulling force capability. Snook and Ciriello[157] have provided data on maximum acceptable pushing and pulling forces. An example of such data is shown in **Table 9-15**. The data suggest significant differences between males and females for peak force capability but small differences for sustained forces (**Table 9-16**).

The coefficient of friction between the shoes and the floor is very important in pushing and pulling activities. First, there is a risk of slipping and falling if the coefficient of friction is low. The static coefficient of friction between the shoes and floor should be at least 0.5 and preferably greater than 0.8.[29] Second, the coefficient of friction affects body posture. With a low coefficient of friction a person would probably stand more erect and thus not be able to use the body weight effectively

Table 9-15	Pushing and pulling static strengths.				
Handle Height (in)	**Pushing Force (lb)**		**Pulling Force (lb)**	
	Males	**Females**	**Males**	**Females**
27	90	35	84	40
43	77	40	57	37
60	64	33	40	31

From Chaffin DB, Andres RO, Garg A: Hum Factors 25:541–550, 1983.

Table 9-16	Maximum acceptable pushing force to accommodate 90% of the workers.	
Workers	**Peak force* (lb)**	**Sustained sorce* (lb)**
90% of males	57	29
90% of females	44	29

*One push of 50 feet every 5 minutes.
From Snook SH, Ciriello VM: Ergonomics 34:1197-1213, 1991.

(leaning forward for pushing and backward for pulling). A change in posture will also affect the compressive force on the spine. Finally, other studies have shown that static pushing and pulling strengths increase by about 50% (from 200 to 300 N for healthy young males) with an increase in the coefficient of friction from 0.3 to 0.6.[50,101]

When pushing objects, a person leans forward. Chaffin, Andres, and Garg[30] showed that 48 inches (120 cm) of horizontal clearance between the hands (or fixture being pushed) and the rearward ankle is required for an average-sized man. Kroemer and Robinson[101] recommended a 66-inch (165 cm) horizontal clearance for a large 95th percentile male. When pulling an object, a person leans backward. Ayoub and McDaniel[10] reported that it is best to place the ball of the forward foot close to or under the handle being pulled, thus allowing the person to lean back significantly.

In summary, the following recommendations are made for pushing and pulling objects:

- Pushing appears to be less stressful than pulling.
- Keep pushing and pulling forces low. The peak force should be less than 45 lb and sustained force less than 30 lb.
- Optimum handle height is approximately 36 inches (about hip height when erect). The range for handle height is 36 to 45 inch.
- Provide a high-friction walking surface and slip-resistant, lightweight shoes with toe protection.
- The surface grade should be less than 4 degrees, preferably less than 2 degrees.
- Good housekeeping is very important. Avoid cracked or broken floors. Maintain wheels.
- Provide adequate room to ensure optimum body posture.

References

1. Adams MA, Hutton WC: The effect of posture on the lumbar spine, *J Bone Joint Surg* Br 67:625-629, 1985.

2. Amendola A: *An investigation of the effects of external supports on manual lifting,* doctoral dissertation, College Station, 1989, Texas A & M University.

3. American Heart Association: *Exercise testing and training of apparently healthy individuals: a handbook for physicians,* Dallas, 1972, American Heart Association.

4. Anderson CK: *A biomechanical model of the lumbosacral joint for lifting activities,* doctoral dissertation, Ann Arbor, 1983, University of Michigan.

5. Anderson CK, Catterall MJ: The impact of physical ability testing on incidence rate, severity rate and productivity. In Asfour SS, editor: *Trends in ergonomics/human factors IV,* New York, Elsevier Science, Inc.

6. Aquilano NJ: A physiological evaluation of time standards for strenuous work as set by stopwatch time study and two predetermined motion time data systems, J Ind Eng 19:425-432, 1968.

7. Arad D, Ryan MD: The incidence and prevalence in nurses of low back pain: a definitive survey exposes the hazards, *Aust Nurses J,* 16:44-48, 1986.

8. Astrand NE: Medical, psychological and social factors associated with back abnormalities and self reported back pain: a cross-sectional study of male employees in a Swedish pulp and paper industry, *Br J Ind Med* 44:327-336, 1987.

9. Astrand PO, Rodahl K: *Textbook of work physiology,* New York, 1977, McGraw Hill.

10. Ayoub MM, McDaniel JW: Effects of operator stance on pushing and pulling tasks, *AIIE Trans* 6:185-195, 1974.

11. Ayoub MM, Selan JL, Liles DH: An ergonomics approach for the design of manual materials-handling tasks, *Hum Factors* 25:507-515, 1983.

12. Barnes RM: *Motion and time study—design and measurement of work,* ed 7, New York, 1980, John Wiley & Sons, Inc.

13. Bartelink DL: The role of abdominal pressure in relieving the pressure on the lumbar intervertebral discs, *J Bone Joint Surg* Br 39:718-725, 1957.

14. Battie MC et al: A prospective study of the role of cardiovascular risk factors and fitness in industrial back pain complaints, *Spine* 14:141-147, 1989.

15. Battie MC et al: Isometric lifting strength as a predictor of industrial back pain, *Spine* 14:851-856, 1989.

16. Battie MC et al: The role of flexibility in back pain complaints within industry: a prospective study, *Spine* 15:768-773, 1990.

17. Bean JC, Chaffin DB, Schultz AB: Biomechanical model calculation of muscle contraction forces: a double linear programming method, *J Biomech* 21:59-66, 1988.

18. Bergquist-Ullman M, Larson U: Acute low back pain in industry, *Acta Orthop Scand Suppl* 170:1-117, 1977.

19. Bigos S et al: Back injuries in industry: a retrospective study, II. Injury factors, *Spine* 11:246-251, 1986.

20. Bigos S et al: Back injuries in industry: a retrospective study, III. Employee-related factors, *Spine* 11:252-256, 1986.

21. Borg G: Psychophysical scaling with applications in physical work and the perception of exertion, *Scand J Work Environ Health* 16(suppl):55-58, 1990.

22. Bourne ND, Reilly T: Effect of a weightlifting belt on spinal shrinkage, *Br J Sports Med* 25:209-212, 1991.

23. Brigham CJ, Garg A: The role of biomechanical job evaluation in the reduction of overexertion injuries: a case study. Paper presented at the twenty-third annual American Industrial Hygiene Association conference, Philadelphia, 1983.

24. Brinckmann P, Biggemann M, Hilweg D: Fatigue fracture of human lumbar vertebrae, *Clin Biomech* 3(suppl 1):1-23, 1988.

25. Bush-Joseph C et al: Influences of dynamic factors on the lumbar spine movement in lifting, *Ergonomics* 31:211-216, 1988.

26. Cady LD et al: Strength and fitness and subsequent back injuries in firefighters, *J Occup Med* 21:269-272, 1979.

27. Caplan PS, Lester LMJ, Connelly TP: Degenerative joint disease of the lumbar spine in coal miners—a clinical and x-ray study, *Arthritis Rheum* 9:693-702, 1966.

28. Chaffin DB: Human strength capability and low back pain, *J Occup Med* 16:248-254, 1974.

29. Chaffin DB, Andersson GBJ: *Occupational biomechanics,* ed 2, New York, 1991, John Wiley & Sons, Inc.

30. Chaffin DB, Andres RO, Garg A: Volitional postures during maximal push/pull exertions in the sagittal plane, *Hum Factors* 25:541-550, 1983.

31. Chaffin DB, Herrin GD, Keyserling WM: Preemployment strength testing: an updated position, *J Occup Med* 20:403-408. 1978.

32. Chaffin DB, Park KS: A longitudinal study of low-back pain as associated with occupational weight lifting factors, *Am Ind Hyg Assoc J* 32:513-525, 1973.

33. Chaffin DB et al: *Pre-employment strength testing in selecting workers for materials handing jobs,* CDC Pub No 99-74-62, Cincinnatti, 1976, U.S. Department of Health and Human Services, National Institute for Occupational Safety and Health.

34. Cox M, Shephard RJ, Corey P: Influence of an employee fitness programme upon fitness, productivity and absenteeism, *Ergonomics* 24:795-806, 1981.

35. Cyron BM, Hutton WC: The fatigue strength of the lumbar neural arch in spondylolysis, *J Bone Joint Surg* Br 60:234-238, 1978.

36. Damkot DK et al: The relationship between work history, work environment and low-back pain in men, *Spine* 9:395-399, 1984.

37. Davis PR, Stubbs DA: Force limits in manual work, part III, *Applied Ergonom* 9:33-38, 1978.

38. Davis PR, Troup JDG: Pressures in the trunk cavities when pulling, pushing and lifting, *Ergonomics* 7:465-474, 1964.

39. Davis PR, Troup JDG, Burnhard JH: Movements of the thoracic and lumbar spine when lifting: a chronocyclophotographic study, *J Anat* 99:13-26, 1965.

40. Dehlin O, Hedenrud B, Horal J: Back symptoms in nursing aides in a geriatric hospital, *Scand J Rehab Med* 8:47-53, 1976.

41. Dehlin O et al: Effect of physical training and ergonomic counselling on the psychological perception of work and on the subjective assessment of low-back insufficiency, *Scand J Rehabil Med* 13:1-9, 1981.

42. Dehlin O et al: Muscle training, psychological perception of work and low back symptoms in nursing aides, *Scand J Rehabil Med* 10:201-209, 1978.

43. Donisch EW, Basmajian JV: Electromyography of deep back muscles in man, *Am J Anat* 133:25-36, 1972.

44. Eastman Kodak Company: *Ergonomic design for people at work,* vol 2, New York, 1986, Van Nostrand Reinhold.

45. Eie N: Load capacity of the low back, *J Oslo City Hosp* 16:75-98, 1966.

46. Eie N, Wehn P: Measurements of the intra-abdominal pressure in relation to weight bearing of the lumbo-sacral spine, *J Oslo City Hosp* 12:205-217, 1962.

47. Eklund JAE, Corlett EN: Shrinkage as a measure of the effect of load on the spine, *Spine* 9:189-194, 1984.

48. Farfan HF, Osteria V, Lamy C: The mechanical etiology of spondylolysis and spondylolisthesis, *Clin Orthop* 117:40-55, 1976.

49. Fiorini GT, McCommond D: Forces on lumbo-vertebral facets. *Ann of Biomed Eng* 4:354-363, 1976.

50. Fox WF: *Body weight and coefficient of friction determinants of pushing capability,* Human Engineering Special Studies Series No 17, Marrietta, GA, 1967, Lockheed Co.

51. Freivalds A et al: A dynamic biomechanical evaluation of lifting maximum acceptable loads, *J Biomech* 17:251-262, 1984.

52. Frymoyer JW et al: Epidemiologic studies of low-back pain, *Spine* 5:419-423, 1980.

53. Frymoyer JW et al: Risk factors in low-back pain, *J Bone Joint Surg Am* 65:213-218, 1983.

54. Garg A: *Basis for guide: biomechanical approach,* scientific support documentation for the revised 1991 NIOSH lifting equation, PO No 88-79303, NTIS Pub No PB91-226274, Springfield, Va, 1991, U.S. Department of Commerce.

55. Garg A: *Basis for guide: epidemiological approach,* scientific support documentation for the revised 1991 NIOSH lifting equation, PO No 88-79303, NTIS Pub No PB91-226274, Springfield, Va, 1991, U.S. Department of Commerce.

56. Garg A: Biomechanical and ergonomic stresses in warehouse operations, *AIIE Trans* 18:246-250, 1986.

57. Garg A, Badger D: Maximum acceptable weights and maximum voluntary strength for asymmetric lifting, *Ergonomics* 29:879-892, 1986.

58. Garg A, Banaag J: Maximum acceptable weights, heart rates and RPE's for one hour's repetitive asymmetric lifting, *Ergonomics* 31:77-96, 1988.

59. Garg A, Beller D: A comparison of isokinetic lifting strength with static strength and maximum acceptable weight with special reference to speed of lifting, *Ergonomics* 37: 1363-1374, 1994.

60. Garg A, Beller D: One-handed dynamic pulling strength with special reference to speed, handle height and angles of pulling, *Int J Ind Ergonom* 6:231-240, 1990.

61. Garg A, Chaffin DB, Freivalds A: Biomechanical stresses from manual load lifting: a static vs. dynamic evaluation, *AIIE Trans* 14:272-281, 1982.

62. Garg A, Chaffin DB, Herrin GD: Prediction of metabolic rates for manual materials handling jobs, *Am Ind Hyg Assoc J* 38:661-674, 1978.

63. Garg A, Funke S, Janisch D: One-handed dynamic pulling strength with special application to lawn mowers, *Ergonomics* 31:1139-1153, 1988.

64. Garg A, Hagglund G, Mericle K: A physiological evaluation of time standards for warehouse operations as set by traditional work measurement techniques, *AIIE Trans* 18(3):235-245, 1986.

65. Garg A, Herrin GD: Stoop or squat: a biomechanical and metabolic evaluation, *AIIE Trans* 11:293-302, 1979.

66. Garg A, Owen B: Reducing back stress to nursing personnel: an ergonomic intervention in a nursing home, *Ergonomics* 35:1353-1375, 1992.

67. Garg A, Owen BD, Carlson B: An ergonomic evaluation of nursing assistants' job in a nursing home, *Ergonomics* 35:979-995, 1992.

68. Garg A, Rodgers SH, Yates JW: The physiological basis for manual lifting. In Kumar S, editor: *Advances in industrial ergonomics and safety IV*. London, 1992, Taylor & Francis: pp. 867-874.

69. Garg A, Saxena U: Effects of lifting frequency and technique on physical fatigue with special references to psychophysical methodology and metabolic rate, *Am Ind Hyg Assoc J* 40:894-902, 1979.

70. Garg A, Saxena U: Maximum frequency acceptable to female workers for one-handed lifts in the horizontal plane, *Ergonomics* 25:839-853, 1982.

71. Garg A, Saxena U: Physiological stresses in warehouse operations with special reference to lifting technique and gender: a case study, *Am Ind Hyg Assoc J* 46:53-59, 1985.

72. Garg A et al: A biomechanical and ergonomic evaluation of patient transferring tasks: bed to wheelchair and wheelchair to bed, *Ergonomics* 34:289-312, 1991.

73. Garg A et al: A biomechanical and ergonomic evaluation of patient transferring tasks: wheelchair to shower chair and shower chair to wheelchair, *Ergonomics* 34:407-419, 1991.

74. Garg A et al: Biomechanical stresses as related to motion trajectory of lifting, *Hum Factors* 25:527-539, 1983.

75. Gilbertons LG, Krag MH, Pope MH: Investigation of the effect of intra-abdominal pressure on the load bearing of the spine, *Trans Orthop Res Soc* 8:177, 1983.

76. Gracovetsky S, Farfan HF, Lamy C: The mechanism of the lumbar spine, *Spine* 6:249-262, 1981.

77. Grew ND, Deane G: The physical effect of lumbar spinal supports, *Prosthet Orthop Int* 6:79-87, 1982.

78. Harman EA et al: Effects of a belt on intra-abdominal pressure during weight lifting, *Med Sci Sports Exerc* 21:186-190, 1989.

79. Hemborg B, Moritz U: Intra-abdominal pressure and trunk muscle activity during lifting, *Scand J Rehab Med* 17:5-13, 1985.

80. Herrin GD, Jariedi M, Anderson CK: Prediction of overexertion injuries using biomechanical and psychophysical models, *Am Ind Hyg Assoc J* 47:322-330, 1986.

81. Hilgen T, Smith LA: The minimum abdominal belt-aided lifting weight. In Karwowski W and Yates JW, editors: *Advances in industrial ergonomics and safety III*, London, 1991, Taylor & Francis: pp 217-224.

82. Horal J: The clinical appearance of low back disorders in the city of Gothenburg, Sweden, *Acta Orthop Scand Suppl* 118:9-109, 1969.

83. Hult L: Cervical, dorsal and lumbar spinal syndromes, *Acta Orthop Scand* 17(suppl), 1954.

84. Hunter GR et al: The effect of a weight training belt on blood pressure during exercise, *J Appl Sports Res* 3:13-18, 1989.

85. Jäger M: *Biomechanisches Modell des Menschen zur Analyze und Beurteilung der Belastung der Wirbelsaule Beider Handhabung von Lasten*, doctoral thesis, Dortmund, Germany, 1987, Universitat Dortmund.

86. Jäger M, Luttmann A: Compressive strength of lumbar spine elements related to age, gender and other influencing factors. *Proceedings of the eighth congress of the International Society of Electrophysiological Kinesiology*, Baltimore, 1990; pp 291-294.

87. Jensen RC: Back injuries among nursing personnel related to exposure, *Appl Occup Environ Hyg* 5:38-45, 1990.

88. Jensen RC: Disabling back injuries among nursing personnel: research needs and justification, *Res Nurs Health* 10:29-38, 1987.

89. Jensen RC: Epidemiology of work-related back pain, *Top Acute Care Trauma Rehabil* 2:1-15, 1988.

90. Kamon E, Ramanathan NL: Estimation of maximal aerobic power using stair climbing—a simple method suitable for industry, *Am Ind Hyg Assoc J* 35:181-184, 1974.

91. Kazarian LE: Creep characteristics of the human spinal column, *Orthop Clin North Am* 6:3-18, 1975.

92. Kellgren JH, Lawrence JS: Rheumatism in miners, part II: x-ray study, *Br J Ind Med* 9:197-207, 1952.

93. Kelsey JL: An epidemiological study of acute herniated lumbar intervertebral discs, *Rheumatol Rehab* 14:144-159, 1975.

94. Kelsey JL: An epidemiological study of the relationship between occupations and acute herniated lumbar intervertebral discs, *Int J Epidemiol* 4:197-205, 1975.

95. Kelsey JL, Hardy RJ: Driving of motor vehicles as a risk factor for acute herniated lumbar intervertebral disc, *Am J Epidemiol* 102:63-73, 1975.

96. Kelsey JL et al: An epidemiologic study of lifting and twisting on the job and risk for acute prolapsed lumbar intervertebral disc, *J Orthop Res* 2:61-66, 1984.

97. Keyserling WM, Herrin GD, Chaffin DB: Isometric strength testing as a means of controlling medical incidents on strenuous jobs, *J Occup Med* 22(5):332-336, 1980.

98. Keyserling WM et al: Establishing an industrial strength testing program, *Am Ind Hyg Assoc J* 41:730-736, 1980.

99. Klein BP, Jensen RC, Sanderson LM: Assessment of workers' compensation claims for back strains/sprains, *J Occup Med* 26:443-448, 1984.

100. Krämer J, Gritz A: Körper-Langenäderungen Durch Druckabhängige Flüssigkeitsverschiebung im Zwischenwirbel-Abschuitt, *Z Orthop*, 118:161-164, 1980.

101. Kroemer KHE, Robinson DE: *Horizontal static forces exerted by men standing in common working postures on surfaces of various tractions*, AMARL Pub No TR-70-114, Dayton, Ohio, 1971, Wright-Patterson Air Force Base, Aerospace Medical Research Laboratory.

102. Kumar S, Godfrey CM: Spinal braces and abdominal supports. In Karwowski W editor: *Trends in ergonomics/ human factors III* New York, Elsevier Science, Inc: pp 717-726.

103. Ladin Z, Murthy KR, DeLuca CJ: Mechanical recruitment of low-back muscles: theoretical predictions and experimental validation, *Spine* 149:927-938, 1989.

104. Lamy C et al: The strength of the neural arch and the etiology of spondylolysis, *Orthop Clin North Am* 6:215, 1975.

105. Lander JE, Simonton RL, Giacobbe JKF: The effectiveness of weight-belts during the squat exercise, *Med Sci Sports Exerc* 22:117-126, 1990.

106. Lawrence JS: Disc degeneration: its frequency and relationship to symptoms, *Ann Rheum Dis* 28:121-137, 1969.

107. Lee K: *Biomechanical modeling of cart pushing and pulling*, doctoral dissertation, Ann Arbor, 1982, University of Michigan.

108. Legg SJ: The effect of abdominal muscle fatigue and training on the intra-abdominal pressure developed during lifting, *Ergonomics* 24:191-195, 1981.

109. Liles DH et al: A job severity index for the evaluation and control of lifting injury, *Hum Factors* 26:683-694, 1984.

110. Lipson SJ: *Orthotic considerations in the management of adult low back pain*, Boston, 1990, Harvard Medical School.

111. Magora A: Investigation of the relation between low back pain and occupation, *Ind Med* 39(11):465-471, 1970.

112. Magora A: Investigation of the relation between low back pain and occupation, *Ind Med* 39(12):504-510, 1970.

113. Magora A: Investigation of the relation between low back pain and occupation, 6. Medical history and symptoms, *Scand J Rehabil Med* 6:81-88, 1974.

114. Magora A, Taustein I: An investigation of the problem of sick-leave in the patient suffering from low back pain, *Ind Med Surg* 38:398-408, 1969.

115. Marras WS, King AI, Joynt RL: Measurements of loads on the lumbar spine under isometric and isokinetic conditions, *Spine,* 9(2):176-187, 1984.

116. Marras WS, Sommerich CM: A three-dimensional motion model of loads on the lumbar spine: I. Model structure, *Hum Factors* 33(2):123-137, 1991.

117. Marras WS, Sommerich CM: A three-dimensional motion model of loads on the lumbar spine: II. Model validation, *Hum Factors* 33(2):139-149, 1991.

118. Marras WS et al: The role of dynamic three-dimensional trunk motion in occupationally-related low back disorders, *Spine* 18(5):617-628, 1993.

119. Mayer TG et al: Objective assessment of spinal function following industrial injury: a prospective study with comparison group and one-year follow-up, *Spine* 10(6):482-493, 1985.

120. Mayer TG et al: Quantification of lumbar function, part II. Sagittal plane trunk strength in chronic low-back pain patients, *Spine* 10(8):765-772, 1985.

121. McCoy MA et al: The role of lifting belts in manual lifting, *Int J Ind Ergonom* 2(4):259-266, 1988.

122. McGill SM, Norman RW: Dynamically and statistically determined low back movements during lifting, *J Biomech* 18(12):877-885, 1985.

123. McGill SM, Norman RW: Partitioning of the L4/L5 dynamic moment into disc, ligamentous and muscular components during lifting, *Spine* 11(7):666-678, 1986.

124. McGill SM, Norman RW: Reassessment of the role of intra-abdominal pressure in spinal compression, *Ergonomics* 30(11):1565-1588, 1987.

125. McGill SM, Norman RW, Sharratt MT: The effect of abdominal belt on trunk muscle activity and intra-abdominal pressure during squat lifts, *Ergonomics* 33(2):147-160, 1990.

126. Milton R et al: Evaluation of low back pain and assessment of lumbar corsets with and without back supports, *Ann Rheum Dis* 40(5):449-454, 1981.

127. Mital A: Comprehensive maximum acceptable weight of lift database for regular 8 hour shifts, *Ergonomics* 27:1127-1138, 1984.

128. Mital A: Psychophysical approach in manual lifting: a verification study, *Hum Factors* 25:485-491, 1983.

129. Moores B: A comparison of workload using physiological and time assessment, *Ergonomics* 14(1):61-69, 1970.

130. Morris JM, Lucas DB, Bresler MS: Role of trunk in stability of the spine, *J Bone Joint Surg Am* 43A(3):327-351, 1961.

131. Nachemson AL: Low back pain: its etiology and treatment, *Clin Med* 78:18-24, 1971.

132. Nachemson AL, Andersson GBJ, Schultz AB: Valsalva manoeuver biomechanics: effects of lumbar trunk loads of elevated intra-abdominal pressure, *Spine* 11(5):476-479, 1986.

133. National Institute for Occupational Safety and Health: *A work practices guide for manual lifting,* technical report No 81-122, Cincinnati, Ohio, 1991, US Department of Health and Human Service, CDC, NIOSH.

134. Ortengren R, Andersson GBJ: Electromyographic studies of trunk muscles, with special reference to the functional anatomy of the lumbar spine, *Spine* 2(1):44-52, 1977.

135. Ortengren R, Andersson GBJ, Nachemson AL: Studies of relationships between lumbar disc pressure, myoelectric back muscle activity and intra-abdominal (intragastric) pressure, *Spine* 6(1):98-103, 1981.

136. Owen BD, Garg A: Assistive devices for use with patient handling tasks. In Das B, editor: *Advances in industrial ergonomics and safety II,* London, 1990, Taylor & Francis; pp 585-592.

137. Owen BD, Garg A: Patient handling tasks perceived to be most stressful by nursing assistants. In Mital A, editor: *Advances in industrial ergonomics and safety I,* London, 1989, Taylor & Francis; pp 775-781.

138. Partridge REH, Duthie JJR: Rheumatism in dockers and civil servants: a comparison of heavy manual and sedentary workers, *Ann Rheum Dis* 27:559-567, 1968.

139. Perry J: The use of external support in the treatment of low-back pain, *J Bone Joint Surg Am* 52A(7):1440-1442, 1970.

140. Petrofsky JS, Lind AR: Metabolic, cardiovascular and respiratory factors in the development of fatigue in lifting tasks, *J Appl Physiol Respir Environ Exerc Physiol* 45(1):64-68, 1978.

141. Pope MH et al: *Occupational low back pain: assessment, treatment and prevention,* St Louis, 1991, Mosby–Year Book.

142. Poulsen E, Jorgensen K: Back muscle strength, lifting and stooped working postures, *Appl Ergonom* 2(3):133-137, 1971.

143. Reddel CR et al: An evaluation of weightlifting belt and back injury prevention training class for airline baggage handlers, *Appl Ergonom* 23(5):319-329, 1992.

144. Ridyard DT: A successful applied ergonomics program for preventing occupational back injuries. In Das B, editor: *Advances in industrial ergonomics and safety II,* London, 1990, Taylor & Francis; pp 125-142.

145. Rodgers SH, Yates JW, Garg A: *The physiological basis of the manual lifting guidelines, scientific support documentation for the revised 1991 NIOSH lifting equation,* technical contract report PO No 86-72315, PB91-226274, Springfield, Va, 1991, US Department of Commerce, National Technical Information Service.

146. Rowe ML: *Backache at work,* Fairport, NY, 1983, Perington Press.

147. Rowe ML: Low back disability in industry: updated position, *J Occup Med* 13(10):476-478, 1971.

148. Rowe ML: Low back pain in industry, *J Occup Med* 11(4):161-169, 1969.

149. Rowe ML: Preliminary statistical study of low back pain, *J Occup Med* 5(7):336-341, 1963.

150. Schultz AB, Andersson GBJ: Analysis of loads on the lumbar spine, *Spine* 6(1):76-82, 1981.

151. Schultz AB et al: Analysis and measurement of lumbar trunk loads in tasks involving bends and twists, *J Biomech* 15(9):669-675, 1982.

152. Schultz AB et al: Loads on the lumbar spine, *J Bone Joint Surg Am* 64A(5):713-720, 1992.

153. Schultz A et al: Lumbar trunk muscle use in standing isometric heavy exertions, *J Orthop Res* 5(3):320-329, 1987.

154. Schultz AB et al: Mechanical properties of human lumbar spine motion segments—part I. Response in flexion, extension, lateral bending and torsion, *J Biomech Eng* 101:46-52, 1979.

155. Seguin J, McGill S: The effect of abdominal belts on passive stiffness of the trunk about three axes. *Proceedings of the twenty-fifth annual conference of the Human Factors Association of Canada,* Hamilton, Ontario, 1992, pp 67–72.

156. Snook SH, Campanelli RA, Hart JW: A study of three preventive approaches to low back injury, *J Occup Med* 20(7):478-481, 1978.

157. Snook SH, Ciriello VM: The design of manual handling tasks: revised tables of maximum acceptable weights and forces, *Ergonomics* 34(9):1197-1213, 1991.

158. Sonada T: Studies on the compression, tension and torsion, and torsion strength of the human vertebral column, *J Kyoto Prefect Med Univ* 71:659-702, 1962.

159. Stubbs DA et al: Back pain in the nursing profession, II. The effectiveness of training, *Ergonomics* 26(8):767-779, 1983.

160. Thomson KD: On the bending movement capability of the pressurized abdominal cavity during human lifting activities, *Ergonomics* 31(5):817-828, 1988.

161. Tichauer ER: *The biomechanical basis of ergonomics,* New York, 1978, John Wiley & Sons, Inc.

162. Troup JDG: Biomechanics of vertebral column, *Physiotherapy* 65(8):238-245, 1979.

163. Troup JDG: The etiology of spondylolysis, *Orthop Clin North Am* 8(1):57-64, 1977.

164. Troup JDG, Edwards FC: *Manual handling and lifting,* London, 1985, Her Majesty's Stationery Office.

165. Troup JDG et al: A comparison of intra-abdominal pressure increases, hip torque and lumbar vertebral compression in different lifting techniques, *Hum Factors* 25(5):517-525, 1983.

166. Valles-Pankratz S: What's in back of nursing home injuries? *Ohio Monitor* 62(2):4-8, 1989.

167. Videman T et al: Low-back pain in nurses and some loading factors of work, *Spine* 9(4):400-404, 1984.

168. Venning PJ, Walter SD, Stitt LW: Personal and job-related factors as determinants of incidence of back injuries among nursing personnel, *J Occup Med* 29(10):820-825, 1987.

169. Walsh NE, Schwartz RK: The influence of prophylactic orthoses on abdominal strength and low back injury in the workplace, *Am J Phys Med Rehabil* 69(5):246-250, 1990.

170. Waters RL, Morris J: Effect of spinal supports on the electrical activity of muscles of the trunk, *J Bone Joint Surg Am* 52A:51-60, 1990.

171. Waters TR et al: Revised NIOSH equation for the design and evaluation of manual lifting tasks, *Ergonomics* 36(7):749-776, 1993.

172. White AA, Gordon SL: Synopsis: workshop on idiopathic low back pain, *Spine* 7:141-149, 1982.

173. Wickström G: Effect of work on degenerative back disease: a review, *Scand J Work Environ Health* Suppl:1-12, 1978.

174. Woodhouse ML et al: Selected isokinetic lifting parameters of adult male athletes utilizing lumbar/sacral supports, *J Orthop Sports Phys Ther* 11(10):467-473, 1990.

175. Wyndham CH et al: The relationship between energy expenditure and performance index in the task of shovelling sand, *Ergonomics* 9(5):371-378, 1966.

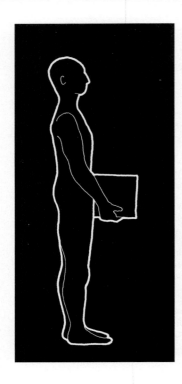

Chapter 10

Postural Considerations and Lifting Limits

Don B. Chaffin

CONTENTS

Many postural problems during lifting can be directly related to the position that the hands need to be located to grasp, move, and position objects in the workplace. Essentially, if objects to be lifted are compact and can be held close to the torso at about hip-to-waist height, the biomechanical stresses on the back and shoulders will be minimized. This was recognized by the expert panels that drafted the 1981 and 1993 National Institute for Occupational Health and Safety (NIOSH) lifting guides.[20] In both the earlier and revised forms of this lifting guide, when the hands of a person performing a lift are close to the torso throughout the lift and the person does not need to bend the torso forward or to the side, a maximum weight can be safely handled (see Chapter 9).

It is unfortunate that technical and economic limitations in most industries do not provide the optimal type of lifting conditions just described. Too often, objects to be lifted are presented to a worker at floor level or on a low shelf. Furthermore, many objects must be lifted to or from a shelf above shoulder height. In addition, it is too often the case that either the shape or size of the object being moved or a separate work surface intrudes into the path of movement and makes it very difficult to keep the hands close to the body throughout the lifting motion.

These types of conditions cause a person to flex and/or twist the torso as well as incur high-moment loadings on the back and shoulders. In other words, the postures one assumes while lifting can only be modified slightly by the lifter (e.g., an informed person will know to step as close as possible to an object before lifting). Many lifting postures are not under the control of the worker but rather are dictated by the layout of the workplace and the size and shape of objects being handled.[4]

This means that to control the risk of low back pain in most industries, the training of workers on how to perform "safe lifting" will only be effective if the working conditions allow recommended lifting techniques to be used. Too often this is not the case. Before a lift training program is initiated, every feasible effort should be made to ensure that the workplace and the objects being handled allow low-stress lifting.

What follows is a kinematic description of job conditions that are known to affect the risk of low back injury in industry. These are presented, along with their biomechanical assessments, both to display how subtle and important small changes can be to the worker and

to illustrate how such conditions can be evaluated with existing biomechanics software. Some practical advice regarding the ergonomics of workplace designs and worker training issues is presented in the last part of this chapter.

LOCATION OF HANDS ON LIFT POSTURES

Several lifting scenarios are described to illustrate the biomechanical effects of hand location when objects of varied weight are lifted. The biomechanical outcomes are predicted by using the University of Michigan's 3D Static Strength Prediction Program (3DSSPP, version 2.0), the logic of which is described by Chaffin and Andersson.[3] In each scenario the predicted L5/S1 compression force and the percentage of male and female workers with expected static strength sufficient to lift the object are reported. For all the analyses, average male and female anthropometry is assumed.

Scenario 1: Lifting Objects from the Floor
When an object to be lifted is on the floor, too often a person must locate the hands under the object (i.e., at floor level) to lift it. If the object is small enough to be lifted between the knees, a person can lower the hands to floor level by assuming many different postures. Two extreme postures are useful to consider. One is the very common "stoop lift" posture wherein the knees are nearly straight and the hips flexed; this allows the torso to lean forward to below horizontal. **Figure 10-1**, *A*, depicts such a posture. In contrast, if a person has the necessary ankle and knee flexibility, the hands can be lowered to the floor by using a "deep squat" posture, depicted in **Figure 10-1**, *B*.

The biomechanical consequences of these two extreme postures have been discussed elsewhere.[1,7,10,15,19] In essence, the deep-squat lift posture has been biomechanically justified for lifting objects that can be brought in very close (less than 9 inches from the ankles) and moved between the knees.

In the simulations depicted in **Figure 10-1**, the hands are assumed to be 9 inches horizontally in front of the ankles with the fingers under the object while applying a vertical lifting force. Two different object weights were used for reference, 25 and 50 lb. The results indicate that the predicted back compression forces are not very different. Because of larger and heavier body segments, the predicted compression values for males performing the 50-lb lifts are higher than the 760-lb L5/S1 disk failure limit referenced by NIOSH,[20] regardless of whether a stoop or squat posture is adopted. It is interesting to note that for both males and females, the predicted anterior-posterior disk shear forces are lower in the deep-squat lift posture than in the stoop lift posture. Although these shear forces have been proposed by some to be an important low back pain risk factor, estimates of their values and corresponding risk levels are not well documented.[17]

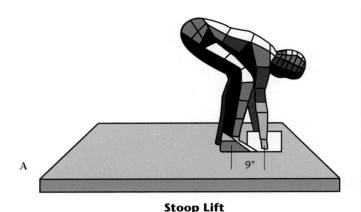

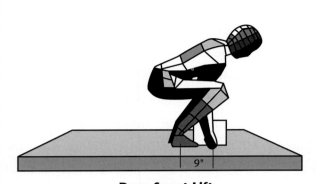

Stoop Lift

25 lb. object	Male	Female
Back Compression (lbs)	621	538
Disc Shear (lbs)	96	83
% Population Strength	94%	88%
Limiting Muscles	Hip Ext.	Hip Ext.
50 lb. object		
Back Compression (lbs)	790	706
Disc Shear (lbs)	121	108
% Population Strength	90%	75%
Limiting Muscles	Hip Ext.	Hip Ext.

Deep Squat Lift

25 lb. object	Male	Female
Back Compression (lbs)	646	557
Disk Shear (lbs)	52	44
% Population Strength	82%	74%
Limiting Muscles	Knee Ext.	Knee Ext.
50 lb. object		
Back Compression (lbs)	803	713
Disk Shear (lbs)	64	57
% Population Strength	76%	64%
Limiting Muscles	Knee Ext.	Knee Ext.

Figure 10-1 Comparison of two different postures used to lift 25- and 50-lb objects from the floor close to the feet. *Ext.,* extension.

One problem with the use of a squat lift posture is that it imposes a high strength demand on the knees (e.g., only about 64% of women would have the knee extension strength to assume the deep-squat posture and lift the 50-lb object as shown). In contrast, the stoop lift posture imposes a large hip and low back extension strength requirement (with only 75% of women capable of lifting 50 lb in the stoop posture). It is concluded that until low back models are further refined to predict spinal shear and ligament tolerances accurately, it is not obvious that there are significant advantages to one specific lift posture over another when the hands are located near the end of the shoes when beginning a lift.

But what happens to lifting postures when an object on the floor is too bulky to easily fit between the knees or is located behind a barrier that restricts getting the object as close to the feet as in **Figure 10-1**? In this situation, where a larger horizontal distance exists between the ankles and hands, the feasible lifting postures become much more constrained.

To illustrate this problem, assume that 25- and 50-lb objects are located such that the hands at the beginning of the lift are now 18 inches in front of the ankles. Placing the hands in this position and maintaining balance while developing the required lifting force, can only be accomplished by assuming a posture that is a "semisquat and stoop" posture, as illustrated in **Figure 10-2**. It requires that the buttocks be positioned poste-

rior to the ankles, thus providing a backward moment about the feet to counteract the forward moment created by upper body mass and the load being lifted. Unfortunately, this posture moves the lower part of the back away from the load being lifted and results in the high predicted L5/S1 disk compression forces depicted in **Figure 10-2**. In this posture, lifting even the 25-lb object becomes questionable and would place some people at risk.

What is clear from this latter comparison is the adverse effect of large horizontal hand displacements when lifting, which cannot be overcome by instructing people to lift in a deep-squat posture with an erect torso. Such a posture is not feasible, because of the limited arm reach capability. One must lean (stoop) the torso forward and rock backward to reach and move the object upward.

If the object can be pulled in and lifted (as opposed to lifted vertically), the load moments and resulting spinal compression forces will be reduced. This latter effect is discussed further by Garg et al.[8] and Danz and Ayoub.[5] Such lifting motions can only be accomplished if there are no barriers to prevent a person from pulling an object in close to the body while lifting.

Scenario 2: Lifting to High Shelves
The task of lifting objects to a high shelf is common in the workplace. The primary reason for this scenario is the cost of floor space in the workplace, which is

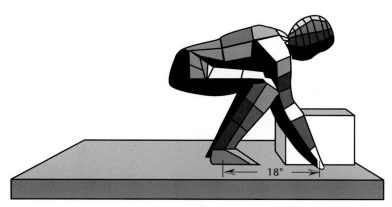

Semi-Squat and Stoop Lift

25 lb. object	Male	Female
Back Compression (lbs)	841	738
% Population Strength	93%	85%
Limiting Muscles	Hip Ext.	Hip Ext.

50 lb. object		
Back Compression (lbs)	1123	1018
% Population Strength	87%	65%
Limiting Muscles	Hip Ext.	Hip Ext.

Figure 10-2 Illustration of the typical semi-squat and stoop posture used to lift objects located on the floor and 18 inches in front of the ankles. *Ext.,* extension.

normally very high. Both the 1981 and revised 1991 NIOSH lifting guides penalize lifting objects to high shelves. From a biomechanical perspective, there are at least two issues. First is the shoulder and arm strength limitation that exists when an object is lifted to a shelf above shoulder height (or about 60 inches). This problem is illustrated in **Figures 10-3**, *A* and *B,* for 25- and 50-lb objects.

In **Figure 10-3**, *A,* the fingers remain under the object being lifted throughout the lift. This hand posture forces the arms to be raised and abducted at the shoulders. The smaller the person, the more abduction required and hence less strength capability. To reduce the arm abduction strength problem, the grip is often released for an instant during the lift and the fingers slid to the side of the object during the lift. This may also be necessary to avoid pinching the fingers against the front of the shelf when the object is set down. As this "regrasp" occurs, an unknown dynamic inertial loading force may be present. This leads to the second issue in these high lifts. The needed regrasp during the lift may cause the object to slip and fall, possibly injuring the feet, or it may dynamically overload the back. The latter issue is more speculative at this time, but a laboratory study by Marras[11] disclosed that unexpected, dynamic impulse loads increase torso muscle cocontractions and thus disk compressions. If the object being lifted slowly is already creating high spinal and muscle forces, the extra dynamic forces imparted during a regrasp may become injurious.

Such an injury scenario is particularly relevant if the high shelf is horizontally distant from the lifter because of a barrier (i.e., another lower protruding shelf, table,

bench top, or conveyor). This situation is depicted in **Figure 10-3**, *B.* In this case, the hands are positioned on handles, however, and therefore the arms do not need to be abducted at the termination of the lift, which lessens the shoulder strength problem, although still a major concern with the 50-lb object (only 16% of women are predicted to be able to lift the 50-lb object in the posture shown in **Fig. 10-3**, *B*). The large horizontal hand location (i.e., 18 inches from the ankles) in **Figure 10-3**, *B,* creates a much greater (by approximately twice) predicted back compression force than that predicted in **Figure 10-3**, *A.* If a dynamic inertial force is superimposed on this static compression force, it could present a significant risk of injury to the low back region even when in an erect posture. Hence there is a need to ensure that higher shelves are not horizontally distant from the lifter and that well-designed handles are provided on heavy and bulky objects.

Scenario 3: Lifting Objects at the Side

If a person needs to carry an object for a long distance, particularly over uneven terrain or up or down stairs, it is helpful if the object can be carried at the side so that it does not interfere with leg motion or vision. If the object has a handle on its top (e.g., luggage) and is tall (i.e., 15 to 25 inches) and narrow (i.e., less than 9 inches), it greatly facilitates the lifting and carrying activities.

But what if the object has no handle and is bulky? Furthermore, assume that the object is on or near the floor and under a shelf or bench. In this situation, to avoid interference with the front of the shelf or bench a person may attempt a side lift. **Figure 10-4** depicts this

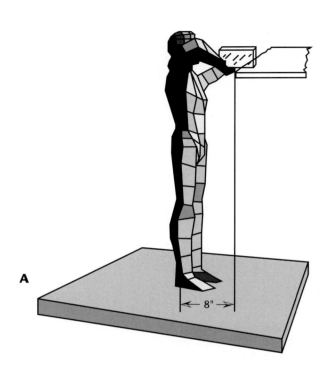

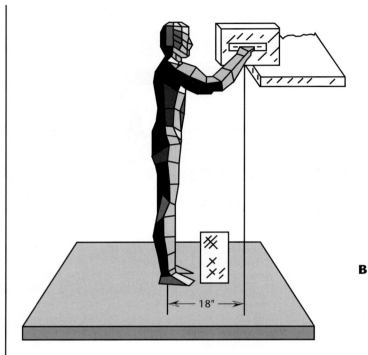

A

B

High Close Lift
(arms abducted)

25 lb. object	Male	Female
Back Compression (lbs)	171	160
% Population Strength	93%	46%
Limiting Muscles	Sh. Ext.	Sh. Ext.
50 lb. object		
Back Compression (lbs)	271	262
% Population Strength	11%	1%
Limiting Muscles	Sh. Ext.	Sh. Ext.

High Far Lift
(arms at sides)

25 lb. object	Male	Female
Back Compression (lbs)	348	331
% Population Strength	98%	94%
Limiting Muscles	Sh. Ext.	Sh. Ext.
50 lb. object		
Back Compression (lbs)	519	517
Population Strength	84%	16%
Limiting Muscles	Sh. Ext.	Sh. Ext.

Figure 10-3 Comparison of lifting objects to high shelves located close, but without handles on the object (**A**), versus to a far shelf, but with handles on the object (**B**). *Sh. Ext.,* shoulder extension.

type of lift posture. To perform this type of lift a person must stoop and twist the torso to the side so that the shoulder is over the object. This allows one arm to extend around the far side of the object and the other arm to cross over the legs to the near side of the object.

Clearly, the postural options available are limited when an object is lifted at the side and the hands must be at or close to the floor. Furthermore, the biomechanical consequences are of major concern. Increased spinal compression force is caused by a larger amount of torso cocontraction than would be expected if the lift were performed in a more symmetric fashion in the sagittal plane.[2,9,16] As shown in **Figure 10-4**, the predicted L4/L5 disk compression force is quite high in the asym-

metric posture shown, in contrast to the sagittal-plane lifts analyzed earlier (see **Fig. 10-1**).

A second biomechanical consequence of asymmetric side-lifting postures is that they induce complex shear forces and axial torque loading on the spinal motion segments.[12,14] Although specific failure limits for these complex stressors have not been promulgated, epidemiologic studies indicate that an increased risk of low back pain exists[13,18] in this type of asymmetric lifting.

Finally, as depicted in **Figure 10-4**, lifting strength is compromised when a side lift is attempted. Garg and Badger[6] disclosed an average 15% decrease in maximal acceptable weights subjects chose to lift at the side as compared with lifts in front of the body. The combina-

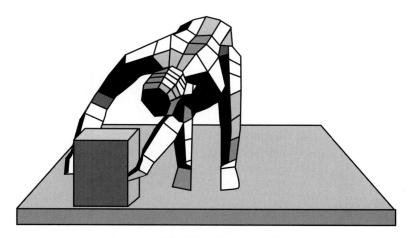

Asymmetric Side Lift from Floor

25 lb. object	Male	Female
Back Compression (lbs)	692	605
L4/L5 A/P Spinal Shear (lbs)	87	79
% Population Strength	85%	59%
Limiting Muscles	R. Hip Ext.	R. Hip Ext.
50 lb. object		
Back Compression (lbs)	914	826
L4/L5 A/P Spinal Shear (lbs)	95	84
% Population Strength	66%	18%
Limiting Muscles	R. Hip Ext.	R. Hip Ext.

Figure 10-4 Illustration of lifting an object on the floor with an asymmetric side-lifting posture. *R. Hip Ext.,* right-hip extension.

tion of biomechanical, epidemiologic, and strength effects resulted in the revised NIOSH guide recommendation that weights lifted at the side of the body be reduced by 30% of the recommended weight lifted in the sagittal plane.

PREVENTING ADVERSE POSTURES DURING LIFTING—ACTIONS NEEDED

It can be concluded that the postures one must use when lifting are dictated to a large extent by the work space layout and the size and shape of the objects being handled. Further, many common working conditions can produce postures that are highly stressful, especially to the low back region. In this context, the first corrective action is to undertake an evaluation of the workplace, with specific emphasis on those lifting tasks that contain one or more of the following adverse postural requirements:

1. Heavy or bulky objects lying on the floor
2. Objects (e.g., boxes) that do not have well designed handles that allow the hands a good power grasp throughout the lift motion
3. Objects that are stored near the back of deep shelves and that cannot be easily pulled close to the body (i.e., where barriers cause large horizontal distances between the torso and object)

4. Objects that are stored near the floor and under or around benches or shelves that force asymmetric lifting postures

Clearly the intent of such evaluations should be to ergonomically redesign (or initially design) the workplace and objects so that a worker is presented packages to be lifted that

1. Allow the person to keep the torso near vertical (i.e., keep the object being lifted close to the body and near hip height)
2. Avoid having to regrasp the object during the lift motion
3. Avoid torso twisting or side bending lifts

If redesign of the work space and/or packages is not feasible, material handling devices (e.g., hoists and articulated arms) may be a good alternative. Although often requiring more time to move an object than necessary when manually lifting, these devices can be very effective in reducing the stresses discussed in Chapter 9.

Finally, all workers involved in lifting objects in industry need to be formally trained (as discussed later in Chapter 17). Such training needs to emphasize the following (as a minimum):

1. Stepping close to object before beginning lifts (even straddling objects if possible) or pulling objects in close before lifting

2. Facing object to balance the load in both hands while lifting
3. Planning (visualizing) the lift trajectory to ensure that the object can be set down close to the body
4. Designating a specific place to set the object down that avoids high lifts and regrasping of the object to reach the set-down area
5. Using correct-fitting gloves to provide a firmer grasp of the object
6. Prearranging objects being lifted so that heavier objects are always at about hip-waist height and easily reached (i.e., close to the torso)
7. Orienting objects long in one dimension so that the largest dimension is vertical
8. If carrying objects, making sure that the walking area is clear and has a uniform, level, high-traction surface
9. Knowing one's load lifting capacity (i.e., strength) and making sure that objects being lifted are not overly stressful—and getting help if needed
10. If lifts are frequent, alternating lifting with lighter work or taking frequent recovery pauses

In summary, postural lifting requirements are only one source of injurious stress to the back in industry. Both ergonomic design and worker training issues must be considered in order to reduce the postural stresses in many different jobs. It is hoped that the preceding will assist in providing one part of a comprehensive program needed to prevent occupational low back pain.

References

1. Anderson CK, Chaffin DB: A biomechanical evaluation of five lifting techniques, *Appl Ergonom* 17:2-8, 1986.

2. Bean JC, Chaffin DB, Schultz AB: Biomechanical model calculation of muscle contraction forces: a double linear programming method, *Biomech* 21:59-66, 1988.

3. Chaffin DB, Andersson GBJ: *Occupational biomechanics,* ed 2, New York, 1991, John Wiley & Sons, Inc.

4. Chaffin DB et al: An evaluation of the effect of a training program on worker lifting postures, *Int J Ind Ergonom* 1:127-136, 1986.

5. Danz ME, Ayoub MM: The effects of speed, frequency, and load on measured hand forces for a floor to knuckle lifting task, *Ergonomics* 35(7-8):833-843, 1992.

6. Garg A, Badger D: Maximum acceptable weights and maximum voluntary isometric strengths for asymmetric lifting, *Ergonomics* 29(7):879-892, 1986.

7. Garg A, Herrin GD: Stoop or squat: a biomechanical and metabolic evaluation, *AIIE Trans* 11:293-302, 1979.

8. Garg A et al: Biomechanical stresses as related to motion trajectory of lifting, *Hum Factors* 25(5):527-539, 1983.

9. Hughes RE, Chaffin DB: Shear force considerations in predicting torso muscle antagonism. *Proceedings of the American Society for Biomechanics annual meeting,* Davis, Calif, 1987.

10. Leskinen TPJ, Stalhammar HR, Kuorinka IAA: A dynamic analysis of spinal compression with different lifting techniques, *Ergonomics* 26:595-604, 1983.

11. Marras WS: Trunk motion during lifting: temporal relations among loading factors, *Int J Ind Ergonom* 1:159-167, 1986.

12. Marras WS, Sommerich CM: A three-dimensional motion model of loads on the lumbar spine: I. Model structure, *Hum Factors* 33(2):123-137, 1991.

13. Marras WS et al: The role of dynamic three-dimensional trunk motion in occupationally-related low back disorders, *Spine* 18(5):617-628, 1993.

14. McGill SM, Norman RW: Dynamically and statically determined low back moments during lifting, *J Biomech* 18:877-885, 1985.

15. Park K, Chaffin DB: A biomechanical evaluation of two methods of manual load lifting, *AIIE Trans* 6(2):105-113, 1974.

16. Pope MH et al: Electromyographic studies of the lumbar trunk musculature during the development of axial torques, *J Orthop Res* 4:288-297, 1986.

17. Potvin JR, Norman RW, McGill SM: Reduction in anterior shear forces on the L4/L5 disc by the lumbar musculature, *Clini Biomech* 6(3):88-96, 1991.

18. Punnett L et al: Back disorders and nonneutral trunk postures of automobile assembly workers *Scand J Work Environ Health* 17:337-346, 1991.

19. Troup JDG et al: A comparison of intra-abdominal pressure increases, hip torque and lumbar vertebral compression in different lifting techniques, *Hum Factors* 25(5):517-525, 1983.

20. Waters TR et al: Revised NIOSH equation for the design and evaluation of manual lifting tasks, *Ergonomics* 36(7):749-776, 1993.

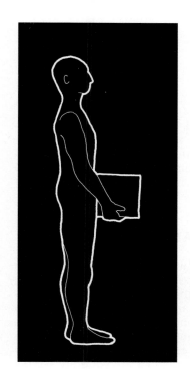

Chapter 11

Whole-Body Vibration

Malcolm H. Pope

CONTENTS

Many authors have related the exposure to whole body vibration (WBV) to low back pain (LBP). Tractor driving has been suggested as a risk factor by Rosegger and Rosegger,[39] Lavault,[26] Christ,[8] Rosegger,[40] Dupuis and Christ,[12,13] Kubic,[25] Köhl,[24] Schultz and Polster,[44] and Frymoyer et al.[14] Christ and Dupuis[9] found that of those with more than 700 tractor driving hours per year, 61% had pathologic radiographic changes of the spine; of those with 700 to 1200 hours, 68% were affected; and of those with greater than 1200 driving hours, 94% were affected. Low back pain paralleled the pathologic changes.

Similar findings are reported for drivers of heavy equipment. Low back pain has been related to the use of earth-moving equipment. Cremona[11] reported a 70% LBP prevalence in operators of heavy equipment. Hilfert et al.[17] found a clear trend of greater pathologic changes on radiographs in drivers of earth-moving equipment. Schmidt[42] compared drivers of heavy trucks and bank employees. Of the truck drivers, 75% had pathologic changes of the spine as compared with 61.1% of the bank employees. Backman[4] found that 40% of bus drivers have LBP, with the prevalence increasing with age. Barbaso[5] also found an increase in the prevalence of both LBP and pathologic changes with age in bus drivers. Kelsey and Hardy[23] investigated the relative risk of herniated nucleus pulposus (HNP) in truck and car drivers. For car drivers, the relative risk was 2.75 and for truck drivers it was 4.67. Heliövaara[16] found that drivers were at a high risk of acquiring herniated lumbar intervertebral disks. His study controlled for age, sex, and place of residence. Of 57,000 people who participated in the baseline examinations, 592 were later discharged from the hospital (during an 11-year follow-up) after having had a herniated lumbar intervertebral disk. When compared with 2140 controls, drivers were found to be at a greater risk for herniated disks.

A review by Seidel and Heide[45] concluded that people who sit in a vibrating environment that is close to or exceeds the exposure limits established by the International Organization for Standardization[21] (ISO) place their musculoskeletal system at risk. In all, their review covers 43,000 workers exposed to WBV and 24,000 controls. The data "indicate an increased health risk of the spine and peripheral nervous system after intense, long-term whole body vibration."[45]

Hulshof and van Zantern[19] also reviewed studies of spine disorders caused by vibration. No study rated highly on all three criteria of quality of exposure data, health effects data, and methodology. Few of the epidemiologic studies were prospective, and none measured vibration exposure limits according to ISO 2631. Subsequently, Magnusson et al,[28] in a comparative epidemiologic study in Vermont and Sweden, found that Vermont truck drivers with the highest ISO vibration exposure also had the highest LBP prevalence. At the same time, they had the highest rate of job satisfaction and the lowest rate of LBP disability.

VIBRATION SIMULATIONS

Mechanical studies have been performed to evaluate the effect of WBV in the seated, standing, and supine postures in both single and multiple directions. The dynamic behavior of the human subject can be determined by acceleration transmissibility and impedance. Using the former method, one compares the output acceleration resulting from the input or driving acceleration. At resonance, the ratio of output to input exceeds unity. For the impedance method, one computes the ratio of the force to move the body to its resulting velocity. This ratio, as a function of frequency, defines the mechanical response. Resonant frequencies are between 4 and 5 Hz, which is usually attributed to the upper torso vibrating vertically with respect to the pelvis, and between 10 and 14 Hz, which represents a bending vibration of the upper part of the torso with respect to the lumbar spine.

Most of the aforementioned studies determined transmissibilities by comparing the output acceleration at the head with the input acceleration at the seat, but they did not measure the relative motion in the lumbar spine. With accelerometers and pins implanted in the lumbar region, Panjabi et al[31] and Pope et al[38] showed that the resonant frequency in the lumbar region of a vertically vibrated, seated operator was 4.5 Hz. However, Panjabi and colleagues found little or no relative motion between L1 and L3. Pope et al[32-34] described tests in which a subject is placed in different controlled sitting postures and the transmissibility and phase angle determined (**Fig. 11-1**). In these studies, pins were placed in the spinous process and an impactor (**Fig. 11-2**) was used to excite the frequencies. The response curves produced in the relaxed and erect postures had the same general form, except that the peaks were more marked in the relaxed posture. A series of cushions were largely ineffective in vibration attenuation.[34]

How does vibration interact with the spine and lead to mechanical changes or material fatigue? Strain energy imparted to the spine results from the work done on the seated operator. That work equals the kinetic energy applied to the driver by the kinetic energy of the vibration. Some simple and revealing mathematical relationships then follow:

$$Work = Kinetic\ energy = 1/2\ mv^2$$

where m = mass and v = velocity, and

$$Velocity = at$$

where a = acceleration and t = time.

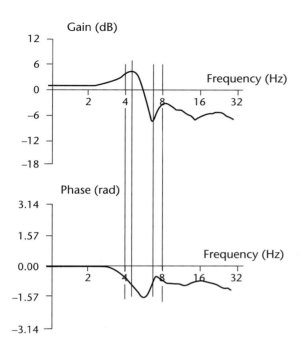

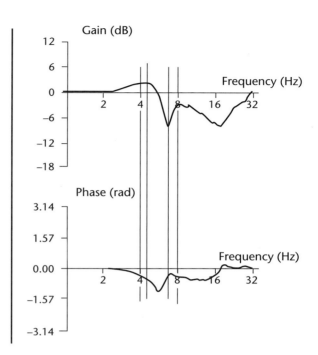

Figure 11-1 The impacting apparatus.

If we then solve the kinetic energy equation by substituting acceleration × time for velocity,

$$\text{Kinetic energy} = 1/2 \; mv^2 = 1/2 \; m(at)^2 = 1/2 \; m(a^2t^2)$$

This reveals a great deal about remediating vibration environments. The energy imparted to the body is a function of the square of the vibration acceleration and the square of the time of exposure to vibration. Therefore, small decreases in either time or vibration acceleration can result in relatively large decreases in the energy transmitted to a worker exposed to the vibration. If either the acceleration or exposure time is decreased by 15%, the energy imparted to the worker is reduced by 28%. If both the acceleration and exposure time are decreased by 15%, the energy imparted to the worker is reduced by 48%. Simple vibration remediations can lead to significant reductions.

MUSCLE RESPONSE AND METABOLIC COST

The electromyographic (EMG) signals of the erector spinae and external oblique muscles were measured by Wilder, Frymoyer, and Pope[49] at each of three vibrational frequencies. Increased activity of the external oblique muscles was found in rotation and lateral bending and during the Valsalva maneuver.

The phasic activity of the erector spinae muscles was measured by Seroussi, Wilder, and Pope.[46] The ensemble-averaged EMG signals were converted to torque by using an in vivo EMG-torque calibration technique. From these data, a phase relationship was established between the input signal to the platform

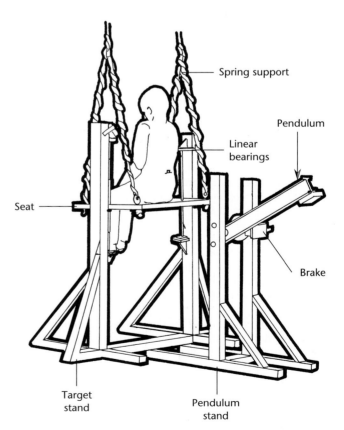

Figure 11-2 Transmissibility and phase of subjects impacted in a relaxed and erect stance.

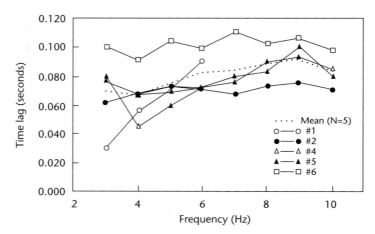

Figure 11-3 Time lag between peak torque and acceleration input.

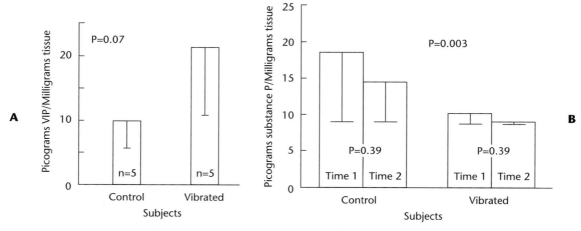

Figure 11-4 A, Tissue vasoactive intestinal peptide levels in rabbit lumbar ganglia. **B,** Tissue substance P levels, time 1 versus time 2.

and the resulting torque. Higher average EMG levels, or muscle torques, were found for the vibration condition. The time lag between the input displacement and the peak torque varied from 30 to 100 ms at 3 Hz and from 70 to 100 ms at 10 Hz (**Fig. 11-3**). At 10 Hz, the muscle contraction tended to coincide with the input signal, or to be 360 degrees out of phase. At all other frequencies, it was out of phase. Seidel and Heide[45] have also monitored the timing of the back muscle response to vibration and found that the muscles are not able to protect the spine.

Bennett, Webb, and Withey[6] showed that oxygen consumption increases with vibration, and Cole and Withey[10] and Webb, Bennett, and Farnile[47] reported increased consumption with an increase in acceleration level. Pope et al[36,37] reported a 14.3% increase in oxygen uptake in both the twisted erect posture and the erect posture.[36,37] Weinstein et al[48] vibrated rabbits at their natural frequency. There was a marked drop in substance P levels with a concomitant increase in vasoactive intestinal polypeptide levels (**Fig. 11-4**). Radioim-

munoassay studies have shown that a significant change in neuropeptides is important in pain response. In studies conducted on a porcine model, Holm and Nachemson[18] demonstrated a loss of nutrition to the intervertebral disk at the first natural frequency, thus suggesting a mechanism by which disks could degenerate with prolonged exposure.

Pope et al[35] measured the levels of back discomfort and von Willebrand factor antigen (vWFAg) in 11 subjects following 25-minute periods of (1) lying down, (2) sitting still and upright, (3) vibrating while sitting, and (4) sitting still and upright. Both back discomfort and vWFAg levels were significantly increased following sitting upright as compared with lying flat and increased further following exposure to vibration. They fell thereafter with a period of sitting upright. These results demonstrate that vibration has a significant effect in increasing back discomfort and the serum levels of vWFAg, in accordance with a hypothesis that vibration may induce vascular damage within the spine.

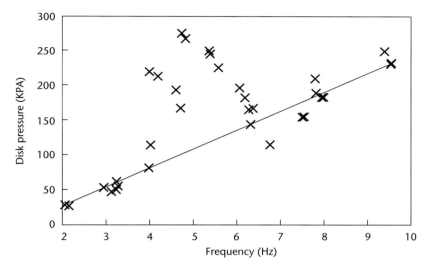

Figure 11-5 Disk pressure as a function of frequency in a vibration study on pigs. *KPA,* disk pressure; *Hz,* frequency.

THE SEATED POSTURE

In most jobs involving WBV, the worker is in a seated position. Numerous studies[20,23,27,29] show a positive relationship between LBP and prolonged sitting, possibly because the pelvis rotates backward and the lumbar spine flattens in the seated position.[1,3,22,41,43]

During unsupported sitting, in vivo disk pressures are about 35% higher than those obtained when subjects are standing.[30] Disk pressures have also been measured when sitting with different back supports.[2] Disk pressures are higher during sitting because the trunk load moment increases when the pelvis is rotated backward and the lumbar spine and torso are rotated forward. Also, the lumbar disk changes shape when the spine curvature is flattened. Inclination of the backrest from vertical to an increase in lumbar support and the use of arm rests resulted in decreased disk pressure.

Vibration also has an effect on intradiscal pressure. Hansson, Keller, and Spengler[15] vibrated pigs longitudinally while they simultaneously obtained measurements of intradiscal pressure. The vibration frequency used varied from 1 to 12 Hz. Intradiscal pressure was sensitive to frequency (**Fig. 11-5**). Disk pressure peaked at 5 Hz and was 2.5 times that at 3 Hz, thus indicating a natural frequency similar to that of the seated human. This result may explain the increased rate of HNP in drivers.

DISCUSSION

Low back pain can have many causes and it is difficult to eliminate some of them. However, many industrial risk factors can be modified to reduce the rate of back disorders. Epidemiologic studies suggest that vibration is an important risk factor for LBP and that many vehicles subject the worker to levels of vibration greater than that recommended by the ISO.[21] The ISO 8-hour fatigue-decreased proficiency (FDP) limit has been shown to not be sufficiently conservative by the work of Bongers and Boshuizen.[7] Workers in occupations where vibration is combined with lifting, pulling, or pushing may be especially prone to back disorders, for example, truck drivers who also load and unload trucks. Workers who are vibrated while in twisted or other awkward postures (i.e., tractor drivers) may be particularly at risk.

Studies indicate that maximum strain occurs in the seated operator's lumbar region at the first natural frequency. In addition, back muscles are not able to protect the spine from adverse loads. At many frequencies the muscle response is so far out of phase that their forces are added to those of the stimulus. The fatigue that is found in muscles after vehicular vibration is indicative of the loads in the muscles. Therefore, it would seem reasonable to recommend avoiding heavy lifting after vibration exposure (i.e., unloading a truck). It would also be advisable for those exposed to prolonged vibration (i.e., long-distance driving) to take frequent rests.

Other job modifications can be considered in attempts to reduce the risks to a driver. A damped seat can attenuate the vibration. Proper ergonomic layout can obviate awkward postures that prestress the spinal tissues. An inclined backrest with lumbar support can also be helpful.

Drivers can be encouraged to reduce vibrations by adapting a smoother driving style. Frequent rests and stretches should also be encouraged. Some studies suggest that lifestyle changes such as reduced smoking, alcohol consumption, and drug use may also be helpful. Only a review of the whole driver and the immediate environment will be truly effective.

References

1. Åkerblom B: *Standing and sitting posture; with special reference to the construction of chairs*, doctoral dissertation, Stockholm, 1948, Nordiska Bokhandeln.

2. Andersson GBJ, Örtengren R: Myoelectric back muscle activity during sitting, *Scand J Rehabil Med Suppl* 3:73-90, 1974.

3. Andersson GBJ, Örtengren R, Nachemson A: The influence of backrest inclination and lumbar support on the lumbar lordosis in sitting, *Spine* 4:45-58, 1979.

4. Backman AL: Health survey of professional drivers, *Scand J Work Environ Health* 9:36-41, 1983.

5. Barbaso E: Sull'incidenza edelle alterazioni della colonna vertebrale nel personale viaggiante di una aienda autotramviaria, *Med Lavoro* 49:630-634, 1958.

6. Bennett MD, Webb R, Withey WR: Personality, performance, and physiologic cost during vibration. *Proceedings of the Physics Society*, London, 1977; pp 75-76.

7. Bongers PM, Boshuizen HC: *Back disorders and whole body vibration at work*, dissertation, 1990, University of Amsterdam.

8. Christ W: Aufbaustörungen der wirbelsäule bei den in der Landwirtschaft tätigen jugendlichen im Hinblick auf das Schlepperfahren, *Grundl Landt* 1:13-15, 1963.

9. Christ W, Dupuis H: Über die Beanspruchung die Wirbelsäule unter dem Einfluss sinusförmiger und stochastischer Schwingungen, Int *Z Angew Phys Arbeitsphysiol*, 22:258-278, 1966.

10. Cole SH, Withey WR: Human response to whole body vibration of different wave forms. *Proceedings of the Physics Society*, 1977, London, 76-77.

11. Cremona E: *Die Wirbelsäule bei den Schwerarbeitern der Eisen- und Stahlindustrie sowie des Bergbaus*. Kommiss. Europ. Germ. Generaldir. Soz. Angelegenheiten Dok, Berlin, 1911 (1972).

12. Dupuis H, Christ W: Uber das Schwingverhalten des Magens unter dem Einflub sinusförmiger und stochastischer Schwingungen, *Int Z Angew Physiol Arbeitsphysiol* 22:149-166, 1966.

13. Dupuis H, Christ W: *Untersuchung der Mögllichkeit von Gesundheitsschädigungen im Bereich der Wirbelsäule bei Schlepperfahrern*, Research report, Bad Kreuznach, Germany, 1972 Max-Planck-Institut für Landarbeit und Landtechnik.

14. Frymoyer JW et al: Risk factors in low back pain: an epidemiologic study, *J Bone Joint Surg Am* 65:213-218, 1983.

15. Hansson T H, Keller TS, Spengler DM: The effect of static and dynamic load on disk pressure in the human lumbar spine. *Proceedings of the Thirtieth Meeting of the Orthopaedic Research Society*, Atlanta, 1984, p 255.

16. Heliövaara M: Occupation and risk of herniated lumbar intervertebral disk of sciatica leading to hospitalization, *J Chronic Dis* 40:259-264, 1987.

17. Hilfert R et al: Probleme der Ganzkörperschwingungsbelastung von Erdbaumaschinen fürern, *Zentralbl Arb Med* 31:152-155, 199-206, 1981.

18. Holm S, Nachemson A: Nutrition of the intervertebral disk, effects induced by vibration. *Presented at International Society for The Study of The Lumbar Spine, Sydney*, 1985.

19. Hulshof C, van Zantern BV: Whole-body vibration and low back pain: a review of epidemiologic studies, *Int Arch Occup Environ Health* 50:205-220, 1987.

20. Hult L: Cervical, dorsal, and lumbar spine syndromes, *Acta Orthop Scand Suppl* 7, 1955.

21. International Organization for Standardization: *Guide for the evaluation of human exposure to whole body vibration*, No ISO 2631 (E), 1985, The Organization.

22. Keegan JJ: Alterations of the lumbar curve related to posture and seating, *J Bone Joint Surg Am* 35:589-603, 1953.

23. Kelsey JL, Hardy RJ: Driving of motor vehicles as a risk factor for acute herniated lumbar intervertebral disk, *Am J Epidemiol* 102:62-73, 1975.

24. Köhl U: Les dangers encourus par les conducterus de tracteurs, *Arch Mal Prof Med Trav Secur Soc* 36:145-162, 1975.

25. Kubik S: Gesundiheitliche Schäden bei Traktoristen. *Proceedings of the International Congress on Occupational Health*, Vienna, 1966, pp 375-377.

26. Lavault P: Quelque aspects de la pathologie du rachis chez le conducteur deu tracteur agricole, *Concours Med* 85:5863-5875, 1962.

27. Lawrence J: *Rheumatism in populations*, London: 1977, Heinemann.

28. Magnusson ML et al: Investigation of the long-term exposure to whole body vibration: a two country study. Winner of the Vienna Award for Physical Medicine. *Presented at the annual meeting of the Austria Society of Physical Medicine and Rehabilitation*, Vienna, Nov, 1992.

29. Magora A: Investigation of the relation between low back pain and occupations: three physical requirements: sitting, standing, and weight lifting, *Ind Med* 41:5-9, 1972.

30. Nachemson AL, Elfström G: Intravital dynamic pressure measurements in lumbar disks. A study of common movements, maneuvers, and exercises, *Scand J Rehabil Med* 2(suppl 1):1-40, 1970.

31. Panjabi MM et al: *In vivo* measurement of spinal column vibration, *J Bone Joint Surg Am* 68:695-703, 1986.

32. Pope MH, Broman H, Hansson T: Factors affecting the dynamic response of the seated subject, *J Spinal Disord* 3:135-142, 1990.

33. Pope MH, Broman H, Hansson T: The dynamic response of a subject seated on various cushions, *Ergonomics* 32:1155-1166, 1989.

34. Pope MH, Broman H, Hansson T: The impact response of the standing subject—a feasibility study, *Clin Biomech* 4:195-200, 1989.

35. Pope MH et al: The effect of vibration on back discomfort and serum levels of von Willebrand factor antigen: a preliminary communication, *Eur Spine J* 3(3): 143-145, 1994.

36. Pope MH et al: The measurement of oxygen uptake under whole body vibration, *Iowa Orthop J* 10:85-88, 1990.

37. Pope MH et al: The metabolic cost of various occupational exposures, *Ergonomics* 30:55-60, 1987.

38. Pope MH et al: The response of the seated human to sinusoidal vibration and impact, *J Biomech Eng* 109:279-284, 1987.

39. Rosegger R, Rosegger S: Health effects of tractor driving, *Agricultural Eng Res* 5:241-276, 1960.

40. Rosegger S: Vorzeitige Aufbraucherscheinungen bei Kraftfahrern, *Z Orthop Ihre Grenzgeb* 108:510-516, 1970.

41. Rosemeyer B: Eine Methode zur Beckenfixierung im Arbeitssitz, *Z Orthop* 110:514, 1972.

42. Schmidt U: *Verleichande Untersuchungen an Schwerlastwagenfahrern und Büroangestellten zur Frage der berufsbedingten Verschleibschäden an der Wirbelsäule und den Gelenken der oberen Extremitäten,* Dissertation, Berlin, 1969, Humboldt University.

43. Schoberth H: *Sitzhaltung. (Sitzschaden Sitzmobel),* Berlin, 1962, Springer-Verlag.

44. Schultz KJ, Polster J: Berufsbedingte Wirbelsäulenschäden bei Traktoristen und Landwirten, *Beitr Orthop Trauma* 26:356-362, 1979.

45. Seidel H, Heide R: Long-term effects of whole body vibration: a critical survey of the literature, *Int Arch Occup Environ Health* 58:1-26, 1986.

46. Seroussi R, Wilder DG, Pope MH: Trunk muscle electromyography and whole body vibration, *J Biomech* 22:219-229, 1989.

47. Webb RDG, Bennett MD, Farnile B: Personality and intersubject differences in performance and physiological cost during whole body vibration, *Ergonomics* 24:245-255, 1981.

48. Weinstein J et al: Neuropharmacologic effects of vibration on the dorsal root ganglion, *Spine* 13:521-525, 1988.

49. Wilder DG, Frymoyer JW, Pope MH: The effect of vibration on the spine of the seated individual, *Automedica* 6:5-35, 1985.

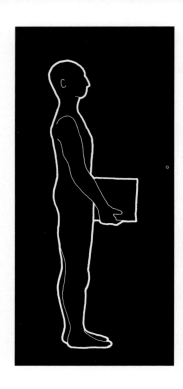

Chapter 12

Adverse Effects of Repetitive Loading and Segmental Vibration

Thomas J. Armstrong
Bernard J. Martin

CONTENTS

The possible effects of repetitive work and exposure to vibration are important health considerations because repetitive work is still an important component of our industrial economy. In many cases, the technology to automate work is not yet available or it is too expensive. In other cases, workers can do the job better or faster than machines. This is particularly true when there are variations in the process, materials, or parts. Some companies have recently shifted from automation back to manual work, so manual work will be an important part of our industrial economy for the foreseeable future.

MANUAL WORK

Manual work entails the exertion of muscles to move or maintain the position of the body or work objects. In some cases, the work object is a part or a product. In other cases it may be a tool or the controls of a machine. In the United States, work is commonly performed for 8 hours per day, 5 days per week, but 10- and 12-hour days and 6 days per week are not uncommon.

Manual work exposes the body to physical stressors that produce physiologic and biomechanical tissue disturbances, as shown in **Figure 12-1**.[5] These disturbances may result in pain, impaired work performance, and other adverse health effects. In most cases these disturbances will subside with time. If, however, the time is too short for complete recovery between successive work periods, these disturbances may begin to accumulate and thereby increase pain and impairment. In extreme cases the pain and impairment can be disabling and persist for days, weeks, months, or years.

The relationship between manual work and adverse health effects is supported by numerous studies of work and health patterns. In his classic 1713 work *De Morbis Artificum (Diseases of Workers)*, Ramazzini[106] wrote:

> Various and manifold is the harvest of diseases reaped by certain workers from the crafts and trades that they pursue. All the profit that they get is fatal injury to their health, mostly from two causes. The first and most potent is the harmful character of the materials they handle. The sec-

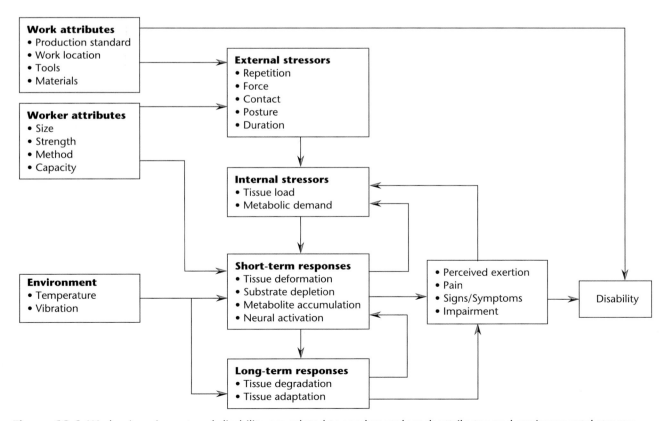

Figure 12-1 Worker impairment and disability are related to worker and work attributes and environmental stresses.

ond, I ascribe to certain violent and irregular motions and unnatural postures of the body, by reason of which, the natural structure of the vital machine is so impaired that serious diseases gradually develop therefrom.

Ramazzini described these disorders in selected occupations. One that is particularly relevant to the contemporary work setting is that of writers and scribes[106]:

> The diseases of persons incident to this craft arise from three causes. First constant sitting, second the perpetual motion of the hand in the same manner, and thirdly the attention and application of the mind. . . . In a word, they lack the benefits of moderate exercise, for even if they wanted to take exercise they have not time for it; they are working for wages and must stick to their writing. . . . Constant writing also considerably fatigues the hand and the whole arm on account of the continual and almost tense tension of the muscles and tendons.

Although workers no longer use the quill pens typical of Ramazzini's time, workers in many contemporary settings are exposed to constant sitting, perpetual motion of the hand, and application of the mind. Keyboard work is a prime example of such work, but examples can be found in the manufacturing sector as well.

In 1893 Gray[38] wrote about the adverse effects encountered by women doing laundry:

> The tendons of the extensor muscles of the thumb are liable to become strained and their sheaths inflamed after excessive exercise, producing a sausage-shaped swelling along the course of the tendon, and giving a peculiar creaking sensation to the finger when the muscle acts. In consequence of its often being caused by such movements as **wringing clothes**, it is known as: washerwoman's sprain.

This condition was described in 1895 by de Quervain[24] and is now referred to as de Quervain's disease. Wringing cloths entails forceful gripping and ulnar wrist deviation. This posture can be found in many jobs that entail the use of hand tools and the finishing and assembly of parts.

Contemporary studies are more specific about both the qualities and quantities of adverse health effects associated with repetitive work. Maeda[74] reported increased cases of neck-shoulder-arm syndromes in Japanese office workers and attributed them to increased "rationalization" of office work in Japan since 1950. Generalizing from 136 cases seen from 1960 to 1969 in his labor hygiene consultation, he argued that affected workers were exposed to unnatural postures and high levels of repetition.

Reports of upper limb disorders increased following passage of worker's compensation laws in the early twentieth century. Obolenskaja and Goljanitzki[92] reported 189 cases of tenosynovitis of the upper extremi-

ties among a group of 700 packers in a tea factory. They suggested that these cases were due to high rates of work consisting of between 7600 and 12,000 exertions per shift. Hammer[44] suggested that human tendons do not tolerate more than 1500 to 2000 exertions per hour. These reports indicate early recognition of the possible adverse health effects of work and the level of risk in specific industries. In addition, they attempt to define repetition and identify a safe critical threshold.

In 1991, Franklin et al[31] presented an analysis of 7926 cases of compensable carpal tunnel syndrome in the state of Washington from 1984 to 1988. The average incidence rates ranged from 0.2 to 25.7 cases per 1000 full-time employees, with the highest rates occurring in jobs that entailed high repetition (job categories "meat, poultry, and fish processing") and the lowest rates in jobs that entailed the lowest levels of repetition (job categories "state employees" and "higher education"). These data support a relationship between repetitive hand work and the risk of upper limb disorders, specifically, carpal tunnel syndrome. No attempt was made to characterize repetition or define a safe critical threshold.

According to the Bureau of Labor Statistics,[16] the incidence of cumulative trauma disorders ranged from 3 to 4 cases per 10,000 private sector workers per year from 1978 to 1984, but then increased steadily to 30 cases per 10,000 workers in 1994. The cause of this increase has been a matter of speculation. Some argue that it is due to increasing work rates to meet increasing national and international competition. Others argue that it is due to increased awareness of these problems by workers, employers, and healthcare providers. Both arguments are probably valid.

Although the observations of Ramazzini and Gray and to a lesser extent Maeda are anecdotal, they demonstrate that the possible adverse health effects of excessive work have been recognized for many years and are not a product of the 1990s. In addition, these observations provide insight into the relationship between work patterns and health patterns; however, the available data are not yet sufficient to determine critical thresholds for design purposes. There are several hurdles to developing models that can be used to establish acceptable exposure: (1) many exposure and health variables must be considered; (2) agreement has not yet been reached on how to measure exposure and health variables; metrics that work well in one study setting do not always work well in another; and (3) it is difficult to control and evaluate all of these variables in a single study.

The health effects of repetitive work include perceived exertion, discomfort, and muscle, tendon, joint, and nerve disorders at various locations of the upper limb. The criteria and threshold for reporting disorders have not yet been standardized, and they vary from one study to another. Some disorders, such as perceived exertion and discomfort, may be harbingers of more serious problems such as a chronic tendon or nerve disorder. Other disorders may actually lead to other disorders, for example, flexor tenosynovitis leading to carpal tunnel syndrome.[69,99] Some health effects are more easily measured than others. This is true for carpal tunnel syndrome and other nerve disorders in which nerve conduction and quantitative sensory testing can be used to objectively quantify certain functional parameters. For many disorders, worker signs and symptoms do not fall into established clinical patterns associated with recognized pathologies. Terms such as "cumulative trauma disorder" or "strain" may be used for lack of a specific diagnosis, or terms such as "tendinitis" or "carpal tunnel syndrome" may be used loosely as a catchall for all hand problems.

Repetition and associated adverse health effects appear to follow a dose-response relationship in which prevalence asymptomatically approaches zero with a decreasing dose and asymptotically approaches 100% with an increasing dose as shown in **Figure 12-2**.[5] In practice, because there is some background level as a result of other factors, the prevalence is almost never zero. Similarly, situations in which the dose is so great that 100% of the work force is affected are very rare. Consequently, most studies only examine part of the dose-response relationship. Also, most studies focus on only one of many possible adverse health effects. The dose-response relationship is often characterized by regression analysis to fit a logistic-response model to observed dose and response data.[60] Dose-response models are potentially useful for designing jobs that entail an acceptable level of risk. Unfortunately, sufficient data are not yet available to determine a dose-response relationship for all possible disorders and all of their possible factors.

The development of a dose-response model requires the identification of groups containing people with different exposure levels. Except for the exposure variable under study, it is important that all other exposure variables be the same, including age, gender, and work experience. As a practical matter, it is very difficult to find such groups that are directly comparable. Often, jobs that require low repetition levels such as machine operators and maintenance are dominated by male workers, whereas jobs that require high repetition levels

such as assembly and sewing are dominated by female workers. It would be hard to separate the differences due to gender from those caused by repetition and force in a comparison of the health patterns of two such groups.

Health effects need to be assessed by using the same objective criteria for all workers. Health effects may be identified from voluntary reports to a healthcare provider or through surveys using questionnaires, interviews, and physical examinations. Voluntary data are affected by the workers' pain and impairment tolerance and their attitude toward the healthcare provider and employer. Workers can be very resourceful in coping with pain and impairment if it jeopardizes their livelihood and may actively try to keep their employer from learning of health problems. This does not mean that such data are not useful, but it does introduce additional variables that may influence the outcome of a study and may make it difficult to compare data from one study with another. Ostensibly, some of these limitations can be overcome by using controlled surveys; however, no agreement has yet been reached on survey instruments for various upper limb disorders. Also, surveys may be influenced by how the survey is conducted, for example, by mail, by interviews, on company time, or on personal time, and how the workers view the investigators. Another problem affecting cross-sectional surveys is that workers who experience problems may self-select a less stressful job or avoid jobs perceived to be stressful. This may reduce the prevalence in strenuous jobs and elevate the prevalence in light-duty jobs.

An example of these biases can be seen in work reported by Nathan, Meadows, and Doyle,[88] who categorized 471 volunteers from 1855 workers in 27 occupations into five graded stress levels with 147, 22, 164, 115, and 23 workers in the various groups. The prevalence of impaired median nerve conduction was reported as 28%, 27%, 47%, 61%, and 39% from the lowest to the highest group. The increasing prevalence of median nerve findings with increasing stress from the first to the fourth levels of stress is consistent with the findings reported by others. The decreasing prevalence from the fourth to the fifth level and the very low participation rate in the fifth level suggest a sampling

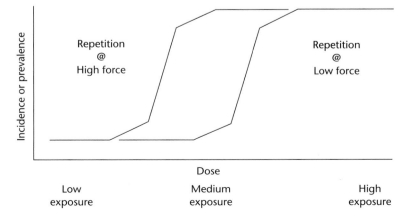

Figure 12-2 Repetition and associated adverse health effects appear to follow a dose-response relationship in which the incidence or prevalence of a given disorder increases with repetition from a background level to a level where all workers will eventually be affected. In this example two cures are shown, one for repetitive exertion in combination with low-force exertion and a second one for repetitive exertion in combination with high forces.

bias. No attempt was reported to balance the study groups by age, gender, or seniority. Silverstein, Fine, and Stetson[115] addressed these issues by using a stratified randomized sample procedure and by selecting equal numbers of persons in each exposure category at each work site. This resulted in four combinations of high and low repetition and high and low force that were balanced as regards age, gender, and years on the job. By conducting a confidential examination of workers on company time they were able to obtain a participation rate of 89.7%. The reported prevalence of carpal tunnel syndrome increased significantly from 0.6% in the low-force, low-repetition job to 5.6%, based on both interview and physical examinations.

A comparison of the Nathan and Silverstein studies demonstrates how outcomes are influenced by the selection of subjects, study sites, and diagnostic criteria and how these factors should be considered in the interpretation of results and conclusions. The ideal study would be a prospective design in which groups of subjects balanced according to all possible personal factors—age, gender, work experience, seniority, recreational activities, natural diseases, etc.—are stratified into groups from low to high for each stressor. All subjects would then be carefully tracked for several years for signs and symptoms of upper limb disorders by using validated diagnostic criteria. Such a study is probably not feasible because populations and work exposures are too unstable. Workers change jobs for reasons other than health, jobs change for economic reasons, and agreement has not yet been reached on valid health effect measures. Consequently, we are left to piece together the dose-response relationship from studies that have examined different populations and work settings, different exposure parameters, and different health criteria.

Epidemiologic studies can be supplemented and guided by our understanding of the underlying biomechanical and physiologic mechanisms. These studies generally involve invasive measures and examine the response of one tissue at one location to a limited, but controlled range of physical stressors. Areas of particularly relevant work include studies of fatigue after sustained and repeated exertion, tendon deformation and adaptation to repetitive loading, and nerve responses to pressure. The mechanisms by which the performance of manual work lead to impairments of the upper limb and worker disability are not fully understood. The literature suggests that biomechanical, physiologic, and psychological processes are involved, as shown in **Figure 12-1**.[5] Work attributes such as production standards, work locations, and tool size and shape, along with worker attributes such as size and behavior, result in external stressors such as repetition, force, contact stresses, and extreme postures. External stressors result in internal stressors such as muscle loads, tendon loads, and metabolic demands. Internal stressors along with worker attributes of capacity result in short-term responses such as increased concentrations of metabolites, decreased

concentrations of substrates, tissue deformation, and nerve stimulation. Short-term responses may lead to long-term responses such as tissue degradation or tissue adaptation, which may increase or decrease individual capacity accordingly. Short- and long-term responses may also result from environmental stressors such as vibration and low temperatures. Responses to environmental stressors may also result in additional force stressors. Short- and long-term responses may result in increased perceived exertion, pain, and signs or symptoms of various upper limb disorders. A disability can develop, depending on the nature of the impairment, work requirements, and worker tolerance. Johansson and Sojka[54] proposed that a stressor that produces a localized disturbance in a muscle may lead to the stimulation of afferent nerve fibers and further stimulation and aggravation via a positive feedback mechanism.

The performance of manual work results in a series of cascading doses and responses in which the response at one level acts as a dose and produces a response at the next.[5] The large number of tissues and mechanisms involved and the variations in worker attributes mean that worker impairments and disabilities may take on many manifestations. Controlled laboratory studies of these responses help to explain the underlying mechanisms; however, care should be exercised in extrapolating from a short-term laboratory study to a lifetime occupational exposure.

Worker behavior and tissue responses may be additionally influenced by environmental stressors such as low temperatures and vibration, which will be discussed in later sections of this chapter. Work methods and tissue disturbances may also be affected by psychological stress from work and non–work-related factors; this may result in altered behavior, including the use of higher than necessary force, and makes the job more stressful. Psychological stresses may also reduce the tolerance of tissues to mechanical and physiologic disturbances and the tolerance of the worker to discomfort.

Although it is not yet possible to establish rigorous design specifications for a given level of risk, together the available studies demonstrate the kinds of problems associated with certain types of work and help to identify extreme situations in which there is likely to be elevated risk to workers. Such studies also provide insight into which factors and aspects of the jobs should be redesigned to prevent injury or facilitate the return to work of an injured worker. Examples of these studies will be described in the following discussion of risk factors for upper limb disorders.

PHYSICAL STRESSORS

Repetition and Force

Study of the relationship between repetition and upper limb disorders requires some way of characterizing repetition. Repetition refers to the temporal aspects of exertion of the body. An exertion can be defined as the production of force to support the gravity, drag, or reaction forces on a body or work object. Force and repetition are related; it is not possible to have an exertion and repetition without force, but it is possible to have repetition with varying degrees of force. Repetition is often expressed as the number of exertions per unit time. Identifying and counting discrete exertions are often unfeasible. Most investigators rate repetition by observations of representative jobs or known work requirements.

Cannon, Barnacki, and Walter[20] compared a group of 30 patients with carpal tunnel syndrome with a group of 90 sex-matched healthy workers and found that the use of vibrating tools was associated with a sevenfold increase in the risk of carpal tunnel syndrome. This was followed by performance of repetitive-motion tasks and by years on the job. Repetitiveness was defined simply as "performance of repetitive motion tasks," without further explanation.

Punnett et al[102] conducted a cross-sectional investigation of hand and arm soft tissue disorders (using a questionnaire) among 162 female garment workers (average age, 43) doing repetitive work and 73 female hospital workers (average age, 41) who did not do repetitive work. The prevalence of symptoms at any site, the shoulder, wrist, or hand, and the prevalence of carpal tunnel syndrome, which ranged from 6.5% to 42%, were all higher than those of the hospital workers, which ranged from 4.3% to 21.9%. Repetitiveness was defined as the number of tasks in the job and the length of time of the work cycle. Both were determined from films of the job.

Silverstein, Fine, and Stetson[115] reported that the prevalence of carpal tunnel syndrome among persons performing highly repetitive, high-force jobs, 5.1%, was significantly higher than that in those performing low-repetition, low-force jobs, 0.6%.[115] The prevalence of carpal tunnel syndrome for workers in the low-repetition, high-force and particularly those in the high-repetition, low-force jobs was elevated, but not significantly. A similar trend was reported for hand and wrist tendinitis in the same population, but the prevalence in the high-repetition, high-force job, 10.8%, was higher than that of carpal tunnel syndrome.[7] Repetition was characterized in terms of cycle time and determined by using observation and work standards. Forces were characterized through observation and surface electromyography.

Viikari-Juntura et al[127] conducted three cross-sectional surveys over a 31-month period of epicondylitis and elbow pain in persons performing jobs considered strenuous: meat cutting and packing and sausage making. They were compared with 289 sex-, age-, and duration of employment–matched persons doing non-strenuous work: managers, maintenance workers, and retail salespersons. The prevalence of symptoms within the last 12 months was 34.9% and 21.2%, respectively, for persons in jobs with high and low levels of strenuous activity. Strenuousness was based on assessment of both

repetition and force and was determined from an analysis of the production standards.

Higgs et al[46] examined differences in subjective and objective measures of upper extremity function in 157 workers performing repetitive tasks in a meat processing plant. Significant impairments were reported in over half of the workers. The highest average impairments were among those whose jobs required the highest number of wrist flexions and extensions per hour. Flexions and repetition per hour were determined from videotapes of selected workers.

Using electrodiagnosis and physical examination, Barnhart et al[10] studied the prevalence of carpal tunnel syndrome in a plant population of 400. They reported a prevalence 15.4% and 31.1% among persons doing jobs with low and high repetition, respectively. Jobs were observed and classified as "highly repetitive" if they entailed repeated or sustained activities that involved flexion, extension, or ulnar deviation of the wrist by 45 degrees; radial deviation of more than 30 degrees; or use of a pinch grip.

Because disorders such as tendinitis and carpal tunnel syndrome develop over long time periods and because they are considered serious medical conditions, it is neither feasible nor desirable to conduct laboratory studies in which they might be induced. Instead, laboratory studies focus on responses that occur over periods of seconds, minutes, hours, or in extreme cases, days. The most frequently studied response is localized fatigue. Localized fatigue is characterized in terms of subjective and objective changes associated with exertion and involves both contractile and noncontractile tissue. Numerous studies have shown increased fatigue with increasing time and static exertion force. Monod[86] showed that endurance has an inverse functional relationship with force. Endurance appeared to decrease from infinity at 15% of maximum strength to zero at 100% of maximum strength. Lind et al[65] demonstrated that forearm blood flow increased with increasing work intensity up to 15% and then decreased with further increases in force. This decrease was attributed to a distortion of the vascular bed and to increasing intramuscular pressure associated with muscle contraction.[52,116] It was suggested that exertions below 15% of maximum strength might be maintained or repeated indefinitely without fatigue; however, later studies showed that fatigue occurs during sustained exertions as low as 5% maximum voluntary contraction (MVC).[117] Bystrom and Fransson-Hall[18] recently showed that 10% MVC was unacceptable for repeated 5-second exertions. This has led to the suggestion that there may not be a safe force level for sustained or highly repetitive work. It may be necessary to schedule work so as to provide distinct recovery periods appropriate for the work being performed.

Basmajian[11] demonstrated that the loads about some joints may be transferred to the ligaments as the muscles fatigue. He suggested that some of the discomfort associated with sustained exertion may be due to sustained or repeated stretching of connective tissues. This accounts for the discomfort in the joints of the upper limb that is associated with carrying a suitcase at the side of the body.

It has been shown that tissues demonstrate viscoelastic properties.[33,37,122] This means that tissue deformations are time as well as force dependent. Consequently, if the recovery time between successive exertions is not sufficient, muscles, tendons, and ligaments will become more and more deformed. At some point these deformations can be expected to interfere with physiologic functions. Kenedi, Gibson, and Daly[59] defined the physiologic limit for skin as the point where deformation is sufficient to occlude cutaneous circulation and result in blanching. An equivalent deformation level has not yet been established for muscles, tendons, and ligaments, but it has been shown that if the recovery time between successive exertions is not sufficient, flexor tendons will continue to lengthen. Goldstein et al[37] found that the rate of creep exceeded the rate of strain recovery in human finger flexor tendons subjected to physiologic loads for 8 seconds and no load for 2 seconds. After 500 cycles, the strain was approximately double that of the first cycle. The creep was negligible when the same loads were applied for 2 seconds with 8 seconds rest.

Recent studies examined the effect of repetitive wrist motion on fluid pressure inside the carpal canal. Using a slit catheter, Szabo and Chidgey[119] measured the intracarpal canal pressure immediately after 30 flexion-extensions of the wrist and then again 10 minutes later. The pressure in 6 healthy subjects immediately returned to the resting level (5 to 8 mm), but the pressure in 17 patients with early to intermediate carpal tunnel syndrome was still elevated (28 mm) 10 minutes following the experiment.

The effects of repeated exertions may be altered by the duration of the exertion, the duration of the work shift, the intensity of the exertion, movement, contact between certain parts of the body and external objects, posture, low temperatures, and vibration.

Duration

Using a case-control study format in which 45 video display unit operators with repetitive strain injuries were compared with 110 job-matched controls, Oxenburgh[93] found no differences between workstations but did find differences in hours of keying. It was found that over 71% of the injured operators spent more than 5 hours per day at their keyboards whereas only 28% of the healthy group spent that much time at their keyboards. In a health hazard investigation by the National Institute for Occupational Safety and Health at a major newspaper, a correlation was found between the percentage of time spent keying and the risk of upper limb disorders.[89] It appears from these data that the risk of upper limb disorders may be reduced by decreasing the number of hours per day spent performing repetitive work. In a longitudinal study of sewing machine opera-

tors working 5- or 8-hour shifts, Waersted and Westgaard[128] showed that shortened work shifts appeared to only delay the onset of adverse health effects, not prevent them. Additional studies are necessary to confirm the effects of 5- versus 8-hour shifts and to investigate the effects of 10- and 12-hour shifts and various break schedules.

Margolis and Kraus[75] obtained an 83% response rate to a mail survey about the carpal tunnel syndrome symptoms of all 1345 checkers who were members of one union local in California. The symptoms of carpal tunnel syndrome were found to increase with the number of hours and years worked. Powell et al[100] reported a linear relationship between miles run per week and overuse injuries in runners. Injury rates exceed 20% per year for women and 15% for men when they exceeded 30 miles per week. MacDonald, Robertson, and Erickson[73] conducted a mail survey of carpal tunnel syndrome symptoms among 7415 dental hygienists in California. Of 2464 questionnaires that were returned, 8.7% reported a history of carpal tunnel syndrome. Significant associations were found between paresthesia and the number of days worked; clumsiness, pain, and burning and the number of days worked per week; and between all symptoms and the number of patients with heavy calculus seen in a day.

It has already been argued that pain and impairment may be cumulative if recovery is insufficient between successive work bouts of a given intensity. It follows that the longer the work is performed, the greater will be the accumulated response. Further research is needed to determine critical response thresholds. Models that integrate responses for given work regimens are needed to evaluate the effects of different work schedules and rates. For example, is there a difference in risk between five 8-hour days and four 10-hour days? It can be argued that if it takes 16 hours to recover from 8 hours of work, then a 14-hour recovery following a 10-hour shift will be inadequate and workers will be at increased risk of impairments and symptoms.

Velocity and Acceleration

Velocity is an attribute of an exertion; therefore it is difficult to separate velocity from repetition. It can range from positive to negative values. Because joint ranges of motion are limited, a given velocity cannot be maintained for more than a few seconds before the joint limits are reached. Cyclic velocity profiles are accompanied by corresponding acceleration profiles and by the accompanying inertial effects. Marras and Schoenmarklin[76] compared wrist postures, velocities, and accelerations between two groups of workers from different industrial plants. The job groups were classified as being at low risk and high risk of cumulative trauma disorders based on incidence rates determined from the Occupational Safety and Health Administration (OSHA) log (0 and 18.4 cases per 200,000 work hours, respectively). Significant differences were found in wrist radial/ulnar deviation, wrist flexion/extension, and forearm supination/pronation velocity and accele-ration between the two groups. For cyclic displacements of a joint, acceleration is related to displacement by the frequency squared and to velocity by the frequency. Thus cycle time, frequency, velocity, and acceleration are all related. Marras and Schoenmarklin suggested that the relationship between acceleration and risk is explained by Newton's second law, force equal to mass times acceleration. Therefore, acceleration increases loading on the tissues of the extremity.

It is possible for a worker to increase the velocity of movement for part of the cycle and to reduce it for another part. Further research is needed to examine the trade-off between increasing velocity and rest time.

Posture

Posture refers to the position of joints and is an attribute of an exertion. Therefore it is difficult to separate posture from repetition. Ramazzini[106] characterized posture simply as natural versus unnatural. Engineers characterize posture in angular units about each axis of rotation with respect to a reference position. The reference position is generally selected as one close to the midpoint of the range of motion that can be easily established. For example, the neutral position of the wrist is typically established with respect to an outstretched hand. Consequently, a three-by-three matrix, or nine variables, is required to characterize the position of the shoulder, elbow, and wrist—excluding the 15 major joints of the hand. Characterization of posture can be simplified by neglecting some axes and categorizing overall hand position. Finger positions are generally characterized in terms of overall hand position, pulp pinch, hook grip, power grip, and so forth. The postures may vary between the beginning and the end of an exertion or job task.

Epidemiologic studies of posture include those by Duncan and Ferguson,[27] who performed a case-control study of 90 male telegraphists with complaints of symptoms in whom occupational cramp or myalgia was diagnosed and 45 unaffected telegraphists of the same sex, age, length of service, and status. Detailed posture observations of shoulder depression, shoulder abduction, shoulder flexion, ulnar deviation, wrist extension, finger extension, mixed extension and flexion, finger flexion, and little finger abduction were performed. It was concluded that keyboard design and work height resulted in work postures that lead to neck and upper limb symptoms in some operators.

Hunting, Laubli, and Grandjean[53] performed medical examinations on a group of persons performing keyboard data entry and a group performing conversation tasks. They concluded that the constrained postures required to use the keyboard/video display terminal and in full-time typists were associated with daily hand, arm, shoulder, and neck pain. Armstrong and Chaffin[4] performed a case-control study of sewing machine operators with diagnosed carpal tunnel syndrome. Operators with carpal tunnel syndrome were found to exert more force and use a pinch grip with an extended wrist posture more frequently than unaffected operators. de Krom et al[22] performed a questionnaire survey of a sex-stratified community-based sample of 715 persons from the population register of Maastricht, The Netherlands, from 1983 to 1985. They found that a duration of activities with a flexed or extended wrist over 5 years was a significant factor in carpal tunnel syndrome. Loslever and Ranaivosoa[68] performed a cross-sectional study of carpal tunnel syndrome and wrist posture and movement. Posture was studied with an electromechanical goniometer, and force was studied by surface electromyography of one to four workers in each of eight hand-intensive industries. The prevalence of carpal tunnel syndrome for both hands was highly correlated with the frequency of flexion, and the use of high force and high or low degrees of flexion appeared to be a greater risk factor than high or low degrees of extension.

Laboratory studies of the possible effects of posture on worker health include those by Brain, Wright, and Wilkinson,[15] Tanzer,[121] Phalen,[99] and Smith, Sonstegard, and Anderson.[118] All concluded on the basis of premortem and postmortem surgical studies and pressure measurements that carpal tunnel syndrome was related to flexion and extension of the wrist and increased pressure on the median nerve. It was further suggested that this pressure plays an important role in the pathogenesis of carpal tunnel syndrome. Szabo and Chidgey[119] reported average fluid pressures inside the carpal tunnel of 5, 15, and 27 mm for neutral, flexed, and extended wrist postures in six normal subjects and 10, 32, and 52 mm for neutral, flexed, and extended wrist postures in patients with carpal tunnel syndrome. Lundborg et al[70] demonstrated that fluid pressure as low as 30 mm was sufficient to produce mild neurophysiologic changes and hand paresthesia after 60 minutes and that 60- and 90-mm pressure was associated with changes after 20 to 30 minutes and 10 to 30 minutes, respectively. These studies demonstrate a dose-response relationship between posture, pressure, and impairment.

Tichauer[123] suggested that the median nerve can be injured by stretching or "yanking," which occurs when the wrist is repeatedly extended in some work tasks. Armstrong and Chaffin[4] proposed a model analogous to a belt stretched around a pulley to characterize acute contact stresses on the finger flexor tendons and the median nerve. Armstrong et al[8] demonstrated that the areas of contact stress corresponded with the proliferation of connective tissue in the median nerve and ulnoradial bursa. These findings reinforced earlier findings by Phalen[99] and Yamagucci.[129] A thickening of the ulnoradial bursa appears to play a role in chronic fluid pressure changes inside the carpal tunnel and the pathogenesis of carpal tunnel syndrome.

The present pulley belt model explains only compression between the flexor retinaculum and the finger flexor tendon when the wrist is flexed or only compression and stretching of the nerve as it is stretched around the flexor tendons when the wrist is extended. It does not account for elevated fluid pressure during flexion and extension or radial and ulnar deviation of the wrist. Further model development is needed to account for changes in carpal canal volume caused by the shape changes that occur with joint movement or displacement of muscle tissue into the carpal canal. Similar models have been proposed for other joint structures such as the shoulder.[43,45]

Although the aforementioned studies demonstrate that impairment may result from prolonged or repeated exertion in some postures and with increasing acceleration, this does not mean that the body should be immobilized. Additional studies are required to determine optimal posture and movement patterns.

Contact Stress

Contact stresses result when the body exerts or rests against objects in the workplace. The average contact stress can be estimated as the force of contact divided by the area of contact. Peak contact stresses with values much greater than average will almost always occur. The irregular shape of the body inevitably results in irregular stress concentrations.

Karlqvist and Bjorksten[58] demonstrated that the location of hand pain corresponded to the location of stress concentrations produced by knife handles. Tannen et al[120] demonstrated similar findings for scissors. These pain patterns were considered an unacceptable response, and no attempt was made to develop a medical diagnosis or investigate the affected tissues. Both investigators focused on the design of tools to alleviate the pain.

Fransson-Hall and Kilbom[32] conducted a systematic study of pain threshold patterns for the hand. They showed that pain increased with greater duration and intensity of pressure and that some parts of the hand were more sensitive to pressure than others.

Lundborg et al[70] studied the effect of fluid pressure on median nerve function inside the carpal tunnel. Median nerve function was measured by nerve conduction studies and two-point discrimination. Fluid pressure was increased by applying pressure on the base of the palm. An intracarpal canal pressure of 30 mm was sufficient to impair nerve function after 60 minutes in some subjects, but the required time decreased to 20 minutes at 90-mm pressure. Similar pressure increases might be produced by pounding with the base of the palm, using a wrist rest on a keyboard, or using certain tools.

Further studies are needed to determine acceptable load pressure–time combinations for other tissues of the upper limb and to develop models of the production of pressure in a given part of the extremity.

Vibration

Vibration is a vector quantity with properties of amplitude and frequency. Standard methods are available for the measurement of resultant or dominant axis acceleration and the frequency of hand-arm vibration exposure.[1] This mechanical stimulus is known to produce a large variety of effects: (1) subjective sensations such as discomfort, numbness, tingling, hypoesthesia (diminished tactile sensitivity), or even movement illusions; (2) disorders affecting the musculoskeletal, vascular, and nervous systems, commonly called hand-arm vibration syndrome, including the so-called vibration-induced white finger syndrome, carpal tunnel syndrome, and peripheral sensory disorders; and (3) degradations in functioning of the motor system that are most frequently expressed by an increase in the tension of active muscles. A detailed review of the effects of "human vibration" can be found in recent publications.[28,40,77,98]

There are numerous reports of a vibratory contribution to upper limb disorders, particularly carpal tunnel syndrome. Rothfleisch and Sherman[114] reported a clinical case series of 16 patients with carpal tunnel syndrome (with 23 affected wrists) from an automobile assembly plant. Over half of the patients were using pneumatic tools at present or had used them in the past with frequencies between 8 and 333 Hz. Dimberg et al[26] reported small (r=.06 to .08) but significant correlations between vibration exposure and musculoskeletal symptoms in the shoulder. Cannon, Bernacki, and Walter[20] reported that the use of vibrating tools was the most significant risk factor for carpal tunnel syndrome in workers in a jet engine manufacturing plant.

It is difficult to separate the adverse effects of vibration from those of other stressors. Vibration exposure results from holding something that vibrates, so vibration exposure is inevitably accompanied by exposure to repetition and force and possibly stressful postures, contact stresses, and low temperatures as well. To assess the relative contribution of vibration to that of repetition and force, data reported by Silverstein, Fine, and Stetson[115] in which the carpal tunnel syndrome prevalence was 5.1% among persons doing highly repetitive and forceful work were stratified on the basis of vibration exposure.[6] It was found that the incidence was approximately twice as great among those who performed high-repetition, high-force jobs with vibration as among those without vibration exposure; however, this difference was not statistically significant because of the reduced sample size. Further studies along this line are needed to determine the relative contribution of vibration with respect to other stressors.

The adverse effects of vibration exposure are essentially multifactorial and result from the interaction of (1) vibration variables, (2) work attributes, and (3) physiologic responses and individual attributes (see **Fig. 12-1**). The complex reactions of the musculoskeletal system to vibration arise from the physical movement of body parts and the responses of the sensory systems generated by such stimulation. The human body does not behave like a passive system, but reacts to vibratory stimulus in many ways. These responses contribute to the multiple mechanisms by which muscle, tendon, and nerve disorders develop in the upper extremities. A scheme of the neurosensory mechanisms that may contribute to vibration-induced musculoskeletal and peripheral nerve symptoms is presented in the following sections. It will be seen that impairments in sensory and sensorimotor functions lead to a vicious circle in which muscle tension is "deregulated" by the predominance of nested positive feedback.

Peripheral Regulation of Muscle Contraction

A simplified scheme of the neuromuscular system of concern is presented in **Figure 12-3, A**. The motoneurons controlling muscle contraction/tension receive a combination of negative and positive feedback from peripheral receptors: the primary and secondary muscle spindle endings acting in parallel with the muscle, the Golgi tendon organs acting in series with the muscle, and various cutaneous mechanoreceptors distributed in skin layers. These receptors provide proprioceptive information about muscle length and the rate of change in muscle length, muscle force, and exteroceptive tactile information, respectively. The messages issued from these receptors are used to control muscle tension at peripheral and central levels. Furthermore, the stretch sensitivity of the muscle spindles is controlled via the γ-system (or fusimotor system). This sensitivity, which corresponds to the gain of the muscle proprioceptive feedback, is adjusted by descending pathways and peripheral reflexive mechanisms principally involving muscle group II (secondary spindle endings) and group III afferents ("pressure pain" receptors) and different joint afferents.[51,56,54,108] It has been observed that these reflex influences acting on the fusimotor system act preferentially as positive feedback increasing spindle sensitivity to stretch.[2,3] Such an action supports the concept that the γ-loop assists α-motor output during muscle contraction.[42] These data show that muscle contraction/tension is regulated by peripheral information from muscle, tendon, and skin integrated by nested feedback mechanisms. Hence this arrangement of the nerve fibers has the potential of increasing the gain of the proprioceptive feedback loop in a "recurrent" manner (perturbation–sensory receptor activation–γ-motoneuron activation–primary spindle activation–increased muscle tension–increased receptor activation, and so forth), as suggested earlier by Johansson and Sojka.[54]

Mechanoreceptors

The sensory information involved in the feedback systems is significantly modified by vibration. Microelectrode recordings of individual afferent nerve fibers reveal the sensory effects induced by vibration. Human studies show that cutaneous,[55,126] articular,[85] and musculotendinous mechanoreceptors[17,109,125] are activated by mechanical vibration. These receptors respond in 1:1 synchrony to the vibratory stimulus up to a certain "cutoff" frequency. Beyond that frequency, they start to respond in a subharmonic mode and then at random.[109,110,125] The frequency "bandwidths" of these receptors are estimated to be about 20 Hz (Golgi, Ib afferents), 60 Hz (secondary spindle endings, group II afferents), 100 Hz (primary spindle endings, Ia afferents), greater than 100 Hz (slowly adapting deep cutaneous receptors), and less than 200 Hz (fast-adapting cutaneous receptors). It is worth noting that these frequencies are within the range of hand tool vibration. Furthermore, the vibration-induced activity of proprioceptive and exteroceptive mechanoreceptors significantly interferes with the sensory messages evoked by natural stimulation such as movement or pressure. As indicated by Ribot-Ciscar[109] and Roll, Vedel, and Ribot,[110] vibration-induced activity of the primary spindle endings can (1) completely mask the response of these receptors to natural changes in muscle lengthening or (2) increase the frequency modulation of the firing of these receptors resulting from movements. In either case, vibration increases the firing frequency of the spindle receptors and increases the global afferent outflow from mechanoreceptors. Also, by modifying the sensory messages, vibration acts at the source of motor regulation systems.

Sensorimotor Systems

MONOSYNAPTIC PROPRIOCEPTIVE REFLEXES

Vibration applied to muscle tendons,[21,63,116,124] body segments,[78,80] or the whole body[112] depresses the Hoffmann reflex and the tendon reflex, which are used to test the integrity of a peripheral regulation loop dedicated to control muscle tension. Both reflexes involve the Ia afferents—α-motoneuron monosynaptic reflex loop (see **Fig. 12-3, B**). The decrease in amplitude of the reflex responses is larger than 90% when vibration is applied to the whole body or a whole limb. This depression of the reflex responses results from an autogenic presynaptic inhibition of the Ia afferents.[9,23,36,87] Studies of vibration frequency effects show that inhibition of the reflex responses is mainly dependent on vibration displacement amplitude in the 20 to 110-Hz frequency range.[78,80]

THE TONIC VIBRATION REFLEX

Paradoxically, inhibition of monosynaptic proprioceptive reflexes coexists with a tonic activity induced in the same muscle by tendon vibration.[21,41,63,82] This response, known as the tonic vibration reflex (TVR), results mainly from the vibration-induced activity of Ia-afferent fibers as shown in **Fig. 12-3, C**,[17,21,110] and is mediated by monosynaptic and spinal polysynaptic pathways.[25,82,113] It appears in both relaxed and contracted muscles. The strength of the TVR can reach up to 10% of the MVC for moderate levels of initial muscle contraction. This reflex response increases with vibration amplitude and is modulated by vibration frequency. This latter modulation in TVR intensity follows an inverted U-shaped curve with a maximum about 100 to 150 Hz.[95,96] Hence the TVR is an involuntary muscle

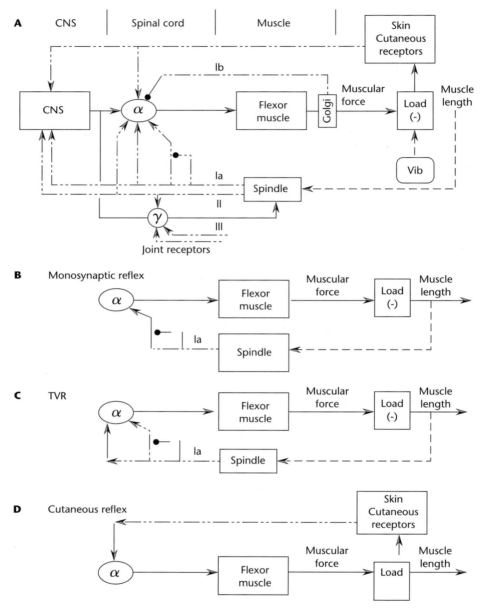

Figure 12-3 Neurosensory mechanisms. Muscle length/tension is regulated by neuromuscular circuits illustrated in a simplified diagram, which includes the γ-system, **A**, Vibration-induced activity of the mechanoreceptor triggers an imbalance between positive and negative feedback that is enhanced by the nested positive γ-loop. The pathways involved in the monosynaptic proprioceptive reflexes, the tonic vibration reflex and the cutaneous reflex, are presented individually in diagrams **B, C** and **D**. The tonic vibration reflex involves both the Ia monosynaptic and polysynaptic pathways; note the presynaptic inhibition mechanism affecting the monosynaptic pathway. The components of the cutaneous reflex are expressed via specific polysynaptic pathways. The symbols denote descending motor pathways (—), afferent pathways (broken lines), excitations (→), inhibitions (—●), and mechanical coupling (——).

activity superimposed on ongoing voluntary muscle contraction and contributes to an increase in muscle tension. Moreover, because of the driving of Ia fibers by the vibratory stimulus, a significant number of motor units contributing to the TVR are synchronized with the vibration cycle.*

CUTANEOUS POLYSYNAPTIC REFLEXES

Cutaneous reflex responses are adaptive sensorimotor activities playing an important protective role (**Fig. 12-3, D**). For example, a noxious stimulus applied to the skin of the hand leads to a reflexive withdrawal of the limb principally organized as a flexion movement. These cutaneous responses are composed of two distinct components associated with the activation of low-threshold tactile fibers and high-threshold cutaneous and nociceptive fibers. When elicited in hand flexor muscles, both components are facilitated by vibration applied to flexor tendons or to the hand.[79,97] This facilitation represents an increase of about 30% of the reflex contraction when the initial muscle contraction is maintained at 10% MVC. The facilitation is significantly larger at 90 Hz than at 200 Hz.[94,97] Thus these results show an increased accessibility of motoneurons to cutaneous information under vibration. They also tend to indicate a decrease in facilitatory influence when vibration frequency increases.

MUSCLE FATIGUE

A decline in the motor unit firing rate as muscle fatigue develops during sustained MVCs is a well-established phenomenon. Recently it has been shown that during brief repeated MVCs, exposure to short periods of muscle tendon vibration (shorter than 20 seconds) can counteract a decline in muscle activity and the motor unit firing rate induced by a fatiguing sustained MVC.[14] However, a fatigue-induced decline in motor output and force is accentuated under prolonged vibration periods during sustained MVCs.[13,14] Also, the rate of muscle fatigue induced by submaximal voluntary contraction of the hand flexor muscles tends to increase in the presence of a TVR elicited by hand vibration.[97]

FORCE CONTROL

As indicated earlier, an increase in muscle tension can result from vibration-induced alteration in the functioning of peripheral mechanisms and from development of the TVR. Radwin, Armstrong, and Chaffin[104] report that hand vibration increases grip exertion while holding loads attached to a vibrating handle.[104] The magnitude of this increase is of the same order as for a twofold increase in load weight for a 49-m/sec^2 vibration at 40 Hz. In addition, this increase is larger at 40 Hz than at 160 Hz. These authors attribute almost all of this increased grip force to the TVR; however, an alteration in the force regulatory pathways may also be involved.

*References 47, 49, 50, 64, 97, 113.

When vibration is applied to the whole body, which does not evoke a TVR, a voluntary increase in foot pressure on a pedal is observed.[34] This increase is obtained when holding a constant torque, repeating torque/rest alternations, or modulating the torque around a given value. An average increase of 16% is measured for a torque range of 10 to 30 Nm and a 2 -m/sec^2 vibration at 18 Hz. Because of the absence of a TVR, this result suggests an alteration in force control within the central nervous system. Also, it suggests that subjects feel less tension under whole-body vibration exposure and tend to compensate for this change in perception. This interpretation is in agreement with a decrease in perceived effort induced by muscle tendon vibration.[83,84] However, Cafarelli and Kosta[19] reported the inverse observation that muscle tendon vibration intensifies the sensation of intramuscular tension during muscle contraction. It is believed that the increased force is explained by (1) the symmetric action of whole-body or limb vibration on agonist/antagonist muscle groups and the ensuing reciprocal interactions[80] and (2) the sensory noise generated by stimulation of the whole body or limb, which accounts for the decrease in the difference between agonist and antagonist afferent messages and a general decrease in the signal-noise ratio. Hence both mechanisms may contribute to decreased force perception, and thus a compensatory increase in tension is observed in the case of global vibration.

Contribution to Disorders of Neurological Mechanisms

From these data it is clear that short-term sensorimotor effects result from vibration-induced activity of musculotendinous and cutaneous receptors. A detailed description of the nature of the mechanisms underlying degradation of motor performance is beyond the scope of the present chapter. Nevertheless, several mechanisms by which vibration contributes indirectly to tissue disorders and muscle fatigue can be proposed. These mechanisms combine with direct insults that weaken tissue tolerance.

ENHANCEMENT OF POSITIVE FEEDBACK LOOPS

First, the TVR, superimposed over ongoing voluntary contraction, increases muscle activity via Ia polysynaptic and monosynaptic (to a lesser extent) pathways as shown in **Figure 12-3**. Second, the gain of this proprioceptive feedback, which can be considered positive feedback in the present case, is likely to increase under the influence of secondary spindle afferents. Indeed, these latter positively affect γ-motoneurons in the same muscles and in synergistic muscles. Although the sensitivity of secondary spindle endings to vibration is lower than that of primary endings, they are strongly activated by this stimulus. Therefore, primary ending firings induced by vibration are further enhanced by the recurrent action of the secondary endings on the fusimotor neurons that increases the sensitivity of the muscle spindles. In addition, γ-motoneurons receive input from the cutaneous and joint receptors activated by the vibration. As a result, a sensory polymodal influence tends to increase spindle sensitivity. At the same time, force control is affected and muscle force exertion increases as a result of a "compensatory" descending command. All these responses act together to increase muscle tension, which in turn enhances the stiffness of the hand-arm system, thus increasing vibration transmission (transmissibility) from the work object to hand-arm tissues.[103,107]

An increase in transmissibility is likely to increase the stretching of muscle spindles, which constitutes another positive feedback. In addition, the activity of some motor units is synchronized with the vibratory stimulus. These muscle fibers are thereby continuously driven by this undesired reflex response during vibration. Moreover, the TVR as well as the voluntary compensatory increase in force is expressed via the recruitment of high-threshold motor units that are fast-fatiguing units. Hence these phenomena contribute to muscle fatigue, a harbinger or precursor of long-term tissue disorders. Because force is a factor in muscle, tendon, and nerve disorders, vibration and the neurologic mechanisms underlying force control are also factors.[105]

Finally, the vibration-induced activity of cutaneous and musculotendinous receptors also alters force control and movement control via long-loop feedback processed by the central nervous system. More specifically, it has been shown that the tactile threshold is elevated by short- and long-term exposure to hand vibration.[71,72,91] Therefore the error in force exertion is aggravated by a reduced sense of touch. Another consequence of vibration-induced activity of mechanoreceptors is the generation of a sensory noise affecting perception. We have shown that pain or discomfort can be attenuated while motor responses are facilitated.[79] Therefore, a masking effect or blurring of perception may impair the subjective assessment of our physical condition under vibration exposure.

The peripheral mechanisms receive certain inputs from the central nervous system that influence their behavior and bind the positive feedback. Some types of peripheral negative feedback play that inhibitory role as well. Renshaw cells activated by muscle contraction and Golgi tendon organs activated by muscle contraction and vibration both have an inhibitory influence on motoneurons as shown in **Figure 12-3**, *A*. Thus this negative feedback will also compete with positive feedback and to some extent limit any increase in muscle tension.

INHIBITION OF NEGATIVE FEEDBACK

An autogenic inhibition of the Ia monosynaptic reflex coexists with the TVR and other positive influences. This means that the gain of the short-loop stretch reflex is reduced. The consequence is a decreased ability of this servomechanism to minimize the influence of perturbations applied to the hand-arm system or, in other words, to adjust muscle stiffness[48,90] and hence mechanical impedance of the limb.[61,62] The net result could be increased strain on the tissues caused by an eventual eccentric stress of large amplitude in response to a perturbation. In the present case, a negative feedback is attenuated.

FREQUENCY EFFECTS

Several studies suggest that alterations in sensorimotor responses induced by vibration tend to decrease significantly with frequency beyond 150 Hz.[94-97,104] This decrease can be attributed to the cutoff in frequency response of the sensory receptors indicated earlier. Because biomechanical effects and resonances of body segments occur mainly in the low and medium frequency ranges (less than 50 to 100 Hz), it seems that high frequencies (greater than 200 Hz) should produce fewer disturbances or impairments. It is hypothesized that in the long term, high-frequency vibration should have fewer adverse effects on health, provided that the displacement amplitude remains below current recommendations.

MUSCLE, TENDON, AND NERVE DISORDERS

The influence of "good" negative feedback opposing perturbations is strongly minimized, whereas that of "bad" positive feedback increasing muscle tension is amplified during vibration exposure. The consequence is a drastic change in the response of the motor system and, more specifically, an increase in force exertion that can reach about 10% MVC. This results in an increase in vibration transmissibility and triggers a vicious circle that increases vibration and force exposure. Hence because force is a recognized factor in muscle, tendon, and nerve disorders, dysfunctioning of neurosensory mechanisms also contributes to muscle, tendon, and nerve disorders. It appears that vibration above 200 Hz has relatively less influence than do lower frequencies on the neurosensory mechanisms. Therefore, from a neurologic perspective, these data may justify increasing tool speed. Frequency should not be increased if it also results in an increased vibration amplitude. A combination of biomechanical and neurosensory models is needed to predict health effects resulting from hand-arm or whole-body vibration exposure.

LOW TEMPERATURE

Low skin temperatures are associated with exposure of unprotected hands and fingers to cold air or cold work objects and with low ambient temperature that can result in reduced peripheral blood flow. Epidemiological studies of low temperature have not yet been performed. Because of its strong vasoconstrictive effect, cold is believed to contribute to the development of pathologies such as the vibration-induced white finger; however, there is no evidence yet to consider cold a pathogenetic factor. Nevertheless, finger temperatures below about 20° C are associated with loss of tactile sensitivity,[39,101] which can result in excessive force exertion and thus aggravate symptoms of nerve impairment. Also, low temperatures induce significant decrements in manual dexterity and tracking tasks.[12,29,35,66,67] Like vibration, low temperatures may result in increased stress on muscles, tendons, and nerves as a secondary effect, and it may affect neurological symptoms.

SUMMARY

Manual work will be an important part of our industrial economy for the foreseeable future. Work requirements such as production standards, work locations, and tool size and shape along with worker attributes such as size and behavior result in external stressors such as repetition, force, contact stresses, and extreme postures. External stressors result in internal stressors such as muscle loads, tendon loads, and metabolic demands. Internal stressors along with worker capacity result in short-term responses such as increased concentrations of metabolites, decreased concentrations of substrates, tissue deformation, and nerve stimulation. If sufficient recovery occurs between successive work periods, short-term responses may lead to tissue adaptation in some cases; if the recovery period is insufficient, tissue degradation may occur. Either response affects individual capacity and tolerance to further work exposure. Environmental stressors such as vibration and low temperatures directly affect tissues and may produce pain and impaired work performance. Impaired work performance may affect how workers do their job and cause workers to exert more force than the minimum specified force. Short-term and long-term responses may result in increased perceived exertion, pain, and signs or symptoms of various upper limb disorders. A disability can develop, depending on the nature of the impairment, work requirements, and worker tolerance. Physical stressors and adverse health effects appear to follow a normal dose-response relationship, but further studies are necessary to determine work design specifications for a given level of risk.

References

1. American Conference of Governemntal Industrial Hygienists: *Threshold limit values for chemical substances and physical agents and biological exposure indices*, Cincinnati, Ohio, 1994.

2. Appelberg B, Johansson H, Sojka P: Fusimotor reflexes in triceps surae elicited by natural simulation of muscle afferents from the cat ipsilateral hind limb, *J Physiol (Lond)*, 329:211-229, 1982.

3. Appelberg B, Johansson H, Sojka P: Fusimotor reflexes in triceps surae muscle elicited by stretch of muscles in the contralateral hind limb of the cat, *J Physiol (Lond)* 363:403-417, 1985.

4. Armstrong TJ, Chaffin DB: Carpal tunnel syndrome and selected personal attributes. *J Occup Med* 21(7):481-486, 1979.

5. Armstrong TJ et al: A conceptual model for work-related neck and upper-limb musculoskeletal disorders, *Scand J Work Environ Health* 19:73-84, 1993.

6. Armstrong TJ et al: Ergonomics and the effects of vibration in hand-intensive work, *Scand J Work Environ Health* 2(13):286-289, 1987.

7. Armstrong TJ et al: Ergonomics considerations in hand and wrist tendinitis, *J Hand Surg 1 [Am]* 12A(5, part 2):830-837, 1987.

8. Armstrong TJ et al: Some histological changes in carpal tunnel contents and their biomechanical implications, *J Occup Med* 26(3):197-201, 1984.

9. Barnes C, Pompeiano O: Inhibition of monosynaptic extensor reflex attributable to presynaptic depolarization of the group Ia afferent fibers produced by vibration of flexor muscle, *Arch Ital Biol* 108:233-238, 1970.

10. Barnhart S et al: Carpal tunnel syndrome among ski manufacturing, *Scand J Work Environ Health* 17:46-52, 1991.

11. Basmajian JV: *Muscles alive: Their functions revealed by electromyography*, ed 4, Baltimore, 1979, Williams & Wilkins; pp 162-169.

12. Bensel CK, Lockhart HM: Cold-induced vasodilatation onset and manual performance in the cold, *Ergonomics* 17(6):717-730, 1974.

13. Bongiovanni L, Hagbarth K, Stjernberg L: Prolonged muscle vibration reducing motor output in maximal voluntary contractions in man, *J Physiol* 423:15-26, 1990.

14. Bongiovanni LG, Hagbarth KE: Tonic vibration reflexes elicited during fatigue maximal voluntary contractions in man, *J Physiol* 423:1-14, 1990.

15. Brain WR, Wright AD, Wilkinson M: Spontaneous compression of both median nerves in the carpal tunnel, *Lancet*, Mar 8:277-282, 1947.

16. Bureau of Labor Statistics: US Department of Labor, 1994.

17. Burke D et al: The response of human muscle spindle endings to vibration during isometric contraction, *J Physiol* 261:695-711, 1976.

18. Bystrom S, Fransson-Hall C: Acceptability of intermittent handgrip contractions based on physiological response, *Hum Factors* 36:158-171, 1994.

19. Cafarelli E, Kosta E: Effects of vibration on static force sensation in man, *Exp Neurol* 74:331-340, 1981.

20. Cannon LJ, Bernacki EJ, Walter SD: Personal and occupational factors associated with carpal tunnel syndrome, *J Occup Med* 23:255-258, 1981.

21. De Gail P, Lance J, Neilson P: Differential effects on tonic and phasic reflexes mechanisms produced by vibration of muscles in man, *J Neurol, Neurosurg, Psychiat* 29:1-11, 1966.

22. de Krom MCT et al: Risk factors for carpal tunnel syndrome, *Am J Epidemiol* 132:1102-1110, 1990.

23. Delwaide P: Le stimulus vibratoire en neurophysiologie clinique: aspects physiologiques et physiopathologiques, *Rev Electroencephalogr Neurophysiol Clin* 4:539-553, 1973.

24. de Quervain: Ueber eine Form von chronischer Tendovaginitis, *Correspondenz-Blatt f Aertzte* 25:389-394, 1895.

25. Desmedt JE, Godaux E: Mechanism of the vibration paradox: excitatory and inhibitory effects of tendon vibration on single muscle motor units in man, *J Physiol* 285:197-207, 1978.

26. Dimberg L et al: The correlation between work environment and the occurrence of cervicobrachial symptoms, *J Occup Med* 31(5), 447-453, 1989.

27. Duncan J, Ferguson D: Keyboard operating posture and symptoms in operating, *Ergonomics* 17(5):651-662, 1974.

28. Dupuis H, Zelett G: *The effects of whole body vibration*, New York, 1986, Springer-Verlag New York, Inc.

29. Dusek R: Effect of temperature on manual performance. In Fisher R, editor: *Production and functioning of the hands in cold climates*, Washington, DC, National Academy of Sciences, National Research Council; pp 63-76.

30. Franklin GM et al: Occupational carpal tunnel syndrome in Washington State, 1984-1988, *Am J Public Health* 81:741-746, 1991.

31. Fransson-Hall C, Kilbom A: Sensitivity of the hand to surface pressure, *Appl Ergonom* 24(3):181-189, 1993.

32. Fung YB: Stress-strain history relations of soft tissues in simple elongation. In Fung YC, Perrone N, Anliker M, editors: *Biomechanics: its foundations and objectives*, Englewood Cliffs, N.J. 1972; pp. 181-208.

33. Gauthier G et al: Effects of whole-body vibration on sensory motor system performance in man, *Aviat Space Environ Med* 52:473-479, 1981.

34. Gaydos HF, Dusek ER: Effects of localized hand cooling versus total body cooling on manual performance, *J Appl Physiol* 12(3):377-380, 1958.

35. Gillies JD, Burke DJ, Lance J: Tonic vibration reflex in the cat, *J Neurophysiol* 34:252-262, 1971.

36. Goldstein SA et al: Analysis of cumulative strain in tendons and tendon sheaths, *J Biomech* 20(1):1-6, 1987.

37. Gray H: *Anatomy, descriptive and surgical*, ed 13, Philadelphia, 1893, Lea Brothers & Co.

38. Green B: The effect of skin temperature on vibrotactile sensitivity, *Perception Psychophys* 21:243-248, 1977.

39. Griffin M: *Handbook of human vibration*, London, 1990, Academic Press, Inc.

40. Hagbarth K, Eklund G: Motor effects of vibratory muscle stimuli in man. In Granit R, editor: *Muscular afferents and motor control, proceedings of the first Nobel symposium*, Stockholm, 1965, Almqvist & Wiksell.

41. Hagberg KE et al: Gamma loop contributing to maximal voluntary contractions in man, *J Physiol*, 380:575-591, 1986.

42. Hagberg M: Local shoulder muscular strain—symptoms and disorders, *J Hum Ergol* 11:99-108, 1982.

43. Hammer AW: Tenosynovitis, *Medi Rec* 140:353-355, 1934.

44. Herberts P et al: Shoulder pain and heavy manual labor, *Clin Orthop* 191:166-178, 1984.

45. Higgs P et al: Upper extremity impairment in workers performing repetitive tasks, *Plast Reconstr Surg* 90(4):614-620, 1992.

46. Hirayama K et al: Separation of the contributions of voluntary and vibratory activation of motor units in man by cross-correlograms, *Jpn J Physiol* 24:293-304, 1974.

47. Hoffer J, Andreassen S: Regulation of soleus muscle stiffness in premammillary cats: intrinsic and reflex components, *J Neurophysiol* 45:267-285, 1981.

48. Homma S, Kanda K, Watanabe S: Integral pattern of coding during tonic vibration reflex. Neurophysiology studied in man. In Somjen G, editor: *Experta medica*, Amsterdam, 1972: pp 345-349.

49. Hori Y, Higara K, Watanabe S: The effects of thiamylal sodium on the tonic vibration reflex in man, *Brain Res* 497:291-295, 1989.

50. Hulliger M: The mammalian muscle spindle and its central control, *Rev Physiol Biochem Pharmacol* 101:1-110, 1984.

51. Humphreys PW, Lind AR: The blood flow through active and inactive muscles of the forearm during sustained handgrip contractions, *J Physiol* 166:120-135, 1963.

52. Hunting W, Laubli T, Grandjean E: Postural and visual loads at VDT workplaces I. Constrained postures, *Ergonomics* 24(12):917-931, 1981.

53. Johansson H, Sojka P: Pathophysiological mechanisms involved in genesis and spread of muscular tension in occupational muscle pain and in chronic musculoskeletal pain syndromes: a hypothesis, *Med Hypotheses* 35:196-203, 1991.

54. Johansson R, Vallbo A: Detection of tactile stimuli. Thresholds of afferent units related to psychophysical thresholds in the human hand, *J Physiol (Lond)* 297:405-422, 1979.

55. Johansson H et al: Different fusimotor reflexes from the ipsi- and contralateral hind limbs of the cat assessed in the same primary muscle spindle afferents, *J Physiol (Paris)* 83:1-12, 1989.

56. Johansson H et al: Reflex actions on the γ-muscle spindle systems of muscles acting at the knee joint elicited by stretch of the posterior cruciate ligament. *Neuro-Orthop* 8:9-21, 1989.

57. Karlqvist L, Bjorksten MG: Design for prevention of work-related musculoskeletal disorders. In Bullock M, editor: *Ergonomics: the physiotherapist in the workplace,* New York, 1990, Churchill-Livingstone; pp 149-181.

58. Kenedi RM, Gibson T, Daly CH: Bio-engineering studies of the human skin II. In Kenedi RM, editor: Biomechanics and related bioengineering topics, Oxford, 1965, Pergamon Press; pp 147-158.

59. Kleinbaum DG, Kupper LL, Muller KE: *Applied regression analysis and other multivariable methods,* Boston, 1988, PWS Publishers.

60. Lacquaniti F, Licata F, Soechting J: The mechanical behavior of the human forearm in response to transient perturbations, *Biol Cybern* 44:35-46, 1982.

61. Lacquaniti F, Soechting J: Changes in mechanical impedance and gain of the myotatic response during transitions between two motor tasks, *Exp Brain Res* 7(suppl):135-139, 1983.

62. Lance JW, Burke D, Andrews C: The reflex effects of muscle vibration. Studies of tendon jerk irradiation, phasic reflex inhibition and the tonic vibration reflex. In Desmedt JE, editor: New developments in EMG and clinical neurophysiology, Basel, Switzerland, 1973, Karger; pp 444-462.

63. Lebedev M, Polyakov A: Analysis of surface EMG of human soleus muscle subjected to vibration, *J Electromyogr Kinesiol* 2:1-10, 1992.

64. Lind AR et al: The circulatory effects of sustained voluntary muscle contraction, *Clin Sci* 27:229-244, 1964.

65. Lockhart JM: Effects of body and hand cooling on complex manual performance, *J Appl Physiol* 50:57-59, 1966.

66. Lockhart JM, Kiess HO, Clegg TJ: Effect of rate and level of lowered finger surface temperature on manual performance, *J Appl Physiol* 60(1):106-113, 1975.

67. Loslever P, Ranaivosoa A: Biomechanical and epidemiological investigations of carpal tunnel syndrome at workplaces with high risk factors, *Ergonomics* 36(5):537-554, 1993.

68. Louis DS: The carpal tunnel syndrome. In Millender LH, Louis DS, Simmons BP, editors: *Occupational disorders of the upper extremity* New York, 1992, Churchill Livingstone International: pp 145-153.

69. Lundborg G et al: Median nerve compression in the carpal tunnel—functional response to experimentally induced controlled pressure, *J Hand Surg* 7(3):252-259, 1982.

70. Lundstrom R: Effects of local vibration transmitted from ultrasonic devices on vibrotactile perception in the hands of the therapist, *Ergonomics* 28:793-803, 1985.

71. Lundstrom R, Johansson R: Acute impairment of the sensitivity of skin mechanoreceptive units caused by vibration exposure of the hand, *Ergonomics* 29:687-698, 1986.

72. MacDonald G, Robertson M, Erickson J: Carpal tunnel syndrome among California dental hygienists, *Am J Dent Hyg* 62:322-328, 1988.

73. Maeda K: Expansion of the occupations which induce neck-shoulder-arm disorders and some problems in taking measures against the disorders—from experience in labor hygiene consultation activities, *Sumitomo Sangyo Eisei* 10:135-143, 1974.

74. Margolis W, Kraus JF: The prevalence of carpal tunnel syndrome symptoms in female supermarket checkers, *J Occup Med* 12:953-956, 1987.

75. Marras WS, Schoenmarklin RW: Wrist motions in industry, *Ergonomics* 36(4):341-351, 1993.

76. Martin B: *Contribution a l'etude de la degradation du fonctionnement des systemes sensori-moteurs liee a l'exposition aux vibrations mechaniques chez l'homme. Role des facteurs neurosensoriels,* dissertation, Marseilles, France, 1989, L'Universite D'Aix-Marseille.

77. Martin B, Roll J, Gauthier G: Spinal reflex alterations as a function of intensity and frequency of vibration applied to the feet of seated subjects, *Aviat Space Environ Med* 55:8-12, 1984.

78. Martin B, Roll J, Hugon M: Modulation of cutaneous flexor responses induced in man by proprioceptive or exteroceptive inputs, *Aviat Space Environ Med* 61:921-928, 1990.

79. Martin BJ, Roll JP, Gauthier GM: Inhibitory effects of combined agonist and antagonist muscle vibration on H-reflex in man, *Aviat Space Environ Med* 57:681-687, 1986.

80. Matthews P: The reflex excitation of the soleus muscle of the decerebrate cat caused by vibration applied to its tendon, *J Physiol* 184:450-472, 1966.

81. McCloskey D: Kinaesthetic sensibility, *Physiol Rev* 58:763-820, 1978.

82. McCloskey D et al: Muscle sense and effort: motor commands and judgments about muscular contractions. In Desmedt JE, editor: *Motor control mechanisms in health and disease,* New York, 1983, Raven Press: pp 151-167.

83. Millar J: Joint afferent fibres responding to muscle stretch, vibration and contraction, *Brain Res* 63:380-383, 1973.

84. Monod H: *Contribution a l'etude du travail statique* [A contribution to the study of static work], J Physiol (Paris) 48: 662-666, 1956.

85. Morin C, Pierrot-Deseilligny E, Hultborn H: Evidence for presynaptic inhibition of muscle spindle Ia afferents in man, *Neurosci Lett* 44:137-142, 1984.

86. Nathan PA, Meadows KD, Doyle LS: Occupation as a risk factor for impaired sensory conduction of the median nerve at the carpal tunnel, *J Hand Surg* [Br] 13B(2):167-170, 1988.

87. National Institute for Occupational Safety and Health: *Health hazard evaluation report: Newsday, Inc,* Rep No HETA 89-250-2046, 1990, NIOSH, Melville, N.Y., 61 pp.

88. Nichols T, Houk J: Reflex compensation for variations in the mechanical properties of muscle, *Science* 181:182-184, 1973.

89. Nishiyama K, Watanabe S: Temporary threshold shift of vibratory sensation after clasping a vibrating handle, *Int Arch Occup Environ Health* 49:21-33, 1981.

90. Obolenskaja AJ, Goljanitzki IA: Die serose tendovaginitis in der Klinic und im Experiment, *Dtsch Z Chir Leipz* 201:388-399, 1927.

91. Oxenburgh M: Musculoskeletal injuries occurring in word processor operators. In Adams A and Stevenson M, editors: *Proceedings of the 21st Annual Conference of the Ergonomics Soceity of Australia and New Zealand,* Sydney, Australia, 1984, CSR, Ltd: pp 137-143.

92. Park H: *Neurophysiological analysis of hand vibration effects on sensorimotor control,* dissertation, Ann Arbor, 1993, University of Michigan.

93. Park H, Martin B: Analysis of the tonic vibration reflex: contribution to muscle stress and muscle fatigue, *Scand J Work Environ Health* 19:35-42, 1993.

94. Park H, Martin B: Contribution of the tonic vibration reflex to muscle stress and muscle fatigue, *Scand J Work Environ Health* 19:35-42, 1993.

95. Park H, Martin B: Cutaneous flexor response alterations as a function of intensity and frequency of vibration applied to the hand, *Scand J Work Environ Health,* vol 20, 1994.

96. Pelmear P, Taylor W, Wasserman D: *Hand-arm vibration. A comprehensive guide for occupational health professionals,* New York, 1992, Van Nostrand Reinhold.

97. Phalen GS: The carpal-tunnel syndrome: clinical evaluation of 598 hands, *Clin Orthop* 83:29-40, 1972.

98. Powell KE et al: An epidemiological perspective on the causes of running injuries, *Physical Sportsmed* 14:100-114, 1986.

99. Provin K, Morton R: Tactile discrimination and skin temperature, *J Appl Physiol* 15:155-160, 1960.

100. Punnett L et al: Soft tissue disorders in the upper limbs of female garment workers, *Scand J Work Environ Health* 11:417-425, 1985.

101. Pyykkö I et al: Transmission of vibration in the hand-arm system with special reference to changes in compression force and acceleration, *Scand J Work Environ Health* 2:87-89, 1976.

102. Radwin RG, Armstrong TJ, Chaffin DB: Power hand tool vibration effects on grip exertions, *Ergonomics* 30:833-855, 1987.

103. Radwin RG, Armstrong TJ, Vanbergeijk E: Hand-arm vibration and work related disorders of the upper limb. In Pelmear PL, Taylor W, and Wasserman DE, editors: *Hand-arm vibration,* New York, 1992, Van Nostrand Reinhold: pp 122-142.

104. Ramazzini B: *De morbis artificum [Diseases of workers],* Chicago, 1713, University of Chicago Press.

105. Reynolds D: Hand-arm vibration: a review of 3 years' research. In Wasserman DE, Taylor W, editors: *Proceedings of the International Occupational Hand-Arm Vibration conference,* 1977, DHEW Pub No 77-170; pp 99-128.

106. Ribot E, Roll JP, Vedel JP: Efferent discharges recorded from single skeletomotor and fusimotor fibres in man, *J Physiol (Lond)* 375:251-268, 1986.

107. Ribot-Ciscar E: *Contribution a l'analyse du codage sensoriel des activites motrices chez l'homme,* these de doctorat, Marseilles, France, 1988, Universite d'Aix-Marseille.

108. Roll JP, Vedel JP, Ribot E: Alteration of proprioceptive messages induced by tendon vibration in man: a microneurographic study, *Exp Brain Res* 76:213-222, 1989.

109. Roll J et al: High frequency activation of myotactic pathway in man and baboon, *Electroencephalogr Clin Neurophysiol* 34:809, 1973.

110. Roll J et al: Effects of whole-body vibration on spinal reflex in man, *Aviat Space Environ Med* 51:1127-1233, 1980.

111. Romaiguère P et al: Differential activation of motor units in the wrist extensor muscles during the tonic vibration reflex in man, *J Physiol* 444:645-667, 1991.

112. Rothfleisch S, Sherman D: Carpal tunnel syndrome—biomechanical aspects of occupational occurrence and implications regarding surgical management, *Orthop Rev* 7:107-109, 1978.

113. Silverstein BA, Fine LJ, Stetson D: Hand-wrist disorders among investment casting plant workers, *J Hand Surg [Am]* 12:838-844, 1987.

114. Sjogaard G, Savard G, Juel C: Muscle blood flow during isometric activity and its relation to muscle fatigue, *Eur J Appl Physiol* 57:327-335, 1988.

115. Sjogaard G et al: Intramuscular pressure, EMG and blood flow during low-level prolonged static contraction in man, *Acta Physiol Scand* 128:475-484, 1986.

116. Smith EM, Sonstegard DA, Anderson WH: Carpal tunnel syndrome: contribution of flexor tendons, *Arch Phys Med Rehabil* 58:379-385, 1977.

117. Szabo RM, Chidgey LK: Stress carpal tunnel pressures in patients with carpal tunnel syndrome and normal patients, *J Hand Surg [Am]* 14:624-627, 1989.

118. Tannen KJ et al: An evaluation of scissors for control of upper extremity disorders in an automobile upholstery plant. In Karwowski W, editor: *Trends in ergonomics/human factors III,* Amsterdam, 1986, Elsevier Science, Inc: pp 631-639.

119. Tanzer RC: The carpal-tunnel syndrome, *J Bone Joint Surg Am* 41:626-634, 1959.

120. Taylor D et al: Viscoelastic properties of muscle-tendon units—the biomechanical effects of stretching, *Am J Sports Med* 18:300-309, 1990.

121. Tichauer ER: Some aspects of stress on forearm and hand in industry, *J Occup Med* 8:63-71, 1966.

122. Van Boxtel A: Selective effects of vibration on monosynaptic and late EMG responses in human soleus muscle after stimulation of the posterior tibial nerve or a tendon tap, *J Neurol Neurosurg Psychiatry* 42:995-1004, 1979.

123. Vedel J, Roll J: Muscle spindle contribution to the coding of motor activities in man. Neural coding of motor performance, *Exp Brain Res* 7(suppl):253-265, 1983.

124. Vedel J, Roll J, Ribot E: Sensitivity of muscular and cutaneous receptors to vibratory stimuli in man. In Frolov KV, editor: *Man under vibration, second international CISM-IFTOMM Symposium,* Moscow, 1985, USSR Academy of Sciences: pp 130-138.

125. Viikari-Juntura E et al: Prevalence of epicondylitis and elbow pain in the meat-processing industry, *Scand J Work Environ Health* 17:38-45, 1991.

126. Waersted M, Westgaard RH: Working hours as a risk factor in the development of musculoskeletal complaints, *Ergonomics* 34:265-276, 1991.

127. Yamaguchi DM: Carpal tunnel syndrome, *Minn Med* 48:22-33, 1965.

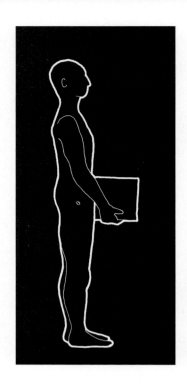

Chapter 13

Slips, Trips, And Falls

Mark S. Redfern
Donald Bloswick

CONTENTS:

Falls cause many injuries in the workplace and occur in all occupations. Historically, injury rates have been highest in the construction trades, yet a significant number of falls also occur in the manufacturing and service industries. Slips, trips, and loss of balance most often lead to fall injuries. Environmental factors such as shoe-floor interface conditions are of primary concern in slips and trips.

Information on the epidemiology, causation, and prevention of falls in the workplace is provided in this chapter. First, the prevalence and severity of fall injuries throughout industry are reviewed in terms of both rates and costs. A second section on causation discusses mechanisms of slips, trips, and falls as they relate to walking on level surfaces and on surfaces that have a change in elevation. Finally, preventive measures used in ergonomically designed workplaces are discussed.

EPIDEMIOLOGY OF FALLS

Injuries Caused by Falls

Slips and falls are a major cause of injuries at work, in public places, and at home. Falls cause about one fifth of all accidental injuries in the United States. Overall, annual healthcare costs associated with fall injuries are over $37 billion and are exceeded only by motor vehicle injuries, which cost about $49 billion.[79] In 1991 the National Safety Council estimated that falls cause about 13% of all occupationally related deaths in the United States (**Table 13-1**) and 17% of all occupationally related injuries (**Table 13-2**).[64] The percentage of fall injuries ranges from 21.9% in construction to 11.7% in manufacturing (see **Table 13-2**). Only overexertion, musculoskeletal injuries, and being struck by an object rank higher. Interestingly, the injury rate from falls at work is comparable to that of nonoccupational falls (18%) reported in the public sector.

Statistics from other countries also indicate that a substantial number of serious injuries are caused by falls. In Great Britain, about 20% (40,000) of all occupational injuries are reportedly due to slips and falls.[55,90]

Table 13-1 Deaths in work accidents.							
	All Ages	**Age**					
Type of Accident		**5-14**	**15-24**	**24-44**	**45-64**	**65-74**	**≥75**
ALL TYPES*	10,500	100	1,900	4,300	2,900	800	500
TOTAL† (%)	100	100	100	100	100	100	100
				100			
Motor vehicle	35.5	0.0	55.0	34.0	34.5	25.0	0.0
Falls	12.7	6.0	8.1	9.1	14.3	20.8	44.4
Electric current	3.6	3.0	4.9	4.7	2.3	0.6	0.2
Fires, burns	3.5	8.0	2.9	3.4	3.2	6.0	3.6
Poison (solid, liquid)	3.4	0.0	1.2	5.7	2.3	1.8	0.0
Drowning	3.2	0.0	4.4	3.9	2.4	1.1	1.6
Air transport	2.4	0.0	0.6	3.8	2.6	0.5	0.4
Water transport	1.7	0.0	2.0	2.2	1.4	0.5	0.4
Poison (gas, vapor)	1.4	0.0	1.6	1.7	1.3	0.8	0.2
Other‡	32.6	83.3	19.3	31.5	35.7	42.9	49.6

All Types are 1990 estimates.
†Percent distribution based on 1988 data (last test year available).
‡Principal types include machinery, struck by a falling object, railway, and mechanical suffocation.
From National Safety Council, Accident facts, 1991, The Council.

Table 13-2	Work injuries involving disability by type of accident and industry division, 1988.								
Type of Accident	All Industries	Agricul-ture*†	Mining†	Construc-tion	Manufac-turing	Transport and Public Utilities	Trade†	Service†	Public Sector
Total (%)	100	100	100	100	100	100	100	100	100
Overexertion	31.3	24.2	24.1	25.1	34.7	31.1	31.1	34.4	29.0
Struck by or struck against	24.0	29.4	26.9	29.0	25.2	18.6	26.7	20.0	19.6
Falls	17.1	17.3	16.0	21.9	11.7	18.3	18.1	19.1	18.1
Bodily reaction	7.6	7.2	5.9	6.6	6.8	8.3	6.9	8.1	10.3
Caught in or be-tween‡	5.2	6.5	10.1	4.1	8.3	4.5	4.4	3.7	2.9
Contact with radia-tion, caustics, etc.	3.1	4.8	5.5	2.6	3.4	2.2	1.8	3.6	4.5
Motor vehicle acci-dent	3.1	2.7	2.7	2.0	1.0	9.6	2.6	3.3	5.2
Rubbed or abraded	2.0	2.9	1.9	3.5	2.6	1.5	1.6	1.4	1.4
Contact with tem-perature extremes	2.0	1.1	2.1	1.8	1.8	0.8	3.3	1.6	1.6
Other, nonclassifi-able	4.6	3.9	4.8	3.4	4.5	5.1	3.5	4.8	7.4

*Excludes farms with fewer than 11 employees.
†Agriculture includes forestry and fishing; mining includes quarrying and oil and gas extraction; trade includes wholesale and retail; and services includes finance, insurance, and real estate.
‡Caught in or between includes caught under; motor vehicle accident includes highway only.
Values are percentages based on 1,047,055 cases involving disability from 14 states from the Bureau of Labor Statistics Supplementary Data System.
Modified from National Safety Council: Accident facts, Chicago, 1991, The Council.

In Scandinavia, slips and falls account for 16% of the accidents at work and home;[53] and Finland reports that 12% of serious injuries are due to falls.[83] In Finland, slipping accidents occur mainly in manufacturing (34%), construction (28%), and transportation (21%).[43]

Historically, falls accounted for over 20% of all injuries that resulted in worker's compensation payments.[89] Construction workers in the United States had the highest rate of compensable injuries from falls, and certain service industries also had high rates.[30] Construction fall injuries occurred among skilled (27%) and unskilled (19%) laborers. Among clerical and transportation workers, falls caused between 8% and 10% of all injuries. Across industries, over 50% of reported falls were due to slips. An additional 24% of reported injuries resulted from trips and missteps.

Gronqvist and Roine[43] analyzed types of injuries caused by falls and found that bone fractures predominated in falls both from heights (47%) and from the same level (59%). However, internal injuries occurred more often in persons who fell from heights (18%) than in those who fell on same-level surfaces (7%). Impacts against the floor or ground and objects on them were associated with over 90% of all reported injuries from falls.

Characteristics of the Workplace

A number of workplace factors have been identified as being directly related to fall injuries and deaths; the characteristics of floor surfaces are major factors (Table 13-3).[40] A floor's slip resistance is believed to be the main determinant of falls on level surfaces. A significant portion of falls occur at changes in elevation while using ladders and stairs. Factors that contribute to falls from elevations are ladder stability, rung and step friction, and balance.

Construction laborers in the United States suffered 37,000 injuries during March 1983,[21] and 11% were caused by falls from elevations. The epidemiology of falls from elevations during home and leisure activities

Table 13-3	Distribution of fatalities and injuries by work surface areas.			
Work Surface Involved	**Estimated Annual**		**Estimated Annual**	
	Injuries	Percentage	Fatalities	Percentage
Floor	53,970	51.4	29	22.0
Ramp	735	0.7	1	0.6
Roof	420	0.4	15	11.0
Platform	8,715	8.3	9	7.0
Walkway	5,355	5.1	6	4.3
Stairs	13,965	13.3	15	11.2
Ladder	11,025	10.5	25	19.0
Scaffold	8,400	8.0	25	18.6
Other	2,415	2.3	2.3	6.3
TOTALS	105,000	100	132	100

From Federal Register *55:13360-13341, 1990.*

has not been as well documented as workplace falls. Nevertheless, there is a basis for the assumption that the relative distribution of same-level to different-level falls is about the same in home and leisure accidents as in the workplace. In 1984, Lund[53] surveyed several epidemiologic studies in which falls between levels both at home and at work consistently amounted to about 43% of all fall accidents. Other studies have also shown that 40% to 45% of all occupational falls occur between levels.[51,69,70,86]

Falls from elevations often cost more than same-level falls and injuries from other types of accidents. Snyder[86] noted that there was a higher percentage of bed disability in falls from elevations than from same-level falls. The Bureau of Labor Statistics[20] reported that 85% of those who survived workplace falls from elevations lost time from work, and that the average time lost was twice that for other work-related injuries. Pater[70] indicated that compensable costs for workplace falls from elevations in New York State averaged $5638 as compared with $4360 for same-level falls. The Center for Excellence in Construction Safety at the University of West Virginia[16] estimates that construction industry falls, many from elevated work surfaces, cost $2.5 billion each year.

Chaffin et al[25] reported that 81% of all fatal falls in California during 1975 were from elevations. Falls from elevations need not be from extreme heights to be serious. Culver[34] indicated that 60% of construction industry fatalities were from 14 m (30 feet) or less and that a fair number were from falls of 3 m (10 feet) or less. Many falls from elevations occurred while ladders were being used.

The Bureau of Labor Statistics[22] noted that in ladder fall accidents resulting in injuries, 26% were from less than 1.2 m (4 feet), 48% were from less than 2.1 m (7 feet), and 71% were from less than 3 m (10 feet). Axelsson and Carter[10] noted that more than 90% of ladder accident victims fell less than 4 m. This emphasizes, as stated earlier, that falls from elevations need not be from extreme heights to cause serious injuries or death.

In 1977 Snyder[86] noted that 31% of construction industry falls in California between 1966 and 1973 involved the use of ladders. Little[52] indicated that at least 10% of occupational accidents associated with work surfaces occurred during ladder use. A Safety Sciences report indicated that of 500 occupational falls studied, 8% occurred while using ladders.[82] In the United States, approximately 100,000 industrial accidents[60] and 200,000 total injuries[6] are associated with ladders annually. In the Swedish construction industry, Axelsson and Carter[10] noted that ladder accidents accounted for nearly 5% of all reported occupational accidents.

Stairs are another type of elevated surface on which many serious accidents occur. The Bureau of Labor Statistics[20] has classified stairs as a major hazard in the workplace and has calculated that 33,000 disabling injuries occur each year from falls on stairs. These falls account for 1.3% of all injuries that lead to disability.[20] Annual reports of stair accidents have increased from 356,000 in 1974 to 540,000 in 1979 and 785,000 in 1982.[71]

Half of those who die from falls down stairs are older than 65 years.[71] The National Bureau of Standards[9] stated in Science Series 120 that "because of the particular vulnerability of the aged, their use of stairs should be minimized whenever possible." The National Safety Council[65] in their 1988 edition of the *Accident Prevention Manual for Industrial Operations* stated that where possible, ramps should be used as a surface between two levels. Safety problems, cost, and accessibility issues in the workplace may make replacement of stairs by ramps fairly common.

Another workplace site where falls often occur is on and about vehicles and equipment. An early study by the Bureau of Motor Carrier Safety[23] found that truck cab ingress and egress accounted for over 40% of slip and fall injuries for a representative sample of motor carriers and that 14% of injuries to drivers resulted from falls as compared with 9% for all motor carrier employees. A study by Safety Sciences[80] found that approximately 20% of driver injuries were associated with falls as compared with 14% associated with moving accidents.

The Construction Safety Association of Ontario (CSAO)[31] published a study in 1980 indicating that 20% of all lost-time accidents among construction industry equipment operators were related to mounting and dismounting equipment. Similarly, Association of American Railroads statistics indicate that activities associated with mounting, dismounting, and climbing on railcars account for 11% of all injuries in the railroad industry.[58] A later study by Safety Sciences[83] found that slips and falls accounted for 27% of all accidents and that falls while climbing on and off vehicles and equipment accounted for 9% of all accidents. Approximately 25% of injuries to drivers of commercial vehicles are caused by slipping, tripping, and falling accidents, and a large percentage of these are associated with vehicle ingress and egress.[66]

Aging and Falls

Because the average age of U.S. workers is increasing, aging effects on human performance are an increasingly important factor in accidents, especially in the area of falls. Falls are the most common type of accident among the elderly;[93] so industry must be made aware of the increased risk of falls for older workers. Problems arise from a reduction in balance and balance recovery in older individuals. The function of three sensory systems involved in balance (visual, vestibular, and proprioceptive) are all reduced, which is what puts older workers at increased risk. The incidence of falls increases exponentially with age.[74] In the elderly population as a whole, 20% to 30% of community dwellers.[13,74] and 40% of institutionalized ambulatory individuals fall each year.[45] Falls are the main cause of accidental death in persons 65 years or older.[62,79] The death rate from falls among the elderly is 12 times greater than for all other ages combined.[79] Eighteen percent of falls among elderly persons require medical attention.[91] The most frequent serious injury from falls in the elderly is hip fracture, with 200,000 hip fractures costing $2 to $7 billion per year in health costs and averaging 21 days of hospitalization.[11,85,93] In a study of 152 falls of elderly persons living at home, 42% occurred while walking on a level surface and 35% occurred during other common activities.[95]

Slips with Recovery

Although not well documented, many injuries occur as a result of a slip without falling. Many times a slip occurs during tasks such as material handling, but stability is recovered in time to prevent a fall. Injury may still result from muscle strain or from being struck by an object. For example, in one industrial study, 37% of nonfalling accidents were reported to involve a slip.[7] In a Finnish study,[42] many amputations were reported to be due to loss of balance resulting from a slip with recovery. Musculoskeletal overexertion injuries also often arise from a slip with recovery. Manning[54] reported that many low back injuries incurred during carrying or lifting were associated with a slip or loss of balance with recovery. Injuries from these types of accidents are not usually reported as being related to a slip. Therefore, the prevalence of injuries due to slips with recovery is undoubtedly underestimated.

CAUSES OF OCCUPATIONAL FALLS

Causes of falls can be explained from a human factors and biomechanics point of view. First, a brief review of normal gait is presented in this section, and then a description of slips and trips during level-surface walking is given on the basis of the biomechanics of gait. Causative factors in falls during changes in elevation are described for ramps, stairs, ladders, and vehicle ingress and egress. Finally, falls from elevated work surfaces are discussed.

Normal Gait

There have been numerous studies of the biomechanics of human gait both on level surfaces and during changes in elevation.[94,97] Of central interest to understanding the biomechanics of slips, trips, and falls are leg trajectories, foot forces, and the relationship between the center of mass of the body and its base of support. Under normal walking conditions, foot trajectories have been shown to be repeatable. Trajectory of the swing foot begins at toe-off, with maximum horizontal velocity occurring just after midswing. Minimum toe clearance between the foot and floor during swing has been shown to be less than 1 cm, whereas its forward velocity is between 4.0 and 5.0 m/sec (**Fig. 13-1**).

Upon heel contact of the swing leg, the center of mass of the body is midway between the feet. Control of balance is therefore being shifted from the back foot to the new lead foot, and a new base of support is formed. At heel contact, the foot is not immediately stationary but often has a forward velocity of approximately 20 cm/sec. This creates a "microslip" of 0.5 to 2.0 cm of the heel at impact in the forward direction.[63,77] This short slipping distance is commonly seen and can be a function of the surface conditions. As surface conditions become more slippery, these microslips become greater.[63,88]

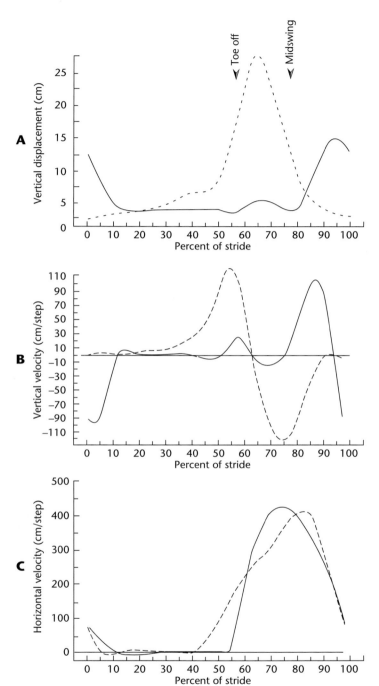

Figure 13-1 Kinematics of the foot during gait as described by trajectories of the toe (*solid line*) and heel (*dashed line*). **A**, Displacements during a step **B**, Vertical velocity. **C**, Horizontal velocity. (Adapted from Winter DA: *The biomechanics and motor control of human gait: normal, elderly, and pathological,* ed 2, Waterloo, Ontario, University of Waterloo Press, 1991.)

Walking creates forces at the feet in the vertical and shear directions. Under normal conditions, foot forces are very repeatable and have the basic shape shown in **Figure 13-2**. Shear forces in the anteroposterior (AP) direction are highest just after foot contact with the ground and during the push-off phase as the body is propelled to the next step. At midstance, when the center of mass passes close to the stance foot, AP shear forces are minimal. The vertical forces are maximum at approximately the same time as the shear forces. The maximum value of the vertical forces tends to be about 1.2 times body weight during normal walking. This maximum occurs at approximately the same time as the shear forces. Shear forces in the lateral directions (not shown in **Fig. 13-2**) are small, generally less than 10% of the normal forces.

Slips on Level Surfaces

Foot slips can occur at both the heel-contact phase and the push-off phase. In terms of foot forces, a slip

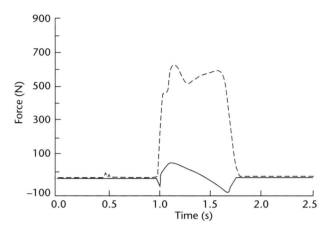

Figure 13-2 Foot forces in the vertical (*dashed*) and anteroposterior shear (*solid*) directions during a step at natural cadence.

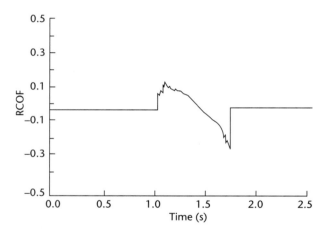

Figure 13-3 Required coefficient of friction (*RCOF*) during a step calculated for the data shown in Figure 13-2.

occurs when the shear forces imposed at the shoe-floor interface exceed the frictional capabilities of that interface. This can happen during either the heel-contact phase or the push-off phase of gait because these are the points where the shear forces are at a maximum. Heel contact is the critical phase in falls. During heel contact, body weight is transferring to the lead foot. Should a slip occur at heel contact, the new base of support is not able to accept body weight. The result is a fall.

The ratio between the horizontal and vertical foot force components (H/V) has been used to understand the biomechanics of slips. This value, also known as the required coefficient of friction (RCOF), can be directly related to the frictional requirements of the shoe-floor interface. **Figure 13-3** shows a typical RCOF curve for normal gait. The AP shear forces are divided by the vertical forces at each point in time in this plot to obtain the RCOF. Note that the RCOF is biphasic with a

maximum in the forward direction at heel contact and a maximum backward direction at toe-off. Again, heel contact is most critical in slips resulting in falls caused by the transfer of weight to the slipping foot. A slip will occur if the RCOF values at heel contact exceed the coefficient of friction (COF) of the shoe-floor interface. The peak of these RCOF values during the heel-contact phase has been used to predict slip potentials for various gait activities.[18,78] The peak RCOF is believed to represent the maximum frictional requirement (in terms of shoe-floor COF) during the task.

The heel-contact event is highly dynamic both in normal gait and during a slip. In fact, slips are common in normal gait at heel contact; however, most are only for a short distance of less than 2 cm.[78,88] These "microslips" do not pose any threat of falling.[72] Slips become uncontrollable in movement leading to falls when they are greater than about 10 cm; this is termed a "slide" by Leamon and Lee.[50] Movements of between 2 and 10 cm that do not result in falls are known as slips with recovery. These events can lead to loss of stability and muscle strains, as will be discussed later in the chapter.

The kinematics of heel contact under load-carrying conditions were investigated by Redfern et al.[78] It was found that heel velocity at heel contact was dependent on subject differences and walking speed, not on the load carried. Walking speed had the largest effect on heel movement, with the average heel velocity at contact ranging from 14 cm/sec at 70 steps per minute to 24 cm/sec at 110 steps per minute. Stride length is also important because stride length is directly related to walking velocity.[40,97]

Trips on Level Surfaces

In contrast to a slip, which is caused by unexpected movement of the base of support, a trip is the result of an unexpected stop of the foot during the swing phase. A sudden stop of the swing foot can cause the center of mass of the body to move far beyond the base of support. A fall occurs when the swing foot is interrupted for a time sufficient to prohibit recovery of the swing leg to establish a new base of support.

As noted earlier, the trajectory of the swing foot has a maximum velocity just after midswing. Toe clearance is also minimal (usually less than 1 cm) at this time (**Fig. 13-4**). Thus an obstacle within the path of the foot need be no higher than 1 cm to potentially cause a trip. As noted by Winter,[97] the center of gravity of the body at the time of minimum toe clearance is at or ahead of the stance foot. Therefore, if a trip were to occur, the forward momentum of the body could not be controlled by the stance leg. The only recovery possible is with the swing leg. It is understandable how minor changes in the flooring surface or obstacles on it can cause trips resulting in falls leading to injury. Work practices that block the worker's vision, such as carrying loads in front of the face, can also increase the chance of trips. The possibility of a recovery during carrying de-

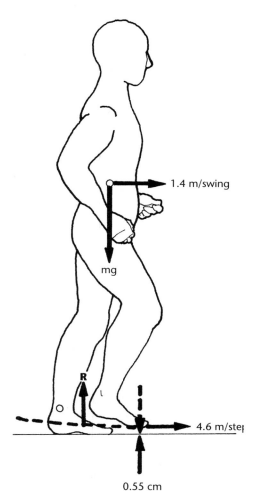

1.4 m/swing

mg

R

l

4.6 m/step

0.55 cm

Figure 13-4 Minimum toe clearance during the swing phase. (From Winter DA: *The biomechanics and motor control of human gait: normal, elderly, and pathological,* ed 2, Waterloo, Ontario, University of Waterloo Press, 1991.)

creases with obstruction height and walking velocity.

Trips can occur even when obstacles are not present, such as when one moves from a walking surface that has a modest COF to a surface with a very high COF, especially when the walker is unaware that the floor conditions vary. In this case the user expects somerelative movement between the shoe and the walking surface. The sudden stop of the foot on the high-COF surface can precipitate a trip or stumble. Trips can also occur at midswing on high-COF floors. Minor changes in foot trajectory can result in the toe contacting the floor at midswing. On high-COF floors, the trajectory can be disrupted and cause a stumble that prohibits proper foot placement.

Age is also a potential factor in tripping accidents. Tripping accidents tend to be more common in the elderly. As previously discussed, minimum toe clearance is less than 1 cm. To avoid falling, the swing foot must

be rapidly repositioned to an appropriate placement. The elderly have a reduced capacity to make these rapid responses.[26] This fact, coupled with their general reduction in visual acuity and balance, places the elderly at higher risk of falls caused by trips.

Falls from Elevated Work Surfaces

Falls from elevated work surfaces are frequently precipitated by the same events that precede slips and falls on level surfaces. These events may be due to a slip of the shoe when the RCOF exceeds the COF between the shoe and the work surface or may be due to a trip caused by the swinging foot being unexpectedly stopped by an obstruction. A major difference between these events on the ground and at an elevation is that there is an increased potential for a significant injury when falling from an elevation. This points out the importance of proper equipment selection, good housekeeping, and proper environmental controls. Causative factors that may differentiate falls on elevated work surfaces from those on level surfaces include inadequate handgrip and contact with hoisted machinery and supplies.

Fall protection equipment is an obvious major factor in preventing falls from elevated surfaces. However, the implementation and choice of equipment can be a problem. Often, workers find that this protection is uncomfortable, and restricts the performance of their job, or is unnecessary. The Bureau of Labor Statistics[19] studied 744 injuries caused by work-related falls from an elevation. Of fall survivors who were working at heights exceeding 3 m (10 feet) every day, 14% stated that the fall protection (belts, harnesses, rails, nets, etc.) was not required, 20% thought that fall protection was not needed, and 46% believed that it was not practical. Almost 50% of the surveyed companies did not require fall protection equipment and 75% did not provide training. Sixteen of the 744 injuries resulted from the improper selection, installation, or use of available fall protection equipment. These results suggest that there is a low awareness on the part of management and workers about the potential severity of falls from elevations and the availability of control measures. Ellis[36] noted that fall protection equipment is often deemed unimportant or inconvenient when working in confined spaces.

Falls from elevated work surfaces may happen during a variety of tasks. In the study mentioned earlier, the Bureau of Labor Statistics[19] determined that 17% of falls occurred during material loading/unloading; 13% during the operation, repair, or cleaning of equipment; and 10% during carpentry tasks. Other assorted tasks included painting, welding, roofing, sheet metal work, and masonry/bricklaying. Twenty-eight percent of the workers said that they were climbing up or down, 13% were walking, 11% were stepping from one surface to another, and 20% were moving backward. The exertion of significant hand force or body movement appears to be associated with falls from elevations.

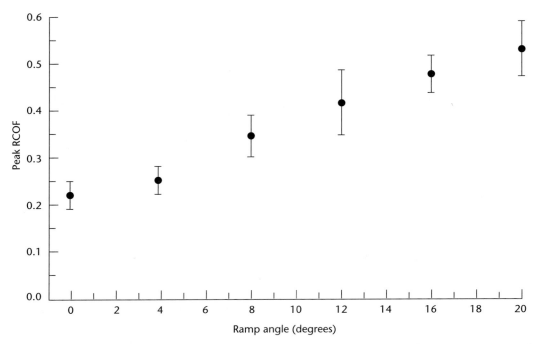

Figure 13-5 Required coefficients of friction (*RCOF*) among subjects for walking down ramps of varying angles.

Falls on Ramps and Stairs

Slips on inclined surfaces are a particular hazard because of the potentially large shear forces. As the ramp angle increases, shear forces along the surface have an increasing gravitational component. In a static case, shear components would increase as the cosine of the angle increases, as pointed out by Grieve,[41,42] and RCOFs to prevent slipping would be expected to increase as the tangent of the ramp angle increases[47] (**Fig. 13-5**). Gait kinematics may change, however, in response to ramp angle increases that could cause foot forces different from those predicted from a simple static analysis. Stride length can affect foot forces and subsequent frictional requirements during gait.[47] Gait speed and foot dynamics may also have an effect.

In a recent study on slip potentials as a function of ramp angle, frictional forces were acquired from a force platform placed within a ramp that was varied at angles from 0 to 20 degrees.[59] Step lengths and walking speeds were also recorded. Peak RCOFs ranged from 0.2 for a flat surface to over 0.6 for a 20-degree incline. Therefore, the use of steep ramps (i.e., 20 degrees) results in an almost threefold increase in the RCOF to prevent slips resulting in falls.

Falls on stairs are caused by a loss of balance or a slip. Most falls on stairs leading to injury occur when descending.[20] Failure to use handrails was also found to be a cause of stair falls. Ellis[35] proposed three factors that contribute to stair falls: stair surface characteristics, human factors, and task characteristics. The major stair design factors are stair width, riser height of 13 to 18 cm (5 to 7 inches), and handrail availability and size (ideally 3.8 cm or 1.5 inches). Another stair design factor

not mentioned by Ellis is the slip resistance of the edges of the stairs. During descent on stairs, high shear forces can be exerted along the edge of the step. Should this area have low slip resistance, a slip off the step could occur. The human factors mentioned by Ellis are speed of descent, age, vision, and any disabilities limiting mobility. Work tasks such as carrying or reaching for objects are also important factors, particularly if they limit vision or the use of handrails.

The biomechanics of walking on stairs indicates the high risk for slips during descent. The foot is located on the step such that the ball of the foot is approximately 3.8 cm from the nose of the step. This places the toe of the shoe beyond the end of the step. Should a slip occur, then a fall is likely. Thus slip resistance on the nose of the stair is critical. Obviously, foot placement is also critical in stair descent. When stairs are not uniform in vertical height, proper foot placement becomes difficult and the fall potential is higher.

Falls from Ladders

The use of ladders has been identified as a cause of falls, particularly in construction and maintenance. In a study of 123 ladder accidents, Cohen and Lin[28] found that 60% of work-related ladder falls occurred while the employee was standing on the ladder, 26% while descending, and 14% while ascending. Approximately 25% of the accidents occurred while performing plant/building maintenance and repair, 25% during building construction, and 18% during vehicle or equipment repair and maintenance. Distribution across ladder types was approximately 57% for step ladders, 30% for extension ladders, 10% for straight ladders, and 3% for other (job-made) ladders. Most workers involved in these accidents had limited work experience. Seventeen percent had less than 1 year of experience and 47% had less than 5 years. Most accidents took place around break time; thus fatigue and inattentiveness may increase the chance of an accident. In a companion study, Cohen and Lin[29] recorded causative factors of accidents related to work conditions, ladder use, and personal and occupational issues. Significant human factors were fatigue, boredom, and uncomfortable posture. Ladder use factors included improper ladder maintenance and improper or defective ladders and slippery support surfaces. Personal issues that were found to increase the likelihood of a ladder accident included lack of prior accident experience and changes in work hours and conditions.

The Bureau of Labor Statistics[22] indicated that in 42% of ladder accidents the user was moving on the ladder and, in 56%, the ladder itself slipped, fell, or broke. The American National Standards Institute[6] found that 22% of ladder accidents involved slipping on the rungs and 56% involved a slip of the ladder.

Specific causative factors associated with ladder accidents were determined by Axelsson and Carter[10] to be tipping of step ladders, sliding of the base of straight ladders, and misstepping on the final step on all ladders. Cohen and Lin[28,29] found that the most common immediate causes of accidents were reaching overhead or overextending to the side (19%); slipping on rungs while descending (14%); misstepping on rungs while descending (10%), frequently while carrying tools or materials; defective or loose ladder parts (9%); being struck by or attempting to catch objects (8%); applying excessive force (7%); leaning the step ladder against a structure (7%); transitioning to/from ladders (6%); and standing on the top rung (6%).

Biomechanical analyses of ladder climbing by Chaffin et al[25] indicate that an increased risk of ladder accidents may result with rung separation greater than 35.6 cm (16 inches), which requires fatiguing exertion when climbing; ladder width less than 60.6 cm (16 inches), which does not allow adequate lateral support; and toe clearance behind the rungs of less than 16.5 cm (6.5 inches), which does not allow the generation of adequate ankle plantar flexion strength. Biomechanical analyses by Bloswick and Chaffin[14] suggest that ladder widths of 38.1 cm (15 inches) and toe clearance of 15.5 cm (6.1 inches) are adequate. Bloswick and Crookston[15] indicate that existing guides on ladders are inadequate and result in the placement of extension ladders at shallow slants that increase the chance that the ladder base will slip. This empiric analysis may explain the high incidence of ladder slip accidents reported.[6,20] The International Occupational Safety and Health Information Centre[46] and the American National Standards Institute (ANSI)[6] suggest that misuse is a significant cause of ladder accidents. In one study, the Bureau of Labor Statistics[22] found that 57% of ladder accident victims were holding onto an object with one or both hands and that 30% had wet, greasy, or oily shoes.

Inadequate training is also a problem. The Bureau of Labor Statistics study found that 60% of ladder accident victims had no training at all in the safe use of ladders. Cohen and Lin[28] found that several victims of ladder accidents were not wearing appropriate footwear or were not properly trained to use ladders.

Falls from Vehicles and Equipment

The causes of falls from vehicles and equipment appear to be a combination of slips, loss of balance, and errors in foot placement. A study of 827 truck driver fall accidents found that nearly 50% involved a foot slip, 25% were caused by a loss of balance, and 20% involved a misstep.[83] These accidents occurred while workers were entering or exiting the cab or climbing on the trailers. Specific activities associated with slip/fall accidents from vehicles and equipment include using/holding tie-down bars (13%); exiting tractors and vehicles (13%); mounting/dismounting tractors, car haulers, and so forth (12%); and securing vehicles and cargo (9%). Most frequently, falls are associated with descending from equipment rather than ascending.[27,33] Bourdioux[66] found that a 9:1 ratio of serious injuries occurred while climbing down as opposed to mounting the equipment.

The effects of whole-body vibration on balance and consequently on falls off equipment are not clear.[32,48,56,57] Vertical whole-body vibrations at frequencies associated with trucks and equipment do not appear to affect standing balance.[32,57] However, anecdotal evidence reveals that many vehicle operators indicate feeling "off balance" after operating heavy equipment for a long period of time. Nonvertical vibrations, exposure duration, noise, and other stressors may play a role.[32] From reported data to date it appears that although vibration may contribute to falls, the key factors in falls from equipment are the biomechanics associated with the design of the egress system.

Steps and handholds are intended to provide the same points of contact as a ladder but must be integrated into the exterior of a vehicle or equipment. This often results in uneven spacing between steps and handholds, so frequent regrasping is necessary. These system characteristics increase the potential for a slip/fall. The need to exert significant force to secure loads on trailers and at the rear of the cab also increases the slip/fall hazard.

PREVENTIONS OF SLIPS, TRIPS, AND FALLS

Level Surfaces

Much work in the prevention of slips and falls has focused on the measurement of "tractive" or slip resistance properties of floors and shoes. Current slip resistance evaluation methods measure the COF of the shoe-floor interface under various conditions such as dry, wet, and oily. These measurements are used by architects, industry, shoe/floor manufacturers, and the legal system as criteria for rating the slip potential of various floor conditions.[70]

The COF is defined as the ratio of the force required to move one surface over another to the total vertical force applied to the two surfaces. Numerous devices have been developed to measure the COF of floor surfaces with various shoe materials. Some of these devices have been tested for usability and reliability.[8,49] The two basic types of devices are static and dynamic recorders. Static COF, the most common measurement for rating slip potential, is defined as the ratio of the horizontal to vertical force measured just before any movement of the shoe material across the floor. The most widely used static COF measurement devices are the James machine, the Drag Sled Tester, the NBS-Brungraber Tester, and the Horizontal Pull Slipmeter. There are a number of less known static testers developed, but they have not been widely accepted. The James machine, developed in the early 1940s, is the most established static COF tester. A minimum COF of 0.5 was established at that time by the Underwriters Laboratory, which used this device with a leather shoe material on floor polishes. Since that time a static COF level of 0.5 has become commonly accepted as "safe" for whatever device is used, with values less than 0.5 becoming gradually more hazardous.[80] This cutoff level was established more by mutual consent than by scientific evidence.[61] One problem in the field of static COF measurement is that different devices do not agree. Static COF measurements vary greatly between devices, particularly under wet, oily, or other contaminant conditions.[17,37]

Although the static COF is routinely used in making evaluations regarding the safety of a floor,[70] its validity under all conditions is questionable.[88] Dynamic COF (DCOF) measures have been shown to be important in slip potential estimations, particularly in walkways.[73,75,88] The DCOF is the shear force required to sustain movement of the shoe material divided by the vertical force. Some DCOF devices that have been used in evaluating the shoe-floor interface are the Horizontal Pull Slipmeter,[37] SATRA Frictional Tester,[73,96] the PSRT,[77] the Finnish slip tester,[44] and the Tortus.[8] The Horizontal Pull Slipmeter and the Tortus are portable devices that can be used in the field. The SATRA, Finnish, and PSRT testers are laboratory-based machines.

Although no thorough comparison tests between these dynamic devices have been reported, there do appear to be differences. These are due to differing shoe configurations, velocities, and vertical forces used by the devices. In general, dynamic measurements can vary greatly from static COFs, with static measures being higher than dynamic ones. Some tests, however, have shown DCOF to actually be higher than the static measures for certain shoe-floor interfaces under specific contaminant conditions. Gronqvist et al[43] developed a classification of slip resistance based on the DCOF. Dynamic floor slip resistance was defined for DCOF as

follows: (1) greater than 0.30 is very slip resistant, (2) 0.20 to 0.29 is slip resistant, (3) 0.15 to 0.19 is unsure, (4) 0.05 to 0.14 is slippery, and (5) less than 0.05 is very slippery. This guideline is much lower than traditional static COF criteria. The DCOF study by Redfern and Bidanda[77] agrees, in general, with the Gronqvist guidelines; however, their classification levels may be low. Redfern and Bidanda[77] indicate that safe DCOF levels should probably be established as greater than 0.3 and probably closer to 0.4. More research into the relationship between slip resistance tests and actual falls is necessary to further establish any firm cutoff levels for DCOF tests.

The debate over which COF measure (static or dynamic) is most appropriate to evaluate floor slipperiness stems from observations of human gait and actual slips. Laboratory experiments have shown that during a slip while walking, the foot never comes to a complete stop but instead continues to move through heel contact.[73,88] Thus the foot slip event is dynamic without a static component. Therefore static COF may not be as relevant as DCOF to the biomechanics of slips during gait. On the other hand, if the foot were initially static, such as during various tasks (lifting, pushing, pulling, or operating a machine), then an argument for the use of a static COF can be made.[38]

Ergonomic design of the floor for fall prevention incorporates the same principles as in other areas of applied ergonomics. First, environmental and worker task constraints must be defined. Next, maintenance, sanitation, and structural requirements are needed. Based on this information, a number of floors can be chosen as possible candidates. Slip resistance tests can then be performed to determine which floors are most slip resistant.

A successful example of ergonomic floor design where slip resistance played an important role is a maintenance balcony in a manufacturing facility. This area had a history of severe falling injuries and redesign was necessary to prevent further injuries. First, environmental contaminants were determined to be mostly water and hydraulic fluid spills. Structural stability in this particular plant required solid steel flooring in this area. Workers performed maintenance tasks on these balconies only infrequently, yet contaminants were usually present. Based on this information, a number of candidate floors were identified and laboratory slip tests using the conditions found in the plant were conducted. The slip tests indicated that two floors outperformed all others tested. These two floors tested equally well for slip resistance, but one was only two thirds the cost of the other and was chosen for its economy. Since the installation of this floor surface on the balconies, fall injuries have been dramatically reduced. Therefore, this floor design has been implemented in other plants as well.

One warning regarding the use of slip resistance testing in floor design should be made. High slip resistance should not be the only ergonomic consideration.

Very high slip resistance can lead to other problems such as trips during midswing. Other ergonomic flooring issues are fatigue from standing and walking on these surfaces for long periods of time, as well as possible knee and hip problems. In the case of the maintenance balconies, workers walked on these surfaces only infrequently and falls were the overwhelming concern. In areas where workers stand for long periods of time, the solution must consider these other ergonomic factors.

Trips

As noted earlier, a trip is caused by a sudden stop of the swing foot so that the center of mass of the body moves forward of the base of support. Trips can best be prevented by work practices that minimize objects of any type on walking and working surfaces and by work practices that prevent the carrying of loads in front of the face. These preventive measures are particularly important on elevated work surfaces and on vehicles where the forward movement beyond the base of support may result in a fall, not to the floor, but to a much lower surface.

Transitions from a low–slip resistance surface to a high–slip resistance surface can also create a trip. Gait patterns appropriate for an area with low to moderate slip resistance can lead to midswing trips, particularly if the floor has a raised surface. These forms of trips should be prevented by minimizing transitions in high-traffic areas and clearly marking them when required.

Elevated Work Surfaces

Because falls from elevated work surfaces are frequently precipitated by the same events that precede slips and falls on level surfaces, the measures to prevent a slip are similar. The provision of a COF adequate to resist the forward slide of the heel during heel strike and to resist a slip at heel strike is of critical importance. This value is dependent on walking velocity, but a nominal static COF value of 0.5 is adequate in most cases. The COF between the shoe and the work surface must remain at a safe level when exposed to contaminants and adverse environmental conditions.

Falls from elevated work surfaces must also be prevented with railings where the worker is at risk of falling. The Occupational Safety and Health Administration (OSHA) general industry standard requires that barriers be provided when there is a drop of more than 1.2 m (47 inches).[67] The exact requirements for the railings required on different types of wall openings and holes, elevated work surfaces, scaffolds, man lifts, and other equipment vary slightly, but railings with a 1.2-m (47-inch) height that have a midrail are generally satisfactory.

In addition to the prevention of slips/falls from an elevated work surface, it is necessary to take measures to protect the worker from the adverse effects of a fall if one occurs. This protection generally takes the form of a personal fall arrest system lifeline and belt or harness connected near the point of operation or a safety net below the operator. The OSHA general industry standard requires that personal fall arrest systems be provided so that the employee will not free-fall more than 1.8 m (6 feet).[68] The OSHA construction standard requires a safety net when workplaces are more than 6.3 m (25 feet) above the next lower surface.[67] Standards and guidelines for fall protection from elevated work surfaces are distributed throughout the OSHA general industry standards, OSHA construction standards, ANSI standards, and other standards and guidelines.[35]

As noted earlier, there is little awareness on the part of management and workers about the potential severity of falls from elevations and the availability of control measures. This indicates that management commitment and worker training are also needed. Bechtel, one of the world's largest engineering and construction firms, makes a special effort to address the proper use of fall protection during new-hire safety orientations and believes that this effort saves lives.[92] Barton-Malow Company, a construction and project management firm in Michigan, and Mortenson, a general contractor in Minneapolis, developed a comprehensive fall protection plan for a joint venture that goes beyond the OSHA standards.[16] The basics of the plan include the following:

- The type of harnesses, belts, and devices workers will use in various situations
- Procedures for assembly, maintenance, and inspection of fall protection systems and equipment
- Safe procedures for handling, storing, and securing tools and materials
- A plan of rescue for injured workers

Ladders

Slip/fall prevention during ladder use must address equipment condition, climbing activity, and work activities performed while on a ladder. Detailed specifications for ladder selection, maintenance, and use are noted in ANSI A14.1 to A14.5[1-5] and in OSHA 1910.25-27.[68] General recommendations for the design and use of ladders can be summarized as follows:

- Orient portable ladders 75 degrees from horizontal.
- For portable ladders, ensure that there is adequate slip resistance between the ladder feet and the ground and between the top of the ladder and the wall or support surface.
- Be sure that there is a minimum of 28 cm (7 inches) of clearance behind the ladder.
- Provide a power grip (finger opposing thumb) whenever possible.
- Provide adequate slip resistance on all hand and foot contact points, and ensure that hands and shoes are not contaminated.
- Ensure that jobs are designed to allow the use of all four limbs and contact of three limbs at all times during the climbing activity.

- Ensure that jobs are designed to allow the user to keep the center of body mass over the feet and not overreach overhead or sideways.
- Ensure that rung separation is consistently 30.5 cm (12 inches).
- Provide ladder cages, wells, platforms, or safety devices (safety line) for fixed ladders of over 6.1 m (20 feet) in unbroken length and platforms or safety devices for fixed ladders of over 9.1 m (30 feet) in unbroken length.
- Provide adequate lighting.
- Train employees in the proper use and maintenance of ladders and the potential hazards involved in their use.

It must again be emphasized that management commitment and employee training are an essential part of any ladder slip and fall prevention program.

Vehicles and Equipment

Climbing and support systems for vehicles and equipment are intended to serve as fixed ladders or fall prevention equipment attached to the exterior of the vehicle. Steps, handholds, and work surfaces that are used for access and movement should incorporate the same safety features as noted earlier for elevated work surfaces and ladders. In reality, this is often quite difficult. Vehicle climbing systems may be required to facilitate lateral as well as vertical movement and are limited as to how far they can extend away from the side of the vehicle. Handholds and work surfaces on equipment must be integrated into the overall design of the trailer.

Guidelines for vehicle and equipment ingress/egress, respectively, are included in 49 CFR 399[24] and SAE J 185.[87] In general, the Bureau of Motor Carrier Safety standard requires that cab ingress/egress systems be designed such that hand force is no more than 35% of body weight, rails allow a full grasp, and the width and depth of steps are 17.7 cm (5 inches). The Society of Automotive Engineers standard for equipment requires that rungs be no more than 40.6 cm (16 inches) apart, handrails be 1.9 to 3.8 cm (0.75 to 1.5 inches) in diameter and no more than 76.2 cm (30 inches) apart, and that steps provide 17.7 cm (5 inches) of toe clearance and be 30.5 cm (12 inches) wide.

Acknowledgement

The authors wish to express their appreciation to Margaret C. Moran for her editorial assistance with this manuscript.

References

1. American National Standards Institute: *American National Standard for ladders–fixed–safety requirements,* ANSI A14.1, 1990.

2. American National Standards Institute: *American National Standard for ladders–portable metal–safety requirements,* ANSI A14.2, 1990.

3. American National Standards Institute: *American National Standard for ladders–portable wood–safety requirements,* ANSI A14.3, 1992.

4. American National Standards Institute: *American National Standard safety requirements for job-made wooden ladders,* ANSI A14.4, 1992.

5. American National Standards Institute: *American National Standard safety requirements for portable reinforced plastic ladders,* ANSI A14.5, 1990.

6. American National Standards Institute: *Rationales for ANSI: A14.1-1981 (wood ladders), A14.2-1981 (metal ladders), and A14.5-1081 (reinforced plastic ladders),* 1983.

7. Andersson R, Lagerlof E: Accident data in new tech Swedish information system on occupational injuries, *Ergonomics* 26:33-42, 1983.

8. Andres RO, Chaffin DB: Ergonomic analysis of slip-resistance measurement devices, *Ergonomics* 28(7): 1065-1079, 1985.

9. Archea J, Collins B, Stahl FI: *Guidelines for stair safety,* (series 120, May 1979), National Bureau of Standards Building Science, Washington D.C.

10. Axelsson P, Carter N: *Measures to prevent portable ladder accidents in the construction industry.* Presented at the fourth International Conference on Slipping, Tripping and Falling, London, 1991.

11. Baker SP, Harvey AH: Falls in the elderly, *Clin Geriatr Med* 501-512, 1985.

12. Reference deleted in proofs.

13. Blake AJ et al: Falls by elderly people at home: prevalence and associated factors, *Age Aging* 17:365-372, 1988.

14. Bloswick DS, Chaffin DB: An ergonomic analysis of the ladder climbing activity, *Int J Ind Ergonom* 6:17-27, 1990.

15. Bloswick DS, Crookston G: The effect of personal, environmental and equipment variables on preferred ladder slant. In Kumar S, editor: *Advances in industrial ergonomics and safety IV,* London, 1993, Taylor & Francis Publishers, Inc; pp. 1015-1020.

16. Britt P: Construction safety: wave goodbye to work-site falls, *Saf Health* 148(3):54-57, 1993.

17. Brungraber RJ: A new portable tester for evaluation of the slip resistance of walkway surfaces, *NBS Tech Note 953,* Gaithersburg, Md, 1977 National Bureau of Standards.

18. Buczek FL, et al: Slip resistance needs of the mobility disabled during level and grade walking. In *Slips, stumbles, and falls: pedestrian footwear and surfaces, ASTM STP 1103,* Philadelphia, 1990, American Society for Testing and Materials; pp 39-54.

19. Bureau of Labor Statistics: Injuries resulting from falls from elevations, Bull No 2195, Washington, DC, 1984, US Department of Labor.

20. Bureau of Labor Statistics: Injuries resulting from falls on stairs, Bull No 2214, Washington, DC, 1984, US Department of Labor.

21. Bureau of Labor Statistics: Injuries to construction laborers, Bull No 2252, Washington, DC, 1986, US Department of Labor.

22. Bureau of Labor Statistics: *Survey of ladder accidents resulting in injuries*, PB83-207985, Washington, DC, 1983, Department of Labor.

23. Bureau of Motor Carrier Safety: *Slips and falls—truck related personal injury accidents*, 1977.

24. Bureau of Motor Carrier Safety: *Step, handhold and deck requirements on commercial motor vehicles*, 49CFR399, 1979.

25. Chaffin DB et al: An ergonomic basis for recommendations pertaining to specific sections of OSHA Standard, 29 CFR 1910, subpart D—walking and working surfaces, Technical report, Ann Arbor, 1978, University of Michigan, Department of Industrial and Operations Engineering.

26. Chen HC et al: Effects of age on available response time on ability to step over obstacles, *J Gerontol Med Sci* (in press).

27. Cohen HH, King K: Analysis of personal injury and illness hazards associated with working in, on, or about commercial motor vehicles. In *Safety sciences*, vol 2, Hazard priorities for the motor carrier industry, vol II, San Diego, 1979 WSA, Inc.

28. Cohen HH, Lin L: A retrospective case-control study of ladder fall accidents, *J Saf Res* 22:21-30, 1991.

29. Cohen HH, Lin L: A scenario analysis of ladder fall accidents, *J Saf Res* 22:31-39, 1991.

30. Cohen HN, Compton DMJ: Fall accident patterns: characterization of most frequent work surface–related injuries, *Professional Saf*, 16-22, 1982.

31. Construction Safety Association of Ontario: *Human factors engineering report on mounting and dismounting construction equipment*, Ontario, 1980, The Association.

32. Cornelius KM, Redfern MS: Postural stability after whole-body vibration exposure, *Int J Ind Ergonom* 13:343-351, 1994.

33. Couch DB, Fraser TM: Access systems of heavy construction vehicles: parameters, problems and pointers, *Appl Ergonom* 12:103-110, 1981.

34. Culver CG: OSHA's goal: build safety into construction, *Saf Health* 146(3):25-27, 1992.

35. Ellis JN: *Introduction to fall protection,* Des Plaines, Ill, 1988, American Society of Safety Engineers.

36. Ellis JN: Plan confined space fall protection before and beyond rescue, *Occup Health Saf* 61(2): 000-000, 1992.

37. English W: Improved tribology on walking surfaces. In Gray BE, editor: *Slips, stumbles and falls: pedestrian footwear and surfaces, ASTM STP 1103* Philadelphia, 1990, American Society for Testing and Materials; pp 73-81.

38. English W: What effect will new federal regulations have on pedestrian safety? *Professional Saf*, March 1992.

39. *Federal Register*: 55:13341-13360, 1990.

40. Grieve DW: Gait patterns and the speed of walking, *Biomed Eng*, 119-122, 1968.

41. Grieve DW: The postural stability diagram (PSD): personal contraints on the static exertion of force, *Ergon* 22(10):1155-1164, 1979.

42. Grieve DW: Slipping due to manual exertion, *Ergonomics* 26(1):61-72, 1983.

43. Gronqvist R, Roine J: Serious occupational accidents caused by slipping. In Nielsen R, Jorgensen R, editors, *Advances in industrial ergonomics and safety V,* London, 1993, Taylor & Francis Publishers, Inc; pp 515-519.

44. Gronqvist R et al: An apparatus and a method for determining the slip resistance of shoes and floors by simulation of human foot motions, *Ergonomics* 32(8):979-995, 1989.

45. Gryfe CI, Amies A, Ashley MJ: A longitudinal study of falls in an elderly population: I. Incidence and morbidity, *Age Aging* 6:201-210, 1977.

46. International Occupational Safety and Health Information Centre: *Ladders*, Geneva, 1966, International Safety Office.

47. James DI: Rubbers and plastics in shoes and flooring: the importance of kinetic friction, *Ergonomics* 26(1):83-100, 1983.

48. Kjellberg A, Wikstrom BO: Whole-body vibration: exposure time and acute effects: a review, *Ergonomics* 28:535-544, 1985.

49. Kulakowski BT et al, Evaluation of performance of three slip resistance testers, *J Testing Evaluation* 17(4):234-240, 1989.

50. Leamon TB, Lee KW: Microslip length and the perception of slipping. *Proceedings of the twenty-third International Congress on Occupational Health*, 1990, p 17.

51. Liberty Mutual Insurance Company: *Research to reality, 1992 annual report*, 1992, Liberty Mutual Insurance Company: pp 18-19.

52. Little AD: *The present status and requirements for occupational safety research*, Report prepared for the National Institute for Occupational Safety and Health, Contract No HSM 099-71-30, 1972, The Institute.

53. Lund J: Accidental falls at work, in the home and during leisure activities, *J Occup Accidents* 6:181-193, 1984.

54. Manning DP: Deaths and injuries caused by slipping, tripping, and falling, *Ergonomics* 26(1):3-9, 1983.

55. Manning DP et al: The incidence of underfoot accidents during 1985 in a working population of 10,000 Merseyside people, *J Occup Accidents* 10:121-130, 1988.

56. Martin B et al: Effects of whole-body vibrations on standing posture in man, *Aviat Space Environ Med* 51:778-787, 1980.

57. McKay JR: *A study of the effects whole-body +az vibration on postural sway*, Rep No AMRL-TR-71-121, Dayton, Ohio, 1972, Wright-Patterson Airforce Base, Aerospace Medical Research Laboratory.

58. McMahon P: Personal communication, Dec 1981.

59. McVay EJ, Redfern MS: Rampway safety: foot forces as a function of rampway angle, *J Am Ind Health Assoc* 55(7):626-634, 1994.

60. Michigan Occupational Safety and Health Act: *MIOSHA Reporter*, July/August, 1980.

61. Miller JM: Slippery work surfaces: towards a performance definition and quantitative coefficient of friction criteria, *J Saf Res* 14(4):120-128, 1983.

62. Morse JM: *Can J Public Health* 77:21-25, 1986.

63. Myung R: *Foot slipperiness and load carrying effects on the biomechanical study of slips and falls.* (dissertation), 1993 Lubbock, Tex., Department of Industrial Engineering, Texas Tech University.

64. National Safety Council: *Accident facts*, Chicago, 1991, The Council.

65. National Safety Council: *Accident prevention manual for industrial operators*, ed 9, Chicago, 1988, The Council.

66. Nicholson AS, David GC: Slipping, tripping and falling accidents to delivery drivers, *Ergonomics* 28(7):977-991, 1985.

67. Occupational Safety and Health Administration: *Safety and health regulations for construction*, No 1926, Washingtion, D.C., 1989, The Administration.

68. Occupational Safety and Health Administration: *Safety and health regulations for general industry*, No 1910, Washingtion D.C., 1992, The Administration.

69. Oregon Department of Insurance and Finance: *Workers' compensation claims characteristics, calendar year 1992*, Portland, Ore., The Department.

70. Pater R: How to reduce falling injuries, *National Safety and Health News*, Oct 1985.

71. Pauls JL: Review of stair-safety research with an emphasis on Canadian studies, *Ergonomics* 28(7):999-1010, 1985.

72. Perkins PJ: Measurement of slip between the shoe and ground during walking. In *Walkway surfaces: measurement of slip resistance*, ASTM STP 649, Philadelphia, 1978, American Society for Testing and Materials.

73. Perkins PJ, Wilson MP: Slip resistance testing of shoes—new developments, *Ergonomics* 26(1): 73-82; 1983.

74. Prudham D, Evans JG: Factors associated with falls in the elderly: a community study, *Age Aging* 10:141-146, 1981.

75. Redfern MS: Factors influencing the measurement of slipperiness, *Proceedings of the Human Factors Society*, San Diego, 1988.

76. Redfern MS, Adams PS: The effect of vertical force on static coefficient of friction. *Proceedings of the Human Factors Society of Canada*, Edmonton, Alberta, 1988.

77. Redfern MS, Bidanda B: Slip resistance of the shoe-floor interface under biomechanically relevant conditions, *Ergonomics* 37(3):511-524, 1994.

78. Redfern MS et al, Kinematics of heelstrike during walking and load carrying: implications for slip testing, *Ergonomics*, (in press).

79. Rice DP et al: *Cost of injury in the US: a report to congress*, San Francisco, 1989, Institute for Health and Aging, University of California and Johns Hopkins University.

80. Rosen SI: *The slip and fall handbook*, Columbia, Md, 1983, Hanrow Press, Inc.

81. Safety Sciences: *Analysis of personal injury and illness hazards associated with working in, on or about commercial motor vehicles*, report prepared for the Bureau of Motor Carrier Safety. contract No DOT-FH-9535, 1979, The Bureau.

82. Safety Sciences: *Occupational fall accident patterns—supplementary data*, report prepared for the National Institute for Occupational Safety and Health, contract No HSM 210-75-0017, 1978, The Institute.

83. Safety Sciences: *VEIIRS: a voluntary employee injury and illness reporting system for the motor carrier industry, vol 2, Final report*, Report prepared for the Bureau of Motor Carrier Safety, contract No. DTFH61-80-C-00186, 1985, The Bureau.

84. Salminen S et al: Falls as serious occupational accidents. Presented at the *fourth International Conference on Slipping, Tripping and Falling*, London, 1991.

85. Schneider EL, Guralnik JM: The aging of America—impact on health care costs, *JAMA* 263(17):2335-2340, 1990.

86. Snyder RG: *Occupational falls*, No UM-HSRI-77-51, Cincinnati, Ohio, 1977, National Institute for Occupational Safety and Health.

87. Society of Automotive Engineers: Access systems for off-road machines, *Recommended Pract J* p 185, 1981.

88. Strandberg L: On accident analysis and slip-resistance measurement, *Ergonomics* 26(1):11-32, 1983.

89. Szymusiac SM, Ryan JP: Prevention of slip and fall injuries, *Professional Saf* 00:11-15, 1982.

90. Thomas: Slipping, tripping and falling accidents at work. Presented at the *fourth International Conference on Slipping, Tripping and Falling*, London, 1991.

91. Tinetti ME, Speechley M, Ginter SF: Risk factors for falls among elderly persons living in the community, *N Eng J Med* 319:1701-1707, 1988.

92. Vastyan J: Making a "big impact" in fall protection, *Occup Health Saf* 61(6):28-33, 1992.

93. Weindruch R, Hadley EC, Ory MG: *Reducing frailty and falls in older persons*, Springfield, Ill, 1991, Charles C Thomas: pp 5-11.

94. Whittle M: *Gait analysis, an introduction*, Oxford, England, 1991, Butterworth-Heinemann.

95. Wild D, Nayak USL, Isaacs B: Description, classification, and prevention of falls in old people at home, *Rheumatol Rehabil* 20:153-159, 1981.

96. Wilson MP: Development of SATRA slip test and tread pattern design guidelines. In *Slips, stumbles, and falls: pedestrian footwear and surfaces*, ASTM STP 1103, Philadelphia, 1990, American Society for Testing and Materials.

97. Winter DA: *The biomechanics and motor control of human gait: normal, elderly and pathological*, ed 2, Waterloo, Ontario, 1991, University of Waterloo Press.

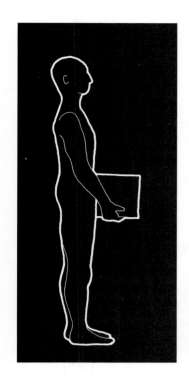

Chapter 14

Introduction to Task Analysis

Jane A. Rajan
John R. Wilson

CONTENTS

Any study of musculoskeletal disorders at work—whether focused on research or intervention—must start from an analysis of the job. This will typically occur when an existing job has been identified—through regular screening, following a complaint, or as a result of a medical report—as presenting a potential risk; alternatively, a job or work station may be assessed as part of a full ergonomics program encompassing an entire department or factory. In all cases, an analysis of what is actually happening in the tasks and jobs (jobs being viewed as composed of tasks and roles) will allow the following:

- Better description of the job and identification of types and levels of risk factors
- Description of those jobs where no or little risk of injury at work is apparent to act as benchmark or reference jobs
- Guidance on what form of intervention to initiate, both generally (e.g., workplace redesign, changed tools, work organization) and specifically within these
- Identification of context and environmental factors that may assist or hinder different forms of intervention
- More complete before/after evaluations of any changes made to the job, tasks, or the workplace

Within ergonomics it is normal practice to carry out a *task analysis* at an early stage of a study. This is, however, one of the most widely misunderstood and misused parts of human-machine systems design. What are reported in the literature as task analyses are often nothing more than mere redescriptions of events. Opinions on the value of task analysis also vary, from those who believe that it is a vital, indeed central part of any ergonomics study to those who wonder what all the fuss is about.

The truth, as often, is somewhere in between. Task analysis, as properly and completely applied, is potentially a valuable part of systems analysis and design and has applications in human factors areas as diverse as training, workplace layout, allocation of function, human reliability assessment, and knowledge acquisition. In the current context, however, what we want to know about is the usefulness of task analysis in the prevention of musculoskeletal injuries. Moreover, if it is useful in this area, we wish to know the most appropriate forms of task analysis.

In this chapter we will first examine how task analysis (or its equivalent) is reported in the applied musculoskeletal disorder literature. Then the body of the chapter will introduce the basic concepts of task

analysis—from description or synthesis, through representation and analysis, to reporting and application. Also, examples of different methods and techniques will be given as appropriate. Finally, we will present some suggested task analyses that use a variety of forms and are based on tasks or jobs with a risk of musculoskeletal injury.

JOB ANALYSIS IN MUSCULOSKELETAL DISORDER STUDIES

Putz-Anderson,[25] in one of the early leading publications of the field, says that "job analysis is not only needed to identify the exposure to risk factors in problematic jobs, but is useful for documenting jobs that illustrate safe levels of task factors and effective work design." With these aims then, he specifies two ways to conduct job analysis—work methods analysis and an ergonomics checklist. To an extent and in the way he describes them, the former might be seen as the task description part of task analysis and the latter as the actual analysis of the tasks.

Work methods analysis, which Putz-Anderson says is particularly appropriate for new or unusually complex jobs, starts with traditional work study (or time-methods study) descriptions where tasks are broken down into fundamental elements (search, grasp, reach, hold, etc.) that are described and timed (sometimes for each limb separately). The work content of each element is then analyzed with respect to potential injury risk, with a brief description of the risk provided for each. He sees the advantage of this approach as breaking a job down into "manageable units" for study. This work methods analysis, although simple and often seen as limited (paradoxically, it is also sometimes seen as taking analysis too far when it becomes micromotion analysis), has provided a basis for some of the process flow and tabular forms of task analysis in use today.

Putz-Anderson's second type of job analysis—checklist administration—might more sensibly be seen as occurring subsequent to task analysis and as embracing the risk evaluation covered in Chapters 2 and 15. He reproduces the Michigan checklist. Two other recent and much more extensive checklist tools are "RULA" (rapid upper limb assessment) from McAtamney and Corlett[21] and the "upper extremity checklist" from Keyserling et al.[16] The latter uses the usual form of additive scoring; RULA tries to be more robust and allow for the inevitable discrepancies of subjective assessment in direct observation by providing a totaling method that is not overly sensitive to small differences in the rating of different work or body parts. Another form of checklist is tabular in nature and, unlike the other two, explicitly recognizes that it is often difficult to assess large elements of a job or even entire jobs. Therefore, Drury et al.[12] devised a form to look in lesser detail at body and limb angles and forces applied for each "task step" that they call a "postural task analysis."

Table 14-1 Upper body and shoulders positions and forces involved during sewing microcycle (steps 1-11: 10 seconds).

Step*	Operation	Position of Left Shoulder	Position of Right Shoulder	Movement Requiring Application of Force	Hand(s) Used to Apply Force	Applied Force (kg)
1	Seize end of trouser leg	Abduction>90°	Adduction, slight flexion	Pull trouser leg along supply bar	Left	0.0015
2	Align two extremities of trouser leg	Abduction>90° external rotation	Adduction	Partially support weight of trouser leg and hook	Left, right	<0.265 (trouser leg) + <0.60 (hook)
3	Press together two lengths, remove hook from supply rack	Abduction, 90°; external rotation	Abduction, 45°	Support weight of trouser leg and hook	Left, right	0.265 + 0.60
4	Place trouser leg under machine and sew	Flexion	Neutral	Partially support weight of trouser leg and hook, press with fingers to advance leg	Left, right	<0.265 + <0.60
				Press on activation pedal		4.3
5	Place hook on receiving bar (during step 4)	Flexion	Neutral	Support weight of hook	Left	0.6
6	Align remaining portion of trouser leg	Slight extension, external rotation	Adduction	Partially support weight of trouser leg	Left, right	<0.265 + <0.60
7	Realign trouser leg at pocket level; place pockets	Abduction, flexion	Slight extension	Press with finger to advance trouser leg	Left	Unknown
				Press on activation pedal and second pedal		
8	Sew remaining portion of trouser leg	Abduction, flexion	Slight extension	Partially support weight of trouser leg	Left, right	4.3 + >10
9	Cut thread	Abduction, flexion	Slight extension	Press with finger to advance trouser leg	Left	Unknown
				Press on activation pedal		4.3
10	Push trouser leg onto bar in front	Flexion, slight abduction	Slight flexion	Pull thread	Left	0.76
11		Flexion, slight abduction	Slight flexion	Push one or several trouser legs with hand	Left	Depends on work technique

From Vezima N, Tierney D, Messing K: *When is light work heavy? Components of the physical workload of sewing machine operators working at piecemeal rates,* Appl Ergon *23:268-276, 1992; with permission from the publisher, Butterworth-Heinemann, Ltd.*
*Steps 7 and 8 concern outer seam operators only.

Table 14-2		Example of a protocol for task analysis.					
Subtask	**Purpose**	**Procedure**	**Feedback**	**Control Problems**	**Display Problems**	**Posture Problems**
Load/unload panel	Production	Move cart of panels to and from workstation. Insert panel. Place on top sheet. Clip in place. Tape down. Remove on completion.	Visual, kinesthetic	Positioning tape with body extended. Arms at maximum reach.	Counting panels by hand—without antilaceration gloves.	Excessive reach, 31 to 38 inches 20 times per setup
Collar on drills	Preparation	Obtain collar and correct drill size. Place in press to specified setting. Remove to WIP for machine.	Visual	Drills lack organization. Boxes underneath shelf		Excessive reach, 31.5 to 38.5 inches
Measure (1 per load)	Quality	Take panel to measurement machine. Take 13 readings using VDT. Log on machine history.	Cognitive visual		Of many thousand holes, only 24 are checked. Off-location holes may not be detected.	Standing work—no chair
Visual inspection	Quality	Move panel to light table. Identifying missing holes.	Visual		400 eye movements with 1-inch travel are required. This task should take 5 min. but inspector takes only 2 min.	Standing work—no chair
Clean drill spindle holder	Maintenance	Once per shift, stop machine. Remove, clean, and replace drill holders. Vacuum. Collect debris.	Visual	Controls difficult to see.	Work area difficult to see.	Excessive reach 31 to 38 inches with a lift to insert into spindle
Add coolant	Maintenance	About once per month.	Visual			
Check gauges	Maintenance	Back of machine. Observe proper readings.	Visual		Gauges difficult to read.	

From Burri GJ, Helander MG: A field study of productivity improvements in the manufacturing of circuit boards, Int J Ind Ergonom *7:207-215, 1991.*
WIP, work in progress; VDT, video display terminal.

The literature on musculoskeletal disorder investigations or interventions seems to contain task analyses that are fairly limited in number and depth. In the following material, a few recent publications are described, somewhat at random. Vezima, Tierney, and Messing[36] report what they call "descriptions of work activities" for sewing machine operators at piecework rates. Before measuring the work stations, the forces exerted by the operators, postures, movements, and production requirements, the work cycle was observed and the stages described; this was presented for a macrocycle, sewing a whole rack of trouser legs, and for a microcycle within this, sewing one leg seam. The simple listing of activities—in sequence order—is subsequently used to aid in the association of postures and forces within activities in a tabular format similar to that used in general task analysis (**Table 14-1**).

In a study of both physical and organizational ergonomics for productivity improvement in the manufacture of printed circuit boards, Burri and Helander[9] show an example of their "protocol task analysis." For each subtask, defined at a fairly gross level in fact, they describe its purpose and procedure, the type of feedback the operator receives, and problems with control (i.e., actions), display (i.e., visual perception), and posture (**Table 14-2**).

Also following a tabular format, Reddell et al[26] assist their study of lumbar injury in airline baggage handlers and subsequent evaluation of a weight-lifting belt by describing the tasks of the personnel in different roles or areas of work. More extensively, Vora, Reynolds, and Corl[37] list the sequence of work activities in an optical disk formatting and cleaning job and, for each, define the operator "subsystems" (sensory or biomechanical) involved. They do, however, head this listing as a task analysis, but one might argue that it is barely a description (**Table 14-3**). Later, when they tabulate design requirements, the existing design, and the proposed design against the four components task, operator, machines, and environment, this may be seen as a form of task analysis (**Table 14-4**).

Dickenson[11] reports the use of both of Putz-Anderson's forms of work analysis,[25] although not explicitly identifying them as such. First, Dickinson uses a simple flowchart to illustrate the activity sequence for two alternative methods of manually bagging chemicals. She also offers a substantial textual description of the activities. This illustrates one debate for task analysis: the relationship between the clarity of a flow diagram or table versus the extent of detail available in text form. In addition, she provides spatial flow diagrams illustrating the movement of materials and the operator on a plan of the workstation. Finally, she uses the United Kingdom Health and Safety Executive's own checklist for manual handling risk factors; this is illustrated in the paper for three linked tasks at once (see **Fig. 14-1**).

There is little consistency in the literature on musculoskeletal injury interventions in terms of views on and the use of "task analysis." Indeed, much of the time what is called a task analysis would not be regarded as such by analysts in other fields. This leaves several questions: would musculoskeletal injury investigations be enhanced by the use of more sophisticated task analysis techniques? Alternatively, is the nature of the problem such that to do more than list tasks before risk factor assessment is to be overzealous? Moreover, is what this community regards as risk factor assessment, using a variety of methods and measures, in fact the equivalent of task analysis techniques used in, say, control room design or human-computer interaction?

In the main part of this chapter we introduce the nature and process of task analysis and then provide a number of examples of the different types of analysis that might be made. In fact, what we are really providing for the reader are examples of task representation. Although we then attempt to assess the utility of different forms of representation/analysis for musculoskeletal disorder investigations, to an extent readers must decide for themselves their utility and practicality in any given situation.

WHAT IS TASK ANALYSIS?

The concept of a task is central to the field of human factors. The study of human activity and involvement with systems invariably requires a study of the tasks that will be carried out by people. Tasks as an entity have existed as long as people have performed work. However, awareness of the need for terminology and concepts relating to the idea of tasks arose as human-machine systems became increasingly complex and industry more advanced. Now, reliability and quality are major issues not just from a hardware point of view but also for the work force, and they can be a major limiting factor in system performance. Therefore, reliable performance of the human systems component must be ensured, and the tasks to be carried out must form a job environment that takes into account the needs, abilities, and skills of the system users. This will be achieved by ergonomics applied within design, such as in task design and design of the human-computer interface.

Concepts and Definitions

Despite the centrality and pervasiveness of tasks in human engineering, no substantial and consistent body of theory focuses on the idea of a task. Although the concept is fundamental and widely used, in only a few cases is it rigorously defined. It is often assumed that the same concept of task is known and understood by all. However, an examination of the literature uncovers huge discrepancies in the scope of what a "task" is assumed to be. For example, three definitions of a task are as follows (see p. 173):

Table 14-3	Task description for disk handling (called "task analysis" by original authors): use of the analysis in design.	

Task Description		**Subsystems Involved**
1	**Disk unloading from rack**	
	1.1 Check that the handling tool is unclamped	S
	1.2 Locate the handling tool on the disk	S/B
	1.3 Clamp the disk	S
	1.4 Remove the disk from the rack	
2	**Preformat disk cleaning**	
	2.1 Loading	
	2.1.1 Locate the disk on the hub	S/B
	2.1.2 Hold the disk in position and clamp the disk on the hub	B
	2.1.3 Unclamp the disk from the tool	B
	2.1.4 Remove the handling tool from the disk	S/B
	2.2 Unloading	
	2.2.1 Locate the handling tool on the disk	S/B
	2.2.2 Clamp the disk	B
	2.2.3 Unlock the hub to release the disk	B
	2.2.4 Remove the disk from the disk cleaner	S/B
3	**Disk formatting**	
	3.1 Loading	
	3.1.1 Open the formatting machine lid	B
	3.1.2 Change the disk orientation to horizontal	B
	3.1.3 Position the spindle to match the index mark on the disk	S/B
	3.1.4 Locate the disk on the spindle (be careful not to touch the formatting head)	S/B
	3.1.5 Unclamp the disk	B
	3.1.6 Remove the handling tool from the disk	S/B
	3.1.7 Lock the disk on the spindle	B
	3.1.8 Close the formatting machine lid	B
	3.2 Unloading	
	3.2.1 Open the formatting lid	B
	3.2.2 Unlock the spindle	B
	3.2.3 Locate the tool on the disk	S/B
	3.2.4 Clamp the disk	B
	3.2.5 Remove the disk from the spindle (be careful not to touch the formatting head)	S/B

Table 14-3	Task description for disk handling (called "task analysis" by original authors): use of the analysis in design—continued.	

Task Description	Subsystems Involved
4 Postformat disk cleaning	
4.1 Loading	
4.1.1 Locate the disk on the hub	S/B
4.1.2 Hold the disk in position and clamp the disk on the hub	B
4.1.3 Unclamp the disk from the tool	B
4.1.4 Remove the handling tool from the disk	S/B
4.2 Unloading	
4.2.1 Locate the handling tool on the disk	S/B
4.2.2 Clamp the disk	B
4.2.3 Unlock the hub to release the disk	B
4.2.4 Remove the disk from the disk cleaner	S/B
5 Disk loading on caddy carrier	
5.1 Load a caddy carrier on the MSA loader	B
5.2 Position the caddy carrier	S/B
5.3 Activate the spindle-elevating switch	S/B
5.4 Locate the disk on the spindle (horizontal orientation)	B
5.5 Unclamp the disk	B
5.6 Remove the handling tool from the disk	S/B
5.7 Slide the caddy carrier on the disk	S/B
Carry the disk from one workstation (machine) to another. This subtask is required after subtasks 1, 2, 3, and 4	B

From Vora PV, Reynolds JL, Corl KG: Design and evaluation of an optical disk handling tool for a cleanroom environment, Appl Ergonom 23:414-424, 1992; with permission from the publisher, Butterworth-Heinemann.
S, sensory; B, biomechanical.

- "Any set of activities occurring about the same time, sharing some common purpose that is recognized by a task performer"[23]
- "Generally speaking, any kind of behavior that can reasonably be labeled with a verb can be called a task"[7]
- "A transfer of information between components *(within a system)*."[34]

These three definitions differ in that their basic focus is on, respectively, a goal-oriented activity, all aspects of human behavior, and abstract rather than concrete behavior.

The wide discrepancy and failure to agree on a common definition would appear to arise from the range of contexts in which a task can occur. The definitions focus on only one particular aspect of a general task model rather than defining a task in a way that would be applicable to all task contexts. For example, the task definitions that focus on physical and observable activity fail to account for tasks that are purely cognitive. To allow a common approach to the issues of analysis, a simple definition of a task is proposed and based on the ideas that a task has a set goal and is purposive and that it is achieved by an action (cognitive or physical in nature).

Table 14-4	Design requirements as addressed by the existing and proposed design of a disk-handling tool.		
Components of TOME	**Design Requirements**	**Existing Design**	**Proposed Design**
Task	Ease in loading/unloading and clamping/unclamping operations	Difficulty in locating the tool on the disk Unclamping operation jerky	Three fixed locators facilitated locating A smooth slider-crack mechanism facilitated clamping/unclamping
Operator	Minimize joint deviations as well as the forces and torques on operator's upper extremities	Wrist deviations extreme (in zone 2 and zone 3) Wrist deviations encouraged while carrying the disk from one station to another because the forces were perpendicular to the disk	Wrist deviations less extreme (essentially in zone 2) Use of the power grip and additional support using the handle reduced wrist deviations
	Reduce the weight of the tool	Tool was lightweight: 1 lb (0.45 kg)	Tool was relatively heavier: 2.3 lb (1.03 kg) Handling of the tool using both hands, however, facilitated handling, and it was not perceived to be heavy
	Minimize demands on sensory (visual) subsystem	Demands on sensory (visual) subsystem because the rack carrying the disks was placed horizontally on the table. Note that this was not a limitation of the disk-handling tool	Demands on the sensory (visual) subsystem reduced by using an inclined rack (30 degree)
Machines	Facilitate handling in both horizontal and vertical orientations	Handling in horizontal and vertical orientation by positioning the hand accordingly	Orientation changed through release R Permitted power grip in both orientations
	Locate the disk on its outside diameter	Located the disk on its outside diameter	Located the disk on its outside diameter
	Eliminate any contact with the surface of the disk	No contact with the surfaces of the disk	No contact with the surfaces of the disk
	Prevent interference with the machine parts, especially the formatting head	No interference with the machine parts	No interference with the machine parts
Environment	Reduce particle (contamination) accumulation	Moving parts not concealed; possibility of contamination accumulation	All the moving parts concealed to prevent contamination accumulation at joints
	Maintain disk in a vertical plane to prevent accumulation of contamination on disk surfaces during carrying	Handling in vertical orientation possible	Handling in vertical orientation possible
	Select wear-resistant tool materials	Nickel-plated aluminum and Teflon used as tool materials	Nickel-plated aluminum, ABS plastic, and Teflon used as tool materials
	Select the tool materials to facilitate cleaning	Facilitated cleaning with isopropyl alcohol	Facilitated cleaning with isopropyl alcohol

As an extension to the concept of a task, much confusion exists over the definition of task analysis, and the term is used to apply to many different approaches to studying tasks. Because there are so many definitions relating to the concept of task and so many methods of task analysis available, it is important to draw some distinctions between the concepts that are used in this area. Three broad categories illustrate different approaches to breaking down task information: job analysis, task analysis, and task description. Task synthesis and task modeling are additional related concepts.

Job Analysis, Task Analysis, and Task Description

Job analysis addresses issues concerning the occupation of an individual by looking at overall duties and responsibilities within the total work context.[27] Task analysis, however, addresses more detailed work issues (or categories of individuals), specifically in the workplace environment. It looks at how individuals work and interact with the system and its interfaces.

Interpretations as to what constitutes a task analysis are loose and varied; in particular, the terms "task analysis" and "task description" are often confused and not clearly defined. In fact they are closely related but different. A task description is a statement of task criteria; it documents the simple elements of observable behavior and concentrates on the physical level of the task only. No quantitative or qualitative judgments are drawn from the task. It is a recording of the operator's observable units of behavior and the simple flow between these. No inferences are made as to the nature of the internal processing or the transformation that takes place between stimulus and response. Task description can be used as a task definition in its own right, but it is more commonly used as a preliminary step in task analysis.

In contrast, task analysis is both descriptive and prescriptive; it takes a task description and adds quantitative or qualitative elements or both to form a statement of human performance requirements that help to specify the human subsystem. However, in science, most analyses are rigorous, and task analysis cannot always be so. In some situations this is a failing, in others an advantage. Whether or not the highly subjective content of task analysis is problematic depends on the context in which it is applied. Not only does task analysis describe the task it analyzes, but it also evaluates, specifies, synthesizes, and interprets the task information.

Selection of a Technique

Task analysis is now firmly established in the ergonomist's repertoire of tools and techniques. However, the choice is such that the average ergonomist can be somewhat daunted by selection from the methods available. Experience suggests that ergonomists tend to favor the use of one or two tried and tested methods, or they develop or adapt a method to suit their own specific needs and applications.

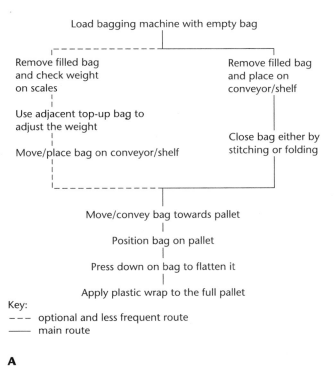

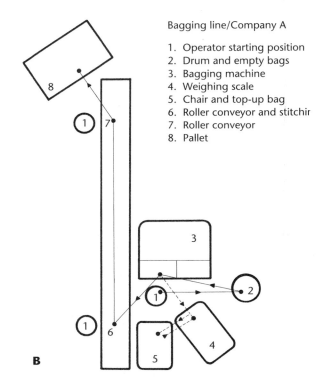

A   **B**

Figure 14-1 A, Simple flowchart. **B,** Spatial flowchart. **C,** Analysis checklist. *(From Dickinson C: Manual handling: an assessment of bag filling operations, Proceedings of Ergonomics in the Process Industries. Institution of Chemical Engineering NW Branch, Symposium No. 5, Winslow, UK, June, 1993, Health and Safety Executive.)*   *Continued.*

Section B: Detailed assessment					
Questions to consider (If the answer is yes, place a check and note the level of risk)	**YES**	**Level of risk**			**Possible Remedial Action** (Make rough notes in this column)
		LOW	**MED**	**HIGH**	
The tasks: do they involve • holding loads away from trunk? • twisting? • stooping? • reaching upwards? • large vertical movement? • long carrying distances? • strenuous pushing or pulling? • unpredictable movement of loads? • repetitive handling? • insufficient rest or recovery? • a work rate imposed by a process?					
The loads: are they • heavy? • bulky/unwieldy? • difficult to grasp? • unstable/unpredictable? • intrinsically harmful (e.g., sharp or hot)?					
The working environment: are there • constraints on posture? • poor floors? • variations in levels? • hot/cold/humid conditions? • strong air movements? • poor lighting conditions?					
Individual capability: does the job • require unusual capability? • hazard those with a health problem? • hazard those who are pregnant? • call for special informantion or training?					
Other factors: Is movement or posture hindered by clothing or personal protective equipment?					
NOTES:					

Figure 14-1, *cont'd* For legend see p. 175.

One reason for this narrow approach is that the possible applications of task analysis are so wide that no one method could cover them all. However, when we examine the dimensions of a task that may need to be analyzed (irrespective of application), it becomes evident that many methods are lacking task information in one or more dimensions. This is not necessarily to the detriment of the method, which may serve its purpose well. However, if a general method of task analysis is to be developed, then these dimensions need to be documented within the analysis. It may be argued that the resulting analysis and representation would be too complex. However, when one considers the complexity of the tasks that are being documented, it becomes evident that this is unavoidable for all but the simplest of tasks.

There are six dimensions that should be considered

for any task analysis that aims to have some general application: *where* (geographic location), *what* (task elements, e.g., the means of interacting with a process, the ways in which tools and equipment are used), *when* (timing and sequence of tasks), *how* (tools and equipment that are used), *why* (the goal[s] of the task), and *who* (the task performer).

An analysis generally cannot document everything within system performance that may influence task performance; these six dimensions encompass the primary factors that relate to task performance. Assumptions that are made about an analysis need to be stated in the accompanying documentation, for example, assumptions about the characteristics of the user population. The analysis would also assume effective human factors design of associated factors that may affect task performance; this may include the social environment and factors such as the motivation of personnel and a well-designed physical environment.

PERFORMING A TASK ANALYSIS

Task analysis is a process by which information about a task is collected and translated into a format that will represent the task or some aspect of the task for the purposes of design or evaluation. The process occurs in a series of distinct stages that are each contingent on one another, although in some methods one or more stages may be merged. The process used is an iterative one, with the iterations occurring within and between stages.

The first stage is always concerned with the information available about the task, and collecting this information is to an extent determined by the goals of the analysis and by the resources available in terms of personnel and access to information about the task. Following this is a process of task description, analysis, and representation. The application for the task analysis will help to decide which of the task analysis techniques available will be the most appropriate. If the analysis is to be used for a large advanced system, the analytic information may need to be fed into a wide range of design areas. In this case, two alternative paths of analysis are open: to carry out the analysis by using a battery of complementary task analysis methods or to carry out a general task analysis that provides a common source of information to feed into other more specific analyses relevant to the applications required. What the analysis is to be used for is ultimately the deciding factor for which methods are used. After a method or several methods have been selected, the analysis can continue in the form of a series of stages (**Fig. 14-2**).

The process of carrying out a task analysis can be very complex because in practice, iteration can occur at any stage of the cycle. This iteration may involve going back one or several stages in the analysis, either to gain more information or to show the analytic information in an alternative form.

Information Collection

The first stage in carrying out a task analysis (having provisionally selected the methods to be used based on the data and resources available) is to gather together all the available information concerning the task. The quality of the information put into the analysis will largely determine the quality of the information produced by the analysis process. Task information may be collected by reference to existing or similar systems or, in the case of a new system, on what has been decided to date by the design team.

Much of the task information will be gathered from people who are involved in the system or similar systems, with the "stakeholders" in the system and their relative importance identified as a means of deciding who to use as a source for system information. This approach ensures that the different viewpoints of managers, operators, and other people in the system are represented and helps to avoid bias in design by ensuring that the needs of all users (rather than just the primary operators of the system) are considered.

A wide range of techniques for collecting information about a task are available, both qualitative and quantitative. The methods used will depend not only on the method(s) of task analysis that are to be used but also on the time and resources available. In addition, the current condition of the system may eliminate the use of certain methods. The methods available can be grouped into four principal approaches to information collection, as shown in **Table 14-5**, which provides an overview of commonly used techniques. For analysis of all but very simple tasks, it is likely that a combination of methods will be employed.

Task Description

Once collected, the information may need some initial organization into a form suitable for task analysis. At this stage, no interpretation is made of the information, but it should be structured in a way that allows it to be interpreted and applied. This stage produces a formal or informal task description (for example, a formal representation that is required as an input into analysis or informal handwritten notes). Sometimes this will be carried out as the data are collected or used as a means of organizing the task data. Alternatively, the task description may constitute a more formal part of the analysis itself.

Task Analysis

If practical constraints allow, the task analysis techniques will have been chosen before the task information or data are collected. Some of the methods and practical issues of carrying out a task analysis are outlined later.

The analysis technique provides a framework for structuring and interpreting the task data. It can be prescriptive as well as descriptive by providing information that can be used for design and evaluation of systems and tasks. However, existing methods of task analysis provide a framework in which to document

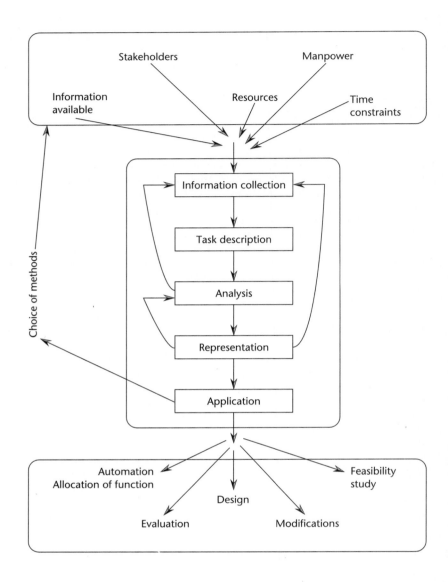

Figure 14-2 Stages in task analysis.

Table 14-5	Information collection for task analysis.	
Type	**Examples**	**Comments**
DOCUMENTATION The documents surrounding a task and its performance can offer a detailed source of data. The task is shown in terms of how it was intended to be performed and documentation can illustrate how the task relates to the wider system purpose	• System specification • Historical records, e.g., incident data • Standards • Job descriptions • Logs • Operating documentation such as procedures, manuals • Health and safety policy	• Show how a task is "meant to be done" • Does not account for informal adaptation to the workplace by personnel • May not be updated as the job is modified or equipment changes and so is out of date • Logs and other documentation completed by personnel may be incomplete • In system design documentation, assumptions made about, e.g., allocation of functions between human and machines

Table 14-5	Information collection for task analysis—continued	
Type	**Examples**	**Comments**

OFF-LINE DATA

This group of information collection techniques involves the derivation of data about the task away from the actual task or at some time after the task has been performed. It includes methods of recording task performance for later analysis and the use of task experts to perform subjective evaluation of the task	• Video techniques • Scenario diagnosis by experts • Critical incident technique (Flanagan, 1954) • Structured and unstructured interviews • Subject matter experts, e.g., table top discussions, retrospective verbal protocols (Bainbridge, 1991) • Walk/talk through	• Recording techniques allow detailed analysis and are useful in an environment where observational measures are too intrusive • Analysis of recorded information is very time consuming • Recorded information allows a detailed examination of the task for analysis and the possibility of repeated observation of the same task • Experts can be questioned in detail and in relation a wide variety of tasks rather than those being performed while data collection is under way • Interviews allow more in-depth questioning while a person is not performing a task concurrently • Away from the task situation, experts may be more prone to forgetting detail • If experts are used, a group or a sample is preferable to avoid bias

TASK SITUATION REPRESENTATION TECHNIQUES

This range of techniques is based on the representation, at varying levels of fidelity, of the task situation	• Simulation • Mock-ups, i.e., static representation (of varying degrees of fidelity) • Physical models, i.e., scale models of the task situation/workplace • Computerized representations	• Highly accurate and realistic representations of the task environment can be used to collect data • Simulation can be expensive and difficult to justify • Events can be represented in real time or manipulated temporally • Rarely occurring events (e.g., emergency situations) can be presented to users of the system • Often used in conjunction with verbal protocols or walk/talk through methods

REAL-TIME OBSERVATIONAL TECHNIQUES

This group of techniques is used to gather task information in an empiric setting while the task in question is being performed	• Observational techniques, e.g., continuous behavior observation, time sampling observation, activity analysis • Mental workload measure, e.g., secondary task technique • Physical task measures, e.g., ECG, cycle time for manual repetitive tasks, frequency of control usage • Concurrent verbal protocols	• Observational data tend to focus on physical and observable task actions • A wide variety of forms exists for recording data collected while observing performance of the task under study, e.g. checklist, running log • A verbal protocol is one of the few methods that aims to gain information on the way personnel make control decisions and may give an insight into the way in which they process information and their mental model of the system

ECG, *electrocardiogram.*

tasks and task-related information. They do not always provide complete tools for design or evaluation. Often an ergonomist or other appropriately qualified specialist is required to interpret the analysis into information that can be usefully applied in design. The effectiveness of the analysis in communicating task information is highly dependent on the following stage of task analysis, that of representing the results of the analysis in a usable form.

Representation

Representation of the analysis is the final form in which it is communicated to the end user, who will generally be a designer or engineer and not the analyst. The representation may be in graphic, symbolic, or textual form, with words used to describe the content of the task elements. The use of natural language to describe and analyze tasks provides a flexibility and accuracy of description not given by any other means. However, the very nature of this flexibility is a source of potential inconsistency among analysts,[4] who may vary in the way in which they approach the task, in attention to detail, and in the exhaustiveness of their analysis. To some extent, this variability between analysts can be overcome by providing a more rigid structure to a task analysis technique. However, variability does not necessarily mean that any one analysis is incorrect, for it may just be an alternative way of representing the task.

This final phase of representing the task is not a trivial one. If a task is complex, the analysis of it will reflect this complexity. It should be remembered that people are intricate and flexible system components and that much of the way in which humans process information and carry out tasks cannot yet be replicated by machines. So it is reasonable to expect a task analysis to be at least as complicated as some of the engineering and systems analyses within the same system. However, particularly as a human factors specialism, task analysis and its representation must aim to follow human factors guidelines with comprehensibility, readability, and the effective use of symbols and signs. Above all, a task analysis must be usable.

APPLICATIONS

Once the analysis is complete, the final stage is its application, generally in the design or evaluation of either an existing or new system. If there is no similar existing system from which task information can be drawn, then the process of task analysis is often labeled "task synthesis," because a view of the task is formed without an existing task basis.

Application is the most important factor in the choice of task analysis method; it determines what information is needed from the analysis and in what form and so also relates to the information collection stage. One important feature of the method is that representation of the analysis is in a format that is suitable for the application and minimizes the chance of misinterpretation. Information should also be presented in a form that other analysts and users can understand. If the analysis has to be changed or updated, it is essential to allow others to relate the documentation of the task to the task analysis method that was used to produce it. What is important is that the analysis provide an accurate representation of the task, be without bias, and be as detailed and complete as the application requires.

A range of applications in which task analysis can be used in relation to the risk of musculoskeletal disorders are available. Some are directly linked to the human factors field, whereas others are on the periphery and allied to other disciplines. Some contribute directly to the design process, and others offer more indirect input. Brief details are given later for three applications of most relevance to musculoskeletal injury interventions—training, work space layout, and workload. (Other potential applications include human reliability assessment, human-machine or human-computer interface design, allocation of function, operator aid and support, personnel selection, and operating procedures and instructions.)

Training

The development of training programs was an early application of task analysis. A task analysis that looks at both the overall goals and the detailed performance of a task gives information for both part-task and whole-task training approaches. The logical breakdown of the task into trainable elements ensures that the task could be taught in a thorough and systematic way. The quality assurance aspect of the analysis also comes into play inasmuch as trained task performance can be evaluated against the standard described in the analysis. The effect of training can only be assessed by the results it produces.

Information that would generally be needed from a task analysis that was to be applied to a training application includes information on the overall goals of the task that cumulatively contribute to the job description; detailed, step-by-step information on how to perform the task to allow systematic training to be developed; and explicit information about the skills that need to be taught to allow the operator to perform the task.

Methods that might be used for training include hierarchical task analysis or an abilities requirements approach (see the next section).

Workspace Design and Workplace Layout

The layout of a workplace is of great importance for the way in which tasks are carried out. Also, the interaction of the user with parts of the system needs to be documented and analyzed for design purposes. There are many factors that affect task performance in the workplace. Most task analysis methods are based on the assumption that these factors are constant and already well designed ergonomically. Such factors include the physical working environment and the social working environment. However, in some situations it is important for these factors to be identified and considered. No methods directly address both the social and physical factors if they simultaneously affect the task, although there are methods that document either the social *or* the physical factors.

Methods to determine the layout of the workplace permit simpler analysis of the task than for other applications. They assess the relative importance and use of different system elements for different parts of a task and allow for design decisions based on this. A task analysis to study workplace design should address (or infer) the following aspects:

1. The layout and design of the workplace and work space—what will help operators perform their tasks effectively; ensure that equipment, information, and the tools needed are at hand; and ensure that a team can function together effectively in the environment
2. The items of equipment that an operator will use in performing the task and thus contribute to their design, with the aim of aiding task performance
3. Information on the relationship between items in the workplace from the point of view of how they are used in the task
4. Restrictions and constraints on the physical environment that limit the design
5. The relationships between tasks, their relationship to different system elements and items of equipment, and their relative importance in the task environment.

A variety of useful methods can be applied within work space design, including link analysis (to analyze physical or operational relationships between interface elements) and job process charts (to represent information exchange between the worker and the system in relation to task elements).

Workload Assessment

Workload can be viewed from several perspectives, including the number of tasks to be performed over time, the sequencing of tasks, the types of tasks to be performed, peaks and troughs in load, and the effort (cognitive or physical) required to be expended on tasks. The concept of workload can refer to the characteristics of the task itself or to the consequences of performing the task (for example, a high workload can have a psychological effect on people). Individual capacity for workload also varies. Assessment of workload in relation to a task can have several practical applications. Assessment of physical workload can help to identify attributes required for personnel selection. This type of factor can also arise in the design of the task itself. For example, if it is repetitive, short-cycle work involving manual material handling, task performance may be improved by allowing self-pacing or by adjusting the design of machinery to make the task less strenuous. The concept of workload also assumes, in a

cognitive sense, time-sharing of tasks. Methods (for example, signal flow graphs) are available that allow this to be documented over time.

From a mental workload point of view, problems can occur if the load is either too low or too high. In modern process control, one of the contradictions of control room operation is that the operator may have long periods of carrying out low-load, repetitive, monitoring tasks interspersed with very high-load decision-making and problem- solving tasks. If low loads are identified, then the task design can be considered and perhaps enhanced to help maintain operator attention, arousal, and motivation. Task analysis indicating high loads allows the potential for two-person operation, job aids, and other aids to be assessed. This too can help personnel selection. The attributes of the operator can be specified to allow appropriate job aids or motivational and job design factors to be designed into the task.

Apart from time and the sequencing of tasks, especially those that are concurrent, it is not possible to specify general factors that are needed within a task analysis method for both physical and psychological workload assessment. Both cognitive and physical tasks need to be specified and factors affecting system performance under different system conditions indicated. Also, with mental workload, often both the normal system operation and system functioning under fault conditions should be analyzed.

METHODS OF TASK ANALYSIS

Taxonomies

Using taxonomies as a means of organizing data has a long history, having originally been developed as a concept by Plato. Many sciences in which data have proven to be vast and confusing have developed taxonomies, for example, atomic tables and zoological classification. Taxonomies are useful because each can have an associated body of knowledge and learning and set applications. Taxonomic methods are one of the most commonly applied approaches to the analysis of tasks, and many other task analysis methods use taxonomy at some point in development of the analysis. Taxonomy offers a means of classifying the elements of a task to organize them for a particular purpose.

An ideal taxonomy would have classes (taxa) that are both mutually exclusive (i.e., no one element could be classified under more than one category) and exhaustive (i.e., every element would clearly fit into a category). However, in practice it is very difficult to achieve such rigor. The first attempts at formalizing task analysis were achieved through the use of task taxonomies. Early taxonomies were based on overtly observable behavior, for example, Gilbreth's micromotion analysis in methods study. These attempts then developed to encompass learning tasks, the information processing approach, and then further toward a taxonomy based on inferences of cognitive behavior, for example, Fleishman's abilities approach.[13] Tasks are usually classified at an

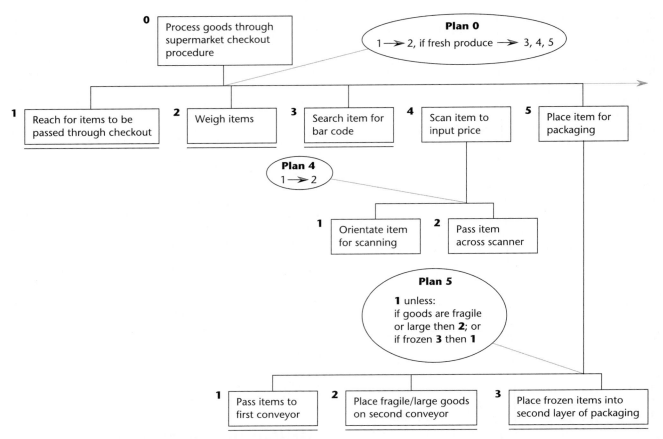

Figure 14-3 Extracts from hierarchical task analysis in tree diagram and tabular form (see Table 14-6), for a laser scanning checkout operation.

ordinal level, although some are divided into a hierarchical taxonomy.

The advantages of taxonomies are that they are a useful vehicle for task breakdown, often very application specific, and can be combined easily with other methods of analysis. The disadvantages are that if categories are not well defined, inconsistencies may arise among analysts, categories are often not mutually exclusive and exhaustive, and it can be difficult to select an appropriate taxonomy.[14]

Hierarchies

A range of task analysis methodologies center around what some of the literature labels the hierarchical nature of tasks. These methods are based on the concept that for a given task, a primary task goal can be identified and then broken down into subgoals or task elements, which in turn can be decomposed into their own subgoals.

The representation of such an analysis is often either tabular or in the form of a tree diagram that provides an explicit representation of the interrelationships of the different task elements (see **Fig. 14-3** and **Table 14-6**). In addition, many other task analysis methods use a hierarchical organization in some form, although it may not be the principal means of task data organization.

The advantages of a hierarchical framework are that it offers a systematic approach to the decomposition of tasks, it is easy to identify where task data are sparse or missing, different levels of analysis can be easily accommodated within the one analytic approach, and it is easy to add further detail to the hierarchy. The disadvantages are that representation solely in the "tree diagram" format restricts the data that can be shown and, although hierarchies clearly show task breakdown in depth, they often do not show so clearly the relationships between task elements on the same level of the hierarchy.[2,5,6,28,31]

Flowcharts/Sequence Diagrams

Various task analysis methods center around a flowchart type of analysis and representation. Most of these methods were developed from the "traditional" flowchart methodologies used in computer programming, systems analysis, and so forth. The method of analysis and the way in which the task is represented are clearly bound together, and it is the representation that largely controls the way the method is applied. Initially, a taxonomy of task elements must be produced, and in the representation, each element of the taxonomy (e.g., decisions or operations) is represented by a different symbol. Similar issues to those arising in the use of

Table 14-6	Extract from a hierarchical task analysis.				
Subordinate	Plan/Operations	Weight Moved and Associated Issues	Reach Distance	View Problems	Perceptual Problems
4. Scan items to input price	1 then 2				
	1. Orientate item for scanning	Weight up to 3 kg for large items, orientation currently difficult if item not positioned with bar code in correct orientation for scanner on input conveyor	Reach to grasp object to orientate for scanning bar code (may be problematic for large items)	Large items may not be easy to manipulate in space to allow bar code to be viewed	Difficult to judge appropriate orientation for awkwardly shaped items
	2. Pass item across scanner	Items above 2 kg have to be regularly moved across scanner and 2-handed operation prohibited by current configuration of checkout	Maximum reach distance for item is 42 cm	View of price indicator in front of cashier can be obscured by bulky items	"Bleep" indicates whether item has been accepted by scanner; however, simultaneous "bleeps" from adjacent checkouts can be mistaken for own and unaccepted items passed

taxonomies apply. The categorization is based on the elements that influence the flow of the task carried out. Sometimes a flowchart representation is accompanied by a tabular format to allow more detail within the representation.

The advantages of the method are that it clearly notes task sequencing and decision points, provides an excellent analysis and representation of procedural tasks, makes feedback loops obvious, and can be used to analyze hypothetical events. The disadvantages are that it is difficult to make explicit the different levels of task detail within the representation, and the methods are difficult to apply to nonsequential tasks.

Flowchart-based methods include job process charts,[32,33] operation sequence diagrams,[8,18] information decision action diagrams,[1] decision flow diagrams,[20] flowcharts for protocol analysis,[5] and input-output diagrams[30] (see **Figs. 14-4 to 14-7**).

Networks

Many of the network approaches to analysis originated from computer science and mathematical modeling applications. They aim to give a representation that presents more of a dynamic model of a task. The analysis methodology is based on the concept of "states" and "transitions," for example, events that cause one state to move to the next.

The advantages of this method are that synchronous and concurrent tasks can be shown, the temporal element of task execution can be included in the analysis, and they have been used to represent the output from verbal protocols. The disadvantages are that task representations can become very complex and difficult to follow and the analysis is presented at one level of description, although hierarchies of "nets" can be used to give a more detailed breakdown.

Particular networks are Petri nets,[24,35] signal flow graphs,[29] and critical path analysis (**Fig. 14-8**).

Task Characteristics and Abilities Requirements Approaches

Several methods approach the analysis of tasks from the point of view of the abilities and skills required to perform the tasks or the characteristics of the task itself rather than an analysis of the elements of the task. Such methods are used primarily in the selection of personnel. One of the more rigorous is Fleishman's task characteristics approach,[13] which is also one of the few validated methods of analysis. It rates a task on a 7-point scale for a range of attributes such as simultane-

Task Description

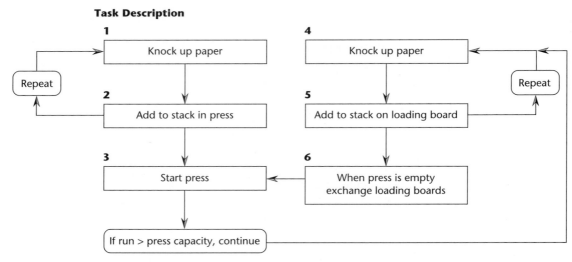

Figure 14-4 Simple flow chart. *(Courtesy Institute for Occupational Ergonomics, University of Nottingham, England.)*

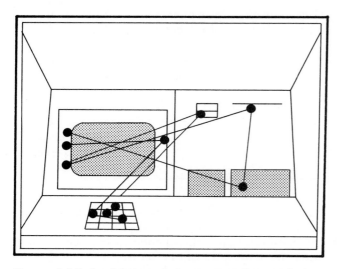

Figure 14-5 Spatial operation sequence diagram for automatic teller machine. *(Johnson GI: Spatial operational sepuence diagrams in usability investigations: contemporary ergonomics. In Lovesey EJ, editor: Proceedings of the Ergonomics Society Annual Conference, 1993, Taylor & Francis.)*

ity of responses, spatial orientation, perceptual speed, and response orientation.

The advantages of this approach are that the methods allow a description of the requirements of the task for comparison with other tasks on a different level, personnel can be "matched" to tasks by using appropriate selection techniques, and tasks can be examined from the point of view of the skills they require. The disadvantage is that the methods look at one very specific aspect of a task only. Particular approaches are abilities requirements[13] and the Position Analysis Questionnaire.[22]

Formal Methods

Over the last decade, a variety of approaches have been developed that take a more formal and rigorous approach to the analysis of tasks. Such methods center mainly on the use of task grammars, for example, the use of a limited vocabulary to describe the task elements, which is then structured by using a set of grammatical rules. Such methods overcome some of the problems of inconsistency caused by the use of natural language in analysis while retaining a degree of flexibility. Their use is principally to assess cognitive tasks in human-computer interface design.

Link Analysis

In an examination of the physical work space and in simple task analysis such as the frequency of performance of a particular task element, several very simple methods of task analysis can be applied. One of these is link analysis. This method involves examination of the links between elements in a system, either concrete or abstract. Examples are the visual links between displays on an interface, which are examined by looking at the eye movements between them, or the physical links between individuals working at different consoles in a control room. Analysis involves identification of the links, the frequency with which they are made, and their relative importance.

The advantages of link analysis are that it is quick and easy to apply, it provides very useful basic information for layout design and evaluation, and the links can be annotated with frequency and criticality information. A disadvantage is that link analysis provides very specific task information that often cannot be used in any other form (see **Figs. 14-9 and 14-10**).[15]

Timeline Analysis

One of the critical elements to be included in a task analysis is the temporal aspect of task performance, yet

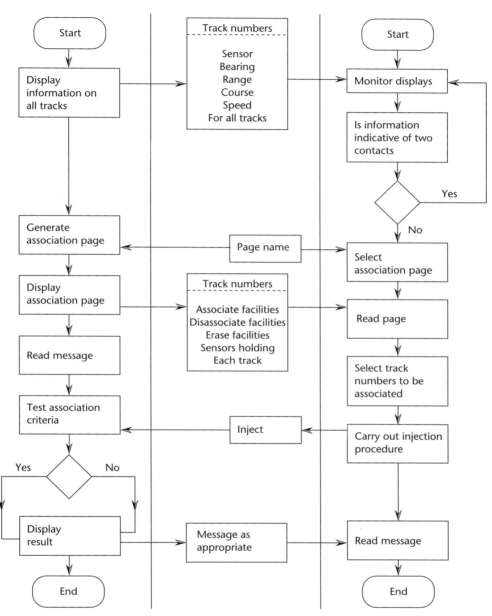

Figure 14-6 Job process chart for a man-computer dialogue concerned with the association of the estimated tracks of vessels. *(Tainsh M: Job process charts and man-computer interaction within naval Command Systems,* Ergonomics *28: 555-565, 1985.)*

it is often this dimension that is omitted and analyses often render only a static representation of a task. Network-based approaches add temporal information, and computer-based simulations such as SAINT[24a] can be used to give a more dynamic dimension to task information. However, timeline analysis provides a simple means of examining the way in which different task elements relate.

A timeline diagram usually takes the form of a graph with two axes, the x-axis representing time and the y-axis representing the different task elements. The method assists in the quantification of workload, the y-axis alternatively being used as a qualitative measure of workload for a given task, and in the allocation of tasks to different team members (**Fig. 14-11**).

The main advantage of the timeline is that it makes the temporal dimension of tasks explicit and it can take as its basis the elements in a task breakdown carried out by a more detailed analysis, which allows it to be more readily integrated with other task analysis methods. As a method, it only addresses the temporal and loading aspects of task performance and thus should usually be employed in conjunction with other methods. It also fails to address the interrelationships between the task

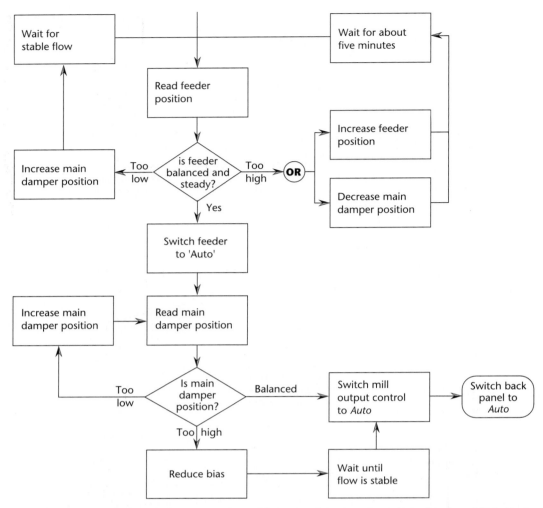

Figure 14-7 Decision-action diagram. *(Kirwan B, Ainsworth LK: A guide to task analysis, London, 1992, Taylor & Francis.)*

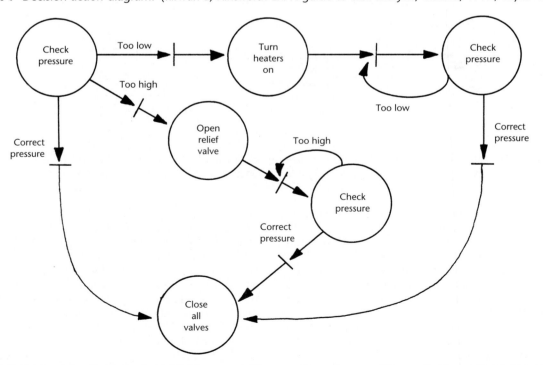

Figure 14-8 Petri net for the task of establishing a specific operating pressure. *(Kirwan B, Ainsworth LK: A guide to task analysis, London, 1992, Taylor & Francis).*

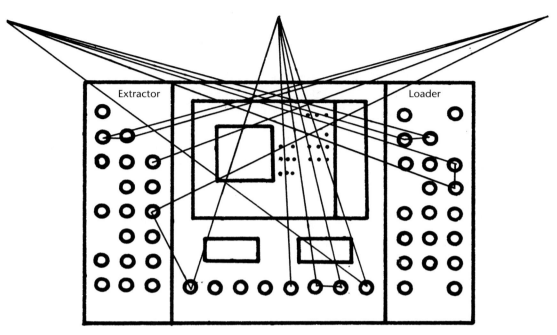

Figure 14-9 Hand/eye movement chart for a control panel. *(Drury CG: Methods for direct observation of performance. In Wilson JR, Corlett EN, editors:* Evaluation of Human Work, ed 2, *London, 1995, Taylor & Francis; p. 45-68.)*

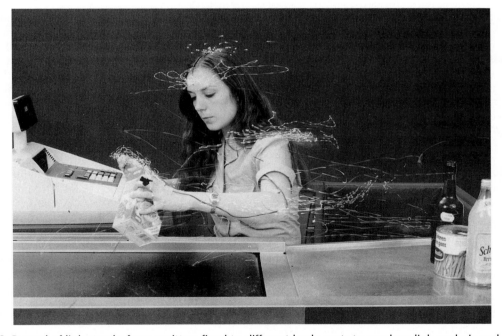

Figure 14-10 Record of light tracks from emitters fixed to different body parts to produce link analysis and then to assess the range of body movements required during checkout operation. *(Strasser H: Evaluation of a supermarket twin-checkout involving forward and backward operation,* Appl Ergonom *21:7-14, 1990.)*

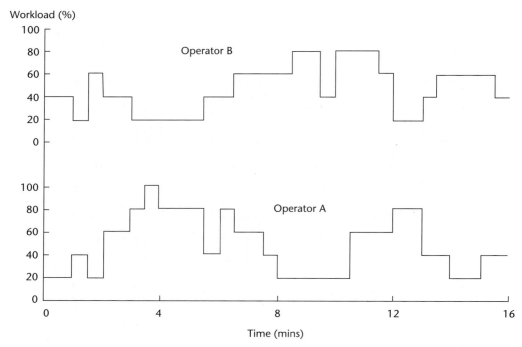

Figure 14-11 Workload analysis. *(Kirwan B, Ainsworth LK:* A guide to task analysis, London, *1992, Taylor & Francis).*

elements and possible external influences on the performance of tasks.[19]

OTHER ISSUES

Although task analysis is commonly used in ergonomics, it is by no means a panacea for human factors analysis and design. A range of issues remain to be addressed to give task analysis credibility and validity as a tool.

Suites of Methods

In a large system analysis or design project wherein the information provided by a task analysis may be used for a variety of applications (such as design of the work space and assessment of workload), one analytic approach is unlikely to provide all the information required. In such a situation it is helpful to use a general analysis, such as a hierarchical breakdown of a task, and then to use this analysis to input into more specific analyses that address issues such as workload. In this way, if the analyses are carried out by several analysts (as is often the case in larger projects), a common basis will have been agreed. When methods are selected so as to complement each other, it is important to ensure that the methods are compatible with one another in terms of the basic task information used for analysis and for subsequent transfer of interpreted information between methods.

Validity

Many task analysis methods rely on the use of natural language to describe the task elements. Although this is a strength, inasmuch as task performance can be expressed very accurately in qualitative terms, it is also a weakness because the analysis is highly dependent on the analyst to ensure accuracy and consistency. With the use of methods that are based on natural language descriptions, however systematic the framework they provide, interrater reliability (the degree to which analysts analyzing the same task independently of each other with the same method produce the same results) can be a problem. More formal methods, which usually take the approach of task grammars where tasks are described with a limited vocabulary (e.g., Task Analysis for Knowledge Description [TAKD][10]) and are constructed by using a predefined grammatical structure, do not provide the same degree of detail that can be useful in examining tasks, although they do produce a higher degree of interrater reliability.

Very few methods of task analysis have been validated by formal studies, although many have gained a high degree of face validity through repeated use and application over a number of years (e.g., hierarchic task analysis[3]). Indeed, methods that use natural language would be very difficult to validate, and in practice, resources necessary to carry out the required repeated task analysis are limited (because it is a very labor-intensive activity).

Translation into Design

Task analysis methods provide a framework and a means of systematically approaching the breakdown of tasks into their constituent elements. However, little or no guidance exists on the translation of this information into practical design recommendations or, indeed, on how to use the information obtained for analysis purposes.

Documentation of Methods

A vast range of task analysis methods heve been reported in the human factors literature; however, very little supporting documentation or guidelines exist to assist the user in applying the methods described, which can be a limiting factor in the selection of methods. Although methods of task description simply provide a framework within which tasks can be structured, it can be more difficult to carry out a more detailed task analysis without a complete step-by-step description of the method.

Accessibility of Information

Task analysis is a labor-intensive activity, and it is important to make the widest and best use of the information produced. This must be in a form accessible to all who might make good use of it, whatever the application. Also, systems evolve throughout their development and life cycle, so it will be helpful if any task analysis can be easily updated and amended.

SUMMARY

Task analysis, although widely misunderstood, has a central role at the outset and then throughout any ergonomics assessment or development program. This is as true for musculoskeletal interventions as for process control room design. Appropriate methods for the former may be a limited subset of the large variety available for use in the latter. Flowcharts, link analyses, and some forms of tabular analysis seem particularly useful for the analysis of work that holds a risk of acute or chronic injury because of posture, repetition, forces applied, or workplace layout. However, some of the newer methods of task analysis,[17] developed more explicitly in an ergonomics or training context, may also have great value for diagnosis and solution generation within interventions to reduce the risk of musculoskeletal disorders at work.

References

1. Ainsworth L, Whitfield D: *Use of verbal reports for analysing power station control skills,* AP Rep 14, Birmingham, U.K., 1983, Applied Psychology Department, Aston University.

2. Annet J, Duncan KD: Task analysis and training design, *Occup Psychol* 41:211-221, 1967.

3. Annet J et al: *Task analysis, training information paper 6,* United Kingdom, 1971, Department of Employment.

4. Astley JA: *Achieving consistency in the use of HF methods for reliability assessment.* In Libberton G, editor: *Proceedings of the 10th Advances in Reliability Technology Symposium,* Bradford, April, 1988, Amsterdam, Elsevier.

5. Bainbridge EA: Analysis of a verbal protocol from a process control task. In Edwards E, Lees F, editors: *The human operator in process control,* London, 1974, Taylor & Francis Publishers, Inc.

6. Beishon RJ: Problems of task description in process control, *Ergonomics* 10:177-186, 1967.

7. Bennett CA: Toward empirical, practical and comprehensive taxonomy, *Hum Factors,* 13:229-235, 1971.

8. Brooks FA: *Operational sequence diagrams,* Proceedings of the first meeting on Human Factors in Electronics, Institute of Radio Engineers, 1960, pp. 33-34.

9. Burri GJ, Helander MG: A field study of productivity improvements in the manufacturing of circuit boards, *Int J Ind Ergonom* 7:207-215, 1991.

10. Diaper D: *Task analysis for human computer interaction,* Chichester, England, 1989, Ellis Horwood.

11. Dickinson C: *Manual handling: an assessment of bag filling operations,* Proceedings of the fifth symposium of Ergonomics in the Process Industries, Wilmslow, UK, June, 1993, Institution of Chemical Engineering.

12. Drury CG, et al: Task analysis. In Salvendy G, editor: *Handbook of human factors,* New York, 1987, J. Wiley & Sons; pp. 370-401.

13. Fleishman EA: On the relation between abilities, learning and human performance, *Am Psychol* 27:1017-1032, 1972.

14. Fleishman EA, Quaintance M: *Taxonomies of human performance,* New York, 1984, Academic Press, Inc.

15. Kantowitz BH, Sorkin RD: *Human factors: understanding people system relationships,* Chichester, England, John Wiley & Sons, Inc.

16. Keyserling WM et al: A checklist for evaluating ergonomic risk factors associated with upper extremity cumulative trauma disorders, *Ergonomics,* 36:807-831, 1993.

17. Kirwan B, Ainsworth LK: *A guide to task analysis,* London, 1992, Taylor & Francis Publishers, Inc.

18. Kurke M: Operation sequence diagrams in systems design, *Hum Factors* 3:66-73, 1961.

19. Laughery KR Sr, Laughery KR Jr: Analytic techniques for function analyses. In Salvendy G, editor: *Handbook of human factors,* New York, 1987, John Wiley & Sons; pp. 329-354.

20. Mallamad SM, Levine JM, Fleishman EA: Identifying ability requirements by decision flow diagrams, *Hum Factors,* 22(1):57-68, 1980.

21. McAtamney L, Corlett EN: RULA: a survey method for the investigation of work-related upper limb disorders, *Appl Ergonom*, 24:91-99, 1993.

22. McCormick EA: Job and task analysis. In Dunette MD, editor: *Handbook of industrial and organisational psychology*, Chicago, 1976, Rand McNally; pp 651-696.

23. Miller RB: Task taxonomy: science or technology? *Ergonomics*, 10:167-176, 1967.

24. Peterson J: *Petri-net theory and the modelling of systems*, New York, 1977, Prentice Hall.

24a.Pritsker AAB, Wortman DB, Seum CS, Chubb GP, Seifert DJ: System Analysis of integrated networks of tasks, SAINT, vol I, Report AMRL-TR-78-126, Wright-Patterson Air Force Base, Ohio 1974, Aerospace Medical Research Laboratory.

25. Putz-Anderson V: *Cumulative trauma disorders*, London, 1988, Taylor & Francis Publishers, Inc.; p. 47.

26. Reddell CR et al: An evaluation of a weightlifting belt and back injury prevention training class for airline baggage handlers, *Appl Ergonom*, 23:319-329, 1992.

27. Rohmert W, Landau K: *A new technique for job analysis*, London, 1983, Taylor & Francis Publishers, Inc.

28. Shepherd A: HTA and training decisions, *Programmed Learning Educ Technol*, 22:162-176, 1985.

29. Sinclair IA et al: Ergonomic study of L.D. waste heat boiler control room, *J Iron Steel Inst*, 204:434-442, 1966.

30. Singleton WT: *Man-machine systems*, Harmondsworth, 1974, Penguin.

31. Stammers R, Shepherd A: Task analysis. In Wilson J, Corlett E, editors: *Evaluation of human work*, ed. 2, London, 1995, Taylor & Francis Publishers, Inc.

32. Tainsh M: Job process charts and man-computer interaction within naval command systems, *Ergonomics* 28:555-565, 1985.

33. Tainsh M: On man-computer dialogues for alpha-numeric status displays for naval command systems, *Ergonomics* 28:683-703, 1982.

34. Teicher WH, Whitehead J: Development of a taxonomy of human performance, MS No 324, 1973 *JSAS Catalogue of Selected Documents in Psychology*, 2, 26-27.

35. Van Biljon WR: Extending Petri-nets for specifying man-machine dialogues, *Int J Man Machine Systems* 28(4):437-458, 1988.

36. Vezima N, Tierney D, Messing K: When is light work heavy? Components of the physical workload of sewing machine operators working at piecemeal rates, *Appl Ergonom* 23:268-276, 1992.

37. Vora PV, Reynolds JL, Corl KG: Design and evaluation of a optical disk handling tool for a cleanroom environment, *Appl Ergonom* 23:414-424, 1992.

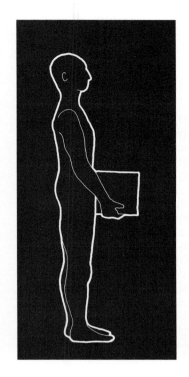

Chapter 15

Task Analysis

William S. Marras

CONTENTS

The objective of an ergonomic workplace analysis is to compare the workplace environment and situation with the known principles and concepts from biomechanics, physiology, and psychology that constitute the ergonomics discipline. To achieve this objective one needs to break a job or task down into manageable units that can be assessed according to known and accepted principles associated with ergonomic design of the work station. This provides one with an organized rationale for selecting and changing the units or components of the task that violate known principles of ergonomics.

Recently an increased emphasis has been placed on ergonomic design of the workplace. This emphasis has been driven by several factors. First, in the United States, the Occupational Safety and Health Administration (OSHA) has developed special emphasis programs centered around ergonomics in industry. OSHA has identified industries that have suffered from extremely high rates of musculoskeletal-related injuries. Some of the largest fines ever levied by OSHA have been issued for ergonomic violations set forth under the general duty clause. Most of these fines were related to cumulative trauma disorders (CTDs) caused by repeated insult to a particular part of the body. Second, industry has recognized that ergonomics results in increases in productivity. When workers perform tasks that do not unduly stress the body, productivity increases and workers are able to produce more with fewer interruptions. Third, quality is directly related to ergonomic influences. When workers can avoid working under painful conditions, the quality of the work and the pride taken in the work increase. Fourth, the Americans with Disabilities Act (ADA) now makes it necessary for employers to prove that denial of employment to an individual is related to the fact that the individual's capabilities are clearly outside the design criteria for the job and that it would be an undue hardship for the employer to tailor the job to the disabled individual. Therefore, this act implies that we should first design jobs so that the majority of workers can be accommodated by the workplace. This can only be accomplished through ergonomic design. Finally, many companies have undertaken ergonomic programs because they are cost effective. Many companies have streamlined their costs extensively over the past decade. However, worker's compensation costs have increased rapidly along with healthcare costs and have made it difficult to compete with foreign manufacturers. Therefore, many industries have found that it is much more cost effective to avoid increased costs associated with ergonomic workplace improvements before an injury occurs as opposed to paying the high cost of rehabilitation after the injury.

OCCUPATIONAL ERGONOMICS PROGRAMS

Ergonomic analyses in industry are typically the responsibility of a plant-level ergonomics team. OSHA has advocated the use of ergonomic processes to control musculoskeletal problems in the workplace.[19] A process implies that the ergonomics activities will continue and are not just a one-time event. Most industrial ergonomics programs used in plants today are participatory in nature. These programs are designed to set up a process where both management and labor work together to identify and correct ergonomic concerns in the manufacturing process. A typical industrial ergonomics program is outlined in **Figure 15-1**. The heart of this process

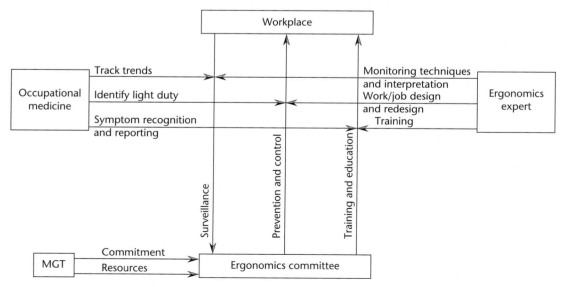

Figure 15-1 Flow chart for an industrial ergonomics process.

at the plant level is the ergonomics committee. This committee is composed of workers who are familiar with the workplace problems and attitudes, as well as process engineers and management representatives who are responsible for specifying the workplace layout. The function of this committee is to evaluate and control the ergonomic risks associated with the workplace. As **Figure 15-1** indicates, ergonomic workplace analyses require that the ergonomics committee interface with the workplace to achieve several objectives. The three main objectives of this committee in performing workplace analyses involve (1) surveillance of the work environment, (2) prevention and control of ergonomics hazards, and (3) training and education of the workers. All these activities are directly associated with workplace analyses. As shown in **Figure 15-1**, both ergonomics experts as well as occupational medicine personnel support the ergonomics committee in achieving these main objectives.

IDENTIFICATION OF ERGONOMIC PROBLEMS THROUGH SURVEILLANCE

The first step in a workplace ergonomic analysis is to determine where the occupationally related musculoskeletal problems are occurring in the plant. The goal of the surveillance component of an ergonomics committee is to help determine which jobs are associated with these problems and to determine the extent or magnitude of the problem. An effective surveillance system also provides a rationale for determining the order or priority in which the ergonomics committee will address the various jobs of interest. The objective is to allow one to tackle immediately those jobs that present the greatest risk of occupationally related musculoskeletal disorders as well as conserve resources for those jobs that represent the greatest risk. A surveillance system also provides a metric by which the ergonomist can judge or track the effectiveness of the ergonomic interventions over time. Surveillance measures can typically take several forms. These measures may consist of workplace injury records, discomfort surveys, physiologic and perceptual tests, checklists, and self-report measures.

The most basic measure of the extent of occupational musculoskeletal disorders can be derived from the available plant medical records. Because these records indicate lost and restricted time as a result of an injury or illness, this measure shows which jobs historically have been related to occupationally related disorders. These jobs are those that have already injured workers and are already costing the company money in worker's compensation, medical, and worker replacement costs. These records can identify those jobs that require immediate attention. In the United States, the Department of Labor requires that most industries keep track of work-related injuries and illnesses by using OSHA 200 logs. These logs, when properly completed, can supply an ergonomics committee with information

about the magnitude of an occupational musculoskeletal disorder. The log reports each incident according to the date of the incident, the employee's name, the occupation of the worker, the department where the injury occurred, and a description of the injury or illness. The number of days associated with the injury or illness must also be reported on this form. The injury or illness rate is typically adjusted or normalized for the number of people exposed to the job. This is accomplished by reporting incidence rates (IRs) that show the number of injuries or illnesses that could be expected for every 100 workers performing the job over the course of a year. An IR is calculated according to the following formula:

$$IR = \frac{Number\ of\ cases/yr \times 200,000\ work\ hours\ per\ plant^*}{Number\ of\ hours\ worked/facility/yr}$$

Because the IR is normalized according to the number of workers exposed to the job, it provides an objective means to compare the risk of musculoskeletal hazards between jobs. In this manner, an ergonomics committee could determine which jobs are experiencing the greatest problem and can then commit more resources to those jobs so that an in-depth ergonomic workplace analysis can be performed. Because OSHA 200 logs must be maintained for at least 5 years, this potentially provides a good historical record of injuries and illnesses in the facility. Similar assessments can be performed by using company medical records. Acceptable IRs can be as high as 6 for a plant,[20] but are often much lower.

There are several factors that can affect the usefulness of these records as a surveillance tool. First, the IR is only as sensitive as the accuracy of the input data. Therefore, it is imperative that the OSHA 200 logs be filled out accurately and consistently. Improper diagnoses, several people (with varying knowledge about the process) filling out the OSHA 200 logs, and poor record keeping can all negatively affect the accuracy and usefulness of the IR as a surveillance tool. The logs are most useful as a surveillance tool when they are recorded as a function of each specific job in the plant. This can provide the ergonomics committee with a means to pinpoint the types of jobs that are most associated with occupational musculoskeletal disorders. If these logs are recorded with enough specificity to the particular job, then IRs can be computed for the job, department, employment classification, and plant. However, if only the employee's department is recorded on the OSHA 200 logs, then pinpointing the specific job responsible for a problem can be difficult.

Once the jobs with high IRs have been considered in a workplace analysis or if, for some reason, the available records do not reveal any trends, the next tool used to help identify the jobs with ergonomic concerns is usually a discomfort survey. When compared with available medical records, discomfort surveys can identify those

*Can also be adjusted to a department, job, and so forth.

jobs that have not been associated with a recordable injury or illness but will become a problem in the future if left unattended. Jobs with high levels of discomfort are typically the second priority in an ergonomic analysis of the workplace, assuming that adequate and accurate medical records are available for all jobs. Discomfort surveys are given to the workers to fill out periodically and are intended for the worker to point out the specific part of the body where discomfort is experienced throughout the workday. An example of an upper extremity discomfort survey is shown in **Figure 15-2**. The worker can shade in the portion of the body that is experiencing pain or discomfort and can also indicate the magnitude of the discomfort for each part of the body. These surveys are then compiled and the trend among and between jobs is studied to identify jobs that should be assigned a high priority for more detailed ergonomic analyses.[7]

There are several worker evaluations that may be used to help assess which jobs in a plant are associated with a risk of musculoskeletal disorders. Most examinations that are practical for the plant environment are perceptual in nature and are designed to determine whether a worker's perceptual ability has been altered (presumably as a result of the job) from a baseline measure. Many of these examinations have been developed to detect upper extremity musculoskeletal disorders in the workplace. For example, several vibrometry systems are now available for plant floor use. These systems stimulate the fingers at different frequencies and are designed to determine whether the sensory system has been compromised, which might be an early warning of a potential ergonomic problem. This would trigger a more in-depth ergonomic analysis. Devices are also available to quickly document on the plant floor the nerve conduction velocity of the worker's median nerve. These devices are also designed to serve as a baseline and screen workers for potential CTDs associated with the workplace. A positive finding in an examination such as this would trigger both a more in-depth clinical examination of the worker as well as a more detailed ergonomic workplace analysis. The sensitivity and specificity of these devices are not well described in the literature.

Surveillance for prioritizing ergonomic workplace analyses can also be accomplished by performing a cursory examination of the workplace. This usually involves either an expert's walk-through examination or the use of a checklist to determine where problem areas may be present. Experts can often compare workplace conditions with accepted ergonomic principles and subjectively determine which jobs require the most immediate attention. Checklists can help guide an ergonomics committee member who is not necessarily an expert in the field of ergonomics to a similar conclusion. These checklists provide a series of questions relating to occupational risk factors.[3] Generally, if more than a predetermined number of responses to these questions are positive, a more involved ergonomic workplace analysis is triggered. However, one must be careful to use these checklists as they are intended. Most checklists are intended as surveillance tools for prioritizing workplace

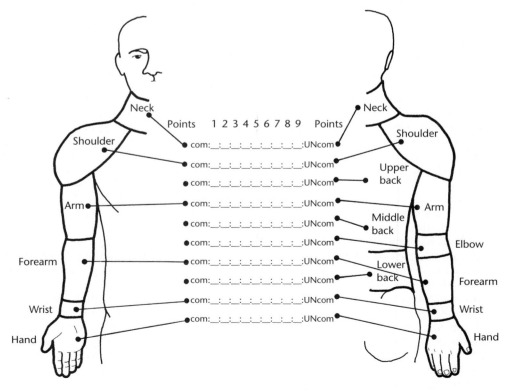

Figure 15-2 Discomfort survey used to identify upper extremity concerns.

analyses. One must be cautious not to use these exclusively to guide corrective action in the workplace because they are not sensitive to the synergistic nature of ergonomic hazards.

Finally, one could gain insight as to which jobs are a priority for more detailed workplace assessment by soliciting input directly from the workers. Self-report mechanisms such as questionnaires, suggestion boxes, and complaint logs could be used. It is necessary to provide at least a basic level of education about musculoskeletal disorders (as indicated in **Fig. 15-1**) to the worker for self-report techniques to work. Worker education should focus primarily on basic ergonomic principles, as well as on symptom recognition. This will enable the worker to know when to report symptoms related to occupational stress and when discomfort may be ignored.

This discussion has shown that there are a large number of techniques available to prioritize and justify more in-depth ergonomic workplace analyses. These techniques vary greatly in their quantitative nature as well as their accuracy. In practice, a combination of these techniques is typically used. It is often not practical to get an accurate picture of risk from the OSHA 200 logs or medical records because many jobs have few workers assigned to the job. Hence a job with one or no injuries and few workers, when normalized for exposure, could artificially inflate or deflate the IR associated with the job. In addition, a large worker turnover associated with a job may mask any problems associated with the job because workers may leave the job before they suffer a recordable injury or illness. Therefore, most ergonomics processes must rely, at least partially, on some of the more subjective surveillance tools such as checklists and discomfort surveys. The ergonomics committee or ergonomist must then use some subjective criterion to weigh the importance of these various techniques and judge the priority of a more in-depth workplace assessment. In-depth workplace analyses can be expensive to conduct as well as time consuming. Therefore, ergonomic resources devoted to in-depth workplace analyses must be rationed according to this surveillance logic.

WORKPLACE TASK ANALYSES

Once a surveillance system has been used to prioritize the problem jobs in a plant and high-risk jobs have been identified, more in-depth workplace analyses are appropriate. Many techniques are available for workplace analysis, and these techniques vary greatly in sophistication, time required to perform the analysis, and level of detail, as well as appropriateness. An ergonomic workplace analysis is intended to accomplish several goals. First, the part(s) of the body at risk must be identified. Second, appropriate analyses must be performed relative to the body parts at risk so that the accepted biomechanic, physiologic, and psychological ergonomic principles involved in the job can be compared with the workplace situation. Finally, once it has been determined how these workplace ergonomic principles relate to the job situation of interest, then potential solutions to the problem can be considered.

Because the body of knowledge associated with ergonomics is varied in its depth of understanding, the appropriate level of detail required in the ergonomic analysis will depend on this level of understanding. Some analysis techniques are very detailed and require knowledge of exact positions of the body and precise measures of velocity or acceleration of the body segments. Other analyses are limited to gross measures such as the amount of weight one is handling or a gross measure of body angle within a 45-degree tolerance. The workplace analysis need only be as detailed as the available knowledge relating to the part of body of interest. In many instances, the accepted means to assess a problem vary from very simplistic to very complicated. In general, the more detailed and quantitative analyses have greater precision and are much more able to definitively assess and control the problem. Quantitative analyses also have the advantage that they can be applied to determine the success of potential solutions. On the other hand, the disadvantage of quantitative workplace analyses is that they can be extremely time consuming and costly to perform. Thus a trade-off exists in ergonomic workplace analyses between the state of ergonomic knowledge, the available time and financial resources, and the level of detail desired.

Regardless of the level of detail required in the ergonomic analysis, it begins with a task analysis of the job in question. The advantage of a task analysis is that it forces the evaluator to consider all aspects of the job that may contribute to the ergonomic risk. Without a task analysis it would be tempting for the ergonomist to suggest solutions that may not remedy the problem inasmuch as it is easy to suboptimize the solution if all tasks and all parts of the body are not considered.

Several methods of performing a task analysis are available, depending on the level of detail desired. The objective of the task analysis is to break down a job into repeatable and manageable units for ergonomic analysis. Traditional time and motion study techniques can serve as a basis for a task analysis. Again, the appropriate task analysis tool depends on the ergonomic principles that one wishes to explore. When using any of these traditional time and motion study tools, the evaluator must decide on an operational definition of each task element based on the degree of detail required for the ergonomic analysis.

The most cursory level of task analysis involves a means to describe the process flow. If the sequence of events is of interest in a task and if the available body of knowledge is such that one does not desire (cannot take advantage of) a high degree of quantification, then a cursory or gross description of the task can be appropriate. A process analysis or flow diagram can be appropriate for this purpose. A process analysis simply divides a task into gross components such as operation, transportation, inspection, or storage without providing any details about the specific components of the operation. However, this analysis does not provide any details about the specific actions performed as a function of these process elements. Such a level of detail may be appropriate for analysis of the workplace based on layout (discussed later).

If a greater level of task detail is desired, an activity chart such as a man-machine chart may be employed. This tool permits the evaluator to break down the process into a series of operations plotted against a time scale. When the interactions of the worker and the tool are included in the activity chart, the assessment is called a man-machine chart. This assessment permits

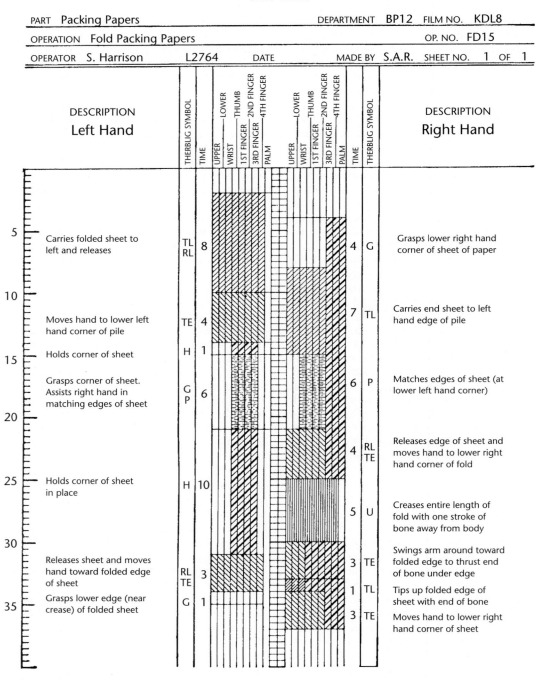

Figure 15-3 A micromotion analysis used to precisely document the activities of both hands during an assembly operation. *(From Barnes RM: Motion and time study: design and measurement of work, ed 7, New York, 1980, John Wiley & Sons.)*

the ergonomist to break up the assessment of the activity in such a way that the time spent in each process can be documented. The level of detail associated with the task is still rather gross in an activity analysis and typically involves major task elements such as "carry box to pallet." The benefit of such an assessment is that it is also possible to get an idea about the physiologic demands of the job because work/rest cycles can be documented with this technique.

When the ergonomist suspects that one of the processes or activities might be associated with an ergonomic risk factor, then that element of the work is subjected to further assessment via an operation analysis. This level of analysis is typically concerned with the specific activities and motions associated with an operation and allows one to analyze the motions used by the worker to perform a task. Motions in this context are operationally defined in terms of the task they facilitate. For example, the level of detail associated with a hand-intensive assembly task may involve operational descriptions such as "release tool" or "grasp part." This level of detail still describes the functions or activities that the worker performs, but at a much finer level of detail that permits the ergonomist to associate a specific operation with any ergonomic risks observed in the work cycle.

One of the most detailed documentations of hand operations involves micromotion studies. In a micromotion study the task elements are broken down into extremely short-cycle operations. The operation is usually filmed or videotaped and the traditional time and motion technique of fundamental hand motion therblig analysis is employed. Therbligs are 17 fundamental operations that can be assigned to a hand-intensive task such as "select," "search," "grasp," or "position" a part. **Figure 15-3** shows a typical micromotion analysis associated with an assembly operation.[2] Task analyses for ergonomic workplace assessments usually use one of these techniques and associate ergonomic principles with each element such as posture of the hand, wrist acceleration, grip force required, and so forth.

POSTURE ANALYSIS

One of the more straightforward ergonomic risk assessment models involves simply tracking the postures that are common during the task of interest. These assessments consider the static (frozen) positions that the workers assume during the job. Posture analyses typically observe a slice of time or a series of slices in time. They usually track the extreme or average postures that are sampled throughout a work period via one of the task analyses mentioned earlier. Posture assessment is typically performed with the assistance of video photography. Workers are videotaped while they perform their jobs and a task analysis is performed at a later time. Once the job is broken up into its specific tasks, the video is reviewed and the posture of the body part of interest is recorded or tallied on a form. Armstrong and

colleagues[1] used this technique to document and analyze the two-dimensional postures of workers' wrists as they performed poultry cutting operations. **Figure 15-4** shows one of these analyses performed by Armstrong et al. The assumption in this study was that deviated wrist postures would increase the risk of upper extremity CTDs. In this case, the videotape was reviewed and paused while the angle of the upper extremity was manually measured with a protractor and documented. As shown in **Figure 15-4**, these postures were summarized over the workday so that various operations could be compared as to how often deviated postures occurred.

Similar techniques have also been used to perform three-dimensional postural studies. These three-dimensional postural studies also rely on videotape that is postprocessed to determine the posture of the worker at different times throughout the work period. These analyses are also static in nature and document the portion of time spent in various postures in a manner similar to two-dimensional analyses. The assumption in these analyses is that deviations from neutral postures place a worker at a greater risk of suffering a musculoskeletal disorder.

In three-dimensional assessments of the workplace, it is much more difficult to accurately assess work postures with video monitoring of the worker. Several methods have been used to accomplish these tasks. Keyserling and Budnick[11] used a mannequin instrumented with potentiometers to replicate the postures observed on the videotape. They froze the videotape while the worker was positioned in the positions of interest and then positioned the mannequin to replicate what was observed on the video. The position information was electronically recorded via the potentiometer-sattached to the mannequin so that quantitative analyses could be performed.

Others have used video digitization to perform similar postural analyses. A three-dimensional postural analysis of the shoulder positions assumed by cashiers working at different-style check stands was performed at the Ohio State University.[16] In this analysis, cashiers wore reflective markers while a video recording of their work activities was collected. A computer-interfaced video motion analysis system was used to track the positions of the markers in three-dimensional space. **Figure 15-5** shows a subject instrumented with markers used to assess shoulder positions on the job. In this analysis the percentage of time throughout a shift that a worker spent with the shoulder in a given position was determined as a function of different check stands. A sample of the results of this study is shown in **Figure 15-6**. In this case it was assumed that the more time the worker spent with the shoulders deviated from the neutral posture, the greater the risk of suffering a musculoskeletal disorder.

As shown earlier, most posture analyses require that the worker be videotaped and an analysis performed at a later time. This analysis is performed by either stopping the videotape at certain postures and manually measur-

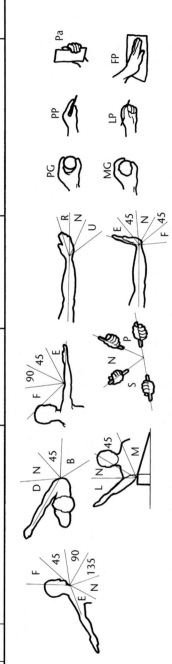

Figure 15-4 Posture analysis system used for assessment of poultry-processing tasks. (*From Armstrong TJ et al: J Am Ind Hyg Assoc, 43:103-115, 1982.*)

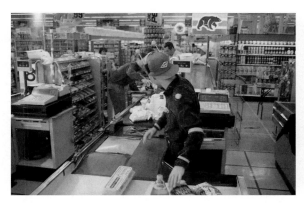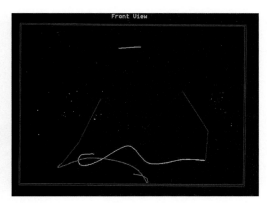

Figure 15-5 Markers placed on the body of a worker tracked by a video analysis system for posture analysis purposes.

ing the body postures of interest on the video monitor, digitizing the position of the worker either manually or automatically, using a video-computer interface, or stopping the video and attempting to recreate the worker posture by using a mannequin or some other means to replicate the posture. These examples have also illustrated that assessment of three-dimensional postures is much more difficult than assessment of two-dimensional postures. The use of video to perform a task analysis and subsequent ergonomic workplace analysis can be fairly straightforward or it can be very difficult, depending on the level of detail required. If the objective of a video analysis is to simply identify gross postural deviations in two-dimensional space without exactly specifying postural angles, the assessment could be performed relatively easily and one need only record the frequency of deviated postures or the time a worker spends in the deviated posture. As the desired level of detail about the posture increases, the amount of time needed to perform the analysis increases markedly. For example, if an indication of the extent of posture deviation is desired, the joint angle must be measured by stopping the video and manually recording the angle of interest or electronically digitizing the position of the joint. Both of these events increase processing time.

If a three-dimensional analysis is desired, processing time is significantly increased. Three-dimensional posture assessments usually require an analysis of at least two video views of the worker, and these views must be time-linked so that the posture in three-dimensional space is assessed at the same points in time. Electronic digitization is typically used to perform this task, but even with a computer interface, this task could require hours to analyze just 1 minute of work. Therefore, one must consider the trade-off between the level of detail one can derive from a workplace assessment, which may involve a large investment in time, and the predictive power of the risk model that will be used to ergonomically assess the job. For example, it may not be wise to invest large amounts of time and resources to perform a detailed three-dimensional posture analysis if the ergonomic literature has not shown a link (significant odds

ratio) between posture and the risk of musculoskeletal disorder for the joint of interest. A case in point would be an analysis of upper extremity disorder risk using posture analysis. One of the problems with posture-related analyses of the upper extremity is that even though there are biomechanical indications that posture increases loading on the body, very few epidemiologic studies validated the notion that the posture is truly related to risk. For example, Hunting, Laubli, and Grandjean[10] produced one of the only studies that have shown that deviations in wrist posture of over 20 degrees in the ulnar plane increase risk to a population of workers.

Posture analyses could also incorporate models of spine loading and body segment strength. Chaffin and associates[4] have developed a static-strength model that can be used to evaluate the risk of musculoskeletal injury caused by manual materials handling. This two-dimensional model assumes that torques are generated about the five major body links during lifting. It also assumes that the strength required to hold the load must exactly counteract the torque imposed about each body link. This model allows one to position the stick figure shown in **Figure 15-7** so that it replicates a work position observed at the work site. The torques estimated to occur around each joint are then compared with a database of male and female static-strength capabilities. This model assumes that if the required torque exceeds the available static strength at the joint, the worker is at risk. The model also performs a simple estimate of spine compression that could be compared with spine tolerance limits as shown in the figure. However, Leamon[12] points out that no evidence has indicated that such models are capable of identifying workplace situations with a risk of occupationally related low back disorder. Thus these types of assessments are intended to be used as gross assessment "guides."

Kinematic Analyses

Kinematic analyses have gained popularity recently because they permit one to evaluate the influence of motion during work. Posture analyses assume that the

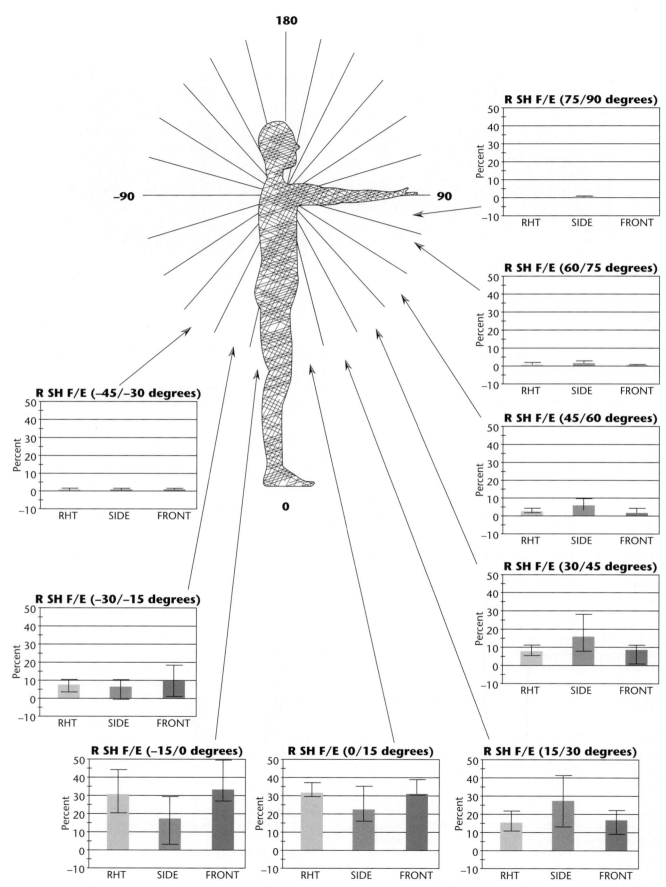

Figure 15-6 Percentage of times workers spend in various positions throughout the workday documented as a function of work station design. *F/E,* flexion extension; *R,* right; *RHT,* right-hand takeaway; *SH,* shoulder.

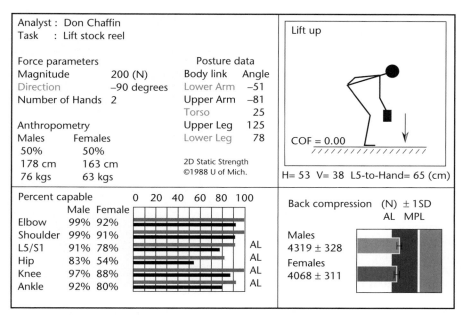

Figure 15-7 Two-dimensional static-strength model used to evaluate required strength and spine loading associated with a task. *(From Chaffin DB et al:* J Am Ind Hyg Assoc *38: 662-675, 1977.)*

worker works in static positions, which often is not the case. Many jobs that lead to musculoskeletal disorders are highly repetitive and involve a large amount of motion. Kinematic analyses provide a means to evaluate the influence of this motion on the risk of musculoskeletal disorder in industry. Thus kinematic analyses represent a more realistic analysis of the work environment. However, interpretation of the significance of these motions has begun to emerge only recently. Marras et al.[17] and Marras and Schoenmarklin[13,14] have identified the types of motions and magnitude of motion that place a worker at an increased risk of suffering a back and wrist disorder, respectively.

In these analyses, motion of the body segments is recorded either by using video or goniometry. Video analyses are appropriate only if the motions of interest are relatively slow. Because normal video records at 30 Hz, this technique is limited by its resolution. Recording at this level would be appropriate for slow motions or simply documenting range of motion. However, if the velocity and acceleration of the body are needed for an analysis, a much greater sampling rate is required. For example, the minimum sampling rate for an estimation of wrist acceleration is 300 Hz. Therefore, unless high-speed video is available, most video analyses of the workplace are limited for kinematic evaluation purposes.

Another significant problem associated with the use of video analyses for kinematic and kinetic analyses is that it is often difficult to record the activities of the worker in the workplace. Three-dimensional analyses require that the worker be recorded by at least two cameras at all times. In work environments it is often difficult to position video cameras around the worker in such a manner that they provide unobstructed views of

the subject by at least two cameras at all times. For example, if lifting analyses are of interest, the worker might lift from bins or machinery might block the camera view of the worker at some point during the lift. Other problems can include poor lighting, mist, or a dirty environment that could result in poor recording quality. When quantitative video analyses are of interest, the sample space must also be calibrated before testing. Typically the calibrated space is only a few cubic meters. Therefore, if the work of interest is performed over several areas or requires the worker to move more than a short distance, estimates of joint positions could be in error. Quantitative video assessments of the workplace could therefore not only be time consuming but could be extremely difficult to perform and may lack the required level of accuracy.

Goniometric measures of motion are often used as an alternative to video, particularly when significant high-order motion components (velocity and acceleration) are of interest. Goniometric systems have the advantage of being able to record and interpret motions on-line because processing of the motion could be performed at the work site. These systems are also adaptable to a variety of work environments and do not suffer from many of the shortcomings associated with the need for line-of-sight recording of the motion of interest as in video. Goniometry also permits the observer to record at different sampling rates, depending on the expected velocity or acceleration of motion. Sampling rates of over 50 KHz are possible with many modern analog-to-digital (A/D) conversion systems.

The disadvantages of goniometric measures in the workplace involve the fact that they are more disruptive to the worker than video recordings are. Goniometric instruments typically require the worker to don equipment that must be securely fastened to the body by tape or straps or even gluing the instrument to the skin. In addition, unless the goniometer is designed extremely well, the instrument may offer some resistance to motion or even restrict the motion of the worker. Thus if the instrument is not designed and properly applied to the worker, ergonomists can alter the very measures that they are trying to measure. The benefit of a kinematic assessment would therefore be greatly reduced if not lost in this ergonomic assessment. In addition, goniometers can provide information only about the part of the body that has been instrumented, and the ergonomist may not have the opportunity to observe how risky motions in one part of the body relate to actions in the workplace unless they are recorded by traditional video means or other goniometric means simultaneously.

Goniometers are most often used to monitor the kinematic characteristics of the back or the wrist in the workplace. Marras et al.[16] used a triaxial back goniometer to monitor over 400 industrial jobs and determine the relationship with the risk of occupationally related low back disorder. The goniometer used to perform this analysis is shown in **Figure 15-8**. This assessment indicated that by recording the moment imposed on the trunk along with the lift rate, twisting velocity, lateral bending velocity, and sagittal trunk angle, ergonomists were 11 times more likely than chance (odds ratio) to pick out the jobs that would be associated with low back disorders. The value of workplace kinematic analyses is clear when one considers that methods used to evaluate lifting risk by static analyses are only 3.5 times more likely than chance to identify high-risk jobs. Similar benefits can be found for wrist goniometric measures. Marras and Schoenmarklin[13,14] used wrist goniometers to monitor the wrist motion patterns of workers involved in jobs with both low risk and high risk of CTD. A worker instrumented with this device is shown in **Figure 15-9**. They found that high wrist acceleration in the flexion/extension plane of the wrist explained (odds ratio, 6:1) why workers in highly repetitive hand-intensive jobs suffered from CTDs above and beyond the traditional risk factors of posture, frequency, and force.

These studies have shown that kinematic variables have the potential to explain more of the risk associated with the workplace than do posture-related variables. This is most likely true because motion can be a powerful biomechanical loading factor. According to Newton's second law of physics, force is a function of mass times acceleration. Therefore, in workplace situations where the work is performed in a rather static posture, analyses may be adequate to assess the work-related risk. However, in circumstances in which the work is performed dynamically and the joints of the body experience appreciable motion, additional and substantial insight into the source of the risk can be gained by performing a kinematic analysis. As demonstrated by Marras et al,[17] significant improvements in risk predict-

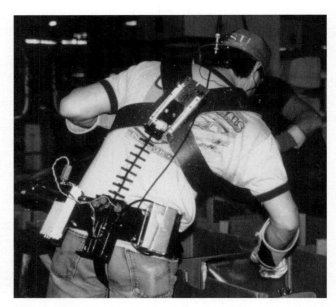

Figure 15-8 The lumbar motion monitor (LMM), a triaxial goniometer to assess workplaces that increase the risk of occupationally related low back disorder. *(From Marras WS et al: Spine 18: 617-628, 1993.)*

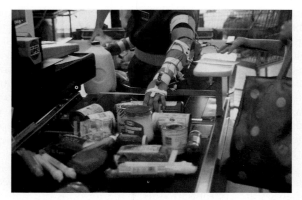

Figure 15-9 Worker instruments with a wrist goniometer used to monitor wrist accelerations during work.

ability can be gained if motion kinematic characteristics are considered along with an analysis of the loads imposed on the body during work. More information regarding both motion and joint loading can be gained from a kinetic assessment of the workplace.

Kinetic Analyses

The next and most detailed and precise level of task analysis detail involves a kinetic analysis of the workplace. Like kinematic analyses, the joint motions experienced by the worker on the job are documented. However, in a kinetic analysis the specific loading pattern experienced by the joint of interest is also predicted. Biomechanical analyses are typically concerned with both external and internal loads imposed on the body. External loads imposed on the body are those caused by the force of gravity acting on a mass such as the weight lifted in a manual materials handling task or the mass of a tool used by a worker. Internal loads are generated within the body as a result of the reaction of the muscles and connective tissues required to counteract the external forces. Because of the biomechanical disadvantage of the internal forces relative to the external forces, the internal forces can be quite extensive. These internal forces can easily be 10 times as great in magnitude as the external force applied to the body. Therefore a great deal of the insight that can be gained with a kinetic analysis is that it can help explain how the body is loaded internally.

The forces imposed on the body are typically derived in many ways. Force plates can be used in such an analysis to derive external force information.[6] Instrumentation can also be added to the interface between the worker and the object that is being manipulated. Danz and Ayoub[5] have instrumented box handles so that force and acceleration information could be measured. Radwin, Masters, and Lupton[21] have placed sensors in the handles of hand tools to derive similar information. However, these techniques require extensive electronic instrumentation and are not usually practical for workplace analyses in the field.

Not only must a kinetic analysis incorporate detailed knowledge of the path of motion of a particular part of the body, but it must also incorporate information about the mass force generation properties of the body. To predict the loading of the joint of interest with this information, a model of internal loading must be included. These models often require extremely detailed information about the motion and force characteristics of the worker and often necessitate force plates and precisely calibrated photographic equipment. An example of such an assessment can be found in work by Freivalds et al,[6] who used ground reaction force and motion information to predict spine loading during lifting. They found that spine compression was greater under dynamic assessment than under static assessment. Kinetic assessments are only as accurate as the model used in conjunction with the workplace measures. Many of the models traditionally used for kinematic analyses assume that the internal forces necessary to support an external load are generated by a single muscle-equivalent internal force. By ignoring the coactivation of the other muscles involved in a task, not only can joint compression be underestimated, but the nature of the loading on the joint could also be misinterpreted.[8] Many models have been developed to overcome this problem. However, most of the models used to account for this coactivation of muscle forces require the use of electromyography (EMG), which makes assessment at the workplace difficult.[9,15,18]

These problems have made kinetic workplace assessments at the work site difficult and rare. Marras et al[16] have performed kinetic analyses of grocery cashiers at different types of check stands in an effort to help understand how shoulder problems might develop when scanning. The usefulness of such assessments is limited because one must make simplifying assumptions about the directions of forces applied to the hand. As this example illustrates, once again one must consider the trade-off between the accuracy of the information one might derive from a kinetic analysis and the cost and effort associated with performing such a detailed workplace analysis. Given today's level of technical sophistication and the limited knowledge of how the body is loaded during work, it is often not worthwhile to perform kinetic analyses. Kinetic techniques are usually feasible only in the laboratory where the testing environment can be highly controlled. In these situations, the task of interest is usually simulated. Hence even with a great deal of precise information derived from a laboratory kinetic ergonomic analysis, the degree of dissimilarity between the workplace and the laboratory environment usually limits the generalizability of the information and assessments.

SUMMARY

This review has shown the variety of means available to analyze a workplace from an ergonomic perspective. Most ergonomic assessments begin by using a variety of surveillance tools to identify the jobs that require and justify attention. Task analyses are then used to determine the part of the job that should be evaluated from an ergonomic perspective. Ergonomic evaluation techniques vary in the level of detail involved in the analysis, the amount of time required to complete the analysis, and the amount of information that can be gained about the risk of musculoskeletal disorder. Any workplace analysis is only as useful as the underlying assumptions or model of risk that is employed. Therefore, one must consider the level of detail necessary for analysis to be a trade-off between the time and cost involved in the analysis, as well as consider the amount of useful information that can be gained from the analysis. Gross task analyses and workplace layout analyses are fast and easy to use but have not been proven effective in explaining a large amount of the risk associated with the work. More detailed task analyses involving kinematic analyses of the motions involved in the task are more effective at identifying and correcting the factors associated with risk; however, they generally involve more processing, more cost, and more time to perform the analysis. Finally, the greatest level of detail, time, and cost is experienced in kinetic analyses, which can evaluate both the motion and force experienced by the body during the performance of work. They require extremely detailed task analyses as well as a means for the assessment of forces imposed on the body. They must also be used in conjunction with an internal loading model designed specifically for the joint of interest. For these reasons, kinetic analyses are usually performed in the laboratory and can suffer from a lack of realism. Hence most practical workplace analyses used today are based on either the layout of the workplace, a gross task analysis, or a kinematic analysis that has been automated for ease of use. The proper choice depends on the amount of useful information that can be extracted from the analysis and used to correct the risky elements of the job.

References

1. Armstrong TJ et al: Investigation of cumulative trauma disorders in a poultry processing plant, *J Am Ind Hyg Assoc* 43:103-115, 1982.

2. Barnes RM: *Motion and time study: design and measurement of work,* ed 7, New York, 1980, John Wiley & Sons.

3. Burke M: *Applied ergonomics handbook,* Chelsea, Mich, 1992, Lewis Publishers.

4. Chaffin DB et al: A method for evaluating the biomechanical stresses resulting from manual materials handling jobs, *J Am Ind Hyg Assoc* 38:662-675, 1977.

5. Danz ME, Ayoub MM: The effects of speed, frequency, and load on measured hand forces for a floor to knuckle lifting task, *Ergonomics* 35(7/8): 833-843, 1992.

6. Freivalds A et al: A dynamic biomechanical evaluation of lifting maximum acceptable loads, *J Biomech* 17(4):251-264, 1984.

7. Goldberg JH, Leader BK, Stuart-Buttle C: Medical logging and injury surveillance database system, *Int J Ind Ergonom* 11(2):107-123, 1993.

8. Granata KP: *An EMG-assisted model of biomechanical trunk loading during free-dynamic lifting,* dissertation, Columbus, 1993, Ohio State University.

9. Granata KP, Marras WS: An EMG-assisted model of loads on the lumbar spine during asymmetric dynamic trunk extension, *Biomechanics* 26:1429-1438, 1993.

10. Hunting W, Laubli T, Grandjean E: Postural and visual loads at VDT workplaces, I. Constrained postures, *Ergonomics* 24(12):917-931, 1981.

11. Keyserling WM, Budnick PM: Non-invasive measurement of three-dimensional joint angles: development and evaluation of a computer-aided system for measuring working postures, *Int J Ind Ergonom* 1(4):251-263, 1987.

12. Leamon TB: Research to reality: a consideration of the validity of various criteria for the prevention of occupationally induced low back pain, *Ergonomics* 37(12):1959-1974, 1994.

13. Marras WS, Shoenmarklin RW: *Quantification of wrist motion in highly repetitive, hand-intensive industrial jobs,* final report, Washington, DC, 1991, National Institute for Occupational Safety and Health.

14. Marras WS, Shoenmarklin RW: Wrist motions in industry, *Ergonomics* 36(4):341-351, 1993.

15. Marras WS, Sommerich C: A three-dimensional motion model of loads on the lumbar spine: I. Model structure, *Hum Factors* 33:123-138, 1996.

16. Marras WS et al: *A biomechanical analysis of grocery scanning operations at three supermarkets,* final report, Washington, DC, 1993, Food Marketing Institute.

17. Marras WS et al: The role of dynamic three-dimensional trunk motion in occupationally-related low back disorders, *Spine* 18(5):617-628, 1993.

18. McGill S, Norman R: Partitioning of the L4-L5 dynamic moment into disc, ligamentous, and muscular components during lifting, *Spine* 11:666-677, 1986.

19. Occupational Safety and Health Administration: *Ergonomics program management guidelines for meatpacking plants,* Washington, DC, 1990, OSHA No 3123, US Department of Labor.

20. Putz-Anderson V, editor: *Cumulative trauma disorders,* Philadelphia, 1988, Taylor & Francis.

21. Radwin RG, Masters GP, Lupton FW: A linear force-summing hand dynamometer independent of point of application, *Appl Ergonom* 22(5):339-345, 1991.

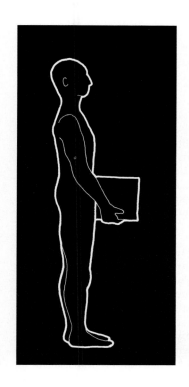

Chapter 16

Workplace Design

Karl H. E. Kroemer

CONTENTS

The design goal of ergonomics, or human factors engineering as it is also called, is to "fit" the work task and the workplace to the human in order to accommodate body size, capabilities, and limitations and subjective preferences.[27] To this end, it is important to identify groups of known stressors so as to avoid them by proper design.

ERGONOMIC PRINCIPLES IN WORK AND WORKPLACE DESIGN

The stressors that cause or aggravate occupational musculoskeletal disorders (OMDs) may, according to the present state of knowledge, be divided into a number of physically defined groups, but with much interaction among them:

Stressor group 1: Body motions. These include the repetitive activities of body segments such as in repeated bending and extending of the trunk in lifting, motions of the arm and shoulder in construction and assembly tasks, motions of the wrist and digits of the hand in assembly or keyboarding, and the like. The extent of such motions may be large or small, and their frequency may vary. In one extreme, the displacement may become zero and result in a maintained ("static") posture of that body segment. The body may also be moved, such as by vibrations transmitted from hand tools.

Stressor group 2: Energy. During occupational work, various amounts of energy may be exerted with various modes of activities. For example, large forces may be maintained over a considerable time, either against objects and tools, such as continued squeezing of the handles of a pair of pliers, or in maintaining a bent-over body posture, such as the neck while working with microscopes. Energy may be transmitted by repeated blows, such as with the palm of the hand to stuff objects into a box, with a hammer to drive nails in construction, or with the fingertips to depress the keys on a computer keyboard. Energy may also be transmitted from an object to the body, such as by vibrating hand tools, including the notorious jackhammer. Physically, the energy may be described in terms of "work" as the integral of force and displacement or as the integral of force (or torque) over time, or it may be described in terms of instantaneous forces, including shocks and impacts.

Stressor group 3: Duration. The relationship of the activities to the time domain is of great importance, as is variability. For example, body motions (stressor group 1) may be changed and/or repeated often or seldom per observation period, such as a minute, an hour, or a work shift, with these "repetitions" staying the same during the work day or changing. Similarly, energy (Stressor Group 2) may remain fairly constant over the workday or other observation period, or may change, possibly with rest periods interspersed.

Clearly, such simplistic terms as *posture, force,* or *frequency* do not sufficiently represent the stressor categories and in fact may mislead because of oversimplification. Furthermore, the stressor categories interact strongly with each other: many combinations are possible among motions, energies, and durations. This fact has been clearly stated by Silverstein, Fine, and Armstrong,[45] who found, with respect to carpal tunnel syndrome, the factors of force and repetition to be strongly associated with the occurrence of that syndrome; the two stressors had a multiplicative effect, together increasing the risk for carpal tunnel syndrome more than five times over the risk associated with either factor alone.

In an attempt to summarize these findings and indicate which activities should be avoided and, more importantly, which ergonomic conditions should be aspired, a listing of generic ergonomic measures to avert common OMDs has been attempted.[23] This list is presented in **Table 16-1.**

DESIGNING TO FIT BODY SIZE

When an object must fit the human body, such as tool handles to hold, protective equipment and clothing to wear, chairs to sit on, and equipment to work with, information about the body size of the user is necessary. Different fitting techniques have been used, some using misleadingly simple body proportion templates. In fact, all "fixed"-design templates may mislead the designer because they assume that all body dimensions (lengths, breadths, depths, and circumferences) can be given as fixed proportions of one body dimensions, usually stature. Obviously, such a simplistic assumption contradicts reality because relationships among body dimensions are neither necessarily linear nor the same for all persons. In spite of the obvious fallacy of the model, "single-percentile constructs" have been generated, especially the 50th percentile phantom of the "average person." Such a ghostly figure does not exist, nor has any human ever been found whose body consisted of all 5th percentile (or 95th or any other fixed percentile) values.

It is necessary to use more refined fitting methods, usually by choosing specific percentiles to determine ranges, or to ensure that the largest person will fit through an opening and that even the smallest can use the equipment. Therefore, one defines the minimally required or largest covered space or zones of conve-

Connective Tissue Disorder	Avoid in General	Avoid in Particular	Do	Design
Carpal tunnel syndrome	Rapid, often repeated finger movements; wrist deviation	Dorsal and palmar flexion, pinch grip, vibrations between 10 and 60 Hz		
Cubital tunnel syndrome	Resting forearm on sharp edge or hard surface			
DeQuervain's syndrome	Combined forceful gripping and hard twisting			
Epicondylitis	"Bad tennis backhand"	Dorsiflexion, pronation		
Pronator syndrome	Forearm pronation	Rapid and forceful pronation, strong elbow and wrist flexion		
Shoulder tendonitis, rotator cuff syndrome	Arm elevation	Arm abduction, elbow elevation	• Use large muscles, but infrequently and for short durations	• The work object properly
Tendonitis	Often repeated movements, particularly with force exertion; hard surface in contact with skin; vibrations	Frequent motions of digits, wrists, forearm, shoulder	• Let wrists be in line with the forearm	• The job task properly
			• Let shoulder and upper part of arm be relaxed	• Hand tools properly ("bend in the tool, not the wrist")
Tenosynovitis, DeQuervain's syndrome, ganglion	Finger flexion, wrist deviation	Ulnar deviation, dorsal and palmar flexion, radial deviation with firm grip	• Let forearms be horizontal or more declined	• Round corners, pad.
Thoracic outlet syndrome	Arm elevation, carrying	Shoulder flexion, arm hyperextension		• Placement of the work object properly
Trigger finger or thumb	Digit flexion	Flexion of distal phalanx alone		
Ulnar artery aneurism	Pounding and pushing with the heel of the hand			
Ulnar nerve Entrapment	Wrist flexion and extension	Wrist flexion and extension, pressure on hypothenar eminence		
White finger, vibration syndrome	Vibrations, tight grip, cold	Vibrations between 40 and 125 Hz		
Neck tension syndrome	Static head posture	Prolonged static head/neck posture		

Table 16-1 Ergonomic means to avoid common musculoskeletal disorders.

Items in the Do and Design columns refer to all connective tissue disorders, except that for neck tension syndrome, head/neck posture should be alternated.
Adapted from Kroemer KHE: Cumulative trauma disorders: their recognition and ergonomic measures to avoid them, Appl Ergonom *20:274-280, 1989.*

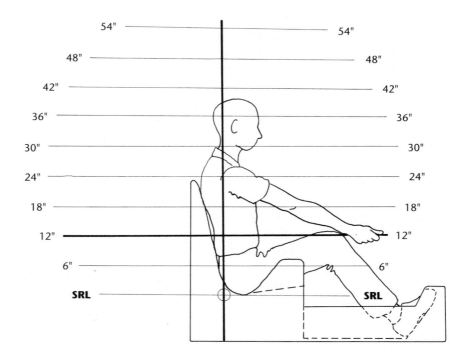

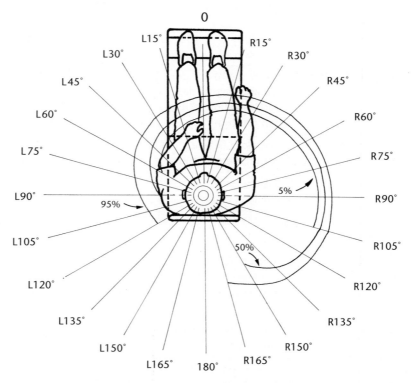

Figure 16-1 Women's grasping reach contours in a horizontal plane 12 inches above the seat. *(From NASA/Webb, editors: Anthropometric sourcebook, 3 vols, NASA Reference Pub 1024, Houston, 1978, National Aeronautics and Space Administration.)*

nience or expediency. An example of work space for the hands is shown in **Figure 16-1**.

"Preferred" working zones are difficult to define because the criteria are not absolute, but depend on the situation, task, and subject. Various "normal working areas" have been reported in the literature since the 1940s, usually in the form of partial spheres around the elbow or shoulder or around the hip or knee.

In many cases it is desirable or even necessary to provide adjustability in the work station, such as in work surface height or seat height, to accommodate different people. Accommodation of persons of various sizes requires that their body dimensions be known. Body dimensions of soldiers have long been of interest for a variety of reasons, among them the necessity to provide uniforms, armor, and equipment. Armies have medical personnel willing and capable of performing body measurements on large samples available on command. Hence, anthropometric information about soldiers is rather complete. For example, the anthropometric data bank of the U.S. Air Force (CSERIAC) contains the data of approximately 100 surveys.

Soldiers are certainly a subsample of the general population, but it is a biased sample because soldiers are youngish, healthy, and neither extremely small nor big. Thus their body dimensions may not truly represent the civilian adult population, although there seem to be no major differences in head, hand, and foot sizes. Unfortunately, such statements are difficult to support because for decades no major survey of the U.S. civilian population has been performed, nor have such surveys been done in other countries. Consequently, at present the only recourse is to use military data to represent the civilian population. For the United States, the survey data of U.S. Army personnel conducted in 1988 are the best. As discussed elsewhere,[27] that survey provides the best available information and is theoretically, as well as demonstrably, by one possible comparison,[36] a good approximation of civilian data. **Table 16-2** presents some selected body dimensions that have been calculated for U.S. civilian adults.

Table 16-2 contains 5th and 95th percentile values, as well as 50th percentiles (averages). Other percentile values can be calculated by following simple statistical procedures, such as those presented by Chaffin and Andersson;[6] Kroemer, Kroemer, and Kroemer-Elbert;[27] and Roebuck.[42]

In general, a useful and correct design procedure entails four steps:

Step 1: *Select those anthropometric measures that directly relate to defined design dimensions.* Examples are hand length related to handle size, shoulder and hip breadth related to escape hatch diameter, head length and breadth related to helmet size, eye height related to the heights of windows and displays, and knee height and hip breadth related to the leg room in a console.

Step 2: *For each of these pairings, determine whether the design must fit only one given percentile of the body dimension or a range along that body dimension.* For example, the escape hatch must be fitted to the largest extreme values of shoulder breadth and hip breadth, with consideration for the clothing and equipment worn; the handle size of pliers is probably selected to fit a smallish hand; the leg room of a console must accommodate the tallest knee heights; and the height of a seat should be adjustable to fit persons with short and with long lower leg lengths.

Step 3: *Combine all selected design values in a careful drawing, mock-up, or computer model to ascertain that they are compatible.* For example, the leg room clearance height needed for sitting persons with long lower leg lengths may be very close to the height of the working surface, which is determined from elbow height.

Step 4: *Determine whether one design will fit all users.* If not, several sizes or adjustability must be provided to fit all users. Examples are one large bed size fitting all sleepers, gloves and shoes coming in different sizes, and seat heights of office chairs being adjustable.

This procedure applies, in principle, whether one uses simple design templates, more sophisticated statistical procedures, or computerized models as part of computer-aided design (CAD) systems. A note of caution is in order, however: computerized systems may use algorithms that are not obvious to the designer, may not follow proper ergonomic principles, or may use incorrect biomechanical dimensions. Use of a computer does not ensure proper human factors engineering because there are three main misuses of computer models:

"Garbage in, garbage out" if the inputs are false
"Garbage out, whatever in" when the model itself is inappropriate
"Garbage use" of the outputs, if misapplied

Only the use of correct input data correctly applied to the correct model will result in proper ergonomic design guidance.

DESIGNING TO FIT BODY POSTURE

One distinguishes three major body working positions: lying, sitting, and standing. Yet there are many other postures, not just transient ones between the three major positions, but postures that are independently important, for example, kneeling on one or both knees, squatting, or stooping, often employed during work in confined spaces such as loading cargo into aircraft, in agriculture, and in many daily activities. Reaching, bending, and twisting body members are usually short-term activities.

| Table 16-2 | Body dimensions of U.S. civilian adults, female/male, in centimeters. |

Dimension	Percentiles						SD	
	5th		**50th**		**95th**			
	Female	**Male**	**Female**	**Male**	**Female**	**Male**	**Female**	**Male**
HEIGHTS								
Standing								
Stature ("height")^f	152.78	164.69	162.94	175.58	173.73	186.65	6.36	6.68
Eye height^f	141.52	152.82	151.61	163.39	162.13	174.29	6.25	6.57
Shoulder (acromial) height^f	124.09	134.16	133.36	144.25	143.20	154.56	5.79	6.20
Elbow height^f	92.63	99.52	99.79	107.25	107.40	115.28	4.48	4.81
Wrist height^f	72.79	77.79	79.03	84.65	85.51	91.52	3.86	4.15
Crotch height^f	70.02	76.44	77.14	83.72	84.58	91.64	4.41	4.62
Sitting								
Height (sitting)^s	79.53	85.45	85.20	91.39	91.02	97.19	3.49	3.56
Eye height^s	68.46	73.50	73.87	79.20	79.43	84.80	3.32	3.42
Shoulder (acromial) Height^s	50.91	54.85	55.55	59.78	60.36	64.63	2.86	2.96
Elbow height^s	17.57	18.41	22.05	23.06	26.44	27.37	2.68	2.72
Thigh height^s	14.04	14.86	15.89	16.82	18.02	18.99	1.21	1.26
Knee height^f	47.40	51.44	51.54	55.88	56.02	60.57	2.63	2.79
Popliteal height^f	35.13	39.46	38.94	43.41	42.94	47.63	2.37	2.49
DEPTHS								
Forward (thumbtip) reach	67.67	73.92	73.46	80.08	79.67	86.70	3.64	3.92
Buttock-knee distance (sitting)	54.21	56.90	58.89	61.64	63.98	66.74	2.96	2.99
Buttock-popliteal distance (sitting)	44.00	45.81	48.17	50.04	52.77	54.55	2.66	2.66
Elbow-fingertip distance	40.62	44.79	44.29	48.80	48.25	52.42	2.34	2.33
Chest depth	20.86	20.96	23.94	24.32	27.78	28.04	2.11	2.15
BREADTHS								
Forearm-forearm breadth	41.47	47.74	46.85	54.61	52.84	62.06	3.47	4.36
Hip breadth (sitting)	34.25	32.87	38.45	36.68	43.22	41.16	2.72	2.52
HEAD DIMENSIONS								
Head circumference	52.25	54.27	54.62	56.77	57.05	59.35	1.46	1.54
Head breadth	13.66	14.31	14.44	15.17	15.27	16.08	0.49	0.54
Interpupillary breadth	5.66	5.88	6.23	6.47	6.85	7.10	0.36	0.37

*Estimated by Kroemer

NOTE: In this table, the entries in the 50th-percentile column are actually "mean" (average) values. The 5th and 95th percentile values are from measured data, not calculated (except for weight). Therefore, the values given may be slightly different from those obtained by subtracting 1.65 SD from the mean (50th percentile) or by adding 1.65 SD to it.
f, above floor; s, above seat; SD, standard deviation.
Adapted from Gordon CC et al: 1988 anthropometric survey of US Army personnel: summary statistics interim report, TR 89/027, Natick, Mass, 1988, US Army Natick Research, Development and Engineering Center.

Table 16-2	Body dimensions of U.S. civilian adults, female/male, in centimeters—continued.							
			Percentiles				**Std. Deviation**	
Dimension	**Female 5th Male**		**Female 50th Male**		**Female 95th Male**		**Female S Male**	
FOOT DIMENSIONS								
Foot length	22.44	24.88	24.44	26.97	26.46	29.20	1.22	1.31
Foot breadth	8.16	9.23	8.97	10.06	9.78	10.95	0.49	0.53
Lateral malleolus height^f	5.23	5.84	6.06	6.71	6.97	7.64	0.53	0.55
HAND DIMENSIONS								
Circumference, metacarpal	17.25	19.85	18.62	21.38	20.03	23.03	0.85	0.97
Hand length	16.50	17.87	18.05	19.38	19.69	21.06	0.97	0.98
Hand breadth, Metacarpal	7.34	8.36	7.94	9.04	8.56	9.76	0.38	0.42
Thumb breadth, Interphalangeal	1.86	2.19	2.07	2.41	2.29	2.65	0.13	0.14
WEIGHT (kg)	39.2*	57.7*	62.01	78.49	84.8*	99.3*	13.8*	12.6*

Work is seldom done when supine or prone, but it does occur, for example, in repair jobs or in low-seam underground mining. Pilots have been put into prone or supine positions in high-performance aircraft to better tolerate the acceleration forces experienced in aerial maneuvers. In some current fighter airplanes and tanks, the pilot or driver is in a semireclining posture.

Sitting and standing are usually presumed to be associated with more or less "erect" posture of the trunk and erect posture of the legs while standing; sitting at work was thought to be "properly" done when the lower parts of the legs were in essence vertical, the thighs horizontal, and the trunk upright. This convenient model of all major body joints at zero, 90, or 180 degrees is suitable for standardization of body measurements, but the "0-90-180 posture" is not one commonly employed, subjectively preferred, or even "healthy" (see the discussion of office furniture later in this chapter).

In terms of physical effort, measured by oxygen consumption or heart rate, lying is the least strenuous posture. Yet it is not well suited to performing physical work with the arms and hands because they must be elevated for most activities that cause high strain.

Standing is a much more energy-consuming posture, but it allows free use of the arms and hands, and if one walks around, much space can be covered. Furthermore, it facilitates the dynamic use of arms and trunk and is thus suitable for the development of large energies and impact forces.

Sitting is, in most aspects, intermediate between these two postures: because body weight is partially supported by a seat, energy consumption and circulatory strain are higher than when lying, but lower than when standing. Arms and hands can be used freely, but their work space is limited if one remains seated. The

energy that can be developed is less than when standing, but given the better stability of the trunk supported on the seat, it is easier to perform finely controlled manipulations. Operation of pedals or controls with the feet is easy in the sitting posture because the feet are fairly mobile and are needed only to stabilize the posture and support the body weight.

The two most important working postures are standing and sitting. It is common experience that in either condition, the most easily sustained posture of the trunk and neck is one in which the spinal column is straight in the frontal view but follows the natural S curve in the side view, i.e., with lordosis (forward bend) in the cervical and lumbar regions and a kyphosis (backward bend) in the thoracic area. Yet maintaining that trunk posture over a long period of time becomes very uncomfortable, mostly because of the maintained muscle tension necessary to keep the body in this position. Also, not being able to move the legs and feet when standing still is very unbecoming because the feet and lower part of the legs swell as a result of the accumulation of body fluids—a problem to which many women are particularly prone. Thus either standing still or sitting still is "unphysiologic"; instead, the posture should be changed often. This includes walking by the standing operator and at least occasionally by the seated person as well and involves motions of the head, trunk, arms, and legs.

Designing for the Standing Operator

Standing as a working posture is used if sitting is not suitable, either because the operator has to cover a fairly large work area or because very large forces must be exerted with the hands, particularly if these conditions prevail only for a limited period of time. Forcing a person to stand simply because the work object is

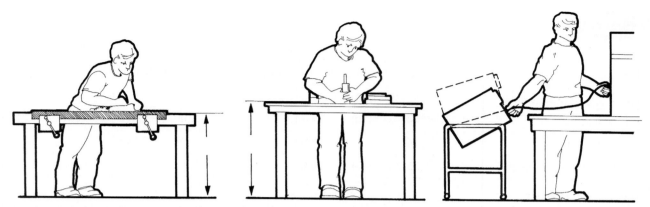

Figure 16-2 Work spaces designed for a standing operator when large forces are required over a large area or work on large objects is required. *(From Kroemer KHE, Kroemer HB, and Kroemer-Elbert KE:* Ergonomics: how to design for ease and efficiency, *Englewood Cliffs, NJ, 1994, Prentice Hall. Used by permission.)*

customarily put high above the floor is often not a sufficient justification. For example, in automobile assembly, car bodies have been turned or tilted and parts have been redesigned so that the worker does not have to "stand and bend" to reach the work object. Examples of work stations designed for standing operators are shown in **Figure 16-2**, according to the need to exert large forces over large spaces, perform strong exertions with visual control, or work with large objects.

The height of the work station depends largely on the activities to be performed with the hands and the size of the object. Therefore, the main reference point is the elbow height of the worker (who, however, is often not standing upright, but bent or reaching). The strongest hand forces and easiest arm mobility are between elbow and hip heights, as a general rule. Therefore, the best height for performing work on objects is near elbow height (with the upper part of the arm vertical) for light or heavy work.[47,49] The support surface (for example, a bench or table) is determined by the working height of the hands and the size of the object on which the person works.

Sufficient room for the feet of the operator must be provided, including enough toe and knee space to move up close to the working surface. Of course, the floor should be flat and free of obstacles. Use of a platform to stand on should be avoided, if possible, because one may stumble over its edge. Although the movements of the body associated with dynamic standing work are basically a desirable physiologic feature, they should not involve excessive bends and reaches, especially not twisting motions of the trunk. People should never be forced to stand still at a work station just because the equipment was originally ill-designed or badly placed, as is unfortunately too often found with drill presses used in continuous work. Also, many other machine tools such as lathes have been so constructed that the operator must stand and lean forward to observe the cutting action and at the same time extend the arms to reach controls on the machine.

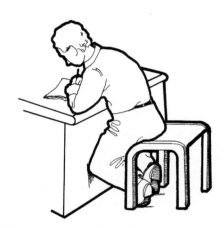

Figure 16-3 Sitting posture contorted because space for the legs is missing

Designing for the Sitting Operator

Sitting is a much less strenuous posture than standing. It allows better controlled hand movements, but coverage of only a smaller area and exertion of smaller forces with the hands. A seated person can easily operate controls with the feet and do so, if suitably seated, with much force. When designing a work station for a seated operator, one must consider the required free space for the legs. If this space is severely limited, very uncomfortable and fatiguing body postures result, as shown in **Figure 16-3**.

The height of the working area for the hands is again mostly determined with respect to the elbows. At about elbow height, with the upper part of the arms hanging, the preferred working area is in front of the body so that manipulations with the fingers are facilitated. Many activities performed by seated operators require close visual observation; this codetermines the proper height of the manipulation area, depending on the operator's preferred visual distance and the preferred direction of gaze. The design principles for accommodating a seated

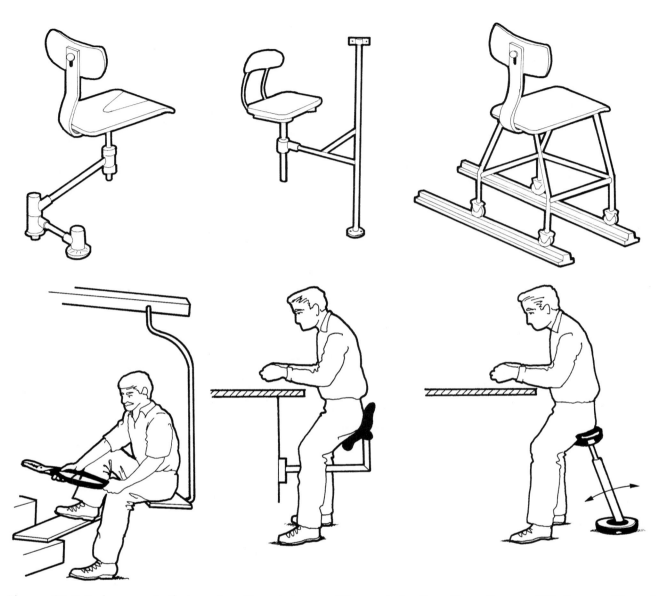

Figure 16-4 Body supports that are transitions between sitting and standing. *(From Kroemer KHE, Kroemer HB, and Kroemer-Elbert KE:* Ergonomics: how to design for ease and efficiency, *Englewood Cliffs, NJ, 1994, Prentice Hall. Used by permission.)*

person are discussed in more detail later in this chapter. In some work stations, sit-stand transitions are suitable, as shown in **Figure 16-4**.

DESIGNING FOR FOOT OPERATION

In comparison to hand movements over the same distance, foot motions consume more energy and are less accurate and slower, but they are more powerful, as one would expect from biomechanical considerations.[20]

If a person stands at work, fairly little force and fairly infrequent operations of foot controls should be required because during these exertions the operator has only the other foot to stand on. For a seated operator, however, operation of foot controls is much easier because the body is largely supported by the seat. Therefore, the feet can move more freely and, given suitable conditions, can exert large forces and energies.

Small forces such as for the operation of switches can be generated in nearly all directions with the feet, with the downward or down-and-fore directions preferred. The largest forces can be generated with extended or nearly extended legs; in the downward direction the force is limited by body inertia, and in the more forward direction force is limited by both inertia and the provision of buttock and back support surfaces. These principles are typically applied in automobiles.

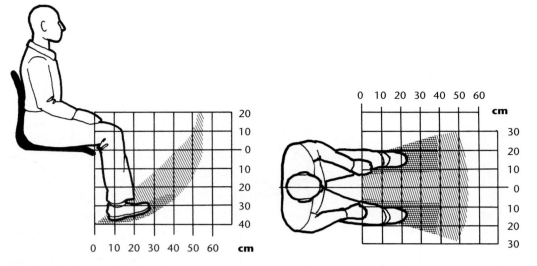

Figure 16-5 Preferred *(crosshatched)* and regular work spaces for the feet of a seated operator. *(Modified from Kroemer KHE: What one should know about switches, cranks, and pedals, Berlin, 1967, Beuth [in German].)*

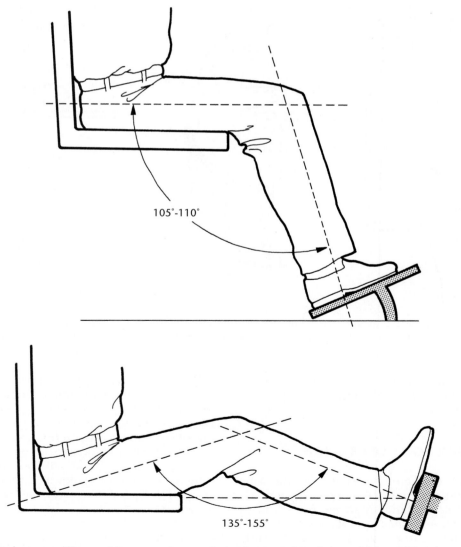

105°-110°

135°-155°

Figure 16-6 Light downward/forward forces can be exerted at knee angles of about 105 to 110 degrees, whereas strong forward forces require knee extension at 135 to 155 degrees. *(Modified from Van Cott HP, Kinkade RG, editors:* Human engineering guide to equipment design (rev. ed.), *Washington, D.C., 1972, U.S. Government Printing Office.*

For example, the operation of a clutch or brake pedal can normally be performed easily with about a right angle at the knee. However, if the power-assist system fails, very large forces must be exerted with the feet. In this case, thrusting one's back against a strong backrest and extending the legs are necessary to generate the needed pedal force (see **Figs. 16-5 and 16-6**).

DESIGNING FOR HAND USE

The human hand is able to perform a large variety of activities ranging from those that require fine control to others that demand large forces. One may divide hand tasks in the following manner:

- Fine manipulation of objects, with little displacement and force. Examples are writing by hand, assembly of small parts, and adjustment of controls.
- Fast movements to an object that require moderate accuracy to reach the target but fairly small force exertion there. An example is hand movement to a switch followed by its activation.
- Frequent movements between targets, usually with some accuracy but little force, such as in an assembly task where parts must be taken from several bins and assembled.
- Forceful activities with little or moderate displacement, such as with many assembly or repair activities, for example, when turning a wrench to tighten a bolt.
- Forceful activities with large displacements, e.g., when hammering.

Accordingly, there are three major types of requirements: for accuracy, for strength exertion, and for displacement. For each of these, certain characteristics of hand movements can be described if one starts from a "reference position" of the upper extremity: the upper part of the arm hangs down, the elbow is at a right angle, the forearm is horizontal and extended forward, and the wrist is straight. In this case, the hand and forearm are in a horizontal plane at approximately umbilicus height.

For *accurate and fast movements,* Fitts' law provides guidance: the smaller the distance traveled and the larger the target, the more accurate is a fast movement. Thus the fingers are able to perform the fastest and most accurate motions. This is followed by movements of the forearm only, which means (when the upper half of the arm is fixed) that either the forearm does a horizontal rotating sweep about the elbow (in fact, about the shoulder joint in which the upper part of the arm twists) or the forearm flexes/extends in the elbow joint. The least accurate and the most time-consuming movements are those in which the upper part of the arm is pivoted out of its vertical reference location. If the hand must be displaced only by short distances from its reference position, pure forearm movements are preferable to those in which the upper half of the arm is also moved out of its hanging position. The space for preferred manipulations is shown in **Figure 16-7**.

Exertion of force with the hands is a more complex matter. Of the digits, the thumb is the strongest and the little finger the weakest. Finger forces depend on the finger joint angles. Gripping and grasping strengths of the whole hand are larger but depend on the coupling used between the hand and the handle (see **Fig. 16-8**). The forearm can develop fairly large twisting torques. Torque about the elbow depends on the elbow angle. Large force and torque vectors are exertable with the

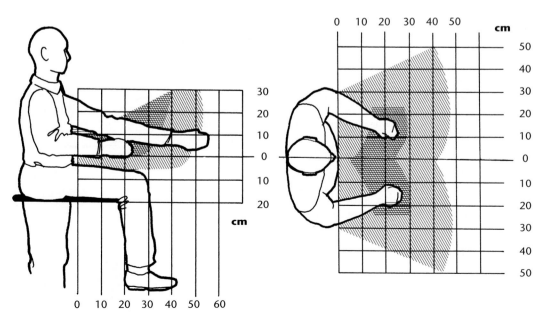

Figure 16-7 Preferred *(crosshatched)* and regular manipulation spaces. *(Modified from Kroemer KHE: What one should know about switches, cranks, and pedals, Berlin, 1967, Beuth [in German].)*

Coupling #1 *Digit touch*
One digit touches an object.

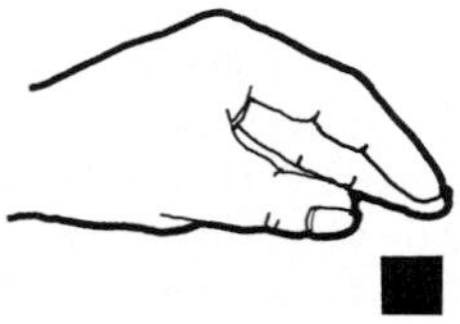

Coupling #2 *Palm touch*
Some part of the palm (or hand) touches the object.

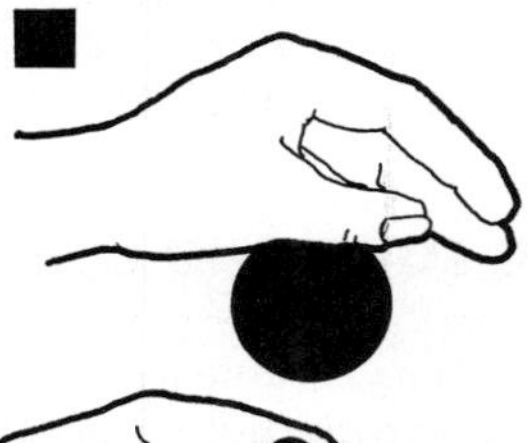

Coupling #3 *Finger palmar grip (hook grip)*
One finger or several fingers hook(s) onto a ridge, or handle. This type of finger action is used where thumb counterforce is not needed.

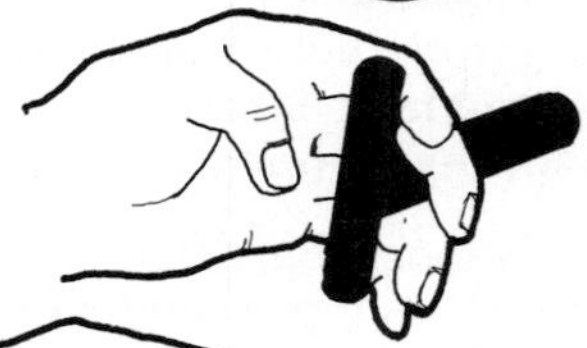

Coupling #4 *Thumb-fingertip grip (tip pinch)*
The thumb tip opposes one fingertip.

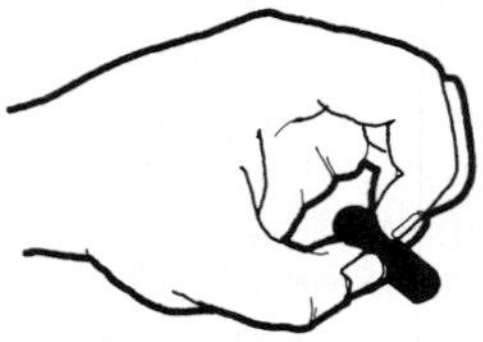

Coupling #5 *Thumb-finger palmar grip (pad pinch or plier grip)*
Thumb pad opposes the palmar pad of one finger (or the pads of several fingers) near the tips. This grip evolves easily from coupling #4.

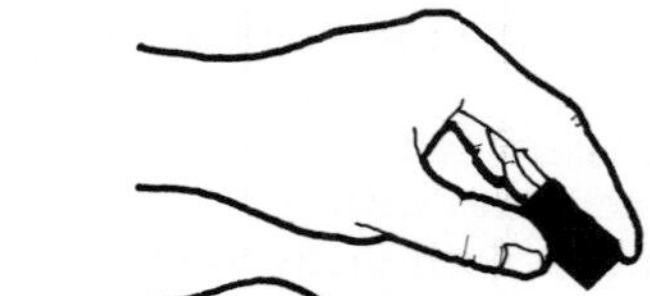

Coupling #6 *Thumb-forefinger side grip (lateral grip or side pinch)*
Thumb opposes the (radial) side of the forefinger.

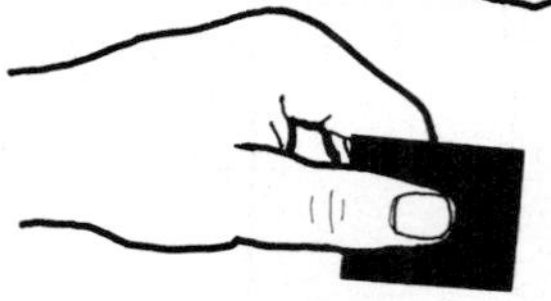

Coupling #7 *Thumb-two-finger grip (writing grip)*
Thumb and two fingers (often forefinger and middle finger) oppose each other at or near the tips.

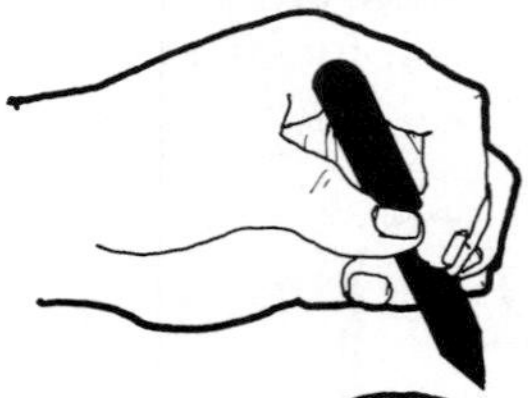

Coupling #8 *Thumb-fingertips enclosure (disk grip)*
Thumb pad and the pads of three or four fingers oppose each other near the tips (object grasped does not touch the palm). This grip evolves easily from coupling #7.

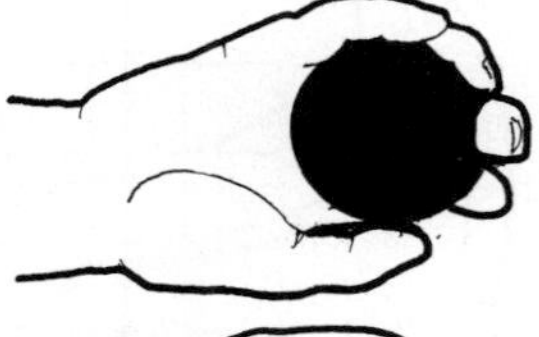

Coupling #9 *Finger-palm enclosure (collet enclosure)*
Most, or all, of the inner surface of the hand is in contact with the object while enclosing it. This enclosure evolves easily from coupling #8.

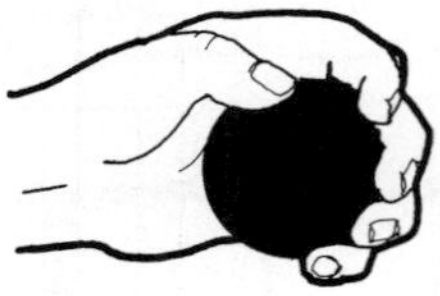

Coupling #10 *Power grasp*
The total inner hand surface is grasping the (often cylindrical) handle, which runs parallel to the knuckles and generally protrudes on one or both sides from the hand. This grasp evolves easily from coupling #9.

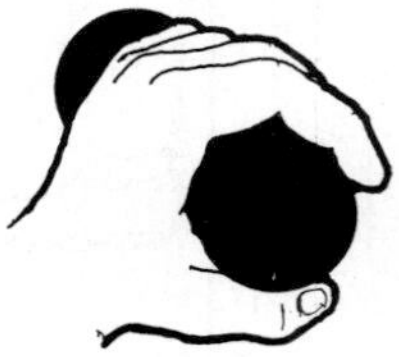

Figure 16-8 Couplings between hand and handle. *(Modified with permission from Kroemer KHE: Coupling the hand with the handle—an improved notation of touch, grip, and grasp,* Hum Factors *28(3), 337-339. Copyright 1986 by Human Factors and Ergonomics Society, Inc. All rights reserved.)*

elbow at about a right angle, but the strongest pulling/ pushing forces toward/away from the shoulder can be exerted with the extended arm, provided that the trunk can be braced against a solid structure. Therefore, forces exerted with the arm and shoulder muscles are largely determined by body posture and body support (**Fig. 16-9**). Details are provided by Kroemer, Kroemer, and Kroemer-Elbert.[27]

DESIGNING HAND TOOLS

Hand tools should fit the contours of the hand, they must be held securely with suitable wrist and arm postures, and they use and amplify strength and energy capabilities without overloading the body. Hence the design of hand tools is a complex ergonomic task.

Hand tools are as old as humanity. They developed from simply using a stone, bone, or piece of wood that fit the hand and served the purpose, to the purposeful development of modern implements (such as screwdrivers, cutting pliers, or power saws) and controls in airplanes and power stations in the twentieth century. A vast literature is available on tool design and is summarized by Greenberg and Chaffin,[17] by Fraser,[12] in a special issue of Human Factors (vol 28, no. 3, 1986), and then by Freivalds,[13] Konz,[22] Chaffin and Andersson,[6] and Mital.[37] The tool must fit the dimensions of the hand, some examples of which are given in **Table 16-2**. More information can be found in publications by Gordon et al,[14] NASA/Webb,[38] Wagner,[51] and particularly Greiner.[18] Chapter 37 in this text discusses tool adaptation for the wrist and hand.

Some hand tools require a fairly small force but precise handling, such as surgical instruments, screwdrivers used by optometrists, or writing instruments. Commonly, the manner of holding these tools has been called "precision grip." Other instruments must be held strongly between large surfaces of the fingers, thumb, and palm. Such holding of the hand tool allows the exertion of large force and torque and has commonly been called the "power grasp." Yet there are many transitions: from merely touching an object with a finger (such as pushing a button) to pulling on a hooklike handle or from holding small objects between the fingertips to transmitting large energy from the hand to the handle. One attempt to systematically arrange the various couplings of hand with handle is shown in **Figure 16-8**.

For the touch-type couplings (numbers 1 to 6 in **Fig. 16-8**), relatively little attention must be paid to fitting the surface of the handle to the touching surface of the hand. Yet one may want to put a slight cavity in the surface of a push button so that the fingertip does not slide off, to hollow out the handle of a scalpel slightly so that the fingertips can hold on securely, or to roughen the surface of a dentist's tool and not make it round in cross section, which would allow it to turn in the hand. Thus design details that facilitate holding on to the tool,

moving it accurately, and generating force or torque play important roles even for small hand tools.

These considerations of "secure tool handling" become even more important for the more powerful enclosure couplings (numbers 8, 9, and 10 in **Fig. 16-8**). These are typically used when large energies must be transmitted between the hand and the tool. The design purpose is to hold the handle securely (without fatiguing muscles and avoiding pressure points) while exerting linear force or rotating torque at the "working end" of the tool.

It is important to distinguish between the energy transmitted to the work object and the energy transmitted between the hand and the handle. In many cases, the energy transmitted to the external object is not the same in type, amount, or time as that generated between the hand and the handle; consider, for example, the impulse energy transmitted by the head of a mallet as compared with the way energy is transmitted between the hand and the handle or the torque applied to a screw with the tip of a screwdriver as compared with the combination of thrust and torque generated by the hand. Therefore, the ergonomist must consider both the interface between tool and object and the interface between tool and hand.

Manually driven tools may be classified as follows, using in part Fraser's listing[12] (note that in each case the operator must "hold" the tool):

- Percussive (e.g., ax, hammer)—human task: swing
- Scraping (saw, file, chisel, plane)—human task: push/pull and hold handle
- Rotating, boring (borer, drill, screwdriver, wrench, awl)—human task: push/pull, turn
- Squeezing (pliers, tongs)—human task: press
- Cutting (scissors, shears)—human task: pull
- Cutting (knife)—human task: pull/push

Power-driven tools may use an electric power source (saw, drill, screwdriver, sander, grinder); compressed air (saw, drill, wrench); smoothed internal combustion (chain saw); or explosive power (bolter, cutter, riveter).

While using manually driven tools, the operator generates all the energy and therefore is always in full control of the energy exerted (with the exception of percussive tools such as hammers or axes), whereas power-driven tools are usually held or moved and the energy to be applied to the outside is largely generated by the auxiliary power. Yet if that tool suddenly experiences resistance, the reaction force may directly affect the operator, often in terms of a jerk or impact that can exceed the person's abilities and lead to injuries. This occurs particularly often with chain saws, power screwdrivers, and power wrenches.[37] A major problem with many powered hand tools is the impacts and vibrations transmitted to the operator, such as by jackhammers, riveters, powered wrenches, and sanders. Impacts and vibrations transmitted to the human, particularly if associated with improper postures, often lead to overuse disorders of the musculoskeletal system.

	Force-plate[1] height	Distance[2]	Force, N	
			Mean	SD
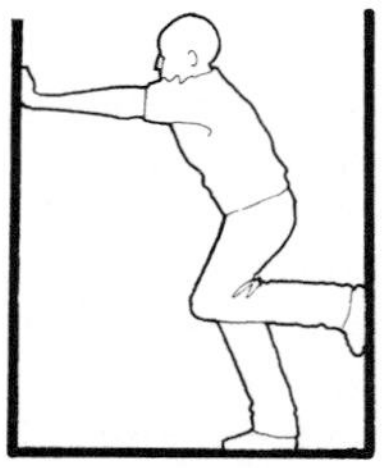	50	80	664	177
	50	100	772	216
	50	120	780	165
	70	80	716	162
	70	100	731	233
	70	120	820	138
	90	80	625	147
	90	100	678	195
	90	120	863	141
	Percent of shoulder height		Both hands	
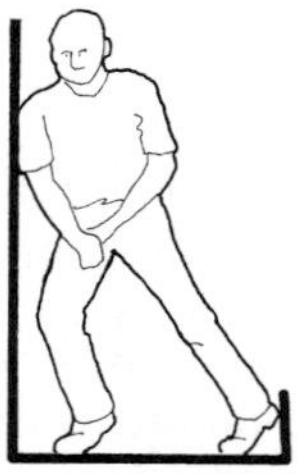	60	70	761	172
	60	80	854	177
	60	90	792	141
	70	60	580	110
	70	70	698	124
	70	80	729	140
	80	60	521	130
	80	70	620	129
	80	80	636	133
	Percent of shoulder height			
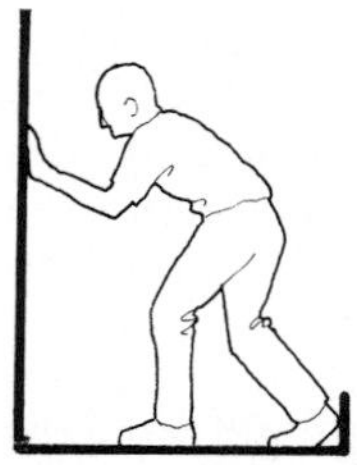	70	70	623	147
	70	80	688	154
	70	90	586	132
	80	70	545	127
	80	80	543	123
	80	90	533	81
	90	70	433	95
	90	80	448	93
	90	90	485	80
	Percent of shoulder height		Both hands	
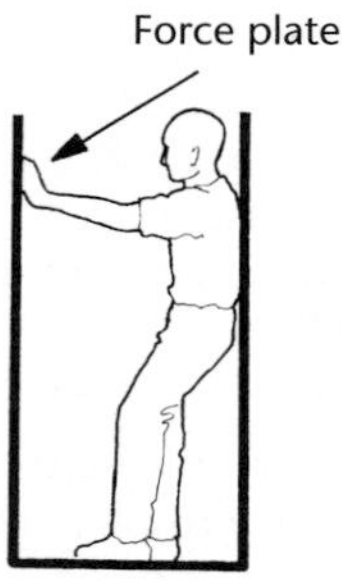			Both hands	
	100 percent of shoulder height	50	581	143
		60	667	160
		70	981	271
		80	1285	398
		90	980	302
		100	646	254
			Preferred hand	
		50	262	67
		60	298	71
		70	360	98
		80	520	142
		90	494	169
		100	427	173
		Percent of thumb-tip reach*		
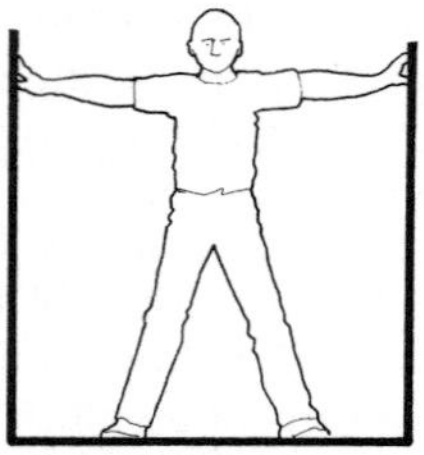	100 percent of shoulder height	50	367	136
		60	346	125
		70	519	164
		80	707	190
		90	325	132
		Percent of span†		

[1] Height of the center of the force plate—20 cm high by 25 cm long—upon which force is applied.
[2] Horizontal distance between the vertical surface of the force plate and the opposing vertical surface (wall or footrest, respectively) against which the subjects brace themselves.

*Thumb-tip reach—distance from backrest to tip of subject's thumb as arm and hand are extended forward.
†Span—the maximal distance between a person's fingertips when arms and hands are extended to each side

N, force; SD, standard deviation

Figure 16-9 Maximal static horizontal push forces that males can exert with the hands and shoulders. *Modified from NASA, editors*: Man-systems integration standards (rev. A), *NASA-STD-3000, Houston, Tex., 1989 NASA.*

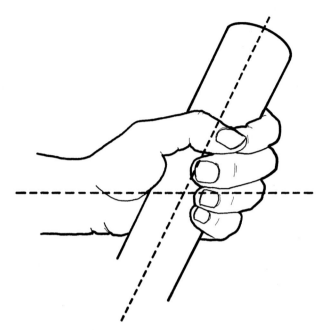

Figure 16-10 "Grip angle."

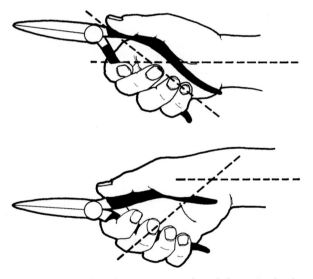

Figure 16-11 Pliers forcing one to bend the wrist (*top*) or allowing a straight wrist (*bottom*).

Proper posture of the hand and forearm while using hand tools is very important. It is a handy rule that the wrist should not be bent but kept straight to avoid overexertion of muscles and tendons and compression of tissue, nerves, and blood vessels. When the wrist is straight, the natural angle between the forearm/wrist and the grasp center of a handle is about 60 degrees, i.e., about 30 degrees ulnarly declined, as opposed to perpendicular (see **Fig. 16-10**). Yet most hand tools are designed as though this were a right angle. Because this is not the case, many common hand tools force the operator to bend the wrist. Such wrist bend should be

incorporated in the handle, as has been proposed by Erwin Tichauer since the 1960s (see **Fig. 16-11**) and recommended in numerous publications since then, as listed by Lewis and Narayan.[31] New technologies allow an assessment of the forces and torques in the hand and the postures in the digit and wrist while manipulations are performed.[52]

Nine of every 10 people, men or women, are right-handed,[18] and some tools are designed to fit only the right hand. Many tools can be used with either the left or right hand, but about 1 in 10 persons prefers to use the left hand and has better skills and more strength available there. Thus it is advisable to provide, if needed, hand tools specifically designed for use with the left hand.

DESIGNING FOR VISION

For many work tasks, the eyes must focus on the work object or the tool or must at least provide general guidance for the manipulation. This is often a problem in repair work or some assembly tasks when either only a small opening is available for manipulation and vision or other objects might interfere with vision.

A particularly difficult ergonomic problem is often associated with microscope use. Many microscopes are so designed that the eye must be kept close to the ocular. This enforces maintenance of the same posture, often over extended periods of time. In addition, the microscope may be so designed or placed that the operator must bend the head and neck to obtain proper eye location in relation to the eyepiece. Significant forward bends of the head and cervical column exceeding 25 degrees from vertical are particularly stressful because the neck extensor muscles must be tensed to prevent the head from pitching forward even more. This "unbalanced" condition also affects the posture of the trunk, and thus both the neck and trunk muscles must be kept in tension over long periods of time. Consequently, complaints by microscope operators about pains and aches in the neck and back areas are frequent. Furthermore, some microscopes have hand-operated controls located high in front of the shoulders. This requires that the hands be lifted to that posture and kept there, also requiring tension in the muscles controlling arm and hand posture. The proper selection of microscopes that allow a variation in eye position with respect to the eyepiece, their arrangements so that the operator need not bend forward, and the proper location of hand controls can alleviate many of the problems found with older microscope work stations.[19,28]

In general, visual targets that require close viewing should be placed in front of the operator in or near the medial plane, 40 to 80 cm ("reading distance") away from the eyes. The angle of the line of sight (from pupil to target) is best between 20 and 60 degrees below the ear-eye line, that is, 0 to 30 degrees below the horizon if the head is held straight (see **Fig. 16-12**).[9,25]

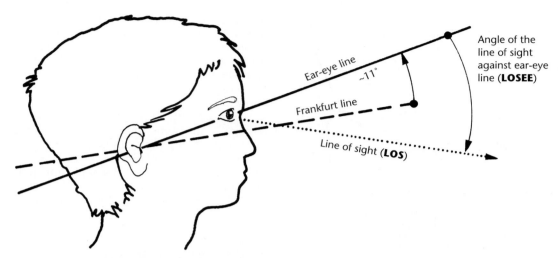

Figure 16-12 Line-of-sight angle against the ear-eye line.

DESIGNING FOR LOAD HANDLING

We all handle loads daily. We lift, hold, carry, push, pull, and lower while moving, packing, and storing objects. The material may be soft or solid, bulky or small, and smooth or with corners and edges; it may come as bags, boxes, or containers, with or without handles. We may handle objects occasionally or repeatedly, during leisure activities, but often as part of our work. On the job, the ergonomic design of material, containers, and work stations can help avoid overexertions and injuries, as should instructions and training on how to "lift properly." For some jobs, the establishment of physical strength requirements may be appropriate.

Manipulation of even lightweight and small objects can contribute to strain because we have to stretch, move, bend, or straighten out body parts while using fingers, arms, trunk, and legs. Heavy loads pose additional strain on the body owing to their weight, bulk, or lack of handles. Apparently, we are poor judges of the biomechanical strain that our bodies experience.[48]

Exerting force and energy in lifting an object with the hand(s) strains the hands, arms, shoulders, trunk, and if one stands, also the legs. The same parts of the musculoskeletal system are under stress in lowering, pushing, and pulling, but the directions and magnitudes of the external and internal force and torque vectors are different. The primary area of physiological and biomechanical concern has been the low back region, particularly the disks of the lumbar spine. In view of this fact, the operative words in the literature have been "low back pain related to lifting." Yet when one considers the musculoskeletal structures within the trunk, a variety of elements may be strained either singly or in combination: the spinal vertebrae, primarily their disk or facet joints; connective tissue such as ligaments and cartilage; and muscles with their tendons. These may all experience "insults," sprains, or

trauma. Compression strain of disks and vertebrae has been primarily studied, but tension is the primary loading of elastic elements such as muscles and connective tissues. Tension strains can be in the form of linear elongation, bending movements, or twisting torque. All structures may be subject to shear.

Loading of the body may come from activities performed on external objects, such as lifting, lowering, pushing, pulling, carrying, or holding; thus the strains may be static or dynamic, of fast onset, and of short or long duration. They may be single or several events; if the same or similar strains reappear, that repetition may be at regular or irregular timing, and the strains may be of similar or dissimilar magnitudes. Body structures can also be strained by just moving the body (according to Newton's second law, force = mass × acceleration) or simply by maintaining a posture by muscle tension without an external load. Any longitudinal contraction of the trunk muscles compresses the spinal column, which is (with some help from intraabdominal pressure) the only load-bearing structure of the trunk.

Aside from sports, the literature has dwelt primarily on the activity labeled "lifting," moving an object by hand from a lower position to a higher one, and on pushing and pulling, carrying, and holding. These events are frequently associated with one-time overloading of body structures and lead to acute trauma injuries. Yet it has long been acknowledged[43] that in many cases low back pain and injuries cannot be traced to a one-time event but are likely to be the result of repeated microtrauma, perhaps accumulated over lifelong working. Hence some or many low back pain episodes and injuries may be related to OMDs.

There are many possible activities, body postures, objects, and work tasks and many structures within the body that might be overly strained. Hence the various types of "training for safe load handling," particularly for lifting, have not been successful, against all expectations and hopes. Yet upon reflection, this is not surprising because it is an attempt to allay the symptoms of the many possible causes instead of removing the causes, acute or cumulative, by proper design of equipment, task, and work procedures.[27]

Nevertheless, several general recommendations should help to reduce the risk of overexertion injuries when lifting.

Lifting Techniques

The "leg lift" has been heavily promoted in training, as opposed to the "back lift." It is normally better to straighten the bent legs while lifting rather than unbending the back. But leg lifts can be done only with certain types of loads, either a load with a small size that fits between the legs or a load with "two handles" between which one can stand (like two small suitcases instead one big case). Large and bulky loads cannot usually be lifted by unbending the knees without body contortion. If one attempts to do so, one may stress the spine disks more than when also slightly unbending the back. Hence proper task and load (container) design is necessary to permit leg lifts. This is covered extensively in Chapters 9 and 10.

The Work Environment

The work environment can be made to contribute to safe manual material activities if it is well designed and maintained.

The *visual environment* should be well lit, clean, and uncluttered and allow good depth perception and discrimination of visual details, differences in contrast, and colors.

The *thermal environment* should be within zones comfortable for the physical work, usually in the range of about 18 to 22° C. Thermal stress resulting from conditions that are too hot or too cold may contribute to material handling safety problems.

The *acoustic environment* should be agreeable, with sound levels preferably below 75 dB. Warning sounds and signals indicating unusual conditions should be clearly perceptible by the operator. High-noise conditions can contribute to an overall straining of the operator and hence affect the safety of material handling.

Good housekeeping helps to avoid injuries. Safe gripping of the shoes on the floor and good support from the chair when seated are necessary conditions for safe material handling. Poor coupling with the floor can result in slipping, tripping, or misstepping. Floor surfaces should be kept clean to provide a good coefficient of friction with the shoes.[7] Clutter, loose objects on the floor, dirt, spills, and so forth can reduce friction and lead to slip and fall accidents, as shown in **Figure 16-13**.

Ergonomic Design of Facility and Equipment

How the job is designed determines the stress imposed by the work on the human material handler. The size of the handled object, its weight, whether it has handles or not, the layout of the task, the kinds of body motions to be performed, the muscular forces and torques to be exerted, the frequency of these efforts, the organization of work and rest periods, and other engineering and managerial aspects determine whether a job is well designed or not and whether it is safe, efficient, and agreeable to the operator.

The layout of the overall work facility, as well as the design of the equipment to be used, contributes to safe and efficient material handling. This includes the organization of the flow of material in general and designing that flow carefully in its details to reduce the involvement of people and to lessen the risk of them becoming injured.

It is the purpose of facility layout, or facility improvement, to select the most economical, safe, and efficient designs for the building, department, and work station. Flowcharts and flow diagrams are easy and well-known tools of the industrial engineer to describe events and activities, to sum up the requirements, and to provide information that leads to redesign or better design in the planning stage of a new facility. Konz[22] and Kroemer, Kroemer, and Kroemer-Elbert[27] provide "recipes" for ergonomic facility design.

Design of Equipment

Ergonomics and human factors research work have provided information on design features that are needed to fit equipment to the human, in particular, to provide safe and efficient working conditions. Much of this information was originally developed for military applications but has found its way into industrial settings as well.

Overall dimensions and space requirements can be derived from human body and reach dimensions, as shown in **Table 16-2**. The purposeful application of such information ensures, for example, that the driver compartment of a lift truck accommodate all driver sizes or that operators not strain themselves when trying to reach an object hanging from an overhead conveyor or attempting to grasp material in the far bottom corner of a transport bin. Of course, one should never design for the "average person" because this ghost does not exist. Instead, one must design for body size ranges, such as from the 5th to the 95th percentile.

Equipment may provide assistance at the workplace to the material handler, or equipment may do the actual transport.

Equipment for assistance at the workplace includes the following:

- Lift tables, hoists, cranes
- Ball transfer tables, turntables
- Loading/unloading devices

Transportation equipment includes the following:

- Nonpowered dollies, walkies, and trucks
- Powered walkies, rider trucks, tractors
- Conveyors of many kinds, trolleys
- Overhead and mobile cranes

Obviously, several of these can be used both at the

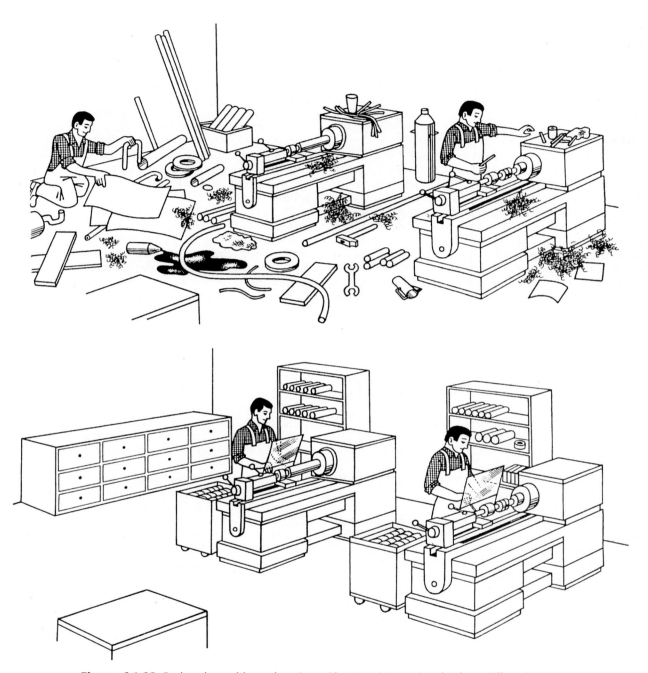

Figure 16-13 Bad and good housekeeping. *(Courtesy International Labour Office, 1988.)*

workplace and for in-process movement, such as hoists, conveyors, and trucks.

Finally, a group of material movement equipment is primarily used for receiving and warehousing:

- Stackers
- Reach trucks
- Lift trucks
- Cranes
- Automated storage and retrieval systems.

All the aforementioned equipment can take over the requirements of holding, carrying, pushing, pulling, lowering, and lifting of materials that would otherwise be performed with the hands of a person. However, whether this will be done by machines depends, aside from economical considerations, on the layout and organization of the work itself. For example, will an operator use a hoist to lift material to be fed into a machine if this is time consuming or awkward? Will a lift table be installed next to an assembly work station if this means removal or relocation of another work station to make sufficient room?[4]

Obviously, facility layout as well as workplace design must be suitable for use of the equipment. Furthermore, the operator must be convinced that it is worthwhile to go through the effort of using a hoist instead of heaving the material by hand.

Equipment must not only be selected to enable the worker to perform the material handling job but must also "fit" the human operator. Ease of use must be considered together with the safety of personnel working with or alongside the equipment. Unfortunately, some material movement equipment such as cranes and hoists, powered and hand trucks, and conveyors show an alarming lack of consideration of human factors and safety principles in their design. The overall worst example is "forklifts," which when lifting, carrying, and lowering a load have that very load obstruct the operator's view. Furthermore, the driver often has only little space to sit and is subjected to vibrations and impacts.

Design of Containers

Containers and trays must be designed to have the proper weight, size, balance, and coupling with the human hand. The container should be as light as possible to add little to the load of the material. Its size and handle arrangement should be such that the center of the loaded tray is close to the body. It should be well balanced, with its weight centered between but below the handholds. Big, heavy, pliable "bags" are usually more difficult to handle than boxes or trays.

Handles on containers or tools should be so designed and oriented that the hand and forearm of the operator are aligned. The operator should not be forced to work with a bent wrist: "bend the handle, not the wrist." Carpal tunnel syndromes and other cumulative trauma problems in the hand and arm are less likely to occur if a person can work with a straight wrist.

The handle should be of such shape and material that squeezing forces are distributed over the largest possible palm area. The handle diameter should be in the range of 2 to 5 cm. Its surface should be slip resistant. Coupling with the hands is better on protruding handles or gripping-notch types, but handhold cutouts or drawer-pull types are acceptable. The location of handles should be according to the scheme shown in **Figure 16-14** for a boxlike object of about 40 × 40 × 40 cm and weighing between 9 and 13 kg.[11]

DESIGNING THE OFFICE WORK STATION

The modern office, often equipped with computers, has little resemblance to the rooms in which male clerks made entries in ledgers or penned letters a hundred years ago. Yet the idea of "sitting upright is healthy" had not changed until it became obvious that people in modern offices sit "any way they like"—apparently without bad health consequences.

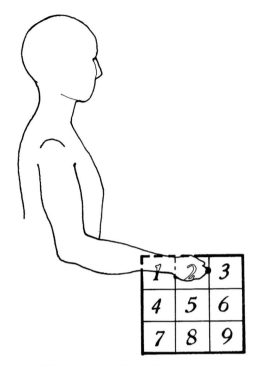

Figure 16-14 Locations of handles in box containers. For lifting and lowering in front of the body, locations 2/2 are best, and 3/8 are acceptable. For work with sideways twisting of the body, locations 6/8 and 8/8 are best for heavy loads, and locations 3/8 and 2/2 are acceptable. *(From Drury CG et al:* Ergonomics *32:467-489, 1989.)*

Different working postures, use of computers in well-lit offices, and changed attitudes give reasons to rethink the recommendations for office furniture design and to facilitate appropriate motor, vision, and behavior interfacing.

Theories of "Healthy" Sitting

In the nineteenth century, several physicians published theories about proper sitting postures and deduced from these theories recommendations for seat and furniture design. Their common concept was that "sitting with an upright trunk means sitting healthily." This idea had remained virtually unchallenged until recently, when various (occasionally even contradictory) theories about healthy postures while sitting at work have been published.

Sitting Upright

The nineteenth century concept was that the spinal column of the sitting person should be "erect" or "upright" (a contradiction in terms because it is actually curved in the side view), similar to that of a "healthy normal upright-standing" person. Special emphasis was placed on maintaining "normal" lumbar lordosis. This posture was believed to put the least strain on the spinal column and its supportive structures, including the musculature. Also, this posture was "socially proper."

Recommendations for the design and use of seats were based on this desired posture. These ideas about suitable posture and furniture were repeated in the literature, apparently without much questioning or contradiction, until the middle of the twentieth century. In retrospect, this is quite surprising given the lack of experimental support for the appropriateness of the upright posture.

Standing or sitting "straight" means that in the lateral view, the spinal column in fact forms an S curve with forward bends (lordoses) in the neck and low back regions and a rearward bulge (kyphosis) in the chest region. Although there appears to be no reason to doubt that this is—in the current evolutionary condition of the civilized human—a "normal" and hence desirable curvature of the spine that keeps the trunk and its organs in acceptable order, how such a posture should be achieved, supported, or even enforced needs to be discussed.

Free Posturing

When one sits down on a hard flat surface, not using a backrest, the ischial tuberosities (inferior protuberances of the pelvic bones) act as fulcrums around which the pelvic girdle rotates under the weight of the upper part of the body. The bones of the pelvic girdle are linked by connective tissue to both the thighs and the lower half of the trunk. Therefore, rotation of the pelvis affects the posture of the lower spinal column, particularly in the lumbar region. If the pelvis rotation is rearward, the normal lordosis of the lumbar spine is flattened. This was deemed highly undesirable by orthopaedists and physiologists. Hence avoidance of backward rotation of the pelvis is a main purpose of many theories of seat design.

Given the tissue connections between the pelvis and thighs, particularly the effects of muscles spanning the hip joint or even both knee and hip joints (e.g., hamstrings, quadriceps, rectus femoris, sartorius, tensor fasciae latae, psoas major), the actual hip and knee angles also affect the location of the pelvis and hence the curvature of the lumbar spine. At a large hip angle, forward rotation of the pelvis on the ischial tuberosities is likely, accompanied by lumbar lordosis. (These actions on the lumbar spine take place if associated muscles are relaxed; muscle activities or changes in trunk tilt can counter the effects.) "Opening the hip angle" is an aim of some theories of seat design.[21]

In 1884 Staffel[46] proposed a forward-declining seat surface to open up the hip angle and thus to bring about lordosis in the lumbar area. Eight decades later, this idea led to a seat pan design with an elevated rear edge that was popular in Europe in the 1960s. More recently, Mandal[34,35] and Congleton, Ayoub, and Smith[8] again promoted that the whole seat surface slope forward and downward. To prevent the buttocks from sliding down the forward-declined seat, the seat surface may be shaped to fit the human underside (Congleton), or one may counteract the downward-forward thrust by either bearing down on the feet (Mandal) or by propping the knees or upper part of the shins on special pads. One may call this posture "semi-sitting" or "semi-kneeling."

Anecdotal evidence and several studies[5,10,29,44] have indicated that some users like this support structure whereas most do not. One of the advantages is the mobility of the trunk, particularly if there is no backrest; among the disadvantages is the tendency to slide off, which is counteracted either by fatiguing leg thrusts or by unpleasant or even painful pressure against the shin pads, and it may be difficult, when trying to stand, to move the legs out of the confined space between the pads and the seat. Although the desired lumbar lordosis might be achieved solely by opening the hip angle to more than 90 degrees and by rotating the pelvis forward, most proponents of the forward declination of the seat pan deem a backrest desirable or necessary. In fact, a well-designed backrest alone could bring about lordosis of the lumbar spine by pushing this section of the back forward. Old wooden school benches simply had a horizontal wood slot at lumbar height that forced the seated pupil to bend the lower part of the back forward to avoid painful contact. There are more subtle and agreeable ways to promote lumbar concavity: a fixed pad[1] or an adjustable lumbar cushion incorporated in the seat back of some car and airplane seats is an example of such design features.

Of course, one can shape the total backrest. Apparently independently from each other, experimental subjects of Ridder[41] in the United States and of Grandjean[15] and his co-workers in Switzerland found rather similar backrest shapes acceptable. In essence, these shapes follow the curvature of the rear side of the human body: at the bottom concave to accept the buttocks, above slightly convex to fill in the lumbar lordosis, then raising nearly straight but declined backward to support the thoracic area, but at the top again convex to follow the neck lordosis. This shape (with more or less pronounced curvatures depending on the designer's assumptions about body size and body posture) has been used successfully for seats in automobiles, aircraft, passenger trains, and cars and for easy chairs; in the traditional office these "first-class" shapes were thoughtfully provided for managers whereas other employees had to use simpler designs such as the miserable small board attached to so-called secretarial chairs.

Relaxed leaning against a declined backrest is the least stressful sitting posture. This is a condition that is often freely chosen by persons working in the office if there is a suitable backrest available: ". . . an impression which many observers have already perceived when visiting offices or workshops with VDT work stations: Most of the operators do not maintain an upright trunk posture. . . . In fact, the great majority of the operators lean backwards even if the chairs are not suitable for such a posture."[16]

Allowing persons to freely select their posture has led in two instances to surprisingly similar results. In 1962, Lehmann[30] showed the contours of five persons "relaxing" under water. Sixteen years later, relaxed body postures observed in astronauts in microgravity were reported by NASA/Webb,[38] shown in **Figure 16-15**. The similarity between the postures under water and in space is remarkable. One might assume that in both cases the sum of all tissue torques around body joints has been nullified. Incidentally or not, the shape of "easy chairs" is quite similar to the contours shown in

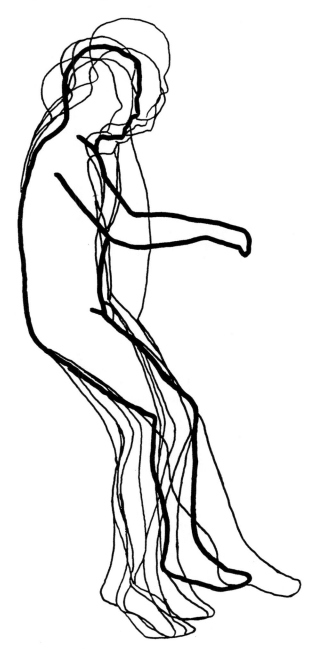

Figure 16-15 Relaxed underwater body postures super-imposed with the relaxed posture in weightlessness. *(From Kroemer KHE, Kroemer HB, and Kroemer-Elbert KE: Ergonomics: how to design for ease and efficiency, Englewood Cliffs, NJ, 1994, Prentice Hall. Used by permission.)*

both figures. Some "executive" computer work stations, sketched in **Figure 16-16**, use similar support shapes, but it is doubtful that such postures and furniture will be used widely in regular offices.

Currently, no one simple theory about the proper, healthy, comfortable, efficient, and optimal sitting posture at work prevails.[3,26,32,33,50] With the idea abolished that everybody should sit upright and that furniture should be designed to this end, the general tenet is that many postures may be comfortable (healthy, suitable, efficient, etc.), depending on one's body, preferences, and work activities. Consequently, it is now generally presumed that furniture should allow many posture variations and permit easy adjustments in its main features, such as seat height and angle, backrest position, or knee pads and footrests, and that the computer work station should also allow easy variations in the location of the input devices and the display. Thus change, variation, and adjustment to fit the individual appear central to well-being. If any label can be applied to current theories about proper sitting, it may be the "free posturing" sketched in **Figure 16-17**.

The "free posturing" design principle has the following basic tenets:

1. Allow the operator to freely assume a variety of sitting (or standing) postures, to easily make work station adjustments, and even to get up and move about.
2. Design for a variety of user dimensions and for a variety of user preferences.
3. Consider new technologies that may develop quickly and should be usable at the work station. (For example, radically new keyboards and input devices including voice recognition may be available soon; display technologies and display placement are undergoing rapid changes.)

Ergonomic Designs of Three Interfaces

One interacts with the work in three interfaces. The first is visual, in which one must look at written material, the keyboard, the computer screen, or the printed output. The second interface is manipulative because the hands operate keys, a mouse or other input device, pen and paper, and a telephone. The third major interface is with the chair where the back, buttocks, and thighs are supported when sitting.

Designing the Visual Interface

In conventional offices, the paper for writing or reading is usually placed on the regular working surface, roughly at elbow height. If an object needs to be looked at more closely, it is lifted to a proper relation to the eyes. For easier reading, a surface inclined to make its angle with the line of sight closer to 90 degrees is often recommended, but the disadvantage of the sloped surface is the sliding or rolling of work materials. Therefore, one usually has a horizontal table or desk surface upon which the various objects are placed at will.

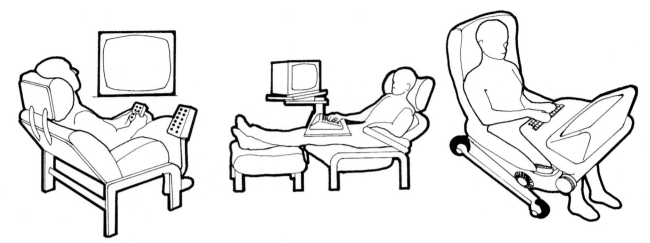

Figure 16-16 Body postures in "executive" computer work stations as adapted from sketches in newspapers.

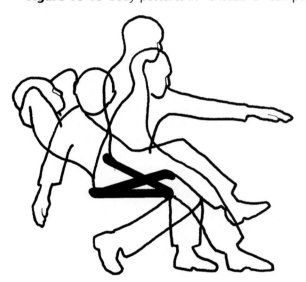

Figure 16-17 "Free posturing." *(Modified from Kroemer KHE: Ergonomic seats for computer work stations. In Aghazadeh F, editor:* Trends in ergonomics/human factors V, *Amsterdam, 1988, Elsevier Science, Inc: pp 313-320.)*

When a *keyboard* is used, there are several visual targets. One is the "printing" area: the platen on a conventional typewriter or the display area on electronic typewriters. This is usually only a few centimeters above the keyboard and located fairly well with respect to human vision capabilities (distance) and preferences (line-of-sight angle), although its display surface (subtended angle) is very small. In many cases a problem has been the placement of a *source document* from which text is copied. To place it flat on a horizontal surface is quite often uncomfortable and makes exact reading difficult. Therefore, various types of document holders have been used that put the source document more vertical and closer to the eyes. Still, often this document

holder is placed far to one side and necessitates a twisted body posture and lateral head and eye movements (**Fig. 16-18**).

Proper placement of all visual targets together is often a problem. First, with the large increase in the number of keys from the typewriter to most *computer keyboards,* many operators scan the keys again, whereas previously typists were able to do their job without looking at the keys. Therefore, the computer keyboard is a rather large, nearly horizontal visual target area usually placed on the work surface. Second, there is the *display area* of the computer monitor (the "screen"), which is commonly placed in front of the operator at about right angles to the line of sight. Third, there is often some sort of *source document* from which information must be gleaned. Its placement causes problems similar to those encountered by typists, but in some cases the source document is fairly large, such as a drawing used in CAD operations.

The placement problem is mostly one of available space within the center of the person's *field of view*. Research has shown that people in a conventional sitting posture prefer to look downward at close visual targets at angles between 10 and 40 degrees below the horizon. They do so by inclining the head forward and rotating the eyeballs downward instead of looking straight ahead. This appears to be a "natural way" of focusing at a near target with the least effort; the more upwards one has to tilt one's eyes, the more difficult it becomes to focus.[25] Thus putting the monitor up high behind the keyboard (often by placing it on the central processing unit of the computer or on a so-called monitor stand) is rather uncomfortable for the viewer. Instead of building a "monitor tower," the screen should be located immediately behind the keyboard, with its lower edge as near as possible to the rear section of the keyboard. A printer may be placed directly on top of the monitor and a source document placed next to it (**Fig. 16-19**).

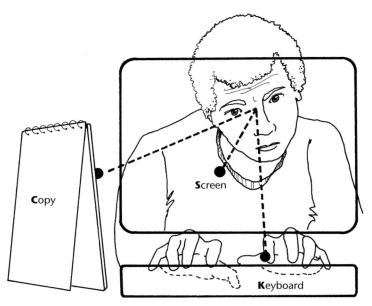

Figure 16-18 The "computer user syndrome." *(From Grant A: Homo-Quintadus, computers and rooms (repetitive ocular orthopedic motion stress),* Optom Vis Sci *67:297-305, 1990. Used by permission.)*

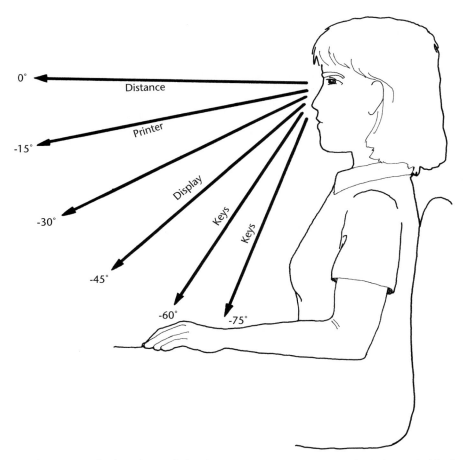

Figure 16-19 Approximate angular locations of visual targets at a computer work station suitable for an upright-sitting person.

Designing the Motoric Interface

On the original typewriter keyboard developed in the 1860s, the keys were arranged in an alphabetic sequence in two rows. The QWERTY layout, patented in 1879, was adopted as an international standard after many modifications in 1966. It has since been universally used on typewriters and then on computers and on many other input devices.

Unfortunately, the traditional typewriter keyboard is still used, largely unchanged, as the major input device for computers. The conventional QWERTY keyboard has several unergonomic features. Keys for letters that frequently follow each other in common text (such as *q* and *u* in English) are spaced apart on the keyboard. This was originally done so that mechanical type bars might not entangle if struck in rapid sequence. Another characteristic is that the "columns" of keys run diagonally from left to right; this was also necessary on early typewriters because of mechanical constraints of the type bars. Yet the keys are arranged in straight sideways "rows," unlike the fingertips. The keyboard must be operated with pronated hands ("thumbs down") because of the horizontal arrangement of the rows of keys. Furthermore, there is a large number of keys, only one of which must be correctly selected to produce the desired character. This requires, cognitively, that a difficult multichoice decision be made, followed by motorically complex use of the arm, wrist, and digit muscles to move the fingertip to the proper key.

"Mechanical" keyboards had strong key resistance and required large key displacement. Hence it was suspected that weak fingers, particularly the little ones, were overworked. Many recommendations for improvements in the traditional keyboard have been proposed in the past. For overviews, see, for example, Alden, Daniels, and Kanarick,[2] Kroemer,[24] and Noyes.[39,40] Suggested improvements, for example, by Dvorak in the 1930s, included relocation of the letters on the keyboard and new geometries of the keyboard, such as curved arrangements of the keys. In 1926 Klockenberg proposed that the keyboard be divided into one half for the left hand and one for the right hand, so arranged that the center sections are higher than the outside sections, thereby avoiding the pronation of the hand required on a flat keyboard. Two keys can be operated simultaneously (chording) to generate one character, thereby reducing the total number of keys.

The letter-to-key allocation on the QWERTY has many often obscure reasons, but it has been retained even for current computer keyboards in spite of many attempts at changes. Redesign concerns not only the placement of keys within the array of keys but also the spatial positioning of the keyboard with respect to the operator. For example, the keyboard may be sloped or (if split) slanted and tilted, as shown in **Figure 16-20**, to facilitate easier motions and better postures of the hand and arm of the user.

Intensive use of state-of-the-art keyboards apparently can lead to OMDs. Not only is this a function of the repetitive energy to tap down keys, but it is also related to the movement of the digits from key to key and associated movements of the wrist and the entire arm. Especially with the large number of keys on current keyboards, extensive movements of the fingertips are often necessary, accompanied by large displacements in the wrist and arm. Up-and-down movements to tap keys are likely to result in flexion/extension of the wrist, which may be partially controlled by providing wrist rests. Yet given large keyboards, the wrist may have to move extensively along the wrist rests, which may feel uncomfortable. The requirement to reach laterally to keys far to the side may result in strong ulnar deviations in the wrist.

Small keyboards can be placed nearly anywhere at the user's convenience, such as on the lap (which was quite difficult with the traditional large keyboard but was nevertheless done by some operators), or they may be incorporated in an armrest, in a glove, or even in the shell of a space suit. New developments may radically change the nature and appearance of keyboards.

The practice of tapping a binary key to generate a single character is an archaic and clumsy way to generate text. Ergonomic redesign of input devices (not only of keyboards but also of mouse, trackball, light pen, etc.) may bring about substantial relief in terms of stresses on the hand/arm/shoulder system. In view of the technical means available, the topic of transferring information to the computer by means drastically different from current input devices is high on the priority list to avoid OMDs. Input by handwriting or by voice is feasible.

Designing Office Furniture

One of the first steps in designing office furniture for proper fit and use is to establish the main clearance and external dimensions that are derived from the anthropometric data of the office workers. There are, of course, many ways to do so. Among them are two alternative strategies to determine major equipment dimensions. One is to keep the major heights constant (in traditional offices, desks and support tables), but to provide fit to persons of different sizes and preferences by seats and possibly footrests that are adjustable in height. The second major strategy is to have all heights adjustable—desks, tables, and seats. If such adjustability is sufficient, footrests would not be needed. In this approach, one starts best with the floor and builds up from there; popliteal height (length of the lower part of the leg) is thought to be the main determinant of seat pan height. The height of the support and work surface should be adjustable so that it can be brought down as low as feasible over the thighs of a sitting person and as high as individually preferred. Thus the added values of popliteal height, thigh thickness, and the thickness of the support structure determine the lowest setting of the support surface. This was not the approach taken in the 1988 American National Standards Institute (ANSI)/ Human Factors Society (HFS) 100 Standard for VDT Work Stations, where a hand/elbow height was arbi-

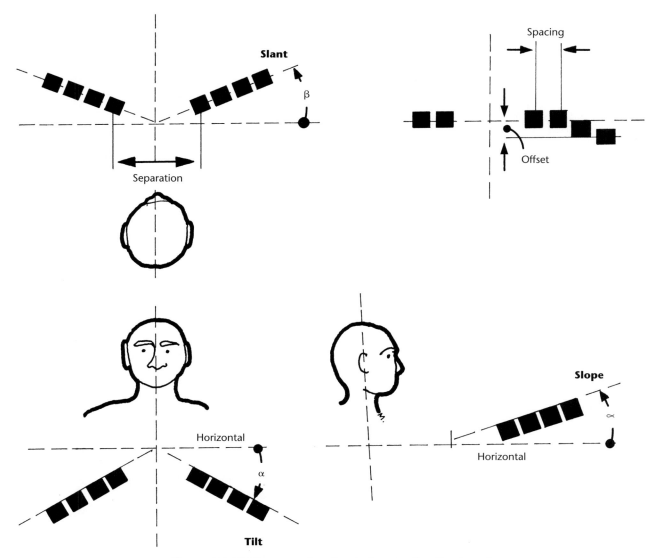

Figure 16-20 Terms to describe design details of keyboards.

trarily presumed from which shoulder height and seat height were sequentially estimated. The procedure of building up from the floor does not require assumptions about body posture and should result in a design that leaves the most freedom to the user for personal adjustments. This is the approach mostly likely to be taken in the 1994 revision of the ANSI/HFS 100 standard.

All components of office furniture, in fact components of all equipment used, must be seen as "parts of an interactive system" where the visual targets (e.g., the monitor), the manipulation areas (e.g., the keyboard), and the body support (e.g., the chair) interact with each other in affecting the postures and habits of the office worker. Furthermore, the work task and the environment (illumination, especially glare, for example) affect the worker. If just one element is ill-placed or, worse, several components are unsuitable, the resulting condition may become unacceptable. For example, **Figure 16-21** shows dropped and elevated wrists while working

on keyboards that are located too high on a table, where the chair cannot be adjusted properly, and where the display is put very high.

The seat itself should be designed according to currently accepted design principles to provide comfortable support and allow change in postures. For this, the seat pan should be able to be tilted both backward and forward, and the backrest should be able to be angled from a nearly upright position to reclining about 30 degrees behind vertical. The backrest should provide full support for the back and preferably include a headrest and an adjustable lumbar support. Armrests, adjustable and perhaps removable, are liked by some and disliked by others. Adjustability in height is, in most situations, a basic requirement. **Figure 16-22** indicates the major adjustment needs in office furniture.

Providing work tasks and equipment that facilitate, almost provoke changing body positions while seated and getting up and moving about frequently are major

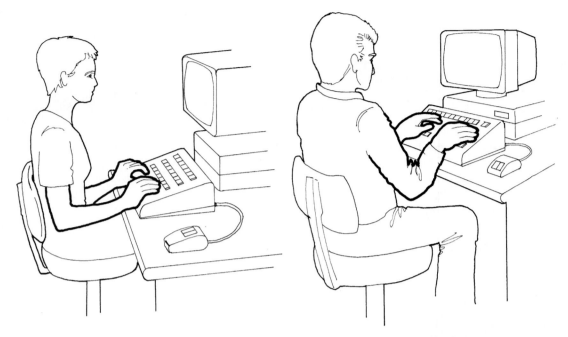

Figure 16-21 Raised and dropped wrists while keyboarding. *(Courtesy Herman Miller, Inc.)*

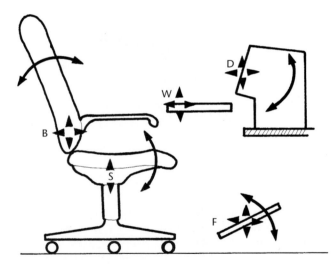

Figure 16-22 Adjustment features of computer work stations.

ergonomic concerns. Occasional but not habitual reaching and stretching are desirable—see **Figure 16-23**—but maintaining contorted postures can lead to overuse disorders.

JOB CONTENT, WORK ORGANIZATION, AND TEAM INVOLVEMENT

Averting OMDs is an important aspect of ergonomic work design. Seven conditions need to be painstakingly avoided:

1. Job activities with many repetitions
2. Work activities that require prolonged or repetitive exertion of muscular force, especially those imparting blows and impacts
3. Putting body segments in extreme positions
4. Work that forces a person to maintain the same posture for long periods of time
5. Pressure from tools or equipment on body tissues
6. Work in which a tool vibrates the body
7. Exposure of the body to cold, including airflow from pneumatic tools

The design and provision of ergonomically appropriate work stations are not sufficient. This must be supplemented by advice on and implementation of their proper use. Suitable movements and postures of the neck, trunk, and wrist, for example, may be facilitated by proper equipment, but they must be accomplished by an operator who uses the equipment to its advantage. Thus it is important that the benefits of proper working habits be appreciated and that workers willingly practice these habits by making full use of adjustment features at the work station.

Many persons like to have autonomy in the performance of their work, to take responsibility for the quality and quantity of their work, and to control their timing. Most prefer to perform larger tasks from beginning to end instead of simply doing specialized tidbits. The ability to receive direct feedback about work performance, best by reviewing one's own work daily supplemented by constructive and positive comments from the supervisor, contributes essentially to the feeling of achievement and satisfaction. Within the limitations set by the requirement that certain work needs to be done,

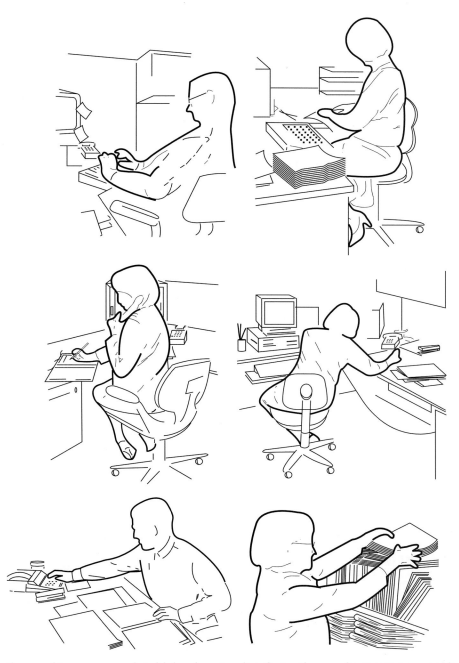

Figure 16-23 Reaching, twisting, and stretching postures in the office. *(Courtesy Herman Miller, Inc.)*

the working person should be free to distribute the workload, both in amount and in pace, according to one's own preferences and needs. Communication with colleagues and social relations are essential, although at individually varying intensities, to well-being and performance.

The organization of working time, particularly the provision of changes in work and rest pauses, is important for many ergonomic reasons. Most people are bored by repetitive, monotonous, and continuous tasks; instead, varying tasks of different lengths should be provided so that each member of the work team has the occasion and cause to move from one task to another or to simply take a break. The "recovery value" of many short rest pauses is larger than that of a few long breaks.

The picture of the "new" designer, engineer, and manager becomes clear. The ergonomist recognizes individual traits as design inputs, sees subjective work habits as normal, expects personal involvement in work outcome, and encourages each member's involvement in decisions about work procedures, work equipment, and the work facility.

Acknowledgment

This chapter uses information contained in our book *Ergonomics: How to Design for Ease and Efficiency,* published in 1994 by Prentice Hall. We thank the publisher for permission to use this material.

References

1. Åkerblom B: *Standing and sitting posture,* Stockholm, 1948, Nordiska Bokhandeln.

2. Alden DG, Daniels RW, Kanarick AF: Keyboard design and operation: a review of the major issues, *Hum Factors* 14:275-293, 1972.

3. Bendix T: Significance of seated-workplace adjustments. In Karwowski W, Yates JW, editors: *Advances in industrial ergonomics and safety III,* London, 1991, Taylor & Francis Publishers; pp 343-350.

4. Bobick TG, Gutman SH: Reducing musculo-skeletal injuries by using mechanical handling equipment. In Kroemer KHE, McGlothlin JD, Bobick TG, editors: *Manual material handling: understanding and preventing back trauma,* Akron, Ohio, 1989, American Industrial Hygiene Association; pp 87-96.

5. Bridger RS, Eisenhart-Rothe CV, Henneberg M: Effects of seat slope and hip flexion on spinal angles in sitting, *Hum Factors* 31:679-688, 1989.

6. Chaffin DB, Andersson GBJ: *Occupational biomechanics,* ed 2, New York, 1991, John Wiley & Sons.

7. Chaffin DB, Woldstad JC, Trujillo A: Floor/shoe slip resistant measurement, *Am Ind Hyg Assoc J* 53:283-289, 1992.

8. Congleton JJ, Ayoub MM, Smith JL: The design and evaluation of the neutral posture chair for surgeons, *Hum Factors* 27:589-600, 1985.

9. Delleman NJ: Visual determinants of working posture. In Mattila M, Karwowski W, editors: *Computer applications in ergonomics, occupational safety and health,* Amsterdam, 1992, Elsevier Science; pp 321-329.

10. Drury CG, Francher M: Evaluation of a forward sloping chair, *Appl Ergonom* 16:41-47, 1985.

11. Drury CG et al: Symmetric and asymmetric manual materials handling; part 1: physiology and psychophysics, *Ergonomics* 32:467-489, 1989.

12. Fraser TM: *Ergonomic principles in the design of hand tools,* Occupational Safety and Health Series No 44, Geneva, 1980, International Labour Office.

13. Freivalds A: The ergonomics of tools, *Int Rev Ergonom* 1:43-75, 1987.

14. Gordon CC et al: *1988 anthropometric survey of U.S. army personnel: summary statistics interim report,* TR 89/027, Natick, Mass, 1989, US Army Natick Research, Development and Engineering Center.

15. Grandjean E: *Physiological design of work,* Thun, Switzerland, 1963, Otto (in German).

16. Grandjean E, Huenting W, Nishiyama K: Preferred VDT work station settings, body postures and physical impairments, *Appl Ergonom* 15:99-104, 1984.

17. Greenberg L, Chaffin DB: *Workers and their tools,* Midland, Mich, 1977, Pendell.

18. Greiner TM: *Hand anthropometry of U.S. army personnel,* Tech Rep TR-92/011, Natick, Mass, 1991, US Army Natick Research, Development and Engineering Center.

19. Helander MG, Grossmith EJ, Prabhu P: Planning and implementation of microscope work, *Appl Ergonom* 22:36-42, 1991.

20. Hoffmann ER: A comparison of hand and foot movement times, *Ergonomics* 34:397-406, 1991.

21. Keegan JJ: Alterations to the lumbar curve related to posture and sitting, *J Bone Joint Surg* 35:589-603, 1952.

22. Konz S: *Work design: industrial ergonomics,* Worthington, Ohio, 1990, Publishing Horizons.

23. Kroemer KHE: Cumulative trauma disorders: their recognition and ergonomic measures to avoid them, *Appl Ergonom* 20:274-280, 1989.

24. Kroemer, KHE: Human engineering the keyboard, *Hum Factors* 14:51-63, 1972.

25. Kroemer KHE: Locating the computer screen: how high, how far? *Ergonom Design* Oct. 7-8, 1993.

26. Kroemer KHE: Sitting at work: recording and assessing body postures, designing furniture for computer work stations. In Mital A, Karwowski W, editors: *Work space, equipment and tool design,* Amsterdam, 1991, Elsevier Science, pp 93-109.

27. Kroemer KHE, Kroemer HB, Kroemer-Elbert KE: *Ergonomics: how to design for ease and efficiency,* Englewood Cliffs, NJ, 1994, Prentice Hall.

28. Krueger H, Conrady P, Zuelch J: Work with magnifying glasses, *Ergonomics* 32:785-794, 1989.

29. Lander C et al: The Balans chair and its semi-kneeling position. An ergonomic comparison with the conventional sitting position, *Spine* 12:269-272, 1987.

30. Lehmann G: *Praktische arbeitsphysiologie,* ed 2, Stuttgart, Germany, 1962, Thieme Medical Publishers.

31. Lewis WG, Narayan CV: Design and sizing of ergonomic handles for hand tools, *Appl Ergonom* 24(5):351-356, 1993.

32. Lueder RK: Seat comfort. A review of the construct in the office environment, *Hum Factors* 25:701-711, 1983.

33. Lueder RK, Noro K, editors: *Hard facts about soft machines: the ergonomics of seating,* London, 1994, Taylor & Francis Publishers.

34. Mandal AC: The correct height of school furniture, *Hum Factors* 24:257-269, 1982.

35. Mandal AC: Work-chair with tilting seat, *Lancet* 1:642-643, 1975.

36. Marras WS, Kim JY: Anthropometry of industrial populations, *Ergonomics* 36:371-378, 1993.

37. Mital A: Hand tools: injuries, illnesses, design, and usage. In Mital A, Karwowski W, editors: *Workspace, equipment, and tool design,* Amsterdam, 1991, Elsevier Science; pp 219-256.

38. NASA/Webb, editors: *Anthropometric sourcebook,* 3 vols, NASA Reference Publ 1024, Houston, 1978, National Aeronautics and Space Administration.

39. Noyes J: Chord keyboards, *Appl Ergonom* 14(1):55-59, 1983.

40. Noyes J: The Qwerty keyboard: a review. *Int J Man Machine Studies* 18:265-281, 1983.

41. Ridder CA: *Basic design measurements for sitting,* Bull 616, Agricultural Experiment Station, Fayetteville, Ariz, 1959, University of Arkansas.

42. Roebuck JA: *Anthropometric methods: designing to fit the human body,* Santa Monica, Calif, 1994, Human Factors and Ergonomics Society.

43. Rowe ML: Low back pain in industry: an updated position, *J Occup Med* 13:476-478, 1969.

44. Seidel B, Windel A: Sitting on "Balans" chairs—subjective assessment of the comfort and the effect on frequencies of complaints. In *Proceedings, 11th Congress of the International Ergonomics Association,* vol 3, London, 1991, Taylor & Francis Publishers; pp 11-12.

45. Silverstein BA, Fine LJ, Armstrong TJ: Occupational factors and carpal tunnel syndrome, *Am J Ind Med* 11:343-358, 1987.

46. Staffel F: On the hygiene of sitting, *Zentrabl Allgemeine Gesundheitspflege* 3:403-421, 1884 (in German).

47. Stier F: The velocity of arm movements, *Int Z Angew Physiol* 18:82-100, 1959 (in German).

48. Thompson DD, Chaffin DB: Can biomechanically determined stress be perceived? In *Proceedings of the Human Factors and Ergonomics Society 37th Annual Meeting,* Santa Monica, Calif, 1993, Human Factors Society; pp 789-792.

49. Ulin SS et al: Effect of tool shape and work location on perceived exertion for work on horizontal surfaces, *Am Indu Hyg Assoc J* 54(7):383-391, 1993.

50. Verbeek J: The use of adjustable furniture: evaluation of an instruction programme for office workers, *Appl Ergonom* 22:179-184, 1991.

51. Wagner C: The pianist's hand: anthropometry and biomechanics, *Ergonomics* 31:97-131, 1988.

52. Yun MH: *A hand posture measurement system for evaluating manual tool tasks.* In Proceedings of the Human Factors and Ergonomics Society 37th Annual Meeting, Santa Monica, Calif, 1993, Human Factors Society; pp 754-758.

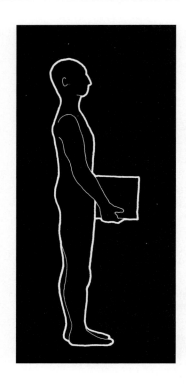

Chapter 17

Education and Training

Margareta Nordin

CONTENTS

Educational efforts are necessary to prevent and treat work-related musculoskeletal disorders. Can an individual work an entire lifetime without the musculoskeletal system being affected or the individual experiencing some kind of symptoms? The answer is probably no. If a work event causes trauma or an injury leading to tissue damage such as a fracture or injury that can be seen in imaging studies, diagnosis and treatment are usually straightforward. Treatment is provided, and if no complication occurs, the fracture will heal in the stipulated time, the employee will return to work, and the company will accept the work-related absenteeism. Most musculoskeletal work-related injuries and disorders do not have a distinct trauma or event related to the perceived pain, however, but rather they may originate from cumulative events at the culmination of which the employee decides to report the exacerbation leading to strong discomfort or pain.[23] The decision to report a cumulative work ailment can be affected by physical, emotional, environmental, or psychosocial issues.

This is the focus of the education and training of occupational health providers in the prevention and treatment of work-related musculoskeletal disorders. It is complex, difficult, and yet rewarding: complex because occupational medicine involves management, often union, and always the employee; difficult because it requires a change in the behavior and health beliefs of the healthcare provider, industry, and patient: and finally, rewarding when we obtain a long-term commitment to the future prevention of disability from all involved parties.

The learning process and health beliefs will be briefly reviewed in this chapter. Thereafter, education and its impact on behavior will be discussed, including a review of the different kinds of educational approaches. Finally, there is a short discussion on the improvement in patient education and counseling and some definitions and measures of success. This chapter is not meant to be exhaustive, but rather it is intended to introduce some concepts about education related to occupational musculoskeletal ailments that need to be discussed.

THE LEARNING PROCESS

The idea of education is to transfer knowledge or a skill to another person or group of individuals. We remember events, people, or those things that interest us. Mood alters our remembrance.[46] In an educational program, the individual is asked to adapt new information. Adaptation is a process that is an equilibrium between assimilation and accommodation. Assimilation is the process by which individuals take new information and incorporate it into their mental schemes and structures.[44] Accommodation relates to the process where we alter or modify these schemes and structures according to the external reality. Assimilation and accommodation are normal processes. The assimilation process will adapt the new information according to its relevance to the individual. Through accommodation, prior knowledge may in turn be modified. When the information received is far beyond the actual level of understanding, we may dismiss it because it cannot be fitted into the existing mental scheme. Nor do we have the capacity to integrate or change it. The adaptation process is idiosyncratic. When designing an educational program, we should understand that the information given may not be adapted in the same way by all participants.

HEALTH BELIEFS

Health beliefs are deeply rooted in culture, tradition, personal theories, fear avoidance, education, and other factors.[25,26,29,59] Giving information is not a one-way process. Giving information to a patient involves both the healthcare professional's and the patient's notions and theories about health and illness.

Studies have shown that a patient's beliefs about illness can differ considerably from those of the healthcare professional.[13,14,36] While teaching, the educator must be sensitive to individuals' beliefs and culture and allow for them to successfully integrate the new information.

"Teaching" imply large knowledge in the subject area. *Good* teaching also implies an understanding of the audience. Popper[45] stated that "patience, time and good will on both sides" facilitates mutual understanding. "Goodwill" here implies the admission that we may learn something from the other person. Bates et al[6] studied chronic pain between Anglo-Americans and native Puerto Ricans as a cross-cultural adaptation. Both groups were patients at pain centers, with approximately 100 patients in each group. Qualitative and quantitative data were collected to gain insight into cultural differences in the experience and adaptation of chronic low back pain. The results yielded a higher intensity of self-reported pain, more pain behavior, and a higher rate of self-reported depression among native

Puerto Ricans. However, no significant difference was found between the two groups in pain interference with work, social, or family activity or in the belief that they would overcome their pain. Similar results were found in a population-based study by Skovron et al.[49] They studied approximately 4,000 adults in Belgium, a bicultural country (French and Flemish) with a uniform healthcare system. Structured personal interviews collected information and explored the relationships of sociocultural and employment factors to the reported experience of low back pain. Their results suggest that sociocultural factors influence the expression of low back pain but not the risk of chronicity.

In the treatment and education of work-related musculoskeletal disorders, Hadler[21] discusses the predicament of a person with regional musculoskeletal symptoms. An individual with musculoskeletal symptoms can seek the advice of a healthcare provider inside or outside the place of employment. An individual who seeks care at the occupational health clinic is considered a claimant insofar as the injury is caused by and related to the performance of the job. Work-relatedness is usually not an issue when an employee seeks care outside the occupational health clinic. The choice of care and the expectation, beliefs, and/or insight are not completely understood. Beliefs and expectations are therefore an important concept in education for the prevention and treatment of work-related musculoskeletal disorders. For example, management in a company may believe that the use of back belts by all manual material handlers will solve all back problems. This is not true.[11] Union leadership may believe that company physicians provide poor care when recommending employees with nonspecific low back pain to return to work as early as possible. This is false.[11] Supervisors may believe that all employees reporting a work-related injury are malingerers. This has not been shown by any study to date. These examples suggest that when an employee reports an injury, caution is necessary to understand why the injury is being reported. Different environments bring about different beliefs. Beliefs are difficult to change. Long-term commitment by all parties involved, including management, union, healthcare providers, and the employee, is necessary to obtain change in the care of work-related musculoskeletal disorders.

EDUCATION AND CHANGE OF BEHAVIOR

Education may not necessarily lead to a change in behavior. Health and sickness behavior is resistant to alteration. A successful educational program must acknowledge the need for frequent and ongoing reinforcement.

Changing habits or behavior rarely happens overnight unless a crisis speeds the process. For example, a car accident may force an individual to use a wheelchair, at least for a period until the injury is healed. Changing health habits such as smoking or overeating

or altering pain behavior comes more slowly. It is a realization building up to a crescendo as an individual just decides to change and does it.[53] We change behavior over time; we get older and sometimes wiser. We change behavior if pain is induced. Work-related, nonspecific musculoskeletal pain is associated with a large component of fear avoidance behavior.[55] Education of the patient is an important tool. Equally important is to educate the healthcare provider and management/union that fear avoidance behavior exists and is treatable. This behavior is not treated by more diagnostic tests or more passive treatment, but by adequate information based on scientific evidence and written material to reinforce the message.

Educational programs that seek to change habits must be designed and discussed with the patient. The program should have a clear definition of what is considered "success," preferably with goals in writing so that all parties understand them. Goals and behavioral changes may conflict in an educational program. For example, we wanted to implement a standardized clinical examination for reported occupational low back pain in a large organization. All parties agreed—the physician, nurses, management, and union. They accepted the goal. However, when the program was implemented, the healthcare provider needed to change the way in which examinations were performed and information was recorded, which now included asking the patient to undress and completing a standardized medical examination form. The clinical examination therefore took longer at first. This procedure conflicted with the number of patients scheduled to be seen in the occupational health center every day. An extensive educational effort by the research team solved the problem, including the establishment of a monthly feedback system that addressed the concerns of all parties, and compliance was obtained.

In the pain behavior domain (pain lasting longer than 7 weeks for nonspecific low backpain, otherwise usually defined as pain present for more than 3 months), the approach is often operant conditioning to change behavior. Education is one component in the concept of functional retraining either by work conditioning or by work hardening (see Chapter 24). When one attempts to change behavior in chronic pain patients, "well behavior" is to be positively reinforced. As for pain behavior, it has been shown that punishment is less effective than rewarding a behavior incompatible with pain behavior.[19,20] Prior experience of the consequences of pain behavior is integrated into the patient's cognitions and feelings about pain. Therefore they may play an important role in the anticipation of reward or punishment. Any pain sensation will be influenced by prior experience and the individual's expectations as to where the consequences will lead. This approach assumes that regardless of why pain behavior occurs (e.g., nociception, adverse effects of disuse, or overguarding), behavior can be changed by education and positive reinforcement. An extensive discussion of the psychological and social factors in the diagnosis and treatment of musculoskeletal disorders is presented in Chapter 6. This biopsychosocial model should be understood when patients are evaluated for apparent confounding obstacles to recovery from work-related symptoms.

PATIENT EDUCATION

The first contact between the patient and the healthcare provider is crucial[4,17] and requires more time. It is here that trust between the two parties is established and patients decide whether they will rely on the treatment or advice proposed. In work-related musculoskeletal conditions, ill-defined symptomatology is often encountered. The impact of communication has been documented to be more important in these conditions, especially communication regarding agreement about the nature of the problem. Studies also show that provider confidence in the diagnosis and optimism about recovery can affect the patient's outcome.[5,11,12,52] In the first encounter, the patient often visits the clinician to retrieve information. Barsky[4] makes the observation that patients "seek not so much palliation or cure, but rather knowledge and education or perhaps even a diagnostic label for their condition." It is in the latter part of this statement that difficulties may arise in work-related musculoskeletal disorders. Abenhaim et al[2] studied more than 2000 back-related worker's compensation cases in the province of Quebec. Those given a specific diagnosis incurred more absenteeism from work.

There could be several reasons for this outcome. The pathophysiology for some diagnoses may be slower (for example, sciatica) than for nonspecific back pain. A specific diagnosis may be dealt with differently on an administrative level or may require additional diagnostic tests and consultations that delay return to work. Labeling a patient with a specific diagnosis can carry the message that the condition is serious and warrants additional time lost from work. For example, a diagnosis of degenerative changes of the spine is classified as a "disease." Thus it is important to reassure patients with nonspecific low back pain that a serious disease is not present but it is a critical component in any discussion of likely diagnoses.[7]

So what should we do as clinicians? What does the patient expect? Pain is both a sensory and an emotional experience.[27] Pain itself is private and perceived only by the individual.[40] In the first encounter with a patient, the clinician can gain useful information by observing the patient's pain behavior. Pain may not be related directly to the degree of tissue damage.[39] The pain expressed in action or words is influenced by a wide range of psychological variables on the process of pain behavior. Patients expressing too much pain in relation to the eventual injury need to be more carefully reassured that the condition is benign if that is the case. Clinicians often have an intuitive grasp of these concepts, but it nevertheless needs to be pointed out that patients with "abnormal" pain behavior need extra reassurance. An increased awareness by the clinician of somatic functioning has been shown to be a predictor of chronic pain, particularly in patients with low back pain.[38] Pain and its control are also discussed at greater length in Chapter 5 of this text.

Deyo and Diehl[17] studied patient satisfaction with medical care for low back pain. The most frequent source of dissatisfaction cited by the patients was failure to receive an adequate explanation for their problems. Patients who perceived less contentment with the encounter wanted more diagnostic tests, were less prone to see the same clinician again, and were also more concerned about a serious illness. A conclusion from this study is the importance of giving the patient an unambiguous message and making sure that the information given was understood. In the recently published guidelines for acute low back pain,[11] the summary of the findings states "that educating patients about back problems may reduce the use of medical resources, decrease patient apprehension, and speed recovery."

Information given by the clinician can furthermore be reinforced by handing out educational material, which is a simple, low-cost intervention with amazingly good results. Roland and Dixon[47] and Symonds et al[51] studied the effect of educational material in randomized control trials. Both studies showed increased patient satisfaction and less healthcare utilization in the follow-up period. Symonds et al[51] also found significantly less absenteeism among patients receiving written information, including fewer stress-related factors, as compared with verbal information about posture and low back pain. It can therefore be concluded that providing information to the patient is crucial, although the optimal content of the information given needs to be studied more.

Computer technologies may provide opportunities for increased access to information on CD-ROM, networks, and interactive sessions tailored to the patient's condition and specific interest.[41] Studies of the use of such tools are currently under way by several research groups.[56] These tools are designed to enhance the clinician's message to the patient and to facilitate decision making by the patient. They may also affect healthcare utilization.

SCHOOLING—A MORE STRUCTURED APPROACH

Back and neck schools provide teaching for a group of patients with similar symptomatology. The group format is thought to provide an economical and efficacious way to transmit information to patients in a supportive atmosphere where patients and instructors can exchange ideas freely. Classes usually comprise 4 to 12 individuals who meet for five to seven sessions consecutively. The term "school" is used to encourage learning and retention of information.[50] Topics included in the back school are typically the causes of injury, anatomy and physiology of the spine, fitness, posture, personal lifestyle, and the relationship between stress and pain.[43] Back schools were very popular during the 1980s, until recently when several reviews and meta-analyses were performed.[16,30,31,35,48] Cohen et al[16] cite 89 publications dealing with back schools. All review papers were inconclusive regarding the efficacy of back school treatment. At most, this type of intervention is marginally effective. A problem with most studies on back school intervention is the poor quality of the study design, including issues of inadequate control groups, the absence of blinded evaluation, faulty statistical methods, poor description of contents, small numbers of patients in each group, noncompliance, and no description of dropouts. Despite the lack of evidence about their efficacy, back schools continue to proliferate. Clinical teams using this type of intervention may want to assess or reassess their success rates when back school is used as the sole mode of clinical treatment for their patients with low back pain, including pain of acute or chronic duration.

COMBINED PROGRAMS INCLUDING EDUCATIONAL EFFORTS

Clinical practice for work-related musculoskeletal disorders commonly uses combined programs including exercises, education, stress management, and other modalities. Increased attention is warranted for these programs. Despite the problem that the contribution of each component is not well understood, the outcome effect is superior in combined programs.* Again, most of the experience and studies have dealt with work-related nonspecific low back pain. However, it seems reasonable to generalize the knowledge gained from these studies to other nonspecific occupational musculoskeletal complaints. The theoretical rationale behind combination programs is that educational concepts can be (1) reinforced by exercises for well-being, (2) practiced for better understanding of the concept, and (3) continuously fed back to the patient for positive reinforcement of "well behavior."

In 1977, Bergquist-Ullman and Larsson[10] performed a randomized controlled trial that included three groups in an occupational setting. They found a significantly shorter duration of sick leave for a combination program including the Swedish back school and an individual workplace visit for each patient as compared with manipulation and short-term diathermy treatment at 1-year follow-up. Unfortunately, the study did not use a blinded evaluator. Choler[15] performed a controlled trial in Goteborg, Sweden, on two urban populations. The Swedish back school was used in combination with fitness training and a work site visit when the team (an orthopaedic surgeon, a nurse, and a physical therapist) deemed it necessary. Patients who had been off work for more than 6 weeks were allowed to participate after a careful standardized evaluation was performed by an orthopaedic surgeon. The study also included an educational program for all primary care physicians in the geographic area. The population and healthcare providers in the control area received no intervention. The results were most encouraging in as much as they were associated with 90% less disability in the intervention group.

A similar approach was used by Lindstrom et al[33,34] in a randomized control trial at the Volvo company in Sweden. The aim of the study was to determine whether an operant-conditioning behavioral approach was effective in blue-collar workers who were sick-listed for more than 8 weeks because of nonspecific low back pain. The program consisted of measurement of functional capacity, a workplace visit, back school education, and an individually designed exercise program. The program was very successful in returning patients to work and significantly reduced long-term sick leave. These last two studies did not use a blinded evaluator, which may have biased the results. Nevertheless, they give an indication that education may contribute to successful outcomes measured as return to work in an occupational setting. Because of the study design, these studies cannot answer to what extent the educational component contributes to success. One observation in the study of Lindstrom et al[33] is that patients in the intervention group continued to improve substantially and significantly in fitness, mobility, and strength until 1 year of follow-up. We can only speculate that the educational component was helpful in convincing the patient that it is safe to move while regaining function. Major educational efforts are one component in functional restoration programs.[9,24,32,37] No studies have yet evaluated the educational component per se in these programs. Treatment programs are reviewed under their respective body segment chapters in Part IV.

IMPROVING PATIENT EDUCATION AND COUNSELING

International interest in patient education and counseling has increased. The first international congress on patient education and counseling, held in Amsterdam in 1977, led to the establishment of a journal, *Patient Education and Counseling*. In 1991 the International Medical Benefit/Risk Foundation was established in Geneva, Switzerland. Their first report on "Improving Patient Information and Education on Medicines" was published in 1993.[28] Although the report is generic in its approach concerning the intake of medicine, it warrants some review. The most important common findings of the survey carried out in Europe, Japan, and North America were as follows: At least 50% of the patients fail to take their medicine properly. The largest gap in patient understanding of prescription medicines is a general lack of awareness and understanding of side effects. The majority of patients still do not ask their physician or pharmacist questions about prescribed medicine.

*References 3,8,11,15,24,33,34,37.

Much needs to be done to foster thinking both by patients and by healthcare providers in terms of the risk and benefits of suggested care. In general, healthcare providers have been ineffective patient educators. Insufficient attention has been given to improving the communication skills of healthcare professionals and to refining these skills in continuing educational programs. Pressure to control costs limits the time that healthcare providers spend consulting patients, regardless of the healthcare system. Finally, patient information and education continue to rely almost exclusively on written material despite problems with literacy and the increasing influence of nonprint communications media everywhere. These findings are important for care providers in occupational settings. In light of continuously shrinking healthcare budgets, an effective healthcare provider may be the only one spending real time educating the patient, distributing materials, setting realistic goals, and ensuring that a treatment plan is understood.

DEFINING SUCCESS OF AN EDUCATIONAL PROGRAM

Return to work is often the desired outcome of a successful program in an occupational environment. This objective should be shared by the employee, management, unions, and also by healthcare providers.

Defining success is not a simple task for an educational intervention. Hall, McIntosh, and Melles[22] studied the impact of perspective on the determination of successful outcomes in four groups in Canada. The groups were the treating staff, the referring physician, the third-party sponsors, and the patients. The outcome measures were ranked for six items: return to work, pain control, functional improvement, increased strength including range of movement, attitude shift, and acquired knowledge. Physicians and patients considered pain control by far the most important. The treating staff and third-party sponsors considered pain control most important for patients who were working, functional improvement most important for patients with work restriction, and return to work most important for patients who were not working. This study underlines the importance of determining the criteria for success before intervention. Success should also be determined by all parties involved. An educational program may be very successful from the patient's perspective but totally ineffective by the third-party sponsors if return to work is not achieved. Much improvement is needed to define success for educational programs related to occupational musculoskeletal impairment. The inconsistency and conflicting results may be a reflection of poor or narrow definitions or unreasonable expectations about the impact of education.

EDUCATION IN PRIMARY PREVENTION

Prevention intervention would be the ideal solution for occupational settings. Primary prevention aims at reducing the injury or illness before it arises. In the area of work-related musculoskeletal disorders, results are inconclusive. There may be several reasons. It is difficult to identify which employees are at risk and motivate individuals in high-risk jobs or individuals who engage in high-risk behavior to change their behavior.[42] In the current working draft on the *Control of Work-Related Cumulative Trauma Disorders,*[3] the prevention effort is described as a process including four distinct components: a surveillance component, a job analysis and design component, a medical management component, and a training component. This document has emphasized the importance of training and education and accentuates the importance of management commitment, the need for a written document describing the eventual program and implementation, the importance of employee involvement, the allocation of resources, and the need for continuous evaluation. Although there is weak evidence of success of primary prevention educational programs, the evidence is encouraging for the process approach in preventing long-term disability.[18,54,58,60]

One of the key components of these programs is to educate management in appropriate ways of responding to employees' complaints and/or reported injuries. The other key component is to have active and open communication between the parties involved and to create a shared "ownership" of ideas, success, and even failures. The shared ownership approach may reduce the risk of making the same mistake over and over again when new educational programs are instituted. Fitzler and Berger[18] trained management in the positive acceptance of low back pain. Employees were encouraged to report low back pain troubles. Company nurses provided in-house conservative treatment that included worker education. One of the goals of this approach was to keep workers on the job by modifying their duties when necessary. The employee was referred to a company physician when needed. Treatment and progress were closely monitored, and the company reduced its compensation cost tenfold over a 3-year period.

A comprehensive primary prevention program was carried out in a telephone plant in Norway.[1,57] The intervention was based on clinical follow-up over a period of 8 years. Commitment was obtained by management and unions, and an ergonomic program including work station design was implemented. This process approach included a large effort in the education of all parties involved and resulted in reduced musculoskeletal sick leave (from 23 days to 2 days) and reduced turnover (from 30% to 8% of total man labor years). Although none of these studies were controlled, they indicate that algorithms with a structured approach and set goal are more successful than unstructured approaches.

SUMMARY

Education and training are important concepts in the management of work-related musculoskeletal disorders. There is weak evidence that education by itself is efficacious for the patient. However, the evidence is strong regarding successful outcomes in combined programs that include educational efforts. In general, there is a need to improve patient education, counseling, and the communication skills of healthcare professionals related to musculoskeletal disorders. Also needed is a definition of what constitutes "successful outcomes" of educational programs. Perhaps the most important message of this chapter is the need for industry to make a long-term commitment to a process-oriented approach in the prevention and treatment of musculoskeletal disorders. This approach should include surveillance, medical management, job analysis and design, and training for all involved parties. Continuous evaluation is recommended, but the goals for a successful outcome must be defined before the program is started and careful measurement tools must already be in place to assess the individual and organizational progress toward those goals.

Acknowledgment

This chapter was partially funded by NIOSH/CDC Grant No. U60/CCU 206153. I am grateful to Judy Trucios for her skillful word processing of this manuscript.

References

1. Aaras A et al: Postural load and the incidence of musculoskeletal illness. In Sauter SL, Dainoff MJ, editors: *Promoting health and productivity in the computerized office,* Philadelphia, 1990, Taylor & Francis Publishers; pp 68-93.

2. Abenhaim L et al: Prognostic consequences in the making of initial medical diagnosis of work-related back injuries, *Spine* 20(7):791-795, 1995.

3. American National Standards Institute: *Control of work-related cumulative trauma disorders, Part I: upper extremities,* Pub No Z-365, New York, 1995, The Institute.

4. Barsky AJ: Hidden reasons some patients visit doctors, *Ann Intern Med* 94:492-498, 1981.

5. Bass MJ et al: The physicians actions on the outcome of illness in family practice, *J Fam Pract* 23(1):43-47, 1986.

6. Bates M et al: A cross-cultural comparison of adaptation to chronic pain among Anglo-Americans and native Puerto Ricans, *Med Anthropol* 16:141-173, 1995.

7. Battie MC, Nordin M: Back school: education and training. In Wiesel SW et al, editors: *The lumbar spine,* ed 2, International Society for the Study of the Lumbar Spine, Philadelphia, 1996, WB Saunders; pp 989-998.

8. Bendix A, Bendix T: *Three different rehab programs for chronic low back pain: a randomized, 2-year questionnaire follow-up study.* Paper presented at the annual meeting of the International Society for the Study of the Lumbar Spine (ISSLS), Helsinki, June 1995.

9. Bendix T, Bendix A: Why intensive rehabilitation of patients with chronic back problems? *Nord Med* 108(12):321-322, 1993.

10. Bergquist-Ullman M, Larsson U: Acute low back pain in industry. A controlled prospective study with special reference to therapy and confounding factor, *Acta Orthop Scand* 170(1):117, 1977.

11. Bigos S et al: *Acute low back problems in adults. Clinical practice guideline No. 14,* AHCPR Pub No 95-0642, Rockville, Md, 1994, Agency for Health Care Policy and Research, Public Health Service, US Department of Health and Human Services.

12. Bush T, Cherkin D, Barlow W: The impact of physician attitudes on patient satisfaction with care for low back pain, *Arch Fam Med* 2:301-305, 1993.

13. Cedraschi C et al: The role of prior knowledge on back pain education, *J Spinal Disord* 5(3):267-297, 1992.

14. Cherkin D, Deyo RA, Berg AO: Evaluation of a physician education intervention to improve primary care for low back pain. I: Impact on patients, *Spine* 16:1173-1178, 1991.

15. Choler U: *Back-pain attempt at a structured treatment program for patients with low-back pain,* SPRI Report 188 Stockholm, 1985, Social Planerings-och Rationaliserings Instiutet Rapport (in Swedish).

16. Cohen JE et al: Group education interventions for people with low back pain: an overview of the literature, *Spine* 19(11):1214-1222, 1994.

17. Deyo RA, Diehl AK: Patient satisfaction with medical care for low-back pain, *Spine* 11(1):28-30, 1986.

18. Fitzler SL, Berger RA: Chelsea program: one year later, *Occup Health Saf* 52:52-54, 1983.

19. Fordyce WE: *Behavioral methods for chronic pain and illness,* St Louis, 1976, Mosby–Year Book.

20. Fordyce WE, Roberts AH, Sternbach RA: The behavioral managment of chronic pain: a response to critics, *Pain* 22:113-125, 1985.

21. Hadler NM: *Occupational musculoskeletal disorders,* New York, 1993, Raven Press.

22. Hall H, McIntosh G, Melles T: *The impact of perspective on the determination of successful outcome: how do you define success?* Abstract presented at Patient Education 200: International Congress on Treatment of Chronic Diseases, Geneva, June 1994.

23. Hall H et al: *The spontaneous onset of back pain.* Paper presented at the annual meeting of the International Society for the Lumbar Spine (ISSLS), Helsinki, June 1995.

24. Hazard RG et al: Functional restoration with behavioral support: a one-year prospective study of patients with chronic low-back pain, *Spine* 14(2):157-161, 1989.

25. Helman CG: Communication in primary care: The role of patient and practitioner explanatory models, *Soc Sci Med* 20:923-931, 1985.

26. Helman CG: Feed a cold, starve a fever—folk models of infection in an English suburban community and their relation to medical treatment, *Cult Med Psychiatry* 2:107-137, 1978.

27. International Association for the Study of Pain, Subcommittee on Taxonomy: Pain terms: a list with definitions and notes on usage, *Pain* 6:249-252, 1979.

28. International Medical Benefit/Risk Foundation: *Improving patient information and education on medicines,* Geneva, 1993, The Foundation.

29. Kay EA, Punchak SS: Patient understanding of the causes of medical treatment of rheumatoid arthritis, *Br J Rheumatol* 27:396-398, 1988.

30. Keijsers JFEM, Bouter LM, Meertens RM: Validity and comparability of studies on the effects of back schools, *Physiother Theory Pract* 7:177-184, 1991.

31. Klingenstierna U: Back schools & educational programs—a review, *Crit Rev Phys Rehab Med* 3(2):155-171, 1991.

32. LaCroix E, Emerson S: Therapy and work hardening for upper extremity disorders. In Millender LH, Louis DS, Simmons BP, editors: *Occupational disorders of the upper extremity,* New York, 1992, Churchill Livingstone International; pp 253-276.

33. Lindstrom I et al: Mobility, strength, and fitness after a graded activity program for patients with subacute low back pain: a randomized prospective clinical study with behavioral therapy approach, *Spine* 17:641-652, 1992.

34. Lindstrom I et al: The effect of graded activity on patients with subacute low back pain: a randomized prospective clinical study with an operant-conditioning behavioral approach, *Physi Ther* 72(4):39-53, 1992.

35. Linton SJ, Kamwendo D: Low back schools—a critical review, *Phys Ther* 67(9):1375-1383, 1987.

36. Lorig KR et al: Converging and diverging beliefs about arthritis: Caucasian patients, Spanish speaking patients and physicians, *J Rheumatol* 11:76-79, 1984.

37. Mayer TG et al: Objective assessment of spine function following industrial injury: A prospective study with comparison group and one-year follow-up, *Spine* 10(6):482-493, 1985, (1985 Volvo Award in Clinical Sciences).

38. McCreary C, Turner J, Dawson E: Emotional disturbance and chronic low back pain, *J Clin Psych* 36:709-715, 1980.

39. Melzack R, Wall P: *The challenge of pain,* Harmondsworth, England, 1982, Penguin.

40. Moffett JA-K, Richardson PH: The influence of psychological variables on the development and perception of musculoskeletal pain, *Physiother Theory Pract* 11:3-11, 1995.

41. Nelson CW: Helping patients decide: from Hippocrates to videodiscs—an application for patients with low-back pain, *J Med Syst* 12(1):1-10, 1988.

42. Nordin M, Weiser S, Halpern N: Education in the prevention and treatment of low back disorders. In Frymoyer J, editor: *The adult spine, principles and practice,* ed 2, New York, 1995, Raven Press.

43. Nordin M et al: Back schools in prevention of chronicity, *Bailliere's Clin Rheumatol* 6(3):685-703, 1992.

44. Piaget J: *The origin of intelligence in the child,* Harmondsworth, England, 1977, Penguin.

45. Popper K: *Knowledge and the body-mind problem,* London, 1994, Routledge.

46. Restack R: *The brain,* Toronto, 1984, Bantam Books; p 192.

47. Roland M, Dixon M: Randomized controlled trial of an educational booklet for patients presenting with back pain in general practice, *J R Coll Gen Pract* 39:244-246, 1989.

48. Schlapback P: Exercise in low-back pain. In Schlapback P, Gerber NJ, editors: *Physiotherapy: controlled trials and facts,* Basel, Switzerland, 1991, Karger; pp 25-46.

49. Skovron ML et al: Sociocultural factors and back pain: a population-based study in Belgian adults, *Spine* 19(2):129-137, 1994.

50. Snook SH, White AH: Education and training. In Pope MH, Frymoyer JW, Andersson G, editors: *Occupational low back pain,* New York, Praeger Publishers; pp 233-244.

51. Symonds T et al: *Can absenteeism due to low back trouble be reduced by psychosocial intervention at the workplace?* Paper presented at the annual meeting of the International Society for the Study of the Lumbar Spine (ISSLS), Helsinki, June 1995.

52. Thomas KB: General practice consultations: is there any point in being positive? *BMJ* 294:1200-1202, 1987.

53. Upton AC, Graber E: *Staying healthy in a risky environment. The New York University Medical Center family guide,* New York, 1993, Simon & Schuster; p 750.

54. Versloot JM et al: The cost-effectiveness of a back school program in industry. A longitudinal controlled field study, *Spine* 17(1):22-27, 1992.

55. Waddell G: Biopsychosocial analysis of low back pain, *Baillieres Clin Rheumatol* 6(3):523-557, 1992.

56. Weinstein J: Presidential lecture. Presentation at the annual meeting of the International Society for the Study of the Lumbar Spine (ISSLS), Helsinki, June 1993.

57. Westgaard RH, Aaras A: The effect of improved workplace design on the development of work related musculoskeletal illnesses, *Appl Ergonom* 16:91-97, 1985.

58. Westgaard RH et al: Muscle load and illness associated with constrained body postures. In Corbett EN, Wilson JR, Manenica I: *The ergonomics of working postures,* London, 1986, Taylor & Francis; pp 5-18.

59. Williams MM et al: A comparison of the effects of two sitting postures on back and referred pain, *Spine* 16(10):1185-1191, 1991.

60. Wood DJ: Design and evaluation of a back injury prevention program within a geriatric hospital, *Spine* 12:77-82, 1987.

PART III

Prevention

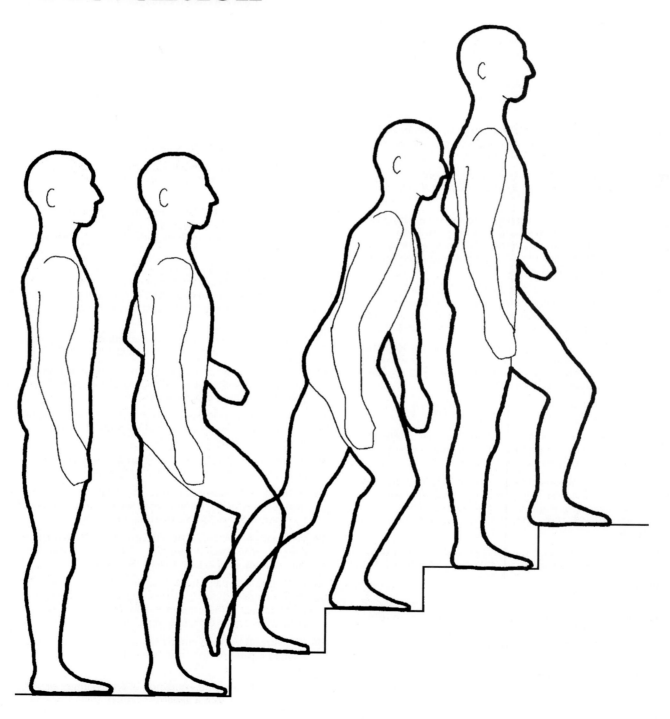

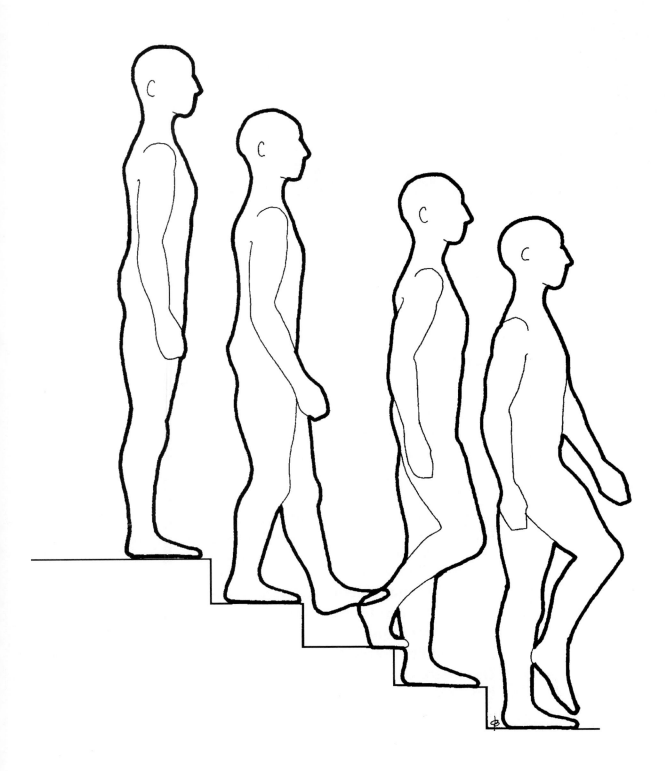

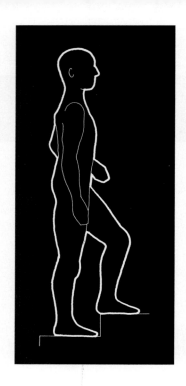

Chapter 18

Prevention

Malcolm H. Pope
Gunnar B.J. Andersson

CONTENTS

The World Health Organization (WHO) divides prevention into three categories: (1) primary prevention, or measures taken to prevent the clinical manifestation of a disease before it occurs, for example, immunizations for childhood infections or the introduction of National Institute for Occupational Safety and Health (NIOSH) limitations to lifting activities on the job; (2) secondary prevention, or measures taken to arrest the development of a disease while it is still in the early asymptomatic stage, for example, the treatment of asymptomatic hypertension to prevent stroke or ergonomic intervention to prevent clinical symptoms in a patient with spondylolisthesis; and (3) tertiary prevention, or measures taken to minimize the consequences of a disease (or injury) once it has become clinically manifested, for example, coronary bypass surgery for a patient with intractable angina or disk excision to treat cauda equina syndrome. Tertiary prevention includes medical and surgical therapy, as well as socioeconomic measures. The Americans with Disabilities Act (ADA) legislates one form of tertiary prevention to a certain degree.

The three classes of prevention are shown in **Figure 18-1**. It should be clear that generally but not always, prevention becomes more difficult and expensive as one moves from primary toward tertiary prevention. It should also be clear that primary and secondary prevention, as well as secondary and tertiary prevention, tend to overlap as they relate to low back pain (LBP), which will be used as an example throughout this chapter.

When prevention is discussed, it is also useful to differentiate between approaches applied to society in general, such as fluoridation of drinking water, and more individual approaches, such as advice against smoking. The first is passive and does not require participation of the individual, whereas the second is clearly active. Compliance will always be an issue when individual approaches are considered. Changes at the workplace can be considered intermediate in that they require both the good intentions of management and the acceptance and compliance of the worker.

Efforts to prevent LBP, particularly in the workplace, have become increasingly important because diagnostic and therapeutic approaches have proved inadequate to curb the soaring incidence and cost of this problem.[3,4] During the past 60 years, a variety of strategies have evolved for predicting and preventing low back injuries and low back disability. Most such methods can be classified as primary, secondary, or tertiary prevention strategies, but there is considerable overlap. In the context of occupational LBP and disability, primary prevention itself involves several distinct elements, including preemployment or preplacement testing of workers, training workers in the safe and effective performance of job tasks, ergonomic job design or job modification, back school education, the use of lifting belts and other corsets, and employee fitness programs. Secondary prevention strategies aim to identify those with mild or recurrent back pain who are at a high risk for low back disability and to intervene appropriately and early enough to change the predicted outcome (i.e., prevent disability). Such interventions may take many forms, including treatment, education, ergonomic counseling, and job modification. Tertiary prevention includes treatment and rehabilitation strategies to minimize the consequences of LBP, reduce the duration of chronicity or disability, restore function, and return people to work. Workplace changes to accommodate workers with back pain can also be labeled tertiary. It should be clear from the aforementioned that primary, secondary, and tertiary prevention issues overlap to some degree in the area of back pain. For those reasons we will divide this chapter further into prevention of LBP in asymptomatic individuals and prevention of disability from LBP in symptomatic workers.

The cost of implementing any given strategy must be weighed against its projected efficacy in preventing back pain or disability. As indicated earlier, prevention strategies can be implemented at different points in the natural history of pain or impairment, after a back pain episode but before chronicity, or after the condition has become chronic. In each instance, the target population

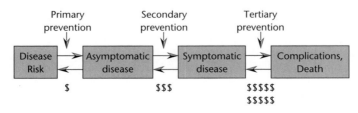

Figure 18-1. The potential course of a disease and the opportunities for prevention.

is unique and the cost-effectiveness of any preventive measure depends on the relationship between its cost and the likelihood of minimizing low back episodes or chronicity.

For instance, if only 5.2% of the working population is likely to experience an impairing low back episode, the likelihood of identifying those individuals by preplacement screening is small; moreover, statistics show that a much smaller percentage can be expected to become permanently disabled. That is, most of these workers will not contribute to the escalating costs associated with low back disorders. It would not be economically defensible, therefore, to invest large numbers of dollars in worker capacity evaluation at this point, and an inexpensive evaluation procedure might be desirable. However, in the case of workers who have experienced LBP in the past or who suffer an LBP episode or injury on the job, a more expensive evaluation procedure might be cost-effective. Such an evaluation would provide a basis for specifying retraining or job redesign criteria that will allow the individual to continue working.

PREVENTION OF LOW BACK PAIN IN ASYMPTOMATIC INDIVIDUALS

To institute true primary prevention of LBP, we should know what constitutes the disease risk. Unfortunately, our knowledge lacks detail. Low back pain is a symptom and not a disease or injury. In spite of our superficial knowledge, there is considerable scientific evidence and common sense knowledge that permit specific suggestions for primary prevention programs. For example, we know that LBP can occur from mechanical trauma, either isolated or repeated. Although we do not know the precise limits at which physical loads become harmful or how individual factors influence those limits, we have developed a great deal of useful information. This knowledge can be used to reduce the physical workload on the lower part of the back.

Six main approaches are used to prevent LBP in asymptomatic individuals:

1. Ergonomics and workplace design
2. Preplacement screening
3. Education and training
4. Fitness programs (back and aerobic exercises)
5. Mechanical supports (lifting belts and corsets)
6. Risk factor modification

Ergonomics and Workplace Design

Job design (and redesign) attempts to prevent LBP by reducing or eliminating work-related risk factors. It has been estimated that up to 25% of low back injuries in industry could be prevented if workplaces were properly designed. Recommendations resulting from ergonomic analyses of workplaces are usually prioritized so as to maximize employee safety and minimize costs to

industry. For example, a typical prioritization scheme might be (1) fix immediately (imminent danger of injury), (2) fix soon (no immediate danger), (3) fix when equipment is shut down, (4) redesign and fix if the cost-benefit ratio is acceptable, and (5) redesign the next time equipment is built or purchased.

Preplacement Screening

Employee screening and selection techniques distinguish those considered fit for the job from those who are not. Screening might include but is not limited to obtaining a medical history, physical examination, and functional capacity testing. Any fitness or functional capacity testing must be based on actual job demands so as not to violate Equal Employment Opportunity Commission (EEOC) and ADA regulations. Also, the development and implementation of a preplacement screening program require careful attention to safety of administration, reliability, practicality, and predictiveness.

Education and Training

Educational programs can help employees become aware of the various risk factors for low back injury and strategies that can be used to minimize the risk. Programs range from simple pamphlets to comprehensive "back school" programs. Most training programs are inexpensive and easy to implement, although training new employees and requiring periodic review can add to the cost. The program contents vary widely but might be designed to provide an understanding of basic anatomy and physiology, mechanisms of injury, concepts of biomechanics and ergonomics, injury prevention procedures, and stress and pain management. In addition, such programs might encourage workers to question the suitability of their work environment, teach new approaches to movement or new techniques for performing tasks, demonstrate the need for physical fitness, and emphasize the workers' responsibility to follow safety guidelines. Separate programs should be developed and implemented for supervisors and managers.

The scientific basis for the effectiveness of education programs has recently been evaluated by Lahad et al and King. King[7] concluded that the evidence of the efficacy of back schools is limited and controversial, whereas Lahad et al[8] found minimal evidence to support the use of educational strategies to prevent LBP. A lack of well-controlled studies contributes to the uncertainty about the value of education, which may be most useful in combination with other prevention strategies or in symptomatic individuals.

Fitness Programs

On- or off-the-job fitness and exercise programs may be effective in reducing the incidence of low back and other musculoskeletal injuries in the workplace. Lahad et al[8] concluded that "there is limited evidence based on randomized trials and epidemiological studies that exercises to strengthen back or abdominal muscles and to improve overall fitness can decrease the incidence and duration of low back pain episodes." In the randomized studies reviewed by Lahad et al,[8] subjects in the intervention groups had fewer days of work lost because of back pain or fewer days with back pain than did controls. None of the studies had a follow-up exceeding 18 months, however. Aerobic exercises appear to be as effective as specific trunk muscle strengthening exercises.

Mechanical Supports (Lifting Belts)

The use of back supports (typically lifting belts) has become a popular prevention strategy in recent years. Their use is based on mechanical concepts, including an increase in intraabdominal pressure, restriction in movements, and general support to the spine. None of these mechanical actions has been worked out. Clinical trials are contradictory, and there currently appears to be insufficient scientific support to recommend the use of back belts for back pain prevention.[8]

Risk Factor Modification

Not knowing enough about risk factors makes this approach difficult. Because occupational factors are considered under job design and redesign, only individual risk factors that are potentially modifiable are considered here. Smoking has been identified as a risk factor in cross-sectional and prospective studies.[8] Obesity is another risk factor less consistently linked to LBP. Smoking cessation and weight loss have not been studied for prevention with appropriate methodology. This is also true for psychological and psychiatric factors.[12] Lahad et al[8] concluded that "although there is no evidence supporting risk factor modification for preventing low back pain (smoking cessation and weight loss), there are other reasons to recommend the interventions."

PREVENTION OF LOW BACK DISABILITY IN SYMPTOMATIC WORKERS

Classic secondary prevention is very difficult because we do not know how to identify asymptomatic "disease" that contributes to LBP in industrial workers. Regular screening programs therefore have limited value. Secondary and tertiary prevention initiatives tend to overlap, particularly with respect to recurrence. Previous LBP, for example, increases the risk of a subsequent episode, and this knowledge is useful in both secondary and tertiary prevention. Most low back school programs should be considered secondary (and tertiary) preventive programs because the person enrolled has already had LBP at one time or another, and back schools were developed with that target group in mind.

It is critically important to consider how to prevent disability in workers with ongoing, chronic, or recurrent LBP. Once an employee has sustained a low back injury or episode of acute LBP, appropriate management of both the medical and compensation aspects of the case becomes critical because the interests and priorities of all those involved may not be the same. The physician seeks to cure the patient by medical intervention; the employer wants to keep the job intact and have the employee return to work as soon as possible; the insurance company wants a quick medical resolution and low compensation liability; and the employee wants to be free of pain and return to normal function, which usually means returning to work as soon as possible. The best injury management model places equal importance on the goals of healing and returning to work. The longer the absence from work, the less likely eventual return to the job. It is likely that psychological factors influence the functional outcome of work-injured employees who cannot return to work within a short period of time. Injury management programs include not only treatment but also such components as case management, early return-to-work programs, job accommodation, and disability prediction.

Surveillance

Surveillance is the ongoing systematic collection, analysis, and interpretation of health and exposure data in the process of describing and monitoring, for example, LBP. The need for occupational health and safety actions can be determined from surveillance data and intervention programs planned, implemented, and evaluated. Passive surveillance involves the use of existing records and data such as Occupational Safety and Health Administration (OSHA) 200 logs and insurance records. Such data are usually immediately available. Active surveillance means that information of importance is actively collected and analyzed. Most commonly, this is done by using a survey questionnaire.

Used appropriately, surveillance can be helpful to determine priority areas for intervention. There is currently no scientific evidence, however, that surveillance reduces the incidence, severity, or cost of back injuries, although anecdotal data suggest that it does. Surveillance is further discussed in Chapter 2.

Case Management

A good injury case management program should include a standardized and coordinated approach to the management of a work injury, a written care plan with goals and timetables for treatment and return to work, and tracking of medical progress. Case management programs should focus on avoiding counterproductive activities and treatments such as inappropriate or delayed initial treatment, prolonged bed rest (or lack of activity), treatment exclusively by drugs, and a failure to consider the potential for reinjury.

Early Return-to-Work Programs

Early return-to-work programs encourage employers to assist the employee in returning to work as soon as possible after an injury. This might involve developing light-duty positions to minimize the risk of reinjury until the employee is fully healed. Programs that keep injured workers on the job, even when they can only perform minor functions, prevent chronicity and long-term disability.

Job Accommodations

Job accommodations can also increase the likelihood of successful return to work after an injury. Three principal ways of accommodating employees who are impaired or disabled are client matching, job restructuring, and job modification. Client matching, the simplest and most efficient way to return a person with a disability to work, involves ensuring that job requirements are consistent with the employee's present abilities. If employees cannot return to their previous jobs, an alternative job is found that they can perform without risk of reinjury. Client matching requires no or minimal job modification. Job restructuring is a "no tech" way of accommodating an injured or disabled worker that involves eliminating or reassigning tasks that the individual cannot perform. For instance, restructuring a job by reassigning heavy lifting tasks to another person would enable a worker with low back injury to return to work sooner and thus to work while recovering from the injury. Job modification and redesign generally imply provision of some type of hardware or assistive device to enable individuals to perform the requisite job tasks. Machinery, equipment, or the job environment can be modified or adapted to enable an injured worker to return to work and prevent subsequent injuries. Occasionally, jobs can be eliminated by changing technology.

Disability Prediction

Developing methods to predict disability early after injury has attracted some interest. For example, Cats-Baril and Frymoyer[2] have worked on the development and testing of a multivariate model by which one can identify patients with low back injury who are at risk of becoming disabled. The model allows for identifying such individuals on their first clinic visit and matching them with the most appropriate and cost-effective treatment strategies. Identification of those at risk for disability is critical for several reasons. As described earlier, individuals who remain out of work for more than 6 months after a low back injury are less likely to return to work. It is this small proportion of patients with LBP that accounts for the largest share of costs. Moreover, if those at risk for disability can be identified before their conditions become chronic, the likelihood of successful rehabilitation can be greatly enhanced.

TREATMENT

Selection of the proper treatment to reduce the chronicity of LBP and prevent recurrence may be the most immediate, practical, and cost-effective preventive possibility, but it is totally redundant if primary prevention is effective. Early recognition of the problem and proper management are important to reduce the number of patients who will become chronic sufferers. Weisel, Feffer, and Rothman[11] showed that early and careful management dramatically reduced the impact of LBP in terms of lost time at work, treatment cost, and direct cost to industry. Recently developed guidelines for the treatment of LBP provide excellent guidance and are discussed in Chapter 22.

The assessment of when a patient can be allowed to return to work safely is based on poorly developed technology. Also yet to be explored is for whom and at what time modifications in the workplace and the work routine can aid in reducing LBP chronicity or recurrence. Even when chronic symptoms have developed, it is important to encourage work activities in some form to avoid all the secondary problems of chronic disability.

Of particular interest when treatment and rehabilitation strategies are chosen, given the natural history of LBP, are interventions that alter the course of chronicity and curtail disability. Low back pain is a symptom, and given the apparent complexity and unpredictability of its onset, as well as the fact that so many people experience back pain at one time or another, there may be little hope of eliminating back pain per se.[10] However, reducing chronicity and, in particular, disability is a realistic and cost-effective goal. For those who have been disabled by back pain for 6 months or more, the chances of a successful return to work without significant intervention are small. Although treatments for LBP have traditionally been disappointing, recent rehabilitation programs aimed at restoration of function, that is, return to work despite LBP, have been shown to be highly successful. Such programs incorporate a comprehensive approach to rehabilitation by attending to the functional, psychosocial, and medicolegal factors associated with illness and recovery.

Mayer et al[9] and Hazard et al[5,6] have reported unprecedented success in returning to work those with chronic disabling LBP as a result of a comprehensive rehabilitation program. Both groups have implemented a program combining functional restoration and counseling, guided by objective measurement of physical function; however, the clinical and socioeconomic settings differed. Mayer et al[9] reported that 87% of program graduates, as compared with 41% of a comparison group, were working 2 years after program participation. Similarly, Hazard et al[6] found, after 1 year, that 81% of program graduates, 40% of program dropouts, and 29% of those denied program participation (by their insurance carriers on the basis of program cost and prior experience with pain centers) were working. Further information about these programs is provided in Chapter 23 of this text.

Psychosocial and behavior techniques also hold promise for the prevention of chronicity. It appears that programs that incorporate these techniques have results superior to those of programs that ignore them.[12] Once back pain has become chronic, psychosocial and behavioral intervention is almost always necessary for successful rehabilitation.

CONCLUSIONS

In spite of the less than concrete scientific evidence on the ultimate effectiveness of any of the proposed preventive routes, all avenues should be explored in light of the magnitude of the LBP problem. Combined prevention programs have proved effective in reducing the frequency of low back complaints, at least in the shorter perspective. Prevention programs should be introduced early, before "bad habits" have developed, and repeated throughout life. Workers should be made aware that they can themselves influence their LBP situation and should be charged with that responsibility. The workplace should be improved as needed and work methods optimized, and workers should not have to exert themselves at or above their actual strength limits. If injured, a program of diagnosis, care, and rehabilitation should be put into immediate effect. This may be unrealistic and optimistic, but it is important to attempt to make a difference in the prevention of LBP. However, we should also be aware that these approaches will not lead to a total extinction of LBP, but will help workers understand its cause(s) and improve our treatment programs.

References

1. Bigos SJ et al: *Acute low back problems in adults. Clinical practice guideline 14*, ACHPR Pub No 95-0642, Rockville, Md, 1994, Agency for Health Care Policy and Research, Public Health Service, US Department of Health and Human Services.

2. Cats-Baril W, Frymoyer JW: Identifying patients at risk of becoming disabled because of low back pain: the Vermont Rehabilitation Engineering Center predictive model, *Spine* 16(6):605-607, 1991.

3. Chaffin DB: Functional assessment for heavy physical labor, *Occup Health Saf* 1:24-64, 1981.

4. Frymoyer JW, Mooney V: Current concepts review: occupational low back pain, *J Bone Joint Surg* 68A(3):469-474, 1986.

5. Hazard RG, Fenwick JW, Kalish SM: Disability exaggeration in patients with chronic low back pain: correlations with psychological factors. Presentation at the annual meeting of the International Society for the Study of the Lumbar Spine, Kyoto, Japan, May 1989.

6. Hazard RG et al: Functional restoration with behavioral support: a one-year prospective study of patients with chronic low back pain, *Spine* 14(2):157-161, 1989.

7. King PM: Back injury prevention programs: a critical review of the literature, *J Occup Rehabil* 3:145-158, 1993.

8. Lahad A et al: The effectiveness of four interventions for the prevention of low back pain, *JAMA* 272:1286-1291, 1995.

9. Mayer TG et al: Objective assessment of lumbar function following industrial injury, *Spine* 10:482-493, 1985.

10. Waddell G: A new clinical model for the treatment of low-back pain, *Spine* 12:632-644, 1987.

11. Weisel SW, Feffer HL, Rothman RH: Industrial low back pain: a prospective evaluation of a standardized diagnostic and treatment protocol, *Spine* 9:199-203, 1984.

12. Weiser S, Cedraschi C: Psychosocial issues in the prevention of chronic low back pain—a literature review, *Baillieres Clin Rheumatol* 6:657-684, 1992.

PART IV

Clinical Evaluation and Patient Care

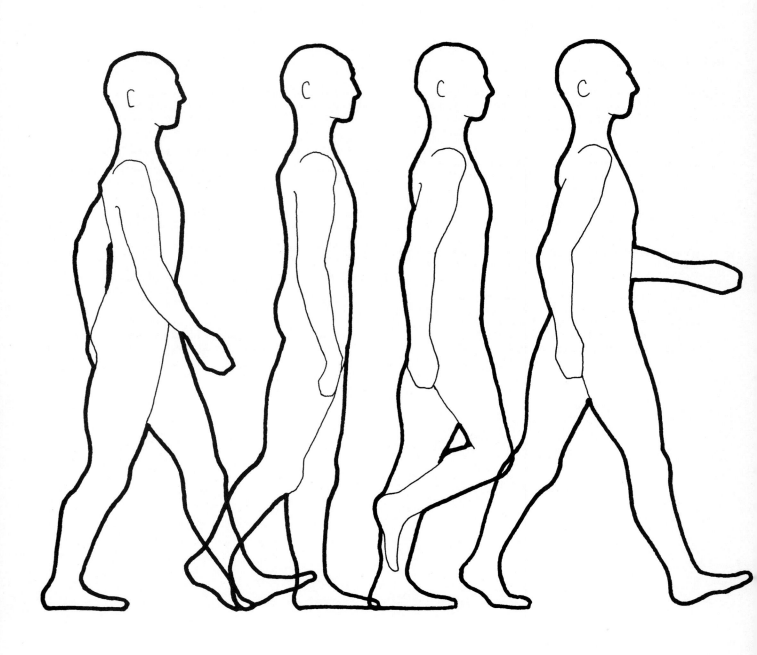

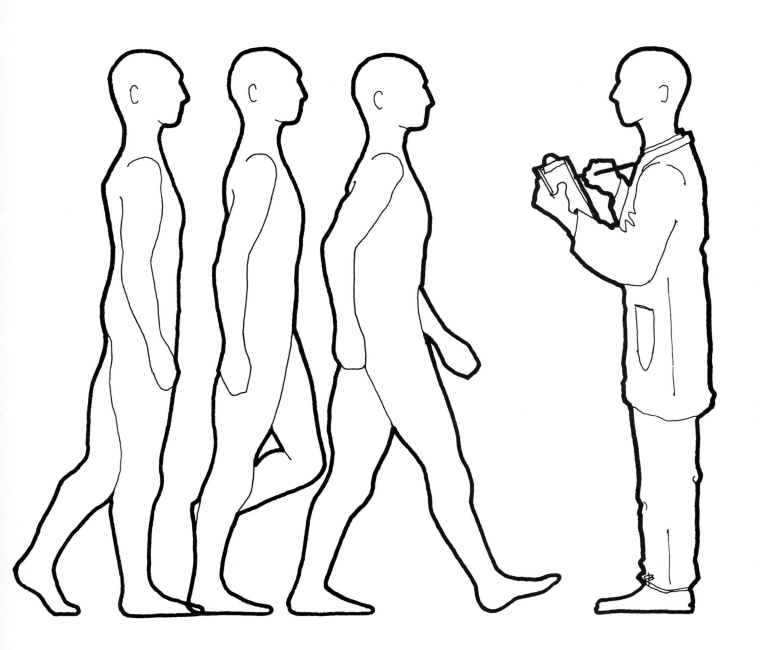

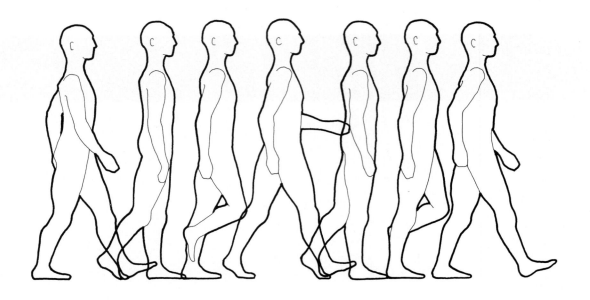

SECTION 1

Low Back

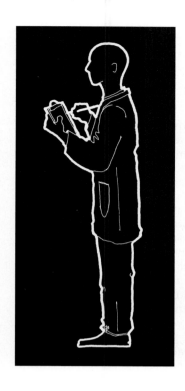

Chapter 19

Epidemiology of the Back

Michele Crites Battié
K. Tapio Videman

CONTENTS

The social and economic impact of back pain and related disability in industrialized countries is well recognized. Back pain is the second leading reason for all physician visits.[24] In addition, back injury complaints are the most expensive category of industrial injury claims[86] and the most common cause of disability in adults under 45 years of age.[70] In response, there are many workplace programs and medical services designed to prevent back problems or minimize their negative consequences. But little progress has been made in alleviating this common condition or its consequences.

When the underlying condition and risk factors for an ailment are understood, prevention and treatment strategies can be rationally based and well directed. In such situations, interventions are likely to be successful. Unfortunately, medical science still lacks information sufficient to guide the prevention and treatment of common back pain. Epidemiologic studies have sought to gain information that could be helpful in guiding these efforts. Epidemiology generally refers to the study of occurrence rates of diseases and, of particular interest, factors associated with disease occurrence or nonoccurrence. The primary goal of such studies is to obtain information about the cause of disease, and it is this aspect of epidemiology that will be the focus of this chapter. However, challenges of the most basic nature have hindered epidemiologic studies of back problems. A primary example is the lack of adequate measures of back symptom–related problems and their environmental determinants.

CHALLENGES FACING EPIDEMIOLOGIC STUDIES OF BACK PROBLEMS

Defining the Problem

Although there is a tendency to approach back pain as though it were a specific disease or injury state, in the vast majority of cases we are dealing with reported symptoms rather than verifiable physical pathology.[87] Miettinen[65] cautions that epidemiologic studies based solely on a complaint have limited value and that inferences to pathology can be misleading. A complaint is an active behavior and, as such, can be influenced by a variety of factors other than physical pathology. Also, there is poor correlation between degenerative changes and the degree of disability. Basic problems encountered in studying pain complaints include qualifying and quantifying the pain experience and controlling the effects of individual and cultural factors on pain perception and interpretation. Studies also can be complicated by uncertain reliability in a person's recall of symptoms,[76] as well as by variations in how researchers define the presence of symptoms.[80]

Moreover, back pain is identified through numerous different reporting systems, primarily health surveys and symptom complaints noted in clinical or workplace settings. In the United States, for example, pain in the workplace becomes known or registered through the filing of an incident report or worker's compensation claim. Taylor[92] has described a complex chain of events that leads to the production of industrial insurance and sickness data and makes it clear that the occurrence of back pain incidents registered in the industrial setting cannot be equated to the occurrence of morbidity. Failure to distinguish between studies of different back-related outcomes such as spine pathology, back symptom complaints, industrial injury claims, absenteeism, and long-term disability may lead to inaccurate conclusions and misleading generalizations. Thus any reviews of study results must consider the type of back-related outcome and the potential biases of the system through which it was registered. An example of the potentially large effect of health system differences was provided by Cherkin et al,[23] who compared rates of back surgery in 11 developed countries and examined the association between these rates and the number of neurologic and orthopaedic surgeons per capita. They found that the rate of back surgery was at least 40% greater in the United States than in any of the other countries investigated and that the U.S. rate was more than four to five times that of England and Scotland. They also found that the rate of back surgery was positively correlated with the number of surgeons per capita (**Fig. 19-1**).

Assessment of Occupational Exposures

In the United States and many other countries, back pain in industrial workers is typically referred to as an "injury." Injury status implies work-related causation, such as from traumatic accidents, overexertion, or structural fatigue of spinal structures caused by, for example, heavy or repetitive loading. It has been argued, however, that the growing problem of back pain in industrialized countries may be based on legislation and sociocultural factors rather than an increase in the incidence or severity of underlying pathology.[61,69,102]

The role of physical loading has been controversial, particularly because heavy occupational loading has declined in recent decades whereas back pain disability has increased. Many cross-sectional studies have reported associations between heavy physical work and low back pain and disability,[45,46,62,78,88,95] but some have not.[25,72,82] Prospective studies have also found mixed results.[15,39,57] Similarly, an increased prevalence of back pain has been shown among sedentary workers in some studies, but not all.[75]

Physical loading associated with work or leisure activity has many dimensions such as frequency, intensity, and duration. Yet adaptation to loading, which is an expected result of regular exercise, has received little

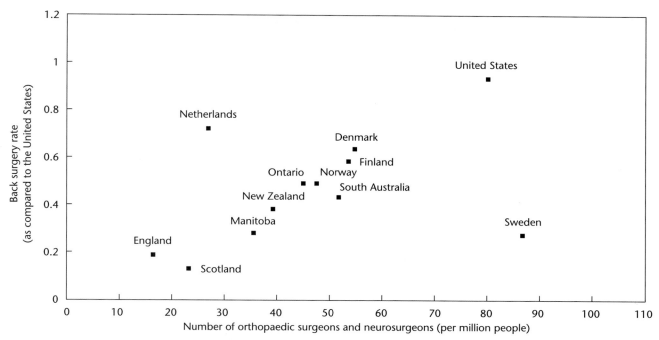

Figure 19-1 Relationship between the relative supply of orthopaedic surgeons and neurosurgeons in a country and the country's back surgery rate. *(From Cherkin DC et al: An international comparison of back injury rates,* Spine *19:1201-1206, 1994.)*

attention in studies of occupational loading. It is often stated that one reason for disability is that work demands exceed the capacity of the worker, although the level of physical demands over prior months is a primary determinant of individual capacity, which should include an adaptation of strength to daily work demands.

It is unclear whether high physical loading is an important factor in the etiology of conditions underlying back symptoms or whether it primarily serves to exacerbate symptoms from already existing conditions. Videman, Nurminen, and Troup[97] controlled for spine pathology and found that a history of back symptoms was correlated with physical loading. This finding supports the belief that loading exacerbates symptoms from existing conditions. The same study found that annular ruptures were more commonly found in subjects who engaged in occupations involving heavy physical loading, which suggests that heavy loading can also lead to increased risk of some structural failures. However, controversy remains as to whether most degenerative changes identified in the spine are the cause of symptoms because such findings are also commonly found in symptom-free persons.*

Occupational exposures that appear frequently on lists of suspected risk factors are *vehicular vibration* and *physical loading involving heavy lifting, bending, twisting, and sustained nonneutral postures.*[2,3,31,51] It is evident that virtually all inhabitants of industrialized countries

*References 19, 20, 42, 43, 81, 104.

are exposed to all these factors during work or leisure time. Exposure is therefore a matter of degree, and reliable, valid methods of measurement are required. Unfortunately, practical tools to quantify the degree of exposure in epidemiologic studies of large populations are not fully developed. Further complicating measurement is that for many outcomes such as structural changes of the spine, there is a need for data on lifetime loading rather than simply current conditions.

Most studies have used the job title as an indicator of occupational loading. Although this is a simple method of estimating occupational exposure, it can be highly inaccurate. The activities and environments of persons with similar job titles can vary substantially, and the loading profiles of workers who remain in one occupation for many years can change greatly. Moreover, most persons hold several different types of jobs during their working years, and their current positions may poorly reflect the physical loading experienced over their working lives. It has also been shown that workers in sedentary jobs tend to engage in more physically loading leisure-time activities than do workers with physically heavy jobs,[48] which can confound attempts to investigate the effects of occupational loading.

Risk Factors versus Risk Indicators

Identifying factors associated with risk can give clues about causation, but an understanding of the basis for associations is required to formulate optimal prevention strategies. For example, Leino[53] showed that greater exercise activity was associated with fewer back symptom reports and back findings, and Videman et al[99] found that former elite athletes had significantly fewer back pain complaints than did nonathletes. If exercise has a protective effect and decreases the risk of back symptoms or spine pathology, then exercise participation could be expected to be beneficial for back pain prevention. However, exercise is also a marker for other healthy lifestyle behavior, as well as higher education, higher life satisfaction, and lower occupational physical demands and psychosocial problems.[83] This means that exercise is marker for other factors that can affect back pain reporting. In view of the fact that physical loading from certain forms of exercise and sports can increase spine pathology,[89,90,97] it is possible that exercise itself may not be directly beneficial and may even have some harmful effects on the spine and that other factors associated with exercise produce the apparent benefits. If this were the case and exercise were only a risk indicator, exercise without other changes in lifestyle would be unlikely to decrease back troubles. Before interventions are planned, it would be important to sort out whether exercise is a risk factor or only an indicator of "healthier" life conditions.

In a review article, Hildebrandt[41] found 24 work-related and 55 individual factors that had been reported by at least one source as associated with low back pain. Most of the work factors were variations of physical loading related to the work tasks and the work environment, as well as accident-related trauma and work content issues. Despite a few additions to the list of suspected risk factors over the past decade or so such as impaired fibrinolysis, smoking, and job dissatisfaction, for the most part there have been few new ideas to help explain the occurrence of back symptoms. Collectively, these factors explain little of the uncertainty in predicting back symptom reports and injury complaints. In a prospective, longitudinal study of back problems in more than 3000 U.S. manufacturing workers, data on more than 50 commonly suspected risk factors explained less that 10% of the uncertainty in predicting who would or would not file industrial back pain complaints.[16]

Retrospective and Cross-Sectional versus Prospective Study Designs

Most of the numerous studies of risk factors have been retrospective or cross-sectional and have investigated the presence or absence of various factors in persons with and without current or previous back problems.[84] Although retrospective studies can be helpful in generating hypotheses about factors that may increase risk, they are prone to bias as well as present a "chicken and egg" dilemma. In addition, many of these studies have relied on insurance company data and employment records, which are often incomplete and categorized for purposes other than research into back problems.[2] Prospective, longitudinal studies are needed to identify and better understand risk factors, but few

have been conducted because of the time and expense typically required. The authors are aware of only 15 such studies: 2 studies of factors associated with hospitalization for herniated disks,[39,44] 6 studies of back symptoms and 1 study of sciatic pain revealed from health surveys,* and 6 studies of industrial back pain reports.†

RISK INDICATORS FOR BACK SYMPTOMS

More than a half-dozen prospective studies have collected baseline information on suspected risk factors, typically through physical examination and questioning, and later the data were analyzed to identify predictors of subsequent back symptoms identified on a follow-up survey **(Table 19-1)**.

Gyntelberg[35] reported the first such study in 1974. He analyzed back-pain complaints in relation to individual physical, demographic, lifestyle, and work-related factors, as well as medical history, in nearly 5000 men employed in a variety of occupations in Copenhagen. Another Danish study of nearly 1000 men and women examined the effects of individual physical, occupational, and medical history factors in greater depth.[14,15] In a subsequent study of nearly 3000 men and women from a variety of occupations in England, Troup and colleagues[94] concentrated on individual physical factors and psychophysical lifting capacity as possible predictors of back pain complaints. Videman, Rauhala, and Asp[98] looked specifically at back pain complaints among Finnish women who had completed their first year of nursing work. Two other Scandinavian studies have reported on individual physical factors associated with back pain complaints, recalled after longer follow-up periods, among military conscripts and metal industry workers.[40,56]

Overall, the studies consistently revealed a history of back symptoms to be a strong indicator of future risk. In view of the fact that recurrence is a widely accepted aspect of the natural history of back symptoms, this finding is not surprising. Other factors having strong associations with future complaints were comorbidities, particularly other types of symptom complaints, measures of psychological distress, and lower socioeconomic status. It is likely that the latter is a marker for a variety of potential risk factors such as occupational exposure, other lifestyle attributes that may increase risk, and generally poorer health.

Other factors that were associated to lesser degrees with back symptoms were greater age, smoking, chronic coughing, heavy occupational physical demands, and in nurses, poor patient handling skill. Although patient handling skill was associated with back pain episodes of sudden onset, it was not associated with back pain of

*References 4, 35, 40, 53-57, 77, 94, 98.
†References 7-9, 13, 17-19, 21, 22, 68, 74, 80.

Table 19-1 Back symptoms on health surveys: results of prospective, longitudinal studies.

Factors Considered	Danish Male Employees,[35] Varied Occupations (5249/?, 1 yr)*	English Employees,[94] Varied Occupations (2891/?, 1 yr)	Copenhagen Residents[14,15] (928/1136 1 yr)		Finnish 1st-Year Nurses[98] (255/255, 1 yr)		Swedish Military Conscripts[40] (999/6824, 2-3 yr)	Finnish Metal Industry Workers[4,53,56] (902/2653, 10 yr)
			First Episode	Recurrent LBP†	Sudden Onset	Gradual Onset		
DEMOGRAPHIC								
Age	↑	↑‡	↓	↑				0
Education			0	0				
Living alone/ divorced	↑		0	0				
Social status	↓↓		↓	↓ (men)				
LIFESTYLE								
Smoking	↓	↑ (women)	↑	↑			↑	0
Leisure-time physical activity	0		0	0				↓ (men)
Sport partici-pation	↓							
Nonwork "physic stress"	↑							
WORK RELATED								
Job classifica-tion			0	0				0
Physical de-mands rating			0	0	↑↑	0		
Physical exertion	↑↑							
Patient han-dling skill					↓↓	0		
Social support/job satisfaction			↓	0				
"Physic stress" at work	↑							↑ (women)
ANTHROPOMETRIC								
Standing height	↑, >181 cm	0	0	0	0	0	↑ (extremes)	
Obesity (rela-tive weight)	0	0	0	0	0	0		0
Leg length inequality			0	0			0	
Scoliosis							0	

Continued.

Table 19-1	Back symptoms on health surveys: results of prospective, longitudinal studies—continued.							
Factors Considered	Danish Male Employees,[35] Varied Occupations (5249/?, 1 yr)*	English Employees,[94] Varied Occupations (2891/?, 1 yr)	Copenhagen Residents[14,15] (928/1136 1 yr) First Episode	Recurrent LBP†	Finnish 1st-Year Nurses[98] (255/255, 1 yr) Sudden Onset	Gradual Onset	Swedish Military Conscripts[40] (999/6824, 2-3 yr)	Finnish Metal Industry Workers[4,53,56] (902/2653, 10 yr)
STRENGTH/ENDURANCE								
Isometric strength		0‡	0	↓ (women)	0	0	0	0
Isometric back endurance			↓ (men)	0				
Sit-up test		0‡	0	↓ (women)	↓	0		0
Psychophysical strength		0‡						
Aerobic capacity	0							
FLEXIBILITY								
Flexion/lateral bending		0‡	↑ (men)	0	0	0		
Extension		0‡						
Length of hamstrings			0	↓ (women)	0	0		
PSYCHOMETRIC								
Health locus of control					0	0		
Personality inventory (MHQ, MMPI)								
Anxiety					↑	0		
Hysteria					0	↑↑		
IQ test							0	

gradual onset, which was the more common complaint. This study of first-year nurses also found that over 50% had experienced back pain before entering the nursing profession, which raises questions about whether primary prevention should be considered before adult work life.[98]

In all the aforementioned studies, back symptoms were found to be very common; the 1-year incidence ranged from 27% to 47%.[35,94] Gyntelberg's summary[35] of the situation still holds true, "Only small differences in risk of low back pain between various groups exist. Therefore, it can be stated that everybody is at high risk, although some groups still have a risk above the high normal." It should be emphasized that the previously mentioned findings were based on reports of pain revealed on follow-up questionnaires or interviews. The symptoms did not necessarily result in visits to healthcare providers, filing of incident reports at the workplace, or time loss from work. They were merely reports from persons who when asked, recalled having had back-related symptoms during a specified period.

RISK INDICATORS FOR INDUSTRIAL BACK PAIN REPORTS

Industrial back "injury" incident reports and claims are specific definitions of back problems to be distin-

Table 19-1	Back symptoms on health surveys: results of prospective, longitudinal studies—continued.						
Factors Considered	Danish Male Employees,[35] Varied Occupations (5249/?, 1 yr)*	English Employees,[94] Varied Occupations (2891/?, 1 yr)	Copenhagen Residents[14,15] (928/1136 1 yr)		Finnish 1st-Year Nurses[98] (255/255, 1 yr)		Swedish Military Conscripts[40] (999/6824, 2-3 yr)	Finnish Metal Industry Workers[4,53,56] (902/2653, 10 yr)
			First Episode	Recurrent LBP†	Sudden Onset	Gradual Onset		
MEDICAL HISTORY								
Back pain history		↑↑		↑↑			↑↑	↑↑
Non–back symptom complaints	↑↑		↑	↑				
Healthcare utilization (for pain)			↑ (men)	↑ (men)				
Respiratory symptoms/ decreased function	↑	↑						

*Number of volunteers/number solicited, follow-up interval.

†LBP, low back pain; MHQ, Middlesex Hospital Questionnaire; MMPI, Minnesota Multiphasic Personality Inventory; ↑, positive association; ↑↑, strong positive association; ↓, negative association; ↓↓, strong negative association; 0, not a predictor.

‡Troup et al found that the use of a test battery including all of these factors slightly enhanced the predictive value of subjects' history of low back pain.

guished from symptom complaints solicited on surveys such as those discussed in the previous section. Most developed countries have systems for filing complaints of work-related injuries and illnesses with their own sets of rules, costs, and benefits. In discussing such systems in the United States, Hadler[36] has emphasized that filing a complaint forces the person to conform to the worker's compensation paradigm. He states that "By definition, work task description is causal. By inference, the illness is a manifestation of major structural damage." We found six prospective, longitudinal studies reported from the United States and Canada that have investigated predictors of industrial back pain reports **(Table 19-2)**. Most have focused on individual physical factors.

Chaffin and Park[22] conducted a study of back incident reports in 411 men and women who engaged in manual lifting in their work at an electronics manufacturing company. The study focused on the effects of occupational lifting and mismatches between individual strength and job requirements. They reported an association between low back pain reporting and jobs with higher lifting strength requirements in terms of position and magnitude of the weight lifted. They also found a higher incidence of back pain reporting in persons who demonstrated less strength on isometric strength testing than that deemed necessary to meet job demands. Strength in excess of job requirements did not appear to have an additional protective effect. However,

only 25 low back incidents were reported among the study group, and the result did not reach statistical significance and awaits verification.

Cady et al[21] later reported on physical fitness as an indicator of risk in 1652 firefighters over a 3-year period. Fitness was defined by a composite score based on aerobic capacity, strength, and flexibility measures. They found that firefighters with low "fitness" levels were about nine times more likely to report a back injury than those in the "most fit" group. However, the few injuries reported among the highly fit were the most serious in terms of cost. The effects of age and other potentially confounding factors were not reported, making interpretation of the results difficult.

Isokinetic lifting strength was investigated as a predictor of low back injury claims among nurses in a more recent study by Mostardi et al.[68] They concluded that lifting strength was a poor predictor of subsequent back symptoms and injury reports. Another prospective study of back injury reports in nurses reported by Ready et al[74] reached similar conclusions about isometric lifting strength and other general fitness parameters. The factors that discriminated most between the nurses who did and did not report subsequent back injuries were previous receipt of compensation pay, smoking status, and poorer job satisfaction. A history of compensation has been associated with work loss caused by back problems in other studies as well.[80]

Table 19-2	Back symptom complaints in the workplace: results of prospective, longitudinal studies.					
Factors Considered	U.S. Aircraft Mfgr. Employees* (3020/4027, 4 yr)†	Electronics Mfgr. Employees[22] (411/?, 1 yr)	Firefighters[21] (1652/1900, 3 yr)	Nurses[68] (171/?, 2 yr)	Nurses[74] (131/574, 1.5 yr)	Canadian Aircraft Mfgr. Employees[80] (269/395, 1 yr)
DEMOGRAPHIC						
Gender	0†					
Age	↓	0				0
Education	0					
ANTHROPOMETRIC						
Standing height	↑ (men)	0			0	
Sitting height	0					
Arm span	0					
Weight	↑ (women)	0			↑	0
Obesity (relative weight)	0				↑	
LIFESTYLE						
Smoking	↑				↑↑	↑
Leisure-time physical activity						0
STRENGTH/ENDURANCE						
Isometric lifting	0	↓ (job matched)			0	
Isokinetic lifting strength				0		
Estimated maximal aerobic capacity	0		↓		0	
Abdominal strength					0	
Composite fitness score	0		↓			
TRUNK FLEXIBILITY					0	
OTHER PHYSICAL EXAMINATION						
Decreased patellar reflex	↑					
Decreased Achilles reflex	0					
Symptoms on SLR	↑↑					

| Table 19-2 | Back symptom complaints in the workplace: results of prospective, longitudinal studies—cont'd. |

Factors Considered	U.S. Aircraft Mfgr. Employees* (3020/4027, 4 yr)†	Electronics Mfgr. Employees[22] (411/?, 1 yr)	Firefighters[21] (1652/1900, 3 yr)	Nurses[68] (171/?, 2 yr)	Nurses[74] (131/574, 1.5 yr)	Canadian Aircraft Mfgr. Employees[80] (269/395, 1 yr)
PSYCHOSOCIAL						
Psychological distress	↑↑					
Health locus of control	0					
Family social support	0					
Stress level				0		
WORK-RELATED						
Social support/job satisfaction	↓↓			↓↓	↓↓	
Perceived physical demands	0					
Maximum weight lifted	0					
MEDICAL HISTORY						
Back pain history	↑↑	↑		↑		↑↑
Prior back-related compensation claim					↑↑	↑↑
Prior MVA					↑	
Healthcare utilization (for pain)	↑↑					

*References 7-9, 13, 16, 17
†Number of volunteers/number solicited, follow-up duration.
↑, positive association; ↑↑, strong positive association; ↓, negative association; ↓↓ strong negative association; 0, not a predictor; SLR, straight leg raise; MVA, motor vehicle accident.
From Battié MC, Videman T: Back pain: epidemiology. In Nordin M, Anderson G, Videman T, editors: Work-related musculoskeletal disorders, St Louis, 1995, Mosby–Year Book.

In the Boeing study, a prospective, longitudinal study of industrial back pain complaints in 3020 aircraft manufacturing workers, isometric lifting strength, maximal aerobic capacity, and range of motion in side bending and flexion were among the factors that were not associated with subsequent complaints. The strongest predictors of future back pain reports, other than having had current or recent back problems at the onset of the study, were negative perceptions of the workplace, including low job task enjoyment and social support, and emotional distress.[16] The only factor from the baseline physical examination that was strongly associated with future reporting was back pain elicited on straight leg raise testing,[7] which probably represents another aspect of recent or current back problems also known to influence future risk. These findings underline the multifaceted nature of back pain reporting in industry.

Although some factors have been identified as risk indicators, their practical value in predicting specifically who will or will not experience or report symptoms is poor. For example, a positive straight leg raise test in the aforementioned study more than doubled the risk of reporting, but fewer than 3% of the subjects had this finding and only one in five of these subjects reported subsequent back pain.[7] This result illustrates the inadequacy of such tests as preemployment or preplacement tools. It was similarly difficult to predict extended disability. In the Boeing study, the factors that contributed to the prediction of extended time loss and that differed significantly between claims of short- and long-term time loss were a low scale 10 score on the Minnesota Multiphasic Personality Inventory (MMPI), indicative of extroversion, and back pain elicited on straight leg raise testing as identified before filing of the back injury claim. Physical capacity measures and the psychological findings commonly seen in chronically disabled patients did not contribute significantly to predicting extended back pain disability in this group of claimants.[17]

A later extension of the Boeing study looked specifically at back incident reports that resulted in the formal filing of industrial insurance claims. Lower job satisfaction and a poorer employee appraisal rating by the employee's immediate supervisor were associated with back injury claims. Given the findings of the earlier analysis of back incident reports, this result was not surprising. A more notable finding of the later analysis was that these psychosocial factors were similarly associated with non–back injury claims as well. It would appear that certain psychosocial factors may predispose to the filing of injury claims, but the study did not provide evidence of significant differences between those who filed back injury claims and those who filed other types of injury claims.[12] Such findings caution against stereotyping persons who file back injury claims as being distinctly different psychosocially from those filing other injury claims. As Leavitt[52] stated, "The unfortunate problem is that stereotypes have consequences. Doubts raised by labels often shape evaluation and treatment of industrial workers in problematic ways, to the extent that their integrity and status as patients is challenged."

RISK INDICATORS FOR SCIATICA AND HOSPITALIZATION FOR HERNIATED DISK

We are aware of two prospective, longitudinal studies that have used hospital discharge data to investigate back-related hospitalization. In a study of World War II U.S. military recruits, military rank and the occupations of craftsman or foreman were associated with higher occurrence rates of hospitalization, whereas rates were lower among clerical occupations.[44] Men who were taller and heavier at the time of their recruitment also had a higher incidence of hospitalization. In a Finnish population-based study of 57,000 men and women followed over an 11-year period, men were 1.6 times more likely than women to be hospitalized for disk herniation.[39] Taller men and women were also more likely to be hospitalized; an association with weight was less clear. The risk of being hospitalized for a herniated lumbar disk or sciatica was lowest in professional occupations and highest among blue-collar workers and motor vehicle drivers.[49]

Riihimäki and co-workers[77] conducted a prospective study of sciatica among concrete reinforcement workers and house painters. During a 5-year follow-up period, 60% of the concrete reinforcement workers and 42% of the house painters had experienced sciatica. The only factors to enter a multivariate model as predictors of these symptoms related to a history of prior sciatica and back "accidents." The relative risk for a person with a history of previous sciatica was 3.4 times that of someone without such a history, and the relative risk related to having had a previous back "accident" was 1.2. Stress was also associated with higher occurrence rates of sciatica during follow-up. Separate analysis of the subset of workers without a history of sciatica before the 5-year follow-up showed that concrete reinforcement workers (with physically heavier jobs) had a relative risk of 1.5 times that of house painters. A history of prior back "accidents" was associated with a relative risk of 1.4.

The apparently high incidence of sciatica reported among concrete reinforcement workers and house painters is supported by another study, which found that in approximately 25% of a general population sample of working-age Finnish men, sciatica had been diagnosed by a doctor at some time.

FACTORS ASSOCIATED WITH SPINAL PATHOLOGY AND STRUCTURAL VARIATIONS

Knowledge of the macropathoanatomy and micropathoanatomy of the spine is limited, particularly as related to the importance of different structural findings. For example, we do not know the clinical value of osteophytes, disk space narrowing, annular ruptures, end-plate changes, intervertebral foramina and spinal canal anthropometry, and facet joint arthrosis. Until recent years, tools have not been available to examine these conditions among the general population. Consequently, studies of factors associated with the pathology of spinal structures have received relatively little attention as compared with studies of the occurrence rates of back symptom reports. Although disk pathology is commonly thought to be responsible for most back symptoms,[67] the specific condition underlying the symptoms remains unresolved for the majority of cases.[87] Also unclear is how to separate degenerative changes caused by physical loading, trauma, and other environmental exposures from age-related degeneration.

In an exceptional study of musculoskeletal findings based on 1000 consecutive autopsies, the occurrence rate of "spondylitis deformans" increased linearly from 0% to 72% between the ages of 39 to 70 years.[38] Although these findings relate to people and work conditions around the turn of the century and the definition of "spondylosis" is not clearly stated, the rapid linear increase is notable. In a review article, Miller, Schmatz, and Schultz[66] reported a similar increase in grades II to III disk degeneration from 0% at age 20 to about 90% at age 70 years. The authors also concluded that radiographic data are corroborated by macroscopic findings.

Frymoyer et al[33] compared the radiographs of three groups of men between the ages of 18 and 55 years: men with no history of back pain, men with moderate back pain, and men with severe back pain. In these three groups the frequency of Schmorl's nodes, claw spurs, disk heights at the L3-4 and L5-S1 levels, the disk vacuum sign, and transitional vertebrae was similar. The radiographic findings that differed in the three groups were traction spurs and/or disk space narrowing between L4 and L5, but these findings did not correlate with occupation, occupational lifting, or whole-body vibration. Riihimäki et al[79] found that concrete reinforcement workers had a relative risk of 1.8 for disk space narrowing as compared with house painters and a relative risk of 1.6 for "spondylophytes." They concluded that heavy physical work enhanced the degenerative process in the lumbar spine.

An autopsy study of 86 subjects by Videman, Nurminen, and Troup[97] showed that occupations that involved sitting, standing, and walking without heavy physical loading were associated with the least degeneration. Workers with heavy physical loading had the highest incidence of annular ruptures, and sedentary work was associated with the highest degree of general disk degeneration.

Genotype may also play an important role in the etiology of degenerative and structural variations of the spine.[11] Specifically, genetic predispositions have been suggested for scoliosis, ankylosing spondylitis, spondylolisthesis, and adolescent disk herniations on the basis of studies of the occurrence rates of these conditions within family members.[64,73,96] Radiographic studies of identical twins have revealed similarities implicating genotype in the development of hyperostosis affecting the ligaments of the spine,[91,93] juvenile lumbar disk herniation,[64] and Schmorl's nodes.[47] However, the sample sizes for these few investigations of identical twins have been very small, ranging from one to seven pairs.

Diskographic, radiographic, and computed tomographic methods are not used for general population studies because of the risks involved, and the value of ultrasonography is limited. Magnetic resonance imaging (MRI) is relatively expensive but safe if standard procedures are followed and can be used to increase our knowledge about the structural changes in the spine and associations with symptomatic conditions. Studies have found increased spinal degeneration among wrestlers, soccer and tennis players, weight lifters, and young gymnasts,[89,90] but these exposures represent extreme loading conditions and are associated with an increased risk of trauma. It is likely that data on MRI findings related to occupational loading will become available in the near future. Biochemical markers related to spine pathology are not yet available for use in epidemiologic research on occupational exposure, but research in this area is progressing.

In summary, the primary suspected explanatory factors for spinal degenerative findings are age, traumatic accidents or injuries, and heavy physical loading (which may include an increased number of injuries). Other suspected factors are vibration, inactivity, postural stresses, and genetic predisposition. It is also possible that chemical exposures accelerate degenerative changes, although with the possible exception of cigarette smoking,[10] evidence of this has not been demonstrated.

FACTORS ASSOCIATED WITH ONSET AND PERSISTENCE OF BACK-RELATED DISABILITY

There is evidence that back symptoms have always been present to some degree among humans and likely will always be. Episodes of these symptoms are, however, typically manageable and relatively short-lived. Of greater concern is the rapid rate of increase in back symptom–related disability. Although most persons recover from back symptoms relatively quickly and experience little disability, approximately 10% of back injury claimants with extended work loss account for approximately 80% of back-related industrial insurance costs.[86] Long-term disability is therefore the outcome that poses the greatest threat not only to the individual but also to society.

Disability is typically represented in the work environment as absenteeism. An examination of factors associated with illness absenteeism led Backenheimer[5] to conclude that "absence behavior is, in considerable measure, a cultural and social phenomenon." He also claimed that "a biological frame of reference is too narrow to explain the condition of being ill." There is growing evidence that these notions also apply to absenteeism and disability from back problems.

Long-term back pain disability is a relatively new phenomenon in the history of Western civilization, and its dramatic growth since World War II suggests that factors other than physical pathology may be influencing its development. This is not to say that back pain is not genuinely experienced by many working people or that severe symptoms do not cause physical limitations of some duration. On the contrary, numerous health surveys indicate that back symptoms are extremely common in both developed and Third World countries.[1,14,71,94,102] However, what appears to have changed in many societies is the public perception of

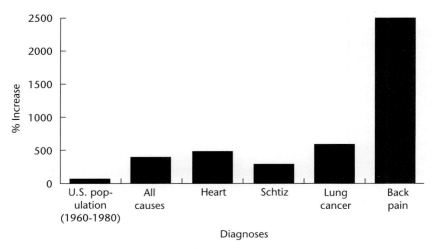

Figure 19-2 Social Security disability insurance awards by diagnosis: percent increase from 1957 to 1976. *Fordyce WE: Back pain, compensation, and public policy. In Rosen JC, Solomon LJ, editors: Prevention in health psychology, Hanover, N.H., 1985, University Press of New England.*

back pain as an "injury" or medical problem and its effect on work life in terms of disability.

One striking example of the tremendous growth in back pain disability seen in many of the developed countries comes from the U.S. Social Security Disability Insurance System, where from 1957 to 1976 the incidence of disability awards increased by approximately 2700%, a rate 14 times that of the population growth **(Fig. 19-2)**.[85] Similarly striking increases in the incidence of disability awards have occurred in Finland, Sweden, and England.[69]

Factors other than just the presence of back symptoms clearly influence back symptom reporting and disability. Of likely importance to the onset and persistence of disability are cultural norms,[1,102] socioeconomic conditions including unemployment rates[100,101] and opportunities for compensation,[34,37,52] emotional distress,[17,19,50] job satisfaction,[17,19] and the physical and social work environment.*

Compensation availability appears to affect the length of disability in the case of both surgical intervention[29,37] and conservative care.[34] Leavitt[52] noted that most studies that have cited an association between compensation and back pain reporting and disability failed to take into account the effects of physical demands of the job; these can affect the outcome and differ significantly between compensation and noncompensation groups. He attempted to disentangle the effects of these factors and found that work-related back symptom reports were associated with more time loss than were non–work-related back symptoms even after controlling for the degree of physical job demands. In addition, a recent related literature synthesis by Loeser, Henderlite, and Conrad[61] concluded that when all other factors are held constant, the existing economic studies imply a positive relationship between the level

*Reference 3, 17, 19, 22, 58-60, 75, 103.

of wage replacement benefits and both the incidence and duration of worker's compensation claims. The relative effect of benefit level appeared to be greater on claims duration than on claims incidence. This would suggest that a key issue may be to determine an optimal wage replacement ratio.

Medical management also has been implicated as a contributor to the growing disability problem. The rise in disability despite advances in medical technology, as well as increasing healthcare costs and utilization, led Frymoyer and Cats-Baril[32] to raise the question, "Have medical professionals of all types become part of the problem rather than part of the solution?"

CONCLUSION AND IMPLICATIONS

In past decades, back-related disability has increased dramatically, raising significant health and economic concerns. This has led back problems to receive much attention from those interested in primary prevention, treatment, and industrial insurance cost containment.

Most programs adopted by employers have aimed at preventing the occurrence of back symptoms or back "injuries." Although such a goal is appealing, there is little evidence to suggest that it is feasible to resolve the problem of work-related back pain and subsequent disability through primary prevention efforts. Effective prevention programs require a clear understanding of risk factors and the ability to alter them. It is evident from the information presented in this chapter that we are limited in our ability to predict who will report back problems, even when multivariate techniques that simultaneously consider several risk indicators are used.

The healthcare system also has failed to resolve this problem despite an increase in healthcare utilization.[32] In their defense, health, safety, and medical professionals have faced an almost insurmountable challenge: to prevent or effectively treat a malady without specific knowledge of the underlying condition or its etiology in the vast majority of cases. This state of knowledge has led to a lack of consensus in the medical management of low back symptoms. Not surprisingly, few treatments have demonstrated an effect beyond the natural history and placebo.[87] The variations in both conservative and surgical treatment practices led to the selection of back pain as one of the first nationally targeted problems for outcomes research in the United States, with funding provided by the Agency for Health Care Policy and Research (AHCPR),[26,27] and a subsequent mandate for the development of clinical practice guidelines.[28] Among the goals of such efforts are the synthesis and dissemination of the findings of medical research and expert opinion to improve the standard of care. The results of the AHCPR study are reported in Chapter 22.

High-quality medical research in part provides the basis for practice guidelines and for optimal decision making among clinicians. The need to elevate standards for research publications became evident from one of the most systematic, comprehensive evaluations of the state of knowledge reported to date by the Quebec Task Force on Spinal Disorders in 1987. Their initial literature search, encompassing the prior 10-year period, identified more than 7000 articles related to low back pain. Yet fewer than 3% of the articles were deemed to be of high scientific quality as judged by a review of the methodology.[87]

In the future it is likely that limited resources will necessitate a greater focus of interventions on factors with clear, strong associations and specific outcomes of interest. For example, if the goal is to decrease back injury claims, we should identify factors specifically related to this outcome, their relative importance, and the magnitude of their effects. Then we can focus on modifying those individual, occupational, or societal factors that appear to most influence back injury claims and are likely to result in the greatest reduction of the problem. For example, on the basis of studies to date of predictors of back injury claims, it might be interesting to examine the effects of interventions that affect various aspects of job satisfaction.

The dramatic increase in the incidence of back pain disability despite generally improved physical work conditions and the lack of clear evidence of a concomitant increase in spinal pathology may provide insight into the current problem. This growth also may be less of a puzzle in that sickness absenteeism and pensions depend only in part on "morbidity" and to a major degree on social security legislation and cultural and psychological factors. Although the role of the physical work environment should not be ignored, the increased incidence of back pain disability suggests a need for a broadened perspective on underlying conditions and risk factors for the development of disability and a closer examination of the effects of sociocultural, legislative, and medical management factors.

References

1. Anderson RT: Orthopaedic ethnography in rural Nepal, *Med Anthropol* 8:46-59, 1984.

2. Andersson GBJ: Epidemiological aspects of low back pain in industry, *Spine* 6:53-60, 1981.

3. Andersson GBJ: The epidemiology of spinal disorders. In Frymoyer W, editor: *The adult spine: principles and practice,* ed 1, New York, 1991, Raven Press; pp 107-146.

4. Aro S, Leino P: Overweight and musculoskeletal morbidity: a ten-year follow-up, *Int J Obes* 9:267-275, 1985.

5. Backenheimer MS: Demographic and job characteristics as variables in absences for illness, *Public Health Rep* 83(12): 1029-1032, 1968.

6. Battié MC, Videman T, Sarna S: *A comparison of risk indicators of osteoarthritis and back-related symptom complaints, hospitalizations, and pensions.* Proceedings of the International Society for the Study of the Lumbar Spine, Marseilles, France, 1993 (abstract).

7. Battié MC et al: Anthropometric and clinical measurements as predictors of industrial back pain complaints: a prospective study, *J Spinal Disord* 3:195-204, 1990.

8. Battié MC et al: A prospective study of the role of cardiovascular risk factors and fitness in industrial back pain complaints, *Spine* 14:141-147, 1989.

9. Battié MC et al: Isometric lifting strength as a predictor of industrial back pain, *Spine* 14:851-856, 1989.

10. Battié MC et al: Smoking and lumbar intervertebral disc degeneration: an MRI study of identical twins, *Spine* 16(9):1015-1021, 1991.

11. Battié MC et al: *Spinal morphology and degenerative changes in identical twins: similarities and differences.* Proceedings of the International Society for the Study of the Lumbar Spine, Chicago, 1992 (abstract).

12. Battié MC et al: *The effect of psychosocial and workplace factors on back-related and other industrial injury claims.* Proceedings of the International Society for the Study of the Lumbar Spine, Marseilles, France, 1993 (abstract).

13. Battié MC et al: The role of spinal flexibility in back pain complaints within industry: a prospective study, *Spine* 15:768-773, 1989.

14. Biering-Sørensen F: Physical measurements as indicators for low-back trouble over a one-year period, *Spine* 9:106-119, 1984.

15. Biering-Sørensen F, Thomsen C: Medical, social and occupational history as risk indicators for low-back trouble in a general population, *Spine* 11:720-725, 1986.

16. Bigos SJ et al: A longitudinal, prospective study of industrial back injury reporting, *Clin Orthop* 279:21-34, 1992.

17. Bigos SJ et al: A prospective study of work perceptions and psychosocial factors affecting the report of back injury, *Spine* 16:1-6, 1991.

18. Bigos SJ et al: *Premorbid risk factors for back pain disability greater than one month.* International Society for the Study of the Lumbar Spine, Chicago, 1992 (abstract).

19. Bigos SJ et al: The value of pre-employment radiographs for predicting acute back injury claims and chronic back pain disability, *Clin Orthop* 283:124-129, 1992.

20. Boden SD et al: Abnormal magnetic-resonance scans of the lumbar spine in asymptomatic subjects, *J Bone Joint Surg* 72:403, 1990.

21. Cady LD et al: Strength and fitness and subsequent back injuries in fire fighters, *J Occup Med* 21:269-272, 1979.

22. Chaffin DB, Park, KS: A longitudinal study of low back pain as associated with occupational weight lifting factors, *Am Ind Hyg Assoc J* 34:513-525, 1973.

23. Cherkin DC et al: An international comparison of back surgery rates, *Spine* 19:1201-1206, 1994.

24. Cypress BK: Characteristic of physician visits for back symptoms. A national perspective, *Am J Public Health* 73:389-395, 1988.

25. Damkot DK et al: The relationship between work history, work environment and low-back pain in men, *Spine* 9:395-399, 1984.

26. Deyo RA, Cherkin D, Conrad D: The back pain outcome assessment team, *Health Serv Res* 25:733-737, 1990.

27. Deyo RA et al: Cost, controversy, crisis: low back pain and the health of the public, *Annu Rev Public Health* 12:141-156, 1991.

28. Edelman B: Federal agency to draft low back pain guidelines, *Orthop Today* 12(4):10, 1992.

29. Flynn JC, Joque MPA: Anterior fusion of the lumbar spine. End result study with long-term follow-up, *J Bone Joint Surg* 61A:1143-1161, 1979.

30. Fordyce WE: Back pain, compensation, and public policy. In Rosen JC, Solomon LJ, editors: *Prevention in health psychology,* Hanover, N.H., 1985, University Press of New England, pp. 390-400.

31. Frymoyer JW: Back pain and sciatica, *N Engl J Med* 318:291-299, 1988.

32. Frymoyer JW, Cats-Baril WL: An overview of the incidences and costs of low back pain, *Orthop Clin North Am* 22:263-271, 1991.

33. Frymoyer JW et al: Spine radiographs in patients with low-back pain, *J Bone Joint Surg* 66A:1048-1055, 1984.

34. Greenough CG, Fraser RD: The effects of compensation on recovery from low back injury, *Spine* 14:947-955, 1989.

35. Gyntelberg F: One year incidence of low back pain among male residents of Copenhagen aged 40-59, *Dan Med Bull* 21:30-36, 1974.

36. Hadler NM: To be a patient or a claimant with a musculoskeletal illness. In Hadler NM, editor: *Clinical concepts in regional musculoskeletal illness,* Orlando, Fla, 1987, Grune & Stratton; pp 7-21.

37. Hanley EN, Shapiro DE: The development of low-back pain after excision of a lumbar disc, *J Bone Joint Surg* 71A(5):719-721, 1989.

38. Heine J: Uber die Arthritis deformans, *Virch Arch Pathol Anat* 260:521-663, 1926.

39. Heliövaara M, Knekt P, Aromaa A: Incidence and risk factors of herniated lumbar intervertebral disc or sciatica leading to hospitalization, *J Chronic Dis* 40:251-258, 1987.

40. Hellsing AL et al: Individual predictability of back trouble in 18-year-old men, *Manual Med* 2:72-76, 1986.

41. Hildebrandt VH: A review of epidemiological research on risk factors of low back pain. In Buckle PW, editor: *Musculoskeletal disorders at work,* London, 1987, Taylor & Francis Publishers; pp 9-16.

42. Hitselberger WE, Witten RM: Abnormal myelograms in asymptomatic patients, *J Neurosurg* 28:204, 1968.

43. Holt EP, Jr: The question of lumbar discography, *J Bone Joint Surg Am* 50:720, 1968.

44. Hrubec A, Nashbold BS: Epidemiology of lumbar disc lesions in the military in World War II, *Am J Epidemiol* 102:366-376, 1975.

45. Hult L: Cervical dorsal and lumbar spinal syndromes, *Acta Orthop Scand Suppl* 17:1-102, 1954.

46. Hult L: The Munksfors investigation, *Acta Orthop Scand Suppl* 16:1-76, 1954.

47. Hurxthal L: Schmorl's nodes in identical twins, *Lahey Clin Found Bull* 15:89-92, 1966.

48. Ilmarinen J et al: Changes in maximal cardiorespiratory capacity among aging municipal employees, *Scan J Work Environ Health* 17 (suppl 1):99-109, 1991.

49. Kelsey JL, Hardy RJ: Driving motor vehicles as risk factor for acute herniated lumbar intervertebral disc, *Am J Epidemiol* 102:63-73, 1975.

50. Klitzman et al: Work stress, non-work stress and health, *J Behav Med* 13:221-243, 1990.

51. *The Lancet* Editorial Reviews: *Risk factors for back trouble,* 8650:1305-1306, 1989.

52. Leavitt F: The physical exertion factor in compensable work injuries. A hidden flaw in previous research, *Spine* 17(3):307-310, 1992.

53. Leino P: Does leisure time physical activity prevent low back disorders? A prospective study of metal industry employees, *Spine* 18(7):863-871, 1993.

54. Leino P: Physical loading and mental stress as determinants of musculoskeletal disorders, *Acta Universitatis Tamperensis* A282:56-60, 1989.

55. Leino P: Symptoms of stress predict musculoskeletal disorders, *J Epidemiol Community Health* 33:293-300, 1989.

56. Leino P, Aro S, Hasan J: Trunk muscle function and low back disorders: a ten-year follow-up study, *J Chronic Dis* 40:289-296, 1987.

57. Leino P, Hasan J, Karppi S-L: Occupational class, physical workload, and musculoskeletal morbidity in the engineering industry, *Br J Ind Med* 45:672-681, 1988.

58. Linton SJ: Risk factors for neck and back pain in a working population in Sweden, *Work Stress* 4:41-49, 1990.

59. Linton SJ, Kamwendo K: Risk factors in the psychosocial work environment for neck and shoulder pain in secretaries, *J Occup Med* 31:609-613, 1989.

60. Linton SJ et al: The secondary prevention of low back pain: a controlled study with follow-up, *Pain* 36:197-207, 1989.

61. Loeser J, Henderlite S, Conrad D: Incentive effects of workers compensation benefits. A literature synthesis, *Med Care* 52:34-59, 1995.

62. Magora A: Investigation of the relation between low back pain and occupation. II. Work history, *Industr Med Surg* 39:504-510, 1970.

63. Matsui H, Tsuji H, Terahata N: Juvenile lumbar herniated nucleus pulposus in monozygotic twins, *Spine* 15(11):1228-1230, 1990.

64. Matsui H et al: Familiar predisposition and clustering for juvenile lumbar disc herniation, *Spine* 17(11):1323-1328, 1992.

65. Miettinen OS: *Theoretical epidemiology: principles of occurrence research in medicine,* New York, 1985, John Wiley & Sons.

66. Miller JAA, Schmatz C, Schultz AB: Lumbar disc degeneration: correlation with age, sex, and spine level in 600 autopsy specimens, *Spine* 13:173-178, 1988.

67. Mooney V, Brown M, Modic M: Clinical perspectives. In Frymoyer JW, Gordon ST, editors: *New perspectives on low back pain,* Park Ridge, Ill., 1989, American Academy of Orthopaedic Surgeons.

68. Mostardi RA, et al: Isokinetic lifting strength and occupational injury: a prospective study, *Spine* 17(2):189-193, 1992.

69. Nachemson AL: Problemets omfatting. In *Ont i ryggen, orsaker, diagnostik och behandling,* Stockholm, 1991, SBU; pp 18-28.

70. National Center for Health Statistics: *Prevalence of selected impairments, United States—1977,* DHHS Pub (PHS) 81-562, series 10, No 134, Hyattsville, Md, 1981, The Center.

71. Nyh S et al: Prevalence of low back pain and other musculoskeletal symptoms in Finnish reindeer herders, *Rheumatology* 20:406-413, 1991.

72. Partridge RE, Duthie JJR: Rheumatism in dockers and civil servants. A comparison of heavy manual and sedentary workers, *Ann Rheum Dis* 27:559-568, 1968.

73. Postacchini F, Lami R, Pugliese O: Familiar predisposition to discogenic low-back pain. An epidemiologic and immunogenetic study, *Spine* 13(12):1403-1406, 1988.

74. Ready AE et al: Fitness and lifestyle parameters fail to predict back injuries in nurses, *Can J Appl Physiol* 18(1):80-90, 1993.

75. Riihimäki, H: Low-back pain, its origin and risk indicators, *Scand J Work Environ Health* 17:81-90, 1991.

76. Riihimäki H, Videman T, Tola S: *Reliability of retrospective questionnaire data on the history of low back trouble.* Proceedings of the International Society for the Study of the Lumbar Spine, Kyoto, Japan, 1989 (abstract).

77. Riihimäki H et al: Predictors of sciatic pain among concrete reenforcement workers and house painters—a five-year follow-up, *Scand J Environ Health* 15:415-423, 1989.

78. Riihimäki H et al: Low back pain and occupation. A cross-sectional questionnaire study of men in machine operating, dynamic physical work and sedentary work, *Spine* 14:204-209, 1989.

79. Riihimäki H et al: Radiographic changes of the lumbar spine among concrete reinforcement workers and house painters, *Spine* 15(2):114-119, 1990.

80. Rossignol M, Lortie M, Ledoux E: Comparison of spinal health indicators in predicting spinal status in a 1-year longitudinal study, *Spine* 18(1):54-60, 1993.

81. Rothman RH: A study of computer-assisted tomography: introduction, *Spine* 9:548, 1984.

82. Sairanen, E., Brüshaber, L., Kaskinen M: Felling work, low-back pain and osteoarthritis, *Scand J Work Environ Health* 7:18-30, 1981.

83. Sarna S et al: Increased life expectancy of world class male athletes, *Med Sci Sports Exerc* 25(2):237-244, 1993.

84. Snook SH: Low back pain in industry. In White AA, Gordon SL, editors: *Symposium on idiopathic low back pain,* ed 1, St Louis, 1982, Mosby–Year Book; pp 23-38.

85. *Social Security Statistical Supplement (1977-1979),* HE 3.3/3:979, Washington, DC, 1979, Government Printing Office.

86. Spengler DM et al: Back injuries in industry: a retrospective study. I. Overview and cost analysis, *Spine* 11:241-251, 1986.

87. Spitzer WO: Scientific approach to the assessment and management of activity-related spinal disorders: a monograph for clinicians. Report of the Quebec Task Force on Spinal Disorders, *Spine* 12(suppl):s12-s15, 1987.

88. Svensson HO, Andersson GBJ: Low back pain in 40 to 47-year-old men: work history and work environment factors, *Spine* 8:272-276, 1983.

89. Swärd L et al: Back pain and radiologic changes in the thoraco-lumbar spine of athletes, *Spine* 15(2):124-129, 1990.

90. Swärd L et al: Disc degeneration and associated abnormalities of the spine in elite gymnasts. A magnetic resonance imaging study, *Spine* 16(4):437-443, 1991.

91. Taketomi E et al: Family study of a twin with ossification of the posterior longitudinal ligament in the cervical spine, *Spine* 17suppl 3:s55-s56, 1992.

92. Taylor PJ: International comparisons of sickness absence, *Proc R Soc Med* 65:577-580, 1972.

93. Terayama K: Genetic studies on ossification of the posterior longitudinal ligament of the spine, *Spine* 14(11):1184-1191, 1992.

94. Troup JDG et al: The perception of back pain and the role of psychophysical tests of lifting capacity, *Spine* 12:645-657, 1987.

95. Valkenburg HA, Haanen HCN: The epidemiology of low back pain. In White AA, Gordon SL, editors: *Symposium on idiopathic low back pain,* St Louis, 1982, Mosby–Year Book; pp 9-22.

96. Varlotta GP et al: Familiar predisposition for herniation of a lumbar disc in patients who are less than twenty-one years old, *J Bone Joint Surg* 73A:124-128, 1991.

97. Videman T, Nurminen M, Troup JDG: Lumbar spinal pathology in cadaveric material in relation to history of back pain, occupation and physical loading, *Spine* 15:728-740, 1990.

98. Videman T, Rauhala H, Asp S: Patient-handling skill, back injuries and back pain. An intervention study in nursing, *Spine* 14:148-156, 1989.

99. Videman T et al: *Elitesport as a predictor of back-related outcomes.* Proceedings of the 1993 American College of Sports Medicine Annual Meeting, Seattle, May, 1993 (abstract).

100. Volinn E, Van Koevering D, Loeser JD: Back sprain in industry. The role of socioeconomic factors in chronicity, *Spine* 16:542-548, 1991.

101. Volinn E et al: When back pain becomes disabling: a regional analysis, *Pain* 33:33-39, 1988.

102. Waddell G: A new clinical model for the treatment of low-back pain, *Spine* 12(suppl):632-644, 1987.

103. Wickström G et al: Previous back syndromes and present back symptoms in concrete reinforcement workers, *Scand J Work Environ Health* 4(suppl 1):47-53, 1987.

104. Wiesel SW et al: A study of computer-assisted tomography: 1. The incidence of positive CAT scans in an asymptomatic group of patients, *Spine* 9:549-551, 1984.

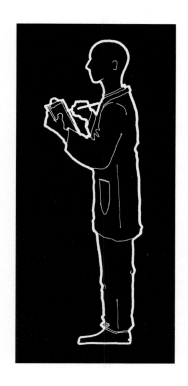

Chapter 20

Clinical Biomechanics of the Spine

Malcom H. Pope

CONTENTS

The spine is an important structure with many conflicting functions. The first function, mobility, provides the motion necessary for the activities of daily living. The second function is one of support for the body segments and any load moments that are applied by the worker. The third function is housing in which the spinal cord and nerve roots are protected. The last function is control, with the muscles acting through the vertebrae to precisely control the posture.

FUNCTIONAL SPINAL UNIT

The functional spinal unit (FSU) consists of two adjacent vertebrae, the interposed vertebral disk, and adjoining ligaments. The motion segment can be divided into anterior and posterior components. The anterior components are the vertebral bodies, the disk, and the attached ligaments; all the remaining structures are posterior components.[19]

The FSU is a structure in which the disk acts as a spring, the facet joints as a pivot, and the posterior ligamentous complex as another spring. Experiments have shown that the FSU exhibits coupled motion in which vertical translation also results in complex movements in other directions. The anterior elements of the FSU have a support function and a function of impact absorption, whereas the posterior elements control motion.

ANTERIOR PORTION

The major structural part of the anterior portion of the FSU consists of the vertebral bodies. These bear mainly compressive loads and are progressively larger caudally as the weight of the upper body increases (**Fig. 20-1**). Therefore, the vertebral bodies in the lumbar region are bigger than those in the thoracic and cervical regions. Compressive strength concomitantly gradually increases from the cervical spine down to the lumbar spine. Overall, the vertebrae are six times stiffer than the disks, three times thicker than the disks, and suffer half the deformation of the disks. The vertebrae are very important in shock absorption. Under compression, end-plate deformation precedes the expelling of hematopoietic contents from the vertebrae themselves.

The vertebrae are an expression of Wolff's law inasmuch as the trabeculae are oriented to resist the vertical compression forces and tensile forces through the spinous and transverse processes caused by muscle and ligament attachments. There is a zone of relative weakness anteriorly because of a lack of trabeculae. Compressive failure, particularly in an osteoporotic individual, occurs in this region.

The other major component of the anterior portion of the FSU is the intervertebral disk. The function of the disk is to distribute loads and restrain excessive motion. The disk is composed of the annulus fibrosus and nucleus pulposus. The annulus is made up of a series of sheets of collagen fibers, with the fibers of one sheet at a 30-degree angle relative to the neighboring sheet. Mathematical models show that with removal of the nucleus, interval stresses ensue as a result of the compressive forces being carried through the annulus. The inner portion of the disk, the nucleus pulposus, is rich in hydrophilic glycosaminoglycans in young adults, but with age the nucleus pulposus becomes progressively less hydrated.

Animal experiments have shown that disks are avascular structures and that end-plate permeability decreases with age, thereby decreasing disk nutrition. Motion is beneficial for intervertebral disks. Solute transport and metabolism are both improved by spinal motion, and intermittent motion is less effective than continuous motion. Aging usually results in disk degeneration.

Degeneration of a disk reduces its proteoglycan content and thus its hydrophilic capacity. As the disk becomes drier, its elasticity and its ability to store energy and distribute loads gradually decrease. The majority of disk herniations occur in the fourth decade of life, and herniations are found in 15% to 30% of autopsy specimens.

The intervertebral disk exhibits creep, which means that the disk will continue to deform under a constant load. This time-dependent behavior comes from the fluid flow of the disk under an applied load and from the inherent viscoelastic behavior of the collagen and proteoglycan matrix. Time-dependent behavior has been demonstrated both in vivo by Keller et al[8] and in vitro by Kazarian.[7] The studies of Eklund and Corlett[3] and Krag, Cohen, and Pope[10] indirectly measured the change in overall height of the subjects. The diurnal loss was about 17 mm. Kazarian[7] noted that a degenerate disk had a higher rate of deformation and the creep curve stabilized sooner.

Virgin[17] was the first to suggest that the nucleus pulposus acts hydrostatically to pressurize the disk and thus stabilize the FSU. In a nondegenerate disk, nucleus pressure is redistributed as tension in the annulus layers. Normal disk pressure is about 1.5 times the compressive load divided by the cross-sectional area. Pressure is higher in the disk center and decreases toward the exterior. Nachemson[15] reports that disk pressure is different in various positions or maneuvers (**Table 20-1**). Andersson et al[1] found in vivo that intradiscal pressure increased linearly with an increase in both trunk load and trunk moment. Disk pressure was found to be high in unsupported sitting but decreases significantly with the use of a backrest inclination greater than 110 de-

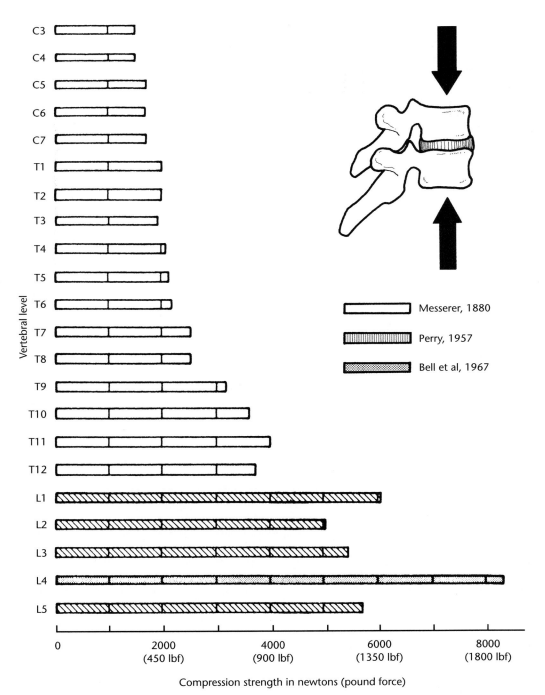

Figure 20-1 Vertebral compression strength at a slow loading rate. *(Modified from White AA, Panjabi MM: Clinical biomechanics of the spine, Philadelphia, 1991, WB Saunders.)*

Table 20-1	Loads on the L3 disk calculated from intradiscal pressure measurements in a 70-kg man.	
Position, Maneuver		**Load (N)**
Supine (awake)		250
Supine (semi-Fowler's)		100
Supine (traction, 500 N)		0
Sitting (unsupported)		700
Standing (relaxed)		500
Coughing		600
Straining		600

grees, with the use of lumbar supports, and with the use of armrests.

The tensile stress in the annulus fibrosus due to disk pressure in the thoracic spine is less than that in the lumbar spine because the higher ratio of disk diameter to height in the thoracic disks reduces the circumferential stress.[11]

POSTERIOR PORTION

The posterior portion of the FSU has a primary role of guiding its movement. The type of motion possible at any level is determined by the orientation of the facets of the FSU to the transverse and frontal planes. This orientation changes throughout the spine (**Fig. 20-2**).

Other structures that influence motion of the spine are the rib cage, which limits thoracic motion, and the pelvis. The cervical spine, the most mobile region of the spine, affords the head a large range of motion, which is necessary for the activities of daily living. Except for the facets of the two uppermost cervical vertebrae (C1 and C2), which are parallel to the transverse plane, the cervical facets are oriented at 45 degrees to the transverse plane and are parallel to the frontal plane (**Fig. 20-2**). The load-bearing function of the facets at all spinal levels is significant. Load sharing between the facets and the disk varies with the position of the spine. The loads on the facets are very high, peaking at about 30% of the total load when the spine is hyperextended.[9] They are also quite high during forward bending coupled with rotation.[4] The facets through the vertebral arches and intervertebral joints play an important role in resisting shear forces. In addition, Farfan[5] showed that 40% of the torsional strength of the FSU comes from the facet joints, and Lorenz, Patwardhan, and Vanderby[12] suggested that 25% of the axial load bearing is from these structures.

LIGAMENTS

The spine ligaments function in conjunction with other elements of the FSU as stabilizers and checkreins. They are tensile elements that can fatigue, and they do contain pain fibers. The overall load deflection curve on the FSU is nonlinear, being reflective of ligament behavior. Extension loads the anterior ligaments and flexion loads the posterior elements.

During flexion, the interspinous ligaments have the greatest strain, followed by the capsular ligaments and the ligamenta flava, whereas in extension the anterior longitudinal ligament bears the greatest strain. During lateral flexion, the contralateral transverse ligament is strained the greatest, followed by the ligamenta flava and the capsular ligaments. The capsular ligaments bear the most strain during rotation. The ligamentum flavum, which connects two adjacent vertebral arches longitudinally, is an exception in its behavior because it contains a large percentage of elastin. The elasticity of this ligament is therefore very high. This allows it to contract during extension of the spine and elongate during flexion. In a neutral position, the ligamentum flavum is under tension as a result of its elastic properties. Because it is located at a distance from the center of motion in the disk, it prestresses the disk and thus adds to overall stability.

KINEMATICS

The range of motion of the spine varies from level to level. White and Panjabi[19] have summarized these data (**Fig. 20-3**). Flexion and extension are about 4 degrees in the upper thoracic, about 6 degrees in the midthoracic, and about 12 degrees in the lower thoracic segments. This increases in the lumbar motion segments to a peak of 20 degrees at L5-S1. Lateral flexion varies from level to level quite markedly but is greatest in the lower thoracic segments and L3-4 (8 to 9 degrees). In the upper thoracic segments the range is 6 degrees. Rotation is greatest in the upper segments of the thoracic spine (9 degrees). The range of rotation is minimal in the lumbar spine because of facet orientation. The lumbar spine is susceptible to injury from rotation.

There have been reports of coupled motion throughout the spine. Coupling refers to a primary motion in one direction leading to a secondary motion in another. For example, C1 moves independently of the rest of the cervical spine, but motion below C1 involves the entire cervical spine. The facets guide the motion, and as a result, flexion-extension is coupled with transverse translation, lateral flexion with rotation (**Fig. 20-4**), and rotation with axial translation. In the thoracic region, rotation is associated with lateral flexion, especially in the upper thoracic region. In this case, the vertebral bodies generally rotate toward the concavity of the lateral curve.[18] Coupling of rotation and lateral flexion

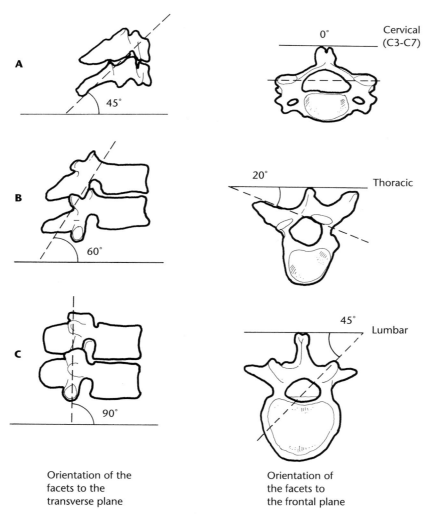

Figure 20-2 Orientation of the facets of the intervertebral joints.[18] **A,** In the lower cervical spine the facets are 45 degrees to the transverse plane and are parallel to the frontal plane. **B,** The facets of the thoracic spine are oriented at 60 degrees to the transverse plane and at 20 degrees to the frontal plane. **C,** The facets of the lumbar spine are oriented at 90 degrees to the transverse plane and at a 45 degree angle to the frontal plane.

occurs in the lumbar spine, with the vertebral bodies rotating toward the convexity of the curve.[13]

KINETICS

The basic building materials of the spine are the vertebral bodies, which take the loads of compression, shear, and bending, and the muscles act as the building blocks in tension. The muscles position and stabilize the spine. Without muscles, the ligamentous spine buckles under loads of as small as 2 kg. In general, the muscle electrical activity electromyographic (EMG) amplitude is directly proportional to the moment arm of the muscle line of action from the center of rotation. We can investigate the role of muscle around the periphery through a free-body analysis in which, mathematically

at least, the body is cut in two and the forces and moments are resolved across that cut surface. Forces are estimated from the EMG signals. In complex postures, very high antagonistic activity occurs. Loads are also produced by body weight, prestress from ligaments, and externally applied loads.

Because the lumbar spine is the main load-bearing area and the most common site of pain, studies have focused on this region. Loads on the cervical spine are mainly produced by the weight of the head, the activity of the surrounding muscles, the inherent tension of adjacent ligaments, and the application of external loads. Investigations in vivo confirm that physiologic loads are lower than those on the thoracic and lumbar spines.

However, quite large loads on the cervical spine have been calculated during neck flexion, particularly in

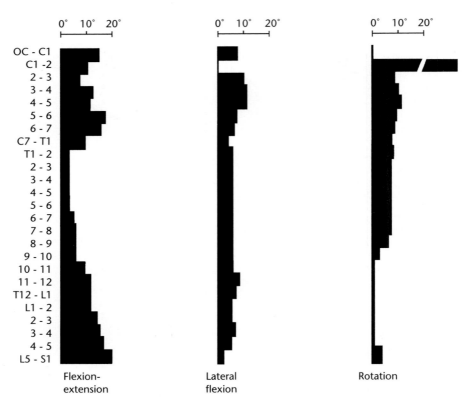

Figure 20-3 A composite of representative values for type and range of motion at different levels of the spine. *(Modified from White AA and Panjobi MM: Clinical biomechanics of the spine, Philadelphia, 1991, WB Saunders Co.)*

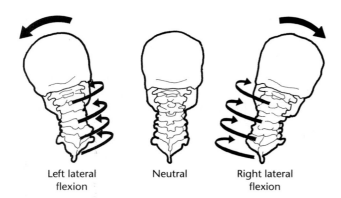

Figure 20-4 Coupled motion during lateral flexion is depicted schematically. When the head and neck are flexed to the left, the spinous processes shift to the right, indicating rotation. The converse is also illustrated. *(Modified from White AA and Panjobi MM: Clinical biomechanics of the spine, Philadelphia, 1991, WB Saunders Co.)*

the lower cervical motion segments. Harms-Ringdahl[6] calculated the bending moments generated around the axes of motion of the atlanto-occipital joint and the C7-T1 motion segment with the neck in flexion, neutral position, and extension (**Fig. 20-5**). The load on the junction between the occipital and C1 was lowest during extreme extension and highest during extreme flex-

ion. The load on the C7-T1 motion segment was low with the neck in the neutral position but tucked in (ranging from an extension moment of 0.8 Nm to a flexion moment of 0.9 Nm). The load increased substantially during slight flexion (reaching 6 Nm).

Moroney, Schultz, and Ashton-Miller[14] studied subjects who resisted loads. Calculation of the maximum (compressive) reaction forces on the C4-5 motion segment ranged from 500 to 700 N during flexion, rotation, and lateral bending and rose to 1100 N during extension.

Body position also affects the magnitude of the loads on the lumbar spine. These loads are minimal during well-supported reclining, remain low during relaxed upright standing, and rise during sitting (**Fig. 20-6**).

Trunk flexion increases the load by increasing the forward-bending moment on the spine. The forward inclination of the spine also makes the disk bulge on the concave side of the spinal curve and retract on the convex side. Hence when the spine is flexed, both compressive and tensile stresses on the disk increase.[1] Nachemson and Elfström[16] and Andersson et al[2] also showed that during relaxed unsupported sitting, the loads on the lumbar spine are greater than during relaxed upright standing. In this position the pelvis is tilted backward and the lumbar lordosis straightens the upper body, thereby creating a longer lever arm for the weight of the trunk.

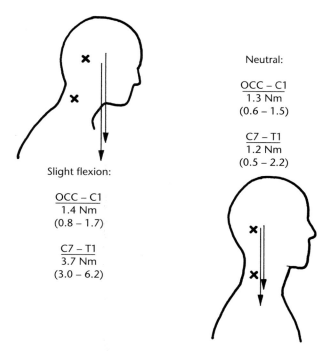

Neutral:

$$\frac{OCC - C1}{1.3 \text{ Nm}}$$
(0.6 – 1.5)

$$\frac{C7 - T1}{1.2 \text{ Nm}}$$
(0.5 – 2.2)

Slight flexion:

$$\frac{OCC - C1}{1.4 \text{ Nm}}$$
(0.8 – 1.7)

$$\frac{C7 - T1}{3.7 \text{ Nm}}$$
(3.0 – 6.2)

Figure 20-5 Extension and flexion moments around the axes of motion of the atlanto-occipital (OCC-C1) joint and the C7-T1 motion segment (marked with *Xs*) are presented for five positions of the head: extreme flexion, slight flexion, neutral, head upright with the chin tucked in, and extreme flexion. Values shown are the medial and range for seven subjects: negative values indicate extension moments. The arrows represent the force vectors produced by the weight of the head. *(Modified from Harms-Ringdahl K: On assessment of shoulder exercise and load-elicited pain in the cervical spine. Biomechanical analysis of load—EMG—methodological studies of pain provoked by extreme position, thesis, 1986, Karolinska Institute, University of Stockholm.)*

The loads on the lumbar spine are lower during supported sitting than during unsupported sitting because part of the weight is supported by the backrest. Backward inclination of the backrest and a lumbar support will further reduce the loads (**Fig. 20-7**).[2]

Because user requirements vary, the kinds of chairs available vary widely. Regardless of use, however, it is

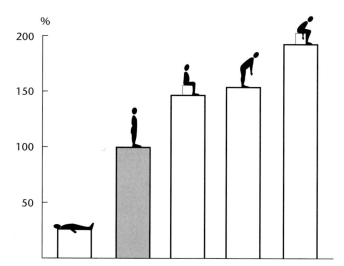

Figure 20-6 The relative loads on the third lumbar disk for living subjects in various body positions are compared with the load during upright standing, depicted as 100%. *(Modified from Nachemson A, Elfström G: Intravital dynamic pressure measurements in lumbar discs: a study of common movements, maneuvers and exercises, Stockholm, 1970, Almquist & Wiksell.)*

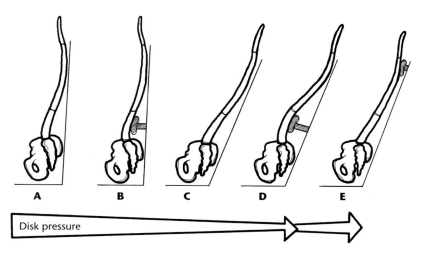

Disk pressure

Figure 20-7 Influence of backrest inclination and back support on loads on the lumbar spine in terms of pressure in the third lumbar disk during supported sitting. **A,** Backrest inclination is 90 degrees, and disk pressure is at a maximum. **B,** The addition of lumbar support decreases disk pressure. **C,** Backward inclination of the backrest to 110 degrees but with no lumbar support produces less disk pressure. **D,** The addition of lumbar support with this degree of backrest inclination further decreases the pressure. **E,** Shifting support to the thoracic region pushes the upper part of the body forward, moves the lumbar spine toward kyphosis, and increases disk pressure. *(Modified from Andersson GBJ, Ortengren R, Nachemson A: Clin Orthop 129:156-164, 1977.)*

important to be able to adjust any chair to meet the basic anthropometric dimensions of the worker. A proper seat height is desirable and should be adjustable for the individual user. The seat surface should be 3 cm to 5 cm below the knee fold when the lower limb is vertical. Foot supports can be used with higher chairs. The width of the seat should be sufficient to accommodate the user. It must be possible to use the backrest, so the seatpan should not be too deep. Pressure should be avoided on the back of the thigh near the knees.

Lifting creates the highest loads on the lumbar spine, and these are the occupational exposures with the greatest incidence of low back pain (LBP) injury reports. The key to prevention is to reduce the load moment, which means reducing either the magnitude of the load, the distance from the body, or both. Therefore, if objects of the same weight, shape, and density but of different sizes are held, the lever arm for the force produced by the weight of the object is longer for the larger object, and the bending moment on the lumbar spine is greater (**Fig. 20-7**).

DISCUSSION

The spine has functions of load bearing, protection of neural elements, and mobility yet stability. The FSU, which is the basic unit, exhibits coupled motion. It is composed of the anterior components (vertebral body, disk, pedicles, and ligament), and the remainder make up the posterior elements. Motion, which is largely controlled by the facet, varies between regimes. Flexion-extension is high in the lumbar spine but rotation is minimal. Loads in the spine are a function of body mass, muscle activity, prestress, and external loads. The latter is particularly important in the lumbar spine.

References

1. Andersson GBJ, Ortengren R, Nachemson A: Intradiscal pressure, intra-abdominal pressure and myoelectric back muscle activity related to posture and loading, *Clin Orthop* 129:156-164, 1977.

2. Andersson GBJ et al: Lumbar disc pressure and myoelectric back muscle activity during sitting. I. Studies on an experimental chair, *Scand J Rehabil Med* 6:104, 1974.

3. Eklund JAE, Corlett EN: Shrinkage as a measure of the effect of load on the spine, *Spine* 9(2):189-194, 1985.

4. El-Bohy AA, King AI: Intervertebral disc and facet contact pressure in axial torsion. In Lantz SA, King AI, editors: *Advances in bioengineering,* New York, 1986, American Society of Mechanical Engineers; pp 26-27.

5. Farfan HF: *Mechanical disorders of the low back,* Philadelphia, 1973, Lea & Febiger.

6. Harms-Ringdahl K: *On assessment of shoulder exercise and load-elicited pain in the cervical spine. Biomechanical analysis of load—EMG—methodological studies of pain provoked by extreme position,* thesis, 1986, Karolinska Institute, University of Stockholm.

7. Kazarian L: Dynamic response characteristics of the human vertebral column: an experimental study of human autopsy specimens, *Acta Orthop Scand Suppl* 146, 1972.

8. Keller L et al: In vivo creep behavior of the normal and degenerated porcine intervertebral disc—a preliminary report, *J Spinal Disorder* 1(4):267-278, 1989.

9. King AI, Prasad P, Ewing CL: Mechanism of spinal injury due to caudocephalad acceleration, *Orthop Clin North Am* 6:19, 1975.

10. Krag MH, Cohen MC, Pope MH: Load-induced changes in human intervertebral disc height in-vivo: a new and closer look, *Orthop Trans* 9(3):516, 1985.

11. Kulak RF et al: Biomechanical characteristics of vertebral motion segments and intervertebral discs, *Orthop Clin North Am* 6:121, 1975.

12. Lorenz M, Patwardhan A, Vanderby R: Load-bearing characteristics of lumbar facets in normal and surgically altered spinal segments, *Spine* 8:122, 1983.

13. Miles M, Sullivan WE: Lateral bending at the lumbar and lumbosacral joints, *Anat Rec* 139:387, 1961.

14. Moroney SP, Schultz AB, Ashton-Miller JA: Analysis and measurement of neck loads, *J Orthop Res* 6(5):713-720, 1988.

15. Nachemson A: Lumbar interdiscal pressure. In Jayson MIV, editor: *The lumbar spine and back pain,* London, 1987, Churchill Livingstone; pp. 191.

16. Nachemson A, Eflström G: *Intravital dynamic pressure measurements in lumbar discs: a study of common movements, maneuvers and exercises,* Stockholm, 1970, Almqvist & Wiksell.

17. Virgin WJ: Experimental investigations into the physical properties of the intervertebral disc, *J Bone Joint Surg* 33B:607-611, 1951.

18. White AA: Analysis of the mechanics of thoracic spine in man. An experimental study of autopsy specimens, *Acta Orthop Scand Suppl* 127:1-105, 1969.

19. White AA, Panjabi MM: *Clinical biomechanics of the spine,* Philadelphia, 1991, JB Lippincott.

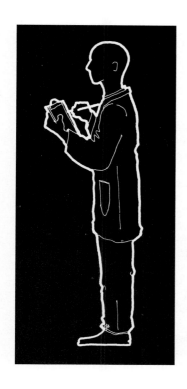

Chapter 21

Clinical Evaluation of the Low Back Region

Dan M. Spengler

CONTENTS

Although patient evaluation and management have been clearly improved by the explosive growth in technology over the past 10 years, the hallmark of patient assessment continues to reside in the fundamentals of the history and physical examination. The information provided in this chapter emphasizes the importance of these basic skills, motivating the reader to continue to improve and update this important basic knowledge area. The focus of the chapter is on the clinical assessment of patients who seek an evaluation of low back pain, with an emphasis on occupational aspects.

HISTORY

For all patients who are examined for an evaluation of low back pain with or without sciatica, a history of the present illness should be completed, including information regarding the nature of the onset of symptoms. In addition, the examiner should document various treatment approaches and the effects of the treatments on symptoms. The reason for the evaluation and any anticipated outcomes must also be understood in advance by both the physician and the patient. For example, if the evaluation is for an independent medical evaluation (IME), the patient needs to understand the purpose of the evaluation and the fact that treatment will not be included because the purpose of an IME is to provide an independent objective assessment for a third party. The evaluation may be to assist another physician in patient management or may be solely to provide an insurance company or a worker's compensation carrier with a diagnosis and recommendations. Historical information, when related to swirling litigation and compensation issues, must usually be more detailed than a history obtained solely to diagnose symptoms and manage a patient. For example, if a patient falls at home and seeks evaluation, the history might be succinct and relate only the type of fall and the distance of the fall. In a contested on-the-job injury encounter, the details may be more important for dispute resolution. Was the fall witnessed? Did the employee return to work? For how long? Is an attorney involved? Who are the physicians or others who have evaluated the patient? Has the employee had a previous injury? Has an impairment been previously recorded? An interview with a patient who is involved in litigation can be facilitated by having the person who is referring the patient summarize the outcomes desired from the consultation. In addition, a succinct summary of the events to date should be provided to serve as a template for review during the interview with the patient. Information provided by the referral source does not replace the need for a good history; it only highlights the issues from another perspective.

On entering the examination room, the doctor must reassure the patient that the evaluation will be thorough. The purpose of the evaluation is generally to establish a diagnosis and outline a plan to reaffirm the diagnosis or to institute treatment to assist the patient with symptom control. This is also the time to inform the patient of the purpose of the examination should the referral be for an IME. Patients may be hostile initially if the physician is viewed as the "company doctor," but this perception can be overcome by informing the patient that although information will be provided to the referral source, the information will be based on an objective evaluation and examination. Patients must also understand that their cooperation is essential in providing a fair and impartial report. In today's managed-care environment, rehabilitation nurses who are employed by the referral source may often accompany the patient and attempt to remain in the examination room during the history and physical examination, but the author believes this to be most inappropriate and the individual should be asked to leave until after the examination. Relatives or spouses may remain with the patient at the discretion of the individual doctor who is performing the evaluation.

The opening aspects of the history should focus on the present illness. The examiner must not lead patients into answers by the use of "closed" questions. For example, "Does your back pain radiate to the posterior of your thigh, calf, and foot?" Patients may often answer yes to these questions even though they may not understand what was asked or the relevance. A much better strategy is to ask the patient to describe the pain. What makes the pain better or worse? These questions can amplify the pain drawing that is gathered before the history and physical examination (**Fig. 21-1**).[9] This tool is helpful to maintain in the patient's file to compare over time or to establish the patient's pain pattern at the time of evaluation.

In addition to the need to record a few notes for later dictation, the physician should also observe the psychological, physical, and emotional behavior of the patient throughout the interview and examination. Loss of eye contact, change in voice tone, or excessive movement on the examining table should be noted because these nonverbal cues may be as important or more important than the actual words spoken. Signs of clinical depression should also be noted because depression can be commonly encountered as both a primary and secondary disorder in patients who complain of low-back pain. Slurred speech or an impressive knowledge of pain medications should also be noted to provide clues for potential medication or alcohol abuse. Medication abuse is quite common (greater than 30%) in patients who complain of chronic back symptoms.[3,11]

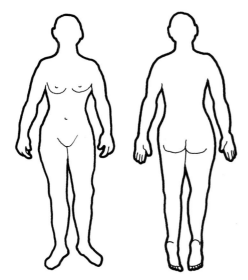

| Numbness ⋮ ⋮ ⋮ | Pins and needles ∷ ∷ |
| Burning ××× | Stabbing /// |

Figure 21-1 Pain drawing for a female patient. *(From Ransford AO, Cairns D, Mooney V:* Spine *1:127-134, 1976.)*

A thorough history of the patient's employment history, length of time on the specific job before injury, and the state or federal government's eligibility requirement for disability benefits may be important background information. If a patient with a poor work history expresses acute low-back pain on the precise day that disability benefits are available, the physician may be legitimately concerned over the significance of any "tissue injury."

Pain patterns should also be noted. Does the pain intensity stay the same throughout the 24-hour day, or is it better or worse in the morning or in the evening? Is the pain predictable or erratic? Is the patient's sleep pattern disrupted because of night pain? Although night pain can be associated with various forms of malignancy, night pain can also reflect clinical depression or be associated with psychosocial issues. The relationship of various activities to the pain complaints should also be discussed. Pain that increases with walking short distances yet disappears rapidly with sitting or lying can represent a typical pain pattern in a patient with lumbar spinal stenosis. Pain descriptors are important, but a clinical diagnosis cannot be advanced solely on the basis of the pain pattern because of the wide variability of clinical symptoms in most disorders that result in low-back pain.

When interviewing a patient with low-back pain that has been present for a significant period of time (more than 3 months), the physician should completely review the patient's systemic symptoms, including fe-

ver, chills, weight loss, lethargy, and any sources of infection whether systemic or not such as a localized cutaneous abscess. Gastrointestinal symptoms are relevant because gastrointestinal disorders can actually occur concomitantly with low-back symptoms and because so many patients take large doses of salicylates or nonsteroidal antiinflammatory agents. Such medications can also lead to significant gastrointestinal bleeding.[8] Genitourinary symptoms are also reviewed because bladder dysfunction can be associated with pressure on the spinal cord or cauda equina. Genitourinary symptoms are more commonly related to other causes than neural compression, but early recognition of a change in bladder habits may signal a subtle increase in pressure on the neural elements.[2] When such symptoms are present, the physical examination should include a well-documented rectal examination. Cystometrograms and a urologic consultation may be necessary to clarify the nature of these problems.[2] Female patients should be questioned regarding any changes in bleeding patterns or pain related to menstruation. Female patients with persisting back complaints should be evaluated by their gynecologist.

Medications taken by the patient should also be recorded. If the patient has been taking multiple medications in the past for back pain, the associated clinical response to the medications should be noted. Other back treatment approaches should also be noted, including the patient's pain-free interval following the intervention (e.g., steroid dose pack, epidural steroid injections, physical therapy).

Psychosocial and economic issues associated with the low back symptoms should be reviewed. Life stressors, litigation, compensation, and other secondary gain parameters would likely not have "caused" the pain, but such issues can certainly maintain the chronicity of symptoms in specific cohorts of patients.[5] This is discussed in greater detail in Chapter 6.

The past medical history should be completed to include any diagnostic assessments, treatment approaches not previously noted, and a list of doctors or others who have evaluated or treated the patient for low-back and other medical problems. The length of any pain-free interval following previous surgical procedures should also be documented. Short-term relief following major surgery may occur after procedures that may not have been clearly indicated. Other causes can include surgery performed at the wrong level, an inaccurate diagnosis, an associated medical disorder with referred low back symptoms, and pain-prone patients who tend to amplify symptoms.

PHYSICAL EXAMINATION

The physical examination permits the physician to objectively assess the patient and record the observations. Findings that can be classified as objective represent the most important parameters. Examples of objective findings would include deep tendon reflexes and circumferential measurements of the calf and thigh to determine swelling or atrophy. Subjective physical examination findings are less helpful and include supine straight leg raising (SLR) (unless done in the sitting position as well) and range of motion. Range of motion is the least reliable of all determinants of the examination.[1] Unfortunately, this parameter is still used, although to a lesser degree, for impairment ratings as suggested in the American Medical Association (AMA) guidelines for impairment. Inappropriate physical examination findings are also important to record inasmuch as the presence of three or more of these findings may alert the physician that the patient may be attempting to amplify the findings for secondary gain.[12] It is important to note, however, that the presence of inappropriate physical findings does not exclude the presence of a pathological process. Therefore, the onus is on the physician to recommend the appropriate diagnostic studies to clarify the diagnosis.

The patient should be suitably attired for the examination to provide for privacy but also facilitate a complete musculoskeletal evaluation. The standard patient gown that is open in back is quite appropriate, together with a sheet for the supine and prone portions of the examination. The physical examination should be complete but also age and complaint related. For example, chest expansion is not an essential portion of the examination in an 80-year-old patient with back pain following a minor fall. On the other hand, chest expansion is clearly important in a 20-year-old male with an insidious onset of low-back pain over a long period of time. Decreased chest expansion (less than 2.5 cm) in such a patient could suggest the diagnosis of ankylosing spondylitis. The physical examination is divided into four components based on the position of the patient, beginning with the patient standing.

Patient Standing

The lumbar spine examination begins with the patient standing. The physician should observe the general configuration of the spine to detect any lateral curvatures, kyphosis, or excessive lordosis. Patients with lumbar paraspinous spasms frequently have a pelvic list that should be noted. In young adult males with low back pain, chest expansion should be measured with a cloth tape because expansion less than 2.5 cm suggests an inflammatory process such as ankylosing spondylitis.

After observing the spine orientation in the erect patient, the physician should ask the patient to flex forward and again analyze the spine. This step of the examination is particularly important in adolescent children to detect early lateral curvatures of the spine.

To assess the range of motion of the lumbosacral spine, the physician should stand behind the patient and observe the lumbar paraspinous muscles. Any eccentric contractions of the musculature suggests lumbosacral paraspinous spasms; limited motion without evidence of such eccentric contractions suggests a lack of patient cooperation.

Forward flexion, lateral flexion, and extension of the lumbar spine should all be observed. Normal patients should be able to nearly touch their toes in the forward direction and the fibular heads in the lateral direction, but extension of the spine is extremely variable. In general, pain increased by flexion suggests lumbar disk abnormalities, and pain with extension suggests degenerative changes involving the posterior elements of the spine, lumbar spinal stenosis, or both. Occasionally, patients with lumbosacral paraspinous spasm will be able to flex forward reasonably normally but will have difficulty returning to the erect position. Such patients may accomplish this move in a two-phase recovery by flexing the knees and extending the hips without motion in the lower back. In older patients, the range of motion of the cervical spine should also be assessed because degenerative osteoarthritis of the cervical spine will occasionally result in low-back complaints.

After observing the range of motion, the physician should percuss the spine to detect any localized tenderness, a subjective reaction. This test has little value if the patient has tenderness at multiple areas, but consistent localized tenderness over the midline of the spine may suggest inflammatory diskitis. The costovertebral angle should be palpated. Tenderness in the costovertebral angle suggests a genital-urinary problem (e.g., pyelonephritis).

Next, patients should be asked to walk on their toes, then heels, to assess the overall strength of the dorsiflexors (L5) and plantar flexors (S1) of the ankle. In particular, the extensor hallucis longus muscles should be observed when the patient is walking on the heels because discrepancies can be detected between this act of walking and later passive strength testing. To assess and detect weakness of the triceps surae group of muscles, which are innervated primarily through the S1 nerve root, the physician should ask the patient to hop several times on the left foot, then on the right foot, and note any discrepancies in the two abilities.

The patient should also be observed while walking in the examining room. Extreme staggering from side to side and other bizarre gait patterns suggest symptom amplification. Patients with true herniated disks often have a gait pattern slightly antalgic on one side, but with no bizarre abnormalities.

Patient Sitting

Next, the patient should sit on the edge of the examining table so that the physician can perform the knee and ankle reflex tests, as well as determine the strength of the extensor hallucis longus muscle. This latter examination is critical in all patients complaining of back and leg pain because many patients have weakness of the extensor hallucis longus but not the tibialis anterior. Weakness of the extensor hallucis longus in a patient who complains of pain in the back and leg suggests involvement of the L5 nerve root. The extensor digitorum brevis muscle should be checked; however, this author remains unconvinced that observation of this muscle has any diagnostic significance in patients

Table 21-1 Nonorganic physical signs in low back pain.		
Category	**Test**	**Comments**
Tenderness	Superficial palpation	Inordinate, widespread sensitivity to light touch of the superficial soft tissues over the lumbar spine is unknown and suggests amplified symptoms
	Nonanatomic testing	Tenderness is poorly localized
Simulation (to assess patient cooperation and reliability)	Axial loading	Light pressure to the skull of the standing patient should not significantly increase symptoms
	Rotation	Physician should rotate the standing patient's pelvis and shoulders in the same plane. This does not move the lumbar spine and should not increase pain
Distraction	Straight leg raising	Physician asks the seated patient to straighten the knee—patients with true sciatic tension will arch backward and complain. These results should closely match those of the traditional recumbent straight leg test
Regional		Diffuse motor weakness or bizarre sensory deficits suggest functional regional disturbances if they involve multiple muscle groups and cannot be explained by neuroanatomy principles
Overreaction		Excessive and inappropriate grimacing, groaning, or collapse during a simple request is disproportionate

Modified from Waddell G. et al: Spine 5:117-125, 1980.

with lumbar disk disease. Asymmetry is often observed in patients who have never had low back pain and/or leg pain.

The most important portion of the sitting examination is the distracting SLR test (**Fig. 21-2**) described in **Table 21-1**. Patients with herniated disks and true symptoms of sciatic tension will arch backward and complain of pain in the buttock, posterior of the thigh, and calf when the symptomatic extremity is straightened. Patients who do not have true sciatic tension will not recognize this as a sciatic tension test and will therefore have no symptoms with the sitting SLR examination. For the patient who complains of neck pain as well as low back pain, the strength and reflexes of the upper extremities can be evaluated with the patient sitting.

Patient Supine

With the patient supine on the examining table, the physician uses a standard tape to measure the true length of the limbs from the anterior superior spine to the medial malleolus on both sides. Although significant discrepancies (more than 2.5 cm) in limb lengths can result in mild compensatory scoliosis and low back discomfort, these associations are uncommon.

The physician should observe the thigh and leg muscles for early signs of muscle atrophy. In addition, the physician should use a cloth tape to measure the circumferences of both thighs one handbreadth above the patella and measure both calves one handbreadth below the patella. Again, discrepancies greater than 2 cm are probably significant and suggest muscle atrophy.

For the standard ipsilateral SLR maneuver, the physician stands to one side of the patient, places the left hand on the patient's patella to extend the knee, places the right hand under the os calcis, and then lifts the leg while keeping the knee extended (**Fig. 21-3**). Patients often describe their discomfort in different locations in the extremity, which makes the results of this standard test less objective. If the patient complains of radicular discomfort during the test, the limb should not be lifted any higher. At that moment, plantar flexion of the ankle should be performed as a distracting test. Because plantar flexion of the ankle should not increase back pain, exacerbation of pain suggests amplification of symptoms by the patient.

The physician should also perform the crossed SLR test by lifting the nonsymptomatic extremity as in the ipsilateral SLR test. If the patient complains of discomfort radiating into the symptomatic extremity when the well extremity is lifted, this test is positive, almost invariably indicating lumbar disk herniation. During both the SLR test and the crossed SLR test, the patient must be allowed to express where the discomfort is

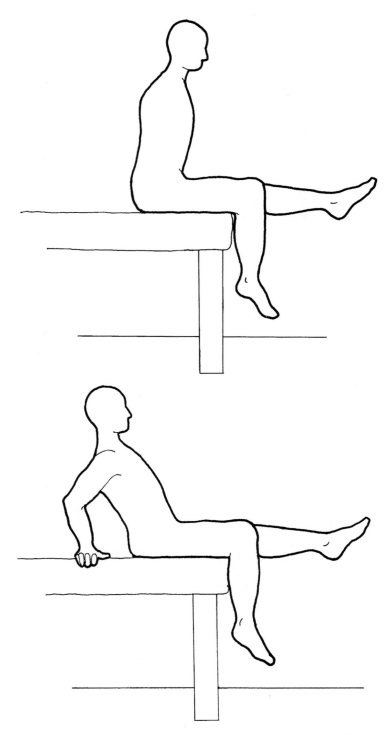

Figure 21-2 Sitting straight leg raising test. The patient at the top demonstrates no evidence of increased sciatic tension when the knee is extended. The patient at the bottom leans back in the "tripod" sign, indicative of true sciatic tension.

occurring. Specifically, asking the patient whether lifting the well extremity causes pain in the symptomatic extremity invalidates the test.

The Patrick's test (**Fig. 21-4**) should then be performed bilaterally. In this test, the shear force applied

across the sacroiliac joint helps detect early abnormalities in the joint. Many patients with osteoarthritis of the hip will complain of buttock pain rather than the classic groin discomfort. Consequently, the hip joint often is overlooked because of the apparent back problem; how-

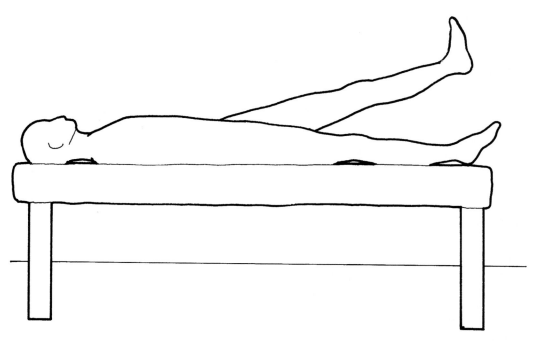

Figure 21-3 Supine straight leg raising (SLR) test. This test must be compared with the sitting SLR test for maximum accuracy to identify sciatic tension.

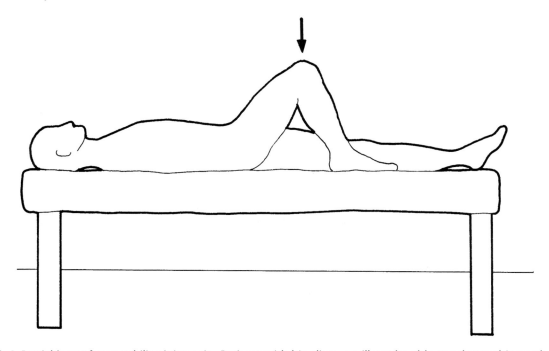

Figure 21-4 Patrick's test for sacral-iliac joint pain. Patients with hip disease will not be able to tolerate this much external rotation without significant pain complaints.

ever, patients with abnormalities of the hip joint cannot tolerate a Patrick's test because of the discomfort when the limb is fully externally rotated into the abducted position. Therefore, while the patient is supine with the limbs extended, the physician should gently rotate the lower extremity both internally and externally, a gradual rotation that allows the physician to pick up early irritability in the hip joint. If internal and external rotations cause pain, the pain may be from the hip joint.

The abdomen should be examined by palpating the four quadrants to detect any intraabdominal masses.

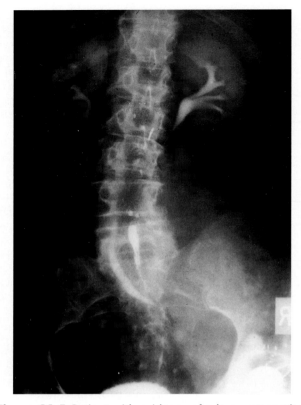

Figure 21-5 Patient with evidence of a large retroperitoneal neoplasm (uterine tumor) eroding into the lumbosacral plexus and causing groin, buttock, and leg pain on the side of the lesion. Note that decompressive laminectomy and total joint replacement were performed within 6 months of this radiograph. Symptoms were misinterpreted to arise from the lumbar spine and then the hip.

Abdominal lesions may erode into the lumbosacral plexus and cause symptoms identical to those of lumbar spinal stenosis or disk disease (**Fig. 21-5**).

The strength of the abdominal muscles should be assessed by having the patient flex the knees while keeping the feet flat on the table and then perform a sit-up. Patients who have extreme difficulty completing even one sit-up are often excellent candidates for a vigorous rehabilitation program. In addition, the patient should be asked to hold the lower extremities 15 cm to 20 cm off the table. In general, a patient with an established herniated disk can easily perform this maneuver, so the primary value of this test is to assess the strength of the abdominal musculature rather than determine the likelihood of a disk herniation.

With the patient supine, the motor strength of the iliopsoas, quadriceps, and hamstrings should be assessed, as well as Babinski's reflexes and proprioception. A sensory examination also should be performed and recorded.

Patient on Side

The supine patient is then asked to turn on one side, to raise the superior extremity, and then to maintain the extremity in the raised position against resistance by the physician (**Fig. 21-6**). In most patients, the gluteus medius is innervated primarily by L5, so patients with L5 radiculopathy often have weak abductors, as do patients with significant hip disease. The trochanter should be palpated to test for trochanteric bursitis. These same tests should be repeated with the patient lying on the opposite side.

With the patient on one side, perianal sensation and buttocks sensation also should be evaluated. All patients over the age of 40 and any patient suspected of a

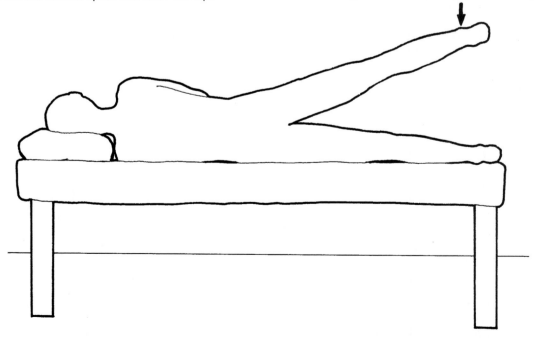

Figure 21-6 Gluteus medius strength testing with the patient on the side and abducting against resistance.

neurologic deficit should have a rectal examination. In males, anal sphincter tone and the size of the prostate may be assessed. Female patients with chronic back pain should have a pelvic examination.

Patient Prone

With the patient prone on the examining table, the lumbar spine and sacrum should then be reexamined for any localized tenderness. A reverse SLR maneuver can be easily accomplished by the physician by simply lifting both of the patient's lower extremities off the table. Next, the patient should flex the knees 90 degrees so that the physician can observe internal and external rotation of the hips. In most patients, the amount of internal and external rotation is quite similar. However, patients with femoral anteversion have excessive internal rotation and limited external rotation. These patients often experience discomfort in the low back area and buttocks during running. When the patient is prone, ankle jerks often are easier to reexamine, and right and left ankle jerks are easily compared. The absence of one or both reflexes should be noted. Finally, the patient should extend first one lower extremity and then the other by using the gluteus maximus muscle. Increased low back discomfort during this maneuver suggests a more superficial myofascial source of the back pain symptoms. Following completion of the history and physical examination, the physician is ready to either begin treatment or refer the patient for imaging studies or other diagnostic studies.

IMAGING STUDIES

Plain radiographs are the most commonly ordered imaging study for a patient who complains of low-back pain. These studies do not need to be ordered in patients who are under the age of 60 unless there is a history of a significant traumatic event or the history and physical examination are suggestive of a systemic disorder. For the routine patient who has acute low-back pain and no significant findings, radiographs can be delayed for approximately 4 weeks while treatment with antiinflammatories and possibly exercise is initiated on an empiric basis. Patients who do not respond to preliminary treatment can be scheduled for additional diagnostic testing if the treatment initially provided is not of benefit. From a cost-effective perspective, routine oblique radiographs do not add to the value of an anteroposterior (AP) and lateral view of the lumbosacral spine and pelvis. The additional cost and radiation exposure for oblique radiographs are not warranted. Should a detailed evaluation of the bony anatomy be considered necessary, localized computed tomography (CT) and three-dimensional reconstruction of the CT images are worthy of consideration. Standing films and lateral flexion-extension views of the lumbosacral spine are indicated when the diagnoses of segmental instability and/or spinal deformity are considered.

Bone scans supplemented with CT reconstruction (single positron emission computed tomography [SPECT]) are of value when an occult bony injury is suspected or if the differential diagnosis includes tumor, infection, or other such conditions. Although a positive bone scan does not lead to a specific diagnosis without additional information, this examination is safe and often represents a worthwhile "screening" study in patients with complex histories and significant pain behavior.

Magnetic resonance imaging (MRI) has jumped to the forefront as the ideal imaging study for a patient with low-back complaints who requires an evaluation of the thoracolumbar spinal canal. Magnetic resonance imaging is safe but costly. In addition, some patients who suffer from claustrophobia are unable to tolerate the study. Because of the ease of obtaining this study, however, many patients are scanned who likely do not need to be. For example, a 35-year-old patient with a 4-week history of sciatica, an absent ankle reflex, and a positive SLR test most likely has a lumbar disk herniation at the L5/S1 level on the symptomatic side. An MRI evaluation should not be ordered unless the patient does not respond to nonoperative management and wishes to pursue operative intervention. Unfortunately, many patients have an MRI performed before a good history and physical examination. Such a strategy wastes valuable healthcare dollars. The other imaging option is lumbar myelography to include the conus, with CT images following the myelogram. The costs for CT/myelograpy and gadoliniumlabeled MRI are quite similar (approximately $1,400.00). Gadolinium-enhanced MRI is reserved for patients who have had previous surgery or who are being investigated with a differential diagnosis that includes infection and/or tumor. In my experience, gadolinium-enhanced MRI is the most reliable method to differentiate scar tissue from recurrent disk herniation in a patient who has had previous lumbar spine surgery (**Fig. 21-7**).[6] A CT scan without contrast should not be used for the isolated purpose of identifying an intervertebral disk herniation.

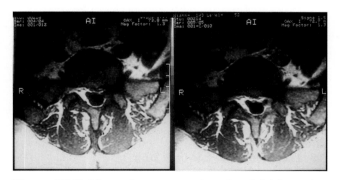

Figure 21-7 Magnetic resonance imaging (plain) on the left and with gadolinium enhancement on the right. Enhancement after gadolinium effectively excludes recurrent disk herniation in this patient. Epidural fibrosis postsurgery resulted in the scar tissue noted in the left epidural space in the pregadolinium image on left.

The CT scan does not afford the opportunity to clearly visualize occult neural tumors in the cauda or conus that can clearly mimic the symptoms of lumbar disk herniation.

To exclude the diagnosis of a retroperitoneal tumor, an abdominal CT scan with contrast or MRI may represent diagnostic options. In addition, ultrasonography and/or intravenous pyelography with a postvoid cystometrogram are indicated when renal disorders are suspected.

Lumbar diskography has been recommended by several authors, but this study should be reserved for the spinal surgeon who has a specific question regarding a specific disk space. Routine use of lumbar diskography has not been shown to be diagnostically effective, let alone cost effective.[7] Most surgeons would agree that if this particular imaging study has a role, it would be to assess the transitional disk space when a lumbar fusion procedure is being considered. If one were considering a fusion from L4 to S1 and the L3 disk space was narrowed, diskography noting the patient's pain response may provide information on the question of extending the fusion to L3 or stopping at L4.[7]

OTHER DIAGNOSTIC STUDIES

Laboratory evaluation should be recommended for patients who are not responding to treatment or who have severe pain. Although many of these tests are indicated in specific situations, a useful screening evaluation for patients with persistent symptoms should include a complete blood count (CBC), sedimentation rate, coagulation survey, SMA-18 (sequential multiple analysis), and a urinalysis. Patients who have evidence for diminished bone density should be more thoroughly evaluated with thyroid studies, protein electrophoresis, urinary calcium, and an evaluation of parathyroid hormone levels. Should one proceed this far in the evaluation, a referral to an endocrinologist with an interest in calcium metabolism is clearly warranted. In young male patients suspected of having ankylosing spondylitis, an HLA-27 antigen study can be ordered.

Selected injection of the lumbar or sacral nerve roots can occasionally provide insight into the pathogenesis of a lumbar radicular problem. The nerve roots must be injected in a controlled setting.[4] Reduplication of a patient's pain syndrome after needle irritation and relief after injection of a small volume of a local anesthetic agent may suggest potential nerve root entrapment. Root injections should be used very selectively because they are not indicated for the majority of patients who have complaints of low-back pain.

Neurological Tests

The electromyogram (EMG) is a safe, accurate diagnostic test that may be used for patients who suffer from acute low-back pain lasting more than 3 weeks or those who suffer from chronic pain. When the test is performed by a competent electromyographer, positive waves on insertion and fibrillation are generally considered objective evidence of nerve root compression. A screening investigation that reveals no fibrillations, positive waves, or other abnormality is a useful negative. In addition, the nerve conduction velocities plus the EMG can assist in ruling out patients who may have peripheral neuropathies. Patients with chronic pain symptoms and give-way weakness but who have normal EMG findings are unlikely to have signficant mechanical compression of nerve roots. The physician must remember, however, that the EMG will not be positive for at least 2 to 3 weeks after a compression event; therefore, a patient may have a normal EMG despite significant compression of a nerve root. The EMG is positive preoperatively in 75% of patients who subsequently undergo surgical intervention for proven disk herniations.[10]

Although EMG is useful, this examination must be considered a diagnostic adjunct and, of course, means little by itself. Careless interpretation of this test can result in inappropriate surgical intervention.

Consultation with a urologist and cystometrography are useful to evaluate patients with urinary-related complaints in addition to back and leg pain. This evaluation must be correlated with the physical examination. If anal sphincter tone is decreased, myelography and surgical intervention should be considered regardless of the results of the cystometrogram. Many hysterical patients or symptom amplifiers will complain of urinary frequency in association with low-back discomfort, a symptom that can be incorrectly interpreted as reflecting significant nerve-root compression. These patients will have normal sphincter tone and an intact bulbocavernosus reflex. Cystometrograms that reveal no evidence of denervation of the bladder are useful and reassuring to both the patient and the physician. Occasionally, more extensive testing with urodynamics may be indicated.

Psychological Assessment

Psychological evaluation is helpful for managing patients who suffer from either acute or chronic low-back pain. All patients who have had at least one failed back surgery should have a psychological assessment. The psychological tests are most accurately interpreted when coupled with a psychological interview. The Minnesota Multiphasic Personality Inventory (MMPI) does not confirm or refute a patient's report of pain, but it does provide information relevant to a patient's readiness to emit pain behavior.[5,10,11] In addition, associated depression and the psychological "cost" of pain to the patient are assessed. A patient's likely response to treatment can also be estimated.

Psychological assessment of a patient who complains of chronic back pain must also include a very thorough psychosocial history. Family members are interviewed, as appropriate, to augment any incomplete areas in the patient's history.

In addition, a complete behavioral analysis is performed on those patients whose pain behavior implicates operant factors.[5] In addition to a thorough interview with a psychologist, the behavioral analysis requires that for 2 weeks the patient keep a pain diary relating pain to events and the time of day, which are very useful data for the physician.[5]

Biopsy

If the physician is concerned about infection or a tumor of the lumbar spine, a diagnostic aspiration biopsy may be performed with a closed-needle technique. The initial biopsy for a soft tissue lesion can be performed through a CT-directed approach. If this is unsuccessful, the Craig needle biopsy system, which uses a large-bore needle under biplane radiographic control, is preferred. Local anesthesia may be possible in patients who are in ill health or patients who have lytic lesions. Most areas of the lumbar spine are readily accessible for this biopsy procedure, although lesions of the thoracic and cervical spine are usually more safely approached through an open biopsy.

Consultations

A patient who suffers from chronic low back discomfort should usually be evaluated by more than one physician. If a physician practices in a multidisciplinary clinic, then the patient who suffers from chronic pain can be conveniently evaluated by an anesthesiologist, psychiatrist, psychologist, neurosurgeon, gynecologist, physiatrist, and other healthcare professionals, including social workers, nurses, and physical therapists. However, the patient-physician relationship should be preserved by having one member of the team serve as liaison to the patient. Therefore, when the total evaluation is completed, the patient's personal physician should synthesize the data and outline the proposed treatment plan.

Patient testing with various dynamometers can on selected occasions be useful in the clinical management of difficult patients. The three-axis dynamometer designed by Isotechnologies, Inc., when used properly, can

---

Differential diagnosis of low-back pain
Trauma
Infections
Inflammations
Neoplasms
Developmental abnormalities
Metabolic diseases
Degenerative disorders
Neurologic disorders
Referred pain
Psychological disorders
Miscellaneous

---

provide confirming evidence for low-effort behavior, which in compensation and litigation patients can be valuable information to more rapidly formulate an appropriate treatment plan and to prevent unwarranted interventions.

DIFFERENTIAL DIAGNOSES

When evaluating patients with complaints of low-back pain, the physician must remain vigilant to identify patients whose symptoms are a result of referred pain unassociated with the intervertebral disk or spinal nerves. In this time of intense focus on cost, the physician must remain dedicated to a proper evaluation for the patient and not cave in to the managed-care bureaucrats who are primarily interested in the cost rather than the quality of care. Patients with low-back pain represent an interesting group. A list of differential diagnoses is provided in the box above. Approximately 2% of patients who come to a low-back specialty clinic will have evidence for neoplasms as the source of the symptoms.[11] An appropriate index of suspicion coupled with the knowledge of appropriate testing will aid the physician in formulating a proper workup.

References

1. Battié MC et al: The role of spinal flexibility in back pain complaints within industry, *Spine* 15 (8):768-773, 1990.

2. Berlic A, Light JK: Function of the conus medullaris and cauda equina in the early period following spinal cord injury and the relationship to recovery of detrusor function, *J of Urol* 148:1845-1848, 1992.

3. Black RF: The chronic pain syndrome, *Surg Clin North Am* 55:999-1011, 1975.

4. Bonica JJ: *The management of pain with special emphasis on the use of analgesic block in diagnosis, prognosis, and therapy,* Philadelphia, 1953, Lea & Febiger.

5. Fordyce WE: *Behavioral methods in chronic pain and illness,* St Louis, 1976, Mosby–Year Book.

6. Hueftle et al: Lumbar spine: postoperative MR imaging with Gd-DTPA, *Radiology* 167:817-824, 1988.

7. Nachemson A: Lumbar discography—where are we today? *Spine* 14(6):555-557, 1989.

8. Pincus T, Griffin M: Gastrointestinal disease associated with nonsteroidal anti-inflammatory drugs, *Am J Med* 91:209-212, 1991.

9. Ransford AO, Cairns D, Mooney V: The pain drawing as an aid to the psychological evaluation of patients with low back pain, *Spine* 1:127-134, 1976.

10. Spengler DM, Freeman CW: Patient selection for lumbar discectomy, *Spine* 4:129-134, 1979.

11. Spengler DM, Loeser JD, Murphy TM: Orthopaedic aspects of the chronic pain syndrome, *Instr Course Lect* 29:101-107B, 1980.

12. Waddell G et al: Nonorganic physical signs in low back pain, *Spine* 5:117-125, 1980.

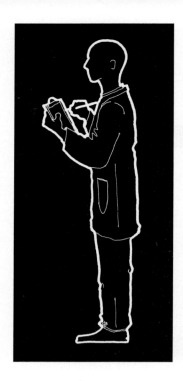

Chapter 22

Treatment of the Acutely Injured Worker

Stanley J. Bigos
Margareta Nordin
Dawn Leger

CONTENTS

Back problems are so prevalent in modern society that the U.S. Department of Health, through the Agency for Health Care Policy and Research (AHCPR), commissioned a multidisciplinary panel of medical experts to assess the literature and develop guidelines for clinical practice. Much of the following chapter is derived from the "Findings and Recommendation Statements" resulting from an extensive methodologically based review of the literature on the guidelines.[5]

Most people will experience low back problems at some time in their lives. National statistics show a yearly prevalence in the U.S. population of 15% to 20%,[2] and more than 50% of working-age people report back symptoms each year.[56,62] Back problems are the most common cause of disability for persons under age 45,[11] with about 1% of the U.S. population chronically disabled and another 1% temporarily disabled at any given time.[2]

There is a high cost associated with back problems for both the patient and society. The economic, societal, and personal costs are believed to be substantial.[2] Beyond the medical costs, lost work time and disability payments can cost up to three times as much as medical treatment.[54] Estimates of the annual societal cost assigned to the back in the United States range from $20 to $50 billion.[44] There are also substantial psychological and social problems for patients with back problems and their families, which add to the difficulties in treatment and recovery.

The AHCPR report was prompted by these factors, but especially by increasing evidence that patients may be receiving inappropriate or suboptimal care. There are marked variations in the use of diagnostic tests, hospitalization, and surgery that imply a lack of consensus about appropriate methods of assessment and treatment of low back problems.[15] Additional studies show that some patients appear more disabled after treatment, especially repeated surgical procedures.[15] In this chapter, low back problems are defined as activity intolerance caused by back pain or back-related leg symptoms.[5]

ASSESSMENT

The initial assessment of a patient with low back problems is of critical importance and should include a focused medical history and a physical examination by a clinician well aware of the potential psychosocial and economic issues that may affect the outcome for a patient limited at work. In some cases, the low back symptoms may be related to a dangerous condition that, however rare, should be eliminated. The assessment first seeks "red flags" to detect possible serious underlying conditions such as a fracture, tumor, infection, or cauda equina syndrome that can be manifested as common back symptoms (**Table 22-1**).

Back symptoms without red flags can be divided into primarily back (nonneurological) or sciatic (neurological) symptoms. This distinction will guide the practitioner in the consideration of special studies for those slow to recover. Special tests are not usually required in the first month of low back symptoms because most patients recover reasonable activity tolerance within 1 month. The initial evaluation also allows the physician to establish a rapport with the patient at the outset, to understand patient expectations, and to become aware of situational factors (psychological or socioeconomic) that can influence the course of treatment and recovery.

Medical History

A few key questions on the medical history can help to rule out serious underlying conditions such as cancer or spinal infection. These include age, history of cancer, unexplained weight loss, immunosuppression, duration of symptoms, responsiveness to previous therapy, pain that is worse at rest, history of intravenous drug use, and urinary or other infection.[5] For spinal fracture, red flags include a history of significant trauma such as a fall from a height; motor vehicle accident for a young patient and lesser trauma to the back; a relatively heavy lift for someone with prolonged use of steroids; or age over 70. The red flags for cauda equina syndrome or severe neurologic compromise include acute urinary retention or overflow incontinence, loss of anal sphincter tone or fecal incontinence, saddle anesthesia (about the anus, perineum, and genitals), or progressive motor weakness in the lower limbs. Many times, simple blood tests rule out back-related tumor or infection.

The physician should look for symptoms of sciatica (leg pain) or neurogenic claudication (walking limitations because of leg pain) in the elderly that suggest possible neurological involvement. Pain radiating below the knee is more likely to indicate a true radiculopathy than is pain radiating only to the posterior of the thigh. Persistent numbness or weakness of the leg(s) increases the likelihood of neurological involvement. Furthermore, cauda equina syndrome is indicated when the patient reports new bladder symptoms, specific dysfunction (urinary retention or overflow incontinence), and/or saddle anesthesia, especially when associated with leg symptoms and weakness. Including pain drawings and visual analog pain rating scales can help document the distribution of pain and intensity of symptoms.[49,61,64]

The physician should be aware of other factors that may influence the reporting of symptoms and treatment outcomes, including elements alluding to any work dissatisfaction, pending litigation, worker's compensation or disability issues, failed previous treatments, substance abuse, and depression relative to education level.*

*References 8, 14, 33, 38, 42, 47, 55.

Table 22-1	Red flags for potentially serious conditions.		

Possible Fracture	Possible Tumor or Infection	Possible Cauda Equina Syndrome
FROM MEDICAL HISTORY		
Major trauma such as vehicle accident or fall from a height	Age over 50 or under 20	Saddle anesthesia
	History of cancer	Recent onset of bladder dysfunction such as urinary retention, increased frequency, or overflow incontinence
Minor trauma or even strenuous lifting (in older or potentially osteoporotic patients)	Constitutional symptoms such as recent fever or chills or unexplained weight loss	
		Severe or progressive neurological deficit in the lower extremity
	Risk factors for spinal infection: recent bacterial infection (e.g., urinary tract infection); IV drug abuse; or immune suppression (from steroids, organ transplantation; or human immunodeficiency virus infection)	
	Pain that worsens when supine; severe nighttime pain	
FROM PHYSICAL EXAMINATION		
		Unexplained laxity of the anal sphincter
		Perianal/perineal sensory loss
		Major motor weakness: quadriceps (knee extension weakness); ankle plantar flexors, evertors, and dorsiflexors (footdrop)

Physical Examination

The basic elements of the physical examination are inspection, palpation, observation including range-of-motion testing, and a specialized neuromuscular evaluation that emphasizes ankle and knee reflexes, ankle and great toe dorsiflexion strength, and the distribution of sensory complaints. For patients with no limb complaints, a simpler examination is sufficient.

In the primary-care setting, for patients with leg symptoms the neurological examination can be conducted with a few tests (**Fig. 22**-1): testing of dorsiflexion strength of the ankle and great toe, with weakness suggesting L5 and some L4 root dysfunction; testing of ankle reflexes to evaluate S1 root dysfunction; testing of light touch sensation in the medial (L4), dorsal (L5), and lateral (S1) aspects of the foot; and the straight leg raising (SLR) test. This short examination will facilitate the detection of most clinically significant nerve root compromise caused by L4-5 or L5-S1 disk herniations, which account for over 90% of all clinically significant radiculopathy due to lumbar disk herniations.[3,25,31,32,52] If there

are other less common L2-3 or L3-4 disk herniations, they will appear in further diagnostic tests that may be ordered if the patient shows no improvement after 1 month. For most patients, no additional diagnostic tests are required and recovery will occur within 1 month after the onset of low back symptoms.[5]

The "red flags" are positive responses to key questions on the medical history or positive findings during the physical examination that suggest the possibility of a serious underlying condition that is causing the acute low back pain. These red flags should prompt immediate additional diagnostic testing and intervention.

The physician's observation of limping or coordination problems can guide specific neurological testing. A patient's inability to heel-walk (L4-5 nerve roots), toe-walk (S1 nerve roots), or do a single squat rise (L3 and L4 nerve roots) provides a baseline for muscle testing. Range-of-motion measurements are of questionable significance given the marked variation among persons without symptoms and their poor correlation to low back symptoms. Severe guarding of lumbar motion in

Nerve root	L4	L5	S1
Pain	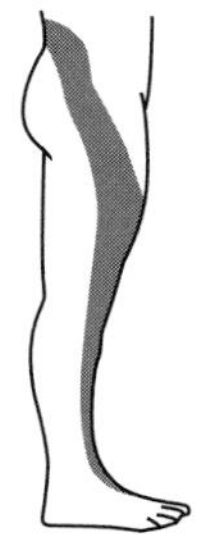	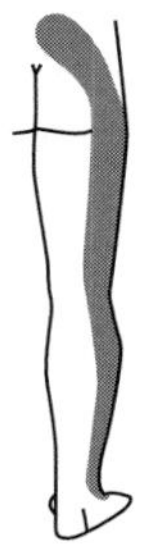	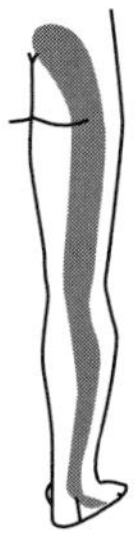
Numbness	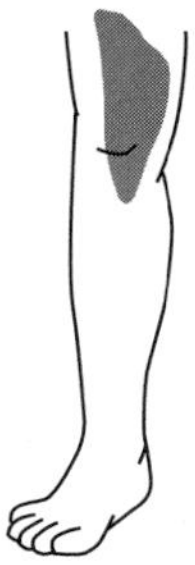	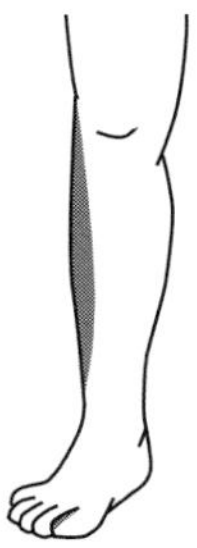	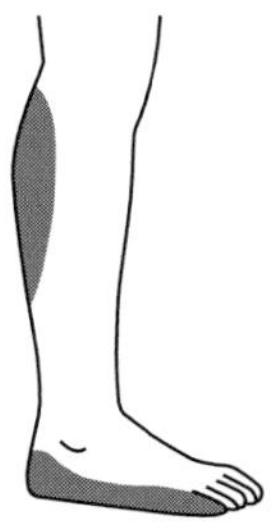
Motor weakness	Extension of quadriceps	Dorsiflexion of great toe and foot	Plantar flexion of great toe and foot
Screening exam	Squat and rise	Heel walking	Walking on toes
Reflexes	Knee jerk diminished	None reliable	Ankle jerk diminished

Figure 22-1 Testing for lumbar nerve root compromise.

all planes may be suggestive of infection, tumor, or fracture, but in the absence of other symptoms, this is simply a nonspecific manifestation of acute low back symptoms.

Inconsistencies in the history and physical examination are evidence of pain behavior and can present a challenge to the physician. For example, closer scrutiny may uncover that the patients perceive themselves to be trapped in jobs where the activity requirement is unrealistic relative to age or health. Patients involved in legal actions or worker's compensation claims may therefore seek medical intervention or advocacy for economic or psychological purposes. The awareness of these behaviors helps prepare the physician for occupation-related problems that may need to be addressed if the patient is slow to recover.

In summary, the medical history and clinical examination are used to classify patients with occupation-related low back symptoms in the lower spine area and/or leg in three working categories:

1. *Potentially serious spinal condition*: tumor, infection, spinal fracture, or a major neurologic compromise

such as cauda equina syndrome as suggested by a red flag (not a low back problem until ruled out)
2. *Sciatica*: back-related lower limb symptoms suggesting lumbosacral nerve root compromise
3. *Nonspecific back symptoms*: symptoms occurring primarily in the back and suggesting neither nerve root compromise nor a serious underlying condition

CLINICAL INTERVENTION

More than 90% of all patients with acute low back problems will return to reasonable activity after 1 month regardless of the treatment they receive.[20,54,65] In the absence of red flags, treatment is similar for most patients with activity intolerance caused by an acute episode of low back symptoms. Assuring the patient that there is no hint of a serious condition and that rapid recovery is expected is of paramount importance. Treatment should include patient education before helping with comfort and activity recommendations. Studies show that providing some educational materials about back problems may reduce the use of medical resources (patients accept the diagnosis and do not insist on additional unnecessary testing),[13] decrease patient apprehension (patients understand and agree with the diagnosis leading to faster recovery),[4] and speed recovery.

Education

An unstructured educational program in which patients are provided with educational information about back problems and given the opportunity to ask questions has been shown to reduce the recurrence of back pain in the year following the intervention.[50] Back schools that offer more structured programs about low back problems have not been shown to be effective in affecting the recovery and recurrence of low back pain among participants.[30,35] Therefore, although it is clear that patients need information and assurance about their problem and recovery, it seems more than adequate to provide that information in an informal setting. The primary physician must generate these positive effects (see box below).

Patient discussion handout #1

BACK PROBLEMS?

The News is Good
Your clinician has not found any dangerous causes for your back problem. Almost everyone has a low back problem at some time. In only 1 person in 200 does the problem have a serious cause. A medical history and physical examination alone are very good at detecting these uncommon cases.

You Should Recover Soon
Nine out of 10 persons with low back problems recover within 1 month, and most recover even sooner. Therefore, an x-ray of your back or other tests at this time would only waste your time. If your recovery happens to be slower than normal, your clinician will then look further for a reason.

Even with back symptoms you may be able to continue your usual activities. But you might have to slow your pace. Strenuous activity or heavy lifting could give you trouble. If you work outside the home, much depends on the kind of work you do. Office work may require few changes. On the other hand, if your job involved heavy labor—like a furniture mover—you will probably have trouble working as usual right away.

Age also makes a difference. As we age, so do our spines. Activities that require speed and strength become harder to do. This happens to many people by age 30, to most people by age 40, and to nearly everyone by age 50. Consider your age as you plan your daily tasks when recovering from a back problem.

You Can Ease Your Discomfort Safely
Your clinician will suggest safe ways for you to be more comfortable as you recover. But staying in bed is not usually the best thing. More than a few days in bed actually weakens your back and could cause your symptoms to last longer. Neither bed rest, medications, nor any other remedies should be expected to do away with *all* the discomfort. It is important to be up and around as much as possible even if you are uncomfortable. The sooner you return to normal daily activities, the sooner your symptoms will disappear.

You May Need to Make Changes in Your Daily Activities
Sitting may not be comfortable. Sitting is not dangerous, but it puts more stress on the back than standing. While recovering, try to spend less time sitting. To make sitting easier, support the curve of your back with a towel or small pillow. If possible, use a chair or other seat with a slightly reclining back.

Lifting. Keep anything you must lift close to the belly button. Lifting a carton of milk or orange juice at arm's length can stress your back more than lifting 30 lbs held close to the body. Also try not to bend forward, twist, or reach when lifting.

Exercising can help your back. Your health provider may suggest safe exercises such as walking, swimming, or riding a stationary bike. If done correctly, these exercises do not stress the back any more than does sitting on the side of your bed (which is not dangerous). What exercising does is keep your back muscles from becoming weakened by not enough activity. In addition, exercise is good for your general health, can speed your recovery, and may help protect you from future back problems. As your symptoms lessen, daily exercise will make it easier for you to resume your normal activities.

Points to Remember
- There is no hint of a serious problem.
- Your back symptoms are the kind that usually disappear within a month. Expect a rapid recovery.
- No medications or other treatments, including home remedies, can be expected to relieve all the discomfort immediately.
- You may need to change some daily activities to keep from irritating your back, but stay active enough to keep from weakening your muscles.
- If you are one of the few who is slow to recover, your clinician will look for the reason. Even if you are slow to recover, there is little chance of a serious reason for your back problem.

Patient Comfort—Medication

Comfort is often the patient's first agenda item. An important component of the treatment of acute low back problems is control of symptoms to avoid the debilitation of too much rest while awaiting spontaneous recovery. The intent is really to provide comfort, but the focus is to avoid long-term activity intolerance. The methods traditionally include oral medications such as acetaminophen and nonsteroidal antiinflammatory drugs (NSAIDs), as well as physical treatment (**Table 22-2**). Studies have not proven the efficacy of many of these methods owing to the rapid rate of spontaneous recovery. If these methods allow the patient to remain active and build activity tolerance through exercise, they can be considered a successful intervention. Although there are side effects associated with the use of these drugs, NSAIDs appear effective in reducing pain in patients with acute low back problems. Acetaminophen is comparable in efficacy and has fewer side effects; therefore the choice of treatment is left to the discretion of the treating physician.[5] The AHCPR panel attempted to determine whether muscle relaxants improved patient outcomes separately and as an adjunct to treatment with NSAIDs, but they were unable to find a statistically significant relationship to determine whether muscle relaxants are more or less effective than

NSAIDs in reducing symptoms. Likewise, the addition of a muscle relaxant did not seem to add to the efficacy of an NSAID. Furthermore, up to 30% of patients are reported to be intolerant of muscle relaxants. Other medications, including opioid analgesics, oral steroids, colchicine, and antidepressants, have not been found to be effective in the treatment of low back symptoms, especially given the potential side effects associated with their use.

Patient Comfort—Physical Treatments

There are conflicting findings about the efficacy of spinal manipulation for the treatment of acute low back pain. Some studies have shown statistically significant short-term effects of manipulation in hastening recovery from low back problems for patients without radiculopathy.[1,51] Manipulation, manual therapy in which loads are applied to the spine by short-lever or long-lever methods, has some effect on patients with acute back problems in the first month of treatment, provided that serious neurological conditions have been screened and ruled out.[24,36] No significant improvements in outcome were shown in studies of patients treated with physical agents and modalities, including ice, heat, ultrasound, massage, cutaneous laser treatment, and electrical stimulation. These modalities may alleviate

Table 22-2 Symptom control methods.

Nonspecific Low Back Symptoms and/or Sciatica	Nonspecific Low Back Symptoms	Sciatica
RECOMMENDED		
Nonprescription analgesics: acetaminophen (safest), NSAIDs (aspirin,* ibuprofen*)		
Prescribed Pharmaceutical Methods	**Prescribed Physical Methods**	
Other NSAIDs*	Manipulation (in place of medication or a shorter trial if combined with NSAIDs)	
OPTIONS		
Muscle relaxants†‡§	Physical agents and modalities† (heat or cold modalities for home programs only)	Manipulation (in place of medication or a shorter trial if combined with NSAIDs)
Opiods†‡§	Shoe insoles†	Physical agents and modalities† (heat or cold modalities for home programs only)
		Few days' rest§
		Shoe insoles†

NSAIDs, *nonsteroidal antiinflammatory drugs.*
Aspirin and other NSAIDs are not recommended for use in combination with one another because of the risk of gastrointestinal complications.
†*Equivocal efficacy.*
‡*Significant potential for producing drowsiness and debilitation; potential for dependency.*
§*Short course (few days only) for severe symptoms.*

some symptoms temporarily and do not present any harmful effects, but they should not be relied on for the treatment of low back pain.[48,68]

Transcutaneous electrical nerve stimulation (TENS) produces continuous pulses of electricity by way of surface electrodes stimulated by a small battery-operated device worn by the patient. This method is geared to provide symptomatic relief for patients with low back problems, but studies have been unable to show a relationship between TENS and the relief of acute low back pain.[16,23]

Shoe insoles and lifts are not believed to have an impact on back symptoms in most cases, and there are conflicting findings about the efficacy of lumbar corsets and back belts. Lumbar corsets and support belts are theoretically designed to treat or prevent low back symptoms by compressing the abdomen (causing increased intraabdominal pressure, which unloads the vertebral column) and acting as a mechanical reminder to decrease bending. Therapeutically, lumbar supports are intended to control pain and protect against injury claims. Although some argue that long-term use of these belts may actually weaken abdominal and back muscles, there is no evidence of either benefit or harm to patients using them.

Traction, when used for low back symptoms, involves the application of intermittent or continuous force along the axis of the spine in an attempt to elongate the spine by either mechanical or manual means. The most common type used for the low back is pelvic traction, in which a snug girdle around the pelvis is attached to weights hung at the foot of the bed. The therapeutic objective of traction for patients with low back problems is to reduce pain, but there is a potential for increased debilitation resulting from prolonged bed rest. Because of the potential problems, the high cost, and inconclusive evidence of its benefits, traction is not recommended for the treatment of acute low back pain.[5]

Biofeedback is another treatment modality that has not been shown to be effective for patients with low back symptoms. Biofeedback involves training patients to control muscular activity according to visual or auditory cues. Results are conflicting in patients with chronic pain.[5]

Patient Comfort—Injection Therapy

Trigger point injections involve the injection of local anesthetic into soft tissues (muscles) near localized tender points in the paravertebral area.[58] The theory that such trigger points are responsible for causing or perpetuating low back pain is controversial and disputed by many experts. Trigger point injections may damage nerves or other tissues or cause infections and hemorrhage, and their efficacy for the treatment of acute low back problems is questionable and unsupported.[10,72] Facet joint injections, on the other hand, involve the injection of local anesthetics and/or corticosteroids into or around facet joints of the lumbar

spine. The therapeutic objective of facet joint injections is temporary relief from motion-limiting pain so that the patient may proceed into an appropriate exercise program.[40] These injections suffer the same potential complications and have not been shown to improve outcomes for patients with acute low back pain.[28] Epidural injections, done primarily in patients with suspected radiculopathy, involve the injection of medication into the epidural space, near the site where the nerve roots pass before entering the intervertebral foramen. The objective is to reduce swelling, inflammation, and pain, but again, the results of numerous studies have not shown any efficacy for patients with acute low back pain. They are invasive, pose rare but serious risks, and are only suggested as an alternative to surgical intervention for patients with acute radiculopathy.

Finally, acupuncture is another method of treating acute low back pain. Acupuncture involves "dry needling" into cutaneous and subcutaneous tissues, muscles, or ligaments according to traditional Chinese meridians. Some rotation of the needles may be done, and electrical stimulation can be added. The therapeutic objective of acupuncture and other dry needling techniques is to reduce pain. The results of many studies are highly contradictory for various types of pain, including chronic low back pain.[59] No studies have been done for acute low back pain, and there are risks of significant complications with this technique. From the literature reviewed, complications include hematomas, infections (hepatitis B and *Staphylococcus aureus*), pneumothorax, and spinal nerve and spinal cord injuries.

Activity Recommendations

Activity recommendations are aimed at keeping patients with acute low back problems as active as possible to avoid debilitation that alone can slow return to work.[37] We now have data to support assuring the patient that it is safe to continue with work activities and that it will not only avoid the debilitation of inactivity but also speed recovery. We now have proof of the importance of continuing to encourage adequate physical activity to avoid debilitation. The overall goal is to disrupt daily activities as little as possible or aid recovery by keeping the patient as active as possible. Bed rest has been a frequently used treatment for acute low back symptoms. The therapeutic hypothesis is to reduce symptoms by reducing intradiscal pressure and pressure on nerve roots. Studies have shown that intradiscal pressures are lowest when subjects are lying supine in the semi-Fowler position, on the back with hips and knees moderately flexed.[44] Unfortunately, as soon as subjects lie on their side, the intradiscal pressure is about 75% to 80% of standing. Because of its debilitating physical and psychological impact, bed rest is a very controversial activity alteration used to help control symptoms. Except in rare cases with extreme pain conditions (including leg pain), a maximum of 2 to 4 days of bed rest may be considered. Deactivation resulting from prolonged bed rest (more than 2 to 4 days) appears to cause significant physiologic effects on general health, bone, and muscle that can jeopardize a comfortable return to normal levels of activity.

Some risk factor studies about low back symptoms point to heavy or repetitive lifting, exposure to whole-body vibration (from vehicles or industrial machinery), asymmetric postures, and postures sustained for long periods of time.[12,19] Other biomedical research has suggested that certain postures and activities increase the mechanical stress on the spine.[9,12,17] Other investigations have not made a clear link between these mechanical stresses as a cause of low back symptoms.[62] However, once symptoms are present, mechanical stresses do correlate with less comfortable tolerance of these activities. When compared with standing, sitting, and postures that involve bending and twisting have been shown to increase mechanical stress on the spine according to pressure measurements in lumbar intervertebral disks.[43] Heavy lifting also appears to increase mechanical stress on the spine, but this stress can be reduced if the lifted object is held close to the body rather than at arm's length.

A "lifting equation" was postulated to calculate reasonable lifting limits for various tasks as part of a guideline developed in 1981 by the National Institute of Occupational Safety and Health (NIOSH)[45] and was revised more recently.[67] The ability of the guideline to reduce the incidence of low back problems has yet to be validated. Other ergonomic guidelines about reasonable lifting have been reviewed by Dul and Hildebrandt[18] and are examined in Chapters 9 and 10 of this text.

Therefore, for patients with acute low back symptoms who cannot tolerate heavy lifting, prolonged sitting, and bending or twisting of the back, a temporary alternative of less mechanically stressful activity can be provided to avoid debilitation while limited from work activities. In recommending activity modifications for patients who work, the clinician may find it helpful to stay within medical jurisdictions and only limit those activities that relate to our best knowledge about the

---

Patient discussion handout #2

SEEKING A REASON FOR SLOW RECOVERY

Special Tests May Be Needed.
If your back problem is slow to recover, your healthcare provider may consider special studies (tests) to find the reason. They may include blood tests, or an imaging study may be needed to view your spine. Nerve tests can help identify certain leg problems. The chances are good that your problem will not be serious. In only 1 person in 200 do low back problems have a serious cause.

Why Wait To Do Special Studies?
You may have read or heard of tests like MRI, CAT scan, or myelography. These are special imaging studies. They use special equipment to provide different views of body structures like your spine. You may wonder why your healthcare provider did not order these tests in the first place. There is a good reason. Imaging studies can be confusing. By themselves, they cannot tell the difference between possible causes of a back problem and common changes in the spine because of aging.

As we grow older, the spine changes. Almost half the population has aging changes in the spine as early as age 35. Yet most people who have such changes will not have a back problem lasting longer than 1 month. Remember that 9 out of 10 people who have low back problems recover within 1 month. For these persons, imaging studies are unnecessary and confusion can be avoided. The tests could show a condition that is not really a problem and has no connection to back symptoms.

Imaging studies are seldom used alone. Surgery is never based on imaging studies alone. The studies could find something that is not really the cause of your problem. Before deciding whether imaging studies are needed, your healthcare provider should review your physical examination carefully. He or she may also do other kinds of tests to find evidence of a problem. Ask your healthcare provider to explain what tests are needed for you.

The table below lists a number of terms that are commonly used to describe (diagnose) the cause of low back symptoms. However, scientific studies have not been able to show a connection between these diagnoses and back symptoms. In addition, there is no evidence that these conditions benefit from surgery or other specialized forms of treatment.

Common Diagnoses Used to Explain Back Symptoms

Annular tear	Adult spondylolysis	Myofascitis
Fibromyalgia	Disk syndrome	Strain
Spondylosis	Lumbar disk disease	Facet syndrome
Degenerative joint disease	Sprain	Osteoarthritis of the spine
Disk derangement/disruption	Dislocation	Subluxation

Continued

Patient discussion handout #2—Continued

When Is Surgery a Choice?

If your back symptoms affect your legs and are not getting better, a herniated lumbar disk (what many people call a "slipped disk") may be the reason. The disk can press on a nerve root in your back and can either irritate the nerve or affect its function. If tests show strong evidence that this is happening, surgery to take the pressure off the nerve root may speed your recovery.

If your healthcare provider tells you that surgery is a possibility, ask about your choices. Ask what would happen without surgery. Before agreeing to surgery, get a second opinion from another healthcare provider. Also, ask about the tests that were done to suggest that surgery is the best approach for your back problems. The table below lists some conditions or diagnoses that sometimes benefit from surgery or other special treatment.

Diagnoses That May Benefit from Surgery or Other Treatment

Leg pain due to herniated lumbar disk. Surgery is sometimes used to relieve pressure on the nerve and can speed recovery if the diagnosis is based on strong evidence. Surgery should not be expected to make the back brand-new.
Leg pain due to spinal stenosis. Spinal stenosis is an uncommon cause of walking limitation in the elderly. It is very rare under the age of 60. Surgery to take pressure off the nerves can improve walking distance and leg pain.
Leg pain with spondylolisthesis. Spondylolisthesis is measurable slippage of one vertebra on another. In extremely rare cases, the slippage may be great enough to affect nerve root function. Surgery is sometimes used to take pressure off the nerve and to fuse the vertebrae to prevent future slippage.
Fracture or dislocation. Surgery is commonly used to repair a fracture or dislocation if the fracture or dislocation affects the spinal nerves.
Spinal arthritis. If the condition is verified by a positive blood test and is not osteoarthritis or degenerative joint disease, nonsteroidal antiinflammatory drugs such as ibuprofen may be used.

Tests Cannot Always Tell You the Cause of Your Symptoms.

Medical science cannot always explain the exact cause of most common low back symptoms. But medical science is very good at finding out whether you have a dangerous condition causing your symptoms. If your problem is not caused by a serious condition, you can continue looking forward to recovery.

Exercise Is Important.

Remember to continue to exercise as you were instructed by your healthcare provider and as described in Handout #1. It is important not to neglect your muscles. Exercise regularly!

Points to Remember:

- Special studies are not needed for early detection and care of low back problems.
- Special studies can mislead if used alone. They can give additional information about a problem if used with other evidence.
- If your healthcare provider suggests surgery, ask what the evidence is for surgery. Ask about your choices and what would happen without surgery. Get a second opinion from another healthcare provider. Your surgeon will understand how important it is for you to be sure.

---

back: lifting, bending or twisting, and sitting (see box above). The nature and duration of limitations will depend on the clinical status of the patient and the physical requirements of the job or the upper limits of the NIOSH lifting guide over at most a 3-month period from the onset of symptoms or an operative procedure. Activity modifications must be time limited and clear for the patient to take to the employer, and they should be reviewed by the clinician on a regular basis. Because nonphysical factors such as emotional distress or low work satisfaction may also affect an individual's symptoms and response to treatment, activity goals can help keep attention focused on the expected return to full functional status and support further physical conditioning to improve activity tolerance.

Various types of exercise programs have been advocated for patients with low back problems. The most commonly studied types focus on back flexion, back extension, generalized strengthening, endurance (aerobic conditioning), stretching, or some combination of these. Most of these exercises can be either taught to the patient for home use or performed under supervision in a clinical setting. The therapeutic objectives of exercise programs for low back symptoms are improvements in conditioning and functioning and fewer or less severe future back problems. Unfortunately, most programs are unproven.

Exercise programs aimed at improving general endurance (aerobic fitness) and specific back muscle conditioning have been shown to benefit patients with acute low back problems,[22,34] although no evidence supports back stretching as an effective treatment for acute low back problems. The AHCPR panel found that patients with acute low back symptoms would benefit from endurance training that can be started early—using exercises that cause minimal mechanical stress on the back by giving set exercise quotas that are gradually increased with time. If symptoms persist, specific trunk muscle conditioning (especially of the back extensors) can be individualized according to the level of activity to which patients wish to return. The early goal of exercise programs is to avoid inactivity-induced debilitation and then to improve comfortable activity tolerance intended to return patients to their highest level of functioning as soon as possible.

The sooner patients return to their normal activity, the less the debilitation that results from the inactivity. Endurance activity alternatives such as walking, stationary biking, swimming, and even light jogging are safe (they present minimal chance of mechanical harm to the spine) alternatives to avoid debilitation or to begin building activity tolerance. It may be helpful to remind patients that even safe activities may increase symptoms slightly at first. Twenty to 30 minutes of such activity may not be comfortable early in a severe episode of low back symptoms, but this does not actually stress the back more than sitting on the side of the bed before rising in the morning.

Additional and continuous education of patients in an activity paradigm about realistic, safe, and comfortable methods and expectations will greatly assist their recovery from an acute low back episode. It should be stressed that inactivity is dangerous to the back as well as to general well-being. Patients should have realistic expectations about their recovery in relation to their age and prior level of fitness, and they should be reassured that additional diagnostic assessment will be considered after 4 weeks if the limitations persist. Patients with a clear understanding of the problem and confidence in the physician have been proven to have a better outcome.[13]

SPECIAL STUDIES AND DIAGNOSTIC CONSIDERATIONS

Because 90% of patients with acute low back problems spontaneously recover, special studies are not required in the first 4 weeks unless "red flags" are detected. Special diagnostic procedures are often considered after 1 month to seek a reason for the slow recovery. There are two kinds of special studies (see **Table 22-3**). First are tests to measure physiologic dys-

function and indicators of infection, inflammation, malignancy, or other systemic illness. Second are tests that provide pictures of a potential anatomic reason for the dysfunction such as a herniated lumbar disk, spinal stenosis, infection, tumor, or abdominal mass. As a result of these tests, intervention such as surgery may be considered (see box on pp. 295 and 296).

Measuring Physiologic Dysfunction

Electromyography (EMG), sensory evoked potentials (SEPs), and thermography are commonly used tests to measure any focal neurologic physiologic dysfunction. Nonneurological diseases are commonly sought through general laboratory screening tests, including the erythrocyte sedimentation rate (ESR), complete blood count (CBC), urinalysis, and bone scan.

Electrophysiologic Tests

Electrophysiologic tests are sometimes helpful in patients with sciatica to evaluate the physiologic functioning of the spinal cord, nerve roots, and peripheral nerves. Needle electromyography (EMG) assesses acute and chronic nerve root dysfunction, myelopathy, and myopathy. H-reflex, a test measuring sensory conduction through nerve roots, mostly assesses S1 radiculopathies. F-wave response, a test measuring motor conduction through nerve roots, is used to assess proximal neuropathies. Surface EMG (which uses surface electrodes instead of needle insertion) seems not to be accurate enough to assess acute and chronic recruitment patterns during static or dynamic tasks. Sensory-evoked potentials assess sensory neurons in peripheral and spinal cord pathways, especially in older patients suspected of having spinal stenosis. These and nerve conduction studies are used to assess acute and chronic peripheral entrapment or general neuropathies that may mimic radiculopathies.

Although these tests have utility for certain patients with particular symptoms that persist over a period of 3 to 4 weeks, test results and their interpretations may vary. It is important that the physician refer patients to a highly skilled diagnostician for electrophysiologic testing because the accuracy of the finding is highly dependent on the skill with which the examination is performed. These procedures are invasive and may cause discomfort to the patient, whose active participation during the testing is sometimes necessary.

Patients with severe leg symptoms of more than 3 to 4 weeks' duration may be appropriate candidates for EMG and H-reflex tests if the physical examination does not provide obvious information about which nerve root(s) is (are) involved. These tests help to document radiculopathy or neuropathy as the cause of symptoms in the lower extremities, identify specific nerve roots that may be compromised, and differentiate between acute and chronic nerve root dysfunction. Test results from needle EMG tests are not reliable before 3 or 4 weeks after the onset of pain. Sensory evoked potentials are believed useful in diagnosing spinal stenosis[57] and

Table 22-3 Contributions of evaluation methods.		
Technique	**Identify Physiologic Insult**	**Define Anatomic Defect**
History	+	+
Physical exam:		
Circumference measurements	+	+
Reflexes	++	++
SLR	++	+
Crossed SLR	+++	++
Motor	++	++
Sensory	++	++
Laboratory studies (ESR, CBC, UA)	++	0
Bone Scan*	+++	++
EMG/SEP	+++	++
X ray†	0	+
CT	0	++++†
MRI	0	++++†
Myelo-CT*	0	++++†
Myelography*	0	++++†

*Risk of complications (radiation, infection, etc.): highest Myelo-CT > Myelogram > Bone scan, X ray or CT least.
†False positive findings up to 30% without symptoms at age 30.
CBC, complete blood cell count; CT, computed tomography; EMG, electromyogram; ESR, erythrocyte sedimentation rate; SEP, sensory-evoked potentials; SLR, straight leg raise; UA, urinalysis.

spinal cord myelopathy. However, F-wave tests and surface EMGs are not considered effective methods of assessing acute low back symptoms.[5]

BONE SCAN

Bone scanning, which involves the intravenous injection of radioactive salts that adhere where bone turnover is most active, can be a helpful screen and facilitate the imaging and detection of occult fractures, infections, and bony metastases of the spine. This method allows the clinician to distinguish between these findings and common benign pathology such as degenerative changes. The imager should, therefore, be asked to identify lesions other than degenerative joint disease, which must usually be confirmed by other diagnostic tests or procedures because of varying efficacy in screening for different pathologies. Bone scanning is moderately sensitive but does not alone specify the diagnosis.

THERMOGRAPHY

Thermography has not been proven effective as a diagnostic tool and is not accurate in predicting the presence or absence of lumbar nerve root compression.

In patients with low back problems, thermography involves measuring small temperature differences between sides of the body and evaluating the patterns on infrared thermographic images of the back and lower extremities. This is a noninvasive procedure that does not involve radiation and has some utility as a physiologic test for documenting the presence or absence of radiculopathy (nerve root compression).[39]

Tests Providing Anatomic Pictures

In addition to radiography, imaging studies are most generally used to obtain pictures of a possible anatomic cause of a measured physiologic abnormality. Imaging studies include plain myelography, magnetic resonance imaging (MRI), computed tomography (CT), CT-myelography, diskography, and CT-diskography. Abnormal findings on anatomic studies such as MRI, CT, myelography, and diskography may be misleading if they are not corroborated with the measured physiologic abnormality pointed to by the medical history or found on physical examination or physiologic tests. A major problem with imaging studies is the difficulty in determining that an anatomic defect, if present, is actually the cause of the symptoms. Many anatomic abnormalities of the lumbar spine are the result of aging

OVERCOMING YOUR BACK PROBLEM

By now, your healthcare provider has given you the news that you can comfortably begin to get back to your daily activities. Even if you required surgery, you can now safely begin a specific, gentle exercise program to condition your body and your back muscles. This program will increase you back's ability to help you do the things you want and need to do.

Start with a simple, safe exercise such as walking, stationary biking, or swimming to build your general stamina. If you have been inactive, you may need to begin slowly and gradually increase your activity each day. Your healthcare provider will make specific recommendations for safe exercises that do not stress your back any more than sitting on the side of your bed. Exercise helps because it

- Trains the muscles that protect your back
- Conditions your whole body
- Stimulates the body to make its own powerful pain killers
- Allows you to do things more comfortably

You will also find out what you can do easily and what takes more effort.

Reality About Back Problems.

Although your recovery seems slow, your symptoms will continue to decrease unless you are inactive. However, your back may never feel as "young" as it once did. This happens to many of us by age 30, most by age 40, and just about everyone by age 50. Back problems are often the **first** sign of aging. You may have noticed that few professional athletes can continue competing beyond age 40. Although some people may be able to resume strenuous activity after back problems as they get older, they usually need to go at a slower pace. Most people need to "shift gears" and make changes in goals and activities as they grow older. Even at a slower pace, exercise will help you to be able to tolerate more of your daily activities.

Once you have had an activity-limiting back problem that lasts for more than a few weeks, there is a 40% to 60% chance of having another back problem within the next few years. However, symptoms are usually not as severe in future episodes as in the first episode.

Success.

As you begin to recover, the goal is to try to prevent back problems from returning or, if they do return, from being severe. Success will depend on two factors. The first is the condition of your protective muscles. The second is the activities you ask your back to tolerate.

Ignoring either of these factors usually means more back problems. For example, a coal miner can expect further problems because mining is so demanding on the back. By contrast, a member of royalty who never needs to stress his or her back but does no conditioning exercises can also expect regular back problems. How well *you* do in the future will depend on what kind of condition you are in and what you ask your back to do. The more easily you and your protective muscles tire, the greater the chance that your symptoms will return. Taking action to condition the protective muscles of your back can reduce your future problems.

Safe Exercises That Are Good For You and Your Back.

Although exercises such as walking, stationary bicycling, or swimming are safe, you may feel some discomfort when you *first* start. After muscles become better conditioned, the soreness goes away. For example, during the winter when the weather is bad and many of us might stay indoors and be less active, the muscles of the back can lose their conditioning. When the first day of spring arrives and many of us go out to the garden, the back may begin to ache when the out-of-condition protective muscles easily tire. Continuing such work daily over a few days or weeks *reconditions* the protective muscles so that they don't tire quite so easily, and the soreness disappears.

Remember that an increase in discomfort in an already painful back is common. But safe exercises (which involve less stress on the back than sitting on the side of the bed) should not harm your back. The shorter the time since beginning the conditioning, the greater the chance of increased soreness.

Conditioning Requires Regular Activity.

Regular activity is essential to obtain the conditioning effect to protect your back. Conditioning is achieved by building up to 30 minutes of continuous walking, stationary cycling, or swimming at a targeted heart rate (see list below) or through jogging for 20 minutes. Conditioning works best if combined with your normal, daily activities both at home and at work. Stay as active as possible and exercise every day.

Your healthcare provider may have suggested ways to modify your daily chores to reduce the chance of irritating your back. Such changes at home or work are usually temporary. They are intended to give you time to improve the condition of your protective back muscles so that you can resume most normal activities. The table on p. 300 offers guidelines to your healthcare provider on work recommendations to allow you reasonable time to recondition your back. Long-term activity tolerance varies greatly from person to person. Age and overall health are also important factors. Regular, mild exercise may be enough for some. Others may be able to return to vigorous activities at a slower pace.

Continued.

Patient discussion handout #3—Continued

Points to Remember:
- Both your level of physical conditioning and the stresses you put on your back will determine how often you will have problems and how severe they become.
- Conditioning usually requires daily work and commitment.
- Be sure your activity goal is realistic and you know what it will take to achieve it. Once you are over your back symptoms or after a month of general conditioning training, your healthcare provider may suggest that you begin doing back muscle, trunk, or extremity exercises to gain further tolerance for specific tasks.
- If you have great difficulty resuming your previous daily routine, you may need to consider whether your old routine is realistic for you now.

Building Exercise Tolerance

1. Try to maintain your daily activity as close to your normal level as possible.
2. As soon as possible, begin walking, riding a stationary bicycle, or swimming. Choose what works for you.
3. Gradually build up to 30 minutes of activity without stopping.
4. Once you can tolerate 30 minutes of activity, establish a target heart rate that will help you to condition your muscles, heart, and respiratory system.
5. Then, your healthcare provider may also recommend some exercises for your back muscles.

Guidelines for Sitting and Unassisted Lifting

Activity	Symptoms and Findings			
	Severe →	Moderate →	Mild →	None‡
Sitting*	20 minutes	→	50 minutes	
Unassisted lifting†				
Men	20 lb	30 lb	60 lb	80 lb
Women	20 lb	25 lb	35 lb	40 lb

*Without getting up and moving around for a few moments.
†Modification of the NIOSH lifting guides, 1981, 1993. Gradually increase unassisted lifting limits to at least 60 lbs (men) and 35 lb (women) by 3 months even with objective findings. Instruct patients to limit twisting, bending, and reaching as much as possible, especially while lifting, and to hold lifted objects as close to the navel as possible.
‡No limitations if the patient requests to go above these levels.

and appear in imaging tests of asymptomatic patients (see Table 22-3). Because of these concerns, researchers stress the importance of not relying too heavily on imaging studies alone for assessment when nerve root compromise is suspected.[27,41,53,55] Findings should be correlated with the medical history, physical examination, and other physiologic methods.

RADIOGRAPHY

Radiographs can be valuable for evaluating patients with "red flags" in the first month of symptoms if there is the possibility of fracture as a result of recent trauma or osteoporosis. Radiographs can also be assistive in finding tumor or infection, but only the CBC and ESR can rule out red flags for cancer or infection. The diagnostic objective of radiography is to reveal the bony and structural abnormalities associated with back symptoms.

Radiography alone is rarely useful in evaluating or guiding treatment of acute low back pain. Plain x-ray films are not effective for diagnosing lumbar nerve root impingement of a herniated disk or spinal stenosis, nor do they add useful clinical information when revealing spinal degenerative changes, congenital abnormalities, spondylolysis, spondylolisthesis, or scoliosis.[7]

COMPUTED TOMOGRAPHY, MAGNETIC RESONANCE IMAGING, MYELOGRAPHY, AND CT-MYELOGRAPHY

Pictures from plain myelography, CT, MRI, and CT-myelography are commonly used in assessing the anatomy of the lumbar spinal canal and its contents. These four tests are used in similar clinical situations,

---

Patient discussion handout #4

WHEN EXERCISE IS NOT HELPING

By now, your healthcare provider has made every effort to seek a medical reason for your continued activity limitation. You are well into the exercise program intended to condition your back for the activities you need to do. Unfortunately, for some people success is less easy and slower to achieve. If this is the case, there are many things to consider.

Age Is Important

Few middle-aged persons have a back that is as strong as it was at 18. Medical science presently cannot reverse the aging process that limits activities requiring both speed and strength. Young people may find it difficult to give up or alter activities that they have been doing for a long time.

Some people continue to look for a "cure" when progress is slow. Such efforts rarely succeed. Consider a basketball star like Larry Bird. Money was surely no object in seeking a cure for his back problem. He could afford the most expensive medical care and conditioning program. Nevertheless, he was forced to retire at age 34. His back could no longer tolerate the physical stress of basketball.

How many athletes in strenuous sports can compete beyond age 35 or 40? Very few! Most of us just adjust our activities as we age, regardless of our occupation or level of physical conditioning, many by age 30, most by age 40, and just about all of us by age 50. Some people continue strenuous activities into their older years, especially if they are able to do it at their own pace. Others may need to consider change.

Be Realistic.

Ask yourself three key questions about your daily activity requirements:

- Can a reasonable exercise program overcome my back problem?
- Will it be possible to continue a more time-consuming exercise program and my usual daily requirements long-term?
- Is there any way I can change my activity requirements now or in the future?

If a reasonable exercise program is not helping you, there are several options: (1) you can choose to put up with discomfort and expect some setbacks, (2) you can begin a more time-consuming conditioning program, or (3) you can change the pace of doing difficult activities. This may include a job change. People may use a combination of the three approaches.

Considering a job change is difficult, especially if back problems continue to limit your ability to do your work. Again, ask yourself this important question: "Is my activity goal realistic, or do I need to look at my options?" A review now might help you avoid a similar dilemma in the near or distant future, especially if your job activities present a problem.

When a job or career change is considered, it is important to gather information from many sources. Some possibilities include private career counselors, local or state employment offices, and veterans' or consumer groups. You may also want to talk to someone working in the field.

Information Is Your Ally.

Whether or not you explore job opportunities alone or with professional help, remember this important point:

Only you can find a way to adjust your life, your job, or your plans in a way that is right for you.

---

provide similar types of information, and are often compared with each other in research studies. There is a lack of a "gold standard" for evaluating the efficacy of these tests alone and in combination, but pictures from these tests can be useful, after 1 month of continuous symptoms, in ruling out tumor, infection, or fracture and in preparation for surgical intervention. Myelography and CT-myelography are invasive and should only be used under special situations for preoperative planning.

There are significant findings from studies comparing the utility of these diagnostic tests for various conditions. These are discussed in detail in the clinical practice guideline.[5] Routine spinal imaging tests are not used during the first month of symptoms except when a red flag is noted in the medical history or physical examination. These tests may be useful after 1 month of symptoms if surgery is being considered for a specific detectable loss of neurologic function or to further

evaluate possibly serious spinal pathology in the presence of red flags. The clinician should remember that relying on imaging studies alone without a reliable measure of physiological dysfunction carries a significant risk of diagnostic confusion.

DISKOGRAPHY

Diskography involves the injection of a water-soluble imaging material directly into the nucleus pulposus of the disk and has two diagnostic objectives: to radiographically evaluate the extent of the disk damage on the diskogram (sometimes with the addition of CT) and to characterize the pain response on disk injection. A symptomatic degenerative disk is considered to be one that disperses injected contrast in an abnormal pattern. Additionally, a painful reaction by the patient is sought to classify the disk as abnormal. This is a risky procedure with many potential complications.

The relationship between positive findings and disease is not clear, nor is the utility of the information collected from this procedure. There seems to be limited evidence that diskography can help identify patients who would benefit from spinal fusion and no evidence that it is helpful in patients with acute low back problems. Other imaging techniques seem preferable and less harmful.

SURGICAL CONSIDERATIONS

Surgery is rarely indicated in the first 4 weeks for acute low back symptoms. This section is presented as an orientation for the primary healthcare provider. The reader is referred to Chapter 21 for more information.

Decompression of nerve roots compressed by a herniated lumbar disk is the only condition for which surgical procedures are commonly considered within the first 3 months of low back symptoms. Surgery for spinal stenosis, which begins gradually in older adults, is rarely considered within this time frame. Except for cases of trauma causing spinal fracture or dislocation, fusion is not usually considered in the first 3 months of symptoms.

Lumbar spine surgery may speed recovery when there are strong indications. In the face of vague indications, surgery may lead to a poorer result than no surgery and necessitate future procedures with greater risks. Surgery is commonly discussed for back symptoms that are unresolved after special studies. Careful consideration should be given to the risks and potential outcomes of surgical treatment for different diagnoses.

Surgery for Herniated Disk

Surgery for herniated disks is invasive and involves the removal of herniated intervertebral disk material that compresses nerve roots. Asymptomatic middle-aged adults commonly have intervertebral disk herniations (usually of the softer central nucleus pulposus through defects in the outer annulus fibrosus) into the neural canal without the entrapment of a nerve root that causes irritation, dysfunction, and leg pain. Standard diskectomy and microscopic diskectomy directly decompress nerve roots, whereas chemonucleolysis (chymopapain injection) and percutaneous diskectomy attempt to do so indirectly. The therapeutic objective is to relieve pressure on nerve roots and reduce pain and possibly weakness and/or numbness in the lower extremities. There are a range of complications associated with the surgery, especially with chymopapain therapy, which has been used less frequently in the United States in recent years.

Lumbar diskectomy may relieve the symptoms faster than continued nonsurgical treatment in patients with severe and disabling leg symptoms (and definite clinical findings of lumbar nerve root compromise) who have not improved after 4 to 8 weeks of nonsurgical treatment. Studies show that there is no difference in long-term outcomes at 4 and 10 years between diskectomy

and conservative care.[69,70] The best results from herniated disk surgery were with direct methods of standard diskectomy and microscopic diskectomy, and in all cases patient preference and expectations play a major role in success of the intervention. Some studies have shown that psychological factors recorded on the Minnesota Multiphasic Personality Inventory (MMPI) were better predictors of surgical outcome than were findings of imaging studies.[53,55]

Surgery for Spinal Stenosis

Spinal stenosis includes any constriction or narrowing of the central spinal canal, lateral recesses, or foramina that results in compression of nerve roots and/or the cauda equina. Surgery for spinal stenosis may include various types of surgical techniques, usually including decompressive laminectomy (sometimes combined with diskectomy and/or spinal fusion) done to alleviate the symptoms of neural compression. Surgery for spinal stenosis is not usually considered in the first 3 months of symptoms. Spinal stenosis is a disease caused by extreme spinal aging, and the most predictable surgical outcome is improved walking tolerance in elderly patients. There are also some younger patients with severe congenital narrowing of the spinal canal who have spinal stenosis symptoms, but this is uncommon. Decisions on treatment should take into consideration the patient's preference, lifestyle, other medical problems, and the risks associated with surgery. Because of the nature of the problem, even good results from surgery will deteriorate over time as the spine continues to age and deteriorate.[29]

Spinal Fusion

Fusion is used for traumatic fractures and dislocation but rarely for common low back symptoms alone within the first 3 months.[26,71] Lumbar spinal fusion surgeries using bone grafts have only been proven helpful in spinal stenosis surgery when slippage and motion are present. The benefit of adding metal devices to produce a rigid connection between two or more adjacent vertebrae has not been proven to be greater than the risk it carries. In fact, the therapeutic objective of spinal fusion surgery for patients with low back pain to prevent any movement in the intervertebral spaces between the fused vertebrae has not been proven to predictably reduce pain and future neurological deficits.[63]

TREATMENT AFTER SPECIAL STUDIES OR SURGERY

Following diagnostic or surgical procedures, the patient can usually be reassured that no dangerous condition jeopardizes reengaging the "activity begets activity tolerance" paradigm by now building comfortable activity tolerance through exercise (see box on p. 299). Postprocedural recommendations emphasize physical reconditioning through gradual exercise to regain tolerance for wanted or needed activity. Symptom-control methods should be used to help make the conditioning process as comfortable as possible.

Conditioning can begin with safe endurance activities to provide a foundation to which specific exercises can be added. Low-stress aerobic conditioning (perhaps 30 minutes per day at a reasonable heart rate) can improve general stamina. Exercises that condition specific extensor and other trunk muscles can begin before general strengthening or specific task training. The importance of *gradual* and *consistent* efforts cannot be overstressed, especially when related to required daily activity such as work. The best activation program is a gradual increase in doing the actual required activity in the workplace. Work recommendations can be graduated over a few months at most to allow time to recondition protective muscles and build specific activity tolerance. If the activity and conditioning recommendations stall temporarily, endurance activities can be emphasized as the least mechanically stressful activity for the back and as an alternative to inactivity, which may further debilitate the patient.

If the patient is having difficulties with reaching the needed activity level, a few simple steps should be taken before considering more specialized or expensive help.

- The history and physical examination can be reviewed to be sure that no "red flags" have arisen.
- Tell the patient of your concern about how realistic the intended activity levels may be until age 65 if they are presently so difficult to attain. This can be an especially emotional issue if related to the return to work.
- Offer to help the patient explore options (see box on p. 301).
- If no efforts are made, tactfully explore nonphysical pressures that may have an impact on any patient's perception of discomfort and progress toward regaining comfortable activity tolerance.
- Offer a counselor to help the patient figure out what other factors may be interfering with recovery.

Nonphysical factors (psychosocial, socioeconomic) are well established as important determinants of patient response to symptoms and care. Frustration commonly leads to the use of specialized help to address these concerns, including psychological counseling and vocational counseling. (See Chapter 6 for additional information.)

CLINICAL ASSESSMENT OF NON-PHYSICAL FACTORS

Nonphysical social, economic, and psychological factors have been reported to be more important than physical factors in affecting the symptoms, response to treatment, and long-term outcomes of patients with chronic low back problems.[66] There are indications that such nonphysical factors may also have an impact on patients with acute low back symptoms. For patients considering surgery, scales 3 and 1 of the MMPI have been found to provide more value than both anatomical and physiological tests, especially in predicting who will do poorly.[53,55] A heightened awareness among clinicians to the way such factors may affect a patient's response to symptoms and treatment is therefore warranted. Work satisfaction and poor work performance reports are two factors that have been identified as predictors for identifying individuals who will report back problems at work.[6] These theories are discussed in greater detail in Chapter 6 of this text.

The clinician can become aware of these nonphysical factors while evaluating and treating patients with low back problems, especially when recovery of activity tolerance following an acute episode of low back symptoms is delayed. More research is needed to define specific means of detecting nonphysical factors as well as intervening in a way that might improve outcomes for those patients slow to recover from acute low back problems.

A clinician can explore possible nonphysical pressures in the course of caring for the patient. The first step comes with any hint of slow progress. The clinician should state concern for what the patient might do if return or long-term continuation of a certain work activity is not possible for any reason. Clinicians should also offer to help the patient seek options and support a decision to return to either the former job or a different job. Once sufficient information is gathered, the patient's decisions become more logical. When a patient makes no effort to seek options, a clinician can raise further legitimate concerns about factors other than back symptoms that might keep someone from seeking counseling. The physician can point out that delays in recovery commonly result from problems other than back symptoms, including illiteracy, depression, and even addiction. This discussion can lead to an explanation of options in treatment when extreme or inappropriate behavior is manifested as acquiescence to disability and pain.

References

1. Anderson R et al: A meta-analysis of clinical trials of spinal manipulation, *J Manipulative Physiol Ther* 15(3):181-194, 1992.

2. Andersson GBJ: The epidemiology of spinal disorders. In Frymoyer JW, editor: *The adult spine: principles and practice,* New York, 1991, Raven Press; pp. 107-146.

3. Aronson HA, Dunsmore RH: Herniated upper lumbar disks, *J Bone Joint Surg [Am]* 45A:311-317, 1963.

4. Bass MJ et al: The physician's actions and the outcome of illness in family practice, *J Fam Pract* 23(1):43-47, 1986.

5. Bigos S et al: *Acute low back problems in adults: clinical practice guideline No. 14,* AHCPR Pub No 95-0643, Rockville, Md, 1994, U.S. Department of Health and Human Services, Public Health Service, Agency for Health Care Policy and Research.

6. Bigos S et al: A prospective study of work perceptions and psychosocial factors affecting the report of back injury, *Spine* 16(1):1-6, 1991.

7. Bigos SJ et al: The value of preemployment roentgenographs for predicting acute back injury claims and chronic pain disability, *Clin Orthop* 283:124-129, 1992.

8. Cats-Baril WL, Frymoyer JW: Identifying patients at risk of becoming disabled because of low back pain. The Vermont Rehabilitation Engineering Center predictive model, *Spine* 16(6):605-607, 1991.

9. Chaffin DB: A biomechanical strength model for use in industry, *Appl Ind Hyg* 3(3):79-86, 1988.

10. Colleé G et al: Iliac crest pain syndrome in low back pain: a double blind, randomized study of local injection therapy, *J Rheumatol* 18(7):1060-1063, 1991.

11. Cunningham LS, Kelsey JL: Epidemiology of musculoskeletal impairments and associated disability, *Am J Public Health* 74:574-579, 1984.

12. Damkot DK et al: The relationship between work history, work environment and low back pain in men, *Spine* 9:395-399, 1984.

13. Deyo RA, Diehl AK: Patient satisfaction with medical care for low back pain, *Spine* 11(1):28-30, 1986.

14. Deyo RA, Diehl AK: Psychosocial predictors of disability in patients with low back pain, *J Rheumatol* 15(10):1557-1564, 1988.

15. Deyo RA et al: Cost, controversy, crisis: low back pain and the health of the public, *Annu Rev Public Health* 12:141-156, 1991.

16. Deyo RA et al: A controlled trial of transcutaneous electrical nerve stimulation (TENS) and exercise for chronic low back pain, *N Engl J Med* 322(23):1627-1634, 1990.

17. Drury CG: Influence of restricted space on manual materials handling, *Ergonomics* 28(1):167-175, 1985.

18. Dul J, Hildebrandt VH: Ergonomic guidelines for the prevention of low back pain at the workplace, *Ergonomics* 30(2):419-429, 1987.

19. Garg A, Moore JS: Epidemiology of low-back pain in industry, *Occup Med* 7(4):593-608, 1992.

20. Goertz MN: Prognosis indicators for acute low back pain, *Spine* 15(12):1307-1310, 1990.

21. Gundewall B, Liljeqvist M, Hansson T: Primary prevention of back symptoms and absence from work. A prospective, randomized, multicentered trial, *Spine* 16(suppl 6):s206-s212, 1993.

22. Hackett GI, Seddon D, Kaminski D: Electroacupuncture compared with paracetamol for acute low back pain, *Practitioner* 232(1443):163-164, 1988.

23. Hadler NM et al: A benefit of spinal manipulation as adjunctive therapy for acute low back pain: a stratified controlled trial, *Spine* 12(7):703-706, 1987.

24. Hakelius A, Hindmarsh J: The comparative reliability of preoperative diagnostic methods in lumbar disk surgery, *Acta Orthop Scand* 43:234-238, 1972.

25. Herkowitz HN, Kurz LT: Degenerative lumbar spondylolisthesis with spinal stenosis, *J Bone Joint Surg [Am]* 73A(6):802-808, 1991.

26. Herron LD, Turner J: Patient selection for lumbar laminectomy and discectomy with a revised objective rating system, *Clin Orthop* 199:145-152, 1985.

27. Jackson RP: The facet syndrome. Myth or reality? *Clin Orthop* 279:110-121, 1992.

28. Katz JN et al: The outcome of decompressive laminectomy for degenerative lumbar stenosis, *J Bone Joint Surg [Am]* 73A(6):809-816, 1991.

29. Keijsers JFEM, Bouter LM, Meertens RM: Validity and comparability of studies on the effects of back schools, *Physiother Theory Pract* 7 (3):177-184, 1991.

30. Kortelainen P et al: Symptoms and signs of sciatica and their relation to the localization of the lumbar disk herniation, *Spine* 10(1):88-92, 1985.

31. Kosteljanetz M et al: Predictive value of clinical and surgical findings in patients with lumbago-sciatica. A prospective study (Part I), *Acta Neurochir* 73(1-2):67-76, 1984.

32. Lacroix JM et al: Low back pain. Factors of value in predicting outcome, *Spine* 15(6):495-499, 1990.

33. Lindström I et al: The effect of graded activity on patients with subacute low back pain: a randomized prospective clinical study with an operant-conditioning behavioral approach, *Phys Ther* 72(4):279-293, 1992.

34. Linton SJ, Kamwendo K: Low back schools: a critical review, *Phys Ther* 67(9):1375-1383, 1987.

35. MacDonald RS, Bell CM: An open controlled assessment of osteopathic manipulation in nonspecific low-back pain [published erratum appears in *Spine* 16(1):104, 199.], *Spine* 15(5):364-370, 1990.

36. Malmivaara A et al: The treatment of acute low back pain—bed rest, exercises, or ordinary activity? *New Engl J Med* 332(6):351, 1995.

37. McNeill TW, Sinkora G, Leavitt F: Psychologic classification of low back pain patients: a prognostic tool, *Spine* 11(9):955-959, 1986.

38. Mills GH et al: The evaluation of liquid crystal thermography in the investigation of nerve root compression due to lumbosacral lateral spinal stenosis, *Spine* 11(5):427-432, 1986.

39. Mooney V: Injection studies. Role in pain definition. In Frymoyer JW, editor: *The adult spine: principles and practice,* New York, 1991, Raven Press; pp. 527-540.

40. Morris EW et al: Diagnosis and decision making in lumbar disk prolapse and nerve entrapment, *Spine* 11(5):436-439, 1986.

41. Murphy KA, Cornish RD: Prediction of chronicity in acute low back pain, *Arch Phys Med Rehabil* 65(6):334-337, 1984.

42. Nachemson AL: Disc pressure measurements, *Spine* 6(1):93-97, 1981.

43. Nachemson AL: Newest knowledge of low back pain. A critical look, *Clin Orthop* 279:8-20, 1992.

44. National Institute for Occupational Safety and Health: *Work practices guideline for manual lifting,* NIOSH Tech Rep No 81-122, Cincinnati, 1981, U.S. Department of Health and Human Services, National Institute for Occupational Safety and Health.

45. Nykvist F et al: Social factors and outcome in a five-year follow-up study of 276 patients with sciatica, *Scand J Rehabil Med* 23(1):19-26, 1991.

46. Postacchini F, Facchini M, Palieri P: Efficacy of various forms of conservative treatment in low back pain: a comparative study, *Neuro-Orthopedics* 6(1):28-35, 1988.

47. Ransford AO, Cairns D, Mooney V: The pain drawing as an aid to the psychologic evaluation of patients with low-back pain, *Spine* 1(2):127-134, 1976.

48. Roland M, Dixon M: Randomized controlled trial of an educational booklet for patients presenting with back pain in general practice, *J R Coll Gen Pract* 39(323):244-246, 1989.

49. Shekelle PG et al: Spinal manipulation for low-back pain, *Ann Intern Med* 117(7):590-598, 1992.

50. Spangfort EV: The lumbar disk herniation, *Acta Orthop Scand Suppl* 142:1-95, 1972.

51. Spengler DM, Freeman CW: Patient selection for lumbar discectomy: an objective approach, *Spine* 4(2):129-134, 1979.

52. Spengler DM et al: Back injuries in industry: a retrospective study. I. Overview and cost analysis, *Spine* 11(3):241-256, 1986.

53. Spengler DM et al: Elective discectomy for herniation of a lumbar disk: additional experience with an objective method, *J Bone Joint Surg [Am]* 72A(2):230-237, 1990.

54. Sternbach RA: Survey of pain in the United States: the Nuprin pain report, *Clin J Pain* 2(1):49-53, 1986.

55. Stolov WC, Slimp JC: *Dermatomal somatosensory evoked potentials in lumbar spinal stenosis.* Paper presented at a joint symposium of the American Association for Electromyography and Electrodiagnosis and the American Electroencephalography Society, 1988; pp. 17-22.

56. Sullivan JGB: The anesthesiologist's approach to back pain. In Herkowitz HN et al, editors: *The spine,* ed 3, Philadelphia, 1992, WB Saunders; pp 1945-1961.

57. ter Riet G, Kleijnen J, Knipschild P: Acupuncture and chronic pain: a criteria-based meta-analysis, *J Clin Epidemiol* 43(11):1191-1199, 1990.

58. Turner JA et al: Patient outcomes after lumbar spinal fusions, *JAMA* 268(7):907-911, 1992.

59. Udén A, Landin LA: Pain drawing and myelography in sciatic pain, *Clin Orthop* 216:124-130, 1987.

60. Vällfors B: Acute, subacute and chronic low back pain: clinical symptoms, absenteeism, and working environment, *Scand J Rehabil Med Suppl* 11:1-98, 1985.

61. Vaughan PA, Malcolm BW, Maistrelli GL: Results of L4-L5 disk excision alone versus disk excision and fusion, *Spine* 13(6):690-695, 1988.

62. Von Baeyer CL et al: Invalid use of pain drawings in psychological screening of back pain patients, *Pain* 16(1):103-107, 1983.

63. Von Korff M et al: Back pain in primary care: outcomes at 1 year *Spine* 18(7):855-862, 1993.

64. Waddell G: Biopsychosocial analysis of low back pain, *Baillieres Clin Rheumatol* 6(3):523-557, 1992.

65. Waters TR et al: Revised NIOSH equation for the design and evaluation of manual lifting tasks, *Ergonomics* 36(7):749-776, 1993.

66. Waterworth RF, Hunter IA: An open study of diflunisal, conservative and manipulative therapy in the management of acute mechanical low back pain, *NZ Med J* 98(779):372-375, 1985.

67. Weber H: Lumbar disk herniation. A controlled, prospective study with ten years of observation, *Spine* 8(2):131-140, 1983.

68. Weber H: The effect of delayed disk surgery on muscular paresis *Acta Orthop Scand* 46:631-642, 1975.

69. White AH et al: Lumbar laminectomy for herniated disk: a prospective controlled comparison with internal fixation fusion *Spine* 12(3):305-307, 1987.

70. Wilkinson HA: Alternative therapies for the failed back syndrome. In Frymoyer JW, editor: *The adult spine: principles and practice,* New York, 1991, Raven Press; pp 2069-2091.

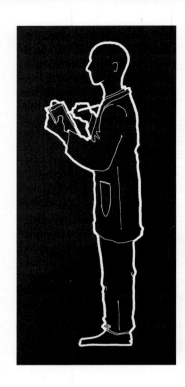

Chapter 23

Rehabilitation of the Worker with Chronic Low Back Pain

Tom G. Mayer

CONTENTS

Rehabilitation of injured workers with spinal disorders creates special problems, much akin to those arising with chronic disability of any musculoskeletal area. Emerging concepts of assessment and care require definition so that the reader may appreciate these concepts in the broader context of all nonoperative assessment, treatment, and prevention.

The first major concept is that the severity of a musculoskeletal injury in the worker's compensation industrial setting is much more dependent on the chronicity of the condition and the disability created than on the inciting event. This observation runs counter to the experience with severe orthopaedic trauma. The vast majority of worker injuries to the musculoskeletal system involve the "soft tissues": "sprains and strains" of musculoligamentous tissues that in most cases have a relatively brief healing period. When healing is incomplete or imperfect and results in permanent impairment of important supporting elements, the socioeconomic cost is dramatically greater in terms of loss of human productivity, direct medical cost, and disability-related indemnity benefits. Most studies demonstrate that the mean cost of low back pain care is more than 10 times greater than the median cost, implying that the relatively small number of chronic cases accounts for most of the social and financial cost.

With the concept of chronological severity in mind, demarcation of treatment into three distinct levels is useful. Primary treatment, which is generally applied in acute cases, is designed for symptom control and most frequently involves the so-called passive modalities (temperature modalities, electrical stimulation, manipulation, etc.). These may be accompanied by low-intensity supervised exercises and education. The vast majority of patients entering the medical system require only this treatment. Secondary treatment is appropriate in the postacute phase and is the first level of reactivation treatment, which at this stage is of medium intensity. Secondary treatment, which generally involves more restorative exercise and education designed to prevent the onset of deconditioning, is usually provided by physical/occupational therapists with consultative psychological, disability management, and physician multidisciplinary services available. Tertiary treatment is appropriate for a small number of chronically disabled patients requiring physician-directed, intensive, interdisciplinary team treatment with multiple professionals on-site and available for the treatment of all participants. Programs are usually organized according to the Commission on Accreditation of Rehabilitation Facilities (CARF) pain management guidelines, but they may follow many diverse patterns. Functional restoration is one of the modes of tertiary treatment with proven outcomes in worker's compensation settings in multiple venues, and as such functional restoration is the focus of this chapter.

Functional restoration involves several concepts not generally considered part of conservative care. The first of these is the concept of deconditioning. From a physical point of view, disuse and immobilization lead to many deleterious effects on joint mobility, muscle strength, endurance, and soft tissue homeostasis. A corollary to this problem is the lack of visual feedback to complex spinal structures, which necessitates a quantification of function technology not specifically required in extremity rehabilitation.

The second major concept involves psychosocial and socioeconomic factors in disability that often accompany chronic and postoperative low back pain. Disability refers to the inability to perform all the usual functions of daily living and is frequently linked to prolonged episodes of severe low back pain. Various treatment interventions are designed to cope with the psychosocial and socioeconomic factors involved in total or partial disability. Psychosocial assessment is often necessary to identify these factors and guide treatment. In addition to psychosocial problems originating because of persistent pain and disability, latent psychopathology may also be activated by these issues. As such, psychiatric interventions including the use of psychotropic drugs and detoxification from narcotic and tranquilizer habituation will often prove necessary.

Finally, primary and secondary treatment alone may be insufficiently effective to deal with chronic dysfunction, and programmatic care delivered by an interdisciplinary team will often prove desirable, if available. Such tertiary approaches will be considered separately.

PHYSICAL AND FUNCTIONAL CAPACITY AND THE DECONDITIONING SYNDROME

Musculoskeletal clinicians have visual access to most parts of the organ system. However, in the spinal anatomy, the small, inaccessible, three-joint complexes that are stacked on each other lend themselves to inspection only with great difficulty. Intersegmental spine movement is difficult to measure, even with biplanar x-ray devices. Multiple small muscles interdigitate over variable numbers of segments, and ligamentous structures may share surprising amounts of load in certain joint positions. Moreover, voluntary dynamic control is attenuated and bilateral comparisons are impossible. Until recently no valid indirect measurement methods were available to assess spine function. In the majority of cases of spine dysfunction not resolving spontaneously, considerable ignorance of pathologic processes is a factor. Currently, however, although absence of direct visualization methodology persists, novel technology for assessing spine function has become part of clinical routine. Yet many clinicians persist in ignoring or refuse to use such technology. In so doing, therapeutic errors are encouraged, outcomes remain unevaluated, and fringe or fad treatments are perpetuated.

The recognition of deconditioning associated with knee meniscal injuries and surgery in World War II and popularized by highly visible football players two decades later led to a therapeutic revolution in combined surgical and rehabilitative treatment of the knee that persists today. Although facilitated by easy visual access to the lower extremity, the concepts translate nicely to spinal disorders. Inactivity leads to loss of general body functional performance ability, as is well recognized by any athlete, with uniform loss of functional capacity. Additionally, the injured area sustains more profound loss of paraarticular soft tissue function and becomes progressively worse as the period of disuse and immobilization increases. These changes create a "weak link" in the localized extremity joint or spinal region, and physical capacity must be measured separately.

In assessing spine function, we have drawn from experience with the extremities in identifying elements of performance that are of value in characterizing extremity physiologic units. Range of motion, strength, neurological status, endurance combined with whole-body aerobic capacity, and activities of daily living are some of the major factors traditionally assessed. Evaluation of extremity neurological function (straight leg raising, lower extremity strength, sensation and reflexes in dermatomal/myotomal patterns) is still viewed by the majority of clinicians as the optimally objective spine functional evaluation; however, these neurological characteristics may be irrelevant for several reasons. First, they are a measure of acute change when noted in relation to surgical pathology. In chronic situations, persistence of neurological changes generally reflects epidural fibrosis or other permanent, noncorrectable anatomic abnormalities. In addition, the neurological deficits, although they emanate from spinal structures, are perceived by the patient as extremity abnormalities producing pain, sensory changes, and weakness of the arms or legs. Consequently, what the clinician currently views as standard "objective" functional tests may provide no useful information to overcome spinal deconditioning.

A critical principle of measurement is the need to be accurate, reliable, and discriminating. Tests also need to be relevant to the physiology being measured. As an example of the latter, an isometric leg lift strength test performed with the back straight in a squatting position probably defines very little about the strength of injured or deconditioned lumbar musculature. Moreover, physics-based principles must be used to evaluate quantitative measurement devices with terms such as "accuracy" and "precision," much as would be used to evaluate the performance of a scale or speedometer. It is not sufficient to identify a device's measurement as "reliable" because very accurate devices may give unreliable data because of normal human variability (which can be accounted for by appropriate normative databases). Similarly, very accurate devices may provide data inca-

pable of being used clinically because of wide fluctuations in human performance caused by a variety of other sources of error. These sources of error may include the human-device interface, training of test administrators, or a "low signal output" by the device relative to the "noise" in the system. Because of a variety of "secondary gain" or fear issues that may impede performance in injured individuals, an effort assessment capability is a desirable concomitant of a device to be used in patients with low back symptoms. Physicians, therapists, and technicians using devices for indirect, objective measurement of spine function should have a basic understanding of quantitative assessment science to allow them to evaluate the merit of each system.

When low back pain disability is assessed, the various psychosocial and socioeconomic components associated with the physical symptoms are likely to make self-report of pain symptoms an unreliable gauge of treatment progression. For this reason, as well as because of the absence of visual feedback to complex trunk joints and musculature, indirect, objective assessment of function is necessary. In fact, such quantitative measures are a necessity for deriving any objective information from the lumbar spine, as compared with extremity rehabilitation, where functional tests may be an adjunct luxury only. Objective, quantitative measurements of function provide the clinician with a definition of patient physical capacity, whereas succeeding tests document changes in performance with treatment. Suboptimal effort demonstrates the degree to which barriers to recovery impede physical performance and lead to changes in psychosocial treatment interventions. Finally, at "maximum medical recovery," quantitative tests outline the patient's work capacity and the functional elements often required as part of an impairment/disability evaluation. The following paragraphs outline the essentials of quantitative functional evaluation (QFE) as used in the standardized functional restoration program implemented at the Productive Rehabilitation Institute of Dallas for Ergonomics (PRIDE). These are the specific physical capacity and functional capacity tests to cover the injured region and whole-person task, respectively, and include the following:

A. **Physical Capacity Testing**
1. RANGE OF MOTION MEASUREMENTS

    Lumbar range-of-motion measurements involve an inclinometer (or gravity/bubble goniometer) to provide angular motion measurements.* This technique involves the placement of an inclinometer over T12-L1 to measure maximum lumbar flexion/extension and a second inclinometer over the sacrum to separate hip motion, thereby deriving true lumbar motion by subtracting the sacral reading from the T12-L1 reading. Although somewhat cumbersome on initial use, proficiency develops rapidly, and newer technology

*References 1, 2, 20, 24, 28, 33, 36, 42, 54, 61.

makes this technique even easier with several computerized inclinometers. Inclinometry provides minimal variability and good interrater reliability. True lumbar motion is derived from the compound motion of the hips and spine, effort is delineated, and the spinal motion pattern is assessable as normal or abnormal.

2. **ISOLATED TRUNK STRENGTH MEASUREMENTS**

   Emerging technology has provided a number of accurate assessment devices for this purpose. These devices actually measure the physical capacity of the lumbopelvic unit, and therefore appropriate isolation of this region is necessary.

   a. **Isometric Technology:** These protocols measure the maximal force a muscle can generate in contraction. Trunk extensor strength, with good pelvic stabilization, is assessed by the Med-X device (Med-X, Ocala, Fla). Training may also be done on this unit, which measures multiportion isometrics but is restricted to a single movement in only one place.

   b. **Isokinetic Technology:** This testing measures dynamic performance by "locking in" the speed and acceleration variables. This makes calculation of both interindividual and intraindividual differences relatively easy. Other dependent variables such as "work" and "power" can be derived from the curves produced. Additionally, an effort factor may be derived through "average points variance," and fatigue and recovery ratios indicative of endurance and recovery after a specific work task may be assessed.[32] Available devices providing these types of measurements include the Cybex TEF unit, Cybex torso rotation unit, the TMC attachment to the Cybex 6000 (Lumex, Ronkonkoma, NY), the Kin-Com device (Chatteck Corp., Chattanooga, Tenn), the Biodex Back attachment (Biodex Co., Shirley, NY), and the Lido Back (Loredan, Inc., Davis, Calif).*

B. **Functional Capacity Tests**

1. **LIFT TESTING**

   a. **Isoinertial Testing:** In isoinertial testing, the velocity is not controlled, but the mass is held constant or progressed. The end point of the test is determined by the subject's self-report of maximum capability, discomfort, or perception of pending injury ("psychophysical test") or by the subject reaching a target heart rate (aerobic test). The Progressive Isoinertial Lifting Evaluation (PILE) offers a standardized protocol with a normative database to assess this capability in an individual.[37-39]

   b. **Isometric Testing:** Distance is kept constant so that force is measured directly, and no actual movement of the lever arm takes place, so the velocity is "0." Several manufacturers produce pieces of equipment that employ this technology.[10,11,48]

   c. **Isokinetic Testing:** Velocity is kept constant and distance is limited to a specific range so that force may be studied dynamically. Ergonomic and anthropometric protocols are used. Effort is assessable through *average points variance,* as in isokinetic joint or regional strength testing. Assessment devices include the Cybex Liftask and the Lido Lift. Both of these units are also capable of alternative isometric protocols.*

2. **AEROBIC CAPACITY TESTING:**

   The following is not intended to be a comprehensive review of aerobic testing but rather a brief overview of different approaches.[8,55] Aerobic capacity tests of the lower and upper portions of the body are basically extremity endurance tests. Their end point is *either* cardiovascular or muscular capacity. Because large lower extremity muscles produce significant cardiovascular load, bicycle ergometry or treadmill tests are frequently used as "stress tests" to screen for cardiac dysfunction. However, in the rehabilitation environment, the limiting factor for performance on lower or upper body ergometry is just as likely to be disuse deconditioning the extremities as it is a loss of aerobic capacity. Distinguishing between these two can be done roughly by identifying the final heart rate; if it is very low at a low work rate, then effort with or without extremity muscular fatigue may be the problem. On the other hand, a high heart rate with a low work rate suggests aerobic capacity rather than extremity muscular deficits; this also documents good effort.

   a. **Bicycle Ergometry Tests:** The use of a stationary bicycle for lower extremity testing is preferred over a treadmill because of the ease of obtaining pulse recordings and the lesser influence of body weight and pain of the workload. Protocols may be intermittent or continuous and involve a progressively increasing workload that is easily calibrated in watts or kilogram-meters. Nomograms based on body weight are available, and the maximum V_{O_2} can be derived from the workload, with an accuracy of $\pm 10\%$. A number of stationary bicycles suitable for this testing are available, with a few having internal computerized programs that automatically calculate the maximum V_{O_2}.

   b. **Arm Ergometry:** The protocol is similar to bicycle ergometry testing and may be used as a primary aerobic fitness test if there is lower extremity dysfunction. However, arm cycling does not stress the cardiovascular and respiratory systems as much as bike or treadmill testing and is more reflective of upper body condi-

*References 7, 13, 14, 19, 29, 35, 40, 41, 46, 47, 56, 57, 59, 60.   *References 12, 22, 24, 25, 30, 53.

tioning. There are several commercially available devices.

3. **EFFORT ASSESSMENT AND CUMULATIVE SCORE:** Effort is assessed on each of the individual tests with a variety of techniques the common denominator of which is a consistency score. On inclinometric mobility, consistency of the true lumbar mobility measurement (sagittal and coronal) is assessed, along with the maximal performance level on three consecutive tests meeting consistency criteria. In addition, a comparison of the pelvic motion component to the straight leg raising component provides a specific assessment of effort in the important lumbar flexion test.[2,3] Dedicated isokinetic machines have the ability to compare a coefficient of variation for curve reproduction not only at the end point of motion but even at multiple performance points along the curve at a high sample rate. These tests of variance permit curve consistency to be expressed with or without regard to performance amplitude, thereby providing an excellent test of curve reliability. Finally, ergometry tests and isoinertial lifting tests may use the heart rate as a measure of effort, as well as a limit for test termination.

At the conclusion of the QFE, physical and occupational therapists evaluate test performance and effort criteria and devise "global effort ratings" for each set of data. At this point the raw data are entered into a custom computer program wherein patient data are compared with normative databases segmented by gender, age, and a weight variable (for selected strength tests) to express patient data as a "percent normal."[35] Thereafter, these "average person" normal expectations may be upgraded or downgraded on the basis of anticipated work and daily activity demands ranging between sedentary and very heavy levels. Finally, through conversion of the data to a series of normative scores, the computer calculates a single "cumulative score" that is a weighted, average score that essentially represents the equivalent of a "grade point average" to give a single measurement of merit. Given that many nonmedical personnel follow the performance of a disabled patient in a rehabilitation environment, such a cumulative score can be very useful in communicating patient progress. A computerized report providing all the aforementioned data on patients with lumbar and/or cervical spinal disorders, along with a physician-generated medical interpretation, is provided with each QFE or Post Program Quantitative Evaluation (PPQE).

BARRIERS TO RECOVERY

Many psychosocial and socioeconomic problems may confront patients recovering from a spinal disorder, particularly if disability from a productive lifestyle is associated with the industrial back pain. The patient's inability to see a "light at the end of the tunnel" may produce a severe situational depression often associated with anxiety and agitation. The back injury itself may be a sign of emotional conflict involving rebellion against authority or job dissatisfaction.[5,6,58] Personality changes may be manifested in anger, hostility, and noncompliance directed at the therapeutic team. Minor head injuries, organic brain dysfunction from age, alcohol, or drugs, or limited intelligence may produce organic cognitive dysfunctions that make patients difficult to manage and refractory to education. A variety of personality disorders such as sociopathy may also complicate treatment.[16,17,21,31,62]

Many chronic spinal disorders exist within a "disability system." Worker's compensation laws were initially devised to protect a worker's income and provide timely medical benefits following industrial accidents. Employers ultimately agreed to this because of a compensatory benefit. In return for providing these worker rights, they were absolved of certain consequences of negligence, and a cost-capped liability set by state statute was included for any injury, no matter how severe. As in any compromise situation, certain disincentives to rational behavior may emerge. One outcome of a guaranteed paycheck while temporary total disability persists is that there may be no clear incentive to an early return to work. A casual approach to surgical decision making and rehabilitation may lead to further deconditioning, both mental and physical, thus making ultimate recovery more problematic. Complicating matters even further is the observation that no group (other than the employer) has verifiable financial incentive to return patients to productivity as soon as possible, although, of course, society has. As a consequence, an odd assortment of health professionals, attorneys, insurance companies, and vocational rehabilitation specialists may have limited motivation to combat foot-dragging on the disability issue. Altering the contingencies may correct some of the problems. However, this assumes that the present system has not already evolved to a near-perfect balance of interests or that legislators will respond to changes in outlook regarding optimal patient care.

Early efforts to distinguish between "functional" (nonorganic) and "organic" low back pain did not meet with success. The complex nature of chronic pain makes it difficult to clearly categorize component factors as purely physical or purely psychological. Instead, chronic pain must be understood as an interactive, psychophysiological behavior pattern wherein the physical and the psychological constantly overlap and intertwine. The focus of psychological evaluation of patients with low back pain must therefore shift away from "functional" versus "organic" distinctions to the identification of important psychological characteristics with behavioral motivators of each patient. These characteristics will obviously have an impact on a patient's disability and response to treatment efforts. Identification of such characteristics will facilitate treatment planning and assist with the prediction of treatment outcome. Although space does not permit an extensive review of the various instruments used for psychological assessment, an analysis of some basic instruments commonly used within the PRIDE system may be useful here:

- *Quantified pain drawing:* The pain drawing provides a nonverbal assessment tool of pain location, severity, and subjective characteristics.[44] Patients are encouraged to freely display all of their pain at all body parts and rate its intensity on a 10-cm line. Scoring uses an overlay that reliably quantifies pain by dividing the human drawing into a series of boxes to yield a score for trunk, extremity, and "outside the body" pain.[9,25] This later dimension is useful for identifying pain magnifiers as well as suggesting the possibility of somatic delusions in rare cases. Such a pain drawing provides an easy and reliable method for documentation of changing pain perception on repeated measures in response to treatment.
- *Million Visual Analog Scale:* This analog scale consists of 15 questions relating to perceptions of pain and disability.[43] Responses are recorded by placing a mark on a 10-cm line that represents an index of severity. Scores are easily obtained by using a ruler or grid. This scale is particularly useful because of its nonverbal form of expression, and its ease of administration and reproducibility make it ideal for monitoring progress through repeated administrations. Extremely exaggerated responses that do not correlate with clinical assessment may also indicate the need for further in-depth psychological evaluation.
- *Beck Depression Inventory (BDI):* The BDI consists of 21 items pertaining to symptoms of depression such as sleep disturbance, sexual dysfunction, weight change, and anhedonia. It is very brief and easy to complete, and it has a cumulative scoring system that takes less than 1 minute to complete. The BDI is designed to identify cognitive factors of depression and, along with the Hamilton Rating Scale for Depression, can provide the clinician with valuable information about the existence and severity of depression in patients with low back pain.[4,49,50,62] The BDI's ease of administration makes it easy to use on repeated visits, offering the clinician a relatively simple means of following depressive symptoms and treatment progress.
- *Minnesota Multiphasic Personality Inventory (MMPI):* The MMPI is one of the oldest and most frequently used indices of psychological functioning. Its first three clinical scales, hypochondriasis, depression, and hysteria, provide valuable information when patients with chronic low back pain are evaluated. Relative elevations in these three clinical scales can alert the clinician to the possibility of important problems such as symptom magnification, poor insight into emotions, and defenses based on denial and somatization tendencies. Many ancillary scales have been developed within the MMPI that also provide specific information pertinent to

chronic low back pain treatment. Notable among these are the McAndrews and ego strength scales. The McAndrews scale helps identify patients with alcoholic or drug-dependent personalities, and may assist the treatment team in preventing drug habituation. The ego strength scale is designed to identify those individuals with limited emotional resources who might lack the motivation and personal responsibility to adequately benefit from an intensive treatment regimen. Many articles document correlations between various behaviors and certain scales, of which these are but a few examples.

- *Other psychological assessments:* The Structured Clinical Interview for DSM-III-R diagnosis (SCID) is an interview test designed to help a trained mental health provider reach a DSM-III-R psychiatric diagnosis. The most important are the axis I and II diagnoses, which occur very commonly in chronic spinal disorders.[51] The Hamilton Depression Inventory is a clinician-administered test that supplements the self-report of the Beck inventory. A nonstructured clinical interview helps clinicians focus on the various critical issues that are the essential barriers to recovery that must be addressed. Many of these may be social (child care or transportation problems) and specifically affect the patient's ability to participate in rehabilitation, or they may involve financial, psychological, legal, and employer-related issues. Similar interviews performed by disability managers are quite useful in evaluating the occupational aspects of ongoing disability, with this role being taken under different training circumstances by occupational therapists, social workers, vocational rehabilitation specialists, or rehabilitation nurses. Tests that evaluate an individual's education and skills, including the Wechsler Adult Intelligence Scale (WAIS-R), are also commonly used in assessment designed to achieve an outcome of returning chronically disabled workers back to a productive lifestyle.

THE FUNCTIONAL RESTORATION PROGRAM

Tertiary treatment uses the physical/functional capacity and psychosocial assessments described in detail earlier to organize a physician-directed, interdisciplinary team treatment approach to restore patients to productivity. Representatives of multiple disciplines are required on site, with all patients having the benefit of access to each specialized group of healthcare providers in an intensive program individualized to the initial assessments.* An additional feature of functional restoration programs is the attention to outcome monitoring for all patients with structured clinical interviews at a minimum follow-up of 1 year. These interviews focus on

*References 8, 18, 20, 22, 23, 40, 41, 52, 57, 59.

specific objective factors of cost and disability.[15,25,27,31,45]

Following the initial assessment, a preprogram phase of treatment is initiated on a once- or twice-weekly basis; the duration and frequency are determined by the degree of deconditioning and psychosocial barriers that would interfere with participation in the 3-week intensive phase. In this phase, physical and occupational therapists are involved primarily in confidence building to overcome the inhibition and fear of injury limiting physical performance and in mobilization and stretching to prepare the patient for the intensive muscle-training portion of the program. Psychologists and disability managers deal with psychological (e.g., depression and/or substance dependence) and social (e.g., financial, transportation, family responsibilities) barriers to program participation, respectively. Utilization cannot exceed 6 weeks but ranges from 2 to 6 weeks and is followed by the program's intensive phase. During this portion of the program the patient participates in a 3-week 10-hr/day program consisting of reconditioning, work simulation, disability management, and a cognitive-behavioral program.[15,25,31,34]

The reconditioning and work simulation aspects of the program involve the use of active (not passive) treatment modalities by physical and occupational therapists. Quantification is necessary for these aspects of the program because they provide the initial levels of exercise from which a progressive resistive program emerges. The indirect assessments confirm functional deficits and psychosocial barriers to effort and lead to a combination of education and exercise training to resolve the deconditioning syndrome. Initial treatment is directed toward mobilizing and strengthening the "weak link" in the biomechanical chain, whereas whole-body work simulation integrates the performance of this link with other parts of the body deconditioned simply by inactivity (see box below).

The cognitive-behavioral multimodal disability management program focuses initially on the diagnosis of psychosocioeconomic barriers to functional recovery in the given individual through the assessment mentioned earlier and then on specific treatments for these problems. The initial treatment may be pharmacologic and involve detoxification from habituating opiate and tranquilizer medications, the prescription of antidepressants, and the use of antiinflammatory medications,

occasionally including major tranquilizers. Remaining treatments include a cognitive, behaviorally based program of education and counseling, including stress management, that is time-limited and aggressively oriented toward sequential goal setting. Failure to meet mutually prearranged goals may result in dismissal from the program (an event currently occurring in about 5% of comprehensive program admissions). In practice, education and counseling account for approximately half of the total program time, with the remainder being spent in physical training.

Finally, just as the quantification of physical function and self-report provides feedback to the staff and patient on individual performance, so too do follow-up outcome measures provide objective statistical confirmation of success in achieving program goals. The PRIDE comprehensive program performs routine 1- and 2-year structured follow-up telephone interviews as a regular part of its ongoing program. The interview includes information on working status, additional surgical/medical/chiropractic treatment, resolution of compensation issues (long-term disability, Social Security Disability, permanent partial/ total disability, etc.), and injury recurrence.[26] The interviews must be performed in the context of possible remaining barriers to full disclosure by the patient, thereby necessitating further investigation through contacts with employers, attorneys, family members, or third-party payers in some cases. Combining the follow-up interview information with preprogram demographic data on the same subjects can provide valid statistical comparisons of the ability of a comprehensive functional restoration program to deal with disability and cost. Because patients with chronic low back pain ultimately account for 80% of the cost of low back pain problems through a combination of medical treatment, lost productivity, indemnity, and government support, program evaluation that includes the involvement of other members of the disability system provides a major resource to clinicians, employers, healthcare planners, and legislators.

Although functional restoration of patients with chronic pain is the area of highest anticipated "bang for the buck" in work-incurred spinal disability, employers and government agencies are often slow to effect change in their policies. Although the Boeing study clearly demonstrates[5,6,58] that job dissatisfaction/personnel relations problems may be the best (or only)

Critical elements of a tertiary functional restoration program

1. Quantification of physical and functional capacity
2. Psychosocioeconomic assessment
3. Physical reconditioning of the injured functional unit
4. Work simulation and whole-body retraining
5. Cognitive-behavioral multimodal disability management program
6. Education and training in work and fitness maintenance
7. Ongoing outcome assessment using objective criteria

predictor of back "injury," use of the medical system to avoid responsibility for good personnel relations has become endemic in some industries. These employers and government agencies may find it easier to ascribe back injury to the "cost of doing business" and pass these expenses to the consumer or taxpayer. An adversarial relationship filled with rancor more often than not alters the status of the patient from an employee to a claimant. Lest we too quickly fall into the trap of labeling an injured worker who seeks redress from perceived punitive employer actions as a "faker" or "malingerer," we must consider the multitude of factors in the evolution of the worker's compensation and personal injury situations themselves.

Although a full discussion of nonmedical legal and administrative issues is a critical adjunct to the rehabilitation of chronically disabled patients, further clarification of these issues can be anticipated elsewhere in this volume. However, it should be clear that employer/employee relationships are critical for the behavior of injured workers. Although in some cases, manipulativeness, opportunism, and low motivation characterize such patients' behavior, their actions are often conditioned by perceived injustice in the essentially adversarial worker's compensation system. Employer-employee conflict is often played out through their respective representatives (the insurance carrier and the plaintiff attorney) in a contest over medical benefits, job retention rights, and disability-related indemnity benefits tied to perceived permanent impairment. The other "players" in the disability system may have a variety of personal and business interests that can diverge in certain critical areas from the best interest of the injured worker. As such, the interdisciplinary team's education on the particular rules of the worker's compensation venue can be an important aspect of treatment to assist the patient in escaping the maze of chronic disability. In this regard, the tertiary care provider is the only disinterested party capable of assisting the patient in formulating a problem-solving solution. In so doing, assessment and tertiary treatment of a chronically disabled worker lead to tertiary prevention in which the most dismal consequence of permanent disability of the young and potentially productive worker is avoided. Because spinal disorders are the primary cause of disability for those under age 45 in most industrialized countries, an average of 25 to 30 years of taxpayer-supported welfare benefits (Social Security Disability Income [SSDI], long-term disability, unemployment insurance, social welfare, food stamps, etc.) can be prevented by the judicious application of tertiary care to workers identified as chronically disabled. Ultimately, the application of tertiary care to the large reservoir of "permanently disabled" patients with low back pain offers a major challenge to society's ability to create jobs and an opportunity to save billions of dollars in unnecessary welfare payments for nonproductivity.

In selected cases, tertiary care may be appropriate even before a maximum normal soft tissue healing period (4 to 6 months postinjury) has been completed with certainty. Although secondary treatment is usually preferable for patients before 4 months of disability, the availability of effective tertiary care with cost-limited and duration-limited programs may make it desirable for selected cases even before 4 months have passed. In particular, with more aggressive employer involvement through transitional work-return programs, with the recognition of early psychosocial stressors potentially leading to enhancement of disability, and with the advent of treatment guidelines to inform healthcare providers and administrative agencies of ways demonstrated to achieve treatment goals, tertiary treatment (at least in a limited form) may be instituted within 6 to 8 weeks of the injury or disability in selected cases. A variety of criteria can be used to distinguish the suitability of secondary or tertiary care in these cases, including the match between physical capacity and job demands, recent prior injury, age, other medical conditions, pre-existing psychosocial barriers, and job availability. Progressive education of healthcare providers in the more advanced concepts of the rehabilitation of injured workers is the best method to advance program effectiveness and ensure quality of care.

SUMMARY

The future lies in finding solutions that involve communication and cooperation between members of the disability system. The injured worker must be given an opportunity for appropriate medical care, reemployment, and compensation for injury meeting legal compensability criteria as provided for other industrial (or personal) injuries. If objective structural documentation cannot provide adequate means for assessing impairment, scheduled or functional assessment-based awards must be considered (wage loss, disability, etc.). At this time, judicious combinations of surgical treatment (if appropriate) and tertiary rehabilitation are becoming more available and should help prevent permanent total disability. Quantification may also lead the way to prevention through worker selection and placement with greater options for work return through the Americans with Disabilities Act (ADA). Prevention programs should be combined with job analysis and redesign following risk assessment, as well as enlightened education of high-risk workers and their personnel managers and supervisors. Combining the services of multidisciplinary occupational health professionals to provide optimal early and late care for the gamut of industrial injuries in a cost-effective manner is the ultimate goal of those who strive to increase the available knowledge through improved structural, physical, and functional capacity assessment technology and through tertiary treatment for workers with chronic spinal disorders.

References

1. Adams M et al: An electroinclinometer technique for measuring lumbar curvature, *Clin Biomech* 1:130-134, 1986.

2. American Medical Association: *Guides to the evaluation of permanent impairment,* ed 3, revised, Chicago, 1990, The Association.

3. American Medical Association: *Guides to the evaluation of permanent impairment,* ed 4, Chicago, 1993, The Association.

4. Beck A, Steer R, Garbin W: Psychometric properties of the Beck Depression Inventory: twenty-five years of evaluation, *Clin Psychol Rev* 8:77-100, 1988.

5. Bigos S et al: Back injuries in industry: a retrospective study II. Injury factors, *Spine* 11:246-251, 1986.

6. Bigos S et al: Back injuries in industry: a retrospective study III. Employee-related factors, *Spine* 11:252-256, 1986.

7. Brady S, Mayer T, Gatchel R: Physical progress and residual impairment quantification after functional restoration, Part II: Isokinetic trunk strength, *Spine* 18:395-400, 1994.

8. Cady L et al: Strength and fitness and subsequent back injuries in firefighters, *J Occup Med* 21:269-272, 1979.

9. Capra P, Mayer T, Gatchel R: Adding psychological scales to assess back pain, *J Musc Med* 7:41-52, 1985.

10. Chaffin D: Human strength capability and low back pain, *J Occup Med* 16:248-254, 1974.

11. Chaffin D, Herrin G, Keyserling W: Pre-employment strength testing: an updated position, *J Occup Med* 20:403-408, 1978.

12. Curtis L, Mayer T, Gatchel R: Physical progress and residual impairment quantification after functional restoration, Part III: Isokinetic and isoinertial lifting capacity, *Spine* 18:401-405, 1994.

13. Davies G, Gould J: Trunk testing using a prototype Cybex II isokinetic stabilization system, *J Orthop Sports Phys Ther* 3:164-170, 1982.

14. Delitto A, Crandell C, Rose S: Peak torque to body weight ratios in the trunk: a critical analysis, *Phys Ther* 69:138-143, 1989.

15. Gatchel R et al: Functional restoration: pitfalls in evaluating efficacy, *Spine* 17:988-995, 1992 (editorial).

16. Gatchel R et al: Millon Behavioral Health Inventory: its utility in predicting physical function in patients with low back pain, *Arch Phys Med Rehabil* 67:878-882, 1986.

17. Gatchel R et al: Quantification of lumbar function. Part 6: The use of psychological measures in guiding physical functional restoration, *Spine* 11:36-42, 1986.

18. Gould J, Davies G, editors: *Orthopedic and sports physical therapy,* St Louis 1985, Mosby–Year Book.

19. Hazard R et al: Isokinetic trunk and lifting strength measurements: variability as an indicator of effort, *Spine* 13:54-57, 1988.

20. Keeley J et al: Quantification of lumbar function. Part 5: Reliability of range of motion measures in the sagittal plane and an in vivo torso rotation measurement technique, *Spine* 11:31-35, 1986.

21. Kinney R et al: *The high prevalence of major psychiatric disorders in chronic low back pain patients: an objective evaluation study.* Proceedings of the annual meeting of the International Society for the Study of the Lumbar Spine, Boston, June 15, 1990.

22. Kishino N et al: Quantification of lumbar function. Part 4: Isometric and isokinetic lifting simulation in normal subjects and low back dysfunction patients, *Spine* 10:921-927, 1985.

23. Langrana N, Lee C: Isokinetic evaluation of trunk muscles, *Spine* 9:171-175, 1984.

24. Loebl W: Measurements of spinal posture and range in spinal movements, *Ann Phys Med* 9:103, 1967.

25. Mayer T, Gatchel R: *Functional restoration for spinal disorders: the sports medicine approach,* Philadelphia, 1988, Lea & Febiger.

26. Mayer T, Gatchel R, Prescott M: Functional restoration socioeconomics outcomes: the PRIDE outcome tracking system, *Spine* (in press).

27. Mayer T, Mooney V, Gatchel R: *Contemporary care for painful disorders: concepts, diagnosis & treatment,* Philadelphia, 1991, Lea & Febiger.

28. Mayer T et al: A male incumbent worker industrial database, Part I: Lumbar spinal physical capacity, *Spine* 19:755-761, 1994.

29. Mayer T et al: A male incumbent worker industrial database, Part II: Cervical spinal physical capacity, *Spine* 19:762-764, 1994.

30. Mayer T et al: A male incumbent worker industrial database, Part III: Lumbar/cervical functional testing, *Spine* 19:765-770, 1994.

31. Mayer T et al: A prospective two-year study of functional restoration in industrial low back injury: an objective assessment procedure, *JAMA* 258:1763-1767, 1987.

32. Mayer T et al: Lumbar trunk muscle endurance measurement: isometric contrasted to isokinetic testing in normal subjects, *Spine* (in press).

33. Mayer T et al: Noninvasive measurement of cervical triplanar motion in normal subjects, *Spine* 18:2191-2195, 1993.

34. Mayer T et al: Objective assessment of spine function following industrial accident: a prospective study with comparison group and one-year follow-up, *Spine* 10:482-493, 1985.

35. Mayer T et al: Optimal spinal strength normalization factors among male railroad workers, *Spine* 18:239-244, 1993.

36. Mayer T et al: Physical progress and residual impairment quantification after functional restoration, Part I: Lumbar mobility, *Spine* 18:389-394, 1994.

37. Mayer T et al: Progressive isoinertial lifting evaluation. An erratum, *Spine* 15:5, 1990.

38. Mayer T et al: Progressive isoinertial lifting evaluation, Part I: A standardized protocol and normative database, *Spine* 13:993-997, 1988.

39. Mayer T et al: Progressive isoinertial lifting evaluation, Part II: A comparison with isokinetic in a disabled chronic low back pain industrial population, *Spine* 13:998-1002, 1988.

40. Mayer T et al: Quantification of lumbar function. Part 2: Sagittal plane trunk strength in chronic low back pain patients *Spine* 10:765-772, 1985.

41. Mayer T et al: Quantification of lumbar function. Part 3: Preliminary data on isokinetic torso rotation testing with myoelectric spectral analysis in normal and low back pain subjects, *Spine* 10:912-920, 1985.

42. Mayer T et al: Use of noninvasive techniques for quantification of spinal range-of-motion in normal subjects and chronic low back dysfunction patients, *Spine* 9:588-595, 1984.

43. Million R et al: Evaluation of low back pain and assessment of lumbar corsets with and without back supports, *Ann Rheum Dis* 40:449-454, 1981.

44. Mooney V, Cairns D, Robertson J: A system for evaluating and treating chronic back disability, *West J Med* 124:370-376, 1976.

45. Nachemson A: Work for all, *Clin Orthop* 179:77-82, 1983.

46. Newton M, Waddell G: Trunk strength testing with iso-machines, Part 1: Review of a decade of scientific evidence, *Spine* 7:801-811, 1993.

47. Newton M et al: Trunk strength testing with iso-machines, Part 2: Experimental evaluation of the Cybex II back testing system in normal subjects and patients with chronic low back pain, *Spine* 7:812-824, 1993.

48. Pederson O, Peterson R, Staffeldt E: Back pain and isometric back muscle strength of workers in a Danish factory, *Scand J Rehabil Med* 7:125-128, 1975.

49. Polatin P: Functional restoration for the chronically disabled low back pain patient, *J Musculoskel Med* 7:17-39, 1990.

50. Polatin P et al: A psychosociomedical prediction model of response to treatment by chronically disabled workers with back pain, *Spine* 14:956-961, 1989.

51. Polatin P et al: Psychiatric illness and chronic low back pain: the mind and the spine—which goes first? *Spine* 18:66-71, 1993.

52. Pope MH, Frymoyer J, Andersson G: *Occupational low back pain,* New York, 1984, Praeger Publications.

53. Porterfield J et al: Simulated lift testing using computerized isokinetics, *Spine* 12:683-687, 1987.

54. Reynolds P: Measurement of spinal mobility: a comparison of three methods, *Rheum Rehabil* 14:180-185, 1975.

55. Schmidt A: Cognitive factors in the performance level of chronic low back pain patients, *J Psychosom Res* 29:183-189, 1985.

56. Smidt G, Blantied P: Analysis of strength tests and resistive exercises commonly used for low-back disorders, *Spine* 12:1025-1034, 1987.

57. Smith S et al: Quantification of lumbar function. Part 1: Isometric and multi-speed isokinetic trunk strength measures in sagittal and axial planes in normal subject patients, *Spine* 10:757-764, 1985.

58. Spengler D et al: Back injuries in industry: a retrospective study I. Overview and cost analysis, *Spine* 11:241-245, 1986.

59. Thompson N et al: Descriptive measures of isokinetic trunk testing, *J Orthop Sports Phys Ther* 7:43-49, 1985.

60. Thorstensson A, Nilsson J: Trunk muscle strength during constant and velocity movement, *Scand J Rehabil Med* 14:61-68, 1982.

61. Waddell G et al: Objective clinical evaluation of physical impairment in chronic low back pain, *Spine* 17:617-628, 1992.

62. Ward N: Tricyclic antidepressants for chronic low back pain: mechanisms of action and predictors of response, *Spine* 11:661-665, 1986.

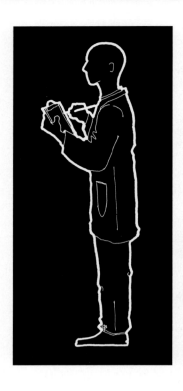

Chapter 24

Workplace Adaptation for the Low Back Region

Shrawan Kumar
Steve Konz

CONTENTS

Low back pain (LBP), a medical enigma of nebulous causation, wreaks economic havoc and social suffering. Its elusive nature and significant impact have frustrated scientists and social policymakers alike. Despite interventions, neither its extent nor its impact has lessened. Attention is gradually being diverted away from it. Increasingly, an attitude that not much has been accomplished in lessening LBP, despite considerable effort, is leading to the realization that it is here to stay. One may therefore accept it as a fact and focus on what can be done in spite of it. A gradual progression from "pain" to "impairment" and from "impairment" to "disability" consideration is all too obvious around us.[48]

LOW BACK PAIN: THE NATURE OF THE PROBLEM

The natural history of LBP and even its broad categorization into subacute, acute, and chronic categories defy scientific precision.[46] In many cases, its insidious onset, relief without medical intervention, recurrence despite all precautions, and eventual chronicity have not only perplexed the medical and scientific community but posed an intellectual challenge even for a scientific conception of the phenomenon. Although many risk factors have been associated with LBP,[26] its etiology remains obscure. Kumar[28] categorized all known risk factors into four broad categories: (1) morphological, (2) genetic, (3) biomechanical, and (4) psychosocial. He stated that whereas morphological and genetic factors are hardly manipulable, the biomechanical and psychosocial factors lend themselves to manipulation. It was, however, conceded that all strategies must take into account the genetic and morphological data for optimal results. Many studies have been conducted to examine the possible impact of different risk factors.[7,9,27,40] However, the human back is like a multilink chain that is only as strong as its weakest link. Unfortunately, the weakest link is most elusive, being different in different people and also different at different times in the same individual because of varying internal and external circumstances. Taking this into consideration, Kumar[26] proposed a quantitative model for overexertion, safety, and risk of injury. The latter harnesses most of the pertinent physical factors for comprehensive handling. Only the future will reveal the success of such an approach in the control of LBP.

LOW BACK PAIN: THE EXTENT OF THE PROBLEM

In spite of the obscurities associated with the etiology, classification, and treatment of LBP, human and economic impacts have been quantifiable with approximations. Chapter 19, on the epidemiology of LBP, gives a comprehensive picture of the problem. Suffice it to say here that LBP is a large social and economic problem. It has only one redeeming feature for being a medical condition—it is a nonfatal affliction. The impact of LBP is much more recognized in Western and industrialized countries, although it occurs in underdeveloped countries alike.[47]

To put the extent of the problem in perspective, a brief description follows. Andersson[1] states that national statistics from the European countries reveal that 10% to 15% of all sickness absence is due to back pain, with the number of workdays lost per worker increasing steadily. A yearly prevalence of 25% to 45% was reported, and chronic back pain was present in 3% to 7% of the adult population. The lifetime prevalence of LBP has been variously reported to be between 70% and 80%. In Canada, LBP has steadily constituted around 27% of all industrial injuries.[43] These have been reported to cost disproportionately higher amounts than all other injuries. In the United States, the yearly prevalence has been reported to be in the 15% to 20% range. Khalil[21] reported that on any given day, 6.5 million people are in bed because of LBP in the United States. At any given time, roughly 75 million Americans have back pain. Webster and Snook[53] reported the cost of LBP in 1989 as incurred by Liberty Mutual, the largest insurer in the United States. They state that LBP constituted 16% of the claims and accounted for 33% of the total expense. Webster and Snook also reported that the mean cost per case of the LBP was $8,300 as compared with $4,100 for all other claims combined, whereas the median cost was $396 ($168 for other claims). In these claim settlements, 34% of the total cost (for LBP) was medical, whereas 66% was indemnity cost (lost time and wages).[53]

No matter which way one looks, LBP is prevalent and expensive. Some of the socioeconomic aspects of our society may accentuate the problem because of alleged secondary gain issue. Medically, a cure for LBP neither exists nor is likely to emerge in the foreseeable future.[11,18,52] No difference in long-term outcome between aggressive and conservative treatments has been identified. We do not seem to be able to control the problem in a significant or meaningful way. We have been able to reduce neither the incidence nor the severity of LBP. It is clearly here to stay. It is therefore of utmost importance to focus on workplace adaptation to reduce human suffering as well as the economic cost. In our endeavor to identify these adaptations, it will be valuable to try to reduce the magnitude and exposure of the identified risk factors to workers, to try to reduce the incidenc of LBP in healthy people, and to allow adaptation in patients with LBP through reduced stress. Such adaptations will be helpful in returning workers to work following injury.

Disability Caused by Low Back Pain

Low back pain is associated with considerable disability that results in work loss. Work loss is the most important social and economic consequence of LBP, although absence from work may be influenced by many factors other than LBP. A direct correlative scale between LBP and between disability and disability and work loss has not been established. However, a simple clinical and subjective assessment of disability[49] has been claimed to have considerable relevance to quality of life as well as industrial performance. This assessment is focused on loss of function rather than pain. The emphasis is on whether an activity can be performed by an individual or whether performance of the activity is restricted because of LBP. Implicit in this assumption is that the restriction must have its onset coincident with the onset of the back pain and must therefore be the functional limitation. The specific criteria used by Waddell et al[49] are as follows:

1. Bending and lifting
2. Sitting
3. Standing
4. Walking
5. Travelling
6. Social life
7. Sleep
8. Sex life
9. Dressing/undressing

The aforementioned criteria combine postural, strength, metabolic, and everyday living activities that are also involved in occupational activities. Low back pain and loss of function through disability are results of biomechanical (kinematic and kinetic) perturbation of the human system. The biomechanical demands on the human systems are dealt with in Chapter 20. However, the functional activities that accentuate these demands at work would therefore be manual material handling, lifting and carrying, prolonged sitting or standing, traveling, bending, and twisting in various ways. It will therefore be most desirable to concentrate on those activities that reduce biomechanical stress on human back and reduce the hazards for initial injury or subsequent recurrence.

ADAPTATIONS: LOW BACK PAIN CONTROL AND PREVENTION

Low back pain has been reported to be a significant problem in the industrial sector with heavy work as well as in sedentary professions.[35,42] Spitzer et al[42] reported the following rank ordering (in descending order) for incidence rates of LBP in Quebec, Canada: forestry, mining, manufacturing, construction, transportation, government, wholesale and retail, service industries, fishing, agriculture, and finance and insurance. However, Magora[35] reported a significant rate of incidence of LBP in bank tellers as well as heavy workers.

Seated Work

In sitting, the load on the intervertebral disk is 140% of what is found in the standing posture.[2] Because the intervertebral disks are avascular, their nutrition is accomplished entirely by a process of diffusion. Intervertebral disks are also viscoelastic materials. The presence of a static load will progressively reduce the water content of the disk. An increased load will accelerate this process. The loss of water from the disk will make the process of diffusion more difficult. Such water loss will then result in reduced oxygen tension and lack of nourishment. This situation is conducive to the process of disk degeneration. Because sedentary occupations involve prolonged exposure to a static load, the process is hastened and the disk is more vulnerable to injuries. Several factors play an important role. Because of the viscoelastic nature of the disk, a constant static load will continue to deform the disk and cause a compression creep. Inasmuch as creep is a time-dependent property, elimination of load will not result in immediate restoration of the preload configuration or the disk water content, thereby prolonging the oxygen- and water-reduced state. Such a state interferes with metabolism of the disk by decreasing the amount of glycosaminoglycans (which have strong affinity for water) and increasing the keratan sulfate content, which is amorphous with far less capacity to imbibe water. In the short term, viscoelastic deformation may also lead to ligamentous laxity and incoordination and potentiate injury through biomechanical perturbations. Over the long term, however, it will lead to the degenerative and permanent changes that are a hazard to the safety of the back. It is therefore of paramount importance that workers in sedentary jobs be encouraged to lead more physically active lives outside of the workplace. In addition, at work they should be encouraged to change posture frequently, move around, and mix nonseated work with seated work. The work space layout, organization of work, working tools, and seat must all be conducive to achieving this goal.

Some jobs that do not allow a person to change posture, stand up, and walk around at periodic intervals should be avoided. These are types of activity in which all the raw materials are delivered to the work station and the finished product is removed either mechanically or manually by someone else. This eliminates the necessity for the worker to either change postures significantly or to get up and move around. An example of such a job could be inspection work where the part to be inspected is moved on a conveyor belt while the inspector remains seated in one position. Such an arrangement not only disallows the opportunity to move around but also effectively ties the worker to the seat because of the incessant arrival of new pieces. For jobs like this, sit-to-stand arrangements may be desirable in which the operator can change posture, obtain back rest, stand up, and do a variety of physical adjustments without losing sight of the oncoming part for inspection. The stools for such work stations should be provided with a seat against which a worker can lean while the legs remain mostly in a standing posture. Furthermore, the support may provide relief for the back, and the feet can be rested. A worker can also stand on one foot while resting the other on the chair stand.

The key component of seated work is a chair. The design of a chair is therefore of paramount importance in affording workers desirable posture features. Currently, many types of chairs on the market are labeled "ergonomically designed." The purchasing departments of industries and people responsible for making decisions must pay special attention in the selection of these chairs. A chair "ergonomically designed" for a given task may not be that well suited for another task. Chair design has long been a contentious issue. Many papers have been written on the subject,* and many chairs have been produced. It is therefore important to carefully and appropriately select or design the seat on which workers are going to sit for a long time. The various aspects of the chair that are frequently considered are seat height adjustability, width of the chair, depth of the seat pan, slope of the seat pan, and other mechanical characteristics such as the base support, the back support, the footrest, and the armrest.

It is not productive to describe the design criteria for a good chair in significant detail because they may vary for different jobs. It is, however, important to emphasize basic principles of seat design that allow for comfortable sitting, change in position by swiveling, and adjustable backrests and armrests.

The problem of sedentary work worsens considerably when prolonged sitting is combined with whole-body vibration such as that experienced by truck drivers.[17,20] It is interesting to note that the natural frequency of many vehicles lies very close to the natural frequency of the human spine (4 to 8 Hz). Such a coincidence of natural frequencies causes resonance and amplification of the amplitude of the motion.[14] In the trucking industry, drivers have to contend with vibratory, sedentary, prolonged exposure and periodic loading and unloading of heavy items on their trucks. These tasks tend to accentuate the musculoskeletal complaints as compared with drivers who only drive and are not responsible for loading and unloading.[45] The solutions for these occupations may entail isolation of vibration either at the source of origin or before reaching the driver seat. The seat must also be designed such that it allows a good and flexible posture. Trucks could be equipped with hoists and dollies to do most of the heavy manual work.

---

*References 5, 6, 12, 13, 16, 33, 34, 36.

MANUAL MATERIALS HANDLING

Manual materials handling involves lifting, lowering, pulling, and pushing of materials and objects. Manual materials handling is quite prevalent in industry. Asfahl[3] reported that for every ton of product, from 80 to 150 tons of materials are handled and moved. It is perhaps for this reason that manual materials handling is associated with the largest number of back injuries. Konz[22] states that 25% of all industrial injuries are associated with manual materials handling. Because of this, 670,000 injuries are caused per year in the United States. Sixty percent of all money spent on industrial injuries is spent on injuries caused by manual materials handling. As a result of these occupational injuries, 93 million workdays are lost per year in the United States alone. These injuries are generally to the musculoskeletal system and involve muscles, ligaments, facet joints, intervertebral disks, and so forth. The injuries may occur in one of two possible modes. First, traumatic injuries occur as a result of one-time forceful exertion. The second type of injury may be the result of a cumulative effect and eventual precipitation of trauma. To avoid injuries caused by manual materials handling, various groups have proposed recommendations for the amount of load that a person can push, pull, carry, or lift. These standards are based on biomechanical, physiological, and psychophysical human responses.

Pulling and Pushing

Depending on the direction of activity, pulling and pushing activities could be resolved into their horizontal and vertical components. Some activities can be entirely in the horizontal and others in the vertical plane. The force that can be exerted by an individual is significantly influenced by the direction and height of the exertion.[30,31] Warwick, Novak, and Schultz[50] showed that, while using both hands, subjects could push an object straight ahead with a force of 29.8 kg but could pull back with a force of only 17.3 kg. The push force to the left and right was 15.9 kg and 17 kg, respectively. Their subjects could lift up 39.4 kg and press down 34.7 kg. Several recommendations for upper force limits for pulling and pushing activities have been published.[37,41] From many studies, a few generalized observations emerge. It is generally agreed that for pulling and pushing activities, two hands are better than one and force capability goes down as the frequency of exertion increases. Pushing at waist level allows people to generate much greater force than pushing at shoulder or knee levels.[31] One must also recognize that the coefficient of friction between footwear and the floor considerably influences the ability of subjects to push or pull.

Job Modifications

Based on the information just presented as well as engineering considerations, various job modifications can enhance the safety of the worker by reducing the level of stress and exposure. Before discarding existing equipment, it may be appropriate to carry out engineering maintenance consisting of lubrication of bearings, wheels, and castors to reduce the amount of friction. It is also desirable to mechanize the jobs that require high-frequency pulling/pushing or carrying over long distances. Some simple examples of reducing the load or stress to the musculoskeletal system are shown in **Figures 24-1** and **24-2**. In **Figure 24-1**, the effect of posture when pushing can be of considerable consequence to the operator.[38] **Figure 24-2** shows the beneficial effect of drum carts (mechanical aids). Clearly some aids are

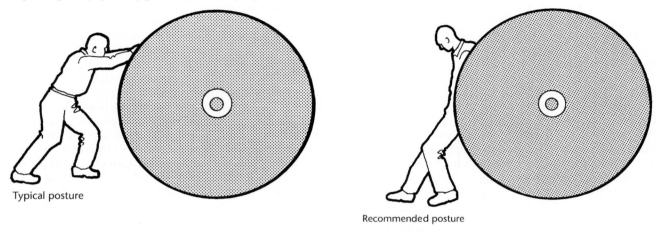

Typical posture

Recommended posture

Figure 24-1 Posture when pushing makes a difference. Ridd[38] reported that peak intraabdominal pressure was 50% less when pushing with the back.

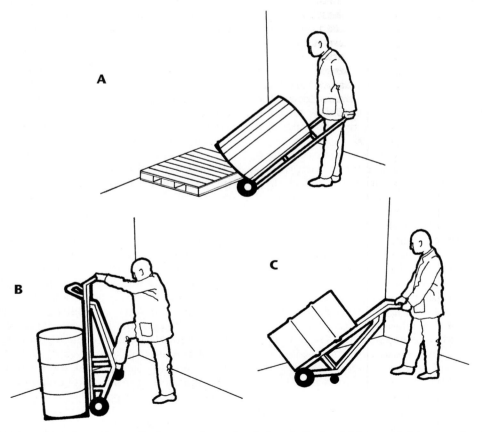

Figure 24-2 Drum carts reduce stress. **A** shows a two-wheeled cart; it should have a latch over the top rim during movement. **B** and **C** show a four-wheeled cart useful for heavier drums. In **B**, the foot can be used to help tip the drum. Note that the hand positions are different in **B** and **C**. Another handle forward of the main handles is also useful when tilting and maneuvering the drum for scales and pallets.

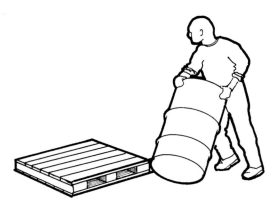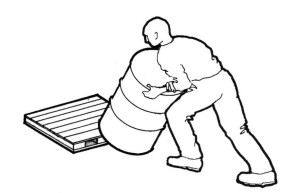

Figure 24-3 Chiming a drum (rotating a tipped drum) requires little effort; with skill, the drum's momentum can be used to move it onto a pallet. A straight push, however, as shown on the right, requires considerable effort. A drum cart is another alternative.

better than others. Oftentimes when mechanical aids or mechanization is unavailable, common sense and the knowledge of biomechanics can be used to reduce the load to the operator. **Figure 24-3** depicts how momentum can help even when a mechanical aid is unavailable.

Holding

Most manual materials handling activities entail a significant dynamic component in moving an object from point A to point B. However, in some jobs, workers hold the object without any movement. In some activities the load to be held may not be external and may involve only maintenance of a static posture. The duration that loads can be held and muscular contractions can be sustained has been the subject of several studies. One of the first studies that reported the relationship between the magnitude of contraction and the duration of hold was by Rohmert.[39] Such maintenance of posture and holding of components are prevalent in auto assembly plants, painting, kitchen work, laundry work, and others.

Carrying

Transporting loads for longer distances (exceeding 10 m) is not uncommon in industries. It is, however, desirable to mechanize all such long-distance carrying. These mechanical aids can be conveyors, lifts, trucks, or any other such device. In the absence of such arrangements, it is better to move materials and objects by pushing on a cart than by carrying on the shoulders. Carrying of a load by humans should be used only as a last resort. In such activities it would be desirable to minimize the momentum of the load on the spine. If human carriage is unavoidable, then job rotation should be implemented to relieve the workers performing the job of carrying.

Carrying objects up and down stairs is especially dangerous because (1) the hands are occupied with holding the object and thus not free to grasp handrails if there is a slip and (2) the object may obstruct vision. Therefore, loads should be moved between levels with hoists, platforms, and elevators and not manually on stairs.[8]

Lifting

The revised National Institute for Occupational Safety and Health (NIOSH) lifting guidelines,[51] the force limits,[10] and the manual materials handling guide[37] follow the approach of recommending maximal weights for specific situations. The revised NIOSH lifting guideline, as well as the manual material handling guide, recommends a maximum load for lift that is modified according to the lifting situation. The basic NIOSH formula is as follows:

$$RWL = LC \times HM \times VM \times DM \times FM \times AM \times CM$$

where:

$$\begin{aligned}
RWL &= \text{recommended weight limit} \\
LC &= \text{load constant} \\
HM &= \text{horizontal multiplier} \\
VM &= \text{vertical multiplier} \\
DM &= \text{distance multiplier} \\
FM &= \text{frequency multiplier} \\
AM &= \text{asymmetry multiplier} \\
CM &= \text{coupling multiplier}
\end{aligned}$$

The NIOSH guideline suggests a load constant of 23 kg. Because of the variation in work situation, this load constant is multiplied by a factor less than 1 to arrive at a recommended load of lifting for a specific situation.

Whereas the foregoing description as well as the original sources of manual materials handling guides will allow one to get a specific solution for a given task, in the following few paragraphs some generic design guidelines without specific numerical recommendations are stated. The principles that follow should be employed in all manual materials handling tasks to reduce the load to the individual and stress on the spine.

WORKER SELECTION

Several studies have shown the significance of the job severity index.[4,19,32] The job severity index is simply the ratio of the task demand in comparison to the person's capability. One approach may therefore be to select workers with large capacities. It is important to consider the capacity of the workers in job-simulated tests. Such a test forces the analyst to measure not only the worker's capacity but also the task requirements.

BENT KNEES VERSUS BENT BACK

Despite a concerted effort to train workers to lift with bent knees and straight backs, the practice has not received any universal acceptance. The logic behind the recommendation has been to reduce the moment arm on the lumbosacral disk, thereby reducing mechanical compression. However, it has been shown that unless the object to be lifted is brought very close to the body, the squat lift can in fact significantly increase mechanical compression on the lumbosacral disk.[9] It has also been shown that the squat method of lifting is associated with significantly higher physiological cost and is more tiring for workers.[29] Another disadvantage of the squat method of lifting is that it causes considerable stress on the knees, which are also a frequent site of mechanical disorders. Therefore a universal acceptance of the squat method of lifting (as opposed to the stoop method of lifting) is neither physiologically nor mechanically sound. It is perhaps for this reason that the acceptance of this method among workers has not been as prevalent as it was initially hoped. Furthermore, if one looks at the statistics of low back injuries associated with lifting over the past 40 years, it is clear that there has been a steady increase in incidence despite many workers in industries following this method of lifting. Sometimes stoop lifting may be preferred, and at other times squat lifting may be preferred. It is important to assess the job as well as the individual performing the job before making a recommendation. Garg et al[15] compared the physiological costs of different methods of lifting. They found that when subjects were allowed to lift any way they wanted, the subjects did not choose either pure stoop or pure squat. Subjects combined the features of both methods in a freestyle lift. The freestyle lift was found to be metabolically least expensive.[15,29] The recommendation would therefore be to use an individual- and task-specific method to minimize stress on spine and reduce the chances of injuries.

SUDDEN AND BALLISTIC MOVEMENTS

Sudden and ballistic movements have a large inertial component. Such inertial forces can exceed the tolerance limits of the human back. In addition, sudden motion may also cause a slip or fall while performing a lift. It is therefore recommended that workers wear shoes with soles having a high coefficient of friction and large contact area. Similarly, the floors must not be smooth and should have a higher coefficient of friction. Data on a force platform[24] indicate that peak forces and torques during lift are very "spiked." The peak force often occurs during initial lowering of the body before the object is even grasped. The accelerations and decelerations during lifting and lowering should be fast enough so that the body gets the benefit of the momentum but not so fast as to cause a jerk that may lead to an injury.

AVOID TWISTING

To maintain symmetry of the human body, the spine is provided with a bilaterally symmetrical arrangement of muscles and ligaments. Any rotation will accentuate the activities in the agonist group of muscles and reduce the contribution of the antagonistic muscles. When manual materials handling is done either in a twisted posture or when the spine is progressively twisted during the lift, the force production in different muscles is continually varied. This accentuates the stress on one group of muscles and ligaments. When the majority of the load is borne by only 50% of the structures, the stress could easily be doubled. This significantly increases the chances of injury. Twisting while bent over such as when taking parts off the floor is bad. A general recommendation is therefore for workers to move their feet instead of twisting their back. However, this may not be followed by the workers as rigorously as desirable, so an engineering approach is recommended that will prevent the need to twist entirely. Such an approach will solve the problem rather than depend on the worker's knowledge, awareness, alertness, and cooperation. **Figure 24-4** shows how the task can be modified to reduce bending and twisting.

MECHANICAL AIDS

The most desirable solution to prevent injuries associated with manual materials handling is to eliminate the need for manual materials handling by using mechanical aids. For example, instead of moving a power tool around the work station, a balancer (**Fig. 24-5**) or manipulator (**Fig. 24-6**) could be used. **Figure 24-7** shows the use of a turntable on a scissors lift to mechanize palletizing. In automation, the operator would be replaced with a palletizer. In some circumstances robots are appropriate. Common machines used to eliminate manual handling are hoists, lift trucks, and conveyors. For loading and unloading trucks, portable and telescopic conveyors can be used. A lever arm can be considered a machine. **Figure 24-8** shows how a tipping aid reduces load on the muscles.

PACKAGING

For job design, an important concept is to keep the load close to the body. To achieve this objective it is important to keep packages small enough so that they can be handled closer to the body. Big, bulky, and awkward packaging increases the moment arm of the load on the spine, thereby increasing the compressive load significantly. Therefore, because of the bulk it may be more difficult to lift 25 kg of feathers than 25 kg of iron. Konz and Coetzee[25] reported that increasing a box's volume up to a 30-cm cube did not bother men but strongly bothered women. Therefore, an important lesson would be to consider the anthropometry of the

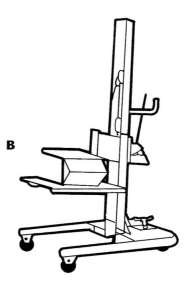

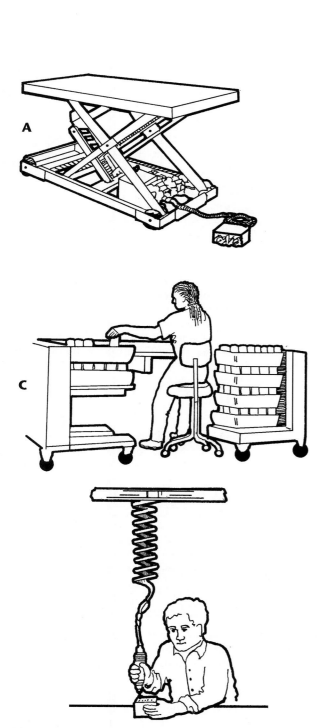

Figure 24-4 Workstation positioners reduce lifting, bending, and twisting. **A**, A scissors lift. **B**, A bin on an adjustable-height cart—useful for temporary work stations such as stocking of shelves. **C**, Self-leveling trucks (similar to cafeteria tray dispensers).

Figure 24-5 Balancers reduce tool weight from pounds to ounces. Note that the balancer is suspended from a job crane to minimize horizontal force as the tool is moved about the workplace. Ulin et al (1993) showed that increased tool weight increased torque at the elbow and shoulder, thereby decreasing comfort of the neck and back as well as the arm.

work population when determining dimensions of the packaging.

COUPLING

Cardboard boxes with cutout holes provide poor coupling because (1) the hand cannot rotate as the object is lifted from the knee to the waist and (2) the cardboard surface area is narrow and tends to concentrate the load on a small area of contact with the hands and thereby cuts the circulation and squeezes the muscles. When the packages to be lifted are larger than the optimal size, it is particularly important to allow for a comfortable handhold. This will permit a relatively risk-free, orderly, and smooth lifting activity that minimizes the chance of injury precipitation.

WORK HEIGHT

Konz[23] states, "drag it, pull it, push it but don't lift it." Wheeled luggage and trash containers are examples. If lifting is necessary, however, it is desirable to do material handling at knuckle height. This also implies that one should not put a load on the floor or work above the shoulders. For example, when cartons are

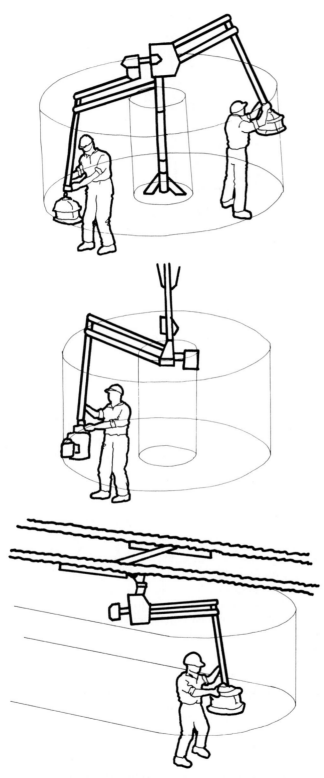

Figure 24-6 Manipulators (balancers with arms) can support tools or can be used to move product around the work stations.

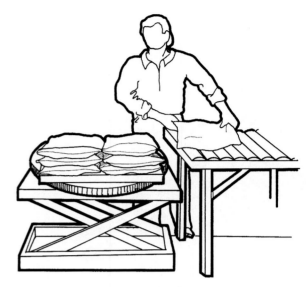

Figure 24-7 Turntables can reduce stress when loading/unloading. The turntable is rotated after a few items are moved. It can be mounted on the floor and a pallet placed on it. If the turntable surface is rollers, ball casters, or an air table, rotation can be manual. If the turntable is mounted on a scissors table (as shown), horizontal transfer can replace lifting/lowering.

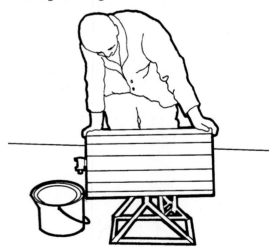

Figure 24-8 Tipping aids permit a drum or carboy to be counterbalanced when pouring. The danger of spills and operator muscle stress are reduced.

loaded from a conveyor, the conveyor height should be adjustable. When cartons are loaded from a pallet, the pallet should be left on the lift truck forks and the fork height periodically adjusted. If the fork lift cannot be tied up, the pallet should be placed on a wheeled lift table. Ayoub, Selan, and Jiang[4] recommend a comprehensive set of guidelines to control and reduce occupational health problems associated with manual materials handling. Their recommendations can be summed up in two statements: (1) eliminate heavy manual materials handling, and (2) decrease the stress to the worker. They recommend the use of mechanical aids such as hoists, lift tables, and conveyors and the provision of best work heights that can be varied to suit the operator and achieve an optimum work arrangement. A reduction of the stress, they suggest, can be achieved by reducing the weight of the object in cases in which it is not possible to split the load between two workers. Reduction of container size and container weight is a desirable goal. They also recommend changing the type of manual materials handling, such as lower the load rather than lift, push the load rather than pull, and pull the load rather than carry. They suggest reducing both the horizontal and vertical distance in reaching for the object and transporting it. Avoiding twisting in both standing and seated work is desirable. Modification of the object to make it easier to handle by using handles, balance containers, and reasonable width are all good design criteria. On the worker side, however, it is also important to provide adequate recovery time by reducing the frequency and allowing for job rotation.

References

1. Andersson GBJ: The epidemiology of spinal disorders. In Frymoyer J et al: *The adult spine,* New York, 1991, Raven Press; pp 107-146.

2. Andersson GBJ, Jonsson B, Ortengren R: Myoelectric activity in individual lumbar erector spinae muscles in sitting: a study with surface and wire electrodes, *Scand J Rehabil Med* 3:91-108, 1974.

3. Asfahl CR: *Industrial safety and health management,* Englewood Cliffs, NJ, 1984, Prentice Hall.

4. Ayoub MM, Selan J, Jiang B: Manual material handling. In Salvendy G, editor: *Handbook of human factors,* New York, 1987. Wiley & Sons.

5. Bendix T, Biering-Sorensen F: Posture of the trunk when sitting on forward-inclining seats, *Scand J of Rehabil Med* 27 (8):873-882, 1983.

6. Bendix T, Hagberg M: Trunk posture and load on the trapezius muscle whilst sitting at sloping desks, *Ergonomics* 27 (8):873-882, 1984.

7. Bigos S, Battié, M: The impact of spinal disorders in industry. In Frymoyer J et al, editors: *The adult spine,* New York, 1991, Raven Press.

8. Chaffin DB: Manual materials handling and the biomechanical basis for prevention of low-back pain in industry—an overview, *Am Ind Hyg Assoc J* 48(2):989-996, 1987.

9. Chaffin DB, Park KS: A longitudinal study of low back pain as associated with weight lifting factors, *Am Ind Hyg Assoc J* 34:513-525, 1973.

10. Davis PR, Stubbs DA: Safe levels of manual forces for young males (1), *Appl Ergonom* 8(3):141-150, 1977.

11. Dvorak J et al: Biomechanics of the craniocervical region: the alar and transverse ligaments, *J Orthop Res* 6:452-461, 1988.

12. Ekland J, Corbett EN: Experimental and biomechanical analysis of seating. In Corbett EN, Wilson J, Manenica I, editors: *The ergonomics of working postures,* London, 1969, Taylor & Francis Publishers; pp 319-330.

13. Floyd WF, Ward JS: Anthopometric and physiological considerations in school, office and factory seating. In Grandjean E, editor: *Sitting posture,* London, 1969, Taylor & Francis Publishers; pp 18-25.

14. Frymoyer JW et al: Risk factors in low-back pain: an epidemiological survey, *J Bone Joint Surg* 65A(2):213-218, 1983.

15. Garg A et al: Biomechanical stresses as related to motion trajectory of lifting, *Hum Factors* 25(5):527-539, 1983.

16. Grandjean E: *Ergonomics of the home,* London, 1976, Taylor & Francis Publishers.

17. Griffin M: *Handbook of human vibration,* San Diego, 1990, Academic Press.

18. Haldeman S: Failure of pathology model to predict pain, *Spine* 15:718-724, 1990.

19. Herrin G, Jaraidi M, Anderson C: Prediction of overexertion injuries using biomechanical and psychophysical models, *Am Ind Hyg Assoc J* 47(6):322-330, 1986.

20. Kelsey J et al: Acute prolapsed intervertebral disc: an epidemiologic study with special reference to driving automobiles and cigarette smoking, *Spine* 9:608-613, 1984.

21. Khalil T: *Ergonomic issues in low back pain: origin and magnitude of the problem.* Proceedings of the Human Factors Society, San Francisco, 1991; pp 820-824.

22. Konz SA: *Facilities design,* New York, 1985, John Wiley & Sons.

23. Konz SA: *Work design: industrial ergonomics,* ed 4, Scottsdale, Ariz, 1995, Publishing Horizons.

24. Konz SA, Bhasin R: Foot position during lifting, *Am Ind Hyg Assoc J* 35(12):785-792, 1974.

25. Konz SA, Coetzee K: *Prediction of lifting difficulty from individual and task variables.* Proceedings of the fourth International Congress on Production Research, Tokyo, 1977.

26. Kumar S: A conceptual model of overexertion, safety and hazard, *Hum Factors* 36:197-209, 1994.

27. Kumar S: Cumulative load as a risk factor for back pain, *Spine* 15(12):1311-1316, 1990.

28. Kumar S: *Functional evaluation of the human back: a research report,* 1991.

29. Kumar S: The physiological cost of three different methods of lifting in sagittal and lateral planes, *Ergonomics* 27(4):425-433, 1984.

30. Kumar S, Dufresne RM, Garand D: Effect of posture on back strength, *Int J Ind Ergonom* 7:53-62, 1991.

31. Kumar S, Narayan Y, Bacchus C: Symmetric and asymmetric two handed push-pull strength of young adults. In Aghazadeh F, editor: *Advanced industrial ergonomics and safety research*, London, 1994, Taylor & Francis; pp 713-719.

32. Liles DH: The application of the job severity index to job design for the control of manual materials handling injury, *Ergonomics* 29(1):65-76, 1986.

33. Lueder RK: Seat comfort: a review of the construct in the office environment, *Hum factors* 25(6):701-711, 1983.

34. Lueder RK: Work station design. In Lueder R, editor: *The ergonomic payoff*, Toronto, 1986, Holt, Reinhart & Winston; pp 142-183.

35. Magora A: Investigation of the relation between low back pain and occupation, *Ind Med* 39(12):504-510, 1970.

36. Mandel AC: Investigation of the lumbar flexion of office workers. In Corbett EN, Wilson J, Manenica I, editors: *The ergonomics of working postures*, London, 1969, Taylor & Francis; pp. 345-354.

37. Mital A, Nicholson A, Ayoub MM: *A guide to manual material handling*, London, 1993, Taylor & Francis Publishers.

38. Ridd J: A practical methodology for the investigation of materials handling problems. In Kvalseth T, editor: *Ergonomics of workstation design*, London, 1983, Butterworth-Heinmann.

39. Rohmert W: Problems in determining rest allowances (Part 1: Use of modern methods to evaluate stress and strain in static muscular work), *Appl Ergonom* 4(2):91-95, 1973.

40. Schultz AB. Andersson GBJ: Analysis of loads on the lumbar spine, *Spine* 6(1):76-82, 1981.

41. Snook SH, Ciriello VM: The design of manual handling tasks: revised tables of maximum acceptable weights and forces, *Ergonomics* 34(9):1197-1213, 1991.

42. Spitzer et al: Scientific approach to the assessment and management of activity-related spinal disorders. A monograph for clinicians. Report of the Quebec Task Force on Spinal Disorders, *Spine* 12 (suppl) 1-559, 1987.

43. Statistics Canada: *Work injuries*, Ottawa, 1991, Statistics Canada.

44. Ulin S, Armstrong T, Snook S, Keyserling M: Examination of the effect of tool mass and work postures on perceived exertion for a screw driving task, *Int J Ind Ergonom* 12:105-115, 1993.

45. van der Beck A et al: Loadings and unloadings by lorry drivers and musculoskeletal complaints, *Int J Ind Ergonom* 12:13-23, 1993.

46. Von Korff M: Studying the natural history of back pain, *Spine* 19 (suppl 18):2041-2046, 1994.

47. Waddell G: A new clinical model for the treatment of low back pain, *Spine* 12(7):632-644, 1987.

48. Waddell G, Allan DB, Newton M: Clinical evaluation of disability in back pain. In Frymoyer J et al, editors: *The adult spine*, New York, 1991, Raven Press.

49. Waddell G et al: Chronic low-back pain, psychologic distress, and illness behavior, *Spine* 9(2):209-213, 1984.

50. Warwick, D, Novak G, Schultz A: Maximum voluntary strengths of male adults in some lifting, pushing and pulling activities, *Ergonomics* 23(1):49-54, 1980.

51. Waters T, Putz-Anderson V, Garg A: *Application Manual for the Revised NIOSH lifting equation*, NIOSH Pub PB94, Rockville, MD, 1994, Department of Health and Human Services.

52. Weber H: Lumbar disc herniation. A controlled, prospective study with ten years of observation, *Spine* 8(2):131-140, 1983.

53. Webster BS, Snook SH: The cost of 1989 workers' compensation low back pain claims, *Spine* 19(10):1111-1115, 1994.

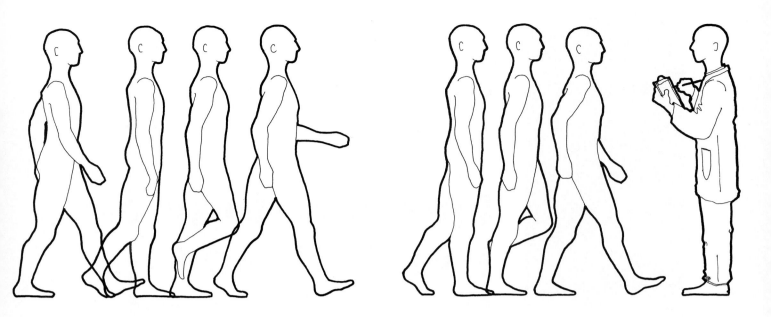

SECTION 2

Neck,
Shoulder, and
Elbow

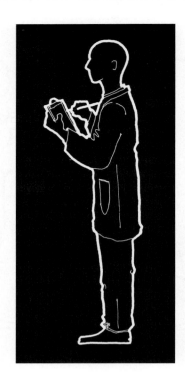

Chapter 25

Epidemiology of the Neck and Upper Extremity

Marianne Magnusson
Malcolm Pope

CONTENTS

As long ago as 1713, neck and shoulder disorders were reported to be related to certain occupations.[82] When compared with other musculoskeletal disorders, disorders of the neck and upper extremity are increasing as seen by the more frequent reporting of these disorders as occupational diseases.[68] The reason for the increase might be the higher degree of automation as a result of improved workplace designs with an emphasis on reducing workload such as heavy lifting and heavy manual work. However, the demands of increasing productivity, which in turn implies the simplification of working tasks, has led to an increased work pace.[99]

CLASSIFICATION OF DISORDERS

Neck and Shoulder

In the international Classification of Diseases,[102] cervical disorders have been classified into three categories: cervical spondylosis, cervical disk disorders, and other disorders of the cervical region. The Finnish version of the World Health Organization (WHO) document included "tension neck syndrome," "syndroma cervicobrachiale," and "syndroma cervicobraciale diffusum." According to the WHO, work-related neck-shoulder disorders have been classified into "occupational diseases," in which there is a direct cause-effect relationship between hazard and disease, and "work-related disease, in which the work environment and the performance of work contribute significantly, along with other factors, to the causation of a multifactorial disease."[101]

The concept of occupational cervicobrachial disorder was adopted in 1973.[6,64] It is defined as "functional and/or organic disturbances resulting from neuromuscular fatigue to doing jobs in a fixed position or with repetitive movement of the upper extremities" and as being of occupational origin. Waris[94] has four categories: cervical syndrome, tension neck syndrome, humeral tendinitis, and thoracic outlet syndrome.

The term "repetition strain injury" was introduced in Australia. It is defined as "a soft tissue disorder caused by muscle overloading from repetitive use or maintenance of constrained postures" and it "occurs among workers performing tasks involving frequent repetitive movements of the limbs or the maintenance of fixed postures for prolonged periods."[14] Cumulative trauma disorder, musculoskeletal injury and disorder, occupational repetitive strain injury, and regional pain syndrome are other terms that describe essentially the same condition.

Elbow

Tennis elbow, also called lateral humeral epicondylalgia or lateral elbow syndrome, is a painful condition of the lateral aspect of the elbow. Cubital tunnel external compression syndrome is a condition caused by the ulnar nerve being compressed at certain elbow flexion angles in a subcutaneous location behind the humeral epicondyle (cubital tunnel). Work-related musculoskeletal ailments of the elbow are rare. The conditions of a painful elbow joint can be worsened by repetitive work, but the primary origins of the disorder should first be attended. The clinical syndrome of this joint will not be covered in this text.[9,24]

EPIDEMIOLOGY

General Population

In general studies that include large sample populations without special demands for neck and shoulder activity, the 12-month prevalence of neck and shoulder disorders was 15% to 18%.[5,95] Disorders of the neck and shoulders are most common among women.[7,23,67,95] In a Swedish study, 50% of the women reported strain injuries from the neck and shoulders, but only 36% of the men did so.[48] Another study reported a 10 times higher rate of sick leave for occupational cervicobrachial disorders in women than sick leave for occupational low back pain in men.[54] A higher rate of tension neck syndromes in women than in men was also reported for industrial workers in the United States.[87]

Women, perhaps even more than men, often work in occupations with repetitive and monotonous work tasks. Many studies have reported an increased prevalence of neck and upper limb disorders in repetitive work.[35,51,62,80,93] In a large Swedish study of 2,537 men and women, 20% of the women and 16% of the men had neck-shoulder problems during the preceding 12 months.[95] The incidence of neck and shoulder problems was found to increase with age and occupational physical load. Takala et al[90] reported a 1-year prevalence of neck and shoulder pain of 18% in women and 16% in men in a Finnish rural population. In a random sample of 855 men and women in Iceland, 65% of the women and 43% of the men had neck or shoulder pain during the previous year.[81] Neck and shoulder pain has been found to be not only interrelated but also related to low back pain; this indicates a susceptibility and a predisposition to musculoskeletal disorders.[65]

Occupational Risk Groups

Musculoskeletal diseases were the major reason for long-term absenteeism in a manufacturing company. Low back pain accounted for the greatest group of all long-term absenteeism at 17.7%, and neck and shoulder pain caused 15.9%. Back disorders were most common in heavy manufacturing workshops, whereas in light manufacturing workshops the most prevalent diseases were related to the neck and shoulder.[54]

Table 25-1	Elbow problems in newspaper workers.		
	All	**Office**	**Production**
12-month prevalence (%)	8	6	12
Missed work (%)	1	1	2
N	906	682	201

From Rosencrance JC, Cook TM, Zimmerman CL: JOSPT 19:267-276, 1994.

Dentists, meat cutters, miners, and "heavy workers" have an increased risk of cervical spondylosis as compared with office workers and farmers.[35] Tension neck syndrome, the most common neck-shoulder disease, reaches a point prevalence of 100% in Japanese film-rolling workers. Keyboard operators had an odds ratio of 3.0 for tension neck syndrome. Females employed in assembly, fish-processing, and ceramics factories, all representing highly repetitive work tasks, had a considerably higher prevalence of neck/upper limb complaints as recorded in a questionnaire, as well as diagnoses at physical examination of the neck and upper limb, than did a control group with more varied tasks.[74]

Neck and shoulder symptoms, without a specific diagnosis or specified symptoms, have been reported in a large number of occupations, including secretaries and office workers,[12,45,46,60,92] dentists,[59,72] sewing machine operators,[89] visual artists and piano players,[18,30] and railway station workers.[15] The yearly prevalence of neck and/or shoulder symptoms for female secretaries and office workers ranged from 45% to 63%; the prevalence for male office workers was considerably lower, 16% to 27%.

Newspaper workers were surveyed in a study of the newspaper industry. Reports of elbow problems are shown in **Table 25-1**.

Musculoskeletal problems have affected instrumental musicians for a long time.[28,29] Lederman and Calabrese[56] noted an increasing number of reports of musculotendinous overuse. Nerve entrapment syndromes have been described in musicians by Lederman,[55] Knishkowsky, and Lederman.[52] Charness et al[19] report that routine electromyography (EMG) and nerve conduction study findings were abnormal in fewer than half of the patients, which attests to the potential for mild ulnar neuropathy to produce disabling symptoms in musicians.

Work-related Factors

Several studies have suggested a relationship between static or repetitive load and disorders in the neck and upper extremity.[33,48,54,63,96] Hagberg and Wegman[35] conducted a metaanalysis of occupational neck-shoulder disorders and found that jobs with highly repetitive shoulder muscle contractions, static muscle work, and work above shoulder level were associated with tension neck syndrome. Several studies have sup-

ported these associations.[4,18,30,75,89] The mechanical load on the shoulders was obvious in all these studies.

Working postures with the neck in extreme flexion increase the load moment three to four times.[38] In this position, however, there is very little muscle activity of the cervical erector spinae muscle, which indicates that the ligaments and joint capsules are exposed to considerable stress.

Working tasks that involve continuous arm movements always generate a static load component.[1,76,88,97,100] The principal muscle to carry this load is the trapezius. The relative load (%MVC) on the upper trapezius has been shown to increase linearly with relative torque in the glenohumeral joint.[32] However, there are large differences between muscles and between flexion and abduction. A given shoulder torque during flexion produces smaller amplitudes in both intramuscular pressure (IMP) and EMG than for the same torque during abduction.[42] With a shoulder abduction of 30 degree, the IMP in the supraspinatus muscle by far exceeds the level at which blood flow is significantly impeded. Therefore, the supraspinatus is extremely vulnerable in work situations with elevated arms.

Kurppa et al,[53] Silverstein,[87] and others have reported that highly repetitive tasks can cause pain and disability in the upper extremity. In many jobs, upper extremity tasks require repetitive contractions of the upper extremity muscles over long periods of time at low contraction intensities and short contraction-relaxation cycles. Edwards[25] has proposed that fatigue and lack of recovery are the elements that can cause injury to the elbow. Byström and Kilbom,[17] in simulations of upper extremity work, concluded that work at a mean contraction intensity of higher than 17% to 21% MVC was not acceptable. The criteria were recovery of blood flow, EMG fatigue index, and subjective ratings. In a later paper, Byström and Fransson-Hall,[16] using the same techniques, suggested that continuous handgrip contractions higher than 10% MVC are to be avoided. These recommendations are conservative, and many industrial jobs exceed them.

Excessive contractions or fatigue can lead to tennis elbow, one of the most common occupational elbow problems. Tennis elbow is characterized by intense pain of the lateral aspect of the elbow exacerbated by grip and more use. Coonrad[20] reports that the main problem is repetition but it is multifactorial in origin. Allander[3] reported a prevalence of 33% in 15,000 subjects. Dimberg,[22] in studies at certain occupational clinics, found that 64% of all cases diagnosed were related to work. Cyriax[21] reported that only 8% of cases were actually related to tennis. However, in a review, Maylack[71] reported that 50% of competitive tennis players will suffer at least one episode of lateral epicondylitis.

Another elbow problem is cubital tunnel external compression syndrome. As the ulnar nerve travels from the brachial plexus to the hand, it is vulnerable to compression at certain elbow flexion angles at a subcutaneous location behind the humeral epicondyle (cubital tunnel). A common occupational risk for cubital tunnel external compression syndrome is resting the elbow on a hard surface for a long period of time. Such problems have been reported in drivers.[2] Mansukhani and D'Souza[70] reported unilateral ulnar neuropathy in diamond workers. The neuropathy was restricted to the arm holding the eyeglass for inspecting the diamonds.

Individual Factors

Musculoskeletal disorders will not develop in all workers performing similar and risky work tasks. Obviously, individual factors influence the exposure-effect relationship. The individual factors most frequently studied or controlled for are sex and age. Some studies have shown that age has an effect on the prevalence of musculoskeletal disorders,[40,51,58,92,95] whereas other studies have shown no such influence.[13] Muscle strength and endurance have an influence on the risk of neck and upper limb disorders. It is obvious that with higher muscle strength, the muscle will be less loaded than in the case of lower strength for the same force exertion. Women in general have lower strength than men, in particular in the upper extremities, and older people are weaker than younger ones.[73] Some studies, however, have shown that women have greater muscle endurance in proportion to their muscle strength than do men.[11,86] This has not been proved for all muscle groups, however. Fatigue and poor strength might thus explain why women have more neck-shoulder disorders than men. It is more likely, however, that more women than men have jobs that involve a high degree of repetitiveness and prolonged static postures of the neck and shoulders.

Poor muscle strength and endurance have been shown to be impaired in patients with neck-shoulder pain. Strength was affected in patients with acute symptoms,[10,54] whereas endurance was impaired in those with chronic conditions as well.[34,88,89] Other studies, however, have failed to show a relationship between neck and shoulder symptoms and strength and endurance.[50] Indeed, the contrary was shown in a prospective study; subjects with high muscle strength in shoulder elevation seemed to be at a higher risk.[44,49] A longitudinal study of motor assembly workers showed that low isometric strength of shoulder muscles was a risk factor for neck and shoulder pain.[47] Hägg, Suurküla, and Kilbom[36] could not show significant relationships between either EMG signs of fatigue during work or isometric strength and the development of muscular disorders during a 2-year follow-up.

A few studies have found certain personality traits to be predisposed to musculoskeletal disorders. The "type A" personality, characterized by competitiveness, impatience, and a feeling of time urgency, has been found to be associated with low back pain[40,41,98] and with neck-shoulder pain.[27,36,85]

Social Factors

Along with recognition of the importance of the physical load, there is a growing awareness of the association between the psychosocial factors, work en-

vironment, and musculoskeletal disorders. Job satisfaction and relations with co-workers and supervisors were the strongest predictors for the development of industry-related back pain in a longitudinal study.[7,8] Monotony, stress, low job satisfaction, lack of control, and low skill requirements characterized a typical light assembly job where young males reported a high rate of back pain.[61,66] Heliövaara[39] also found monotony and time pressure to be highly related to musculoskeletal symptoms. In a study of occupational drivers, the group that had the highest incidence of both back pain and neck and shoulder pain reported the highest stress level and lowest job satisfaction.[65] The same study also found a strong relationship between back pain and neck and shoulder pain, which indicates that one or several musculoskeletal disorders can develop in predisposed individuals. Tola et al[92] found that moderate or poor job satisfaction and physical loading factors were significant risk factors for neck and shoulder pain. Bergenudd et al[7] found that women with a history of shoulder pain were less satisfied with their jobs than were women who did not experience pain. Psychological stress at work may thus contribute to the development of musculoskeletal disorders. In particular, the combination of high work demand and low control seems to play an important role in the development of musculoskeletal complaints.[40,41]

PATHOMECHANISMS

Workload

Mechanical stress on musculoskeletal tissues is the common causative factor in musculoskeletal disorders. Normally, the tissues adapt to mechanical stress, that is, tissues strengthen with increased stress and weaken with less stress.[91] When the stress exceeds the limit of adaption, pathologic changes may occur in the tissue. However, the risk of symptoms developing may also increase when the physical stress is very low.[99] Hagberg, Kvarnström, and Wegman[34,35] suggest three possible pathomechanisms for muscle pain as a result of physical load: (1) mechanical failure, (2) local ischemia, and (3) energy metabolism disturbances. *Mechanical failure* of the muscles is typically the cause of the muscle soreness that occurs 24 to 48 hours after heavy physical exertion. The pain is due to rupture of the Z disks and outflow of metabolites from the muscle fibers, which directly or through edema activate pain receptors. *Local ischemia* produces an accumulation of metabolites within the muscle that is typically a result of static or repeated muscular contraction or repeated muscular injuries.

Energy metabolism disturbances occur when energy demand exceeds production. The resulting development of muscle pain may be delayed up to 48 hours, because of the prolonged replenishment of intracellular glycogen stores. Edwards[25] proposed another model for pathological change in the muscle following occupational injury. He suggested that occupational muscle pain might be a consequence of a conflict between motor control of the postural muscular activity and that needed for movement or exertion.

Some studies have been conducted to provoke pain or discomfort in the shoulder-neck region. Hagberg[32] studied the immediate and long-term effect of continuous repetitions of shoulder flexions with and without weights for 1 hour or until exhaustion. He found that all subjects had pain localized to the descending part of the trapezius muscle directly after the experiments. In 14 of the 18 experiments, the subjects had pain 24 hours later, and after 48 hours tenderness occurred in the trapezius muscle and the rotator cuff insertions.

Harms-Ringdahl and Ekholm[37] studied the effect of prolonged extreme flexion of the neck and found that pain was experienced after 15 minutes and increased with time. Interestingly enough, the pain disappeared within 15 minutes, but in 9 of the 10 subjects, pain recurred the same evening or the following morning and lasted for up to 4 days. Lee and Waikar[57] found a correlation between EMG root-mean-square values and discomfort ratings in subjects simulating microscope work for 4 hours.

Muscular Fatigue

Muscular fatigue is related to the force of the active muscle, that is, fatigue develops faster with higher relative muscle force. Some muscle groups are more fatigable than the neck and trunk extensor muscles.[31,79,83] Limits to muscular load for constrained work lasting 1 hour or more have been proposed by

Jonsson[43]: static muscular load should not exceed 2% to 5% MCV, the mean load level should be limited to 10% to 14% of MCV, and peak loads should be within 50% to 70% MCV. Muscular fatigue and muscle "overuse" are further discussed in Chapter 8.

Entrapment

Radial tunnel syndrome, also known as resistant tennis elbow, is seen in workers who have to perform multiple repetitive motions, especially wrist extensions with or without force. The mechanism behind the condition is entrapment of the radial nerve and involves its sensory branch.

PREVENTION

According to Hagberg and Wegman,[35] the occupationally related etiological fraction of neck and upper extremity injuries is high, and therefore a relatively large number could be prevented. Some studies have been able to prove that intervention in working conditions is successful.[78] Rehabilitation of neck and upper limb disorders, however, often fails when not combined with improvements in the work environment.[26,77] Only a few studies have been able to describe an exposure-effect relationship. To make prevention successful, future studies are needed on the quantification of physical exposure as well as the importance of psychosocial factors.

References

1. Aarås A, Westgaard RH: Further studies of postural load and musculoskeletal injuries of workers at an electromechanical assembly plant, *Appl Ergonom* 18:211-218, 1987.

2. Abdel-Salam A, Eyres KS, Cleary J: Driver's elbow: a cause of ulnar neuropathy. *J Hand Surg [Br]* 16B:436-437, 1991.

3. Allander E: Prevalence, incidence and remission rates of some common rheumatic diseases and syndromes, *Scand J Rheumatol* 3:145-153, 1974.

4. Amano M et al: Characteristics of work actions of shoe manufacturing assembly line workers and a cross-sectional factor-control study on occupational cervicobrachial disorders, *Jpn J Ind Health* 30:3-12, 1988.

5. Anderson JAD: Shoulder pain and tension neck and their relation to work. *Scand J Work Environ Health* 10:435-442, 1984.

6. Aoyama H et al: Recent trends in research on occupational cervicobrachial disorder. *J Hum Ergol, 8,* 39-45, 1979.

7. Bergenudd H et al: Pain in middle age. A study of prevalence and relation to occupational work load and psychosocial factors, *Clin Orthop* 231:234-238, 1988.

8. Bigos SJ et al: A prospective study of work perceptions and psychosocial factors affecting the report of back injury, *Spine* 1:1-6, 1991.

9. Binder AI, Hazleman BL: Lateral humeral epicondylitis—a study of nature history and the effect of conservative therapy, *Br J Rheumatol* 22:73-76, 1983.

10. Bjelle A, Hagberg M, Michaelson G: Occupational and individual factors in acute low back shoulder-neck disorders among industrial workers, *Br J Ind Med* 38:356-363, 1981.

11. Björkstén M, Jonsson B: Endurance limit of force in long-term intermittent static contractions, *Scand J Work Environ Health* 3:23-27, 1977.

12. Björkstén M, Jonsson B: Musculoskeletal disorders among medical secretaries, *Arbete och Hälsa* 34, 1987 (in Swedish).

13. Brisson C et al: Effect of duration of employment in piecework on severe disability among female garment workers, *Scand J Work Environ Health* 15:329-334, 1989.

14. Browne CD, Nolan BM, Faithful DK: Occupational repetition strain injuries. Guidelines for diagnosis and management, *Med J Aust* 140:329-332, 1984.

15. Brulin C et al: Musculoskeletal disorders in railway workers in Finland, Norway, and Sweden, *Arbete och Hälsa* 23, 1988 (in Swedish).

16. Byström S, Franson-Hall C: Acceptability of intermittent handgrip contractions based on physiological response, *Hum Factors* 36 (1):158-171, 1994.

17. Byström S, Kilbom, Å: Physiological response in the forearm during and after isometric intermittent handgrip, *Eur J Appl Physiol* 60:457-466, 1990.

18. Chang WS et al: Occupational musculoskeletal disorders of visual artists. A questionnaire and video analysis, *Ergonomics* 30:33-46, 1987.

19. Charness ME et al: Occupational cubital tunnel syndrome in instrumental musicians, *Neurology* 37 (suppl):115-120, 1987.

20. Coonrad RW: Tennis elbow, *Instr Course Lect* 35:94-101, 1986.

21. Cyriax JH: The pathology and treatment of tennis elbow, *J Bone Joint Surg [Am]* 18A:921-938, 1936.

22. Dimberg L: *Lateral humeral epicondylitis (tennis elbow) among industrial workers*, Stockholm, 1983, Swedish Work Environment Fund (research report).

23. Dimberg L et al: The correlation between work environment and occurrence of cervicobrachial symptoms, *J Occup Med* 31:447-453, 1989.

24. Doherty M, Preston B: Primary osteoarthritis of the elbow, *Ann Rheum Dis* 48:743-747, 1989.

25. Edwards RHT: Hypotheses of peripheral and central mechanisms underlying occupational muscle pain and injury, *Eur J Appl Physiol* 57:275-281, 1988.

26. Ekberg K et al: Cross-sectional study of risk factors for symptoms in the neck and shoulder area, *Ergonomics* 38(5):971-980, 1995.

27. Flodmark BT, Aase G: Musculoskeletal symptoms and type A in blue collar workers, *Br J Ind Med* 49:683-689, 1992.

28. Fry HJH: Overuse syndrome in musician, *Med J Aust* 146:390, 1987.

29. Fry HJH: Overuse syndrome in musician. 100 years ago. An historical review, *Med J Aust* 145:620-625, 1986.

30. Grieco A et al: Muscular effort and musculoskeletal disorders in piano students: electromyographic, clinical and preventive aspects, *Ergonomics* 32:697-716, 1989.

31. Grunow L, Rosenburg R, Kramer H: Vergleich des Kraft-Zeit-verlaufs beiisometrischer Daueranspannung des Rückenstreckapparates und der Armbeugemuskulatur bei maximal möglicher Willküranspannung, *Z Gesamte Hyg* 31:205-208, 1985.

32. Hagberg M: Electromyographic signs of shoulder muscle fatigue in two elevated arm positions, *Am J Phys Med* 60:111-121, 1981.

33. Hagberg M: The role of the work environment in shoulder and neck discomfort, *Arbetsmiljöfonden Stockholm*, 1988 (in Swedish).

34. Hagberg M, Kvarnström S: Muscular endurance and electromyographic fatigue in myofascial shoulder pain, *Arch Phys Med Rehabil* 65:522-525, 1984.

35. Hagberg M, Wegman DH: Prevalence rates and odds ratios of shoulder-neck diseases in different occupational groups, *Br J Ind Med* 44:602-610, 1987.

36. Hägg GM, Suurküla J, Kilbom Å: Predictors of work related neck and shoulder problems. A longitudinal study of female assembly workers, *Arbete och Hälsa*, 10, 1990, (in Swedish).

37. Harms-Ringdahl K, Ekholm J: Intensity and character of pain and muscular activity levels elicited by maintained extreme flexion position of the lower-cervical–upper-thoracic spine, *Scand J Rehabil Med* 18:117-126, 1986.

38. Harms-Ringdahl K et al: Load moments and myoelectric activity when the cervical spine is held in full flexion and extension, *Ergonomics* 29:1539-1552, 1986.

39. Heliövaara M et al. Determinants of sciatica and low-back pain, *Spine* 16 (6):608-614, 1991.

40. Holmström EB, Lindell J, Moritz U: Low back pain and neck-shoulder pain in construction workers; occupational workload and psychosocial factors. Part 1: Relationship to low back pain, *Spine* 17:663-671, 1992.

41. Holmström EB, Lindell J, Moritz U: Low back pain and neck-shoulder pain in construction workers; occupational workload and psychosocial risk factors. Part 2: Relationship to neck and shoulder pain, *Spine* 17:672-677, 1992.

42. Järvholm U: *On shoulder muscle load. An experimental study of muscle pressures, EMG and blood flow*, doctoral thesis, Göteborg, Sweden, 1990, Göteborg University.

43. Jonsson B: Measurement and evaluation of local muscle strain in the shoulder during constrained work, *J Hum Ergol* 11:73-88, 1982.

44. Jonsson BG, Persson J, Kilbom Å: Disorders of the cervicobrachial region among female workers in the electronics industry: a two-year follow up, *Int J Ind Ergonom* 3:1-12, 1988.

45. Kamwendo, K: *Neck and shoulder disorders in secretaries. Prevalence, risk factors, and neck school intervention*, doctoral dissertation, Lund, Sweden, 1991, Lund University.

46. Kemmlert K, Kilbom Å: Neck-shoulder disorders associated with work situation. An evaluation using questionnaires and work place visit, *Arbete och Hälsa* 17:1-92, 1988 (in Swedish).

47. Kilbom Å: Isometric strength and occupational muscle disorders, *Eur J Appl Physiol* 57:322-326, 1988.

48. Kilbom Å, Broberg E: Health hazards related to ergonomic work conditions, *Women Health* 13:81-93, 1988.

49. Kilbom Å, Persson J: Work technique and its consequences for musculoskeletal disorders, *Ergonomics* 30:273-279, 1987.

50. Kilbom Å, Persson J, Jonsson BG: Disorders of the cervicobrachial region among female workers in the electronics industry, *Int J Ind Ergonom* 1:37-47, 1986.

51. Kivi P: Rheumatic disorders of the upper limbs associated with repetitive occupational tasks in Finland in 1975-1979, *Scand J Rheumatol* 13:101-107, 1984.

52. Knishkowsky B, Lederman RJ: Instrumental musicians with upper extremity disorders. A follow up study, *Med Probl Perform Arts* 1:85-99, 1986.

53. Kurppa K et al: Incidence of tenosynovitis or peritendinitis and epicondylitis in a meat processing factory, *Scand J Work Environ Health* 17 (1):32-37, 1991.

54. Kvarnström S: Occurrence of musculoskeletal disorders in a manufacturing industry, with special attention to occupational shoulder disorders, *Scand J Rehabil Med, Suppl* 8:1-112, 1983.

55. Lederman RJ: Nerve entrapment syndromes in instrumental musicians, *Med Probl Perform Arts* 1:45-48, 1986.

56. Lederman RJ, Calabrese LH: Overuse syndrome in instrumentalists, *Med Probl Perform Arts* 1:7-11, 1986.

57. Lee KS, Waikar WL: Physical stress evaluation of microscope work using objective and subjective methods, *Int J Ind Ergonom* 2:203-209, 1988.

58. Leino P: Symptoms of stress predict musculoskeletal disorders, *J Epidemiol Community Health* 43:293-300, 1989.

59. Letho T: *Health of the dentist with reference to work-related and individual factors,* doctoral thesis, Turku, Finland, 1990, Publications of the Social Insurance Institution (ML:99).

60. Linton SJ, Kamvendo K: Risk factors in the psychosocial work environment for neck and shoulder pain in secretaries, *J Occup Med* 31:609-613, 1989.

61. Lundberg U et al: Psychological and physiological stress responses during repetitive work at an assembly line, *Work Stress* 3(2):143-153, 1989.

62. Luopajärvi T et al: Prevalence of tenosynovitis and other injuries of the upper extremities in repetitive work, *Scand J Work Environ Health* (suppl):3:48-55, 1979.

63. Maeda K: Occupational cervicobrachial disorder and its causative factors, *J Hum Ergol* 6:193-202, 1977.

64. Maeda K, Horiguchi S, Hosokawa M: History of the studies on occupational cervicobrachial disorder in Japan and remaining problems, *J Hum Ergol* 11:17-29, 1982.

65. Magnusson M et al: Investigation of the long-term exposure to whole body vibration: a 2-country study. Vienna Award for Phys Med 1992, *Eur J Phys Med Rehabil* 3:28-34, 1993.

66. Magnusson M et al: The loads on the lumbar spine during work at on assembly line in a car factory. The risks for fatigue injuries, *Spine* 15:774-779, 1990.

67. Mäkelä M et al: Prevalence, determinants, and consequences of chronic neck pain in Finland, *Am J Epidemial* 11:1356-1367, 1991.

68. Malker B, Blomgren UB: *Occupational diseases 1985,* Stockholm, 1989, National Board of Occupational Safety and Health, and Statistics Sweden (in Swedish).

69. Malker HSR et al: Occupational musculoskeletal disorders. Identification of risk by ISA statistics, *Arbete och Hälsa* 29:1-122, 1990 (in Swedish).

70. Mansukhani KA, D'Souza C: Ulnar neuropathy at the elbow in diamond sorters, *Indian J Med Res* 94:433-436, 1991.

71. Maylack FH: Epidemiology of tennis, squash, and racquetball injuries, *Clin Sports Med* 233-243, 1988.

72. Milerad E, Ekenvall L: Symptoms of the neck and upper extremities in dentists, *Scand J Work Environ Health* 16:129-134, 1990.

73. Murray MP et al: Shoulder motion and muscle strength of normal men and women in two age groups, *Clin Orthop* 192:268-273, 1985.

74. Ohlsson K: *Neck and upper limb disorders in female workers performing repetitive industrial tasks,* doctoral thesis, Lund, Sweden, 1995, Lund University.

75. Ohlsson K, Attewell R, Skerfving S: Self-reported symptoms in the neck and upper limbs of female assembly workers. Impact of length of employment, work pace, and selection, *Scand J Work Environ Health* 15:75-80, 1989.

76. Onishi N et al: Shoulder muscle tenderness and physical features of female industrial workers, *J Hum Ergol* 5:87-102, 1976.

77. Parenmark G, Alffram PE, Malmkvist AK: The significance of work tasks for rehabilitation outcome after carpal tunnel surgery, *J Occup Rehabil* 2:89-94, 1992.

78. Parenmark G, Malmkvist AK, Örtengren R: Ergonomic moves in an engineering industry: effects on sick leave frequency, labour turnover and productivity, *Int J Ind Ergonom* 11:1-10, 1993.

79. Petrofsky JS, Phillips CA: The strength-endurance relationship in skeletal muscle: its application to helmet design, *Aviat Space Environ Med* 53:365-369, 1982.

80. Punnett L et al: Soft tissue disorders in the upper limbs of female garment workers, *Scand J Work Environ Health* 11:417-425, 1985.

81. Rafnsson V et al: Muskuloskeletala besv'r bland islänningar, *Nord Med* 104:104-107, 1989.

82. Ramazzini B: *De morbis artificum,* ed. 2, New York, 1964, Hafner Publishing (Translated by WC Wright and originally published in 1713).

83. Rohmert W et al: A study stressing the need for a static postural force model for work analysis, *Ergonomics* 29:1235-1249, 1986.

84. Rosencrance JC, Cook TM, Zimmermann CL: Active surveillance for the control of cumulative trauma disorders: working modes in the newspaper industry, *JOSPT* 19(5):267-276, 1994.

85. Salminen JJ, Pentti J, Wickström G: Tenderness and pain in neck and shoulders in relation to type A behaviour, *Scand J Rheumatol* 20:344-350, 1991.

86. Sato H, Ohashi J: Sex differences in static muscular endurance, *J Hum Ergol* 18:53-60, 1989.

87. Silverstein BA: *The prevalence of upper extremity cumulative trauma disorders in industry,* doctoral thesis, Ann Arbor, 1985, University of Michigan.

88. Sjogaard G et al: Physical workload and musculoskeletal disorders in sewing machine-operators. In Adams SA et al, editors: *Ergonomics International 88.* Proceedings in the tenth congress of the International Ergonomics Association, Sydney, Ergonomics Society of Australia; pp 384-386.

89. Sjogaard G et al. *Shoulder-neck problems in sewers: an epidemiologic and work physiologic investigation,* Copenhagen, 1987, Arbetsmiljofondet (in Danish).

90. Takala EP et al: Seasonal variation in neck and shoulder symptoms, *Scand J Environ Health* 18:257-261, 1992.

91. Tipton CM, Vailas AC, Matthes RD: Experimental studies on the influence of physical activity on ligaments, tendons and joints: a brief review, *Acta Med Scand (suppl)* 711:157-168, 1986.

92. Tola S et al: Neck and shoulder symptoms among men in machine operating, dynamic physical work and sedentary work, *Scand J Work Environ Health* 14:299-305, 1988.

93. Viikari-Juntura E: A life-long prospective study on the role of psychosocial factors in neck-shoulder and low-back pain, *Spine* 16:1056-1061, 1991.

94. Waris P: Occupational cervicobrachial syndromes: a review, *Scand J Work Environ Health* 5(3):3-14, 1979.

95. Westerling D, Jonsson BG: Pain from the neck and shoulder region and sick leave, *Scand J Soc Med* 8:131-136, 1980.

96. Westgaard RH, Aarås A: Postural muscle strain as a causal factor in the development of work-related musculoskeletal illnesses, *Applied Ergonom* 15:162-174, 1984.

97. Westgaard RH, Bjorklund R: Generation of muscle tension additional to postural load, *Ergonomics* 30:911-923, 1987.

98. Wickström G et al: Type A behaviour and back pain, *Work Stress* 3:203-207, 1989.

99. Winkel J: Why is there an increase in the occupational disorders? *Nord Med* 104:324-327, 1989 (in Swedish).

100. Winkel J, Oxenburgh M: Towards optimizing physical activity in VDT/office work. In Sauter S, Dainoff M, Smith M, editors: *Promoting health and productivity in the computerized office: models of successful ergonomic interventions,* London, 1990, Taylor & Francis Publishers; pp 94-117.

101. World Health Organization: *Identification and control of work-related diseases. Report of a WHO Expert Committee,* WHO Tech Rep Series 714:9, Geneva, 1985.

102. World Health Organization: *International Classification of Diseases. Manual of the international statistical classification of diseases, injuries, and causes of death,* vol 1, Geneva, 1977, The Organization.

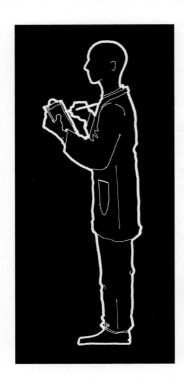

Chapter 26

Biomechanics of the Neck

Jiri Dvorak
Aaron Sandler
James A. Antinnes

CONTENTS

The biomechanics of the cervical spine is determined by the shape of the vertebral bodies and the orientation of the zygapophyseal joints and can accordingly be divided into three sections:

- Upper cervical spine: occiput, atlas, axis
- Lower cervical spine: C2/C3 to C7
- Cervical-thoracic junction: C7 to the third thoracic vertebra (**Fig. 26-1**)

The primary aim of the clinician treating a patient with neck pain is to find the region or even segment responsible for pain symptoms. Because the intersegmental nerve root anastomosis makes it almost impossible for a patient suffering from neck pain to localize the exact origin of pain,[11,12,27] the clinician must base the diagnosis on functional and palpatory examinations of the cervical spine. To do this correctly requires analysis and interpretation of normal and disturbed motion patterns based on a knowledge of clinical biomechanics and an understanding of developmental anatomy.

The natural aging process results in many changes in the cervical spine that must be taken into account in the clinical assessment, especially as related to range of motion. It is well established that range of motion decreases with age, mainly in the middle and lower segments of the cervical spine.[4] This is due to the ongoing transformation process of the intervertebral disk and the development of uncovertebral joints[14,30]; later it may also be due to development of osteoarthritis of the zygapophyseal joints.

In the first two decades of life, the uncovertebral spaces of the lower part of the cervical spine begin to undergo a lifelong transformation into uncovertebral joints. This transformation is a response to the compressive force of the weight of the head, which the upright posture of the body requires the cervical spine to support (**Fig. 26-2**).[14,29,30] The result is the formation of lateral tears of the disk annulus beginning in the second decade of life (**Fig. 26-3**). These lateral tears continue to develop into the medial center part of the disk until, in the third decade, complete transverse tears commonly occur (**Fig. 26-4**).[29] The resulting space in the middle of the intervertebral disk partially takes over the function of the zygapophyseal joints during the second and third decades. (At this stage, the nucleus pulposus dries out, appearing on radiographs as a narrowing between the vertebrae of the lower cervical spine, which provides a

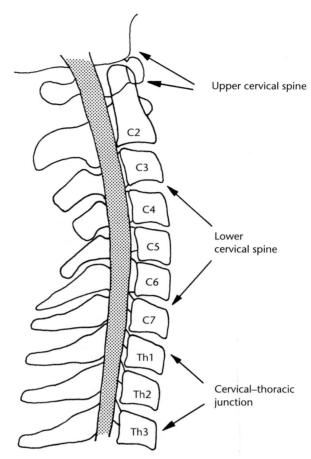

Figure 26-1 Sections of the cervical spine.

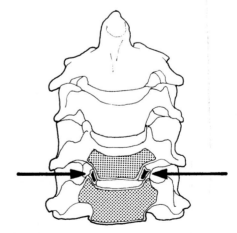

Figure 26-2 Drawing of the uncovertebral joints. *(From Luschka H: Die halbgelenke des menschlichen körpers, Berlin, 1858, Reimers.)*

convenient way for the clinician to monitor these changes.)

This new space within the disk significantly reduces the load-absorbing function of the intervertebral disk in the cervical spine. To support the load of the head, a transformation of the uncovertebral joints starts to occur.[29] Instead of the original pointed shape, the uncovertebral processes now become flat with a shape like that of a cow horn (**Fig. 26-5**) and take over the load of the cranial vertebrae. The overall result is a natural transformation of the structure and shape of the uncovertebral processes that is probably responsible for much of the decreased range of motion that accompanies aging and must be taken into account in any clinical assessment of the cervical spine.

In the first two decades of life the surfaces of the articular processes are covered by a thin layer of cartilage, with the uneven surfaces filled in by a synovial fold in the joint capsule. This synovial fold has been described by Penning and Töndury[22] as meniscoid. It is found within the entire cervical spine (**Fig. 26-6**) and again degenerates or atrophies with increasing age.

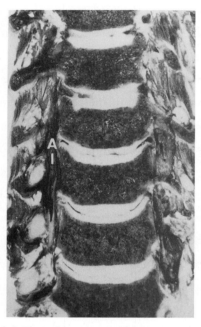

Figure 26-4 Frontal section of the cervical spine of a 33-year-old male. In the three lowest segments, each intervertebral disk shows a complete transverse tear; however, the upper two levels have only lateral tears. *(From Töndury G, Theiler K: Entwicklungsgeschichte und Fehlbildungen der Wirbelsäule, ed 2, Stuttgart, Germany, 1990, Hippokrates-Verlag.)*

Figure 26-3 Frontal section of the cervical spine of a 9-year-old child. Remnants of cartilage are still present. The arrow points to a space in the lateral part of the intervertebral disk at level C3-C4.

A

B

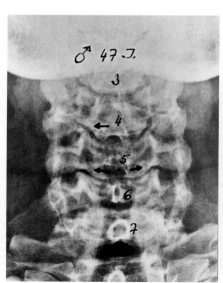
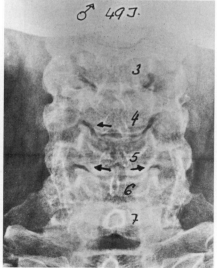

Figure 26-5 Cow horn–like shapes (*arrow*). Changes of the uncovertebral disks at the C4-5 and C5-C6 levels of the same subject at the age of 47 years (**A**) and 49 years (**B**). At the same level on the lateral views, anterior and posterior osteophytes are starting to form (**C** and **D**) and narrow the intervertebral foramen at the C5-C6 level (**E** and **F**).

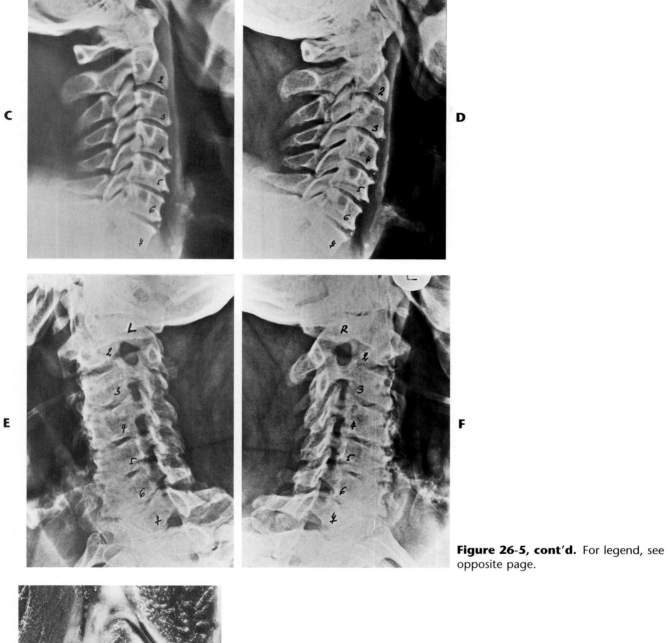

Figure 26-5, cont'd. For legend, see opposite page.

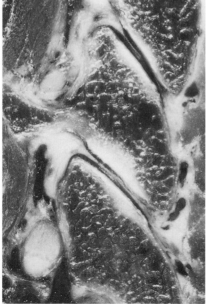

Figure 26-6 Parasagittal section of the intervertebral joints (zygapophyseal joints) at the level of C4 and C6. The articular processes show an inclination of approximately 45 degrees. The arrow points to the synovial folds in between the intervertebral joint surfaces, which have been described by Töndury as meniscoid. *(Courtesy Professor Doctor W. Rauschning, Uppsala, Sweden.)*

UPPER CERVICAL SPINE: OCCIPUT/C2

The upper cervical spine, which consists of the occiput, atlas, and axis, is responsible for most of the axial rotation and some of the flexion-extension and lateral bending of the head. In addition to allowing large rotations, it must be stable enough to support the weight of the head and protect the delicate spinal cord and intervertebral arteries from injury and is therefore quite a complicated structure. Possible motion in the atlantooccipital and atlantoaxial joints is determined by the orientation of the articular processes. The occipital condyles are an oval-shaped, bean-like form with a sagittal orientation of the joint axis of 28 degrees on average (**Fig. 26-7**).[8,10] The frontal orientation of the joint axis (**Fig. 26-8**) averages 124 degrees in males and 127 degrees in females.[9,28]

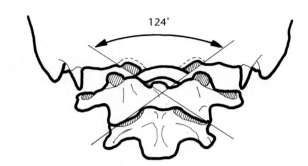

Frontal orientation of joint axis

Figure 26-8 Frontal orientation of the occipital condyles according to Stoff. *From Stoff E: Zur Morphometric des oberen Kopfgelenks,* Verh Anat Gesch Jena *70:575, 1976.*

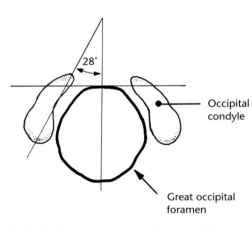

Figure 26-7 Sagittal orientation of the occipital condyles is 28 degrees on average. *(From Ingelmark BE: Acta Anat (Basel) 6:1-48, 1947.)*

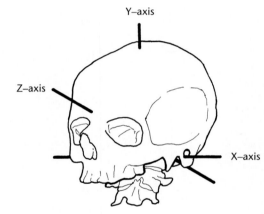

Figure 26-9 Possible joint axis of the upper cervical spine according to Knese. *From Knese KH: Kopfgelenk, Kopfhaltung und Kopfbewegung des menschen,* Z Anat Entwickl *114:67-107, 1949.*

Table 26-1	Possible movements in the atlanto-occipital joint according to different authors.		
Occipto-C1 Joint	**Flexion/Extension (Total)**	**Side Bending (One Side)**	**Axial Rotation (One Side)**
Fick (1904)	50	30-40	0
Poirer and Charpy (1926)	50	14-40	0
Werne (1957)	13	8	0
Penning (1978)	35	10	0
Dvorak et al (1985)	—	—	5.2
Clark et al (1986)	22.7	—	4.8
Dvorak et al (1987)	—	—	4
Penning and Wilmink (1987)	—	—	1
Panjabi et al (1988)	24.5	5.5	7.2

The motion axis of the atlanto-occipital joints has been described by Knese[9] (**Fig. 26-9**). The atlanto-occipital joints are described as a spheroid articulation. They are connected with a tight joint capsule that limits the movements possible. The dominant movement in the atlanto-occipital joint is flexion and extension of approximately 22 to 24 degrees according to the author. Lateral bending, again according to the author, is between 5 and 10 degrees. The idea of axial rotation in this joint has long been rejected; however, newer investigations by Dvorak and Panjabi[7] show axial rotation in both in vitro and in vivo studies. A summary of movements possible in the atlanto-occipital joint is shown in **Table 26-1**.

The atlantoaxial joint consists of four joint spaces: the two atlantoaxial lateral joints, the atlantoaxial median joint (between the anterior arch of the atlas and the dens axis), and a joint between the posterior surface of the dens and the transverse ligament, which is connected to the anterior joint space. From the medial part arises a large synovial fold in the lateral atlantoaxial joint (**Fig. 26-10**).[4] This joint capsule is loose, which allows for a great deal of motion. It is here that most of the axial rotation occurs. The movements possible in the atlantoaxial joints are summarized in **Table 26-2**.

Motion within the upper cervical spine, especially in the atlantoaxial joint, is mainly limited by ligaments that, with exception of the tectorial membrane, consist

Table 26-2	Summary of possible motions at the atlanto-axial joint according to various authors.		
C1-2 Joint	Flexion/Extension (Total)	Side Bending (One Side)	Axial Rotation (One Side)
Fick (1904)	0	0	60
Poirer and Charpy (1926)	11	—	30-80
Werne (1957)	10	0	47
Penning (1978)	30	10	70
Dvorak et al (1985)	—	—	32.2
Clark et al (1986)	10	—	14.5
Dvorak et al (1987)	—	—	43.1
Penning and Wilmink (1987)	—	—	40.5
Panjabi et al (1988)	22.4	6.7	38.9

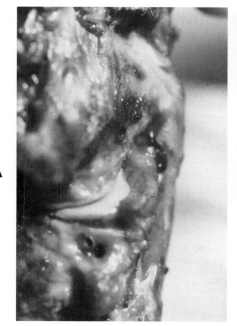
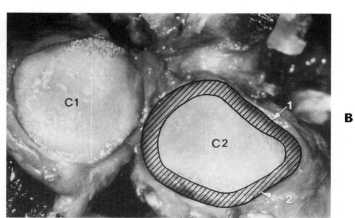

Figure 26-10 Dissection of normal left atlanto-axial meniscoid from a fresh cadaveric specimen (**A**); the surface is covered with meniscoid (**B**).

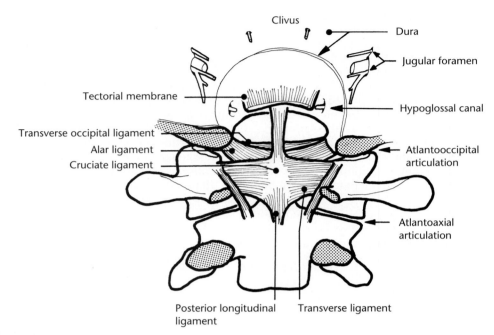

Figure 26-11 Ligaments of the upper cervical spine, posterior view. *(From Lang J:* Klinische Anatomie der Halswirbelsäule, *New York, 1991, Georg Thieme Verlag.)*

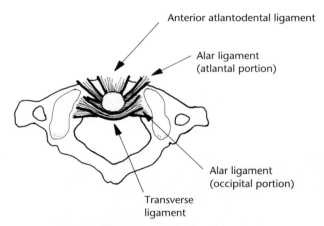

Figure 26-12 Drawing of the ligaments of the upper cervical spine (axial dissection). *(From Dvorak J et al:* Spine *13:748-755, 1988.)*

of non-stretchable collagen fibers.[25,26] The tectorial membrane, which consists of elastic fibers, inserts at the great occipital foramen and distally joins the posterior longitudinal ligament. The biomechanical properties of the tectorial membrane have been studied by Oda et al,[17] who documented their large elasticity.

The cruciate ligament (**Fig. 26-11**) has the important function of restricting potentially dangerous anterior gliding of the atlas during flexion movement of the head while still allowing the atlas to turn freely around the dens during axial rotation. It consists of two main parts: a horizontally oriented transverse ligament and vertically oriented longitudinal fibers. The transverse ligament inserts at the medial portion of the lateral mass of the atlas. The caudal fibers are occasionally fixed at the base of the dens and may additionally stabilize the dens (**Fig. 26-12**). At the level of the dens is a thin layer of cartilage covering the transverse ligament,[5] which allows the ligament to move more freely and protects it from damage caused by friction. The transverse ligament consists exclusively of collagen fibers with an interesting fiber orientation similar to a folding lattice (**Fig. 26-13**). This allows extensive stretching of the ligament during axial rotation without damage to the fibers. In vitro experiments show failure of the transverse ligament to occur between 170 and 700 N.[5]

The main limiting structures for the upper cervical spine are the alar ligaments. Consisting exclusively of nonstretchable collagen fibers, the alar ligaments connect the dens axis with the occipital condyles and the anterior arch of the atlas (**Fig. 26-12**).[1,3,13] Occasionally a loose connection is also found between the basis of the dens axis and the anterior arch of the atlas[3]; this has been described by Von Barrow as the atlantodental anterior ligament. According to Werne,[31] alar ligaments are of great importance in limiting axial rotation (**Fig. 26-14**), a belief that has been confirmed by newer investigations.[5,18] In conjunction with the tectorial membrane, the alar ligaments also limit flexion of the occiput. During lateral bending (**Fig. 26-15**), the alar ligament is responsible for forced rotation of the second vertebra.[5,31] The apical ligament has no functional meaning and is actually a rudiment of the chorda dorsalis.[10]

Clinical analysis of upper cervical spine motion can

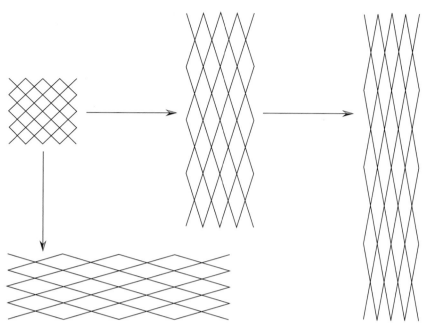

Figure 26-13 The orientation of the collagen fibers of the transverse ligament is similar to a folding lattice and allows extensive stretching of the ligament during flexion and axial rotation without damage to the fibers.

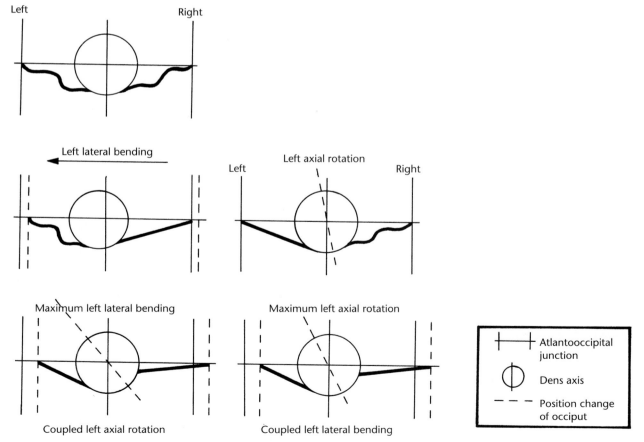

Figure 26-14 Drawing of possible movements in the atlanto-axial joint during axial rotation of the head according to Werne. *From Werne S: Studies in spontaneous atlas dislocation,* Acta Orthop Scand Suppl *23:80, 1957.)*

Left lateral bending   Right lateral bending

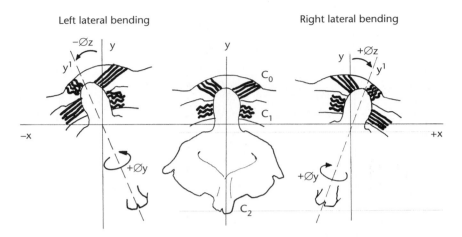

Figure 26-15 Function of the alar ligaments during side bending of the head. *(From Dvorak J et al: Spine 13:748-755, 1988.)*

Left lateral bending   Right lateral bending

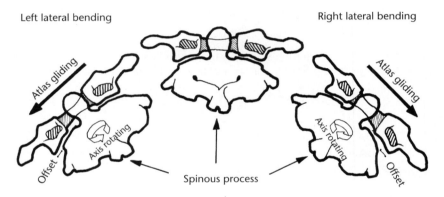

Spinous process

Figure 26-16 Forced rotation of the axis and gliding of the atlas in the direction of bending as seen from functional radiographs in the anteroposterior view. *(From Reich C, Dvorak J: Manual Med 2, 1986.)*

be done through the use of functional radiographs. In the AP view, lateral bending can be assessed.[24] Physiological movements, gliding of the atlas in bending direction, and forced rotation of the axis are presented in **Figure 26-16** as seen on functional radiographs. Axial rotation is currently assessed through measurements of functional computed tomographic (CT) scans and may in the future be tested by functional magnetic resonance imaging (MRI)(**Figs. 26-16** and **26-17**).[2,6]

LOWER CERVICAL SPINE

The anatomic structures of the motion segments of the lower cervical spine are different from those in the upper cervical spine. Their particularities include the uncovertebral joints, which support part of the axial load once the intervertebral disk loses its elasticity due to age-related transformations.[14,29,30] The articular processes of the cervical spine are inclined approximately 45 degrees from the horizontal plane (**Fig. 26-18**), with

steeper inclinations in the lower segments. The transverse processes hide and protect the spinal nerve and vertebral artery.

The motion segments are connected and stabilized by ligaments, anteriorly by the anterior longitudinal ligament (**Fig. 26-19**) and dorsally by the posterior longitudinal ligament. The density of nociceptive and mechanoreceptive innervation of the posterior longitudinal ligament is high in comparison to other cervical spine ligaments and the disk.[16] This results in a very sensitive ligament that indirectly controls the innervation of neck muscles through nociceptive and mechanoreceptive reflexes.[34] The laminae are connected by the strong ligamentum flavum, which consists almost exclusively of elastic fibers and is a major limiting structure in flexion movement.

The dominant motion in the lower cervical spine is flexion-extension. Different parameters can be measured with flexion-extension x-ray views, including segmental rotation, translatory movement, and the location of the center of rotation (**Fig. 26-20**).[7] Because a

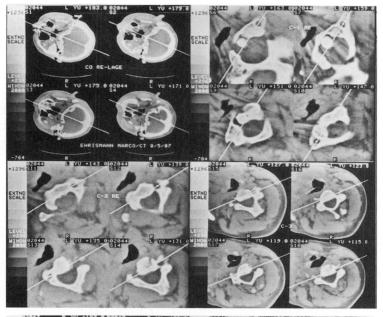

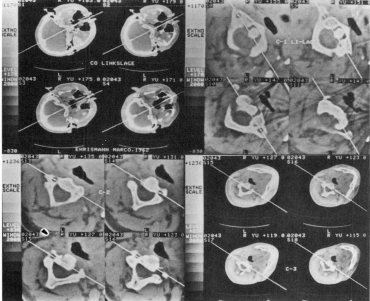

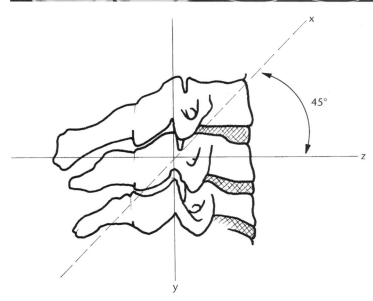

Figure 26-17 Functional computer tomographic scan of the upper cervical spine during axial rotation within the atlantoaxial and atlantooccipital joints.

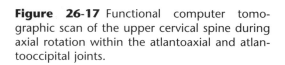

Figure 26-18 Orientation of the articular processes of the lower cervical spine in the frontal plane. *(From White AA, Panjabi MM:* Clinical biomechanics of the spine, *ed 2, Philadelphia, 1990, JB Lippincott.)*

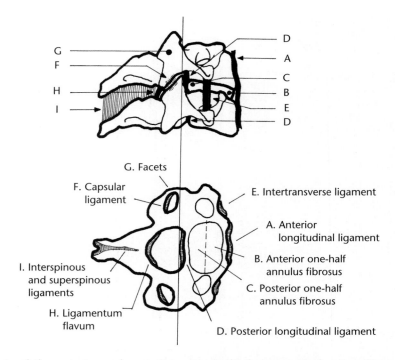

Figure 26-19 Ligaments of the anterior and posterior parts at the lower cervical spine. *(From White AA, Panjabi MM: Clinical biomechanics of the spine, ed 2, Philadelphia, 1990, JB Lippincott.)*

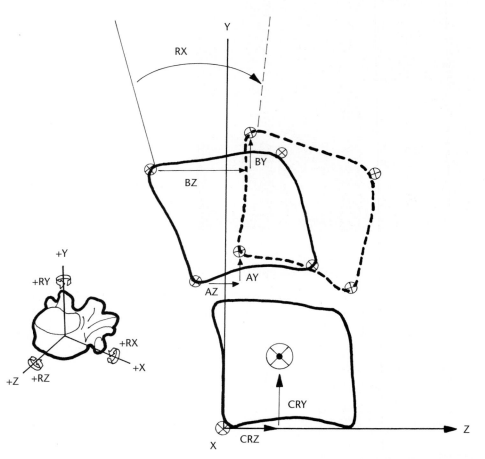

Figure 26-20 Parameters for measurement of segmental motion using computer-assisted methods. RX is the rotation about the x-axis; CRY and CRZ are the centers of rotation of the Y and Z rotations, respectively; AY, AZ, BY, and BZ are the translations of point A in the Y and Z directions and point B in the Y and Z directions, respectively.

significant motion difference exists between actively and passively performed movements, the use of passively performed radiographs has been recommended in diagnosing segmental instability, such as can occur after trauma (**Fig. 26-21**).[6,7] The first description of the center of rotation in healthy adults came from Penning's mea-surements[22] of flexion and extension radiographs. The center of rotation has been determined with computer-assisted methods[7] and has confirmed Penning's findings (**Fig. 26-22**). **Table 26-3** shows the relevant data on flexion-extension movements of healthy adults for in vitro and in vivo examinations. **Table 26-4** presents data

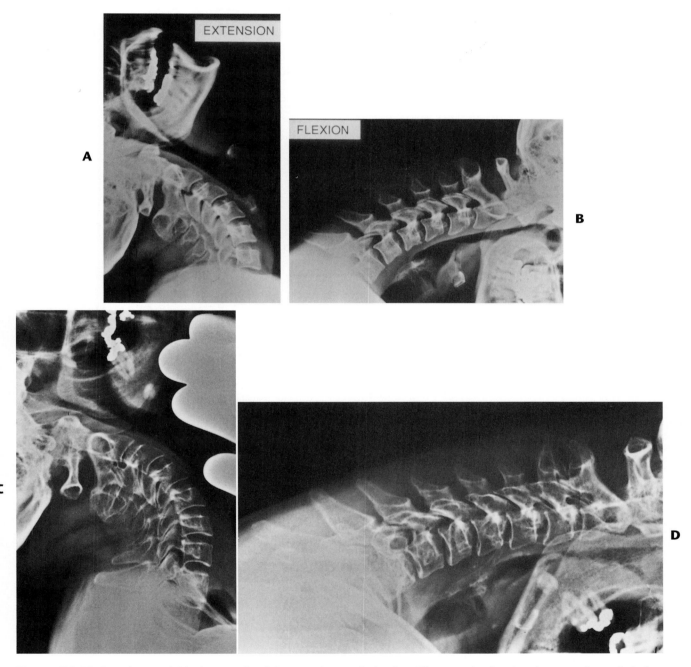

Figure 26-21 Female, aged 51, 1 year after injury to the cervical spine. The examination has been performed during active and passive motion (**A-D**) and measured according to Penning's method (**E** and **F**). According to the functional diagram, there is a significant difference in segmental motion, especially that related to segments C3-C4 and C6-C7. Drawing the vertebral bodies on a transparent paper (**G**) makes the difference obvious. *(From Dvorak J et al: Spine 13:748-755, 1988.)*

Continued.

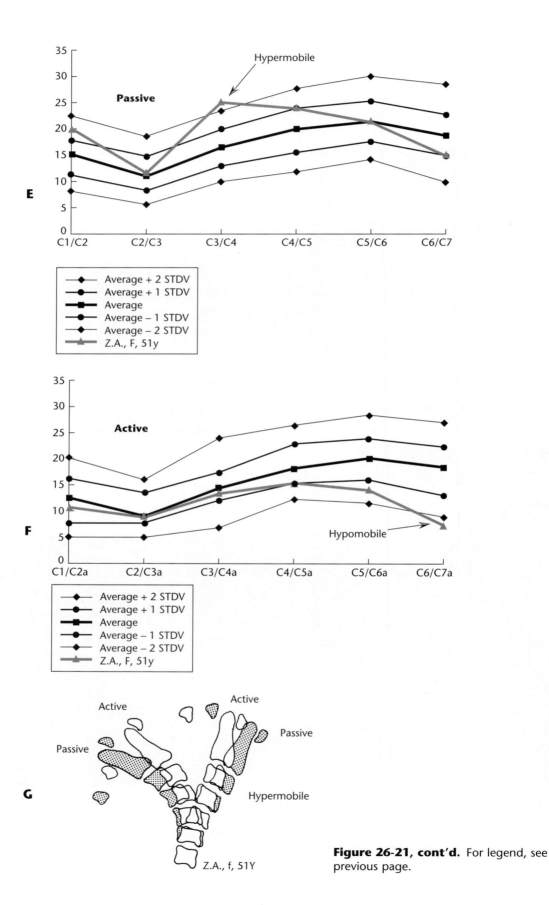

Figure 26-21, cont'd. For legend, see previous page.

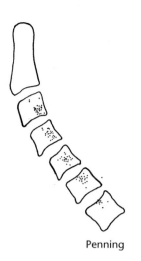
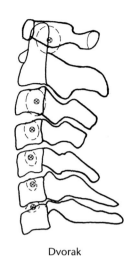

Penning   Dvorak

Figure 26-22 Determination of the center of rotation by graphic method (*Penning, 1960*) and by using computer-assisted methods on a normal population. *(From Dvorak J et al: J Orthop Res 9:828-834, 1991.)*

| Table 26-3 | Summary of flexion-extension movements of healthy adults in vivo and in vitro. |

Flexion/Extension (Total)	Dvorak (1988) (In Vivo/Passive)	Dvorak (1988) (In Vivo/Active)	White and Panjabi (1978)	Penning (1978) (In Vivo/Active)
C2-C3	10.0	12.0	8.0	12.0
C3-C4	15.0	17.0	13.0	18.0
C4-C5	19.0	21.0	12.0	20.0
C5-C6	20.0	23.0	17.0	20.0
C6-C7	19.0	21.0	16.0	15.0

| Table 26-4 | Averages and standard deviations of rotations, translations, and coordinates of center of rotation as measured by computer-assisted methods. |

Parameter*	C1-2	C2-3	C3-4	C4-5	C5-6	C6-7
RX (deg) Male	15.4 6.1	11.7 3.1	16.0 2.5	20.1 2.8	21.5 3.9	21.0 4.0
RX (deg) Female	12.9 3.4	12.3 3.0	18.3 4.7	22.1 3.9	24.1 4.0	21.8 3.5
AZ (mm)	−3.8 1.6	2.4 0.9	3.2 1.0	3.6 1.2	2.9 1.1	2.0 0.9
AY (mm)	6.2 2.3	1.8 0.8	2.3 1.0	2.9 0.7	3.2 0.8	3.1 0.8
BZ (mm)	−1.4 1.4	6.9 1.7	8.5 1.8	10.0 1.9	9.8 1.9	8.4 1.9
BY (mm)	8.1 3.0	3.0 1.3	3.6 1.2	4.2 1.0	4.3 1.0	3.9 0.9
CRZ (mm)	−4.1 4.2	4.0 3.5	4.3 2.7	6.0 2.2	6.4 1.8	6.4 2.5
CRY (mm)	30.0 5.6	9.4 4.8	9.7 3.4	10.4 2.8	12.9 2.5	17.2 2.1

*See Figure 26-20 for definitions.

on rotation, translation, and center of rotation as measured by computer-assisted methods on a healthy population.[7]

Lysell[15] describes the so-called top angle, or segmental arch, as being flat at the level of C2 and steep at the lower cervical spine. Motion of the upper segments during flexion-extension is therefore fairly horizontal, whereas motion of the lower segments is more like that of an arc (**Fig. 26-23**).

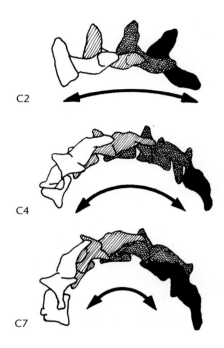

Figure 26-23 Segmental arch of the top angle according to Lysell.[15] The flatter the articular surfaces, the flatter the top angle of the motion segments and vice versa.

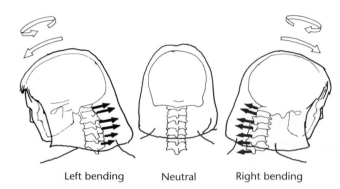

Left bending   Neutral   Right bending

Figure 26-24 Coupled axial rotation during lateral bending of the head. (*From White AA, Panjabi MM: Clinical biomechanics of the spine, ed 2, Philadelphia, 1990, JB Lippincott.*)

Table 26-5a	Values of main lateral bending according to various authors.		
Main Side Bending (One Side)	**Moroney (1988) (In Vitro FSU)**	**Penning (1978) (In Vivo/Active)**	**White and Panjabi (1978)**
C2-C3	4.7	6.0	10.0
C3-C4	4.7	6.0	11.0
C4-C5	4.7	6.0	11.0
C5-C6	4.7	6.0	8.0
C6-C7	4.7	6.0	7.0

Table 26-5b	Values of coupled axial rotation according to various authors.		
Coupled Axial Rotation (One Side)	**Dvorak (1987) (In Vivo/Passive)**	**Penning (1978) (In Vivo/Active)**	**White and Panjabi (1978)**
C2-C3	3.0	3.0	9.0
C3-C4	6.5	6.5	11.0
C4-C5	6.7	6.8	12.0
C5-C6	7.0	6.9	10.0
C6-C7	5.4	5.4	9.0

Lateral bending of the cervical spine is normally coupled with axial rotation to the same side.[15,33] This means that the spinal processes are moving in a direction opposite the motion (**Fig. 26-24**). This coupled motion is of clinical importance because palpation of the spinal processes can serve as an indirect indicator of disturbed function in motion segments. The lateral bending of the cervical spine below the first cervical vertebra has been variously reported by different researchers. According to Penning,[21] the lateral bending is 35 degrees, whereas White and Panjabi[33] report between 4 and 10 degrees per motion segment. Axial rotation, as measured with functional CT scans, is between 3 and 7 degrees[2,23] but an in vitro study[19] had results a little higher, between 8 and 12 degrees. **Table 26-5** summarizes the segmental motions for lateral bending with coupled axial rotation according to the different authors.

References

1. Cave AJE: On the occipito-atlanto-axial articulations, *J Anat (Lond)* 68:416, 1934.

2. Dvorak J, Hayek J, Zehnder R: CT-functional diagnostics of the rotatory instability of upper cervical spine. Part 2: An evaluation on healthy adults and patients with suspected instability, *Spine* 12:726-731, 1987.

3. Dvorak J, Panjabi MM: Functional anatomy of the alar ligaments, *Spine* 12:183-189, 1987.

4. Dvorak J et al: Age and gender-related normal motion of the cervical spine, *Spine* 17(105):5393, 1992.

5. Dvorak J et al: Biomechanics of the craniocervical region: the alar and transverse ligaments, *J Orthop Res* 6:452-461, 1988.

6. Dvorak J et al: Functional radiographic diagnosis of the cervical spine: flexion/extension, *Spine* 13(7):748-755, 1988.

7. Dvorak J et al: In vivo flexion/extension of the normal cervical spine, *J Orthop Res* 9:828-834, 1991.

8. Ingelmark BE: Ueber den cranicervicalen Uebergang beim Menschen, *Acta Anat (Basel)* 6:1-48, 1947.

9. Knese KH: Kopfgelenk, kopfhaltung und kopfbewegung des menschen, *Z Anat Entwickl* 114:67-107, 1949.

10. Lang J: Craniocervical region, osteology and articulations. *Neuroorthopedics* 1:67-92, 1986.

11. Lang J: *Klinische anatomie der halswirbelsäule*, New York, 1991, Georg Thieme Verlag.

12. Lang J, Bartram CT: Ueber die Fila articularia der Radices ventrales et dorsales des menschlichen Rückenmarkes, *Gegenbaurs Morphol* 128:417-462, 1982.

13. Ludwig K: Ueber das Lig. alare dentis, *Z Anat Entwickl Gesch* 116:442, 1952.

14. Luschka H: *Die halbgelenke des menschlichen körpers*, Berlin, 1858, Reimers.

15. Lysell E: Motion in the cervical spine. An experimental study on autopsy specimens, *Acta Orthop Scand Suppl* 123:1-61, 1969.

16. Mendel T, Wink CS, Zimny ML: Neural elements in human cervical intervertebral discs, *Spine* 17(2): 132-135, 1992.

17. Oda T et al: Role of tectorial membrane in the stability of the upper cervical spine, *Clin Biomech* 7(4):201-207, 1992.

18. Panjabi MM et al: Effects of alar ligament transection on upper cervical spine rotation, *J Orthop Res* 9:584-593, 1991.

19. Panjabi MM et al: Three-dimensional movements of the upper cervical spine, *Spine* 13(7):726-730, 1988.

20. Penning L: *Functioneel rontgenonderzoek bij degenerative en traumatische afwijkingen der laag-cervicale bewegingssegmenten*, 1960, University of Groningen, The Netherlands.

21. Penning L: Normal movement of the cervical spine, *AJR Am J Roentgenol* 130:317-326, 1978.

22. Penning L, Töndury G: Entstehung, Bau und Funktion der meniskoiden Strukturen in den Halswirbelgelenken, *Z Orthop* 98:1-14, 1964.

23. Penning L, Wilmink JT: Rotation of the cervical spine: a CT study in normal subjects, *Spine* 12:732-738, 1987.

24. Reich C, Dvorak J: The functional evaluation of craniocervical ligaments in sidebending using x-rays, *Manual Med* 2, 1986.

25. Saldinger PF: *Histologische Untersuchung des kraniozervikalen Bandapparates im Hinblick auf Weichteilverletzungen der Halswirbelsäule*, Diss. med., Bern, 1987 (Leitung J. Dvorak).

26. Saldinger PF et al: Histology of the alar and transverse ligaments, *Spine* 15:257-261, 1990.

27. Simmons E, Marzo J, Kallen F: Intradural connections between adjacent cervical spinal roots, *Spine* 12(10):964-968, 1987.

28. Stoff E: Zur Morphometrie des oberen Kopfgelenks, *Verh Anat Gesch Jena* 70:575, 1976.

29. Töndury G, Theiler K: *Entwicklungsgeschichte und Fehlbildungen der Wirbelsäule*, (ed 1), Stuttgart, Germany, 1958, Hippokrates-Verlag.

30. Töndury G, Theiler K: *Entwicklungsgeschichte und Fehlbildungen der Wirbelsäule*, (ed 2), Stuttgart, Germany, 1990, Hippokrates-Verlag.

31. Werne S: Studies in spontaneous atlas dislocation, *Acta Orthop Scand Suppl* 23:80, 1957.

32. White AA, Panjabi MM: *Clinical biomechanics of the spine*, ed 2, Philadelphia, 1990, JB Lippincott.

33. White AA, Panjabi MM: The basic kinematics of the human spine, *Spine* 3:12-20, 1978.

34. Wyke B: Neurological mechanisms in the experience of pain, *Acupunct Electrother Res* 4:27-35, 1979.

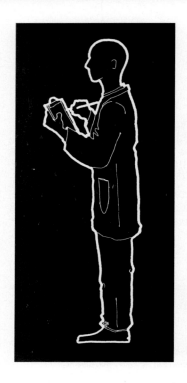

Chapter 27

Biomechanics of the Shoulder

Malcolm H. Pope
David G. Wilder

CONTENTS

The shoulder is the first part of a complex mechanical chain linking the shoulder to the fingers, the main components of which are given in **Table 27-1**. Many occupational tasks require a high level of neuromuscular coordination of these components. Frequently these are complex three-dimensional movements (e.g., kinematics) of the glenohumeral, acromioclavicular, and sternoclavicular joints and the scapulothoracic articulation. Previous investigations of shoulder kinematics, ligamentous function, and muscle function (electromyographic [EMG] analysis) will be reviewed in this chapter.

KINEMATICS OF THE SHOULDER

Kinematics is the study of motion without consideration of the forces producing the motion. The motion is usually expressed in relation to a fixed bony landmark. However, these are difficult to define with precision. The kinematics of the shoulder involves complex interactions of the glenohumeral, acromioclavicular, and sternoclavicular joints and the scapulothoracic articulation.

The eulerian coordinate system and the screw displacement axis system in shoulder kinematics have been reviewed by Morrey and An.[21] The eulerian system has the advantage of presenting joint kinematics in a coordinate system that is aligned with the anatomical planes of motion at the shoulder.

Joint kinematics is described as either two-dimensional (planar) or three-dimensional (spatial) motion (**Fig. 27-1**). In planar motion (three degrees of freedom), kinematics is often described by instantaneous centers of rotation (ICR). Walker[31] used the method of Rouleaux to calculate the ICR for the glenohumeral articulation from plane radiographs. Morrey and An[21] have used the ICR to describe planar glenohumeral motion as sliding, spinning, and rolling (**Fig. 27-1**). Planar motion of the glenohumeral joint can be described by a combination of any of these three different motions. Sliding is pure translation of the humeral head relative to the glenoid. Therefore, the contact point of the humeral head does not change whereas that of the glenoid does. For spinning, isolated rotation of the humeral head occurs without translation. The contact point on the humeral head changes, whereas the ICR on the glenoid remains fixed. During spinning, the ICR of glenohumeral joint rotation is located at the center of curvature of the humeral head. In a rolling motion, the humeral head has contact with the glenoid without spinning or sliding, and the ICR is located at the glenohumeral contact point.

Six degrees of freedom are required to define the spatial position of a joint. Morrey and An[21] have described how, in the glenohumeral joint, the position of the humerus relative to the glenoid is dependent on the order of the three angular rotations about each orthogonal axis, and they have defined a convention for the order of glenohumeral joint rotation. The screw-axis system may be used to describe three-dimensional kinematics if at least three reference points on the rigid body are measured. This technique is not dependent on the reference coordinate system, and data from different sets can be compared. This technique is rarely used, however, because the kinematic descriptors are not related to anatomic reference planes and are difficult for the clinical community to interpret.

Many different experimental measurement techniques have been used to characterize the complex kinematics of the shoulder and constituent joints. These have included protractor-type goniometers, electrogoniometers,[7] accelerometers,[23] photography,[5] ultrasonography,[17] sonic digitization,[6] the 6–degree-of-freedom electromagnetic position sensor,[1,2,8] planar X-ray,[14,16,27] and stereoradiography.[18] Only the x-ray measurements and the 6–degree-of-freedom electromagnetic position sensor have been able to provide accurate evaluations of joint kinematics in vivo. The latter technique has allowed inclusion of the dynamic effects of the shoulder musculature.

The classic work of Inman, Saunders, and Abbott[16] in 1944 employed the direct x-ray measurement technique to study abduction movement of the shoulder. However, many investigators have pointed out the limitations of these techniques: ionizing radiation and limited accuracy. Poppen and Walker[27] used planar radiography to measure humeral head movement on the glenoid fossa during abduction of the arm in the scapular plane. Motion is mostly rotational, but from 0 to 30 degrees and often to 60 degrees of abduction, the humeral head moved from an inferior to a superior position about 3 mm, indicative of some rolling and/or sliding. With additional elevation, the humeral head exhibited almost pure rotation relative to the glenoid, thereby indicating a spinning motion of the humeral head on the glenoid. These kinematic components are observed in the normal shoulder as a result of compression of the humeral head into the glenolabral socket.[27] In some patients with shoulder pathology (rotator cuff tear, instability, degenerative arthritis), an abnormal gliding motion of the humeral ball occurred with abduction. For subjects with normal shoulder joints, the scapula rotated externally with abduction. From 0 to 30 degrees, most of the abduction was due to glenohumeral rotation. After 30 degrees, abduction of the humerus on the glenoid and scapula rotation on the thorax were equally involved in humeral head movement.

Table 27-1	Main components of the shoulder.		
Bones	**Joints**	**Ligaments**	**Muscles of Pectoral Girdle**
Scapula	*Synovial*	Glenohumeral (capsular)	*Scapulohumeral and claviculohumeral*
	Glenohumeral	Superior	Superficial group
Clavicle	Acromioclavicular	Medial	Deltoid (anterior middle, posterior)
	Sternoclavicular	Inferior	Pectoralis major (clavicular head)
Humerus			Deep group
	Bone-muscle articulation	Coracohumeral	Rotator cuff muscles
Sternum	Scapulothoracic		Subscapularis
		Coracoacromial	Supraspinatus
			Infraspinatus
		Acromioclavicular (capsular)	Teres minor
			Other
		Coracoclavicular	Teres major
		Conoid	
		Trapezoid	*Scapuloradial*
			Biceps (long and short heads)
		Costoclavicular	
			Scapuloulnar
		Sternoclavicular (capsular)	Triceps (long head)
		Interclavicular	*Thoracohumeral*
			Latissimus dorsi
			Pectoralis major (sternocostal head)
			Thoracoscapular
			Serratus anterior
			Pectoralis minor
			Trapezius (upper, middle, lower)
			Levator scapulae
			Rhomboid group
			Thoracoclavicular
			Subclavius

From Zuckerman JD, Matsen FA: Biomechanics of the shoulder. In Nordin M, Frankel VH, editors: Biomechanics of the musculoskeletal system, *Philadelphia, 1989, Lea & Febiger.*

Howell et al[14] used planar radiographs to measure the position of the humeral head relative to the glenoid in the horizontal plane. In the horizontal plane there was almost pure rotation of the humeral ball relative to the glenoid. Howell and Kraft[13] used similar horizontal-plane radiographs to study subjects with labrum defects. They found that the rotational glenohumeral articulation was maintained by the mechanical restraint formed by the articular surface of the glenoid, labrum, and glenohumeral capsule-ligament. It was suggested that the rotator cuff was not required for normal glenohumeral kinematics.

The acromioclavicular joint, a small synovial articulation between the distal end of the clavicle and the proximal aspect of the acromion of the scapula, permits scapular motion. Inman, Saunders, and Abbott[16] found that the scapula rotates posteriorly relative to the clavicle about a transverse axis that passes through the joint. They also found that during shoulder abduction and forward flexion, the total clavicular elevation at the joint is 20 degrees and that this occurs in the first 30 degrees and the last 45 degrees of arm elevation.

The range of sternoclavicular joint motion was found by Inman, Saunders, and Abbott[16] to be about 40 degrees of arm elevation in both the frontal and sagittal planes; 36 degrees of clavicular evaluation occurred through the first 90 degrees, and beyond 90 degrees, clavicular motion was negligible. Rotation about the long axis of the clavicle was approximately 40 degrees.

Except for its attachment through the acromioclavicular and sternoclavicular joints, the scapula is without connection to the thorax. This allows for a wide range

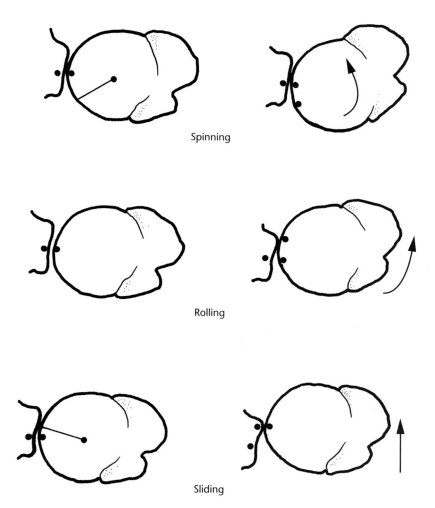

Spinning

Rolling

Sliding

Figure 27-1 Planar glenohumeral articulation. Included are spinning, rolling, and sliding motions. These motions may occur either in isolation or in combination. *(Used with permission from Zuckerman JD, Matsen FA: Biomechanics of the shoulder. In Nordin M, Frankel VH, editors: Biomechanics of the musculoskeletal system, Philadelphia, 1989, Lea & Febiger.)*

of scapular motion. Inman, Saunders, and Abbott[16] examined arm elevation in the frontal and sagittal planes and found that about two thirds of the motion (120 degrees) took place at the glenohumeral joint and one third (60 degrees) at the scapulothoracic articulation. The 2:1 ratio of glenohumeral-to-scapulothoracic motion remained quite constant between subjects.

The planar radiographic measurement technique is obviously useful for evaluating glenohumeral and scapulothoracic kinematics in vivo. However, this technique has limited accuracy. The reported accuracy of planar measurements range between 1 and 5 mm,[18] depending on the technique used. In addition, the technique is not accurate if a significant amount of motion occurs out of the plane of the film. Terry et al[29] have demonstrated that any attempt at simple planar motion of the glenohumeral joint results in coupled or out-of-plane motion.

To overcome the problems associated with the planar technique, Kärrholm[18] has used the stereoradiographic technique in vivo. Tantalum markers were implanted and used as digitization landmarks to facilitate a high degree of resolution for a complete 6–degree-of-freedom evaluation of shoulder kinematics. Högfors et al[12] were able to demonstrate that the relative displacement between the humerus, scapula, and clavicle exhibits similarities between individuals and was insensitive to small hand loads. The shoulder rhythms for arm elevation in the scapular plane were observed to be similar to those previously described with the planar technique.

Harryman et al.[8] have performed an in vitro investigation of the glenohumeral joint by using a 6–degree-of-freedom position and force sensors. They used bone pins to rigidly attach an electromagnetic position sensor to the humerus and scapula of subjects with normal shoulder joints.[24] The humeral head translated anteriorly with passive glenohumeral flexion, and posterior translation occurred with glenohumeral extension. External rotation produced posterior translation of the humeral ball relative to the glenoid.

Substantial translation of the humeral head relative to the glenoid has resulted from standard clinical examination of glenohumeral laxity, which suggests that isolated glenohumeral laxity may not be an indication for surgical intervention. Laxity is synonymous with clinical instability, which represents an abnormal range of motion caused by a stretched ligament. The humeral head translates similarly with anteriorly, posteriorly, and inferiorly directed loading.

THE SHOULDER MUSCULATURE

The human shoulder joint is composed of 17 muscle units that control the composite thoracoscapulohumeral articulation.[33] This includes the anterior, middle, and posterior deltoid as well as the upper, middle, and lower trapezius (**Table 27-1**). The deltoid is a very large muscle with a large lever arm and therefore great ability to produce torque in the shoulder joint. The rotator cuff muscles attach very close to the axis of rotation and provide joint compression. A minimum of two opposing muscles is required to control even the simplest functional movement. The agonist muscle, the prime mover, initiates the desired contraction. The antagonist muscle either decelerates joint motion caused by the agonist or acts as the prime mover in the opposite direction. A synergist muscle provides an additive contribution.

Dynamic EMG studies of the deltoid and the four rotator cuff muscles (infraspinatus, teres minor, subscapularis, and supraspinatus) during forward elevation, flexion, and abduction have shown that they are all active throughout the full range of motion (**Fig. 27-2**).[3,15,16,24,26] At the initiation of abduction, the dominant direction of the deltoids' pull is vertical, and large vertical shear forces are created. Because the supraspinatus muscle is horizontally oriented at 70 degrees to the glenoid fossa, compression is the dominant force generated. Sigholm et al[28] used EMG techniques to determine muscle load in three parts of the deltoid: the infraspinatus, the supraspinatus, and the upper trapezius. Muscle force was heavily dependent on arm elevation and hand load. Humeral rotation and elbow flexion had little effect. Herberts et al[11] report that rotator cuff tendinitis is present in over 16% of workers doing tasks that require high loads with arm elevation (e.g., shipyard workers). Supraspinatus tendinitis, as well as neck pain in the vicinity of the upper trapezius, is common in many industries.[4,9] In most subjects, fatigue was quickly evident in the upper trapezius and supraspinatus in 90 degrees of abduction.

Herberts, Kadefors, and Broman[10] analyzed the effect of shoulder and elbow position on muscle fatigue

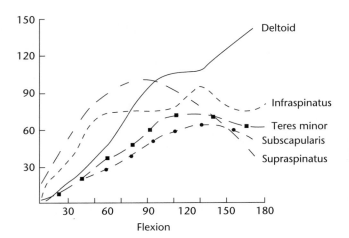

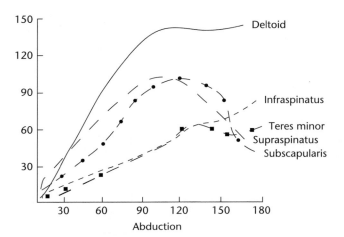

Figure 27-2 Relative electrical activity of the deltoid and rotator cuff during flexion (*top*) and abduction (*bottom*). The vertical scale is in microvolts. (*Reproduced with permission from Perry J: Muscle control of the shoulder. In Rower C, editor: The shoulder, New York, 1988, Churchill Livingstone Internationl; pp 17-34.*)

and found that muscle fatigue was present in the anterior and middle deltoid, supraspinatus, infraspinatus, and upper trapezius for overhead and shoulder-level work. They also found that the infraspinatus had the highest localized fatigue levels of all muscles tested.

The combined effect of rotator cuff synergistic action is to create a net compressive force. The compressive force is the major contributor to shoulder joint stability in the midrange of motion.[30] The ligaments and other static restraints come into play only at the extremes of motion.[19] Inman et al[16] calculated that the maximum compressive force occurs at 90 degrees of elevation. Poppen and Walker[27] found that the resulting compressive force increased linearly with abduction to reach a maximum of 0.89 times body weight at 90 degrees abduction. Beyond this, the resultant force decreases to 0.4 times body weight at 150 degrees abduction.

Although EMG analysis offers the apparent advantage of measuring the contribution of each muscle to joint behavior, this technique has limitations in estimating muscle force output. The relationship between muscle force and the EMG signal changes in a nonlinear relation with the contraction level, the length of the muscle, and the contraction velocity.[25] Surface electrodes have been used in most studies but have problems with signal cross talk from surrounding muscle groups. The effect of a muscle on a joint force can only be computed if the distance of the muscle from the instantaneous center is known. This is difficult in the shoulder because the distance of each muscle from the ICR changes as a function of shoulder position.

An approach that has been advocated to prevent shoulder injuries is to match worker strength with the work demands. Walmsley and Szybbo[32] investigated the concentric isokinetic torque of the shoulder internal and external rotator muscles. The greatest torque for the external rotator muscles was found at 90 degrees of shoulder flexion, whereas for the internal rotator muscles the greatest torque was at the neutral position. Kuhlman et al[20] found the isokinetic and isometric peak torques to be similar. Strength decreased with increasing age and was less in women. These factors should be considered in prevention.

CAPSULAR AND LIGAMENT FUNCTION

O'Connell et al[22] measured strain by using Hall effect transducers on the three glenohumeral ligaments during external rotation torques at 0, 45, and 90 degrees of abduction. The superior and middle glenohumeral ligaments were highly strained in the lower range of abduction, whereas the inferior glenohumeral ligaments carried the most strain in the last half of abduction. Terry et al[29] measured in vitro forces by mounting liquid mercury strain gauges on the three glenohumeral ligaments and the capsule. The glenohumeral ligaments carried force in abduction, extension, and external rotation or any combination of these. The posterior capsule was loaded in abduction, flexion, and internal rotation. The coracohumeral ligament was taut in flexion and extension.

SUMMARY

The shoulder joint is really four distinct articulations, and motion of the joint requires coordination between the articulations. The most important articulation is the glenohumeral joint, which is largely a ball-and-socket joint, but it does exhibit some gliding. Electromyographic studies have demonstrated high muscle forces with arm elevation and holding loads in the hands. This fits well with observations of epidemiologic studies, in which elevated arms are associated with a variety of shoulder problems. Fatigue data show great promise in defining postures and load limits for workers.

References

1. An KN et al: Application of a magnetic tracking device to kinesiological studies, *J Biomech* 21:613-620, 1988.

2. An KN et al: Three-dimensional kinematics of glenohumeral elevation, *J Orthop Res* 9:143-149, 1991.

3. Basmajian JV, DeLuca CJ: *Muscles alive: their functions revealed by electromyography,* Baltimore, 1985, Williams & Wilkins; pp 223-289.

4. Bjelle A, Hagberg M, Michaelsson G: Clinical and economic factors in prolonged shoulder pain among industrial workers, *Scand J Work Environ Health* 5:205-210, 1979.

5. Engen JJ, Spencer WA: Method of kinematic study of normal upper extremity movements, *Arch Phys Med Rehabil* 49:9-12, 1968.

6. Engin AE: Kinematics of human shoulder motion. In Mow VC, Ratcliffe A, Woo SL-Y, editors: *Biomechanics of diarthroidal joints,* vol 2, New York, 1990, Springer-Verlag, New York; p 405.

7. Engin AE: On the biomechanics of the shoulder complex, *J Biomech* 13(7):575-590, 1980.

8. Harryman DT et al: Translation of the humeral head on the glenoid with passive glenohumeral motion, *J Bone Joint Surg* 72A:1334-1343, 1990.

9. Herberts P, Kadefors R: A study of painful shoulder in welders, *Acta Orthop Scand* 47:381-387, 1976.

10. Herberts P, Kadefors R, Broman H: Arm positioning in manual tasks. An electromyographic study of localized muscle fatigue, *Ergonomics* 23:655-665, 1980.

11. Herberts P et al: Shoulder pain and heavy manual labor, *Clin Orthop* 191:166-178, 1984.

12. Högfors C et al: Biomechanical model of the human shoulder joint—II. The shoulder rhythm, *J Biomech* 24:699-709, 1991.

13. Howell SM, Kraft TA: The role of the supraspinatus and infraspinatus muscles in glenohumeral kinematics of anterior shoulder instability, *Clin Orthop* 263:128-134, 1991.

14. Howell et al: Normal and abnormal mechanics of the glenohumeral joint in the horizontal plane, *J Bone Joint Surg AM* 70A:227-232, 1988.

15. Howell SM et al: Clarification of the role of supraspinatus muscle in shoulder function, *J Bone Joint Surg* 68A:195-201, 1986.

16. Inman VT, Saunders M, Abbott LC: Observations on the function of the shoulder joint, *J Bone Joint Surg* 26A:1-30, 1944.

17. Jerosch J, Marquardt M, Winkelman W: Der Stellenwert der Sonographie in der Beurteilung von Instabilitaten des glenohumeralen Gelenkes, *Z Orthop* 128:41-45, 1990.

18. Kärrholm J: Roentgen stereophotogrammetry, review of orthopaedic applications, *Acta Orthop Scand* 60(4):491-503, 1989.

19. Kronberg M, Nemeth G, Broström LA: Muscle activity and coordination in the normal shoulder. An electromyographic study, *Clin Orthop* 257:76-85, 1990.

20. Kuhlman JR et al: Isokinetic and isometric measurement of strength of external rotation and abduction of the shoulder, *J Bone Joint Surg* 74A(9):1320-1333, 1992.

21. Morrey BF, An KN: Biomechanics of the shoulder. In Rockwood CA, Matson FA, editors: *The shoulder*, Philadelphia, 1989, WB Saunders; pp 208-245.

22. O'Connell PW et al: The contribution of the glenohumeral ligaments to anterior stability of the shoulder joint, *Am J Sports Med* 18:579-584, 1990.

23. Padgaonkar AJ, Kreiger KW, King AI: Measurement of angular acceleration of a rigid body using linear accelerometers, *J Appl Mech* 42(3):552-556, 1975.

24. Perry J: Muscle control of the shoulder. In Rower C, editor: *The shoulder*, New York, 1988, Churchill Livingstone International; pp 17-34.

25. Perry J, Bekey GA: EMG-force relationships in skeletal muscle, *CRC Crit Rev Biomed Eng* 7:1-22, 1981.

26. Perry J, Glousman R: Biomechanics of throwing. In Nicholas JA, Hershman EB, editors: *The upper extremity in sports medicine*, St Louis, 1990, Mosby–Year Book.

27. Poppen NK, Walker PS: Normal and abnormal motion of the shoulder, *J Bone Joint Surg* 58A:195-201, 1976.

28. Sigholm G et al: Electromyographic analysis of shoulder muscle load, *J Orthop Res* 1:379-389, 1984.

29. Terry GC et al: The stabilizing function of passive shoulder restraints, *Am J Sports Med* 19:26-34, 1991.

30. Vanderhooft E et al: Glenohumeral stability from concavity-compression: a quantitative analysis, *Orthop Trans* 16:774, 1992.

31. Walker PS: *Human joints and their artificial replacements*, Springfield, Ill., 1977, Charles C Thomas.

32. Walmsley RP, Szybbo C: A comparative study of torque generated by shoulder internal and external rotator muscles in different positions and at varying speeds, *J Orthop Sports Phys Ther* 6:217-222, 1987.

33. Zuckerman JD, Matsen FA: Biomechanics of the shoulder. In Nordin M, Frankel VH, editors: *Biomechanics of the musculoskeletal system*, ed 2, Philadelphia, 1989, Lea & Febiger.

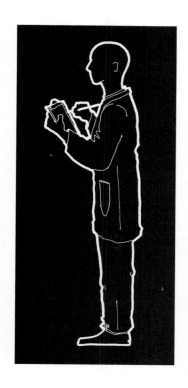

Chapter 28

Clinical Evaluation of the Neck and Shoulder

Frances Cuomo
Jess H. Lonner
Jeffrey M. Spivak
Joseph D. Zuckerman

CONTENTS

Coordinated movement of the neck, shoulder, and elbow is essential to integrated function of the entire upper extremity, including the hand. Symptoms related to these specific areas are often vague and clinically difficult to diagnose. Numerous associated musculoskeletal disorders have been identified, such as tendinitis and nerve entrapment syndromes, and have been found to be related to repetitive and forceful use of the upper extremity in a wide variety of occupations.[2,29] The pathology may easily become chronic when prompt diagnosis is eluded and treatment delayed. Because symptoms may overlap, it is important to discern between referred pain and that arising locally. Sound knowledge of local anatomy and appreciation of the salient features of the history and physical examination are crucial to the formulation of an accurate diagnosis, treatment regimen, and plan for prevention, especially with regard to work-related injuries and cumulative trauma disorders.

CLINICAL EVALUATION OF THE NECK

History

In questioning a patient with regard to neck and/or radiating arm pain, specific details concerning the occupation, the injury, the pain itself, and associated symptoms all play an integral role in the initial assessment.

Specific occupations are considered high risk for neck pain, such as typists and data processors, who are forced to maintain certain neck positions and body postures for prolonged periods of time. Work associated with prolonged vibration exposure, frequent lifting, and long periods of driving predisposes to lumbar disorders and may also be associated with cervical disk disease.[19,23] Psychological factors such as worker satisfaction with the job and feelings about the supervisor can be important inasmuch as job dissatisfaction has been shown to be associated with poor outcomes from work-related injuries.[8,11,12] Patients should always be questioned about any past history of neck pain or injury that may have predisposed them to further pain with only minimal provocation. Also important is any history of past compensation claims with or without associated time off work.

The exact circumstances of any injury should be fully elucidated. Direct trauma must be distinguished from indirect injury caused by twisting, rapid flexion/extension, or isometric strain. Associated injuries must all be documented, including head trauma, loss of consciousness, upper extremity injury, and additional lowback or midback pain.

The main pain complaints must be fully characterized at the initial evaluation. The onset of pain may have immediately followed the injury, or it may have been delayed, with the patient returning to work for some time before the onset of symptoms. Maximal pain may have come on suddenly, or it may have evolved progressively over time. The location of the pain and any radiation must be documented. Is it constant or intermittent? The intensity of the pain and whether it varies over time should be explored. Radiating radicular pain from neural compression, such as that due to a herniated cervical disk, is often worse with maneuvers such as coughing, sneezing, or bearing down for a bowel movement, all of which increase intracranial pressure. Patients with this type of pain often report the pain decreased with abduction of the arm, which relaxes the brachial plexus and nerve roots, and such patients occasionally maintain the arm in abduction.

Neck pain caused by muscular spasm and soft tissue injury (cervical strain) is often accompanied by occipital headaches and radiation of pain laterally to the trapezius and caudally to the thoracic paraspinal musculature. Associated symptoms of radicular pain from nerve root compression include numbness, paresthesias (tingling or "pins and needles"), and weakness in the involved upper extremity. Symptoms of cervical spinal cord compression include loss of upper extremity and hand coordination, changes in balance and gait pattern, and diffuse weakness (cervical myelopathy). Loss of bladder and bowel control is a late finding in spinal cord compression, but it should be ruled out in any patient complaining of traumatic neck or radiating arm pain.

With all this information, a sense of the injury is often ascertained only after the initial interview. Posterior neck pain, with or without headaches and without radiation or symptoms in the extremities, is unlikely to represent an acute disk herniation; rather, it is more likely to be caused by an underlying cervical strain or soft tissue injury or even a fracture. On the other hand, unilateral neck pain with radiation along the arm and forearm to the middle finger that worsens with coughing and sneezing and is relieved by arm abduction more likely than not is due to an acute posterolateral cervical disk herniation. Neck pain accompanied by progressive upper and lower extremity weakness and difficulty walking may represent an underlying instability, cervical spondylosis with stenosis, or a large central disk herniation, all of which can cause spinal cord compression and produce symptoms of cervical myelopathy.

Physical Examination

Physical examination of a worker with a potential neck injury or disorder involves testing all four extremities as well as the neck, and it is recommended that the patient be undressed except for undergarments and an examination gown. Simple anterior inspection may reveal head rotation and facial asymmetry caused by long-standing torticollis. New-onset neck stiffness with fixed rotation or a lateral bend may represent underlying rotatory subluxation of the atlantoaxial joint or an involuntary attempt to enlarge the posterior neural foramen of a nerve root compressed by an acute disk herniation. A short neck with a low hairline may be a sign of Klippel-Feil syndrome (congenital fusion of one or more cervical vertebrae); limited neck motion is the third part of the classic clinical triad seen with this syndrome.

Palpation of the posterior of the neck may reveal midline tenderness, more indicative of possible bony, ligamentous, or disk pathology. Paraspinal tenderness is commonly due to spasm, which may or may not have an underlying structural lesion. Trapezial and periscapular tenderness is often a product of muscle spasm as well. Palpation of the anterior muscular and glandular soft tissues of the neck should also be included, especially for complaints of anterior neck pain, which is uncommon in cervical spine pathology.

Range of motion of the neck, including flexion/extension, rotation, and lateral bending, should be carefully assessed. Both active and passive ranges should be recorded, as well as particularly painful motions that may or may not cause a guarding response. The normal range of the flexion/extension arc is 80 to 90 degrees and can be measured as deviation from neutral (facing straight ahead) when viewed laterally. Also, many examiners will record the minimal distance from chin to chest with flexion and the mouth closed. Lateral rotation of the cervical spine is tested by having the patient bring the chin as far around as possible in an attempt to touch the shoulder. Normal lateral rotation is about 75 degrees to each side and should be symmetric. Lateral bending is tested by asking the patient to bring the ear down to the shoulder. Average lateral bending is 60 to 70 degrees and should also be symmetric.

A detailed neurological examination is done to assess for specific deficits and signs of myelopathy caused by spinal cord compression. An examination of the cranial nerves (II to XII) is done to rule out intracranial pathology. Extraocular movements are tested to assess oculomotor (III), trochlear (IV), and abducens (VI) nerve function. Masseter muscle testing examines the trigeminal nerve (V). The facial nerve (VII) is tested by examining grimace or the ability to maintain the mouth closed while puffing the cheeks with air. Gross hearing assessment is done to check acoustic nerve (VIII) function. Uvular symmetry and gag reflex testing assess the glossopharyngeal (IX) and vagus (X) nerves. The accessory nerve (XI) supplies the sternocleidomastoid and trapezius muscles, and their functions (contralateral neck rotation and ipsilateral shoulder elevation, respectively) are assessed by resistive muscle testing. Finally, normal and symmetric tongue movements confirm the function of the hypoglossal (XII) nerve.

Evaluation of upper extremity sensation, motor strength, and reflexes should be done in a systematic way to localize findings to specific root levels (**Fig. 28-1**). Sensation to light touch is assessed on the lateral aspect of the arm (C5), the lateral (radial) aspect of the forearm and thumb (C6), the middle finger (C7), the little finger and medial (ulnar) aspect of the forearm (C8), and the medial aspect of the arm (T1). Key motor units tested for root level include the deltoid and biceps (C5); wrist extensors (C6); triceps, wrist flexors, and finger extensors (C7); finger flexors (C8); and intrinsics (C8 and T1). Normal reflexes commonly elicited include the biceps (C5, partial C6), brachioradialis (C6), and triceps (C7).

Lower extremity strength and sensation should also be examined to rule out the weakness and sensory changes commonly seen with spinal cord compression. Hyperreflexia of the knee and ankle jerks, clonus, and an extensor plantar response (positive Babinski sign) all point to upper motor neuron involvement and myelopathy common with significant spinal cord compression. In the upper extremities, a pectoralis reflex and a positive Hoffmann sign can often be elicited in cases of significant cervical spinal cord compression. A Hoffmann sign is considered positive if rapid extension of the middle finger (using a flicking motion) in a relaxed hand causes a reflex flexion response of the index finger and thumb (**Fig. 28-2**). The Hoffmann sign may be normal in a small percentage of people, but it is usually bilateral when normally present.

Specific signs and provocative tests indicative of certain cervical pathologies have been described. Lhermitte's sign is described as electric shock–like pain radiating from the posterolateral region of the neck down the back and extremities with extremes of neck flexion and/or extension (**Fig. 28-3**). It is found in 25% of patients with myelopathy due to cervical spondylosis and can also be present in patients with central disk herniations. Spurling's sign is radicular pain elicited by neck extension and ipsilateral rotation with applied axial compression of the head and neck (**Fig. 28-4**). If positive, it implies cervical root compression at the intervertebral foramen, either by degenerative changes or by an acute posterolateral disk herniation. In the shoulder abduction sign, the patient has the affected arm abducted at the shoulder, often with the elbow flexed and the hand holding the head (**Fig. 28-5**). The patient reports this as the position of most pain relief, with increased pain on attempted return of the arm to the side. Abduction is believed to relax the roots contributing to the brachial plexus, thus alleviating the pain. The converse, or radiating arm pain relieved by shoulder abduction, is also a positive shoulder abduction sign and is indicative of cervical root compression.

Diagnostic Testing

The main use of diagnostic testing is to confirm the clinical impression based on the history and physical examination. The specific anatomic level(s) and type of pathology can be visualized as well.

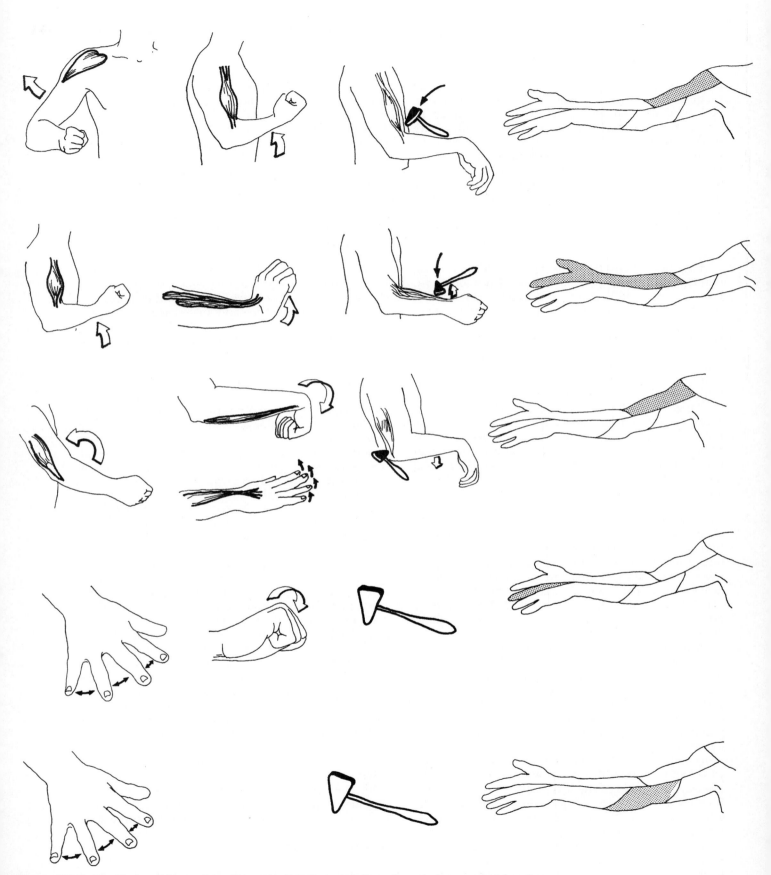

Figure 28-1 Specific localizing points of examination for evaluation of cervical nerve root function.

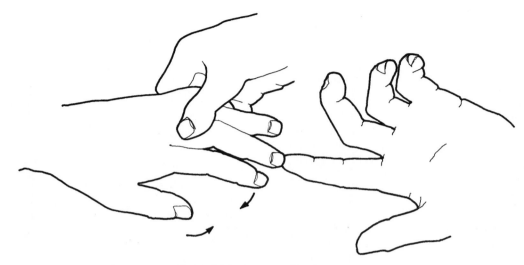

Figure 28-2 The Hoffmann sign.

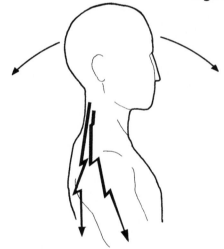

Figure 28-3 Lhermitte sign.

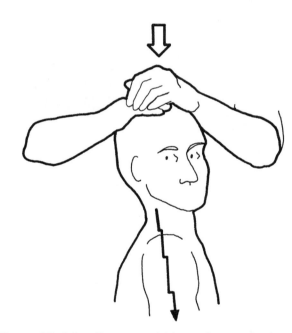

Figure 28-4 Spurling test, which produces radicular arm pain with neck extension, ipsilateral rotation, and manual compression.

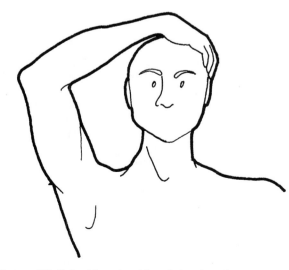

Figure 28-5 Positive shoulder abduction sign.

For neck pain alone, plain radiographs are indicated whenever a history of trauma has been elicited and the pain has been persistent for 4 to 6 weeks despite symptomatic treatment. Plain films are also indicated for neck pain associated with fevers or chills or accompanied by unexplained weight loss, in patients aged 60 and over, and in patients with any history of tumors. Lateral radiographs are the most useful projection for

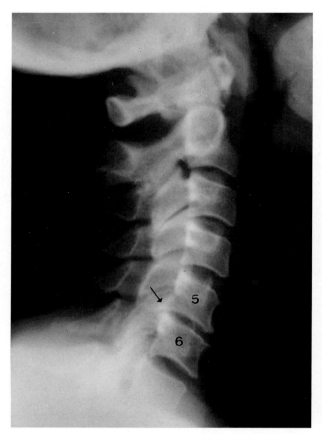

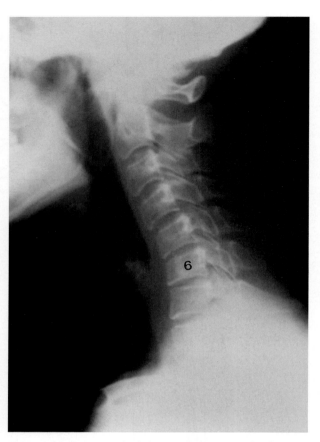

Figure 28-6 Lateral cervical radiograph. The overall alignment and lordotic curve are normal. The arrow shows moderate cervical spondylosis, specifically posterolateral osteophytes, at the C5-C6 level.

Figure 28-7 Reversal of the normal cervical lordosis with actual kyphosis from C5 to C7 in a 39-year-old worker with acute neck and arm pain following an overhead lifting injury.

evaluating anatomy and alignment (**Fig. 28-6**). All seven cervical vertebrae must be visualized on the lateral radiograph. Degenerative changes are common on plain radiographs and do not necessarily identify the source of the patient's pain.[22] A loss of the normal cervical lordosis seen on the lateral radiograph is common in acute disk herniations because the involuntary flexion helps to open the posterior neural foramina (**Fig. 28-7**). In older patients, odontoid fractures may be sustained even after relatively minor trauma. Full visualization of this region includes an open-mouth anteroposterior (AP) film, and tomograms may be necessary to fully rule out this injury.

Voluntary flexion and extension lateral radiographs are indicated in cases of significant neck injury with pain and normal x-ray findings to rule out instability due to traumatic ligamentous disruption. They are also used to rule out instability in cases of atlantoaxial subluxation of greater than 3 mm (anterior atlantodens interval as seen on the lateral radiograph) and in patients in whom subaxial subluxations are noted. Anteroposterior oblique radiographs are useful to assess the neural foramina, which may be narrowed because of degenerative disease of the uncovertebral joints at the

posterolateral disk margin or the facet joints along the posterior border of the neural foramen (**Fig. 28-8**).

Magnetic resonance imaging (MRI) of the cervical spine is indicated to assess the neural elements in all cases of myelopathy and cases of persistent radiculopathy despite an initial course of nonoperative treatment. Disk herniations can easily be seen, as well as spinal canal stenosis and compression of the spinal cord (**Fig. 28-9**, A and B).[17] Magnetic resonance imaging can also be useful for examination of the vertebrae and to rule out tumor or infection when plain radiographs are suggestive of vertebral pathology (**Fig. 28-10**). Regardless of the indication, it must be remembered that radiographic abnormalities must correlate with the clinical findings and history if they are to be considered significant. In asymptomatic volunteers, MRI examination revealed cervical disk herniations, bulges, or foraminal stenosis in 19% of subjects; cervical disk degeneration was noted in 25% of subjects under 40 years of age and in 56% of those over the age of 40.[3]

Technetium-99 bone scanning is indicated in patients who primarily have neck pain that is persistent despite at least 6 weeks of appropriate nonoperative treatment and have normal plain radiographs. In this

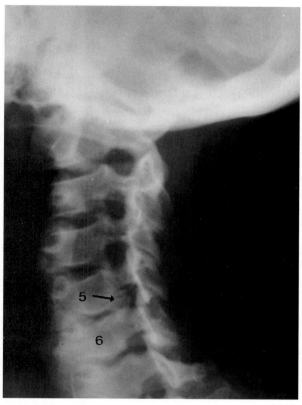

Figure 28-8 Oblique radiograph of the same patient as in Figure 28-6 showing significant narrowing of the C5-C6 foramen from degenerative uncovertebral spurs (*arrow*).

setting, a bone scan may be indicated to rule out a stress fracture, tumor, or infection as causes of the neck pain. In addition, gallium-67 citrate or indium-labeled white blood cells can be used to increase the specificity of bone scanning for infection.

Diskography involves the injection of sterile fluid (usually with contrast material) into the nuclear portion of the disk space under pressure to anatomically define this space. The role of diskography in the diagnosis and localization of neck pain remains controversial.[5,26] The procedure may be useful in localizing discogenic neck pain. Even those who believe strongly in the usefulness of diskography point to it mainly as a provocative test where results are considered positive if typical pain is elicited with injection of the disk space. Because of this, many orthopedists prefer to do the test themselves to be able to personally evaluate the patient's pain response. Computed tomographic (CT) scanning following diskography can be useful to assess specific anatomy of the annular pathology.

With the use of MRI scanning, the role of the myelogram in a diagnostic workup of neck pain is limited. The myelogram and postmyelogram (intrathecal contrast) CT scan remain essentially preoperative studies, able to best assess individual nerve root compression as failure of the nerve root sleeve to fill with dye.

Electrodiagnostic studies, including electromyography (EMG) and nerve conduction velocity studies, are useful in documenting specific levels of cervical root compression and in differentiating cervical radiculopa-

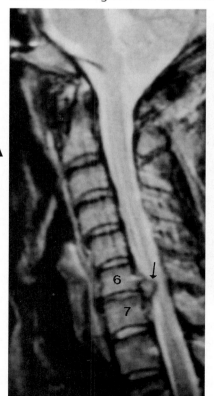

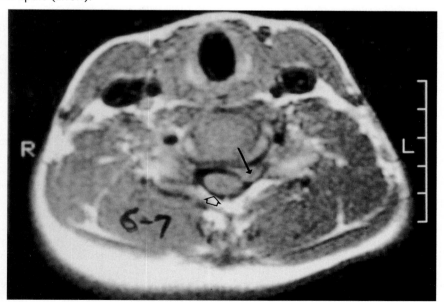

Figure 28-9 Magnetic resonance images showing a large left-sided C6-C7 disk herniation in a 29-year-old worker with sudden onset of neck and left arm pain radiating to the middle finger. The thin arrows show the extruded disk material, and the wider, open arrow points to the spinal cord. **A,** Sagittal image. **B,** Axial image.

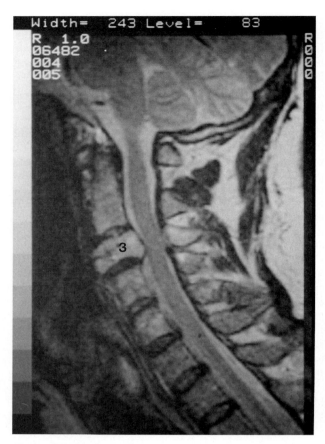

Figure 28-10 Sagittal magnetic resonance imaging showing pathologic fracture of C3 in a 46-year-old male with a 2-month history of neck pain. The diagnosis of plasmacytoma was made via CAT scan–guided needle biopsy.

thy from a peripheral compressive neuropathy. These tests can also be useful in distinguishing acute radiculopathy, which has more potential for recovery, from chronic radiculopathy, where weaknesses are less likely to improve.[6]

THE SHOULDER

History

Complaints related to the shoulder are approached in an organized, methodical manner, with care taken to not focus too quickly on a specific complaint so as to avoid missing a more generalized or related condition. At the initial assessment, identification of personal and work-related risk factors is essential. Age, dominance, occupation, and the chief complaint should begin every history because these are the major contributors in the interview to the establishment of an accurate diagnosis. For example, a 40-year-old carpenter complaining of pain in the overhead position is a signal for the physician to further evaluate for rotator cuff pathology, as opposed to a 20-year-old gymnast complaining of a feeling of the shoulder "slipping out" in the abducted

and externally rotated position, in which case one would suspect ligamentous instability.

When complaints are industrially related, exploration into the exact nature of the task and how often it is performed may further elucidate occupational risk factors that can predispose or aggravate the current condition. How often and how quickly the task is carried out should be noted. Certain tasks have been particularly associated with upper extremity tendinitis, most notably those involving repetitive work with the arm in a forward elevated position.[14,15,24,25] High-risk occupations for shoulder pathology include assembly workers, punch press operators, welders, dentists, and interpreters for the deaf. Other work-related risk factors include high force, awkward joint posture, direct pressure, vibration, and prolonged constrained postures.[31] Examples include acromioclavicular joint synovitis manifested as localized tenderness and pain on adduction. This disorder is associated with repeated lifting and with direct trauma secondary to carrying heavy objects such as piping or lumber on the shoulder.[31]

A detailed work history with documentation of prior claims, time off work, and whether litigation is in process constitute valuable information because secondary gain can play a significant role in the prognosis. Patients should always be questioned with respect to previous injuries and preexisting conditions that may be related to the present condition. Within the work history, just as important as the task performed is the mechanical and psychological environment in which the task is performed. The presence of a draft, work at a height, the positioning of equipment/tools, and the use of gloves, in addition to the degree of stress involved, may all play a role in the multifactorial etiology of repetitive strain disorders. In a comparison study of data processors with and without upper limb symptoms, Ryan and Bampton[33] postulated that work posture, work organization, and work social climate were all implicated in the development of pain syndromes and that focusing on one area alone would not be effective.

Symptoms of pain, instability, and loss of motion account for the majority of complaints about the shoulder. Radiation of symptoms versus noting maneuvers that elicit pain, the presence of night pain, and neck and opposite shoulder pain can aid in differentiating between referred pain and local pathology. Bilateral shoulder pain that is worsened by hyperextension or rotation of the neck but not by glenohumeral motion is most often due to cervical spine pathology as opposed to an intrinsic shoulder disorder. The onset of pain, be it gradual or sudden, can help identify whether an acute injury has occurred as opposed to disorders of a more chronic etiology. It is important to note the location, intensity, and character of the pain, the presence of radiation, and associated symptoms in addition to aggravating and relieving factors. These features will likely suggest the origin of the pain when the pain occurs, and its duration can help one to gain insight into the severity of the problem. Pain at night and at rest, a need for analgesics, interference with activities of daily living, or simply discomfort with rigorous activity or sports describes the spectrum of intensity the patient may be experiencing. Localized pain that is intense enough to disrupt sleep and cause limitation of simple overhead activities is most commonly due to rotator cuff pathology. However, infection, arthritis, and frozen shoulder syndrome can less frequently be manifested in a similar manner. Pain on carrying heavy packages at the side or when pushing a revolving door open is more indicative of pain secondary to instability of the glenohumeral joint. When pain radiates down the arm into the hand and posterior of the scapula and is associated with paresthesias, it is more likely to be caused by a cervical radiculopathy than by intrinsic shoulder pathology.

If an acute injury is reported, details of its mechanism and the position of the arm at the time force was applied should be ascertained. Direct trauma is more likely to cause muscular contusion or fracture, whereas forced abduction and external rotation often result in anterior capsule and ligamentous stretching or dislocation. Feelings of subluxation or crepitus at the time of injury with an inability to continue working secondary to immediate pain attests to the severity. If a fall has occurred, the height of the fall and the type of surface onto which the patient fell and which body part struck first should be recorded. A fall onto the top of the shoulder often results in varying degrees of acromioclavicular separation whereas falls onto the outstretched hand can easily result in proximal humeral fractures.

Physical Examination

Even with the most thorough history, the physician may or may not have a clear sense of the underlying problem. Therefore, a systematic, meticulous approach to the physical examination is required to avoid missing subtle findings and arriving at an inaccurate or incomplete diagnosis. A thorough examination of the neck and cervical spine, as detailed earlier, must be included in the evaluation of all potential shoulder problems.

The initial component of physical examination of the shoulder should involve general inspection of the patient. This phase begins with watching removal of the patient's shirt, with care taken to exhibit appropriate decorum in respecting patient modesty. A patient may use his contralateral upper extremity to splint or cradle the involved limb. When undressing, patients with frozen or painful shoulders tend to remove their unaffected limbs from the shirt sleeves first to avoid excessive rotation of the affected shoulder. Much of the remainder of the examination can be performed with the patient either sitting upright or standing erect.

The shoulder should be inspected for signs of asymmetry caused by either muscle wasting, soft tissue swelling, or bone or articular incongruities. Muscle spasm involving the trapezius or paracervical muscles may also cause asymmetry, perhaps due to nerve root pathology[16] or muscle fatigue related to postural or high load demands.[4,18,32] Deltoid atrophy may be associated with general disuse of the shoulder, or it may be related to axillary nerve pathology; it is best noted from an ante-

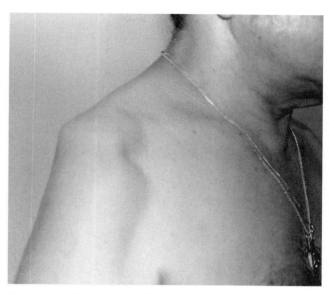

Figure 28-11 Severe axillary nerve palsy manifested as deltoid atrophy, squaring off of the shoulder, and inferior subluxation of the humeral head.

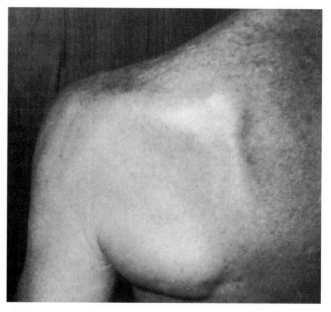

Figure 28-12 Supraspinatus and infraspinatus atrophy noted from behind; the atrophy was secondary to a long-standing rotator-cuff tear.

rior vantage point and is characterized by squaring off of the involved shoulder (**Fig. 28-11**). Atrophy of the supraspinatus or infraspinatus muscles is best visualized from behind (**Fig. 28-12**). This is most commonly seen in association with rotator cuff tears but may also be related to supraspinatus nerve entrapment neuropathy or C5 nerve root pathology. Prominence of the clavicle may suggest clavicle fracture or malunion, as well as

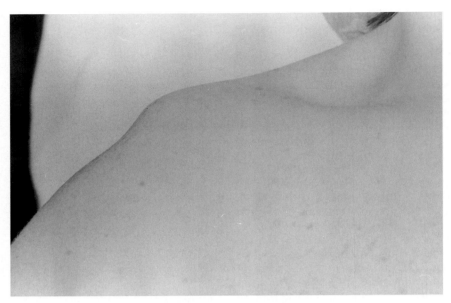

Figure 28-13 Acromioclavicular separation with complete loss of articulation of the joint surfaces and prominence of the distal end of the clavicle.

acromioclavicular joint dislocations (**Fig. 28-13**). Swelling is unusual but may be seen in cases of subacromial bursitis or extravasation of synovial fluid in massive rotator cuff tears. Posterior dimpling or a "sulcus" may suggest anterior shoulder dislocation.

The next step in a comprehensive examination of the shoulder is palpation of the bony and soft tissue elements. Tenderness or crepitus about the clavicle suggests fracture or nonunion, particularly if this is consistent with details of the history. Acromioclavicular joint tenderness is found in cases of arthritis and may be seen in those whose occupations require carrying heavy loads on their shoulders like lumber or postal bags,[27,31,35] or in case of instability secondary to traumatic ligamentous disruption. Tenderness on palpation over various anatomic landmarks can provide important clues leading to a diagnosis: tenderness of the anterior of the acromion may be a subtle indicator of rotator cuff impingement; tenderness about the greater tuberosity may be seen in cases of rotator cuff tears, supraspinatus tendinitis, or fracture; tenderness over the bicipital groove, which is found between the greater and lesser tuberosities, is suggestive of bicipital tendinitis; and tenderness over the posterior joint line beneath the posterior of the acromion may represent glenohumeral arthritis. Anterior joint or capsular tenderness is more representative of soft tissue injury after anterior shoulder dislocation or subluxation.[16] Local warmth is a nonspecific indicator of inflammation and is seen in conditions such as inflammatory arthritides or infection. Anesthesia or hypoesthesia in the dermatome overlying the middle deltoid suggests injury to the axillary nerve from either traction, compression, or demyelination.

Joint motion, both active and passive, must be assessed. It is important to understand the two basic components of shoulder elevation: glenohumeral and scapulothoracic. It is generally held that the former accounts for the initial two thirds and the latter for the initial third of elevation, but reports vary from ratios of 2:1 to 5:4, with the scapulothoracic component increasing with elevation.[16,20,28] To assess the relative contributions of each, the scapula should be stabilized by holding the inferior scapular angle. Adhesions or rotator cuff derangement will likely alter the normal fluid pattern of glenohumeral motion, and a greater proportion of the arc of motion will, by compensating, become scapulothoracic.

The Society of American Shoulder and Elbow Surgeons has recommended that four planes of shoulder motion be assessed in all patients: total forward elevation (both active and passive), active and passive external rotation with the elbow at the side, external rotation with the arm abducted 90 degrees, and internal rotation behind the back (active or passive because these will generally be about the same).[16] Abduction and internal rotation are best examined with the patient sitting upright on the examination table. Forward elevation and external rotation should most accurately be examined with the patient both upright and supine to ensure that compensatory movements of the spine are eliminated. Limited active arc of motion may have a musculotendinous or neurological etiology, or it may have a basis in pain. Limited passive motion suggests a mechanical block as in adhesive capsulitis, malunion of fractures, loose bodies, or arthritis within the glenohumeral joint.

When assessing forward elevation, the practitioner should view the patient from a lateral position and reference the angle of the arm with the posterior of the thorax. External rotation, both active and passive, is best assessed with the arm at the side and the elbow

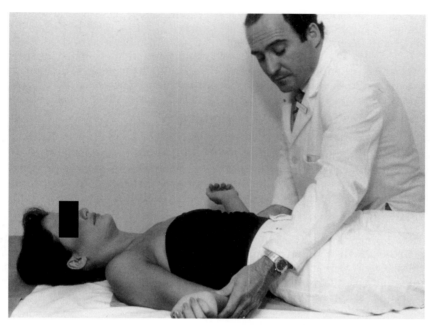

Figure 28-14 External rotation of glenohumeral joint is assessed with the patient supine to prevent torso rotation. The elbow is flexed to 90 degrees with the arm at the side.

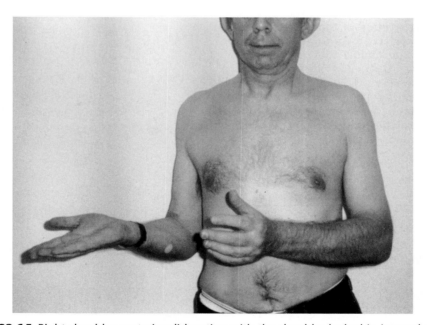

Figure 28-15 Right shoulder posterior dislocation with the shoulder locked in internal rotation.

flexed 90 degrees (**Fig. 28-14**). A deficiency in active external rotation is generally representative of neurologic or rotator cuff derangement, but it may also be seen in adhesive capsulitis or in patients with mechanical blocks such as locked posterior dislocations (**Fig. 28-15**). Testing external rotation with the arm abducted 90 degrees may be helpful, particularly in patients performing repetitive overhead activities such as throwing or welding. Symptoms suggestive of capsulolabral defi-

ciencies, greater tuberosity pathology, and instability are elicited in this position.

Testing internal rotation is generally performed with the patient sitting upright. The patient is asked to reach around the back while internally rotating (and slightly extending) the shoulder. The level reached by his outstretched thumb is recorded. This is commonly documented as the buttock, sacrum, iliac crest, and then the exact lumbar or thoracic spinous process reached. Generally, active and passive range of motion in this plane is similar. Limitations are again suggestive of subacromial pathology such as rotator cuff derangement or a frozen shoulder.

Muscle strength testing is essential to assess the competence of the musculotendinous complexes about the shoulder, as well as identify possible peripheral or central neuropathology such as cervical stenosis or peripheral compressive neuropathy. In this regard, a thorough understanding of the structure of the brachial plexus and innervation patterns more peripherally is critical. Clearly, a suggestion of cervical pathology will stimulate a more thorough neurologic examination. When muscle strength is recorded, the universal system of grading should be followed. This system grades muscle strength on a scale from 0 to 5, with the opposite and presumably normal limb used as the control for comparison (**Table 28-1**). It is important to realize that in the presence of pain, the accuracy of motor strength recording may be called into question.

The primary motor functions tested are forward flexion, abduction, external rotation, and internal rotation. These are tested by resisting the particular plane of motion. Forward flexion is primarily the role of the anterior head of the deltoid muscle (axillary nerve, C5-C6), with secondary flexors including the biceps and coracobrachialis muscles (musculocutaneous nerve, C5-C7) and the clavicular portion of the pectoralis major muscle (lateral pectoral nerve, C5-C6). Abduction tests the strength of both the middle third of the deltoid muscle (axillary nerve, C5-6) and the supraspinatus muscle (suprascapular nerve, C5). The supraspinatus muscle may be isolated by abducting the arm 90 degrees, maximally pronating the forearm with the thumb down, and testing the abduction strength with the arm in the plane of the scapula. External rotation strength principally assesses the infraspinatus muscle (supras-

capular nerve, C5-C6) and teres minor muscle (axillary nerve, C5-C6). The posterior deltoid (axillary nerve, C5-C6) also has a secondary role here. Internal rotation strength testing evaluates the integrity of the subscapularis muscle or nerve (C5) and is tested with the arm at the side, elbow flexed 90 degrees, and resistance provided against the patient's forearm as the shoulder is internally rotated.

In patients with documented or suspected glenohumeral instability—the most common type being anterior—the simplest test, particularly in the absence of anesthesia, is the "apprehension test." In cases of anterior instability, this is performed with the examiner standing behind the patient's involved shoulder. The arm is abducted 90 degrees and the arm externally rotated as the humeral head is levered anteriorly with gentle pressure from behind (**Fig. 28-16**). This will produce a sense of apprehension in patients as they sense impending shoulder subluxation or dislocation. Poste-

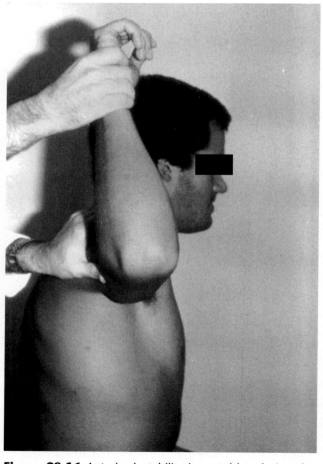

Figure 28-16 Anterior instability is tested by placing the shoulder in 90 degrees of abduction and external rotation while attempting to level the humeral head out anteriorly with gentle posterior pressure. Apprehension and pain are indicative of positive responses.

Table 28-1	Muscle grading.
Muscle Gradations	**Description**
5 (normal)	Complete ROM against gravity with full resistance
4 (good)	Complete ROM against gravity with some resistance
3 (fair)	Complete ROM against gravity
2 (poor)	Complete ROM with gravity eliminated
1 (trace)	Evidence of muscle contraction; no joint motion
0 (absent)	No contractility

ROM, *range of motion.*

rior instability is less common but may be seen, particularly in patients with seizure disorders. Apprehension may be tested as a posteriorly directed force is applied to a humerus that is flexed and internally rotated. Patients with inferior instability may have their symptoms reproduced by applying longitudinal, downward traction on the arm. In these cases, an inferior "sulcus sign" will also exist (**Fig. 28-17**).

In patients without gross shoulder instability, actual glenohumeral translation may be difficult to produce on examination without the benefit of anesthesia. Nevertheless, this should be assessed in all patients. Instability may be tested with the patient sitting upright or lying supine. The scapula is stabilized with one hand and the humeral head grasped with the other. Anterior and posterior translatory loads are applied to evaluate anterior and posterior instability, respectively. Then a longitudinal axial load is applied to the elbow to observe whether there is a component of inferior instability with the production of an inferior "sulcus." Anterior and posterior instability may also be tested with the patient supine. The arm is abducted 20 degrees, an axial load is applied, and anterior and posterior stresses are exerted. It is important to compare these findings with those in the opposite shoulder because some degree of instability may be expected even in normal shoulders, particularly in patients with generalized hyperlaxity.

Several provocative tests can be used to elucidate rotator cuff derangement: the so-called impingement tests. Two classically used impingement tests exist. The Neer test consists of forced forward elevation of the arm.[23] Pain is evoked as the inflamed supraspinatus tendon impinges against the inferior border of the anterior of the acromion (**Fig. 28-18**). In the Hawkins impingement test, the arm is forward-flexed 90 degrees and then forcibly internally rotated. Pain is evoked as the inflamed supraspinatus tendon is impinged against the coracoacromial ligament.

Pain caused by bicipital tendinitis may be elaborated by two frequently employed tests: Yergason's test and Speed's test. The former consists of actively supinating the forearm against examiner resistance with the elbow flexed 90 degrees. The latter involves forward elevation of the arm against resistance with the elbow extended and forearm supinated. Both tests, if positive, will elicit pain in the region of the bicipital groove. It should be noted that this diagnosis is often a component of the impingement syndrome and most likely does not exist as an isolated entity.

In addition to the detailed neurologic examination outlined earlier, a careful vascular examination should be performed to rule out vascular compression in the neck as the source of claudicant shoulder pain—the so-called thoracic outlet syndrome. Distal pulses should

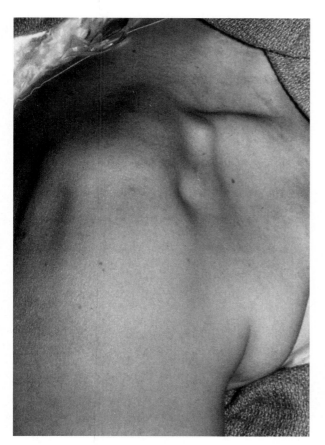

Figure 28-17 Inferior ligamentous laxity exhibited by an inferiorly subluxed humeral head with downward traction on the humerus with the arm at the side.

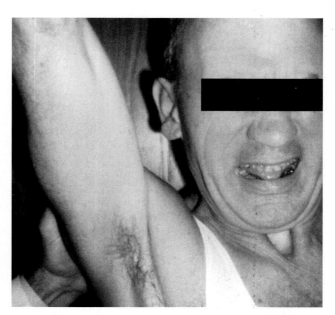

Figure 28-18 Positive impingement sign as described by Neer with forced forward elevation of the arm causing the supraspinatus to impinge on the undersurface of the acromion.

routinely be palpated. Several tests have a time-honored role in the diagnosis of vascular insufficiency. Perhaps the most commonly used is Adson's maneuver or one of its several modifications. The examiner palpates the radial pulse and abducts the ipsilateral arm 90 degrees while extending and externally rotating the shoulder with the patient turning the head to the opposite side. A diminishing peripheral pulse signifies proximal compression and is a positive test. It is critical to identify the source of vascular compression, including an accessory rib, Pancoast's tumor, fibrous bands, or clavicular malunion, so that proper steps in management may be taken.

Diagnostic Testing

The practitioner will generally establish the diagnosis after a thorough history and comprehensive physical examination. Most imaging tests are performed to confirm the physician's clinical impression. However, inevitably in some cases the diagnosis remains unclear and further investigation is warranted.

The mainstay of imaging remains the plain radiograph. In general, all patients with complaints referable

to the shoulder should receive a routine series of at least three radiographs as initial screening. This consists of AP, scapular lateral, and axillary radiographs of the shoulder with the beam centered over the glenohumeral joint. It is important to follow meticulous guidelines when shooting these radiographs and keep in mind that the glenoid is rotated anteriorly approximately 35 to 40 degrees (**Fig. 28-19**). A true AP radiograph in the scapular plane is taken with the posterior aspect of the affected shoulder against the cassette and the opposite shoulder rotated anteriorly approximately 40 degrees. The AP radiograph in internal rotation will show the greater tuberosity en face; external rotation will show it in profile. Both will show different aspects of the humeral head. The distance between the humeral head and the acromion process should be assessed in these views. In cases of massive rotator cuff tears, the normal interspace, averaging 10 mm, may diminish as the humeral head migrates cephalad, and a break in the inferior calcar line may be seen[9] (**Fig. 28-20**). Also considered routine in trauma situations is the scapular lateral (or "Y") view, in which the scapula is seen tangentially. This is an anterior oblique projection taken

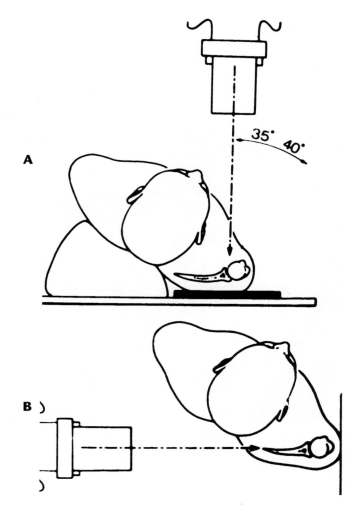

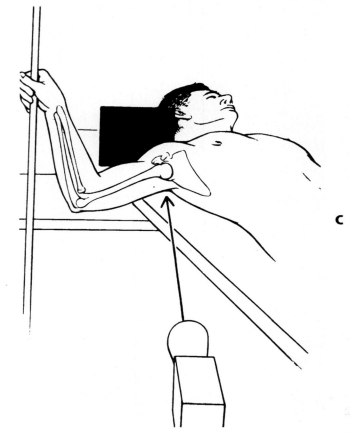

Figure 28-19 Technique for obtaining scapular anteroposterior **A**, lateral **B**, and axillary **C** views of a trauma series required on all patients.

with the patient rotating the involved shoulder 60 degrees toward the central beam.[9] Its value lies in identifying shoulder dislocations, as well as fractures of the humeral head or neck or scapula.

In the axillary view, the patient is positioned supine with the arm abducted. A horizontal x-ray beam is directed in towards the axilla. This projection visualizes the relationship between the humeral head, glenoid, coracoid, and acromion (**Fig. 28-21**). It is a key projection for identifying shoulder dislocations as well as any associated glenoid avulsion fractures (bony Bankart lesion) or impression fractures of the humeral head (Hill-Sachs lesion) (**Fig. 28-22**). The relative position of the anterior aspect of the acromion with respect to the clavicle should be assessed, particularly in cases of impingement syndrome. Anterior protrusion of the anterior process of the acromion beyond the anterior limits of the clavicle has been shown to predispose to impingement.[9,36]

The "outlet view" represents a lateral projection into the subacromial space. It is an ideal projection for assessing the slope of the acromion which has been shown to have an impact on the development of impingement syndrome (**Fig. 28-23**). It is taken with the patient standing and the affected shoulder rotated 60 degrees toward an x-ray beam angled 10 to 15 degrees caudad.[9]

A specialized AP radiograph angled 15 degrees cephalad is a valuable tool for imaging the distal and middle aspects of the clavicle and acromioclavicular joint. As such, this projection is used to assess clavicle fractures, acromioclavicular joint sprains, acromioclavicular joint arthritis or spurring (a source of rotator cuff impingement), or distal clavicle osteolysis (common to weight lifters).[9]

Magnetic resonance imaging, which has become the imaging modality of choice in the majority of centers for identifying most soft tissue pathology about the shoulder, has rendered arthrography almost obsolete, although MRI is more costly. Both T1 and T2 sequencing are performed so that subtle disorders are not overlooked.[34] Imaging includes axial, coronal, and sagittal oblique projections.

Magnetic resonance imaging is clearly indicated in evaluation of the rotator cuff in cases of impingement syndrome or suspected cuff tears, particularly when conservative measures such as nonsteroidal antiinflammatory medications, occupational therapy, and possibly subacromial steroid injections have failed to relieve the patient's symptoms. Subacromial bursitis and supraspinatus tendinitis will result from long-standing impingement. Eventually the inflammatory changes within the substance of the rotator cuff may progress to the point where degenerative tears ensue. It is important in these circumstances to differentiate the pain and weakness resulting from tendinitis versus cuff tear because the treatment for each will obviously differ. Magnetic resonance imaging will often also show the source of cuff impingement such as an osteophyte from the undersurface of the acromioclavicular joint, acromioclavicular joint hypertrophy, or a downward-beaking acromion that may be associated with a subacromial spur (**Fig. 28-24**).

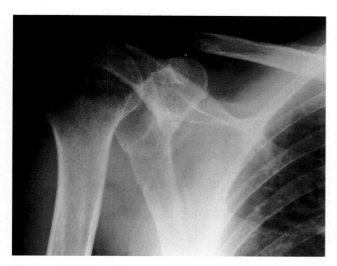

Figure 28-20 In the presence of massive rotator cuff tears, a high-riding humeral head is noted with decreased acromiohumeral distance and a break in the inferior calcar margin.

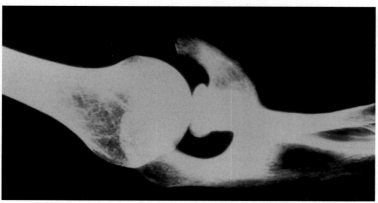

Figure 28-21 Axillary view crucial for determining the position of the humeral head in relation to the glenoid.

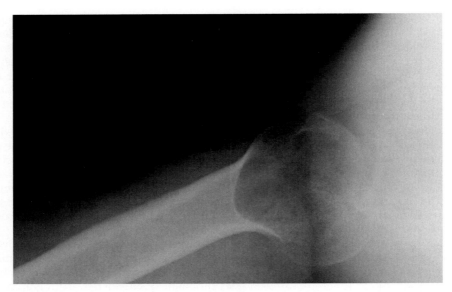

Figure 28-22 Locked posterior dislocation with a humeral head impression fracture.

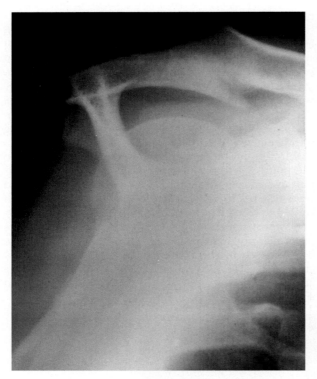

Figure 28-23 Supraspinatus outlet view with a large subacromial spur causing impingement.

Other indications for MRI include evaluation of shoulders with glenohumeral instability to detect labral tears or tears of the capsular tissues. Although infrequent, in cases of violent traumatic anterior shoulder dislocations, the subscapularis tendon may be torn either directly off its insertion on the lesser tuberosity or in its midsubstance. In the latter case, MRI will potentially show retraction at the site of the tear, or in chronic cases, calcific deposits may be seen in the substance of the subscapularis muscle or tendon.[35] The tendon of the long head of the biceps can be imaged on axial cuts as it sits in the bicipital groove. Absence of the tendon in this landmark would imply rupture and subsequent retraction (which may be obvious on clinical examination) or subluxation, as may be seen in a congenitally shallow bicipital groove or after trauma.[35] Bicipital tendinitis is often a more proximal phenomenon and is difficult to image by MRI. Finally, MRI has a role in the diagnosis of avascular necrosis of the humeral head and should be considered in certain high-risk groups such as deep sea divers, sicklers, or steroid users in the setting of shoulder pain even without radiographic findings.

Although it has been replaced by MRI in many centers, arthrography continues to have a role in the diagnosis of disorders of the shoulder.[10] It entails injection of either contrast alone or contrast followed by the injection of room air into the glenohumeral joint. Then various x-rays views are taken to assess different components of the shoulder. The technique has a time-honored role in the diagnosis of complete rotator cuff tears and may in fact be more accurate than MRI in determining the presence of a full-thickness cuff tear (**Fig. 28-25**). Like MRI, the arthrogram may also be used to visualize the long head of the biceps tendon, thereby diagnosing rupture, tenosynovitis, or subluxation. Lesions of the glenoid labrum and adhesive capsulitis may also be assessed by arthrography, especially when followed by CT scanning.

Computed arthrotomography has a role that is, at the current time, incompletely defined. This modality may be superior to other imaging techniques in defin-

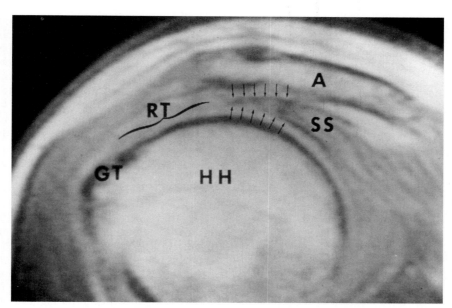

Figure 28-24 Magnetic resonance image of the right shoulder revealing a full-thickness rotator cuff tear (*RT*) with a retracted supraspinatus tendon (*SS*) underneath the acromion (*A*). The greater tuberosity (*G*) is also shown.

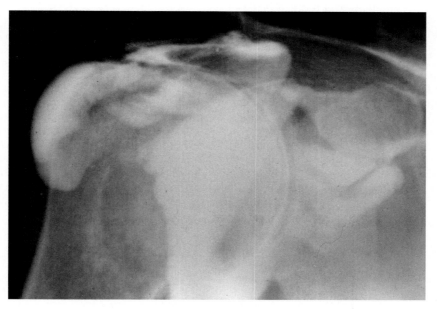

Figure 28-25 Arthrogram documenting a full-thickness rotator cuff tear with dye extravasating into the subacromial space and laterally to the greater tuberosity.

ing subtle capsular lesions or labral tears, particularly in cases of poorly documented shoulder instability.[7]

Technetium bone scanning has a limited role in the evaluation of problems related to the shoulder, but it may be of use in the evaluation of adhesive capsulitis or in ruling out occult infection, tumor, or avascularity in the presence of persistent symptomatology.[8]

Lidocaine injection tests serve a vital role with regard to problems of the shoulder in that they can be

valuable diagnostic tools when the precise diagnosis is in question. For instance, at times it may be difficult to localize the source of symptoms to the acromioclavicular joint, the subacromial space, or the glenoid labrum. In these situations, selective lidocaine injection could be of obvious benefit. The subacromial space is the most frequently injected region. Amelioration of symptoms will point to rotator cuff tendinitis or tear as the culprit; conversely, if symptoms persist, the source of pain is

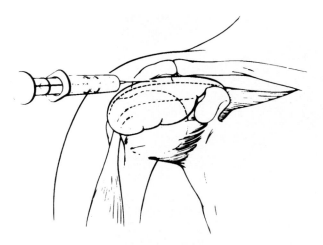

Figure 28-26 Subacromial lidocaine injection test via a lateral approach is extremely valuable in the diagnosis of impingement.

elsewhere, although the subacromial space may be responsible at least in part. Various techniques for injection have been described; nevertheless, it is always important to follow strict sterile technique to minimize the risk of infection. The subacromial space can be injected from a lateral approach with relative ease (**Fig. 28-26**). Downward traction may be applied to the arm to help widen the interval between the humeral head and the acromion. The acromioclavicular joint is also a frequent source of pain. It is easily palpated between the distal clavicle and the acromion. A needle can be directed into the joint from its superior aspect. Often pathology in this joint is associated with impingement of the rotator cuff, and selective injection here may help clarify the severity of the pain referable to this joint.[8]

Other studies may be included in an evaluation of the shoulder, including routine blood tests like a complete blood count, erythrocyte sedimentation rate, rheumatoid factor, antinuclear antibody, and blood chemistry analysis, to exclude inflammatory arthritides or infection in suggestive cases. Additionally, adhesive capsulitis is more likely in diabetic patients, hence the importance of assessing serum glucose levels.

Electromyographic and other nerve conduction studies have a definite role in distinguishing central from peripheral neuropathy, as well as in investigating the possibility of a neural basis of muscle wasting or weakness when intrinsic myotendinous pathology is ruled out.

CONCLUSION

The problem of shoulder and neck pain in the industrial setting has reached epidemic proportions.[1,13,20,21,25] Historical review, however, indicates that this is not a problem peculiar to the mechanization of society. Detailed reference to musculoskeletal problems affecting the labor force can be found dating back to 1713 in a description by Ramazzini:[30]

Various and manifold is the harvest of diseases reaped by workers from the crafts and trades they pursue. The first cause I ascribe to the nature of the materials they handle. The second to certain violent and irregular motions and unnatural postures by which the structure of the vital machine is so impaired that serious diseases develop therefrom.

In confronting a patient with neck or shoulder complaints related to the workplace, the physician has a simple goal: prompt diagnosis and expeditious institution of appropriate treatment. This is a critical component to returning the patient to work and restoring a potentially threatened sense of self-worth. This task requires a sound understanding of the regional anatomy of the neck and shoulder as well as an appreciation for the host of disorders that commonly affect this area.

References

1. Aaras A, Westgaard RH, Stranden E: Postural angles as an indicator of postural load and muscular injury in occupational work situations, *Ergonomics* 31:915-933, 1988.

2. Armstrong T, Silverstein B: Upper extremity pain in the workplace: role of causality. In Hadler N, editor: *Clinical concepts in regional musculoskeletal illness*, New York, 1987, Grune & Stratton.

3. Boden SD et al: Abnormal magnetic resonance imaging scans of the cervical spine in asymptomatic subjects: a prospective investigation, *J Bone Joint Surg* 72A:1178-1184, 1990.

4. Chaffin DB: Localized muscle fatigue—definition and measurement, *J Occup Med* 15:346, 1973.

5. Cloward RB, Busaid LL: Discography. Technique, indications, and evaluation of normal and abnormal discs, *AJR Am J Roentgenol* 68:552-564, 1952.

6. Eisen A, Hoirch M: The electrodiagnostic evaluation of spinal root lesions, *Spine* 8:98-106, 1983.

7. El-Khoury GY, Renfrew DL: Computed arthrotomography of the shoulder. In Seeger LL, editor: *Diagnostic imaging of the shoulder*, Baltimore, 1992, Williams & Wilkins.

8. Fitzler SL, Berger RA: Attitudinal change: the Chelsea back program, *Occup Health Saf* 51:24-26, 1982.

9. Gold RH, Bassett LW: Disorders of the shoulder: plain radiographic diagnosis. In Seeger LL, editor: *Diagnostic imaging of the shoulder*, Baltimore, 1992. Williams & Wilkins.

10. Goldman AB: Shoulder arthrography. In Seeger LL, editor: *Diagnostic imaging of the shoulder,* Baltimore, 1992, Williams & Wilkins.

11. Greenwood JG: Work related back and neck injury cases in West Virginia, *Orthop Rev* 14:53-61, 1985.

12. Gyntelberg F: One year incidence of low back pain among residents of Copenhagen aged 40-59, *Dan Med Bull* 21:30-36, 1974.

13. Hagberg M: Occupational and musculoskeletal stress and disorders of the neck and shoulder: a review of possible pathophysiology, *Int Arch Occup Environ Health* 52:269-278, 1984.

14. Hagberg M: *Work-associated complaints in the neck and shoulders,* Stockholm, 1982, Swedish Work Environment Fund (in Swedish).

15. Hagberg M: Work load and fatigue in repetitive arm elevations, *Ergonomics* 24:543-555, 1981.

16. Hawkins RJ, Bokor DJ: Clinical evaluation of shoulder problems. In Rockwood CA, Jr, Matsen FA, editors: *The shoulder,* Philadelphia, 1990, WB Saunders.

17. Hedberg MC et al: Gradient echo MR imaging in cervical radiculopathy, *AJR Am J Roentgerol* 150:683-689, 1988.

18. Herberts P et al: Shoulder pain and heavy manual labor, *Clin Orthop* 191:166-178, 1984.

19. Hult L: Cervical, dorsal, and lumbar spinal syndromes, *Acta Orthop Scand Suppl* 17:1-102, 1954.

20. Inman VT, Saunders JB, Abbott LC: Observation of the function of the shoulder joint, *J Bone Joint Surg* 26A:1-30, 1944.

21. Jarvholm U et al: The effect of arm support on supraspinatus muscle load during simulated assembly work and welding, *Ergonomics* 34:57-66, 1991.

22. Kellgren JH, Lawrence JS: Osteoarthrosis and disk degeneration in an urban population, *Ann Rheum Dis* 17:388-397, 1958.

23. Kelsy JL et al: An epidemiologic study of acute prolapsed cervical intervertebral disc, *J Bone Joint Surg* 66A:907-914, 1984.

24. Kvarnstrom S: Occurrence of musculoskeletal disorders in a manufacturing industry, with special attention to occupational shoulder disorder, *Scand J Rehab Med Suppl* 8:1-112, 1983.

25. Loupajarvi T et al: Prevalence of tenosynovitis and other injuries of the upper extremities in repetitive work, *Scand J Work Environ Health* 5:48-55, 1979.

26. Meyer RR: Cervical discography: a help or hindrance in evaluating neck, shoulder, arm pain? *AJR Am J Roentgenol* 90:1208-1215, 1963.

27. Neviaser JS: Adhesive capsulitis and the stiff and painful shoulder, *Orthop Clin North Am* 11:327-331, 1980.

28. Poppen NK, Walker PS: Normal and abnormal motion of the shoulder, *J Bone Joint Surg* 58A:195-201, 1976.

29. Putz-Anderson V, editor: *Cumulative trauma disorders: a manual for musculoskeletal disorders of the upper limbs,* Philadelphia, 1988, Taylor & Francis Publishers.

30. Ramazzini B: *Treatise on the diseases of workers,* New York, 1964, Hafner Publishing (Translated by WC Wright; originally published in 1713).

31. Rempel DM, Harrison RJ, Barnhart S: Work-related cumulative trauma disorders of the upper extremity, *JAMA* 267:838-842, 1992.

32. Rohmert W et al: Effects of vibration on arm and shoulder muscles in three body postures, *Eur J Appl Physiol* 59:243-248, 1989.

33. Ryan G, Bampton M: Comparison of data process operators with and without upper limb symptoms, *Community Health Studies* 12(1):63-68, 1988.

34. Seeger LL: Magnetic resonance imaging of the shoulder. In Seeger LL, editor: *Diagnostic imaging of the shoulder,* Baltimore, 1992, Williams & Wilkins.

35. Wells JA et al: Musculoskeletal disorders among letter carriers, *J Occup Med* 25:814-820, 1983.

36. Zuckerman JD et al: The influence of caracoacromial arch anatomy on rotator cuff tears, *J Shoulder Elbow Surg* 1:4-12, 1992.

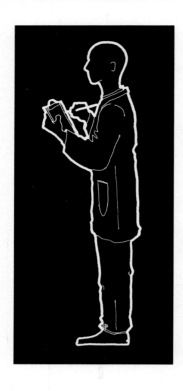

Chapter 29

A Diagnostic and Treatment Algorithm of the Cervical Spine

William C. Lennen
Sam Wiesel

CONTENTS

Anumber of conditions can cause symptoms of neck pain with or without associated arm or shoulder pain (see box p. 380). Neck pain as a clinical syndrome is common and can be seen in both the presence and the absence of a history of trauma or positive radiographic findings. Some of the more important musculoskeletal disorders associated with neck pain are covered in detail in this chapter. These disorders include neck strain, acute herniated disk, cervical degenerative disk disease (including spondylosis with and without myelopathy), rheumatoid arthritis, and hyperextension injuries.

Each of these diagnostic entities are defined in detail, including pertinent history and physical characteristics, as well as radiographic findings. In addition, a treatment rationale is discussed for each. Finally, a diagnostic and treatment algorithm is presented that will integrate each of the previously discussed clinical entities into a usable format.

NECK SPRAIN

Neck sprain (cervical strain) is one of the most common disorders the practicing physician may need to evaluate. The term *sprain* is in actuality a misnomer. As opposed to a hyperextension injury, this syndrome often occurs in the absence of a distinct traumatic episode in the vast majority of patients. It consists of nonradiating pain or discomfort in the neck region along with associated loss of range of motion. Neck pain as an isolated complaint is attributed to abnormalities in structures innervated by the sinovertebral nerve.[2] This nerve innervates the posterior longitudinal ligament, the epidural vasculature, the dura, and the spinal periosteum. The facet joints are innervated by branches of the posterior primary ramus at each spinal level.

The pain associated with cervical strain is often a dull aching pain that is exacerbated by movement. In addition, a component of referred pain may be involved. This is not, however, true radicular pain secondary to mechanical compression of a nerve root. The area of the referred pain is generally to other mesenchymal structures derived from a similar sclerotome during the process of embryogenesis. More common referred patterns include the posterior of the shoulder, the occipital area, the scapular region, and the anterior chest wall, also known as cervical angina pectoris.[18]

Once again, the history generally does not consist of a traumatic event. The pain may start after a night's rest or simply by turning the head. After the onset of pain has been determined, the frequency, quality, and precise distribution should be ascertained. It is also essential to avoid missing early myelopathy. Careful questioning should therefore address subtle long-tract signs, including bowel or bladder dysfunction and gait abnormalities. Clinically, the pain may begin as a headache, or more often it may be located in the lower to middle base of the neck. The etiology of the pain is thought to be derived from the soft tissues of the cervical spine, including the ligamentous structures and/or the surrounding musculature.[15]

Physical examination of the patient will usually reveal only some local tenderness lateral to the bony spine. The loss of motion in individual patients is variable and tends to directly correspond with the intensity of the pain. True muscular spasm, defined as continuous muscular contraction, is rare, except in severe cases of torticollis in which the head is tilted to one side.

Radiographic studies in neck strain are usually normal. For this reason, plain films are generally not warranted on the first office visit. If the pain does persist for more than 2 weeks, however, a radiograph should be obtained to rule out other more serious causes of neck pain such as instability or neoplasia.

The prognosis for patients with cervical strain is excellent because the natural history of this disorder is complete resolution of all symptoms over a period of several weeks. Therapy consists primarily of rest and immobilization, often with the use of a soft cervical orthosis.[15] Certain medical interventions such as antiinflammatory agents and/or muscle relaxants may aid in the acute phase of pain management, but they do not appear to alter the natural course of the syndrome.

Cervical traction has been used for many years, but opinions vary regarding its effectiveness. Traction should not be prescribed before plain films are obtained to rule out fracture, tumor, and infection. The use of cervical traction is absolutely contraindicated in the presence of rheumatoid arthritis, osteoporosis, infection, cord compression, and malignancy. Traction can be manual or mechanical. Manual traction allows for more interaction between the patient and therapist. If home traction is to be used, low-weight traction (5 to 10 lb) pulling is preferred with the supine patient in slight flexion at the neck.[1] The primary benefit from traction may consist of immobilization inasmuch as some evidence indicate that at least 25 lb is necessary to actually distract the vertebrae.

Although no good randomized, prospective clinical trials have studied their efficacy, trigger point injections do seem to empirically work well. The purpose of trigger point injection is to decrease inflammation in a specific anatomic area. The results appear to be superior the more localized the trigger point. These injections can be repeated at 1- to 3-week intervals.[18]

Causes of neck and neck-related pain syndromes

LOCALIZED NECK DISORDERS
   Osteoarthritis (apophyseal joints, C1-C2-C3 levels
      most often)
   Rheumatoid arthritis (atlantoaxial)
   Juvenile rheumatoid arthritis
   Sternocleidomastoid tendinitis
   Acute posterior cervical strain
   Pharyngeal infections
   Cervical lymphadenitis
   Osteomyelitis (staphylococcal, tuberculosis)
   Meningitis
   Ankylosing spondylitis
   Paget's disease
   Torticollis (congenital, spasmodic, drug involved, hys-
      terical)
   Neoplasms (primary or metastatic)
   Occipital neuralgia (greater and lesser occipital
      nerves)
   Diffuse idiopathic skeletal hyperostosis
   Rheumatic fever (infrequently)
   Gout (infrequently)

LESIONS PRODUCING NECK AND SHOULDER PAIN
   Postural disorders
   Rheumatoid arthritis
   Fibrositis syndromes
   Musculoligamentous injuries to the neck and shoul-
      der
   Osteoarthritis (apophyseal and Luschka)
   Cervical spondylosis
   Intervertebral osteoarthritis

   Thoracic outlet syndromes
   Nerve injuries (serratus anterior, C3-4 nerve root,
      long thoracic nerve)

**LESIONS PRODUCING PREDOMINANTLY SHOULDER
PAIN**
   Rotator cuff tears and tendinitis
   Calcareous tendinitis
   Subacromial bursitis
   Bicipital tendinitis
   Adhesive capsulitis
   Reflex sympathetic dystrophy
   Frozen shoulder syndromes
   Acromioclavicular secondary osteoarthritis
   Glenohumeral arthritis
   Septic arthritis
   Tumors of the shoulder

**LESIONS PRODUCING NECK AND HEAD PAIN WITH
RADIATION**
   Cervical spondylosis
   Rheumatoid arthritis
   Intervertebral disk protrusion
   Osteoarthritis (apophyseal and Luschka joints, inter-
      vertebral disk, osteoarthritis)
   Spinal cord tumors
   Cervical neurovascular syndromes
      Cervical rib
      Scalene muscle
      Hyperabduction syndrome
      Rib-clavicle compression

From Wiesel SW et al: Neck pain, *ed 2, Charlottesville, Va, 1992, The Michie Company; pp 60-61.*

ACUTE HERNIATED DISK

A herniated disk occurs when the nucleus pulposus protrudes through the fibers of the surrounding annulus fibrosus.[14] Stookey,[16] as well as Rothman and Marvel,[14] have described types of soft disk herniations (**Fig. 29-1**). Infraforaminal herniation is the most common, with production of dermatomal radicular symptoms. Herniations occurring posterolaterally will produce predominantly motor signs and symptoms. As opposed to the lumbar region, disk herniations occurring centrally may cause myelopathy because of the presence of the cord in the cervical region.

Most disk herniations occur around the fourth decade of life while the nucleus pulposus remains gelatinous. The most common levels for herniation are at the C6-C7 and C5-C6 levels. Those at the C7-T1 and C3-C4 levels are uncommon, and those at the C2-C3 level are extremely rare. Not every disk herniation is symptomatic. The presence and severity of symptoms depend on the individual spinal reserve capacity, the presence or absence of associated inflammation, the size of the herniated fragment, as well as the presence of concomitant disease processes such as uncovertebral joint osteophytes.

In general, a herniated disk will affect the nerve root of the next lowest cervical level. According to this rule, a C3-C4 disk will affect the C4 nerve root, a C4-C5 disk will affect the C5 nerve root, and so on. The radicular symptoms will then correspond to the involved nerve root. In addition, as previously stated, a herniated disk may cause some long-tract signs because of the presence of the spinal cord at the cervical level.

Most patients have symptoms consisting primarily of arm pain. Although the pain may begin in the neck region, the pain radiates down into the shoulder, arm, forearm, or hand along a clearly defined dermatome. The onset of pain may be gradual, although acute tearing or snapping sensations may occur. The arm pain may vary in intensity from a dull cramping pain in the arm with use to pain so severe as to preclude use of the extremity. In addition, attacks of sharp pain may radiate

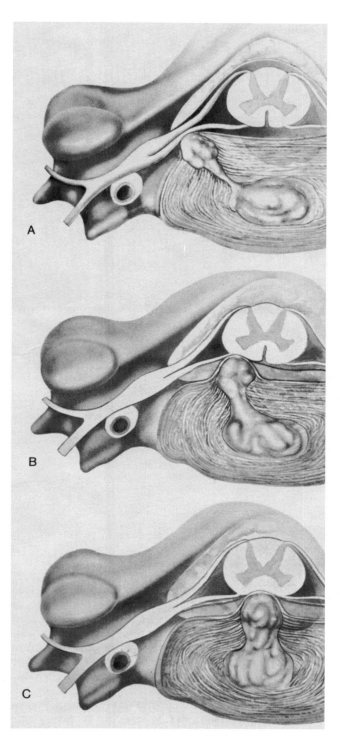

Figure 29-1 Types of soft disk herniations. *(From Boden SD et al: The aging spine: essentials of pathophysiology, diagnosis, and treatment, Philadelphia, 1991, WB Saunders.)*

into the hand and fingers with associated paresthesias. Pain severe enough to awaken the patient at night is not uncommon.

Extrinsic pressure on the vascular structures or peripheral nerves is the most likely imitator of disk herniation causing radiculopathy. Chest and shoulder pathology must also be ruled out (e.g., apical carcinoma of the lung with encroachment of the brachial plexus with or without Horner's syndrome).

Physical examination may reveal some decreased motion of the neck that may be so severe as to be manifested as frank torticollis. Any maneuver (such as the Valsalva maneuver) that stretches the involved nerve root may recreate the pain pattern. Spurling's test, in which the neck is extended, may often make the pain worse by narrowing the involved intravertebral foramina further. Additionally, coughing, shoulder abduction, and axial compression tests are often positive in patients with compression radiculopathy. The axial compression test is performed by placing an axial load on a patient whose head is flexed laterally and slightly rotated. A positive finding consists of worsening or reproduction of radicular symptoms. The shoulder abduction relief test is positive if radicular symptoms are decreased when a sitting patient elevates one hand above the head with the elbow flexed to 90 degrees and the shoulder abducted to 90 degrees.[3] An axial manual traction test is performed with the patient supine. A positive finding consists of a decrease or complete absence of radicular symptoms when 20 to 30 lb of axial traction is applied.

In addition to these tests, neurological findings are generally abnormal. Sensory examination may reveal subjective changes in sensation.[8] This portion of the neurological examination is the least helpful, however, because the results are often difficult to interpret and the examination requires a coherent and competent patient to be of any value. Motor and reflex changes are the most helpful. Henderson, Hennessy, and Shuey[8] found a demonstrable motor deficit in 65% of 846 patients with cervical radiculopathy. Likewise, they also found diminished deep tendon reflexes in 71% of their patients.

The specific motor and deep tendon reflex changes noted depend on the cervical nerve root that is compressed by the herniated disk (**Table 29-1**). With involvement of the third cervical nerve root (i.e., herniation of the C2 disk), pain will radiate up the neck posteriorly to the suboccipital region, as well as toward the mastoid and the pinna of the ear. No demonstrable motor or reflex deficit will be present. Compression of the fourth cervical nerve root will also not result in any demonstrable motor or reflex deficit. Despite the fact that the C4 nerve root supplies the diaphragm, fluoroscopic studies have not shown any abnormalities in diaphragm functioning in those patients with known C4 radiculopathy. The pain will generally radiate to the base of the neck and to the superior aspect of the scapula.

Table 29-1		Cervical radiculopathy symptoms and findings.
Disk Level	**Nerve Root**	**Symptoms and Findings**
C2-C3	C3	*Pain:* Back of neck, mastoid process, pinna of ear *Sensory change:* Back of neck, mastoid process, pinna of ear *Motor deficit:* None readily detectable except by EMG *Reflex change:* None
C3-C4	C4	*Pain:* Back of neck, levator scapulae, anterior of chest *Sensory change:* Back of neck, levator scapulae, anterior of chest *Motor deficit:* None readily detectable except by EMG *Reflex change:* None
C4-C5	C5	*Pain:* Neck, tip of shoulder, anterior of arm *Sensory change:* Deltoid area *Motor deficit:* Deltoid, biceps *Reflex change:* Biceps
C5-C6	C6	*Pain:* Neck, shoulder, medial border of scapula, lateral aspect of arm, dorsal part of forearm *Sensory change:* Thumb and index finger *Motor deficit:* Biceps *Reflex change:* Biceps
C6-C7	C7	*Pain:* Neck, shoulder, medial border of scapula, lateral aspect of arm, dorsal part of forearm *Sensory change:* Index and middle fingers *Motor deficit:* Triceps *Reflex change:* Triceps
C7-T1	C8	*Pain:* Neck, medial border of scapula, medial aspect of arm and forearm *Sensory change:* Ring and little fingers *Motor deficit:* Intrinsic muscles of hand *Reflex change:* None

EMG, *electromyography.*
From Boden SD et al: *The aging spine: essentials of pathophysiology, diagnosis, and treatment, ed 1,* Philadelphia, *1991,* WB Saunders; *p. 46.*

In contradistinction to the third and fourth cervical nerve roots, the fifth through eighth cervical roots will generally demonstrate motor, reflex, and/or sensory abnormalities when compressed. Compression of the fifth cervical nerve root may demonstrate decreased sensation in the area of the autonomous distribution of the axillary nerve, namely, the lateral aspect of the deltoid. Motor loss will result in weakness of the deltoid, although the supraspinatus, infraspinatus, and some of the elbow flexors may likewise be affected. Clinically, the patient has difficulty with motions requiring abduction of the arm for overhead activities such as combing hair. The pain radiates from the side of the neck to the top of the shoulder. The biceps reflex may be diminished.

With involvement of the sixth cervical nerve, the pain radiates from the neck down the lateral aspect of the arm and forearm into the radial side of the hand and down into the tips of the index and long fingers, as well as the thumb. Numbness may be located on the dorsum of the hand and the autonomous distribution for the sixth nerve root, the tip of the index finger. Loss of the biceps reflex is an early sign of compression of this nerve root, as is demonstrable weakness of the biceps muscle. Other muscles that may also be weakened by C6 involvement include the supinator, infraspinatus, extensor pollicis, and extensor carpi ulnaris.

With compression of the seventh cervical nerve root, the patient will often complain of pain radiating from the lateral reason of the neck down the back of the arm, along the posterolateral aspect of the forearm, and into the middle finger. Sensory changes can be found in the tip of the middle finger, the autonomous zone for C7. Motor and reflex changes center primarily around the triceps muscle. With compression of the seventh nerve, the triceps reflex will be diminished. Likewise, muscle weakness of the triceps will be elicited. The patient may not be aware of the true severity of the weakness of the triceps despite the fact that it is the main extender of the elbow. Elbow extension can still be performed in the presence of severe triceps weakness with the assistance of gravity. Weakness will be noted by the patient in activities that require forceful extension of the elbow, such as in the backhand stroke of racquet sports. Other weaknesses that may be more difficult to identify include weakness of the pectoralis major, pronator, wrist and finger extensors, and latissimus dorsi.

Involvement of the eighth cervical nerve root generally results in pain below the wrist in the ulnar border of the hand and the little finger. The sensory changes will likewise be in this distribution, particularly the tip of the little finger. No reflex can demonstrate an eighth nerve root compression, although the flexor carpi ulnaris reflex may be decreased. The motor function of C8 primarily involves the intrinsic musculature of the hand. Patients will generally complain of loss of fine motor skills and grip strength. Rapid atrophy of the interosseous muscles can occur because of their small size. This atrophy may result in rapid loss of fine hand movements.

The diagnosis of an acute herniated cervical disk is made primarily from the history and physical examination as detailed earlier. Plain films may be normal and are nondiagnostic. Occasionally, disk space narrowing is seen at the involved interspace, or oblique films may show foraminal narrowing. Plain films are useful primarily for ruling out other causes of arm and neck pain such as instability and neoplasia. Other diagnostic tests such as electromyography (EMG) or myelography are not useful as screening tests and should be used more to confirm diagnoses based on a detailed history and physical examination. In addition, the routine use of computed tomography (CT) or magnetic resonance imaging (MRI) is not warranted. These sensitive studies may reveal disk bulges that are not clinically significant, possibly leading to unnecessary surgical procedures. Once again, they need to be correlated with the symptoms and physical findings.

The primary mode of treatment for an acute herniated disk is rest and immobilization. Strict bed rest at home with the exception of bathroom privileges should be prescribed. The patient should remain at bed rest for 2 weeks while wearing a soft cervical orthosis at all times during this period. The cervical orthosis improves the chance that the patient will remain at rest. The collar must fit properly and hold the head in a neutral to slightly flexed position. If the neck is held in hyperextension, the patient will often be uncomfortable and therefore noncompliant in its use. Once the acute pain starts to subside, the patient should be weaned slowly from the orthosis and likewise increase activity gradually. If the patient complies with the bed rest and immobilization, the use of analgesics is often not necessary. Occasionally, a brief course of analgesic medicine may be required in severe cases. Benzodiazepines and muscle relaxants can act as central nervous system depressants. As such, they have a limited role in the treatment of acute herniated disk disease.

Drug therapy does, however, have an important role in combination with rest and immobilization. Antiinflammatory medications such as aspirin and other nonsteroidals may play a role by decreasing some of the inflammation. As discussed earlier, it is believed that inflammation does play a part in the production of radicular symptoms inasmuch as the resulting arm pain is produced by a combination of pressure from the ruptured disk and inflammation around the involved nerve root. Most of these medications can have adverse gastrointestinal side effects but can generally be tolerated well for brief periods of time. The patient should be educated on these side effects, however, and be instructed to stop taking them immediately should side effects occur. Routine use of oral systemic steroids is not necessary but may prove useful in the more refractory cases. In this case, a tapering dose schedule over a period of 7 days can be used.

Injections of local anesthetic and steroid into the cervical epidural space may provide some pain relief. This again is based on the premise that inflammation plays a significant role in the production of radicular symptoms. This procedure, however, requires considerable experience and technical competence and is not entirely without a risk of complications. Some authors have had limited success with this procedure, but we do not routinely use cervical epidural steroids.

Indications for surgical intervention in the treatment of an acute herniated disk include persistent radicular pain unresponsive to at least 3 months of conservative therapy, progressive neurologic deficit, static neurologic deficit in the presence of radicular-type pain, and radiographic studies such as CT or MRI with a myelogram confirmatory of clinical signs and symptoms (**Fig. 29-2**).

The prognosis for patients with an acute herniated cervical disk is generally very good.[4] If patients are compliant with the rest and immobilization program as outlined, most will be able to return to work within a period of 1 month, at least under light-duty conditions. **Figure 29-3** shows a flowchart for the treatment of neck pain. This chart is applicable to both cervical strain and acute herniated disk disease because initially both groups are treated in a similar fashion with similar conservative measures. Most patients will get better within 6 weeks with this conservative protocol. If symptomatic improvement is not achieved after 6 weeks, the two groups should then be addressed separately. The two groups consist of those who have neck pain as a primary complaint (i.e., cervical strain) versus those with arm pain (brachialgia) as the primary symptom (i.e., acute herniated disk disease).[17]

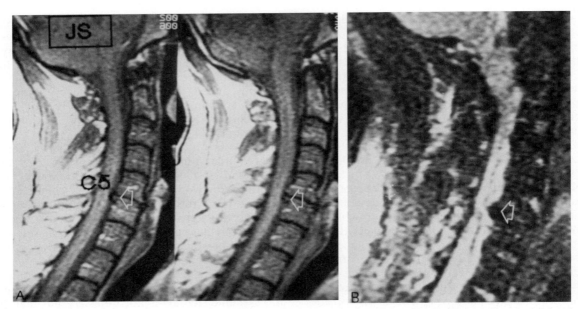

Figure 29-2 Magnetic resonance images of a 45-year-old male with unilateral C6 rediculopathy. **A,** Midsagittal view showing more pathologic anatomy than a parasagittal view of the unaffected side (*arrows*). **B,** Parasagittal view of the affected side showing hard disk pathology (*arrow*). *(From Boden SD et al: The aging spine: essentials of pathophysiology diagnosis, and treatment, Philadelphia, 1991, WB Saunders.)*

CERVICAL DEGENERATIVE DISK DISEASE

Cervical degenerative disk disease can produce a number of syndromes in concert with cervical spondylosis, including (1) isolated cervical spondylosis, (2) cervical spondylosis with myelopathy, (3) cervical spondylosis with radiculopathy, (4) cervical spondylosis with myeloradiculopathy, and (5) cervical spondylosis with associated visceral or vascular encroachment.[4] Radiculopathy secondary to spondylosis will not be discussed separately because it does not significantly differ from radiculopathy secondary to acute herniated disk disease as previously described. Cervical spondylosis may result in the formation of large anterior osteophytes that either impinge on the esophagus and produce difficulty in swallowing or impinge on the vertebral artery and produce symptoms of vertebrobasilar insufficiency.

Spondylosis

Cervical spondylosis is a term used to describe the chronic process of degenerative changes that occur as part of natural aging. These include changes in the vertebral body, intervertebral disk, uncovertebral joints of Luschka, zygapohyseal joints, ligamentum flavum, dura, and soft tissues. With this occur intervertebral disk degeneration, disk space collapse, and spinal canal and foraminal osteophyte formation, as well as hypertrophy of the facets, lamina, ligamentum flavum, and dura.

These changes are seen in varying degrees in patients with spondylosis, as well as to a lesser extent in asymptomatic elderly individuals. These changes can also produce a wide variety of clinical signs and symptoms depending on the severity of each of these changes.

Along with the achievement of an erect posture, the human cervical spine has been able to develop a high degree of mobility and flexibility. It has paid the price for this mobility with an almost universal propensity for degenerative change. Cadaveric studies have revealed that nearly everyone will demonstrate some degree of degenerative change in the cervical spine by age 55. However, not everyone will have clinically symptomatic complaints. Friedenberg and Miller[7] have shown a lack of correlation between symptoms and degenerative changes seen on plain radiographs of the cervical spine. These changes become clinically significant only when directly related to clinical symptoms.

The primary causative factor for cervical spondylosis appears to be age-related changes that occur in the intervertebral disks, including loss of annulus fibrosus elasticity, desiccation of the nucleus pulposus, and narrowing of the disk space with or without associated disk rupture. Secondary changes then occur and include facet overriding, increased motion, osteophyte formation, inflammation of synovial joints, and microfractures. These changes can then result in the different clinical syndromes previously described.

Historically, the typical patient with cervical spondylosis will be over 40 years of age and have a

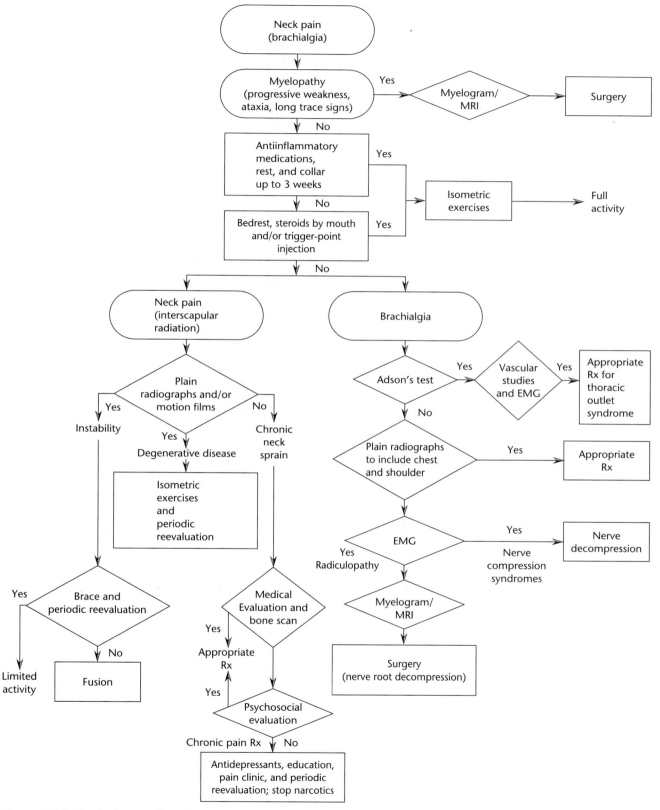

Figure 29-3 Cervical spine algorithm. *(From Wiesel SW et al: Neck pain, Charlottesville, Va, 1988, The Mitchie Company.)*

complaint of neck ache. Referred pain patterns are not uncommon, however, with true sclerotomal referral patterns. These include shoulder pain, suboccipital referred pain, occipital headaches, intrascapular pain, anterior chest wall pain, or other nonspecific symptoms such as blurred vision and tinnitus.

Physical examination of a patient with cervical spondylosis often reveals little in the way of objective clinical findings. Neurological findings are generally normal in isolated spondylosis without radiculopathy or myelopathy. Some decrease in motion of the cervical spine may be evident. Point palpation may reveal some tenderness along the midline of the neck, as well as some tenderness in areas of referred pain.

Plain radiographs are primarily obtained to rule out more serious causes of neck pain. Plain films in the anteroposterior, lateral, and oblique planes will reveal varying degrees of change, including disk space narrowing, osteophyte formation, foraminal narrowing, facet degeneration, or instability patterns. Once again, these changes do not directly correlate with the presence or severity of clinical symptoms.

The mainstay of therapy for patients with cervical spondylosis is conservatism. In the presence of acute exacerbation of symptoms against a background of chronic disease, rest and immobilization are generally beneficial. Aspirin or other nonsteroidal antiinflammatory medications may also be helpful for acute exacerbations and may be needed on a chronic basis to abate symptoms. As previously described, trigger point injections may also be of value both diagnostically and therapeutically. A soft cervical orthosis may assist in resting and immobilizing the cervical spine. Cervical isometric exercises and changes in the patient's daily activities such as work habits, sleeping positions, and driving of automobiles may be useful adjuvant therapies in the treatment of these chronic patients. The use of manipulative techniques and traction protocols is generally not recommended for this patient population.

Spondylosis with Myelopathy

When the previously described degenerative changes of the cervical spine become so severe as to impinge on the spinal cord, a pathologic process termed *myelopathy* is produced. Spinal cord and nerve root compression produces *myeloradiculopathy*. Radiculopathy has already been described in detail in relation to acute herniated disk disease and will not be addressed further here.

Those patients with developmental cervical stenosis are more prone to the development of spondylitic myelopathy at a younger age. Etiological factors in the reduction of canal reserve volume include hypertrophy of the ligamentum flavum, facets, lamina, and dura with redundant annulus fibrosus, foraminal osteophyte compression of radicular vessels, vertebral osteophyte cord compression, tethering of the cord by dentate ligaments, and finally, ossification of the posterior longitudinal ligament or ligamentum flavum.[1] A reduction

in volume of the spinal canal can result in direct canal compression as well as intrinsic or extrinsic ischemia. Edward and LaRocca[5] have demonstrated that development of myelopathy with spondylosis is almost certain with canal diameters of less than 10 mm. Patients with canals 10-mm to 13-mm in diameter are at risk, those with canals 13 to 17 mm canals are myelopathic prone, and myelopathy rarely develops with canal diameters greater than 17 mm.

In addition to these static considerations, dynamic changes in the cervical spine may result in myelopathy.[16] Penning and van der Zwaag described the pincer mechanism in 1966. In this mechanism, the spinal cord becomes compressed between the anterosuperior margin of the lamina of the inferior vertebrae and the posteroinferior osteophyte (i.e., hard disk disease) of the superior level. Flexion of the spine causes stretching of the cord over vertebral body osteophytes, with extension possibly resulting in retrolisthesis of one vertebral body on another or buckling of the hypertrophied ligamentum flavum. All these dynamic changes can cause compression of the cord as it passes through the cervical canal.

Clinically, most patients are between 40 and 60 years of age when initially seen, with males more often affected. In fewer than 5% of patients with cervical spondylosis does myelopathy develop. Although a history of trauma may occasionally be given, the onset is more often insidious. Acute myelopathy generally reflects a central soft disk herniation producing a high-grade block. The natural history is one of deterioration initially, followed by a plateau in deficit lasting for several months. The exact clinical picture is variable, with a patchy distribution of deficits. This distribution depends on the number of levels involved and the severity of cord impingement at each level.

Typically, patients will have a gradual onset of peculiar sensations (numbness and paresthesias) with associated weakness and clumsiness. Lower extremity symptoms may precede those in the upper extremity and include gait disturbances, peculiar leg sensations, weakness, hyperreflexia, spasticity, and clonus. Upper extremity findings that may initially be unilateral often progress to bilaterality. These include hyperreflexia, a brisk Hoffmann sign, and muscle atrophy, particularly of the hand intrinsics. Abnormalities in micturition are seen in approximately one third of cases and connote a more severe cord impingement. Sensory changes are a less reliable sign of myelopathy.[10] Spinothalamic tract signs may be seen with disturbances in pain and temperature sensation in the upper extremities, thorax, or lumbar region. These may be characterized by a stocking glove distribution. Dorsal column function can be affected with resultant vibratory and proprioceptive disturbances. Impingement on the dorsal division of the nerve root may produce unusual dermatomal sensory changes.

Spondylosis with nerve root compression has been divided into four categories by Ferguson and Caplan.[6]

These include (1) lateral or radicular syndrome, which consists of a spondylitic radiculopathy without myelopathic symptoms; (2) medial or spinal syndrome, in which upper motor neuron signs are predominant; (3) combined medial and lateral syndrome with a combination of both cord and root involvement; and (4) vascular syndrome, which represents an acute vascular episode unaffected by surgical intervention.

In addition, a number of different syndromes have been described primarily on the basis of the spinal cord tracts affected in the myelopathic process. These include (1) Brown-Sequard syndrome with ipsilateral motor dysfunction, contralateral pain, and temperature dysfunction one to two levels below the motor involvement; (2) central cord syndrome with upper extremity involvement greater than lower extremity involvement; (3) transverse lesion syndrome, which occurs most commonly with involvement of the posterior columns, spinal thalamic tracts, and corticospinal tracts; (4) brachialgia cord syndrome with upper extremity radicular symptoms and long-tract signs; and finally (5) the motor system syndrome with corticospinal tract involvement and weakness of both the upper and lower extremities.

The differential diagnosis for patients with cervical spondylitic myelopathy includes such disorders as multiple sclerosis, amyotrophic lateral sclerosis, spinal cord tumors, syringomyelia, disk herniation, intracranial lesions, low-pressure hydrocephalus, and subacute combined degeneration. Each of these should be ruled out with an appropriate history and physical examination as well as diagnostic studies.

Plain radiography in these patients will generally demonstrate typical degenerative findings, including spinal canal narrowing by prominent posterior osteophytes, variable foraminal narrowing, disk space narrowing, facet joint arthrosis, and instability. Magnetic resonance imaging can demonstrate structural as well as parenchymal changes (**Fig. 29-4**). The myelogram is also of value in demonstrating the typical washboard appearance (**Fig. 29-5**) with multiple anterior and posterior dye column defects.[15] The posterior defects are produced by facet joint arthrosis and ligamentum flavum buckling. In contrast to the previously described syndromes of neck strain, acute herniated disk disease, and spondylosis without myelopathy, in which the mainstay of treatment is conservative therapy, the treatment of myelopathy is primarily surgical. In a patient who is a poor surgical candidate because of concomitant medical conditions, conservative measures such as immobilization and rest with a cervical orthosis are viable options.[13] In general, however, management of patients with myelopathy centers around surgical decompression of the spinal canal and prevention of further spinal cord impingement and vascular compromise.

Studies looking at the natural history and prognosis of cervical spondylitic myelopathy are confusing and often difficult to compare because of the lack of a universal classification system. Some common factors can be identified, however. The age at onset and duration of symptoms before the onset of treatment are prognostic factors. Increased age at diagnosis and delay in treatment for longer than 1 year are poor prognostic indicators. Most of the patients in these series had periods of nonprogression, or plateau phases, interspersed with periods of rapid deterioration. A minority of patients had a steady progression of the disease with resultant severe disability. Conservative therapy rarely reverses the myelopathy. Treatment of these patients is therefore surgical. Progression of the myelopathy after surgical decompression is uncommon. Both anterior and posterior surgical procedures have been reported to lead to improvement in the myelopathy of patients with cervical spondylosis.

RHEUMATOID ARTHRITIS

Approximately 2% to 3% of the general population is affected with rheumatoid arthritis. Of these, 86% will show radiographic evidence of cervical spine disease and 60% will have clinical signs and symptoms of cervical spine involvement.[9] Cervical spine involvement is a reflection of the erosive inflammatory changes characteristic of this systemic disease process.

Involvement of the cervical spine consists of three distinct syndromes: (1) atlantoaxial instability, (2) basilar invagination, and (3) subaxial instability. Atlantoaxial instability is the most common of these syndromes. Ranawat[12] has shown that these syndromes tend to occur in combination. He found that 60% of his patients had atlantoaxial instability, 16% had basilar invagination, and 60% had subaxial instability. Risk factors for the development of atlantoaxial instability include prolonged systemic steroid use, long disease duration, older age, and erosive peripheral joint involvement.

Patients with cervical spine involvement secondary to rheumatoid arthritis will often have neck pain localized to the middle posterior area of the neck and occipital region. Range of motion may be limited and crepitance or sensations of frank instability may be present. Neurological changes can be variable and are often difficult to interpret in rheumatoid patients, who may have severe involvement of the upper and lower extremities. Physical examination should be performed very carefully to rule out upper motor neuron signs such as hyperreflexia and spasticity, as well as the presence of abnormal reflexes such as the Babinski and Hoffmann signs. Brain stem involvement by compression of the invaginated dens and/or associated pannus can result in symptoms of vertebrobasilar insufficiency. Other nonspecific findings may include the onset of bowel or bladder incontinence or retention, development of spasticity, and a change in ambulatory status.

Evaluation of patients with any of these clinical symptoms should first begin with plain radiographs of the cervical spine. Common findings include osteope-

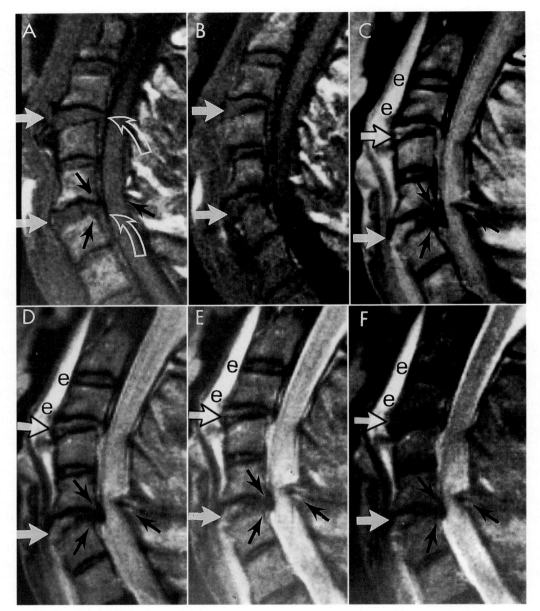

Figure 29-4 A, 500-ms TR/17-ms TE sagittal image in a patient who sustained a cervical extension injury. Note the disruption of the anterior longitudinal ligament at multiple levels (*solid white arrows*), as well as the traumatic disk herniations (*open arrows*). Pinching occurs at the C5-6 level (*black arrows*). **B,** A parasagittal 500-ms TR/17-ms TE image shows anterior longitudinal ligamentous disruption (*arrows*), as well as prevertebral soft tissue swelling. **C,** The midline sagittal 2000-ms TR/30-ms TE 7-mm image demonstrates ligamentous disruption (*white arrows*), prevertebral edema (*e*), and pinching at C5-6 (*black arrows*). The canal compromise appears more serious on this 7-mm sagittal image, most likely because of a partial volume effect from the lamina laterally. **D,** A 2000-ms TR/60-ms TE midline sagittal image shows similar findings, again with prevertebral edema (*e*), ligamentous disruption (*white arrows*), and some increase in signal intensity of the spinal cord at the site of compression (*black arrows*). **E,** and **F,** 2000-ms TR/90- and 120-ms TE images with similar findings, although the increased signal intensity within the spinal cord secondary to edema is more obvious on those more T2-weighted scans. The absence of any significant focal areas of decreased signal intensity indicates a relative absence of intramedullary hemorrhage (contusion) and a more favorable prognosis. Despite the initially severe neurologic deficit, this patient eventually recovered significant function. *(From Modic MT, Masaryk TJ, and Ross JS: Magnetic resonance imaging of the spine, ed 2, St Louis, 1994, Mosby–Year Book.)*

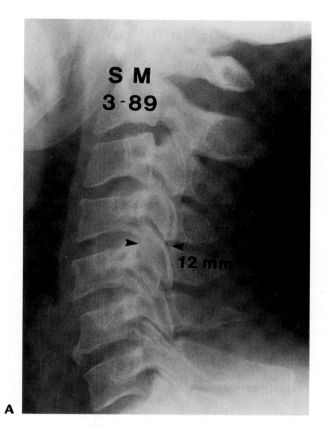

A

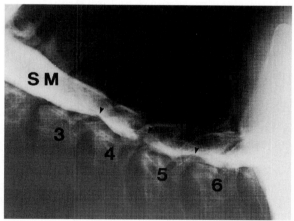

B

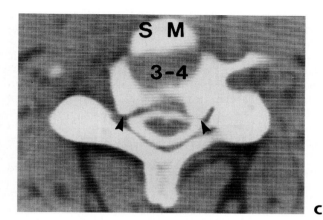

C

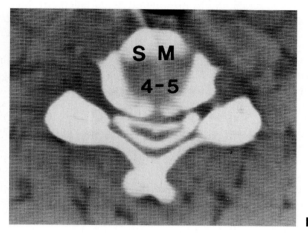

D

Figure 29-5 A, Lateral roentgenogram of a 43-year-old man with complaints of left shoulder pain, gait abnormality, and leg weakness. He had mild spondylotic changes and a congenitally narrow cervical canal (12 mm). **B,** Lateral myelogram showing significant extradural defects at C3-4, C4-5, and C5-6. **C,** A computed tomographic myelogram shows large uncovertegral spurs (*arrows*) plus soft disk material protruding at C3-4. **D,** Severe spinal cord flattening at C4-5 from the disk and an osteophytic ridge. *(From White AH and Schofferman JA: Spine care, vol 2, St Louis, 1995, Mosby–Year Book.)*

nia, facet erosion, disk space narrowing, and subluxation of the lower cervical spine (stepladder). Atlantoaxial instability is determined on the basis of dynamic flexion-extension views of the cervical spine. An atlantoaxial interval of less than 3.5 mm is considered normal. Surgical intervention is generally recommended for a distance greater than 7 to 8 mm.[18]

Basilar invagination occurs with upward migration of the odontoid process into the foramen magnum with resultant brainstem impingement. Radiographic evaluation includes a measurement of the distance from the tip of the odontoid to beyond MacGregor's line. This is seen on the lateral view of the cervical spine and represents a line drawn from the tip of the hard palate to the posterior base of the foramen magnum. Normally, the dens should not protrude more than 3 mm above this line. Protrusion more than 8 mm in females or 9.7 mm in males may be an indication for surgery. Likewise, the Wakenheim line, which is drawn along the cranial surface of the clivus, should be tangential to or intersect the tip of the odontoid. With cranial settling, the tip of the dens will be posterior to this line. A

CT scan is useful in determining the relationship of the bony elements with each other as well as in relation to the spinal cord.

Subaxial subluxations are also evaluated on dynamic flexion-extension views of the spine. Significant subluxation is defined as translation of one vertebral body on another of 3.5 mm or more or disk space angulation of 11 degrees or more.[17]

The great majority of these patients can be managed conservatively despite the fact that cervical spine involvement will develop in a significant number of patients. The mainstay of nonoperative therapy is a hard cervical orthosis (i.e., Philadelphia collar). This produces symptomatic relief without actually affecting the atlantoaxial interval. Medical treatment of these patients plays a crucial role in nonoperative management. Medications such as high-dose aspirin, methotrexate, chloroquine, and oral steroids are often administered under the supervision of a rheumatologist.

Prognostically, these patients tend to do very well with conservative measures, and only a small percentage of patients die of medullary compression from significant atlantoaxial disease. Atlantoaxial disease gradually worsens with time, with only 2% to 14% of patients exhibiting progressive neurological symptoms.[9]

To summarize, surgical intervention should be considered in the presence of (1) more than 3.5 mm of mobile subaxial subluxation on flexion-extension views, (2) atlantoaxial subluxation greater than 8 mm in the presence of spinal cord compression on flexion-extension radiographs, or (3) cranial settling indicative of basilar invagination in the presence of radiographic evidence (MRI) of cord compression. Additionally, in the absence of these findings, the presence of a progressive neurologic deficit would be a strong indication for surgical intervention.

HYPEREXTENSION INJURIES

The majority of hyperextension injuries to the cervical spine result from rear-end automobile accidents.[10] This causes an acceleration hyperextension injury in the driver of the struck car. Falls and sports injuries contribute to the remainder of the hyperextension injuries. This injury has great economic considerations. The term "whiplash injury" was introduced by H. E. Crowe in 1928, and since that time, this injury has become a major source of litigation potential.

The pathophysiology behind a hyperextension injury involves an injury to the soft tissues of the neck region.[11] Usually the driver of the struck automobile is relaxed and unaware of the incipient collision. When struck from behind, the automobile accelerates forward acutely. If no headrest is present, the driver's head is thrown back and the neck forced into hyperextension as the torso continues onward with the automobile. The sternocleidomastoid, scalenes, and longus coli muscles are stretched beyond their elastic limit and are severely stretched or torn. Tears of the longus coli muscles may be associated with a concomitant tear of the sympathetic trunk and result in Horner's syndrome. Further hyperextension may result in injury to the esophagus or larynx with subsequent difficulty in swallowing and hoarseness, respectively. Additionally, injury to the anterior longitudinal ligament may result in hematoma formation with cervical radiculitis or injury to the intervertebral disk. Also, when the head is thrown backward, the jaw generally lags behind, thus resulting in injury to the tempomandibular joint as the jaw falls open. When the head recoils forward, the skull may strike the driver's wheel or windshield and result in a head injury.

Hyperextension injuries in elderly patients with preexisting cervical spondylosis may acutely compress the spinal cord as the already limited spinal reserve volume is overcome. This cord compression can take the form of frank paralysis or the central cord syndrome.

Patients with a hyperextension injury are generally examined 12 to 24 hours after the initial traumatic event. It is at this point that the patient will start to feel stiffness in the neck, as well as pain at the base of the neck made worse by motion. The pain becomes progressively worse, and eventually the slightest head or neck movement will elicit severe pain. The anterior cervical musculature may be tender to palpation, and the patient may have hoarseness, dysphagia, or pain with chewing or opening of the mouth. Pain may radiate into both shoulders or arms and upward into the base of the skull. Other pain patterns may include the anterior of the chest, interscapular region, and vertex of the skull.

The potential for a closed-head injury even in the absence of visible head trauma should not be forgotten. Concussion can occur secondary to mechanical deformation during the acceleration-deceleration phase of the injury. This may result in headache, photophobia, mild transient confusion, fatigue, tinnitus, or transient concentration abnormalities.

Physical examination must be complete from head to toe so that other associated injuries are not be overlooked. The potential for a chance fracture of the lumbar spine exists if the patient was wearing a lap-type seatbelt. The head should be examined for any evidence of a closed head injury. A unilateral dilated pupil may suggest an injury to the sympathetic chain as it travels along the longus coli muscles with resultant Horner's syndrome. It may also indicate significant intercranial pathology in a patient with an altered level of consciousness. Temporomandibular joint tenderness should be assessed as well as suboccipital tenderness, which may indicate that the head struck the top of the seat.

A careful and thorough neurological examination should be performed. Again, particular attention should be paid to elderly patients. These individuals may have baseline spinal stenosis secondary to cervical spondylosis with resultant cord injury or central cord syndrome.

If any objective neurologic deficit is identified, further diagnostic tests are necessary. These include CT scanning and/or MRI. Computed tomography is better at providing bone detail, whereas MRI will better demonstrate soft tissue disruption such as intervertebral disk protrusion.

In most cases of hyperextension injury, only soft tissue disruption occurs. Plain radiographs should be obtained, however, to rule out unsuspected facet dislocations, facet fractures, odontoid fractures, or spinous process fractures. In most cases, these films will be normal or may show some straightening of the cervical spine. As noted, other diagnostic studies should be obtained as the history and physical findings dictate (e.g., head CT). Treatment involves primarily rest and immobilization. Rest consists of a soft cervical orthosis that assists in relieving muscle spasms and prevents quick movements of the head. Collar wear beyond 2 to 4 weeks should not be encouraged because this may result in weakening of the neck musculature and in turn development of a long-term psychoneurosis. Strict bed rest may be necessary for 3 to 5 days if the symptomatology is severe. Heat in the form of hot soaks or heating pads may be useful. Although narcotics should be avoided, medical therapy in the form of nonnarcotic analgesics, nonsteroidal antiinflammatory medications, and muscle relaxants is helpful. Activity should be restricted according to the severity of symptoms.

Characteristically, improvement should occur after 2 weeks of treatment as outlined earlier. If improvement does not occur, an additional 2 weeks of rest and immobilization should be prescribed with the addition of home cervical traction. Low-weight traction consisting of 7 to 10 lb for 20 to 30 minutes per day will generally give symptomatic improvement. Persistence of symptoms past 4 weeks should alert the physician to search for another etiology. If headaches persist, a CT scan of the head should be obtained to rule out a closed head injury. If arm or shoulder pain persists, CT of the spine and/or EMG should be performed.

In general, symptoms should be resolving by 6 weeks, although complete resolution may take as long as 1 year. Persistence of symptoms beyond 6 weeks or severity equal in intensity to that in the initial period may alert the physician to secondary gain from pending litigation, and a compensation neurosis should be suspected. The physician should certainly rule out any significant pathology by a careful history, physical examination, and appropriate diagnostic tests before assigning this diagnosis to a patient. The physician should not, however, overtreat the patient and encourage a retreat into a life of incapacitating neck pain.

The point at which the patient is able to return to the workforce is dependent on both the severity of the hyperextension injury and the type of work the patient is involved in. Patients involved in heavy manual labor may require 3 to 4 weeks of treatment before returning to work, whereas those in less demanding positions may be able to return after only 2 weeks of treatment.

Limitations on the work performed should consist of no lifting of objects heavier than 50 lb, no bending, and no prolonged periods of stooping. These should be in effect for the first 1 to 3 weeks back to work. The prognosis is generally good for complete recovery, depending on the severity of the injury. Occasionally, a 5% to 10% disability rating is appropriate in an honest patient in whom symptoms persist during hard manual labor.

CERVICAL SPINE ALGORITHM

The goal for patients with neck pain is to obtain an accurate diagnosis and administer the correct therapy at the appropriate time. The previously presented clinical entities have been organized into a standardized approach. A graphic display of this decision-making process is presented in **Figure 29-3** in the form of an algorithm.

Entry into the algorithm begins with evaluation of those patients seen for neck pain with or without associated arm pain. Patients with a history of trauma and associated fractures and/or dislocations are excluded. The first task is a thorough medical history and physical examination to rule out the presence of cervical myelopathy, as discussed earlier.

Once a myelopathic process is confirmed, surgical intervention should be considered in a timely fashion. The best results are obtained with only 1– to 2–mortar unit involvement and relatively short duration of symptoms.[1] Further studies, including myelography or MRI, should be performed to precisely define the neural compression. Adequate surgical decompression should then be performed.

Once cervical myelopathy is ruled out, the majority of patients should then be started on a course of conservative management. All patients are treated the same in this regard, regardless of the etiology of the neck pain. Initially, this nonoperative management will consist primarily of immobilization and drug therapy. A well-fitted soft cervical collar should be worn for 24 hours per day to prevent awkward positioning and movements during sleep as well as during wakeful hours. In addition, antiinflammatory medications, analgesics, and muscle relaxants will improve patient comfort.

The majority of patients will symptomatically improve with this protocol within approximately 10 days and should then start to be weaned over the next 2 to 3 weeks. Additionally, their level of activity should be gradually increased, and they should start a series of exercises aimed at strengthening the paravertebral musculature. If the condition remains unimproved, patients should continue full-time collar wear and pharmacologic management.

If no significant improvement in symptoms is seen after 3 to 4 weeks, a trigger point injection at the point of maximum tenderness should be considered. This is performed with a combination of 10 mg of corticosteroid and 3 to 5 ml of lidocaine. If this is likewise not successful at 4 to 5 weeks, a trial of home cervical traction may be considered.

A total period of 6 weeks of conservative management of patients with neck pain should be pursued. The majority of patients will respond to this program and return within 2 months to their previous life style. If, on the other hand, the symptoms fail to resolve within 6 weeks of conservative therapy, the patients are then divided into two groups depending on whether the neck pain is predominant or arm pain (brachialgia) is the primary component.

For those patients whose main complaint is neck pain and for whom conservative therapy for 6 weeks has failed, plain radiographs, including flexion-extension films, should be obtained. A number of these patients will be found to have evidence of instability. The criteria for objective instability include horizontal translation of one vertebra on another of 3.5 mm or an angular difference of 11 degrees between adjacent vertebrae. The majority of these patients will do well with nonoperative management consisting of education and bracing. Those who do not may require segmental spinal fusion. A second group of patients will be found to have changes characteristic of degenerative disease. Radiographic findings include osteophyte formation, loss of intervertebral disk height, narrowing of the neural foramina, and zygapophyseal joint osteoarthritis. As previously mentioned, degeneration of the cervical spine may be a normal part of the aging process. The difficulty arises in determining which of the degenerative changes are clinically significant. The most significant change has been found to be narrowing of the intervertebral disk height, particularly at C5-C6 and C6-C7.[7] Treatment of these patients consists primarily of antiinflammatory agents, support braces, and trigger point injections. During quiet periods, isometric exercises should be used. Reexamination is necessary to monitor for the development of myelopathic symptoms or signs.

The great majority of patients will have normal plain films. These patients will have a preliminary diagnosis of neck strain. After failure to improve with conservative therapy, these patients should have a thorough medical evaluation, as well as a bone scan, to rule out infection, neoplasia, or inflammatory arthritides as the etiology of the neck pain. If this workup proves to be negative, they should then undergo psychosocial evaluation and receive treatment, if appropriate, for depression or substance dependence, both of which can frequently be found in patients with neck pain. If the psychosocial findings prove to be normal, the patient is considered to have a diagnosis of chronic neck pain. Treatment therefore consists of thorough education and support, as well as detoxification from narcotics and the institution of an exercise program. Antidepressant agents may prove to be useful, and frequent reevaluations are necessary to avoid overlooking any serious pathologic process.

Another major group of patients in this algorithm are those patients in whom arm pain is the predominant symptom. The etiology of this pain may be either direct pressure from a herniated disk or inflammation about a nerve on a hypertrophic bone (hard disk disease).[14] Other causes of extrinsic compression of the vascular or nervous structures supplying the upper extremity may also imitate brachialgia and must therefore be ruled out. This includes pathologic processes of the chest and/or shoulder region. A thorough history and physical examination, including an Adson test, shoulder examination, and Tinel's test of the carpal, cubital, and ulnar tunnels, should be performed. Based on the results of this examination, appropriate studies should be performed. If Adson's test is positive, vascular studies and EMG should be performed to evaluate causes of thoracic outlet syndrome. Compression of the brachial plexus may occur secondary to vascular structures, cervical ribs, muscular or fibrous bands, or neoplastic processes. Additionally, an apical lung carcinoma can cause brachial plexus compression with or without Horner's syndrome from sympathetic chain involvement.

If plain films of the chest and shoulder are negative and fail to reveal a source of extrinsic compression, EMG studies should be performed. If these are indicative of peripheral nerve compression, surgical decompression at the site should be performed. In the presence of radicular symptoms, a myelogram or MRI should be performed, and if the results are consistent with the neurologic deficit, history, and physical findings, surgical decompression of the nerve root should be undertaken. In the presence of these findings, conservative treatment will result in persistent symptoms.

This algorithm is applicable to all patients with nonspecific neck or arm pain and provides a rational approach to the therapeutic and diagnostic sequence of events in these patients. The goal of this approach must always be to appropriately treat the etiology of the pain while avoiding unnecessary tests and therapeutic interventions and at the same time minimizing the chance of overlooking other serious pathologic processes manifested as neck or arm pain.

References

1. Boden SD et al: *The aging spine: essentials of pathophysiology, diagnosis, and treatment,* ed 1, Philadelphia, 1991, WB Saunders.

2. Connell MD, Wiesel SW: Natural history and pathogenesis of cervical disc disease, *Orthop Clin North Am* 23:369-380, 1992.

3. Davidson RS et al: The shoulder abduction test in the diagnosis of radicular pain in cervical extradural compressive monoradiculopathies, *Spine* 6:441-446, 1981.

4. DePalma AP et al: The natural history of severe cervical disc degeneration, *Acta Orthop Scand* 43:392-396, 1972.

5. Edward WC, LaRocca SH: The developmental segmental sagittal diameter in combined cervical and lumbar spondylosis, *Spine* 10:43-49, 1985.

6. Ferguson RJL, Caplan LR: Cervical spondylotic myelopathy, *Neurol Clin* 3:373-382, 1985.

7. Friedenberg ZB, Miller WT: Degenerative disc disease of the cervical spine, *J Bone Joint Surg* 45A:1171-1178, 1963.

8. Henderson CM, Hennessy R, Shuey H: Posterior lateral foraminotomy for an exclusive operative technique for cervical radiculopathy: a review of 846 consecutively operated cases, *J Neurosurg* 13:504-512, 1983.

9. Lipson SJ: Rheumatoid arthritis of the cervical spine, *Clin Orthop* 182:143-149, 1984.

10. McNab I: Acceleration injuries of the cervical spine, *J Bone Joint Surg* 46A:1797-1799, 1964.

11. McNab I: The whiplash syndrome, *Orthop Clin North Am* 2:289-403, 1971.

12. Ranawat CS et al: Cervical spine lesion in rheumatoid arthritis, *J Bone Joint Surg* 61A:1003-1010, 1979.

13. Roberts AH: Myelopathy due to cervical spondylosis treated by collar immobilization, *Neurology* 16:951-959, 1966.

14. Rothman RH, Marvel JP: The acute cervical disc, *Clin Orthop* 109:59-68, 1975.

15. Rothman RH, Simeone FA: *The spine,* ed 2, Philadelphia, 1982, WB Saunders.

16. Stookey B: Compression of spinal cord and nerve roots by herniation of nucleus pulposus in the cervical region, *Arch Surg* 40:417-432, 1940.

17. Wiesel SW, Feffer HL, Rothman RH: The development of a cervical spine algorithm and its perspective application to industrial patients, *J Occup Med* 27:272-276, 1985.

18. Wiesel SW et al: *Neck pain,* ed 2, Charlottesville, Va, 1992, The Michie Company.

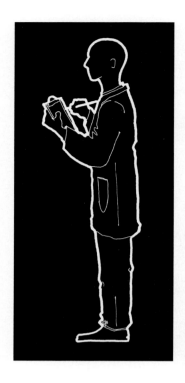

Chapter 30

Treatment of Shoulder Disorders

Paul H. Marks
Freddie H. Fu

CONTENTS

Disorders of the shoulder girdle are very common and can limit participation in vocational, recreational, and professional activities. Developing an approach to the management of shoulder disorders relies on appropriate history taking, physical examination, and imaging. This chapter outlines the treatment of most common shoulder problems, including rotator cuff pathology; instability; fracture and dislocations of the sternoclavicular joint, clavicle, acromioclavicular joint, and proximal end of the humerus; frozen shoulder; and degenerative joint disease.

ROTATOR CUFF DISEASE IN THE SHOULDER

In an older patient who complains of shoulder pain, the diagnosis of rotator cuff disease must be considered. This entity is very common and important. In 1934, Codman's classic publication[32] summarized 25 years of observations on the musculotendinous cuff and its components. Coleman also discussed ruptures of the supraspinatus tendon and performed the first repair of the cuff in 1909. Although there have been recent advances in diagnosis and imaging of the rotator cuff, current views and treatments are quite similar to concepts proposed 50 years ago.

Anatomy and Function

The components or musculotendinous units of the rotator cuff are known to function as dynamic stabilizers for the glenohumeral joint. Electromyographic (EMG) and biomechanical studies have demonstrated the role of the rotator cuff in providing support of the capsule and preventing excessive anterior and posterior movement. Studies have suggested that the rotator cuff contributes between one third and one half of the power of the shoulder in abduction and at least 80% of the power in external rotation.[30]

The rotator cuff which consists of the subscapularis, supraspinatus, infraspinatus, and teres minor, functions to approximate the humeral head to the glenoid cavity. The supraspinatus assists the deltoid in abduction, whereas the subscapularis, infraspinatus, and teres minor serve to depress the humeral head during elevation of the arm. Depression of the humeral head during elevation of the arm helps to avoid impingement. The infraspinatus and teres minor function to externally rotate the arm. These muscle actions may also reduce the strain on the inferior glenohumeral ligament with the arm abducted and essentially rotated.[28] In this position they serve to pull the humeral head posteriorly.

The subscapularis internally rotates the arm. It serves as an effective restraint to external rotation and anterior translation of the humeral head with the arm at the side of the body; however, it is ineffective in doing so with the arm abducted to 90 degrees.[138] At 90 degrees of abduction, the subscapularis lies above the equator of the humeral head and cannot reinforce the anterior aspect of the shoulder.

The vascular anatomy of the cuff tendons has been reported by many authors. Most have concluded that the supraspinatus has a "critical zone" that is prone to calcium deposits and potential rupture.[95] Rathbun and MacNab[114] found that filling of the cuff vessels was dependent on the position of the arm at the time of injection. They documented poor filling of the supraspinatus tendon near its attachment to the greater tuberosity and suggested that tendon failure may be caused by "constant pressure from the head of the humerus which tends to wring out blood supply to the tendon when the arm is held in the resting position of adduction and neutral rotation."[114]

The long head of the biceps may be considered a part of the rotator cuff. It attaches to the supraglenoid tubercle of the scapula. This structure is positioned to function as a humeral head depressor. It also guides the humeral head as it is elevated.[131] The concomitant tears that occur in the rotator cuff and biceps tendon attest to the close functional relationship between these two structures.

Neer stated that "impingement of the rotator cuff beneath the coracoacromial arch has been recognized as one of the causes of chronic disability of the shoulder." Anatomically, this problem occurs during elevation of the arm anterior to the scapular plane. He attributed pathologic changes of the rotator cuff to mechanical impingement and believed that most rotator cuff tears were due to attritional tears from a narrow supraspinatus outlet.[25,97] Additionally, Neer discussed associated alterations on the undersurface of the anterior third of the acromion, the coracoacromial ligament, and in time the acromioclavicular joint. He described three different stages of impingement. Stage I usually occurs in patients less than 25 years old. Pathology is characterized by edema and hemorrhage. The clinical course is reversible and conservative treatment is suggested. Stage II is seen in the 25-year-old to 40-year-old age group. Pathology includes fibrosis and tendinitis. These patients have activity-related pain and treatment may be surgical if there is no response to rehabilitation. Stage III disease typically occurs in patients greater than 40 years old. Pathology in this group includes acromioclavicular spurs and full-thickness cuff tears. These patients have progressive disability and are often candidates for acromioplasty and repair.

Bigliani, Morrison, and April[16] reported on a morphologic study in which the variation in shape of the acromion was correlated with tears of the rotator cuff. They described three types of acromion. Type I has a flat profile, type II has a smooth curve, and type III has an angular curve or "hook type" of acromion. The latter type was noted to be present in higher frequency with complete tears of the rotator cuff.

Neer has suggested an important role of the rotator cuff in maintaining a so-called watertight joint space and allowing continuation of the normal synovial fluid mechanics that maintain cartilage nutrition and may prevent secondary osteoarthritis.[99]

The scapulothoracic joint must also be considered when rotator cuff problems are managed. The scapula sits on the posterior-lateral aspect of the thorax. It is angled approximately 30 degrees anterior to the frontal plane. As a result of this, abduction of the arm relative to the scapula occurs 30 to 40 degrees anterior to the frontal plane. Abduction of the arm in the scapular plane places the rotator cuff muscles in their most efficient position and reduces tension on the joint capsule.

The scapula is approximated to the thorax by the scapulothoracic muscles. These include the upper, middle, and lower trapezius, serratus anterior, rhomboideus major and minor, levator scapulae, pectoralis minor, and subclavius. These muscles must function to position and stabilize the scapula during movement of the arm.

Innman, Saunders, and Abbott[65] described scapulohumeral rhythm as the coordinated motion between the scapula and humerus that occurs when the arm is elevated through its full range. During the first 30 degrees of elevation of the arm, motion primarily occurs at the glenohumeral joint and the scapula is said to be setting. Elevation of the arm beyond this occurs in a 2:1 ratio of glenohumeral to scapulothoracic motion. The total arc of elevation is a result of approximately 120 degrees of motion of the glenohumeral joint and 60 degrees of motion of the scapulothoracic joint. Motion of the scapulothoracic joint occurs as a result of elevation and rotation at the sternoclavicular and acromioclavicular joints.

Normal scapulohumeral rhythm is important for normal function of the shoulder girdle; it allows for maintenance of the length-tension relationship of the rotator cuff muscles, which allows them to function efficiently throughout the full arc of motion. Additionally, proper movement of the scapula positions the glenoid under the humeral head to enhance glenohumeral stability. Poor motion and positioning of the scapula have been linked to impingement and rotator cuff problems.

Classification of Injury

Cuff tendon failure can be classified by various criteria. These include partial- or full-thickness tears, acute or chronic injury, and traumatic or degenerative etiology. The cuff pathology is almost always near the tendon insertion. It nearly always occurs in the supraspinatus component of the rotator cuff, because this is the area that is subject to mechanical impingement against the coracoacromial arch. A full-thickness tear extends from the bursal through to the humeral aspect of the cuff. A partial tear may involve the bursal or the humeral side of the tendon. Acute tears occur suddenly and are found in only a relatively small portion of patients with rotator cuff pathology. Chronic tears are more common and are usually insidious in onset. It should be noted that the size of the complete tear can also be used to describe the pathology. A "massive tear" is the term used by Cofield[33] to describe a defect more than 5 cm in diameter.

The incidence of full-thickness rotator cuff tears has been documented in various cadaver studies as being between 5% and 26.5%.[102,147] The incidence of cuff pathology has also been documented in clinical subjects. Age has been found to correlate with incidence.[94] Moseley found that the incidence rose dramatically with the age of the patient. Traumatic cuff tears have also been found in patients with anterior-inferior dislocations. Arthrographically documented tears were seen in 30% in the fourth decade and 60% in the sixth decade.[110]

Recently, the role of secondary impingement and eccentric overload has been recognized in the pathogenesis of rotator cuff injuries in throwing athletes.[66] It is hypothesized that in throwing athletes, weakness and fatigue of the rotator cuff results in overload of the passive restraints. This results in laxity and subluxation of the glenohumeral joint and leads to secondary impingement. Additionally, the rotator cuff muscles are eccentrically overloaded as they attempt to stabilize the head of the humerus in the glenoid cavity. Repetitive eccentric overloading of the rotator cuff results in inflammation and injury to the rotator cuff tendons.

CLINICAL PRESENTATION

History

The majority of patients with rotator cuff pathology are over 40 years of age. Fifty percent of patients will recall a traumatic incident that initiated the symptoms. They usually do not describe a major injury. One can usually elicit a history of recurrent "bursitis" and/or "tendinitis"; these episodes often resolve with rest or other conservative measures. With time, there is increasing shoulder discomfort. This is noted with forward elevation and external rotation of the arm against resistance. Patients may have complaints of nocturnal discomfort, particularly when sleeping on the affected side. With movement, patients may describe crepitus.

Physical Examination

The physical findings may be related to the underlying pathology. Crepitus would relate to the lack of smooth surfaces in the subacromial space. Weakness of flexion, abduction, and external rotation relates to loss of the tendinous attachment to bone. Upward riding of the humeral head on deltoid contraction results from a loss of the depressor action of the rotator cuff, and this further exacerbates impingement and cuff degeneration.

Partial tears of the rotator cuff may cause pain with motion, crepitus, and stiffness. A complete tear may reveal a palpable defect of the cuff. As previously noted, associated tendinitis of the biceps may be present, and this should be documented.

The patient should be examined for impingement signs. Specifically, this includes full forward flexion with pain at terminal motion, otherwise known as the Neer impingement sign. Pain may also be elicited with the Hawkins' test, a provocative test that elicits pain from impingement by bringing the arm into forward flexion, adduction, and internal rotation, thus driving the supraspinatus insertion into the coracoacromial arch and creating pain. The acromioclavicular joint can be stressed with cross-chest adduction. Stability of the biceps tendon should be elicited. Bicipital pathology tests include those of Speed and Yerguson. Speed's test reproduces pain with resisted forward elevation of the humerus against an extended elbow. The pain is localized to the bicipital groove area. Yerguson's test reproduces pain over the bicipital groove with resisted supination of the forearm with a flexed elbow. Muscle strength testing about the shoulder is part of the neurological examination and should be documented.

Differential Diagnosis

When assessing a patient with a suspected tear of the rotator cuff, one should consider other underlying pathologies in the differential diagnosis. These include cuff tendinitis, bursitis, frozen shoulder, cervical spondylosis, suprascapular neuropathy, snapping scapula, acromioclavicular or glenohumeral arthritis, and glenohumeral instability.

Methods of Treatment

Despite rotator cuff pathology, not all patients will be symptomatic, so aggressive treatment is not indicated in an asymptomatic shoulder. In a symptomatic shoulder, the goals of treatment are elimination of pain, restoration of function, and prevention of recurrence or progression.

Nonoperative Treatment

Nonoperative modalities of treatment include physical therapy, rest, elimination of aggravating activities, and administration of antiinflammatory medications and steroid injections. In one study, 44% of the patients with arthrogram-proven rotator cuff tears were shown to respond to nonoperative treatment.[134]

Successful nonoperative management of impingement and rotator cuff injuries requires an understanding of the anatomy and biomechanics of the shoulder girdle and an appreciation of the underlying etiology. Treatment is based on the patient's signs and symptoms at examination. Progression should be based on the response to treatment. General goals for the rehabilitation of an individual with rotator cuff pathology are listed in the box on this page.

Patients with acute signs and symptoms complain of constant pain at rest that is referred distally over the

---

Goals of rotator cuff problems

Control pain
Restore motion
Improve rotator cuff function
Strengthen scapular muscles
Correct posture
Resume function
Prevent recurrence

---

deltoid insertion, and they generally exhibit decreased motion with pain before resistance with passive testing.

During this phase, the focus of treatment is on pain control. This includes the use of relative rest to avoid those activities that aggravate the symptoms. Additionally, the patient is encouraged to position the arm in abduction in the scapular plane. This reduces pain and prevents "wringing out" of the rotator as described earlier. Pain-relieving modalities are used and may include ice, moist heat, and transcutaneous electrical nerve stimulation (TENS). Gentle mobilization and range-of-motion exercises are performed to prevent loss of motion and development of a stiff shoulder.

Patients in the subacute phase have intermittent pain that is more localized to the shoulder. The pain may be aggravated by repeated movements. Motion may be limited and resisted testing may be weak and painful. During this period, treatment continues to consist of relative rest, and modalities can be used to decrease pain and promote healing. The intensity of exercise can be progressed. The focus is on restoration of the normal motion necessary for function of the individual. Full range of motion must be restored, with particular emphasis on restoration of external rotation. External rotation is necessary so that the greater tuberosity can clear the acromion as the arm is elevated overhead. Joint mobilization techniques should be used if glenohumeral mobility is decreased. Often the posterior capsule is tight and requires stretching. Stretching exercises can also be used to increase motion. Joint mobilization should be avoided for patients with hypermobility. For these patients, the focus of treatment should be on the development of dynamic stabilization. This requires strengthening of the rotator cuff as well as proprioceptive exercises to retrain the muscles to dynamically stabilize the glenohumeral joint. Finally, strengthening of the axioscapular muscles (serratus anterior, trapezius) is important to establish normal scapulothoracic motion and decrease the role of scapulothoracic dyskinesia in impingement biomechanics.

Strengthening exercises begin with isometrics with the shoulder positioned in 30 to 45 degrees of abduction in the scapular plane. Active and light progressive resisted exercises are initiated as tolerated. These should specifically strengthen the rotator cuff muscles. Several studies have demonstrated maximum EMG activity in the rotator cuff muscles with a variety of exercises.[18,137] The supraspinatus may be strengthened by performing abduction in the scapular plane with the arm internally rotated, but caution must be taken to avoid further impingement with this exercise. Additionally, the supraspinatus may be strengthened by performing prone horizontal abduction with the arm abducted to 100 degrees in the frontal plane and maximally externally rotated. The infraspinatus may be strengthened by performing prone horizontal abduction with the arm abducted to 90 degrees in the frontal plane and externally rotated. The teres minor may be strengthened by prone external rotation with the arm abducted to 90 degrees. The subscapularis may be strengthened by performing internal rotation with the arm at the side. Both eccentric and concentric phases of the rotator cuff exercises are emphasized. Adding excessive resistance to these exercises should be avoided because it will only result in substitution by larger muscles of the shoulder complex. These exercises must be performed precisely without substitution in order to develop specific muscles of the rotator. Internal and external rotation with the arm at the side of the body will not fully develop the rotator cuff. Strengthening exercises for the scapular muscles should also be included. Particular emphasis should be placed on strengthening the middle and lower trapezius as well as the serratus anterior.

Successful treatment of rotator cuff injuries is dependent on an understanding of the underlying anatomy and biomechanics, as well as an appreciation of the underlying etiology. Treatment must be appropriate for the patient's stage of inflammation. A knowledge of the functional demands placed on the shoulder is also necessary. Signs of overly aggressive treatment must be recognized and include increased pain greater than 2 hours after treatment and/or regression of motion or strength. If the patient's symptoms do not improve after 3 to 6 months, further investigation with imaging modalities as discussed before is indicated. Some would suggest that nonoperative treatment should continue, but only about 50% of such patients will respond.

Operative Treatment

Samilson and Binder[127] outlined the following indications for operative repair: (1) a patient "physiologically" younger than 60 years, (2) a clinically or arthrographically demonstrable full-thickness cuff tear, (3) failure of the patient to improve with nonoperative management for a period not less than 6 weeks, (4) a need to use the involved shoulder in overhead activities in the patient's vocation or avocation, (5) full passive range of motion, (6) a patient's willingness to exchange decreased pain and increased external rotator strength for some loss of active abduction, and (7) the ability and willingness of the patient to cooperate.[127]

Currently, anterior acromioplasty with limited detachment of the deltoid appears to be the most direct, least harmful, and most effective procedure for persistent rotator cuff tendinitis. Ellman[42] has documented an 88% satisfactory result rate in patients who have chronic impingement treated by arthroscopic acromioplasty. Simple debridement of partially torn rotator cuffs has allowed an 85% rate of return to activity in a group of patients treated by Andrews, Broussard, and Carsons.[7]

Recently, Burkhart[26] has published results of arthroscopic treatment of massive rotator cuff tears. He treated 10 patients with painful, massive, complete tears involving primarily the supraspinatus with arthroscopic acromioplasty and rotator cuff debridement. All patients except one had normal preoperative motion and strength. These patients maintained adequate mechanics of the glenohumeral joint during abduction because there is a balance of two important force couples.[112] The first force couple is in the coronal plane and consists of the rotator cuff and deltoid such that the rotator cuff maintains a fixed fulcrum for rotation of the deltoid during abduction. The second force couple acts in the transverse plane and consists of a balance between the anterior and posterior portions of the rotator cuff that allows the humeral head to maintain centering during rotation of the glenohumeral joint. This study showed that normal shoulder function is possible with massive unrepaired rotator cuff pathology.

For the vast majority of cuff tears that come to operative management, an open approach is used. The extent of the rotator cuff tear is ascertained at the time of surgery, and the torn edges of the rotator cuff are identified. The following sequence has been suggested for closure: (1) resection of the bursal scar, (2) identification of the tear, (3) assessment of tissue mobility, (4) mobilization of the rotator cuff, and (5) planning for closure, either side to side or in most cases to a trough in bone.[76] Concomitant acromioplasty is performed in these patients. Recent long-term results of this technique have been reported by Bigliani et al.[17] In patients with an average follow-up of 7 years, 85% had satisfactory results with adequate pain relief, and 92% could raise the arm above the horizontal plane.

Many techniques have been described for massive tears that cannot be treated as just outlined. These options include accepting the defect, moving local tissue into the deficient area, and inserting a free graft of local or distant tissue, that is, either an allograft, xenograft, or prosthetic material.[34] Latissimus dorsi transfer for the treatment of massive tears of the rotator cuff has been described by Gerber et al.[49,51] In cases with good subscapularis function but irreparable defects in the external rotator tendons, restoration of approximately 80% of normal shoulder function was obtained.

Postoperative Care

Postoperative care following surgery on the rotator cuff is dependent on the status of the deltoid, the size of the repair (i.e., small versus massive), the ability to mobilize tissue, and the safe range of motion achieved at surgery. Therefore, postoperative care must be individualized to the patient and the procedure rather than everyone being treated with a standardized protocol.

Immediate postoperative care following rotator cuff surgery should protect the healing structures, control pain, and restore range of motion. For small tears, the arm is generally immobilized at the side for 4 to 6 weeks with a deltoid-splitting technique. Pain-relieving modalities can be used to improve comfort. Passive range-of-motion exercises are begun immediately postoperatively and performed several times per day in the range prescribed by the surgeon. Once sufficient healing has occurred (i.e., at 4 to 6 weeks), active assisted and active range-of-motion exercises can be initiated. Strengthening exercises using isometrics can also be initiated at this time.

Postoperative management following the repair of massive tears in which the deltoid was detached includes immobilization for up to 6 weeks. Generally an abduction pillow is used to reduce tension on the postoperative repair. Modalities are used to control pain as necessary. Passive range of motion is performed for the first 6 weeks. The safe range of motion achieved at surgery must be communicated by the physician to the therapist. Active assisted and active range-of- motion exercises are delayed for 6 weeks to ensure adequate tissue healing. Isometric strengthening exercises are usually delayed until 12 weeks after surgery.

Once sufficient time for healing has passed, the patient is gradually progressed through the rehabilitation program. Initial emphasis is on restoring the motion necessary for normal function of the shoulder complex. Attention is directed at reestablishing normal scapulohumeral rhythm. Additionally, strengthening exercises focus on developing the rotator cuff and scapular muscles. Functional activities are incorporated to allow gradual resumption of function. The patient must be willing to accept some limitation in level of function.

In patients who complain of shoulder pain, pathology of the rotator cuff is important to consider because of the large spectrum of disease from impingement to complete and massive tears of the rotator cuff. Many patients may respond to nonoperative therapy, although slightly fewer than 50% may fall into this group. After careful history taking and physical examination, the majority of patients can initiate a course of nonoperative management. In those patients who do not respond, imaging of the cuff is the next appropriate step in the algorithm. In patients with simple tendinitis or impingement, conservative management is continued. If symptoms persist, acromioplasty, either open or with endoscopic techniques, can be considered. Patients with complete disruption or full-thickness disruption may be candidates for other operative approaches as outlined earlier. The most direct and simple repair technique is often the most appropriate: progression from direct tendon repair, to repair of bone, to transposition of local tissue, to grafting. Postoperative support should vary according to need. Physiotherapy after surgery is a vital part of the treatment protocol.

SHOULDER INSTABILITY

A rational approach to surgical management of instability should be based on an understanding of the definition of successful repair and an appreciation of the reasons for failure. Successful surgery is traditionally defined as elimination of recurrence of instability. According to this definition, up to a 97% rate of excellent results has been reported with a large variety of procedures.*

Both operative and nonoperative treatment must be based on an appreciation of the spectrum of glenohumeral instability. A classification system for shoulder instability should include the following factors: frequency of occurrence, etiology, direction of instability, and degree of instability. One can distinguish between traumatic, recurrent instability and atraumatic, recurrent instability. The former occurs as a result of a single episode of macrotrauma, is usually unilateral, is less responsive to a rehabilitation program, and has the Bankart lesion as the most common primary pathology. The latter may occur as the result of repetitive microtrauma (e.g., swimming or throwing), may be bilateral, is responsive to a therapy program, and has excessive capsular laxity as the most common primary lesion. Voluntary instability is found in a subset of individuals with atraumatic instability. These patients can be further subdivided into two groups. Group I patients with voluntary instability have an arm position–dependent instability that is usually posterior but may be anterior. These patients usually respond to rehabilitation and do not have an underlying psychiatric disturbance. If they remain refractory to conservative treatment, they may be well managed by surgery. Group II patients have the ability to selectively contract muscles to create a dislocation. Some of these individuals have an underlying psychiatric disturbance and use their instability as a trick to control their environment.[123] These individuals are not candidates for surgical treatment and are better managed by psychiatric counseling and conservative rehabilitation.

There is a spectrum of glenohumeral instability in which subluxation and dislocation represent degrees of injury to the capsulolabral structures. Dislocation is defined as complete separation of the articular surfaces, and subluxation represents increased humeral head translation within the glenoid to a degree beyond normal tissue laxity. Because the parameters of normal glenohumeral translation have not yet been fully defined,[128] clinical subluxation is defined as detectable glenohumeral translation with accompanying symptoms. The increased use of arthroscopy has led to the characterization of an additional group within this spectrum of instability. This group appears to be throwing athletes in whom symptomatic labral tears or attrition

*References 1, 2, 6, 14, 22, 23, 29, 40, 44, 67, 78-81, 83, 84, 90, 93, 100, 103, 116, 122, 130, 135

develops secondary to increased glenohumeral translation without clinical subluxation.[4,5,9]

Appreciation of the direction of instability is critical to selection of a successful approach to treatment. Traditionally, 95% of all instability has been observed to be simple anterior instability; however, there has been increasing recognition of significant posterior instability in athletes who are loose-jointed individuals.[8,48] Posterior instability is usually subluxation inasmuch as dislocation occurs only with rarer, traumatic episodes.[48] Since Neer and Foster's paper[103] on multidirectional instability (MDI), there has been an increasing awareness of both atraumatic and traumatic capsular laxity occurring in more than one direction. The main direction of instability is usually anterior, although inferior instability appears to be the hallmark of this diagnosis.[6,36,46,100,103] Traditional procedures that treat anterior capsular laxity by Bankart repair or capsular plication will not adequately manage the associated components of inferior and/or posterior instability. In the worst scenario, these procedures can actually lead to instability in the opposite direction.

Failure of the operative approach may occur at any point in the course of treatment and may be due to either physician or patient error or a combination of the two. For a successful outcome, the diagnosis, surgical procedure, and rehabilitation must be individualized and appropriate in each case.

A correct diagnosis is critical in categorizing the instability and recommending the appropriate form of treatment. For example, a misdiagnosis of impingement or failure to recognize a concomitant rotator cuff tear in a patient over the age of 50 may lead to failure despite a technically adequate anterior stabilization procedure. Additionally, a Bankart procedure that ignores the inferior component of capsular laxity in a patient with MDI will fail.

Assuming a correct diagnosis, a variety of technical pitfalls are encountered with each type of stabilization procedure. Appropriate anterior capsular tension must be restored, and procedures that overtighten the anterior capsule or subscapularis tendon may result in serious functional limitation of external rotation. In some cases this may lead to osteoarthritis or exacerbation of posterior instability in patients with unrecognized MDI.[57,149]

Knowledge of the regional anatomy or an inadequate exposure will predispose to an inadequate repair and possible neurovascular injury.[117] Assuming the correct diagnosis and correct procedure, the failure of patient compliance or inappropriate rehabilitation may result in limited range of motion or recurrence of instability.

To avoid complications of treatment, it is critical to be both sensitive and specific in the initial diagnostic assessment of the individual's shoulder complaints. Both the degree and direction of any instability must be accurately determined, and any associated fractures, neurovascular injury, or concomitant rotator cuff pathology must be identified.

IMPINGEMENT SYNDROME

Impingement syndrome may occur either as an isolated entity or in combination with instability.[57,146] Hawkins and Hawkins[57] identified several patients whose untreated impingement syndrome was the cause of their ongoing pain after anterior shoulder stabilization. This should not be confused with the common finding in patients with anterior instability of pain located posteriorly in combination with clinical findings consistent with impingement syndrome.[58,140] This impingement pain is likely a secondary phenomenon related to repetitive traction and compression of the rotator cuff during subluxation or to overwork of the rotator cuff muscles in an attempt to maintain the humeral head centered in the glenoid in the setting of capsular insufficiency. Jobe et al[67,126] described this overlap in the literature, and Altchek et al[6] observed a 20% incidence of impingement symptoms in individuals with surgically confirmed anterior-inferior MDI.

In most cases it is possible to correctly diagnose impingement syndrome from the history and examination; however, if this evaluation is inconclusive, examination under anesthesia (EUA) and arthroscopic inspection will assist in clarification of the diagnosis.

Anterior shoulder instability in a patient older than 40 years of age is a unique situation that deserves special consideration if complications and failure of treatment are to be avoided. The association of concomitant anterior shoulder dislocation and rotator cuff tear has been reported by numerous orthopaedic surgeons.* This concomitant injury may be missed if one is not attentive. Moreover, there is an increased risk for adhesive capsulitis in this older group of patients if early range of motion is not begun following reduction of a dislocation.

The incidence of an associated rotator cuff tear in this group has been reported to be as high as 70% to 90%.[60,87,88] Most recently, Neviaser et al[105] and Hawkins et al[60] have increased our understanding of this problem. Anterior dislocation in an older individual may result in disruption of a rotator cuff that has undergone age-related attrition. The anterior capsulolabral structures are spared.[60,115] McLaughlin[85] and subsequently Craig[37] have termed this the "posterior mechanism" of anterior shoulder instability.

In older patients with persistent external rotation and abduction weakness following the reduction of an anterior dislocation, physicians should avoid the trap of assuming an axillary nerve injury as the etiology.[37,105] The overall incidence of clinically significant axillary nerve injury in this setting has been reported to be in the range of 9% to 18%.[19,118] Neviaser et al observed an incidence of 7.8% for axillary nerve injury in association with rotator cuff tear after anterior dislocation. A suprascapular nerve injury is rare in the setting of anterior dislocation.[37]

*References 32, 59, 86, 87, 88, 105, 133.

In general, older patients have a lower rate of recurrence of instability after an initial episode of anterior instability.[124] This is particularly true if there is an associated fracture of the greater tuberosity that reduces the range of motion of the joint and muscle strength.[88,118] In older patients with an unrecognized rotator cuff tear, pain and weakness appear to be more common problems than recurrent instability.[60,105]

In a separate group of older patients, recurrent anterior shoulder instability develops as the result of an excessively redundant anterior capsule and no rotator cuff tear.[72] These individuals typically demonstrate the stigmata of generalized ligamentous laxity, including thumb to forearm; hyperextension of the elbow, knee, and metacarpal joints; a history of easy bruising, hernias, and scar spreading; and excessive skin laxity. These features should be documented during the examination.

An approach to treating older individuals (>45 years) following an initial shoulder dislocation is based on classifying such patients into three groups:

Group I: If after reduction no significant weakness of external rotation or abduction is found, immobilization should be continued no longer than 7 to 10 days. A gentle range-of-motion program should begin and progressive supervised therapy should follow. Failure to move the shoulder early in these patients can result in marked limitation of motion.

Group II: Patients with persistent pain and external rotation and abduction weakness will likely have an associated rotator cuff tear. Early arthrography and EMG should be performed to confirm this fact and to rule out any associated axillary nerve injury. Conservative treatment in this setting will usually result in a poor outcome.[57] Early repair of the rotator cuff generally yields good results, and surgery performed after a delay in diagnosis may be fraught with difficulty because the cuff tissues may become extensively scarred and difficult to mobilize.[60,105] If the patient does have an associated axillary nerve injury, we would still perform an early repair of the cuff, although final function will likely be determined by return of axillary nerve function.

Group III: Recurrent instability in older patients may be due to either a rotator cuff tear or excessive capsular laxity.[60,72,105] Labral lesions may occur but are less common in this group. Examination will usually reveal those patients with generalized ligamentous laxity, but an arthrogram is essential to clarify the status of the rotator cuff. It is prudent to know the pathology before surgery is attempted because most cuff pathology is best treated through an anterior superior approach with an acromioplasty whereas anterior capsulolabral pathology is managed through a deltopectoral interval approach. It should be noted that Neviaser et al[105] observed a significant subscapularis tear in all cases of recurrent instability.

Fracture of the greater tuberosity, the second most common associated fracture after the Hill-Sachs lesion,

occurs in about 10% of all anterior dislocations.[85] In most cases this fracture reduces anatomically with reduction of the glenohumeral joint and recurrence of shoulder instability is actually less than if no fracture were present.[85] Displacement of the greater tuberosity fragment more than 1 cm may result in residual impingement and blocked external rotation. In these cases, surgical reduction and fixation may be necessary.

A glenoid rim fracture may occur with anterior dislocation and continued displacement of the anterior glenoid articular surface of greater than 25% to 35% will result in recurrent instability.[11,75,120] Computed tomography (CT) will demonstrate this clearly, and surgical reduction and fixation may be necessary if residual displacement is greater than 2 mm.

The axillary nerve is the most commonly injured neurovascular structure, with the reported incidence ranging from 5% to 33% in first-time dislocators.[19,122] Both a motor and sensory examination should be performed before and after any reduction maneuver because complete motor paralysis may occur without any detectable hypoesthesia. Any residual neurological deficit persisting longer than 3 to 4 weeks should be evaluated by EMG.[19] Most patients spontaneously recover over a 6-week period inasmuch as the majority of these injuries are neuropraxic in nature.

The axillary artery is occasionally damaged with anterior dislocation because it is relatively fixed as it passes beneath the pectoralis minor and over the subscapularis.[38,68,85,118] This is particularly the case in older individuals, in whom atherosclerosis may render the vessels less compliant to displacement. Clinical findings include severe pain, expanding hematoma, and diminished peripheral pulses; an arteriogram should be performed urgently in such cases because timely repair is crucial to a successful outcome.

Failure to recognize the voluntary aspect of a patient's instability may result in the failure of any procedure for recurrent instability. Rowe, Pierce, and Clark[123] described a typical patient in this group as an adolescent with an underlying psychiatric problem, without any prior history of significant trauma, who can voluntarily dislocate his shoulder and who has essentially normal radiographic findings. As already noted, group I patients are typically emotionally stable individuals with positional instability.[48] Group I patients represent a subset of atraumatic, voluntary instability, and if they fail to respond to conservative management, an operative procedure that reduces the excessive capsular laxity is a reasonable alternative. It is crucial to sort out this group from those in group II, who have a muscular-control type of voluntary instability that may be used as a trick to control the environment. These individuals are managed by psychiatric counseling and rotator cuff strengthening exercises.

The spectrum of MDI includes those individuals with excessive ligamentous laxity (atraumatic type), those with instability resulting from repetitive overhead activities with extremes of motion (microtrauma type), and those with instability following violent trauma (macrotrauma type).[6,132]

Recognition of MDI is critical because traditional stabilization procedures such as the Bankart or Bristow operations will fail to adequately address the inferior component of instability.* Moreover, too tight an anterior repair in this setting may actually aggravate the posterior component of MDI.[58,149]

The diagnosis of MDI is based on the history as well as the classic finding of a significant "sulcus sign." In addition, 50% of these individuals will usually have stigmata of generalized ligamentous laxity.

Up to 50% to 70% of these individuals will respond well to a rehabilitation program aimed at rotator cuff strengthening if it is coordinated with activity modification. This is in contrast to young individuals with posttraumatic, unidirectional, anterior recurrent instability, who often require surgery.[27]

Missed, unreduced anterior dislocation may occur in elderly patients, individuals with substance abuse, individuals with seizure disorders, and unconscious, multiply injured patients.[55,125] Unlike missed posterior dislocations that go unrecognized because of a failure to perform an adequate radiograph, missed anterior dislocations are usually due to a failure to perform any radiograph.[55] The chronicity of the dislocation must be established. If an anterior dislocation is less than 6 weeks old and no concomitant osteoporosis or history of steroid use is present, an attempt at mild, gentle closed reduction may be made under general anesthesia.[55] In cases with chronic, unreduced dislocations older than 6 weeks, open reduction and stabilization are recommended. In these cases, an axillary radiograph will confirm the diagnosis; however, CT will give valuable information about the status of the humeral head and glenoid. It is helpful to have this information before surgery because significant bone loss of the anterior glenoid or posterolateral humeral head may necessitate supplemental bone grafting. In older individuals, an arthrogram may also be appropriate to rule out an associated cuff injury.

An anterior surgical approach through the deltopectoral interval is recommended. If necessary for exposure, the superior 1 cm of the pectoralis major insertion may be detached. The anterior 1 cm of the conjoined tendon insertion at the level of the coracoid process can be divided. The subscapularis is usually contracted and fibrotic along with the capsule and rotator cuff, and the axillary nerve may be stretched tightly across the anterior glenohumeral joint. This must be kept in mind during release of these tight anterior structures. Following release of the subscapularis and capsule, it is often necessary to remove granulation tissue within the joint before the humeral head is reduced. Following reduction and repair of the capsule, early motion is preferred rather than spica immobilization advocated by some surgeons.[55] Management of glenoid bone deficiency and large Hill-Sachs lesions is discussed later.

*References 6, 46, 50, 83, 100, 103, 113, 118, 119, 132.

In cases in which the dislocation is older than 1 year or when the Hill-Sachs lesion is larger than 50% of the articular surface, the humeral head may no longer be viable and a hemiarthroplasty may be the best alternative treatment. In these cases, placement of the prosthesis in greater than the normal retroversion of 30 degrees (50 to 60 degrees) will help prevent recurrence of anterior instability.

Although most procedures have a success rate in excess of 95% in providing stability to the shoulder, no single surgical technique is perfect. In general, procedures that do not address specific pathology should not be employed in the primary surgery setting. An individualized approach to each situation is recommended, because a variety of pathological lesions may be present in different patients.

The optimum technique, as defined by Cofield, Kavanaugh, and Frassica,[35] would be one with the following characteristics: low recurrence rate, low complication rate, low reoperation rate, low rate of osteoarthritis (uses no hardware), no limitation of motion, anatomic treatment of pathology, and no technical difficulty. Because no one procedure satisfies all these criteria, we will present specific pitfalls and their management for a variety of common anterior stabilization techniques.

EXAMINATION UNDER ANESTHESIA AND DIAGNOSTIC ARTHROSCOPY

It is essential to confirm both the direction and the degree of instability by EUA before any surgical procedure. This will aid in the decision of which operative approach and procedure to use. One should perform a drawer test on the shoulder to assess the amount of anterior, posterior, and inferior translation of the humeral head in the glenoid. Anterior and posterior translation is assessed with the shoulder at 90 degrees' abduction and neutral rotation and is graded on a scale of +1 to +3 (+1 is movement of the humeral head to the rim but not over it, +2 represents humeral head dislocation over the glenoid rim with spontaneous reduction when pressure is released, and +3 is frank dislocation of the humeral head that does not reduce spontaneously).[6] One should not be surprised to find increased posterior translation along with anterior translation when a patient with suspected anterior instability is examined because injury to the ligaments on both sides of the joint may occur with an anterior dislocation.[107,128]

Inferior instability is assessed by the presence of a "sulcus sign." This test is performed with downward traction on the adducted arm, and the degree of acromiohumeral interval separation is noted.[140] The "sulcus sign" is graded on a scale of +1 to +3 (+1 is 0 to 1 cm, +2 is 1 to 2 cm, +3 is greater than 2 cm).[6] Arthroscopic inspection may occasionally be useful in these patients, although office examination, history, and an EUA usually confirm the diagnosis. Most labral lesions below the equator of the glenoid are associated with a deficient inferior glenohumeral labrum.

SURGICAL PROCEDURES FOR INSTABILITY

The classic Bankart procedure[13,111] and its modifications[67,122,135] anatomically repair a detached glenoid labrum together with the inferior and middle glenohumeral ligaments.

Several variations in handling of the subscapularis deserve mention. Thomas and Matsen[135] have described a technique first proposed by Ellison. The subscapularis and capsule are both divided laterally, with medial retraction allowing repair of the Bankart lesion with the joint in an inside-out fashion. This approach is useful in revision cases in which extensive scarring is found medially at the glenoid.

Jobe and Glousman[67] have recommended longitudinal division of the subscapularis muscle with preservation of its lateral insertion on the lesser tuberosity. This approach is designed to minimize scarring and shortening of the muscle in a throwing athlete. Several potential problems with this approach include limited inferior exposure in cases in which a capsular shift might be necessary and the potential for injury to the axillary nerve and brachial plexus if longitudinal splitting is carried too far medially.

To repair the Bankart lesion once the sutures are well placed through the bony anterior glenoid rim, the lateral capsule is repaired to the rim. A potential error here is to not address any concomitant capsular laxity. The standard Bankart procedure handles capsular laxity by placing the sutures more laterally through the lateral capsular flap. The T-plasty repair pulls the inferior portion of the capsule superiorly before placement of the sutures through the capsule.

The inferior capsular shift procedure as originally described by Neer and Foster[103] is designed to treat excessive capsular laxity occurring with MDI. It has been used successfully and involves detachment of the capsule laterally along its humeral attachment with a superior-lateral shaft of the inferior flap and then an inferior-lateral shift of the superior flap.[39,46] Repair of an associated Bankart lesion is performed first, and failure to address this lesion has been associated with failure of the procedure.[81] Inferior detachment of the capsule laterally along the humeral neck probably involves less risk to the axillary nerve than does a medial paraglenoid capsulotomy incision; however, there is still significant risk with inferior dissection, and Neer[100] observed three cases of axillary nerve neuropraxia early in his experience. To avoid this potential complication, the inferior flap should be developed by placing stay sutures in the capsule and pulling superiorly while applying progressive external rotation. An elevator is placed inferiorly and used to remove any muscle from the capsule before its division. If the axillary nerve cannot be palpated and its exact location is not precisely known, it should be visualized before division of the inferior capsule.

A T-plasty procedure can be performed to manage capsular laxity and concomitant labral detachment simultaneously.[6] The basic goal of the T-plasty is to restore proper tension in the inferior glenohumeral ligament by advancing this structure superiorly and medially. At completion of the capsular repair, external rotation with the arm at the side should be in the range of 35 to 45 degrees without undue tension on the repair.

The Bristow procedure and its modifications basically involve fixation of the coracoid process and attached conjoined tendon to the scapular neck through a split in the subscapularis tendon.* The procedure theoretically functions by provision of an anterior bone block, formation of a dynamic musculotendinous sling, and partial tenodesis of the inferior third of the subscapularis tendon. It does not directly address pathological lesions such as labral detachment or capsular laxity.

Although the Bristow procedure has a success rate comparable to that of other procedures, it is generally accepted to be a poor alternative for stabilization in athletes involved in overhead sports, because it may limit external rotation.[14,61,79,80] The orthopaedic literature has documented a high incidence of complications with this procedure.[10,12,43,149]

The major risk with the Bristow procedure is injury to the musculocutaneous nerve (MCN).[12,15,45,117,149] This complication is usually due to inadequate knowledge of variations in regional anatomy or poor surgical technique.[117] Significant variations in anatomy of the conjoined tendon and MCN may be encountered.[45,117] The MCN, in most cases, enters the coracobrachialis muscle at a distance of 5 or more cm distal to the coracoid process; however, in 5% of cases it may also be as close as 2.5 cm from the tip of the coracoid.[12,45,117] If the nerve is observed to enter the muscle at 2.5 cm or closer to the coracoid process, the Bristow procedure should not be performed. Finally, staple fixation may impinge or rupture the biceps tendon with improper placement.

The Putti-Platt procedure treats anterior instability by shortening the subscapularis in a "vest-over-pants" technique to limit external rotation.[23,62,78,108] The subscapularis is detached 2.5 mm medial to its insertion, and the capsule and subscapularis are then sutured to the glenoid rim with the arm in internal rotation. The main complication of this procedure is loss of function from excessive limitation of external rotation, and in the extreme case, this may result in secondary glenohumeral arthritis caused by excessive constraining forces on the articular surfaces.[56] Instability may also result if the patient has unrecognized MDI.[57]

In the duToit capsulorraphy procedure, a staple is used to effect a Bankart-type repair, and complications stem from problems with staple fixation and placement.[21,41,130] Injury to the articular surface and loosening of the staple have been reported.[150] Metal devices are mentioned here for their historical role in the development of arthroscopic Bankart repairs.

---

*References 2, 3, 10, 14, 22, 29, 30, 40, 44, 53, 61, 63, 64, 77, 79, 80, 82, 89, 106, 129, 136.

The enthusiasm for arthroscopic stabilization of anterior shoulder instability is based on the assumption that limited disruption of the anterior soft tissues will result in a better functional outcome. This is particularly relevant to young throwing athletes who require full external rotation and power. Although short-term studies are encouraging, long-term data supporting this assumption are not available.

The technique, which was originally popularized by Johnson,[69] uses a dual-pronged staple and attempts to reproduce the duToit capsular staple–Bankart repair arthroscopically.[4,41,140] Since then, modified techniques have included the use of a removable rivet,[144] modified staple capsulorrhaphy,[52] cannulated screw and ligament washers,[148] and suture Bankart repair.[4,31,91,92]

The ideal patient is an individual with posttraumatic, recurrent anterior unidirectional instability with labral detachment below the level of the equator of the glenoid. Patients with MDI are not candidates for this procedure. Routine examination of patients under anesthesia is performed before the procedure. Individuals with a significant sulcus sign are treated with an open capsular procedure.

One can use a suture technique in which absorbable sutures are placed through the inferior glenohumeral ligament and a Bankart repair is achieved through transscapular drill holes.[4,31,91,92] Drill holes are placed above the equator on the anterior scapular neck to allow restoration of tension in the inferior glenohumeral ligament as it is pulled superiorly and medially with the repair. More recently, the use of a biodegradable cannulated tack to avoid problems associated with hardware or drilling across the scapula has been discussed.[139]

No matter what form of fixation is used, it is essential to adequately prepare the anterior scapular neck to ensure a bleeding bony bed for the repair. When a motorized burr is used, care should be taken not to slip over the glenoid rim and injure the articular surface. Injury to the suprascapular nerve is a theoretical risk with pin placement through the scapula. Excessive lateral penetration of the pins should be avoided.[92]

In conclusion, many pitfalls and complications are potentially encountered in surgery for shoulder instability. The shoulder surgeon must have an organized approach to diagnosis and treatment. If surgery is contemplated, the procedure must be tailored to the individual patient and must deal with the underlying pathology.

FRACTURES AND DISLOCATIONS ABOUT THE SHOULDER

Fractures and dislocations about the shoulder are very common injuries. These injuries are best classified by anatomic location for the purpose of discussion. Shoulder girdle injuries are located at the sternoclavicular joint, clavicle, acromioclavicular joint, proximal end of the humerus, and scapula. An associated neurovascular injury may or may not be present.

Sternoclavicular Joint

Most often sternoclavicular dislocations do not cause any significant functional disability.[25] An anterior dislocation is usually asymptomatic and does not require any treatment. Posttraumatic ankylosis of the sternoclavicular joint can cause pain and disability. Compression of the mediastinal structures can occur with posterior dislocations of the sternoclavicular joint. In general, anterior injuries can be treated conservatively and posterior injuries may require some intervention.

Surgical management of chronic sternoclavicular dislocations may include soft tissue reconstruction, arthrodesis, resection of the medial aspect of the clavicle, and resection combined with costoclavicular ligament reconstruction.

Clavicle

Clavicular fractures account for greater than 60% of shoulder girdle fractures. The middle third of the clavicle is involved in 82% and the distal third in 15%.[121] Nonunion of the clavicle is relatively uncommon and reported in 1.8% of those patients treated nonoperatively.[121] If a nonunion does occur, most often it is minimally symptomatic. One study has determined that atrophic nonunions are less likely to become symptomatic than are hypertrophic nonunions.[145] In a study by Johnson and Collins,[68] 26 clavicular nonunions treated nonoperatively resulted in 23 excellent results, 2 good results, and 1 poor result. Rowe[121] has noted spontaneous uniting of apparent nonunions as long as 5 months from the time of injury. Only patients with significantly symptomatic nonunions and malunions should be offered reconstructive surgery.

Malunion of the middle third of the clavicle, if symptomatic, can be managed with osteotomy and bone grafting. This is supplemented with internal fixation. Nonunions can be managed by excision of the pseudoarthrosis, reduction, bone grafting, and internal fixation with promising results.[71,101] Distal clavicular nonunions, which can result after type II distal clavicle fractures, have been treated by excision of the distal fragment and/or open reduction and internal fixation. The results of excision cannot be recommended.[68] Neer[98] has documented some success with transacromial wire fixation. The fixation is removed after union has occurred.

Acromioclavicular Joint

Of shoulder girdle dislocations, 9% involve the acromioclavicular joint. Fifty percent are complete grade III or higher dislocations with disruption of the conoid and trapezoid components of the coracoclavicular ligaments.[121]

The majority of acute acromioclavicular injuries can be treated nonoperatively: application of ice over the first 24 hours, possibly a sling for comfort, and resumption of activity at approximately 1 week if tolerated. Posterior displacement of the clavicle is uncommon and may require surgery to reduce the clavicle. It may be wedged into the angle between the acromion and the spine of the scapula. One may attempt a closed reduction by displacing the shoulder posteriorly to widen the distance between the acromion and sternum.

Treatment of injuries that involve complete separation of the acromion and clavicle is controversial. Some have attempted closed reduction with pressure by tape or a splint, but significant problems with the skin have been noted when these techniques are used.

Surgery for acute grade III lesions has included many techniques:[96] direct acromioclavicular joint stabilization with ligament repair; clavicle stabilization by attachment to the coracoid, as with a Bosworth screw, wire, Dacron tape,[54] silk sutures, or absorbable suture; and resection of the outer end of the clavicle and coracoclavicular ligament stabilization with the coracoacromial ligament.[141]

The majority of patients with chronic acromioclavicular subluxations or dislocations are asymptomatic or minimally symptomatic and respond well to nonoperative management. Occasionally, acromioclavicular subluxations become symptomatic.[99] Degenerative joint disease or osteolysis of the distal end of the clavicle may develop. These problems can be assessed with an acromioclavicular view on plain radiographs and by injection with local anesthetic to confirm the diagnosis with pain relief.

Proximal Humerus Fracture Dislocations

The classification of proximal humeral fractures is based on the absence or displacement of each of four major segments: the humeral head, the greater and lesser tuberosities, and the humeral shaft. The Neer classification is most commonly used and considers the segment displaced if there is greater than 45 degrees of angulation or 1 cm of displacement. It should be noted that all patients with a suspected fracture of the proximal end of the humerus require a shoulder trauma series of radiographs. This includes anteroposterior, lateral, and axillary views. The treating physician must exclude concomitant dislocation of the humeral head. A complete vascular and neurologic examination must be performed and documented.

Treatment considerations include the patient's age, functional demands, dominance, expectations, anticipated compliance, degree of segment displacement, and bone quality. The majority of these fractures can be managed with protective immobilization and early range of motion. This is, of course, based on the aforementioned factors and includes fracture stability. In a prospective randomized study of proximal humerus fractures (minimally displaced), Kristiansen, Angermann, and Larsen[74] compared 1 and 3 weeks of immobilization before starting physical therapy. Shorter immobilization resulted in better functional results during the first 3 months. After 6 months, the results in both groups were essentially the same.

Fractures that are more significantly displaced require reduction. This can be accomplished by closed means or with open reduction and internal fixation. Occasionally, prosthetic replacement is preferred. Available internal fixation includes tension band wires, screws, percutaneous pins, plates and screws, and intramedullary nailing.

Two-part lesser tuberosity fractures are often associated with posterior glenohumeral dislocation. Smaller fragments can be treated nonoperatively: larger fragments may require open reduction and internal fixation. Two-part greater tuberosity fractures may include a tear of the rotator cuff. This will require open reduction and internal fixation with either a tension band wire or screw and repair of the rotator cuff tear. Two-part fractures of the anatomic neck are uncommon and carry a significant risk of osteonecrosis. Flatow, Bigliani, and April[45] published a series of 12 two-part greater tuberosity fractures that were treated surgically by open reduction and internal fixation with a heavy nonabsorbable suture and careful repair of the rotator cuff. All fractures healed, and early range of motion resulted in good or excellent results in all patients.

Two-part surgical neck fractures can be either impacted or completely displaced and unstable. Options for treatment include closed reduction, with or without percutaneous pinning, or open reduction and internal fixation. Kowalkowski and Wallace[73] published a series of 22 displaced fractures treated with closed percutaneous Kirshner wire stabilization of the surgical neck. Significant problems in obtaining adequate reduction as well as migration of the smooth pins were encountered. Unsatisfactory results were more common in the older age group (greater than 50 years old).

In three-part fractures, closed reduction is often difficult to maintain and therefore open reduction is required. Tension-band wiring can often be used because it incorporates the rotator cuff in the repair. If the fracture is severely comminuted or the bone osteoporotic, a hemiarthroplasty can be considered, especially in elderly patients.

In young patients with a four-part proximal humerus fracture, an attempt at open reduction and internal fixation is considered despite the high risk of osteonecrosis. If reconstruction is not possible or the patient is elderly and has poor bone stock, a hemiarthroplasty is preferred.

As discussed earlier, it is important to eliminate the presence of concomitant dislocation of the humeral head. Isolated dislocations without fracture can be seen. Many posterior dislocations of the humeral head are missed and recur chronically. These patients most often complain of decreased range of motion. They may or may not complain of pain. Articular impression fractures can often best be imaged with CT scanning. In general, closed reduction can be considered if the injury is less than 6 weeks old; after 6 weeks, open reduction is required. Treatment of the articular impression defect is based on the percentage of head involvement. If the defect is less than 20%, it will generally be stable after a period of immobilization. If the defect is between 20% and 40%, a transfer procedure into the defect may be required, as well as possibly a subscapularis transfer for posterior dislocations or infraspinatus transfer for anterior dislocations. A hemiarthroplasty may be used if the defect is greater than 40% of the head or if significant degenerative changes are present.

Frozen Shoulder

Frozen shoulder—also termed *adhesive capsulitis*—has many underlying causes. It can be seen in association with other shoulder pathologies, for example, posttraumatic, postsurgical, and rotator cuff pathology. It is also associated with other disease entities, including insulin-dependent diabetes mellitus, parkinsonism, cardiovascular disease, and thyroid disease.

Most patients have an insidious onset of pain and stiffness. The vast majority of patients demonstrate a gradual decrease in pain and return of motion over time. There may be improvement for up to 18 months. Treatment consists of gentle physical therapy, antiinflammatory medication, and occasional use of cortisone injections intraarticularly and subacromially. If the patient does not respond after 6 months, consideration may be given to manipulation under anesthesia. More recently, arthroscopic release and debridement have been proposed.[143] Open surgical release is rarely indicated and may in fact worsen the problem. Ozaki et al,[109] however, reported on 17 patients treated surgically for recalcitrant adhesive capsulitis. These patients showed significant contracture of the coracohumeral ligament and rotator interval. Resection of these structures relieved pain and restored motion.

DEGENERATIVE JOINT DISEASE OF THE SHOULDER

Degenerative joint disease of the shoulder can occur secondary to a number of different underlying pathologic conditions. The glenohumeral joint requires prosthetic replacement less often than other major joints. Osteoarthritis of the glenohumeral joint is uncommon, and patients with rheumatoid arthritis can most often be managed nonoperatively with regard to the shoulder. Degenerative joint disease may develop after fracture of

the proximal humerus and subsequently require treatment. In rare cases, proximal humerus fractures may necessitate prosthetic replacement.

Any of the aforementioned pathological entities may be an indication for shoulder replacement. It is, however, most useful for diseases in which the proximal humeral subchondral bone has become distorted and the articular surface destroyed. All patients should pursue a nonoperative course of management initially. Should symptoms persist or progress symptomatically, surgical intervention can be contemplated.

Although shoulder prosthetic systems have improved, the patient may be a candidate for arthrodesis. This can be considered in a younger, active patient with degenerative arthritis, joint sepsis, or loss of deltoid and rotator cuff function or as a salvage procedure following failed total-joint arthroplasty.

The humeral component is designed to preserve metaphyseal bone stock and provide adequate fixation. The glenoid component is often not required, particularly if the rotator cuff is intact or repairable. Hemiarthroplasty is usually considered in younger patients with osteoarthritis, posttraumatic conditions without glenoid loss, rotator cuff pathology, or osteonecrosis. In many patients with more extensive osteoarthritis and rheumatoid arthritis involvement, glenoid resurfacing has improved pain relief. The glenoid most commonly is cemented into position. In younger patients with good bone stock, consideration is given to uncemented glenoid fixation with bone ingrowth. Recent results of survivorship analysis have predicted a 27% failure rate.[24] Other studies have reported excellent pain relief with total-shoulder arthroplasty.[47,142]

CONCLUSION

In attempting to treat the myriad of shoulder problems, the orthopaedist must first make an accurate diagnosis. The goals of treatment include controlling symptoms, improving function, and preventing recurrence, if possible. A systematic approach to management includes appropriate conservative modalities and surgical intervention, if necessary. Future concerns must address cost-effectiveness, standards of care, and outcome research.

References

1. Aamouth GM, O'Phelan EH: Recurrent anterior dislocation of the shoulder: a review of 40 athletes treated by subscapularis transfer (modified Magnusson-Stack procedure), *Am J Sports Med,* 5:188-190, 1977.

2. Akermak C et al: Results of of the Bristow repair: sports participation after surgery. In Bayley I, Kessel L, editors: *Shoulder surgery,* Berlin, 1982, Springer-Verlag; pp. 92-94.

3. Allman F et al: Symposium on sports injuries to the shoulder, *Contemp Surg* 7(3):70-109, 1975.

4. Altchek DW, Skyhar MJ, Warren RF: Shoulder arthroscopy for shoulder instability, *Instr Course Lect* 36:187-198, 1989.

5. Altchek DW et al: Arthroscopic labral debridement. A three year follow-up study, *Am J Sports Med* 20:702-706, 1992.

6. Altchek DW et al: T-plasty anterior repair for anterior and inferior instability of the shoulder, *J Bone Joint Surg* 73A:105-111, 1991.

7. Andrews JR, Broussard TS, Carson WG: Arthroscopy of the shoulder in management of partial tears of the rotator cuff: a preliminary report, *Arthroscopy* 1(2):117-122, 1985.

8. Andrews JR, Carson WG: The arthroscopic treatment of glenoid labrum tears in the throwing athlete, *Orthop Trans* 8:44, 1984.

9. Andrews JR, Carson WG Jr, Mcleod WD: Glenoid labrum tears related to the long head of the biceps, *Am J Sports Med* 13:337-341, 1985.

10. Artz T, Huffer JM: A major complication of the modified Bristow procedure for recurrent dislocation of the shoulder, *J Bone Joint Surg* 54A:1293-1296, 1972.

11. Aston JW, Gregory CF: Dislocation of the shoulder with significant fracture of the glenoid, *J Bone Joint Surg* 55A:1531-1533, 1973.

12. Bach BR et al: An unusual neurological complication of the Bristow procedure: a case report, *J Bone Joint Surg* 70A:458-460, 1988.

13. Bankart ASB: The pathology and treatment of recurrent dislocation of the shoulder joint, *Br J Surg* 26:23-29, 1938.

14. Barry TP et al: The coracoid transfer for recurrent anterior instability of the shoulder in the adolescent, *J Bone Joint Surg* 67A:383-386, 1985.

15. Bigliani LU, McCann PD, Dalsey RM: *An anatomic study of the suprascapular nerve.* Presented at the annual meeting of the American Shoulder and Elbow Surgeons, Las Vegas, Feb 12, 1989.

16. Bigliani LU, Morrison DS, April EW: The morphology of the acromion and its relationship to rotator cuff tears, *Orthop Trans* 10:216, 1986.

17. Bigliani LU et al: Operative repair of massive rotator cuff tears: long term results, *J Shoulder Elbow Surg* 1(3):120-130, 1992.

18. Blackburn TA et al: EMG analysis of posterior rotator cuff exercises, *J Natl Athl Train Assoc* 25:40-45, 1990.

19. Blom S, Dahlback L: Nerve injuries in dislocation of the shoulder joint and fractures of the neck of the humerus, *Acta Chir Scand* 136:461-466, 1970.

20. Reference deleted in proofs.

21. Boyd HB, Hunt HL: Recurrent dislocation of the shoulder. The staple capsulorrhaphy, *J Bone Joint Surg Am* 47A:1514-1520, 1965.

22. Braley WG, Tullos HS: A modification of the Bristow procedure for recurrent dislocation of the shoulder, *Am J Sports Med* 13(2):81-86, 1985.

23. Brav EA: An evaluation of the Putti-Platt reconstruction procedure for recurrent dislocation of the shoulder, *J Bone Joint Surg* 37A:731-741, 1955.

24. Brenner BC et al: Survivorship of unconstrained total shoulder arthroplasty, *J Bone Joint Surg* 71A:1289-1296, 1989.

25. Brown JE: Sternoclavicular dislocation, *Am J Orthop* 3:134, 1961.

26. Burkhart SS: Arthroscopic treatment of massive rotator cuff tears, *Clin Orthop* 267:45-56, 1991.

27. Burkhead WZ, Rockwoood CA Jr: Treatment of instability of the shoulder with an exercise program, *J Bone Joint Surg* 74A:890-896, 1992.

28. Cain PR et al: Anterior stability of the glenohumeral joint: a dynamic model, *Am J Sport Med* 15:144-148, 1987.

29. Cameron JC, Hall M, Courtney BC: The Bristow procedure for recurrent anterior dislocation of the shoulder, *J Bone Joint Surg* 67B:327, 1985.

30. Carol EJ et al: Bristow-Latarjet the repair for recurrent anterior shoulder instability: an eight year study, *Neth J Surg* 37(4):109-111, 1985.

31. Caspary RB: Arthroscopic reconstruction for anterior shoulder instability, *Techniques Orthop* 3(1):59-66, 1988.

32. Codman EA: *The shoulder: rupture of the supraspinatus tendon and other lesions about the subacromial bursa*, Brooklyn, NY, G Miller & Co, Medical Publishers.

33. Cofield RH: Rotator cuff disease of the shoulder, *J Bone Joint Surg* 67A(6):974-79, 1985

34. Cofield RH: Subscapular muscle transposition for repair of chronic rotator cuff tears, *Surg Gynecol Obstet* 154:667, 1982.

35. Cofield RH, Kavanaugh BF, Frassica FJ: Anterior shoulder instability, *Instr Course Lect* 34:210-227, 1985.

36. Cooper RA, Brems JJ: The inferior capsular shift for multidirectional instability of the shoulder, *J Bone Joint Surg* 74A:1516-1521, 1992.

37. Craig EV: The posterior mechanism of acute anterior shoulder dislocations, *Clin Orthop* 190:212-216, 1984.

38. Curr JF: Rupture of the axillary artery complication dislocation of the shoulder, *J Bone Joint Surg* 52B:313-317, 1970.

39. Detrisac DA, Johnson LL: *Arthroscopic shoulder anatomy: pathologic and surgical implications*, Thorofare, New Jersey, 1986, Slack.

40. DeWaal D et al: A comparison of the results of the Bristow-Latarjet procedure and the Bankart/Putti-Platt operation for recurrent anterior dislocation of the shoulder, *Acta Orthop Belg* 51:831-892, 1985.

41. DuToit GT, Roux D: Recurrent dislocation of the shoulder. A 24 year study of the Johannesburg stapling operation, *J Bone Joint Surg* 38A:1-12, 1956.

42. Ellman H: Arthroscopic subacromial decompression: analysis of one-to-three year results, *Arthroscopy* 3(3):173-181, 1987.

43. Fee JJ, McAvoy JM, Dainko EA: Pseudoaneurysm of the axillary artery following a modified Bristow operation: report of a case and review, *J Cardovasc Surg* 19:65-68, 1978.

44. Ferlic DC, DiGiovine NM: A long-term retrospective study of the modified Bristow procedure, *Am J Sports Med* 16:469-474, 1988.

45. Flatow EL, Bigliani LU, April EW: An anatomic study of the musculocutaneous nerve and its relationship to the coracoid process, *Clin Orthop* 244:166-171, 1989.

46. Foster CR: Multidirectional instability of the shoulder in the athlete, *Clin Sports Med* 2(2):355-367, 1983.

47. Friedman RJ et al: Non-constrained total shoulder replacement in patients who have rheumatoid arthritis and class-IV fractures, *J Bone Joint Surg* 71A:494-498, 1989.

48. Fronek J, Warren RF, Bowen M: Posterior subluxation of the glenohumeral joint, *J Bone Joint Surg* 71A:205-216, 1989.

49. Gerber C: Latissimus dorsi transfer for treatment of irreparable tear of the rotator cuff, *Clin Orthop* 275:152-160, 1992.

50. Gerber C, Ganz R: Clinical assessment of instability of the shoulder: with special reference to anterior and posterior drawer tests, *J Bone Joint Surg* 66B:551-556, 1984.

51. Gerber C et al: Latissimus dorsi transfer for the treatment of massive tears of the rotator cuff, *Clin Orthop* 232:51-61, 1988.

52. Gross MR: Arthroscopic shoulder capsulorrhaphy: does it work? *Am J Sports Med* 17:495-500, 1989.

53. Halley DK, Olix ML: A review of the Bristow operation of recurrent anterior shoulder dislocation in athletes, *Clin Orthop* 106:175-179, 1975.

54. Harrison WE Jr, Sisler J: Reconstruction of the AC joint using a synthetic fascial graft, *J Bone Joint Surg* 56A:1313, 1974.

55. Hawkins RJ: Unrecognized dislocation of the shoulder, *Instr Course Lectures* 34:258-263, 1985.

56. Hawkins RJ, Angelo RC: Glenohumeral osteoarthrosis. A late complication of the Putti-Platt repair, *J Bone Joint Surg* 72A:1193-1197, 1990.

57. Hawkins RH, Hawkins RJ: Failed anterior reconstruction for shoulder instability, *J Bone Joint Surg* 67B:709-714, 1985.

58. Hawkins RJ, Kennedy VC: Impingement syndrome in athletes, *Am J Sports Med* 6:151-158, 1981.

59. Hawkins RJ, Koppert G: The natural history following anterior dislocation of the shoulder in the older patient, *J Bone Joint Surg* 64B:255, 1982.

60. Hawkins RJ et al: Anterior dislocation of the shoulder in the older patient, *Clin Orthop* 206:192-195, 1986.

61. Helfet AJ: Coracoid transplantation for recurring dislocation of the shoulder, *J Bone Joint Surg* 40B:198-202, 1958.

62. Hoveluis L, Gavle JJ, Frein LH: Recurrent anterior dislocation of the shoulder: results after Bankart and Putti-Platt operation, *J Bone Joint Surg* 61A:566-569, 1979.

63. Hovelius L et al: Bristow-Latarjet procedure for recurrent anterior shoulder subluxation and dislocation, *Am J Sports Med* 9:283-287, 1981.

64. Hovelius L et al: The coracoid transfer for recurrent anterior dislocation about the shoulder, *J Bone Joint Surg* 65A:926-934, 1983.

65. Inman VT, Saunders JB, Abbott LC: Observations on the function of the shoulder joint, *J Bone Joint Surg* 26:1-30, 1944.

66. Irrgang JJ, Whitney SL, Harner CD: Nonoperative treatment of rotator cuff injuries in throwing athletes, *J Sport Rehab* 1:197-222, 1992.

67. Jobe FW, Glousman RE: Anterior capsulolabral reconstruction. In Tibone JE editor: *Techniques in orthopedics*, Frederick, Md, 1989, Aspen Publications; pp. 29-35.

68. Johnson EW Sr, Collins HR: Nonunion of the clavicle, *Arch Surg* 87:963, 1963.

69. Johnson LL: *Arthroscopic management for shoulder instability: stapling.* Presented at the annual meeting of the Arthroscopic Association of North America, Atlanta, February 1988.

70. Reference deleted in proofs.

71. Jupiter J et al: Non-union of the clavicle. Associated complications and surgical management, *J Bone Joint Surg* 69A(5):753-760, 1973.

72. Kinnet JG, Warren RF, Jacobs B: Recurrent dislocation of the shoulder after age fifty, *Clin Orthop* 149:164-168, 1980.

73. Kowalkowski A, Wallace WA: Close percutaneous K-wire stabilization for displaced fractures of the surgical neck of the humerus, *Injury* 2:209-212, 1990.

74. Kristiansen B, Angermann P, Larsen TK: Functional results following fractures of the proximal humerus: a controlled clinical study comparing two periods of immobilization, *Arch Orthop Trauma Surg* 108:339-341, 1989.

75. Kummel BM: Fractures of the glenoid causing chronic dislocation of the shoulder, *Clin Orthop* 69:189, 1970.

76. Kunkel SS, Hawkins RJ: Rotator-cuff repair utilizing a trough in bone, *Techniques Orthop* 3(4):51-57, 1989.

77. Latarjet M: A propos du traitment des luxations recidivantes de s'epaule, *Lyon Clin* 49:994-997, 1954.

78. Leach RE et al: Results of a modified Putti-Platt operation for recurrent shoulder dislocation and subluxation, *Clin Orthop* 164:20-25, 1982.

79. Lombardo SJ: The modifed Bristow-Laterjet procedure, *Techniques Orthop* 3(4):12-22, 1989.

80. Lombardo SJ et al: The modified Bristow procedure for recurrent dislocation of the shoulder, *J Bone Joint Surg* 58A:256-261, 1976.

81. Loomer R, Fraser J: A modified Bankart procedure for recurrent anterior-inferior shoulder instability. A preliminary report, *Am J Sports Med* 17:374-379, 1989.

82. Mackenzie DB The treatment of recurrent anterior shoulder dislocation by the modified Bristow-Laterjet procedure, *S Afr Sports Med J* 65:325-330, 1984.

83. Matsen FA III, Zuckerman JD: Anterior glenohumeral instability, *Clin Sports Med* 2(2):319-338, 1983.

84. Mackenzie DB: The Bristow-Helfet operation for anterior recurrent dislocation of the shoulder, *J Bone Joint Surg* 62B:273-274, 1980.

85. McLaughlin HL: Dislocation of the shoulder with tuberosity fracture, *Surg Clin North Amer* 43:1615, 1963.

86. McLaughlin HL: Injuries about the shoulder and arm. In McLaughlin HC, editor: *Trauma*, Philadelphia, 1959, WB Saunders; pp. 233-296.

87. McLaughlin HL, Cavallaro WV: Primary anterior dislocation of the shoulder, *Am J Surg* 80:615-620, 1950.

88. McLaughlin HL, MacLellan DI: Recurrent anterior dislocation of the shoulder. A comparative study, *J Trauma* 2:191-201, 1967.

89. Mead NC: *Bristow procedure* Letter presented at the Spectator Society, July 9, 1964.

90. Miller LS et al: The Magnuson-Stack procedure for recurrent glenohumeral dislocation, *Am J Sports Med* 12:133-137, 1984.

91. Morgan CD: *Arthroscopic Bankart suture repair—2 to 5 year results*. Presented at the annual meeting of the American Shoulder and Elbow Surgeons, Las Vegas, Feb 12, 1989.

92. Morgan CD, Bodenstab AB: Arthroscopic Bankart suture repair: technique and early results, *Arthroscopy* 3(2):111-122, 1987.

93. Morrey BF, Janes JM: Recurrent anterior dislocation of the shoulder: long-term follow-up of the Putti-Platt and Bankart procedure, *J Bone Joint Surg* 58A:252-257, 1976.

94. Moseley HF: *Ruptures of the rotator cuff*, Springfield, Ill, Charles C Thomas.

95. Moseley HF, Goldie I: The arterial pattern of the rotator cuff of the shoulder, *J Bone Joint Surg* 45B(4):780-789, 1963.

96. Mumford EB: Acromioclavicular diagnosis—a new operative treatment, *J Bone Joint Surg* 23:799-802, 1941.

97. Neer CS: Anterior acromioplasty for the chronic impingement syndrome in the shoulder, *J Bone Joint Surg* 54A(1):41-50, 1972.

98. Neer CS: Fractures of the distal third of the clavicle, *Clin Orthop* 53:43, 1960.

99. Neer CS: Impingement lesions, *Clin Orthop* 173:70-77, 1983.

100. Neer CS: Involuntary inferior and multidirectional instability of the shoulder: etiology, recognition, and treatment, *Instr Course Lect* 34:232-238, 1985.

101. Neer CS: Non-union of the clavicle, *JAMA* 172:1006-1011, 1960.

102. Neer CS, Craig EV, Fukuda, H: Cuff-tear arthropathy, *J Bone Joint Surg* 65A:1232-1244, 1983.

103. Neer CS, Foster CR: Inferior capsilar shift for involuntary inferior and multidirectional instability of the shoulder, *J Bone Joint Surg* 62A:897-908, 1980.

104. Neer CS, Rockwood CA Jr: Fractures and diagnoses of the shoulder. In Rockwood CA Jr, Greer DP, editors: *Fractures in adults*, vol 1, ed 2, Philadelphia, 1984, JB Lippincott; p. 675.

105. Neviaser RJ, Neviaser TJ, Neviaser JS: Concurrent rupture of rotator cuff and anterior dislocation of the shoulder in the older patient, *J Bone Joint Surg* 70A:1308-1311, 1988.

106. Nielson AB, Nielson K: The modified Bristow procedure for recurrent anterior dislocation of the shoulder. Results and complications, *Acta Orthop Scand* 53:229-232, 1982.

107. Norris T: Diagnostic techniques for shoulder instability, *Instr Course Lect* 34:239-257, 1985.

108. Osmond-Clark H: Habitual dislocation of the shoulder: the Putti-Platt operation, *J Bone Joint Surg Br* 30B:19-25, 1948.

109. Ozaki J et al: Recalcitrant chronic adhesive capsulitis of the shoulder. Role of contracture of the coracohumeral ligament and rotator interval in pathogenesis and treatment, *J Bone Joint Surg* 71A:1511-1515, 1989.

110. Pettersson G: Rupture of the tendon aponeurosis of the shoulder joint in anterior inferior dislocation, *Acta Chir Scand* 77 (suppl):1-184, 1942.

111. Perthes: Uber operation bei habitueller schulterluxation, *Deutsche Zeitschr Chir* 85:199-277, 1906.

112. Poppen NK, Walker PS: Forces at the glenohumeral joint in abduction, *Clin Orthop* 135:165-170, 1978.

113. Protzman RR: Anterior instability of the shoulder, *J Bone Joint Surg* 62A:909-918, 1980.

114. Rathbun JB, MacNab I: The microvascular pattern of the rotator cuff, *J Bone Joint Surg* 52B:540-553, 1970.

115. Reeves B: Experiments on tensile strength of the anterior capsular structures of the shoulder in man, *J Bone Joint Surg* 50B:858-865, 1968.

116. Regan WD et al: Comparative functional analysis of the Bristow, Magnusson-Stack, and Putti-Platt procedures for recurrent dislocation of the shoulder, *Am J Sports Med* 17:42-48, 1989.

117. Richard RR et al: Injury to the brachial plexus during Putti-Platt and Bristow procedure. A report of eight cases, *Am J Sports Med* 5:374-380, 1987.

118. Rookwood CA: Subluxation and dislocation about the shoulder. In Rockwood CA, Green DP, editors: *Fractures in adults*, Philadelphia, 1984, JB Lippincott; pp. 722-860.

119. Rockwood CA Jr: Subluxation of the shoulder: the classification, diagnosis and treatment, *Orthrop Trans* 4:306, 1979.

120. Rowe CR: Prognosis in dislocations of the shoulder, *J Bone Joint Surg* 38A:957-977, 1956.

121. Rowe CR: An atlas of anatomy and treatment of mid clavicular fractures, *Clin Orthop* 58:29, 1968.

122. Rowe CR, Patel D, Southmayd WW: The Bankart procedure: long-term end-result study, *J Bone Joint Surg* 60A:1-16, 1978.

123. Rowe CR, Pierce DS, Clark JG: Voluntary dislocation of the shoulder. A preliminary report on a clinical electromyographic and psychiatric study of twenty-six patients, *J Bone Joint Surg* 55A:445-460, 1973.

124. Rowe CR, Sakellarides HT: Factors related to recurrences of anterior dislocation of the shoulder, *Clin Orthrop* 20:40-47, 1961.

125. Rowe CR, Zarins B: Chronic unreduced dislocations of the shoulder, *J Bone Joint Surg* 64A:494-505, 1982.

126. Rubenstein DC et al: Anterior capsulolabral reconstruction of the shoulder in athletes, *J Shoulder Elbow Surg* 1:229-237, 1992.

127. Samilson RL, Binder WF: Symptomatic full thickness tears of the rotator cuff: an analysis of 292 shoulders in 276 patients, *Orthop Clin North Am* 6(2):449-466, 1975.

128. Schwartz RC et al: Capsular restraints to anterior-posterior motion of the abducted shoulder, *Orthop Trans* 12:727, 1988.

129. Shively J, Johnson J: Results of the modified Bristow procedure, *Clin Orthop* 187:150-153, 1984.

130. Sisk TD, Boyd HB: Management of recurrent anterior dislocation of the shoulder: duToit-type or staple capsulorrhaphy, *Clin Orthop* 103;150-156, 1974.

131. Slatis P, Aalto K: Medial dislocation of the tendon of the long head of biceps brachii, *Acta Orthop Scand* 50(1):73-77, 1979.

132. Skyhar MJ, Altchek DW, Warren RF: Shoulder instability in athletes. In Nicholas J, Hershman, editors: *The upper extremity in sports medicine*, Philadelphia, 1990, Mosby–Year Book; pp 181-212.

133. Stevens JH: Dislocation of the shoulder, *Surgery* 83:84-103, 1926.

134. Takagish N: Conservative treatment of the ruptures of the rotator cuff, *J Jpn Orthop Assoc* 52:781-787, 1978.

135. Thomas SC, Matsen FA III: An approach to the repair of avulsion of the glenohumeral ligaments in the management of traumatic anterior glenohumeral instability, *J Bone Joint Surg* 71A:506-513, 1989.

136. Torg JS et al: A modified Bristow-Helfet-May procedure for recurrent dislocation and subluxation of the shoulder. Report of 212 cases, *J Bone Joint Surg* 69A:904-913, 1987.

137. Townsend H et al: Electromyographic analysis of the glenohumeral muscles during a baseball rehabilitation program, *Am J Sports Med* 19(3):264, 1991.

138. Turkel SJ et al: Stabilizing mechanisms preventing anterior dislocation of the glenohumeral joint, *J Bone Joint Surg* 63A:1208-1217, 1981.

139. Warner JJP, Warren RF: Arthroscopic Bankart repair using a cannulated absorbable fixation device, *Operative Techniques Orthop* 1(2):192, 1991.

140. Warren RF: Subluxation of the shoulder in athletes, *Clin Sports Med* 2(2):339-354, 1983.

141. Weaver JK, Dunn HK: Treatment of acromioclavicular injuries, especially complete acromioclavicular separation, *J Bone Joint Surg* 54A:1187, 1972.

142. Weiss AP et al: Unconstrained shoulder arthroplasty: a five year average follow-up study, *Clin Orthop* 257:86-90, 1990.

143. Wiley AM: Arthroscopic appearance of frozen shoulder, *Arthroscopy* 7:138-143, 1991.

144. Wiley AM: Arthroscopy for shoulder instability and using a technique for arthroscopic repair, *Arthroscopy* 4:25-30, 1988.

145. Wilkins RM, Johnston RM: Ununited fractures of the clavicle, *J Bone Joint Surg* 65A:773-778, 1983.

146. Willis JB, Meyn MA Jr, Miller EH: *Infraspinatus transfer for recurrent anterior dislocation of the shoulder*. Presented at the annual meeting of the American Academy of Orthopaedic Surgeons, Las Vegas, Feb 27, 1981.

147. Wilson CL, Duff GL: Pathologic study of degeneration and rupture of the supraspinatus tendon, *Arch Surg* 47:121-135, 1943.

148. Wolf EM: Arthroscopic anterior shoulder capsulorrhaphy, *Techniques Orthop* 3:67-73, 1988.

149. Young C, Rockwood CA: Complications of failed Bristow procedure and their management, *J Bone Joint Surg* 73A:969-981, 1991.

150. Zuckerman JD, Matsen FA: Complications about the glenohumeral joint related to the use of screws and staples, *J Bone Joint Surg* 66A:175-180, 1984.

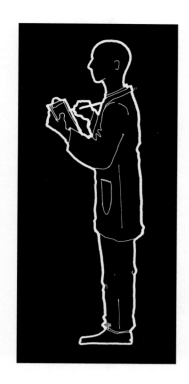

Chapter 31

Workplace Adaptation

Thomas J. Armstrong

CONTENTS

Previous chapters (8, 16, 26, and 27) show that deviation of neck, shoulder, and elbow postures from neutral positions is associated with adverse health effects such as fatigue and chronic muscle, tendon, and nerve disorders. The effects of these disorders range from minor discomfort and degraded performance to disability. Available data suggest that the time of onset of adverse effects decreases with increasing exertion duration, frequency, and force. This does not mean, however, that some postures can or should be maintained indefinitely without interruption. Also, it does not mean that brief exposures to extreme posture are not desirable.

The relationship between certain work activities and adverse health effects is referred to as the "dose-response" relationship (see Chapter 12). The dose-response relationship provides insight into how work can be designed to minimize the risk of possible adverse health effects or to facilitate the return to work of persons in whom an adverse effect may have developed. Unfortunately, sufficient data are not yet available to specify job designs that provide a specific level of risk. For example, it cannot be said how many times a group of workers can exert a horizontal force of 50 N to engage the bit of a powered screwdriver weighing 15 N at an elevation of 1.5 m before unacceptable health effects would develop in a given fraction of them. It is extremely important that the work equipment and procedures be evaluated at all stages of design and implementation.

Workplace adaptation entails three basic steps:[14]

1. Evaluation of the proposed or existing job
2. Specification of adaptations
3. Evaluation of adaptations

It may be necessary to repeat one or more of these steps one or more times to achieve a desired level of control.

EVALUATION

Evaluation entails (1) documentation of the process, equipment, procedures, and environment and (2) evaluation of stressors, including posture, force, duration, and frequency.[1,7] The documentation is performed from available job descriptions, time studies, workplace inspections and measurements, equipment specifications, and interviews with workers and supervisors. This information is then used to identify stressful postures and forces necessary to reach, hold, and use work objects, as well as the duration and frequency of these exertions. The boxes on p. 413 and 414 and **Figures 31-1** and **31-2** illustrate evaluation summaries of two jobs: claims processor and assembler.

An evaluation of stressful postures and forces entails examining each step of the operation for extreme neck, shoulder, and elbow postures and forces (see **Fig. 31-3**). These elements should be recorded along with their duration, frequency, and cause. For example, in the claims processor job described in the box opposite, extreme reaches to the workers' side are required 80 times per day to get unfinished files and 80 times per day to put aside finished files. Workers must reach over the files and rotate their forearms to use the keyboard six hours per shift. In the assembler job described in the box on p. 414, the workers must reach for parts beside and behind them 2,400 times per 8-hour shift; they must elevate their elbow above shoulder height and rotate their forearm 14,400 times per shift, and so forth.

The analysis should also include an inspection of infrequent or irregular elements. For example, in the claims processor job (see box p. 413), 3 out of 10 claims are set aside to await additional information that must be retrieved by telephone. In the assembler job (see box p. 414), 1 out of 12 screws is defective and requires additional movements and time to replace. By their very nature, it may be hard to identify irregular elements from existing job descriptions or observations. Often they are identified via worker and supervisor interviews.

SPECIFICATION OF ADAPTATIONS

The causes of the physical stressors should be apparent from the work evaluation. The tabulation of stressors and their causes illustrated in the boxes on p. 413 and 414 provides a systematic format for developing possible adaptations. This format also provides insight into how the overall stressfulness of the job will be affected by the proposed control measures and how one adaptation may affect other stressors. For example, in the box on p. 413 it can be seen that the claims processors are exposed to 2 hours of a stressful shoulder-neck posture per day to hold the phone handset. It can also be seen that a headset or a bracket attached to the handset could reduce this exposure. Yet another adaptation might be passing uncompleted files to another worker who does all of the phoning; however, this solution could result in increased keyboard times and other undesirable effects.

Reaching for documents is associated with cart location and design. It follows that locating the carts close to the workers' side and modifying them with a fold-down side would reduce reaching. Because these reaches occur an average of only once every 3 minutes, it can be argued that this work element is by itself unlikely to produce adverse health effects; however, it can also be argued that when combined with other factors, this

Sample documentation and analysis of "claims processor" job for identifying and controlling shoulder and neck stressors.

TITLE
Claims processor

STANDARD
Complete 80 claims per day

EQUIPMENT
Computer, keyboard, 13-in. color monitor and claim processor software
Desk
Staple remover
Stapler
Telephone with handset
Adjustable-height chair
Carts for holding files

METHOD
1. Get file from cart—place on lap in front of keyboard
2. Remove staples
3. Sort documents
4. Perform keystrokes to open file
5. Perform keystrokes to update file

6. Call for information as necessary—3 calls per 10 claims
7. Perform keystrokes to close file
8. Staple documents
9. Stamp and date file
10. Place finished file in cart
11. Note: occasionally claims processor cannot finish file and will set it aside at the front of desk until someone calls back with necessary information

MATERIALS
Files weighing 5-50 N

ENVIRONMENT
Inside
Overhead fluorescent lights with diffusers

WORKER
Skilled male and female keyboard operators
Fifth percentile female to 95th percentile male stature

Ergonomic Stressors

Stressor	Proposed Adaptation
POSTURE Reaching for unfinished files (80 times/shift) Reaching over file on lap to use keyboard (6 hr/shift) Looking down at file (4 hr/shift) Extending the neck to see monitor through bifocals (2 hr/shift) Reaching to put aside finished files (80 times/ shift) Inward forearm rotation and wrist deviation to position hands over keyboard (6 hr/shift) Holding phone between neck and shoulder (2 hr/shift)	Provide access for carts so that it can be positioned to minimize reaching Provide adjustable tray to hold file above keyboard Provide corrective lenses that do not require worker to extend neck Investigate variable geometry keyboard to reduce forearm rotation Provide headset for phone Investigate adjustable keyboard holder Investigate wrist rest Provide adjustable monitor holder
FORCE Lifting files weighing up to 50 N from cart to lap (80 times/shift) and from lap to cart (80 times/shift)	Provide access for cart so that it can be positioned to minimize reaching Investigate drop side for cart

Continued

Sample documentation and analysis of ''assembler'' job for identifying and controlling shoulder and neck stressors

TITLE
Assembler

STANDARD
Assemble 2,400 pumps per 8-hr shift

EQUIPMENT
Assembly line (1 m above floor level)
Power screwdriver suspended above line
Rack and bin for holding parts

METHOD
1. Get motor assembly from bin (weight, 40 N) and position on subassembly
2. Get handful of screws with one hand
3. Get screwdriver with other hand
4. Position screw in screwdriver ⎫ ×6
5. Drive screw (1 out of 12 screws ⎭ is defective and must be backed out and replaced)

ENVIRONMENT
Inside
Overhead fluorescent lights with diffusers

WORKER
Males and females
Fifth percentile female to 95th percentile male stature

Ergonomic Stressors

Stressor	Proposed Adaptation
POSTURE Reaching for motor assemblies located to side and behind worker (300 times/hr) Reaching for parts located to side and behind worker (300 times/hr) Reaching for screwdriver located overhead (300 times/hr) Driving 1800 screws/hr with pistol-shaped driver requires elevation of elbow and forearm rotation Reaching upstream and downstream to keep up with production line (50% of time, but 90% of time when bad screws are encountered)	Position trays close to worker and production line to minimize reaching Unload trays one corner at a time and then rotate tray 90 degrees to minimize reaching Adjust tool suspender to minimize tension and locate tool as close as possible to point of use Investigate use of in-line tool with articulating arm to control torque Investigate indexing production line in which work object stops until released by worker Position work object as close to edge of production line as possible to minimize reaching Investigate quality control program to avoid defective screws that take extra motions to try to and reject
FORCE Lifting motor assemblies weighing 40 N from bin (300 times/hr) Pulling down power tool into work position (300 times/hr)	Investigate small hoist or air balancers to facilitate transferring motors to line See above recommendations for tool suspender

reaching could result in an adverse effect or could aggravate an existing case. An analysis of the low cost associated with parking the carts close to the workers versus the possible cost of medical treatment and lost work for disabled workers would support locating carts close to the workers. Such an analysis would probably also support a modification of the cart with drop sides.

Workplace adaptations may involve modification of

• Work processes

• Work standards
• Design of methods
• Workplace layout
• Equipment
• Training

Work processes refer to the technologies used for completing the work objectives. In the claims processor example (box, p. 413), the technologies are keyboards and telephones. Alternative technologies include scan-

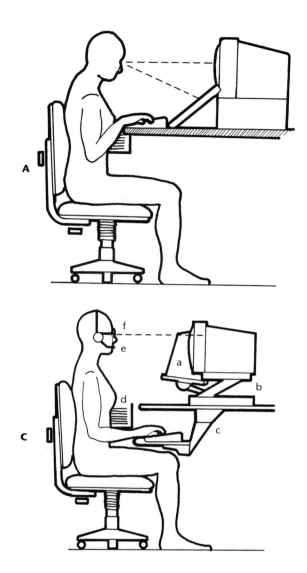

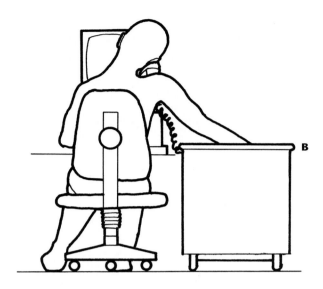

Figure 31-1 A, Illustration of a claims processor job. **B,** Major stresses include reaching for documents, holding the telephone, reaching for the keyboard, looking down at documents, and reaching to get and put aside documents. **C,** Possible claims processor job interventions include an adjustable document holder (*a*), adjustable monitor holder (*b*), adjustable keyboard holder (*c*), drop-side cart (*d*), headset for phone (*e*), and optically correct glasses (*f*).

ners and electronic mail. In the assembler example (box, p. 414), the technologies include threaded fasteners; alternative technologies include clips and adhesives.

Work standards refer to the quantity and quality of work produced in a given time. In the claims processor example, the standard is 80 claims per 8-hour shift; in the assembler example, the standard is 2400 motor assemblies per 8-hour shift. The work standard is an important factor in how many times per day workers must assume a given posture or exert a given force. Reducing work standards is generally considered an adaptation of last resort; however, it may be shown that the lost productivity is more than offset by the reduced cost of medical treatment and lost work for a disabled worker.

Work methods refer to the procedures or sequence of movements used to perform the job. In the assembler example, the method entails getting motors from a bin, placing them on the line, and driving six screws. A methods change to reduce reaching would be to unload one corner of the bin and then rotate it 90 degrees so that the workers are always working from the corner closest to them. A methods change may also require an equipment change and worker training.

Workplace layout refers to the position of equipment and work objects in the workplace. In the claims processor example, the workplace layout includes the position in space of the carts with files, the keyboard, the monitor, the phone, and the active file with respect to the worker. Adaptations include repositioning the carts to reduce reaching, adding equipment to allow repositioning of the keyboard, and supplying adjustable docu-

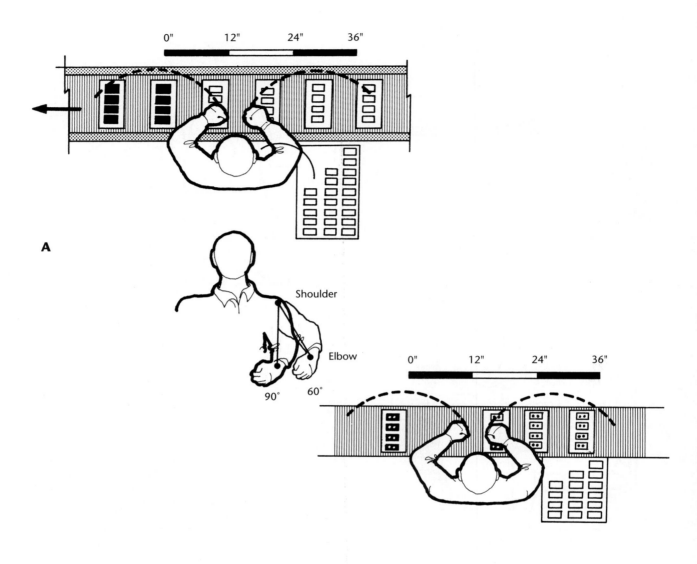

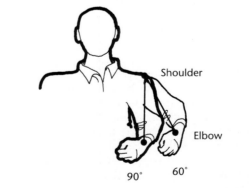

Figure 31-2 A, Work station layout for a line worker. **B,** Proposed interventions for the line worker example include using a narrower conveyor to reduce reaching over line "dead space," using an indexing line so that the worker does not have to "chase" the assemblies, and using a smaller box of parts mounted on a turntable to reduce reaching to the side and behind the worker.

ment and monitor holders. In the assembly example, adaptations include equipment to reposition the parts bin and adjustment of the suspender so that the tool can be positioned to minimize reaching.

Anthropometric data may be used to estimate reach distances.[3,11] Average link length proportions can be used with population stature data to estimate vertical, horizontal, and lateral reach limits (see **Fig. 31-4**). Caution should be used in interpreting reach predictions based on link length data. A reach distance based on *average proportions and a given percentile stature* may correspond to a different *percentile reach*. Work locations should be made as adjustable as possible to accommodate individuals and should be tested with user tri-

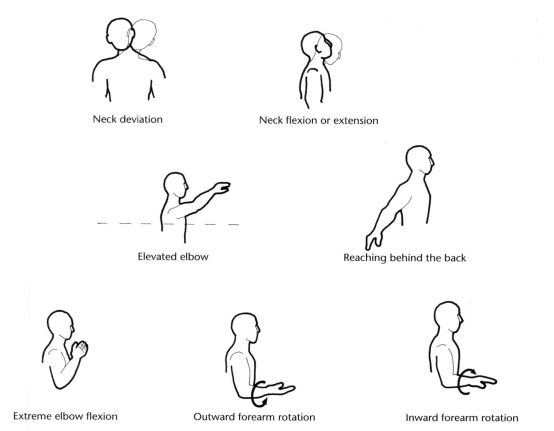

Figure 31-3 Shoulder and neck stressors include extreme neck, shoulder, and elbow postures and force *(Modified from Armstrong TJ: Hand Clin 553-565, 1986.*

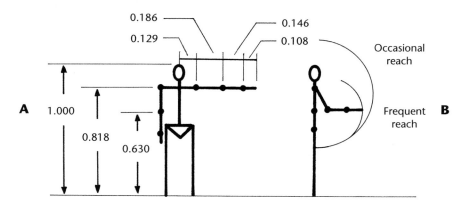

Figure 31-4 Average link length proportions **A**, can be used with population stature data to estimate vertical, horizontal, and lateral reach limits, **B**, The outer arc represents maximum reach without bending. The inner arc represents maximum reach without bending and not flexing the shoulder more than 30 degrees to minimize loads on shoulder tissues.

als.[8,12,14] Reach data for U.S. civilian populations are available from U.S. National Health surveys.[13]

Equipment refers to hardware such as tools to drive fasteners or shape and smooth surfaces, containers, jigs, fixtures for holding parts, and seating to support the worker. A proposed adaptation in the claims processor example includes modification of the cart; adjustable holders for the keyboard, monitor, and files; and a headset for the phone. In the assembly example, equipment changes include an in-line screwdriver with articulating arm, an indexing assembly line, and a turn-table for the parts bin.

Training entails instructing workers on the hows and whys of arranging and performing their work. In the claims processor example, it should be explained to the workers where they should position the carts and why this is necessary to prevent possible shoulder problems. Follow-up training and evaluations should be performed to determine whether the workers understand and follow the specified procedures. If procedures are not followed, further evaluations should be performed to determine why they are not followed.

The design of adaptations should draw on all available resources. Available resources will vary from one situation to another, depending on the size and type of industry. Possible resources include

- Job designers—engineers, facilities people, setup people
- Safety and health personnel—doctors, nurses, industrial hygienists, safety personnel
- Supervisors
- Workers or work representatives
- Purchasing
- Sales and technical representatives from suppliers
- Catalogs, brochures, technical specifications
- Scientific papers, books, magazines

In general, the team approach is the most effective way to mobilize the resources necessary to develop and implement workplace adaptations. On occasion, however, the problems are conspicuous and the solution is clear so organizing a special team is not merited.

Development of adaptation is not an exact process. Consequently, all adaptations should be evaluated to ascertain their effectiveness.

EVALUATION OF ADAPTATIONS

Ideally, adaptations should be evaluated in terms of their effects on upper limb disorders. Unfortunately, such evaluations are difficult. Upper limb disorders develop over long periods of time. To determine the effect of a given adaptation on the occurrence of disorders would require identification of a group of several hundred workers, implementation of the adaptation in a random subset of these people, and some kind of comparison adaptation in the others.[6] The population would then have to be tracked for 1 or more years. Unfortunately, such studies are extremely difficult and expensive. It is difficult to find large groups in which adaptations can be randomly assigned. Work activities are generally dictated by production schedules that may cause the work population to shrink or swell. In addition, non–health-related factors may cause a turnover in the work population. Although evaluation of health patterns is an important means of identifying workers and jobs that merit further evaluation and assessing an overall program, in most cases it provides only limited feedback about specific adaptations.

Adaptations can be evaluated by using the same methods that were used for the initial job evaluations. This analysis should begin as the adaptations are developed on paper and continue through the prototype, pilot testing, and implementation phases.[8] In some cases it may be possible to identify and evaluate other jobs at that work site or other work sites where the proposed adaptations have already been implemented. In other cases it may be necessary to develop prototypes and conduct pilot testing on a small number of the proposed interventions. Worker feedback can be obtained through interviews; however, care should be taken to avoid leading questions.[9] The questions should be structured in such a way as to provide guidance on how to enhance the adaptation. For example, one of the proposed adaptations for the assembly job was the use of another tool and locating it to minimize reaching. In this case, workers could be permitted to try several tools and then rank them in order of preference. They could also be asked to try the tools at several locations and rate them on a scale of 0 to 10 where 0 is "too low," 5 is "just right," and 10 is "too high."[2,12] Even though these measures do not ensure that future shoulder, neck, or elbow problems will not develop, they do provide a basis for selecting a work configuration that minimizes stress on the worker.

Discomfort patterns can also be used to evaluate work designs before and after they are implemented.[4,5,10] Workers are shown pictures of the body and asked to identify and rate areas of discomfort. Discomfort patterns provide information about many parts of the body, as well as those parts likely to be affected by the stress of concern and the proposed adaptation. Often, the variation from within and between workers is considerable, and rigorous statistical conclusions may not be possible.

SUMMARY

The available data are not yet sufficient to develop design specifications that can be used to achieve a given level of risk of neck, shoulder, and elbow disorders; however, the data do provide insight into some of the things that can be done to reduce risk. Control of disorders entails three basic steps: (1) evaluation of the job to determine the frequency, duration, and cause of extreme reaches and forces; (2) specification of adaptations; and (3) evaluation of the adaptations. It may be necessary to repeat these steps before the desired level of control is achieved. Development of workplace adaptations should be integrated into an ongoing program that includes health surveillance, job surveys, evaluation of affected workers and jobs, medical management, training, and a team approach with participation from all levels of the organization.

References

1. Armstrong TJ: Ergonomics and cumulative trauma disorders, *Hand Clin* 2(3):553-565, 1986.

2. Armstrong TJ, Punnett L, Ketner P: Subjective worker assessments of hand tools used in automobile assembly, *Am Ind Hyg Assoc J,* 51(12):639-645, 1989.

3. Armstrong TJ et al: Repetitive trauma disorders: job evaluation and design, *Hum Factors* 28(3):325-336, 1986.

4. Corlett EN, Bishop RP: The ergonomics of spot welders, *Appl Ergonom* Mar: 23-31, 1978.

5. Harms-Ringdahl K: On assessment of shoulder exercise and load-elicited pain in the cervical spine. Biomechanical analysis of load—EMG—methodological studies of pain provoked by extreme position, *Scand J Rehab Med* (suppl) 14:1-40, 1986.

6. Hennekens CH, Buring JE, Mayrent SL, editors: *Epidemiology in medicine,* Boston, 1987, Little, Brown.

7. Keyserling WM, Armstrong TJ, Punnett L: Ergonomic job analysis: a structured approach for identifying risk factors associated with overexertion injuries and disorders, *Applied Occup Environ Hyg* 6(5):353-363, 1991.

8. McClelland I: Product assessment and user trials. In Wilson JR, Corlett, EN, editors: *Evaluation of human work: a practical ergonomics methodology,* New York, 1990, Taylor & Francis; pp. 218-247.

9. McCormick E: Job and Task Analysis. In Salvendy G, editors: *Handbook of industrial engineering,* New York, 1982, John Wiley & Sons; pp. 2.4.1-2.4.21.

10. Saldana N et al: A computerized method for assessment of musculoskeletal discomfort in the workforce: a tool for surveillance, *Ergonomics* 37(6):1097-1112, 1994.

11. Ulin SS, Armstrong TJ, Radwin RG: Use of computer aided drafting for analysis and control of posture in manual work, *Appl Ergonom* 21(2):143-151, 1990.

12. Ulin SS et al: Effect of tool shape and work location on perceived exertion for work on horizontal surfaces, *Am Ind Hyg Assoc J* 54(7):383-391, 1993.

13. US Dept. of Health, Education and Welfare: Weight and height of adults 18-74 years of age: United States, 1971-1974 *Vital Health Stat* 11(211), Hyattsville, Md., 1979, National Center for Health Statistics.

14. Wilson JR: A framework and a context for ergonomics methodology. In Wilson JR, Corlett EN, editors: *Evaluation of human work: a practical ergonomics methodology,* London, 1990, Taylor & Francis; p. 6.

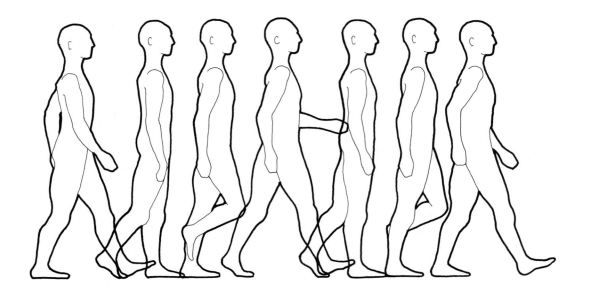

SECTION 3

Wrist and Hand

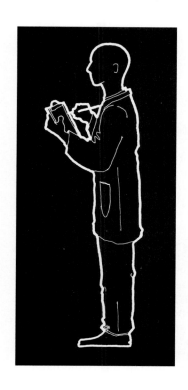

Chapter 32

Epidemiology of Wrist and Hand Disorders

David Rempel
Laura Punnett

CONTENTS

The findings of epidemiologic studies that address workplace and individual factors associated with hand and wrist musculoskeletal disorders are summarized in this chapter. From an epidemiologic point of view, this topic is problematic because although many specific hand and wrist disorders such as carpal tunnel syndrome (CTS) and hand-arm vibration syndrome are recognized, no criteria for case definitions are universally accepted. More data are available for CTS than for other hand and wrist disorders because of its relatively well defined pathology and available diagnostic methods such as nerve conduction velocity testing.

These disorders are not new; epidemics and clinical case series of work-related hand and wrist tendinitis were reported throughout the 1800s and early 1900s.[19,78] Although prospective studies were too few to prove causation of specific factors, within the last 20 years a number of well-designed, cross-sectional studies have focused on the hand and wrist. Those studies consistently identify certain key risk factors at the same time as they point to the multifactorial nature of work-related hand and wrist disorders. The etiology of these disorders is probably influenced by both biomechanical and work organizational factors; reporting and clinical progression are also likely affected by the worker's perception of the work environment and by medical management. A conceptual model of this complicated relationship, adapted from Armstrong et al,[5] is presented in **Figure 32-1**. The model is based on epidemiologic studies and pathophysiologic mechanisms clarified in laboratory studies.

Healthcare providers should use this information to prevent loss of function in their patients and reduce the overall incidence of hand, wrist, and other musculoskeletal disorders in the workplace.

FREQUENCY, RATES, AND COSTS

National incidence rates of work-related hand and wrist disorders in the United States are not easy to assess because of the difficulty in attributing causation and the sparse data on background incidence and prevalence. Annual incidence rates of all work-related repeated-motion disorders reported by U.S. private employers to the Bureau of Labor Statistics are shown for 1978 to 1993 in **Figure 32-2**. Approximately 55% were hand or wrist disorders, a percentage also reported in industrial studies[55] and studies from other countries.[43] The dramatic rise after 1983 may be partially explained by industry underreporting on the Occupational Safety and Health Administration (OSHA) 200 log, a factor that was partially rectified after OSHA levied large fines against some meat processing and automobile manufacturers for underreporting in the early 1980s. A similar rise in work-related hand/forearm problems has been observed in other countries such as Finland,[43] Australia,[7] and Japan.[62]

Rates of hand and wrist symptoms and associated disability among working adults were assessed by a 1988 national interview survey of 44,000 randomly selected U.S. adults (National Health Interview Survey).[64] Of those who had worked any time in the past 12 months, 22% reported some finger, hand, or wrist discomfort that fit the category "pain, burning, stiffness, numbness, or tingling" for 1 or more days in the past 12 months. Only one quarter were due to an acute injury such as a cut, sprain, or broken bone. Nine percent reported having prolonged hand discomfort, that is, discomfort of 20 or more days during the last 12 months or 7 or more consecutive days that was not due to an acute injury. Of those with prolonged hand discomfort, 6% changed work activities and 5% changed jobs because of the hand discomfort.

Administrative records (e.g., worker's compensation) are frequently used to estimate incidence rates, but the data are extremely problematic to interpret because of varying decision rules that may have no clinical value in defining a "case." For example, Fine et al[27] evaluated multiple records for the same time period at two U.S. automobile plants. Within each facility the magnitude of the incidence rates of hand and arm disorders varied dramatically between data sources: the rates were 10 times higher in the worker's compensation records than in the OSHA 200 log and 10 times higher in the plant medical records than in the compensation data. Nevertheless, the relative ranking of the departments within each plant was similar, regardless of which data source was used.

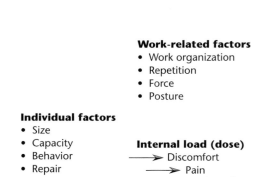

Work-related factors
• Work organization
• Repetition
• Force
• Posture

Individual factors
• Size
• Capacity
• Behavior
• Repair

Internal load (dose)
→ Discomfort
→ Pain
→ Disorder
→ Disability

Figure 32-1 A possible model of the relationship between exposure to work, worker attributes, and the development of chronic musculoskeletal disorders of the hands and wrist. Internal loads and individual capacity result in a reversible, cascading series of events ranging from minor mechanical or biologic disturbances to tissue damage and disability. *(Modified from Armstrong TJ et al:* Scand J Work Environ Health *19:73-84, 1993.)*

The incidence of work-related CTS and factors predicting disability have been assessed on a large scale in Washington State. A review of 7926 worker's compensation claims for CTS from 1984 to 1988 yielded an industry-wide incidence rate of CTS claims of 1.74 per 1000 full-time employees.[28] Rates up to 20 cases per 1000 full-time employees were observed in shellfish, fish, and other meat packing industries. Industries with the highest rates of occupational CTS are presented in the box below. The box also shows a high correspondence with the occupations in Finland having the highest rates of hand, wrist, and forearm disorders despite some geographic differences in industry.

Approximately 40% of all the Washington State workers with CTS went on to surgical treatment.[1] Of these, the mean duration of lost time was 4 months. The length of time lost from work was not associated with demographic factors (age, gender, wage) or case severity, as assessed by clinical staging or nerve conduction values. Most (67%) returned to the same job, 15% found a different job, and 3 years after surgery, 18% had not returned to work. Workers from jobs with elevated rates of CTS or jobs involving repetitive hand activity were less likely to return to the same job. Similarly, a predictor of poor long-term outcome after surgery is a return to repetitive or physically demanding work.[2,53]

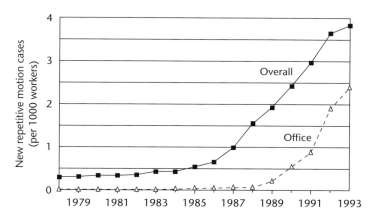

Figure 32-2 Incidence rates (per 1000 full-time employees) of repeated-motion disorders for all U.S. private-sector workers from 1978 to 1993. The lower curve (----) is the incidence for industries with primarily office work (finance, insurance, and real estate). Approximately 55% are hand/wrist disorders. *(From Bureau of Labor Statistics, 1978–1993.)*

Industries with the highest incidence rates of carpal tunnel syndrome from the Washington State workers' compensation system from 1984 to 1988 and occupations with the highest rates of hand, wrist, and forearm disorders in Finland from 1975 to 1979.

Carpal tunnel syndrome: Washington State workers' compensation	Hand, wrist, and forearm disorders: Finland reports of occupational disorders
Oyster, crab, clam packing	Butcher
Meat, poultry dealers	Packer
Packing house	Food industry worker
Fish canneries	Sawmill worker
Carpentry	Shoe maker
Fruit and vegetable canning	Seamstress
Egg production	Food processors
Box, shook, pallet, bin manufacturing	Electrical mechanic
Sawmills	Serial production worker
Steel-casting foundries	Textile worker
Logging	Paper industry worker

Data from Franklin GM et al: Occupational carpal tunnel syndrome in Washington State, 1984-1988, Am J Pub Health *81:741-746, 1991; and Kivi P: Rheumatic disorders of the upper limbs associated with repetitive occupational tasks in Finland in 1975-1979,* Scand J Rheumatol *13:101-107, 1984.*

Few data are available to assess the long-term financial and functional impact on patients and society, and the data that currently exist vary among states and change with time. In 1992, California's largest worker's compensation carrier reported an average medical and compensation cost per CTS claim of $18,000.[14] In Washington State between 1987 and 1989, the comparable cost was $8,200.[1]

DISORDER TYPES AND THEIR NATURAL HISTORY

The box below lists some hand and wrist disorders identified in occupational epidemiologic studies. Nonspecific hand/wrist pain is the most common problem, followed by tendinitis, ganglion cysts, and CTS.[35,47,55,73] In their early stages, these disorders may be manifested by nonspecific symptoms without signs or laboratory findings. It is important to remember that symptoms in the hand may be due to nerve or vascular lesions further up the arm.

In high-risk workplaces, rates of nonspecific symptoms, tendinitis, and CTS, when measured, appear to track each other; that is, specific disorders usually do not occur in isolation. For example, in a pork processing plant, the rank order of hand and wrist problems as a percentage of all morbidity was nonspecific hand/wrist pain, 39%; CTS, 26%; trigger finger, 23%; trigger thumb, 17%; and DeQuervain's tenosynovitis, 17%.[56] Similar ratios of disorders have been observed in manufacturing workers,[6,55,73] food processors,[45,47] and computer operators.[9,35]

For the purposes of this chapter, tendinitis includes hand, wrist, and distal forearm tendinitis or tenosynovitis and trigger finger. Tendinitis occurs at discrete locations, the most common site being the first extensor compartment (DeQuervain's disease), followed by the

---

Examples of disorders of the hand and wrist observed in workplace studies

Nonspecific hand and wrist pain or paresthesia
Tendinitis
   Tenosynovitis
   Finger tendinitis
   Wrist tendinitis
   Stenosing tenosynovitis
Carpal tunnel syndrome
Ganglion cysts
Hand-arm vibration syndrome
Osteoarthritis
Hypothenar hammer syndrome
Guyon tunnel syndrome
Gamekeeper's thumb
Digital neuritis

---

five other pulley sites on the extensor side of the hand and three on the flexor side. The diagnosis is based on the history, symptom location, and palpation and provocative maneuvers on physical examination. No association of tendinitis with age has been found, but a bimodal curve with seniority has been described; for example, work-related tendinitis was higher among workers with less than 3 years of employment, which may be due to a healthy worker effect.[55]

In cross-sectional workplace studies, the prevalence of ganglion cysts, as assessed by physical examination, is 2% to 3%.[9,35,55] Whether these rates are higher among those performing repetitive hand activity versus those performing tasks with low repetitiveness is unknown.

There are no universally accepted diagnostic criteria for CTS. Some consider an abnormal nerve conduction study a gold standard.[36,42,58] However, relying exclusively on nerve conduction studies can lead to reporting very high prevalence rates, 28%[58] and 19%[8] in low-risk working populations. A case definition incorporating typical symptoms and signs has been proposed by the National Institute for Occupational Safety and Health (NIOSH) for surveillance purposes[17]; however, the usual signs have relatively poor sensitivities and specificities.[29,36,42] This definition may therefore have limited value in distinguishing CTS from other hand disorders. Hand diagrams completed by patients have a good predictive value when filled out by patients referred to an electrodiagnostic center,[41] but not in a workplace study.[30] Only in the later stages are weakness and thenar atrophy noticeable features. In approximately 25% of cases, CTS is accompanied by other disorders of the hand or wrist.[65]

Few studies have evaluated how osteoarthritis of the hand and wrist relates to work.[33,84] Hadler et al[33] assessed the hands of 67 workers at a textile plant in Virginia. Significant differences in finger and wrist-joint range of motion, joint swelling, and x-ray patterns of degenerative joint disease were observed between three different hand intensive jobs; the observed differences were reported to match the pattern of hand usage.

Hand-arm vibration syndrome, or vibration white finger disease, occurs in occupations involving many years of exposure to vibrating hand tools.[59] This is a disorder of the small vessels and nerves in the fingers and hands that is manifested as localized blanching at the fingertips with numbness on exposure to cold or vibration. The symptoms are largely self-limited if vibration exposure is eliminated at an early stage,[22,31] but with continuing exposure, the condition becomes irreversible.

Hypothenar hammer syndrome, or occlusion of the superficial palmar branch of the ulnar artery, has been associated in clinical series and case-control studies with habitually using the hand for hammering[46,61] and with exposure to vibrating hand tools.[40] The mean length of exposure before seeking medical attention was 20 to 30 years.

Small case-control studies or clinical series have described factors associated with less common disorders such as gamekeeper's thumb,[15,60] digital neuritis, and ulnar neuropathy at the wrist.[73]

Individual Factors

Good data on individual risk factors such as age and gender are available only for CTS. In general population studies and clinical case series, the average age of patients with CTS is approximately 55 years.[10,65,75,85] In contrast, the mean age for "occupational" cases, based on the Washington State worker's compensation study, is 37.5 years.[28] Furthermore, as displayed in **Figure 32-3**, the incidence increases with age in the general population but does not appear to do so in the occupational cohort. Age explained only 3% of the variability in median nerve latency in a cross-sectional study of an industrial cohort.[58]

In a similar manner, gender appears to play a greater role in population-based studies of CTS than in industrial studies. In regional population studies and clinical series, the incidence of CTS is higher in females than males by a factor of 2.2:1 to 3.7:1,[10,65,75,85] whereas in workplace studies, when employees perform similar hand activities, the ratio is much closer to unity at 1.2:1.[28,58,73] Carpal tunnel syndrome can be a sequela (usually self-limiting) of pregnancy[23]; however, the role of other female reproductive factors such as oophorectomy, hysterectomy,[11,16,20,66] or the use of oral contraceptives[69] is less certain. The overall implications are that when hand activities are taken into account, the differences between working men and women are not particularly prominent and hormonal influences likely account for relatively little morbidity when ergonomic exposures are high.

Other individual factors with strong associations to CTS are diabetes mellitus,[65,75,85] rheumatoid arthritis,[65,75,85] and obesity.[20,25,58,80,82] For other factors, the associations are based on single studies or the studies present conflicting results: thyroid disorders,[35,65] vitamin B_6 deficiency,[3,24,54] wrist size and shape,[4,12,32,39] and general deconditioning.[58]

WORK-RELATED FACTORS

The box below summarizes the characteristics of work that have been associated with elevated rates of hand and wrist symptoms and specific disorders like CTS and tendinitis. Although the associations are almost all based on cross-sectional studies of different design and method, these same risk factors continue to appear with remarkable consistency. **Tables 32-1** and **32-2** summarize selected studies of wrist and hand tendinitis and CTS that include a control group. Several recent reviews have evaluated the extent to which CTS is associated with work.[34,76]

Work factors associated with disorders of the hands and wrists

Repetition
Force
Posture extremes
Vibration
Mechanical contact
Duration of work
Work organization

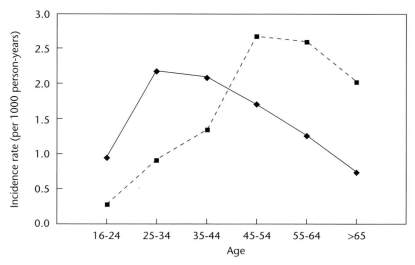

Figure 32-3 Population age-specific incidence rates of carpal tunnel syndrome for Rochester, Minnesota, from 1961 to 1980 (----) (N=1016)[75] as compared with work-related incidence rates for the Washington State worker's compensation system from 1984 to 1988 (...) (N=7926).[28]

Table 32-1	Selected controlled epidemiologic studies evaluating the association between work and wrist, hand, or distal forearm tendinitis[a]			
Authors	**Exposed Population**	**Control Population**	**Rate in Exposed (%)**	**Rate in Control (%)**
Kuorinka et al, 1979	90 scissors makers	133 shop attendants	18	14
Luopajarvi et al, 1979[b]	152 bread packaging	133 shop attendants	53[c]	14
Silverstein et al, 1986[d,e]	**Industrial**	**Industrial**		
	143 low force/high rep	136 low force/low rep	3?	1.5
	153 high force/low rep	136 low force/low rep	4?	1.5
	142 high force/high rep	136 low force/low rep	20[c]	1.5
McCormack et al, 1990	**Manufacturing**	**Manufacturing**		
	369 packers/folders	352 knitting workers	3.3[c]	0.9
	562 sewers	352 knitting workers	4.4[c]	0.9
	296 boarding workers	352 knitting workers	6.4[c]	0.9
Kurppa et al, 1991[b,f]	102 meat cutters	141 office workers	12.5?	0.9
	107 sausage makers	197 office workers	16.3[c]	0.7
	118 packers	197 office workers	25.3[c]	0.7

[a]Case criteria are based on history and physical examination.
[b]All exposed and control subjects are female.
[c]Significant difference from control.
[d]Adjusted for age, sex, and plant.
[e]Analysis includes other disorders, although tendinitis was most common.
[f]Cohort study with a 31-month follow-up.

Table 32-2	Selected controlled epidemiologic studies evaluating the association between work and carpal tunnel syndrome*				
Authors	**Exposed Population**	**Control Population**	**Criteria**	**Rate in Exposed (%)**	**Rate in Control (%)**
Silverstein et al, 1987†	**Industrial** High force/high rep	**Industrial** Low force/low rep	History and physical examination	5.1‡	0.6
Nathan, 1988§‖	22 keyboard operators	147 admin/clerical	Electrodiagnostic	27	28
	164 assembly line	147 admin/clerical	Electrodiagnostic	47	28
	115 general plant	147 admin/clerical	Electrodiagnostic	38	28
	23 grinders	147 admin/clerical	Electrodiagnostic	61‡	28
Barnhart, 1991§	106 ski manufacturing repetitive jobs	67 ski manufacturing nonrepetitive jobs	Electrodiagnosis and signs	15.4‡	3.1

*Diagnoses are based on history and physical examination or nerve conduction study.
†Control for age, gender, and years on job.
‡Significantly different from control group.
§Control for age and gender.
‖Low participation rate and limited exposure assessment.

Studies using crude measures of exposure have reported associations between repetition and hand/wrist pain and disorders. In a study relying exclusively on nerve conduction measurements, median nerve slowing occurred at a higher rate among assembly line workers than among administrative controls.[34,57] Although no systematic assessment of exposure was carried out, assembly line workers were believed to have more repetitive work than the control group. The rate of persistent wrist and hand pain was higher in garment workers performing repetitive hand tasks than in the control group of hospital employees.[66] Persistent wrist pain, or pain that lasted most of the day for at least 1 month in the last year, occurred in 17% of the garment workers and 4% of hospital controls, whereas persistent hand pain occurred in 27% of garment workers and 10% of the controls. Others have observed a similar link between high hand/wrist repetition and CTS[8,18,83] and tendinitis.[45] The link to repetition may be that these are jobs that require high velocity or acceleration of the wrist or repeated postural stress.[52]

Rates of wrist tendinitis among scissors makers were compared with those of shop attendants in department stores in Finland. Examinations and histories were standardized and performed by one person. The rates between the groups were not significantly different; however, among the scissors makers, the rate of tendinitis increased with increasing number of scissors handled.[44] Luopajarvi et al[47] compared packers in a bread factory with the same control group. The packers' work involved repetitive gripping, up to 25,000 cycles per day, with maximum extension of the thumb and fingers to handle wide bread packages. Approximately half of the packers had wrist/hand tenosynovitis as compared with 14% among the controls. The most common disorder of the hand or wrist was thumb tenosynovitis, followed by finger/wrist extensor tenosynovitis. Carpal tunnel syndrome was diagnosed in four packers and no controls.

The force that is applied to a tool or materials during repeated or sustained gripping is also a predictor of the risk for tendinitis and CTS. For example, in a study of the textile industry, the risk of hand and wrist tendinitis was 3.9 times higher among packaging and folding workers than among knitters.[55] The packing and folding workers were considered to be performing physically demanding work as compared with the knitting workers. Armstrong and Chaffin[4] observed that women with CTS applied more pinch force during production sewing than did their job-matched and sex-matched controls. It is possible that those with CTS altered their working style as the carpal tunnel syndrome progressed; however, it is unlikely that they would increase the pinch force because this would also trigger symptoms. In a study by Moore and Garg[56] at a pork processing plant, in the jobs that involved high grip force or long grip durations such as Wizard knife operator, snipper, feeder, scaler, bagger, packer, hanger, and stuffer, almost every employee was affected. Others have observed a similar relationship with work involving sustained or high force grip in grinders,[57] meatpackers and butchers,[25,45] and other industrial workers.[78,81] Years of exposure to both repetitive wrist movement and "heavy load on the wrist" were strongly associated with CTS.[83]

The most comprehensive study of the combined factors of repetition and force was a cross-sectional study of 574 industrial workers by Silverstein et al.[4,73,74] Disorders were assessed by physical examination and history and were primarily tendinitis followed by CTS, Guyon tunnel syndrome, and digital neuritis. Subjects were classified into four exposure groups based on force and repetition. The "high-force" work involved a grip force averaging more than 4 kg force whereas "low-force" work involved less than 1 kg of grip force. The "high-repetition" work involved a repetitive task in which either the cycle time was less than 30 seconds (greater than 900 times in a workday) or more than 50% of the cycle time was spent performing the same kind of fundamental hand movements. The high-risk groups were compared with the low-risk group after adjusting for plant, age, gender, and years on the job. The odds ratio of all hand/wrist disorders for high force alone was 5.2, and that for high repetition alone was 3.3; this increased to 29 for jobs that required both high force and high repetition. The identical analysis of just CTS revealed an odds ratio of 1.8 for force, 2.7 for repetition, and 14 for the combined high-force, high-repetition group. A metaanalysis of Silverstein's data pooled with Luopajarvi's study results concluded that for high-force, high-repetition work, the common odds ratio for CTS was 15.5 (95% confidence interval [CI], 1.7 to 141) and for hand/wrist tendinitis it was 9.1 (95% CI, 5 to 16).[76] Estimates of the percentage of CTS cases among workers who perform repetitive or forceful hand activity that can be attributed to work range from 50% to 90%.[34,77]

Work involving increased wrist deviation from a neutral posture in either the extension/flexion or ulnar/radial direction has been associated with CTS and other hand and wrist problems.[37,78,79] De Krom et al[20] conducted a case-control study of 156 subjects with CTS versus 473 controls randomly sampled from the hospital and population registers in a region of the Netherlands. After adjustment for age and sex, a dose-response relationship was observed for increasing hours of work with the wrist in extension or flexion. No risk was observed for increasing hours performing a pinch grasp or typing, although methodologic limitations may have obscured such associations. Some studies of computer operators have linked awkward wrist postures to the severity of hand symptoms,[26] risk of tendinitis or CTS,[71] and arm and hand discomfort.[21,38,70]

Prolonged exposure to vibrating hand tools such as chain saws has been linked in prospective studies to hand-arm vibration syndrome.[22,31] The risks are primarily vibration acceleration, amplitude, and frequency; hand coupling to tool; hours per day of exposure; and years of exposure. Based on existing studies, however, no clear vibration acceleration/frequency/duration threshold has been found that would protect most workers. Therefore, medical surveillance is recommended to identify cases early while the disease can still be reversed.[59] Nonetheless, both the American National Standards Institute (ANSI) and the International Standards Organization (ISO) have promulgated guidelines limiting the duration of exposure as a function of acceleration and frequency. The use of vibrating hand tools may also increase the risk of CTS,[16,68,72,83] either by direct nerve injury or by indirectly increasing applied grip force through a reflex pathway.[67]

Prolonged or high-load localized mechanical stress over tendons or nerves from tools or from resting the hand on hard objects has been have been associated with tendinitis[79] and nerve entrapment[37,65] in case studies.

The average total hours per day that a task is repeated or sustained has been a factor in predicting hand problems.[48,51] For example, an increase in hours of computer use has been a predictor of increased symptom intensity or increased rate of disorder in computer operators.*

Work organizational (e.g., work structure, decision control, workload, deadline work, supervision) and psychosocial factors (e.g., job satisfaction, social support, relationship with supervisor) appear to have some influence on hand and wrist symptoms among computer users. Among newspaper reporters and editors, work organizational factors modified the expected relationship between work station design and hand and wrist symptoms. Symptom intensity increased as keyboard height increased among those with low decision latitude but not among those with high decision latitude.[26] In another study of newspaper employees, the risk of hand and wrist symptoms was increased among those with increasing hours on deadline work and less support from the immediate supervisor.[9] Among directory assistance operators at a telephone company, high information processing demands were associated with an elevated rate of hand and wrist disorders.[35] On the other hand, in an industrial setting, Silverstein, Fine, and Armstrong[73] observed no effect of job satisfaction. Work organizational factors are the most difficult to interpret in cross-sectional studies because psychosocial problems may develop in the workplace after and as a consequence of employees' symptoms and unsuccessful efforts to obtain job modifications or other accommodation.

*References 9, 13, 26, 38, 49, 63.

SUMMARY

Although variability exists between industries, hand and wrist disorders account for most work-related upper extremity musculoskeletal disorders. These disorders are costly to the worker, employer, and the worker's compensation system; however, a full accounting of their financial impact has yet to be done. Hand and wrist problems may present in any number of ways, from the most common presentation of nonspecific hand symptoms to discrete entities such as hand-arm vibration syndrome or DeQuervain's tenosynovitis. However, if the symptom rates are high in a work population, so are the rates of specific disorders.

The lack of prospective studies and an uncertainty of the pathophysiologic mechanisms involved limit our ability to definitively identify causative factors. Nonetheless, current studies point to a multifactorial relationship between work and these disorders. Some disorders such as tendinitis and CTS are clearly associated with work involving repetitive and forceful use of the hands, postural stress, and vibration. For other disorders such as ganglion cysts and osteoarthritis, the relationship to work is not well studied. Symptom severity and disorder rates—or at least their reporting—appear to be influenced by work organizational factors such as decision latitude and cognitive demands. Carpal tunnel syndrome has been linked to individual factors in population-based studies and clinical case series. However, in workplace studies, when workplace exposure is high and quantified, individual factors play a limited role relative to workplace factors.*

*References 4, 16, 26, 38, 35, 74.

References

1. Adams ML, Franklin GM, Barnhart S: Outcome of carpal tunnel surgery in Washington State workers' compensation, *Am J Ind Med*, 25:527-536, 1994.

2. Al-Qattan MM, Bowen V, Manktelow RT: Factors associated with poor outcome following primary carpal tunnel release in non-diabetic patients, *J Hand Surg [Br]* 19B:622-625, 1994.

3. Amadio PC: Pyridoxine as an adjunct in the treatment of carpal tunnel syndrome *J Hand Surg [Am]* 10A:237-241, 1985.

4. Armstrong TJ, Chaffin DB: Carpal tunnel syndrome and selected personal attributes, *J Occup Med* 21:481-486, 1979.

5. Armstrong TJ et al: A conceptual model for work-related neck and upper-limb musculoskeletal disorders, *Scand J Work Environ Health* 19:73-84, 1993.

6. Armstrong TJ et al: Investigation of cumulative trauma disorders in a poultry processing plant, *Am Ind Hyg Assoc J* 43(2):103-116, 1982.

7. Bammer G: VDUs and musculoskeletal problems at the Australian National University. In Knave B, Wideback PG, editors: *Work with display units 86*, Amsterdam, 1987, Elsevier Science Publishers BV.

8. Barnhart S et al: Carpal tunnel syndrome among ski manufacturing workers, *Scand J Work Environ Health* 17:46-52, 1991.

9. Bernard B et al: *Health hazard evaluation report: Los Angeles Times*, NIOSH Rep No 90-013-2277, Washington, DC, 1993, US Department of Health and Human Services, Public Health Service, Centers for Disease Control, National Institute for Occupational Safety and Health.

10. Birbeck MQ, Beer TC: Occupation in relation to the carpal tunnel syndrome, *Rheumatol Rehabil* 14:218-221, 1975.

11. Bjorkqvist SE et al: Carpal tunnel syndrome in ovariecto-mized women, *Acta Obstet Gynecol Scand* 56:127-130, 1985.

12. Bleeker MQ et al: Carpal tunnel syndrome: role of carpal canal size, *Neurology* 35:1599-1604, 1985.

13. Burt S et al: *Health hazard evaluation report: Newsday,* NIOSH Rep No 89-250-2046, Washington, DC, 1990, US Department of Health and Human Services, Public Health Service, Centers for Disease Control, National Institute for Occupational Safety and Health.

14. California State Compensation Insurance Fund: Personal communication, 1993.

15. Campbell CS: Gamekeeper's thumb, *J Bone and Joint Surgery* 37B(1):148-149, 1955.

16. Cannon LJ, Bernacki EJ, Walter SD: Personal and occupa-tional factors associated with carpal tunnel syndrome, *J Occup Med* 23:255-258, 1981.

17. Centers for Disease Control: Occupational disease surveillance—carpal tunnel syndrome, *MMWR Morb Mor-tal Wkly Rep* 38:485-489, 1989.

18. Chiang HC et al: The occurrence of carpal tunnel syn-drome in frozen food factory employees, *Kao Hsiung J Med Sci* 6:73-80, 1990.

19. Conn HR: Tenosynovitis, *Ohio State Med J* 27:713-716, 1931.

20. de Krom M et al: Risk factors for carpal tunnel syndrome, *Am J Epidemiol* 132:1102-1110, 1990.

21. Duncan J, Ferguson D: Keyboard operating posture and symptoms in operating, *Ergonomics* 17:651-662, 1974.

22. Ekenvall L, Carlsson A: Vibration white finger: a follow up study, *Br J Ind Med* 44:476-478, 1987.

23. Ekman-Ordeberg G, Salgeback S, Ordeberg G: Carpal tun-nel syndrome in pregnancy: a retrospective study, *Acta Obstet Gynecol Scand* 66:233-235, 1987.

24. Ellis J et al: Clinical results of a cross-over treatment with pyridoxine and placebo of the carpal tunnel syndrome, *J Clin Nutr* 32(10):2046-2070, 1979.

25. Falck B, Aarnio P: Left-sided carpal tunnel syndrome in butchers, *Scand J Work Environ Health* 9:291-297, 1983.

26. Faucett J, Rempel D: VDT-related musculoskeletal symp-toms: interactions between work posture and psychoso-cial work factors, *Am J Ind Med* 26:597-612, 1994.

27. Fine LJ et al: Detection of cumulative trauma disorders of upper extremities in the workplace, *J Occup Med* 28:674-678, 1986.

28. Franklin GM et al: Occupational carpal tunnel syndrome in Washington State, 1984-1988, *Am J Public Health* 81:741-746, 1991.

29. Franzblau A et al: Workplace surveillance for carpal tun-nel syndrome: a comparison of methods, *J Occup Rehabil* 3:1-14, 1993.

30. Franzblau et al: Workplace surveillance for carpal tunnel syndrome using hand diagrams, *J Occup Rehabil* 4:185-198, 1994.

31. Futatsuka M, Ueno T: A follow-up study of vibration-induced white finger due to chain-saw operation, *Scand J Work Environ Health* 12:304-306, 1986.

32. Gelmers H: Primary carpal tunnel stenosis as a cause of entrapment of the median nerve, *Acta Neurochir* 55:317-320, 1981.

33. Hadler N et al: Hand structure and function in an indus-trial setting, *Arthritis Rheum* 21:210-220, 1978.

34. Hagberg M, Morgenstern H, Kelsh M: Impact of occupa-tions and job tasks on the prevalence of carpal tunnel syndrome, *Scand J Work Environ Health* 18:337-345, 1992.

35. Hales TR et al: Musculoskeletal disorders among visual display terminal users in a telecommunications company, *Ergonomics* 10:1603-1621, 1994.

36. Heller L et al: Evaluation of Tinel's and Phalen's signs in diagnosis of carpal tunnel syndrome, *Eur Neurol* 25:40-42, 1986.

37. Hoffman J, Hoffman PL: Staple gun carpal tunnel syn-drome, *J Occup Med* 27:848-849, 1985.

38. Hunting W, Ldubli T, Grandjean E: Postural and visual loads at VDT workplaces, *Ergonomics* 24:917-931, 1981.

39. Johnson EW et al: Wrist dimensions: correlation with me-dian sensory latencies, *Arch Phys Med Rehabil* 64:556-557, 1983.

40. Kaji H et al: Hypothenar hammer syndrome in workers occupationally exposed to vibrating tools, *J Hand Surg [Br]* 18B:761-766, 1993.

41. Katz JN et al: A self-administered hand symptom diagram for the diagnosis and epidemiologic study of carpal tun-nel syndrome. *J Rheumatol* 3:1-14, 1990.

42. Katz JN et al: Validation of a surveillance case definition of carpal tunnel syndrome, *Am J Public Health* 81:189-193, 1991.

43. Kivi P: Rheumatic disorders of the upper limbs associated with repetitive occupational tasks in Finland in 1975-1979, *Scand J Rheumatol* 13:101-107, 1984.

44. Kuorinka I, Koskinen P: Occupational rheumatic diseases and upper limb strain in manual jobs in a light mechani-cal industry, *Scand J Work Environ Health* 5:39-47, 1979.

45. Kurppa K et al: Incidence of tenosynovitis or peritendini-tis and epicondylitis in a meat processing factory, *Scand J Work Environ Health* 17:32-37, 1991.

46. Little JM, Ferguson DA: The incidence of hypothenar hammer syndrome. *Arch Surg* 105:684-685, 1972.

47. Luopajarvi T et al: Prevalence of tenosynovitis and other injuries of the upper extremities in repetitive work, *Scand J Work Environ Health* 5:48-55, 1979.

48. MacDonald G: Hazards in the dental workplace, *Am J Dent Hyg* 61:212-218, 1987.

49. Maeda K, Hunting W, Grandjean E: Factor analysis of lo-calized fatigue complaints of accounting-machine opera-tors, *J Hum Ergol,* 11:37-43, 1982.

50. Reference deleted in proofs.

51. Margolis W, Kraus JF: The prevalence of carpal tunnel syndrome symptoms in female supermarket checkers, *J Occup Med* 29:953-956, 1987.

52. Marras WS, Schoenmarklin RW: Wrist motions in industry, *Ergonomics* 36:341-351, 1993.

53. Masear VR, Hayes JM, Hyde AG: An industrial cause of carpal tunnel syndrome, *J of Hand Surg [Am]* 11A:222-227, 1986.

54. McCann J, Davis R: Carpal tunnel syndrome, diabetes and pyridoxal, *Aust J Med* 8:638-640, 1978.

55. McCormack RR Jr et al: Prevalence of tendinitis and related disorders of the upper extremity in a manufacturing work force, *J Rheumatol* 17:958-964, 1990.

56. Moore JS, Garg A: Upper extremity disorders in a pork processing plant: relationships between job risk factors and morbidity. *Am Ind Hyg Assoc J* 55:703-715, 1994.

57. Nathan PA, Meadows KD, Doyle LS: Occupation as a risk factor for impaired sensory conduction of the median nerve at the carpal tunnel, *J Hand Surg [Br]* 13B:167-170, 1988.

58. Nathan PA et al: Obesity as a risk factor for slowing of sensory conduction of the median nerve in industry, *J Occup Med* 34:379-383, 1992.

59. National Institute of Occupational Safety and Health: *Criteria for a recommended standard. Occupational exposure to hand-arm vibration,* DDHS Pub No 89-106, Cincinnati, 1989, The Institute.

60. Newland CC: Gamekeeper's thumb, *Orthop Clin North Am* 23(1):41-48, 1992.

61. Nilsson T, Burstrvm L, Hagberg M: Risk assessment of vibration exposure and white fingers among platers, *Int Arch Occup Environ Health* 61:473-481, 1989.

62. Ohara H, Aoyama H, Itani T: Health hazards among cash register operators and the effects of improved working conditions, *J Hum Ergol* 5:31-40, 1976.

63. Oxenburgh M, Rowe S, Douglas D: Repetitive strain injury in keyboard operators, *J Occup Health Saf Aust N Z* 1:106-112, 1985.

64. Park CH et al: Health conditions among the currently employed: United States, 1988. National Center for Health Statistics, *Vital Health Stat* 10:186, 1993.

65. Phalen GS: The carpal-tunnel syndrome, *J Bone Joint Surg* 48A:211-228, 1966.

66. Punnett L et al: Soft tissue disorders in the upper limbs of female garment workers, *Scand J Work Environ Health* 11:417-425, 1985.

67. Radwin RG, Armstrong TJ, Chaffin DB: Power hand tool vibration effects on grip exertions, *Ergonomics* 30:833-855, 1987.

68. Rothfleisch S, Sherman D: Carpal tunnel syndrome: biomechanical aspects of occupational occurrence and implications regarding surgical management, *Orthop Rev* 7:107-109, 1978.

69. Sabour M, Fadel H: The carpal tunnel syndrome, a new complication ascribed to the pill, *Am J Obstet Gynecol* 107:1265-1267, 1971.

70. Sauter SL, Scheifer LM, Knutson SJ: Work posture, work station design, and musculoskeletal discomfort in a VDT entry task, *Hum Factors* 33:151-167, 1991.

71. Seligman P, Boiano J, Anderson C: *Health Hazard Evaluation of the Minneapolis Police Department,* 1986, Springfield, Va, NIOSH HETA 84-417-1745, US Department of Commerce, National Technical Information Service.

72. Seppalainen AM: Nerve conduction in the vibration syndrome, *Scand J Work Environ Health* 6:82-84, 1970.

73. Silverstein BA, Fine LJ, Armstrong TJ: Hand wrist cumulative trauma disorders in industry, *Br J Ind Med* 43:779-784, 1986.

74. Silverstein BA, Fine LJ, Armstrong TJ: Occupational factors and carpal tunnel syndrome, *Am J Ind Med* 11:343-358, 1987.

75. Stevens JC et al: Carpal tunnel syndrome in Rochester, Minnesota, 1961 to 1980, *Neurology* 38:134-138, 1988.

76. Stock SR: Workplace ergonomic factors and the development of musculoskeletal disorders of the neck and upper limbs: a meta-analysis, *Am J Ind Med* 19:87-107, 1991.

77. Tanaka S et al: The US prevalence of self-reported carpal tunnel syndrome, *Am J Public Health* 84:1846-1848, 1994.

78. Thompson A, Plewes L, Shaw E: Peritendinitis crepitans and simple tenosynovitis: a clinical study of 544 cases in industry, *Br J Ind Med* 8:150-160, 1951.

79. Tichauer E: Some aspects of stress on forearm and hand in industry, *J Occup Med* 8:63-71, 1966.

80. Vessey MP, Villard-MacInosh L, Yeates D: Epidemiology of carpal tunnel syndrome in women of childbearing age. Finding in a large cohort study, *Am J Epidemiol* 19:655-659, 1990.

81. Welch R: The causes of tenosynovitis in industry, *Ind Med* 41:16-19, 1972.

82. Werner RA et al: The relationship between body mass index and the diagnosis of carpal tunnel syndrome, *Muscle Nerve* 17:632-636, 1994.

83. Wieslander G et al: Carpal tunnel syndrome (CTS) and exposure to vibration, repetitive wrist movements, and heavy manual work: a case-referent study, *Br J Ind Med* 46:43-47, 1989.

84. Williams WV et al: Metacarpo-phalangeal arthropathy associated with manual labor (Missouri metacarpal syndrome), *Arthritis Rheum* 30:1362-1371, 1987.

85. Yamaguchi D, Liscomb P, Soule E: Carpal tunnel syndrome, *Minn Med J* 1965; pp 22-23.

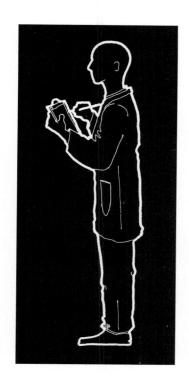

Chapter 33

Biomechanics of the Wrist and Hand

K. N. An

CONTENTS

The human hand is a relatively mobile, three-dimensional structure capable of conforming to the shape of manipulated objects. The biomechanical structure of the hand can be considered a linkage system of intercalated bony segments balanced by muscle and tendon forces and joint constraints. Reviewed here will be the normal range of joint motion and potential strength of the hand, and then more basic biomechanical considerations of muscle-tendon function and joint stability will be discussed. It is hoped that this information will be useful in better understanding work-related disorders.

MOTION

The fingers and thumb consist of phalanges articulated at the interphalangeal (IP) joints. Within the physiologic range of motion, the IP joints can be considered hinge joints that allow flexion-extension motion. In a normal hand, each IP joint has at least 90 degrees of motion. The proximal phalanx articulates with the metacarpal at the metacarpophalangeal (MP) joints. The MP joints are usually considered universal joints, allowing not only flexion-extension but also abduction-adduction motion. Again, in a normal hand the range of flexion-extension is about 90 degrees and that of abduction-adduction is 20 to 30 degrees.

The wrist joint connects the digits of the hand to the radius and ulna of the forearm. The wrist joint is a composite articulation of eight carpal bones. The range of wrist motions required to comfortably perform activities of daily living consists of a total of 60 degrees of wrist extension, 54 degrees of flexion, 40 degrees of ulnar deviation, and 17 degrees of radial deviation. The majority of the hand placement and range-of-motion tasks could be accomplished with 70% of the maximum range of wrist motion. This converts to 40 degrees each of wrist flexion and extension and 40 degrees of combined radial-ulnar deviation.

STRENGTH

The potential strength of various joints in the hand and wrist in normal subjects has been studied with dynamometers. Normal pinch strengths ranged from 3 to 10 kg and grasp strengths from 20 to 40 kg. The wrist position and size of the grasped object have a significant influence on grip strength. Grip strength as a function of wrist joint position has been studied extensively. A self-selected wrist position of 35 degrees of extension and 7 degrees of ulnar deviation has been identified as the position in which maximum grip strength could be generated.[9] For a given size of an object, the grip strength is significantly reduced when the wrist position deviates from this self-selected position.

The strength of the wrist joint is in the range of 10 to 20 Nm of flexion, 6 to 10 Nm of extension, 10 to 18 Nm of radial deviation, and 10 to 20 Nm of ulnar deviation.

TENDON EXCURSION

The ability to control the movement of an individual digit of the hand depends very much on the anatomic arrangement of the musculotendinous complex. The magnitude of tendon excursion during joint movement for a given task would also be important for assessing possible overuse injury caused by cumulative trauma.

For the finger and thumb, the pulley structures on the palmar side of the digits restrain bowstringing of the digital flexor during joint flexion. Alteration of such a pulley system in the hand will disturb the relationship between tendon excursion and joint angular displacement and thus joint function. Parameters have been defined from the curves of tendon excursion and joint motion for comparing tendon-pulley-joint interactions under normal and abnormal conditions.[8] The range of movement of the joint produced by a given standardized amount of excursion is called the *effective range of motion. Absolute tendon excursion* is excursion from full extension to 90 degrees of flexion, as measured with the flexor tendon set at its normal length in the neutral position. Division of the pulley would result in bowstringing and the addition of slack to the tendon system, which had to be taken up before any joint motion could occur. This amount of tendon slack is termed *bowstring laxity.* By subtracting the bowstring laxity from absolute tendon excursion, *relative tendon excursion* is defined.

The biomechanical functions of the musculotendinous complex could be reflected by the relationship of tendon excursion and joint angular displacement. The rate of change in tendon excursion as the joint rotates is equal to the moment arm of the associated muscle or tendon for that specific joint motion.[4] The moment arm defines not only the effectiveness of the tendon in joint rotation but also the mechanical advantage of the tendon in resisting external loads. The larger the moment arm, the higher the torque and rotation angle generated for the same amount of muscle force and excursion. A determination of the potential moment arm contributions of muscles can provide insight into the balance of forces at a joint for planning tendon transfers or designing orthotics to assist in providing mobility or stability while minimizing loss of function.

For example, tendon excursion and joint rotation angles of the wrist are measured by using an electric

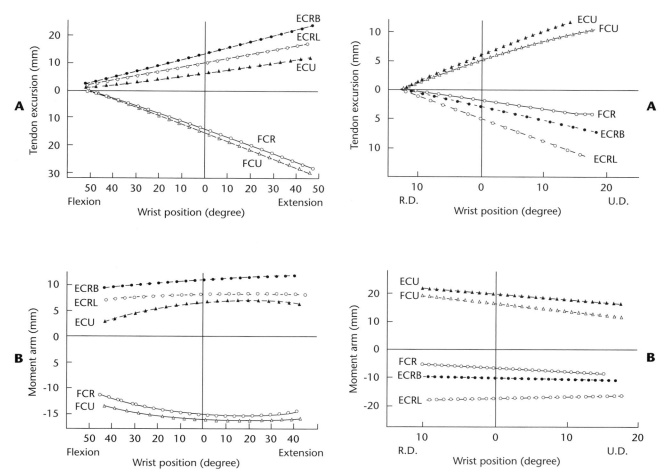

Figure 33-1. *(Left)* Tendon excursion and moment arm of the five wrist motor tendons during flexion-extension motion. **A,** Tendon excursion. The wrist joint was moved from full flexion to full extension passively. **B,** Moment arms calculated from **A.** The flexors and extensors show the different directions of the moment arm. Extensors show the plus moment arm, and flexors show the minus moment arm; *(Right)* Tendon excursion and moment arm of the five wrist motor tendons during radial-ulnar deviation. **A,** Tendon excursion. The wrist joint was moved from radial deviation *(RD)* to ulnar deviation *(UD)* passively. **B,** Moment arms calculated from **A.** The ulnar side tendons show the plus moment, and the radial side tendons show the minus moment. *(From Horii E, An KN, Linscheid RL:* J Hand Surg *18(1):83-90, 1993.)*

potentiometer and an electromagnetic tracking device, respectively.[1] The instantaneous moment arms of each tendon are then calculated from the slope of the curve between the tendon excursion and the joint angular displacement. Calculated tendon moment arms are found to be consistent throughout a full range of flexion-extension and radioulnar deviation motion and correspond closely to the anatomic location and orientation of the tendons (**Fig. 33-1**).

MUSCLE AND JOINT FORCES

The potential force generated by a muscle depends on its size and architecture. Three anatomic parameters

of muscle morphology have been recognized to be important in defining the biomechanical potential of the muscle:[5] : (1) muscle fiber length is related to the potential range of physiologic excursion of the tendon and muscle; (2) the physiologic cross-sectional area of a muscle is proportional to its maximum tension potential; and (3) physically, the product of the force and distance is work; therefore, the muscle mass or volume has been considered to be proportional to the work capacity of the muscle.

In addition, potential force generation is further regulated by the velocity of shortening or lengthening of the muscle and the muscle length at the time of contraction. It is well known that potential muscle force generation depends on the muscle length at contraction. Usually, an optimum length at which maximum contractile force is generated can be found. The force potential of muscle with contraction at either a shorter or longer muscle length will be less. The arrangement of the muscle fiber architecture will further influence the characteristics of the muscle contraction.[7] It has been demonstrated that parallel muscle fibers produce a length-tension curve with maintained force throughout a wider range of excursion than do muscles with a shorter fiber pennate structure, which produce sharply peaked curves. The index of muscle architecture, defined as the ratio of muscle fiber length to muscle belly length, has been used to define such characteristics.

The orientation or constraint of muscles or tendons crossing a joint determines the characteristics of excursion and the moment arm. In general, the larger the moment arm, the better the mechanical advantage for the same amount of tendon or muscle force. On the other hand, the larger the moment arm, the more tendon excursion expected for the same amount of joint rotation. The excursion of the tendon eventually affects the muscle length of contraction and ultimately determines the potential force generation according to the muscle length-tension characteristics.

The size and shape of the object to be grasped determines the joint configuration of the thumb and fingers involved in grasp function. The corresponding moment arms of both the intrinsic and extrinsic muscles at a particular joint configuration determine the mechanical advantage, tendon excursion, and corresponding muscle length. Therefore, as discussed earlier, the size and shape of the object are important considerations in determining the power and strength of the grasp. Furthermore, the extrinsic muscles of the fingers and thumb originate from the forearm. Wrist joint motion will therefore create excursion of these tendons and modify the muscle contraction characteristics because of the length-tension relationship. Thus grasp power and strength are regulated by wrist joint configuration as well.

Because of the relatively smaller moment arms or mechanical advantage of the muscles and tendons across the joints as compared with those of externally applied forces at the tip of the digits, the muscle force required to balance grip or pinch functions is much higher. For example, in the tip and pulp pinch function, the forces of the flexor profundus and sublimis are about one to two times the force at the tip of the digits. The associated forces in the intrinsic muscles are in the range of 0.5 to 1.5 times the applied forces.[2,3] Accordingly, with such a magnitude of muscle and tendon forces, the compressive and shear forces across the finger joints are found to be quite significant (**Fig. 33-2**).

FORCE THROUGH WRIST CARPAL JOINT

When the hand is used, a tremendous amount of force is encountered at the wrist joint. The distribution of the forces among the carpal bones has great potential for injury to the associated bone and soft tissue. Cumulative trauma with compression of the lunate, for example, has been thought to result in avascular necrosis of the lunate (Kienböck's disease). It has been postulated that excessive and uneven loading is experienced by the lunate between the lunate fossa of the radius and the compressible triangular fibrocartilage of the ulna. The overall force transmitted from the proximal row of carpal bones to the distal radioulnar joint has been examined by numerous investigators. Although the findings have not been in complete agreement and are probably dependent on the measurement technique, trends of certain important characteristics have been quite consistent.

On average, 15% to 20% of axial wrist joint force is transmitted by the distal end of the ulna, and 80% to 85% is transmitted through the radius in the neutral position (**Fig. 33-3, A**).[6] The effect of joint position and forearm rotation on the percentage of load transmission across the radius and ulna has also been recognized. At the midcarpal joint, 30% of the total force was transmitted through the scaphotrapezial joint, 19% through the scaphocapitate joint, 31% through the lunocapitate joint, and 21% through the triquetrohamate joint with the wrist in the neutral position. With the wrist loaded, the carpal bones translate in the ulnar direction, down the inclined slope of the distal end of the radius (**Fig. 33-3, B**). In addition, tensions in the intercarpal liga-

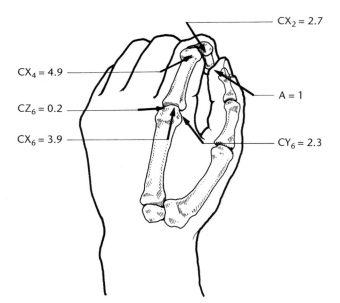

Figure 33-2. Resultant joint forces during tip pinch function of one unit force, that is, *A*=1. Forces represent the actions of the proximal segment applied onto the distal segment crossing the joint. *(From An KN, Cooney WP III: Biomechanics, section II, The Hand and Wrist. In Morrey BF, editor:* Joint replacement arthroplasty, *New York, 1991, Churchill Livingstone International; pp. 137-146.)*

ments are also observed when the wrist is loaded (**Fig. 33-3, C**). Interaction of the carpal bones is conceptually analogous to a Rubic's cube in which motion in one segment directly affects the position of another segment.

JOINT CONSTRAINT AND STABILITY

Joint constraint and stability are provided by the joint articular surfaces, the capsuloligamentous structures, and the musculotendinous units. Primary joint stability is related to balance of the muscle and tendon forces to an externally applied force. On the other hand, the capsuloligamentous structures appear to play the role of initial stabilizer against instantaneous loading and provide a second line of defense in maintaining joint stability. The collateral ligaments of all the joints in the hand and the intercarpal ligaments in the wrist are important soft tissues for joint constraint. The locations and orientations of the ligament lines of action determine their characteristics in resisting loads on the joint. For example, the radial collateral ligament (RCL) and the ulnar collateral ligament (UCL) are the primary ligaments of the MP joint. The RCL originates from the radial-dorsal aspect of the metacarpal head, with insertion into the radial-volar aspect of the proximal pha-

lanx. Therefore, the RCL is found to be the primary ligament in resisting ulnar deviation and pronation of the proximal phalanx at the MP joint. On the other hand, the UCL is the primary constraint in resisting radial deviation and supination of the proximal phalanx. The relative contribution of each of the ligaments in resisting joint displacement has been studied by sequential sectioning or removal of the individual ligaments (**Fig. 33-4**). The reduction of the load after removal of each ligamentous structure represents the contribution of the ligament.

SUMMARY

Work-related injuries are commonly encountered in the hand. Because of the nature of hand function, a tremendous amount of tension and repetition is experienced by the tendon and intrinsic muscles. The amount of tension may not be high enough to cause great damage to the tendon and muscle. However, these tensions could create compressive and frictional forces on the tendon and adjacent tissues when the tendons run around the pulley, bony surface, or other soft tissues. These compressive and friction forces could potentially be the causative forces leading to cumulative trauma disorders of the bone and soft tissue.

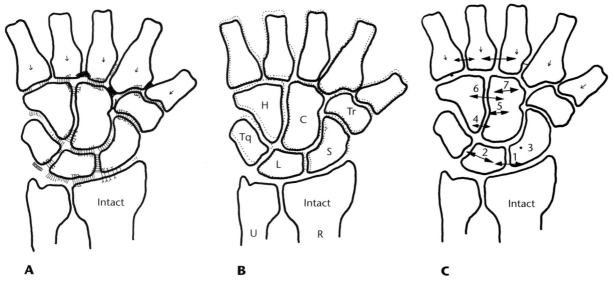

Figure 33-3. A, Each arrow represents the cumulative compressive force vector between adjacent bones and between the carpal bones and distal ends of the radius and ulna. These joint compressive forces or pressures within the carpus are calculated by this model when all the joints and ligaments are intact and axial loads are applied along the metacarpals. **B,** Predicted displacements of the carpal bones under the loading condition shown in **A.** Slight ulnar translation is present as a result of a component of force tangential to the radial articular surface. Carpal bone displacement must be considered when the concentration of the force vector across articular surfaces is analyzed. The dotted line represents the unloaded position and the solid line represents the loaded position of the carpus: *S,* scaphoid; *L,* lunate; *Tq,* triquetrum; *Tr,* trapezium/trapezoid; *C,* capitate; *H,* hamate; *R,* radius; *U,* ulna. **C,** Each arrow represents the calculated tension for the different carpal ligaments under the same loading condition: *1,* palmar radiolunate ligament; *2,* dorsal radiotriquetral ligament; *3,* palmar radiocapitate ligament; *4,* palmar capitatotriquetral ligament; *5,* dorsal scaphotriquetral ligament; *6,* palmar/dorsal hamatocapitate ligaments; *7,* flexor retinaculum. *(From Horii E, Garcia M, et al: J Hand Surg [Am] 15A(3):393-400, 1990.)*

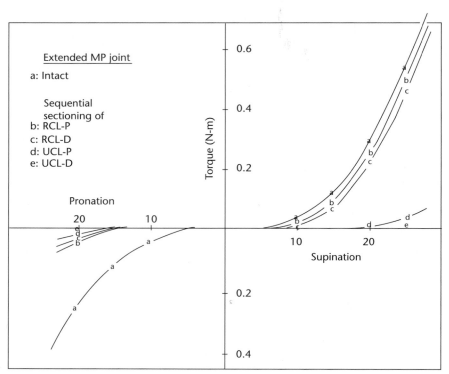

Figure 33-4. Load-displacement curves were obtained by measuring the restraining torques when the metacarpophalangeal joints were displaced in supination and pronation. Curve *a* represents the torques with the entire capsule-ligament complex intact. Curves *b* and *c* represent the torques when the palmar and dorsal portions of the radial collateral ligament (RCL) were sectioned, respectively. Curves *d* and *e* represent the restraining torques when the palmar and dorsal portions of the ulnar collateral ligament were sectioned, respectively. The difference in load between each curve for a given displacement indicates the contribution of that particular sectioned element. For example, the difference in load between curves *a* and *b* represents the contribution of the palmar portion of the RCL. *N-m*, newton-meter. *(From An KN, Cooney WP III: Biomechanics, section II, The Hand and Wrist. In Morrey BF, editor:* Joint replacement arthroplasty, *New York, 1991, Churchill Livingstone International; pp. 137-146. Copyright 1993 by Mayo Foundation.)*

References

1. An KN, Berger RA, Cooney WP: *Biomechanics of the wrist,* New York, 1991, Springer-Verlag.

2. An KN, Cooney WP: III: Biomechanics. Section II: The hand and wrist. In Morrey BF, editor: *Joint replacement arthroplasty,* New York, 1991, Churchill Livingstone; pp. 137-146.

3. An KN et al: Forces in the normal and abnormal hand, *J Orthop Res* 3:202-211, 1985.

4. An KN et al: Tendon excursion and moment arm of index finger muscles, *J Biomech* 16:419-425, 1983.

5. Chao EYS et al: *Biomechanics of the hand. A basic research study,* Singapore, 1989, World Scientific.

6. Horii E et al: Effect on force transmission across the carpus in procedures used to treat Kienböck's disease, *J Hand Surg [Am]* 15A(3):393-400, 1990.

7. Kaufman KR, An K N, Chao EYS: Incorporation of muscle architecture into muscle length-tension relationship, *J Biomech* 22:943-948, 1989.

8. Lin GT et al: Functional anatomy of the human digital flexor pulley system, *J Hand Surg [Am]* 14A:949-956, 1989.

9. O'Driscoll SW et al: The relationship between wrist position, grasp size, and grip strength, *J Hand Surg* 17:169-177, 1992.

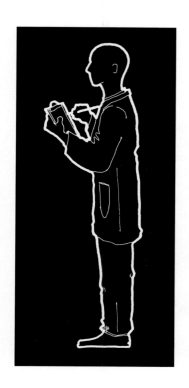

Chapter 34

Clinical Evaluation of the Wrist and the Hand

Michael S. Bednar

CONTENTS

The ability to manipulate objects with the hands is one of the major differences that sets humans apart from other species. Because of the intimate relationship between work and use of the hand, the hand is vulnerable to a variety of injuries.

Evaluation of the hand and wrist should focus on the anatomic structures that are most likely injured.[1] The organ systems of the hand may be divided into skeletal, musculotendinous, nervous, vascular, and skin and subcutaneous tissue. In evaluating each of these systems, the examiner should rely on a directed history and careful physical examination, including observation, light and deep palpation, and diagnostic maneuvers.[2]

HISTORY

On initial examination, the examiner should ask the patient to describe the chief complaint in one or two sentences. The patient's age, hand dominance, sex, and occupation should be noted. If an injury has occurred, the time and place are noted. In addition, the mechanism of injury, including the position of the hand and wrist at the time of the injury, as well as the magnitude of the forces involved, is elicited in an attempt to anticipate the structures that may have been injured. For instance, a fall onto a hyperextended wrist in a patient 18 to 25 years old is suggestive of a scaphoid fracture, whereas the same mechanism of injury in an older individual may lead to a distal radius fracture.

Patients should then be asked to detail the difficulties they are having with their hand and wrist at this time, including pain, paresthesia, weakness, and difficulties with motion. The past medical history is pertinent regarding an injury to the same hand in the past and/or previous treatments. Patients should also be questioned about medical conditions, including diabetes, inflammatory arthritides, renal disease, thyroid disease, and pregnancy.

With a careful history, the correct diagnosis can be made in approximately 90% of cases.

PHYSICAL EXAMINATION

Bones and Joints

The wrist is composed of 10 bones forming three distinct joints (**Fig. 34-1**).[3] The distal radioulnar joint (DRUJ) is the articulation of the ulnar head with the sigmoid notch of the radius. Along with the elbow, this joint is responsible for forearm pronation and supination. The main stabilizer of the DRUJ is the triangular fibrocartilage complex (TFCC) (**Fig. 34-2**). The radiocarpal joint is composed of the articulation of the scaphoid and lunate with the radius. This space is continuous with the ulnocarpal joint, the articulation of the remaining portion of the lunate and triquetrum with the ulna through the TFCC. The third joint is the midcarpal joint, the articulation between the proximal carpal row (scaphoid, lunate, and triquetrum) with the distal carpal row (trapezium, trapezoid, capitate, and hamate). The radiocarpal and midcarpal joints each provide approximately half of the flexion/extension and radial/ulnar deviation. The eighth carpal bone, the pisiform, is a sesamoid bone of the flexor carpi ulnaris (FCU) and does not contribute to wrist motion.

The carpal bones are held in position by intrinsic

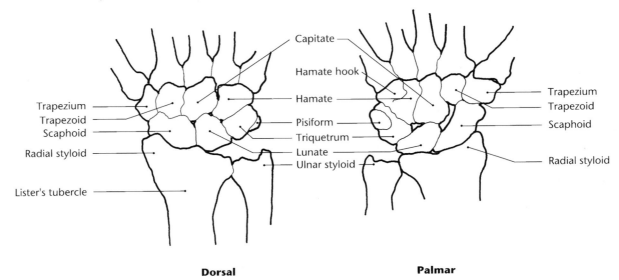

Dorsal   **Palmar**

Figure 34-1 Dorsal and palmar view of the wrist showing skeletal anatomy. (*From Reckling FW, Reckling JB, Mohn MP, editors:* Orthopaedic anatomy and surgical approaches, *St. Louis, 1990, Mosby–Year Book; pp. 112–129.*)

and extrinsic ligaments (**Fig. 34-3**). Intrinsic ligaments connect the individual carpal bones. The most clinically important intrinsic ligaments are the scapholunate, lunotriquetral, and deltoid (between the proximal and distal rows). The extrinsic ligaments join the radius and ulna to the carpus. These ligaments are stronger on the palmar side than on the dorsal side and are better seen from within the wrist joint.

Before palpation, the range of motion of the wrist is recorded. Pronation and supination are measured by asking the patient to hold a pencil in a clenched fist with the elbow flexed to 90 degrees. The angle between the pencil and the humerus is recorded. The normal

range of pronation/supination is 80/80. Flexion/extension and radial/ulnar deviation are measured between the forearm and the third metacarpal. Normal flexion/extension is 80/70 and normal radial/ulnar deviation is 20/30. The patient is first asked to actively move the joint, and the examiner then passively moves the joint. If passive and active motion are limited and equal, the problem is most likely due to joint stiffness. If the passive joint motion is substantially greater than the corresponding active motion, the problem is most likely due to the musculotendinous unit.

The examination of the wrist may be divided into four quadrants: radial, dorsal, ulnar, and palmar. In each

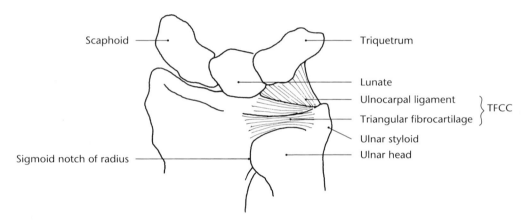

Figure 34-2 Dorsal view of the wrist showing the triangular fibrocartilage complex (*TFCC*)—triangular fibrocartilage and the ulnocarpal ligament. *(From Reckling FW, Reckling JB, Mohn MP, editors: Orthopaedic anatomy and surgical approaches, St. Louis, 1990, Mosby–Year Book; pp. 112–129.)*

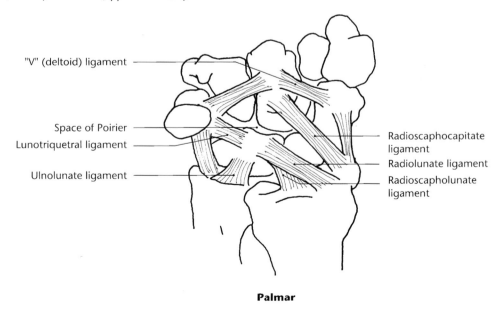

Palmar

Figure 34-3 Palmar view of the wrist showing the volar ligaments. The radioscapholunate ligament is thought to be the most important stabilizer of the proximal pole of the scalphoid. Note the space of Poirier, a weak area over the capitolunate articulation. *(From Reckling FW, Reckling JB, Mohn MP, editors: Orthopaedic anatomy and surgical approaches, St. Louis, 1990, Mosby–Year Book; pp. 112–129.)*

quadrant the bony and soft tissue structures should be examined for swelling, overlying redness, point tenderness, and crepitus. Examination of the soft tissues will be discussed in later sections.

The bony structures in the radial zone include the radial styloid, the scaphoid, the scaphoid tubercle, the trapezial tubercle, and the carpometacarpal (CMC) joint of the thumb. The radial styloid is found by palpating the distal end of the radius to its radial tip. When the wrist is ulnarly deviated, the body of the scaphoid is palpated just distal to the tip of the radial styloid. Tenderness in this region, called the radial snuffbox, is suggestive of a scaphoid fracture. The scaphoid tuberosity is palpable by sliding palmarly from the scaphoid body until the radial pulse is palpated. The first bony structure palpated distally is the tuberosity at the distal end of the scaphoid.

Identification of the scaphoid tuberosity is essential in performing the Watson maneuver, a technique to evaluate competence of the scapholunate ligament. With the patient facing the examiner, the patient's flexed elbow rests on a table. The examiner's right thumb is placed on the scaphoid tuberosity and the patient's wrist is ulnarly deviated. The examiner applies pressure from the palmar aspect of the tuberosity and radially deviates the wrist. Radial deviation causes the scaphoid to flex. If the ligament is incompetent, the examiner feels a "pop" and the patient experiences discomfort as the scaphoid subluxes dorsally.

The last joint to be palpated on the radial side of the wrist is the thumb CMC joint. The metacarpal should be palpated proximally until a depression is detected at the joint line. The right CMC joint is stressed as the examiner secures the patient's wrist with the right hand while grasping the base of the metacarpal between the left thumb and index finger. The metacarpal is displaced volarly as well as radially and ulnarly. Pain and crepitus with this maneuver suggest degenerative arthritis of the wrist.

The structures on the dorsum of the wrist are identified in relation to Lister's tubercle. This bony prominence lies approximately 1 cm proximal to the wrist joint along a line drawn from the radial border of the middle finger. The proximal scaphoid and the scapholunate ligament lie in line with Lister's tubercle. These structures are best palpated by flexing the wrist. Approximately 1 cm distal to this is a second depression that marks the midcarpal joint, the articulation of the head of the capitate with the proximal carpal row. The CMC joints of the index and middle fingers are located more distally. A bony spur, called a carpal boss, can develop at this joint and cause local pain and swelling.

An examination of the ulnar side of the wrist should include the DRUJ, the ulnar styloid, the TFCC, the pisiform, and the lunotriquetral joint. Stability of the DRUJ is tested by palmarly and dorsally stressing the distal end of the ulna in neutral rotation, pronation, and supination. Laxity, crepitus, and pain are noted.

The ulna is then palpated to its tip. Pain just distal to the ulnar styloid is suggestive of TFCC pathology. The pisiform is found lying within the FCU and is stressed to identify evidence of pisotriquetral arthritis. The lunotriquetral joint is then examined. When examining the right wrist, the examiner places his right thumb on the pisiform. The left thumb is placed over the dorsum of the patient's lunate. The thumbs are then compressed. Pain on the ulnar side of the wrist is suggestive of a tear of the lunotriquetral ligament.

Because most of the bony structures on the volar side of the wrist are deep to the flexor tendons, only the hook of the hamate is readily palpable. It is located 1 cm distal and 1 cm radial to the pisiform. Tenderness over this structure is suggestive of fracture.

Just distal to the hook of the hamate are the CMC joints of the ring and small fingers. Unlike the relatively immobile CMC joints of the index and middle fingers, these joints have 15 degrees and 30 degrees, respectively, of flexion and extension.

The bones and joints of the hand are more accessible to palpation than are the bones of the wrist. The active and passive range of motion of the metacarpophalangeal (MP), proximal interphalangeal (PIP), and distal interphalangeal (DIP) joints is measured. Average normal values are MP, 0/85; PIP 0/110; DIP, 0/65. In the thumb, motion of the MP and interphalangeal joints can vary and should be compared with that of the contralateral side.

The remainder of the hand examination is tailored to the region causing the most pain. Each of the bones in the region is palpated for tenderness. Pain on palpation is sought along the radial and ulnar aspects of the joint because this suggests an injury to the collateral ligament. Metacarpophalangeal joint collateral ligaments are tested by placing the joint in full flexion to tighten the ligament and then stressing the joint in the direction opposite the painful side. The PIP joint is laterally stressed in slight flexion. The most common collateral ligament injury is disruption of the ulnar collateral ligament of the thumb MP joint, often termed a gamekeeper's or skier's thumb. This ligament is tested by radially stressing the thumb MP joint in approximately 30 degrees of flexion.

Muscles and Tendons

The musculotendinous units are divided into extrinsic muscles, which take their origin in the forearm, and intrinsic muscles, with origins in the hand. Examination of these structures should determine whether they are in continuity, whether they are under active control, and whether they are inflamed. A thorough understanding of the topographical anatomy and function of each musculotendinous unit is required to evaluate these points.

None of the muscles that move the wrist inserts into a carpal bone except for the FCU, which inserts into the pisiform. Therefore, the wrist extrinsics travel with the finger extrinsics to insert into the hand. As the tendons pass across the wrist, they are held close to the joint by a retinaculum, which may act as a point of constriction and inflammation (**Fig. 34-4**).

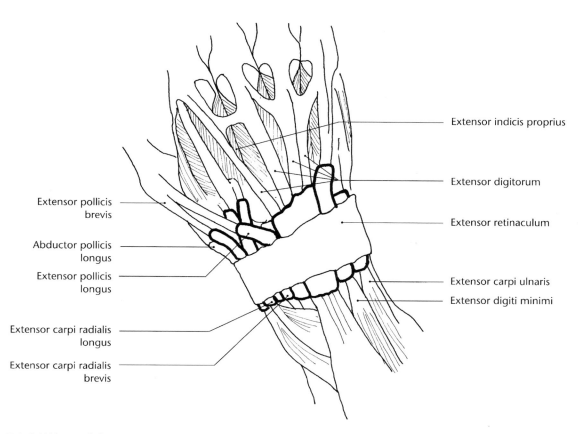

Figure 34-4 Wrist and finger extensors. *(From Reckling FW, Reckling JB, Mohn MP, editors:* Orthopaedic anatomy and surgical approaches, *St. Louis, 1990, Mosby–Year Book; pp. 112–129.)*

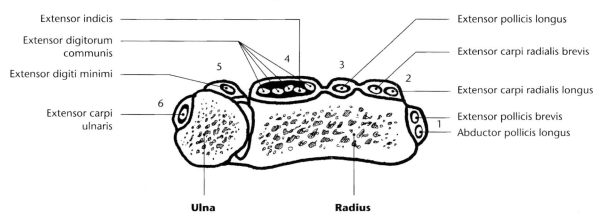

Figure 34-5 The six dorsal compartments of the wrist (cross section of a pronated right wrist viewed distal to proximally). *(From Reckling FW, Reckling JB, Mohn MP, editors:* Orthopaedic anatomy and surgical approaches, *St. Louis, 1990, Mosby–Year Book; pp. 112–129.)*

Examination of the tendons at the wrist begins with an inspection to identify regions of localized redness and swelling. Palpation should proceed in a systematic fashion. The six dorsal compartments of the wrist are shown in **Figure 34-5**. On the radial aspect of the wrist, the contents of the first dorsal compartment, the abductor pollicis longus (APL) and the extensor pollicis brevis (EBP) tendons, are best palpated with radial abduction

of the thumb. The APL inserts into the base of the thumb metacarpal and the EPB into the proximal phalanx. As they pass through the extensor retinaculum just proximal to the radial styloid, the tendons may become inflamed, a condition termed DeQuervain's stenosing tenosynovitis. The pain of this condition is accentuated and the diagnosis confirmed by the Finklestein maneuver. The thumb is tucked inside the fin gers in a clenched-fist position and the wrist is ulnarly deviated.

The extensor pollicis longus (EPL) from the third dorsal compartment is located on the ulnar side of Lister's tubercle, a bony prominence on the dorsum of the radius just proximal to the radiocarpal joint. The contents of the second dorsal compartment, the extensor carpi radialis longus and extensor carpi radialis brevis, are deep to the EPL and difficult to palpate. Spontaneous rupture of the EPL may occur from rheumatoid arthritis or following a distal radius fracture. Although the EPL primarily inserts into the distal phalanx of the thumb, a rupture of the tendon leads to diminished extension at the MP joint and loss of hyper

extension at the interphalangeal joint. The EPB, the primary extensor of the MP joint, is often not strong enough to fully extend the MP joint when the EPL is absent. Because some residual extension of the interphalangeal joint is maintained by the intrinsic muscles of the thumb, the diagnosis should be suspected when the EPL tendon cannot be palpated even if thumb interphalangeal extension is preserved.

The dorsum of the wrist contains the contents of the fourth dorsal compartment, the extensor digiti communis and the extensor indicis proprius, as well as the fifth compartment, which contains the extensor digiti minimi. At the wrist level, these tendons are located between Lister's tubercle and the ulnar head. Distally,

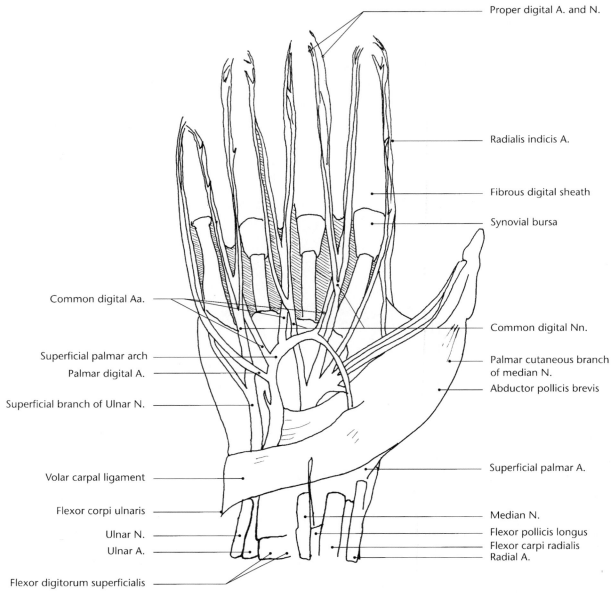

Figure 34-6 Palmar anatomy of the hand. *(From Reckling FW, Reckling JB, Mohn MP, editors:* Orthopaedic anatomy and surgical approaches, *St. Louis, 1990, Mosby–Year Book; pp. 112–129.)*

they pass across the dorsum of the hand to insert into fingers. The one unique function of the finger extrinsic extensors is extension of the MP joints. This is tested by having the patient make a fist and then actively extending the MP joints while keeping the PIP and DIP joints flexed.

The ulnar side of the wrist contains the contents of the sixth dorsal compartment. The extensor carpi ulnaris tendon is palpable in a groove in the ulnar head just radial to the ulnar styloid, particularly when the patient extends and ulnarly deviates the wrist. If a tear occurs in the sheath, when the patient begins this position in pronation and then supinates and flexes the wrist, the tendon will sublux from its groove.

On the flexor surface (**Fig. 34-6**), the FCU tendon is palpable with wrist flexion at its insertion into the pisiform. A common site of pain involving this structure is insertion of the FCU into the pisiform. In the middle of the flexor surface is the palmaris longus (PL). The PL is absent in approximately 20% of patients. It can be palpated by asking patients to touch their thumb tip to the tip of their small finger while flexing the wrist. The PL is an important landmark because the median nerve is deep to it and the palmar cutaneous branch of the median nerve lies just radial to the tendon. The extrinsic digital flexor tendons are located in the central

flexors of the wrist. In this location, the flexor digitorum superficialis (FDS) is superficial to the flexor digitorum profundus (FDP). The FDP inserts into the distal phalanx of each finger and is the sole structure capable of active DIP flexion (**Fig. 34-7**). The integrity of the FDP is tested by holding the finger extended and asking the patient to flex the DIP joint. The FDS splits at the level of the MP joint and passes deep to the FDP to insert into the middle phalanx and produce PIP flexion. The integrity of the FDS tendon is tested by holding all other fingers extended and asking the patient to flex the PIP joint of the finger being tested. By holding the uninvolved fingers extended, the patient is unable to flex the PIP joint by using the FDP because the FDP tendon arises from a common muscle mass. The last deep extrinsic finger flexor is the flexor pollicis longus (FPL). After coursing through the deep, radial aspect of the carpal tunnel, the FPL inserts into the distal phalanx of the thumb.

As the tendons course through the hand and fingers, they are held next to the bone by a series of pulleys (**Fig. 34-8**). Irritation of the tendons at these points of constriction may cause tenosynovitis. A trigger finger occurs when the inflammation becomes so enlarged that the tendon has difficulty passing under the pulley and either triggering or locking results. The A-1 pulley is the

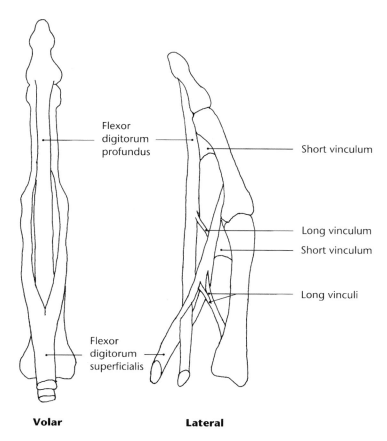

Flexor digitorum profundus

Short vinculum

Long vinculum
Short vinculum

Long vinculi

Flexor digitorum superficialis

Volar   **Lateral**

Figure 34-7 Flexor digitorum superficialis and flexor digitorum profundus. *(From Reckling FW, Reckling JB, Mohn MP, editors:* Orthopaedic anatomy and surgical approaches, *St. Louis, 1990, Mosby–Year Book; pp. 112–129.)*

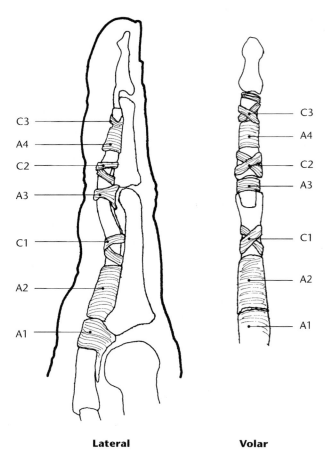

Lateral   **Volar**

Figure 34-8 The digital bursa has ben stripped away to show individual pulleys and their relationship to joints and phalanges (*A,* annular; *C,* cruciate). *(From Reckling FW, Reckling JB, Mohn MP, editors: Orthopaedic anatomy and surgical approaches, St. Louis, 1990, Mosby–Year Book; pp. 112–129.)*

leading edge of the flexor sheath, located at the MP joint, and is the most common location for triggering in the fingers and thumb.

The flexor carpi radialis is located just ulnar to the radial artery. The tendon passes from the forearm into a tunnel composed of a ridge from the trapezium and a portion of the transverse carpal ligament. Inflammation of the tendon in this tunnel may lead to point tenderness of the tendon approximately 1 cm distal to the radial styloid.

Nerves

Sensory and motor function in the hand and wrist is predominantly supplied by the median, ulnar, and radial nerves. The median nerve courses beneath the volar antebrachial fascia and PL to enter the carpal tunnel (**Fig. 34-6**). The nerve shares this space, which is surrounded by bone on three sides and the transverse carpal ligament palmarly, with the four FDS tendons, four FDP tendons, and the FPL tendon. After exiting the

carpal tunnel, the motor branch supplies the abductor pollicis brevis, opponens pollicis, and half of the flexor pollicis brevis muscles. The rest of the nerve supplies the lumbricals to the index and middle fingers, as well as sensation to the palmar aspect of the thumb, index and middle fingers, and the radial border of the ring finger (**Fig. 34-9**). The tip of the index finger has the region of purest median nerve innervation with the least crossover from other nerves.

The ulnar nerve enters the wrist ulnar to the ulnar artery in Guyon's canal, the superficial space between the pisiform and the hook of the hamate (**Fig. 34-6**). The ulnar nerve divides into a sensory and motor branch. The sensory nerve supplies the small finger and the ulnar border of the ring finger, with the purest area of sensation at the tip of the small finger (**Fig. 34-9**). The motor branch supplies the hypothenar muscles (abductor digiti minimi, flexor digiti minimi, opponens digiti minimi), volar and dorsal interossei, ring and small finger lumbricals, adductor pollicis muscle, and half of the flexor pollicis brevis muscle.

The radial nerve–innervated muscles are in the forearm. The sensory portion courses along the radial aspect of the forearm to supply the dorsal skin of the thumb, index and middle fingers, and radial border of the ring finger (**Fig. 34-9**). The area of purest radial nerve sensation is the dorsal first web space.

The ability to test sensation is dependent on the cooperation and understanding of the patient. Gross sensation is tested by lightly touching each of the fingers without the patient looking. The patient is asked to identify which finger is being stroked. More definitive evaluation is performed by testing static or moving two-point discrimination. Two blunt probes such as the ends of a paper clip are initially set 15 mm apart. The ends are then longitudinally touched to the radial or ulnar aspect of the finger tip until skin blanching is produced. Without watching, the patient should be able to distinguish being touched with one point or two. The distance between the points is incrementally decreased to 5 mm. The ability to distinguish at this level indicates normal sensation. Reliability at any level is assumed when two correct responses are elicited out of three attempts.

The other essential aspect of neurologic testing is the motor examination. The presence of atrophy is noted. Strength against resistance is measured and recorded by the British rating scale. In this system, 5 is normal strength, 4 is diminished strength, 3 is resistance against gravity, 2 is motion with gravity eliminated, 1 is muscle flicker, and 0 is no movement. More objective, although less specific measurements can be made by determining grip and pinch strengths with dynamometers. Grip strength can be measured at five different grip size settings. Because grip is harder when the meter is placed at very narrow and very wide distances, a bell-shaped curve of grip strengths should be produced. Failure to produce a normal pattern should raise questions about patient compliance and the validity of the test.

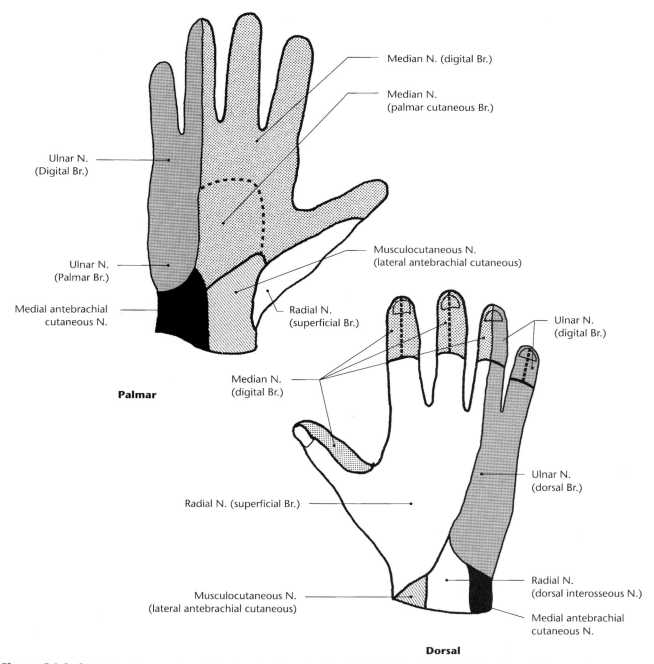

Median N. (digital Br.)

Median N.
(palmar cutaneous Br.)

Ulnar N.
(Digital Br.)

Ulnar N.
(Palmar Br.)

Medial antebrachial
cutaneous N.

Musculocutaneous N.
(lateral antebrachial cutaneous)

Radial N.
(superficial Br.)

Palmar

Median N.
(digital Br.)

Ulnar N.
(digital Br.)

Ulnar N.
(dorsal Br.)

Radial N. (superficial Br.)

Radial N.
(dorsal interosseous N.)

Musculocutaneous N.
(lateral antebrachial cutaneous)

Medial antebrachial
cutaneous N.

Dorsal

Figure 34-9 Cutaneous innervation of the hand. *(From Reckling FW, Reckling JB, Mohn MP, editors:* Orthopaedic anatomy and surgical approaches, *St. Louis, 1990, Mosby–Year Book; pp. 112–129.)*

Particular importance is given to examining the most distal muscle innervated by a nerve. The abductor pollicis brevis muscle is the last innervated by the median nerve. The muscle is tested for bulk by asking the patient to touch the tip of the thumb to the tip of the ring finger. Muscle bulk on the radial border of the thumb metacarpal is examined (**Fig. 34-6**). A normal bulge extends well past the bone. If some loss is noted, mild atrophy is present. If the muscle is even with the

bone, moderate atrophy is denoted. Severe atrophy is present when the muscle excavates below the bone.

The last muscle innervated by the ulnar nerve is the first dorsal interosseous muscle. Atrophy is noted along the radial border of the index metacarpal and the patient has difficulty abducting the index finger against resistance. Other signs suggest loss of ulnar-innervated functions. Froment's sign is hyperflexion of the thumb interphalangeal joint in lateral pinch. Normally, the thumb is firmly held against the radial border of the index finger in pinch by the adductor pollicis. With ulnar neuropathy, the FPL substitutes and produces the flexion. Another finding in ulnar neuropathy is Wartenberg's sign. Because of the inability to actively adduct the small finger, patients will complain that their small finger gets caught when trying to put their hand in a pocket.

Specialized tests may detect nerve irritability. Tinel's sign designates the paresthesia produced in the distribution of the nerve when the skin over the nerve is tapped. Irritability may be caused by complete or partial laceration, neuroma, or chronic compression. The Phalen maneuver tests the median nerve at the wrist, because pressure in the carpal tunnel is increased with wrist flexion and extension. With the elbows straight, the wrists are flexed to their maximal extent and held for 1 minute. A positive test occurs if numbness and tingling are elicited within 60 seconds. Both the time to onset and the distribution of symptoms should be recorded.

The Vascular System

Blood is supplied to the hand and wrist predominantly through the radial and ulnar arteries (**Fig. 34-10**). In the hand, the ulnar artery becomes the superficial palmar arch, which courses palmar to the nerves and tendons and supplies the common digital arteries. The radial artery becomes the deep palmar arch after giving off the princeps pollicis artery to the thumb. Interconnections between the superficial and deep arches are present in most but not all hands.

The Allen test evaluates the arterial supply to individual fingers. Both the radial and ulnar arteries are occluded at the wrist by the examiner. The patient then tightly flexes and extends the fingers to exsanguinate the hand. With the fingers in a relaxed position, pressure is relieved from the radial artery. Notations are made of which fingers become pink and the time taken to restore the circulation. The process is then repeated to evaluate the ulnar artery.

Injuries to the vessels are common. Complete arterial lacerations will bleed less than partial lacerations because of more complete vasoconstriction of the severed artery. An aneurysm of the ulnar artery may occur between the pisiform and hook of the hamate, resulting in the hypothenar hammer syndrome. The most common injury mechanism is secondary to repeated blows using the heel of the hand. If the aneurysm is sufficiently large, the ulnar nerve may become compressed, leading to paresthesia of the ring and small fingers.

Another vascular disorder is vasospasm. When the fingers are exposed to cold, an exaggerated pallor of the digits known as Raynaud's phenomenon may occur, with or without cyanosis. The diagnosis can be established by placing the involved fingers in cold water and

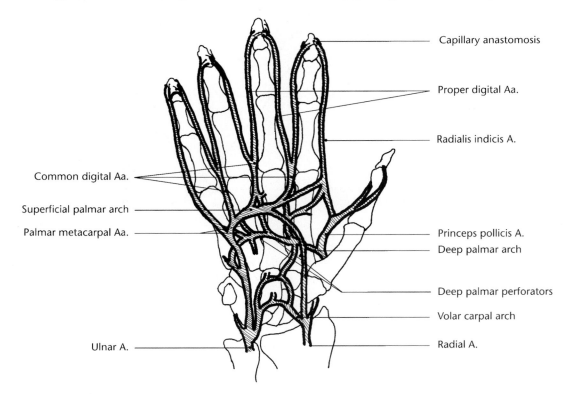

Capillary anastomosis

Proper digital Aa.

Radialis indicis A.

Common digital Aa.

Superficial palmar arch

Palmar metacarpal Aa.

Princeps pollicis A.
Deep palmar arch

Deep palmar perforators

Volar carpal arch

Ulnar A.

Radial A.

Figure 34-10 Most common pattern of arterial supply to the hand. Note the radial artery and deep palmar arch. *(From Reckling FW, Reckling JB, Mohn MP, editors: Orthopaedic anatomy and surgical approaches, St. Louis, 1990, Mosby–Year Book; pp. 112–129.)*

observing the skin response. Raynaud's phenomenon may be idiopathic (primary) or secondary to connective tissue disorders, neurologic disorders, or blood dyscrasias.

Skin and Subcutaneous Tissue

The mobility of the skin on the dorsum of the hand is far greater than the mobility on the palmar surface. The fibrous septi and palmar aponeurosis firmly link the palmar skin to the deep structures and thus enhance grip. This anatomic difference explains many observations seen on physical examination.

After injury, the skin and subcutaneous tissue should be examined for scars, erythema, abrasions, lacerations, skin loss, ecchymosis, and swelling. These observations should be drawn on a sketch of the hand entered in the medical record. Because most of the venous and lymphatic drainage of the fingers and hand occurs through the loose dorsal tissue, hand swelling is usually more pronounced dorsally, even when the pathologic process is palmar. Discrete, well-localized swelling is more indicative of an isolated process such as an inflamed joint or tendon sheath. Diffuse swelling suggests trauma or infection.

The most frequent pathologic process involving the palmar fascia is Dupuytren's disease. This thickening and contracture of the fascia may lead to the formation of cords. As the cords contract, it becomes increasingly difficult to straighten the fingers or thumb. A skin pit or nodule most commonly forms over the palmar aspect of the MP joint. Examination should note the distribution of cords and the degree of joint contracture of the MP and PIP joints.

Examination of the skin may provide insight into the integrity of the deeper structures. The presence of ulcers and the color and temperature of the skin as compared with the opposite side are indicators of vascular changes. Dry skin and loss of dermal ridges may be related to denervation.

Finally, it should be remembered that the hands are exposed to a variety of potentially injurious elements, including the sun. Suspicious skin lesions should be examined to rule out squamous cell carcinoma, basal cell carcinoma, and melanoma. Although uncommon, squamous cell carcinoma is the most common malignant tumor of the hand.

References

1. American Society for Surgery of the Hand: *The hand: examination and diagnosis,* ed 2, New York, 1983, Churchill Livingstone International.

2. Hoppenfeld S: *Physical examination of the spine and extremities,* Norwalk, Conn, Appleton-Century-Crofts; pp 59-104.

3. Reckling FW, Reckling JB, Mohn MP, editors: *Orthopaedic anatomy and surgical approaches,* Philadelphia, 1990, Mosby–Year Book; pp 112-129.

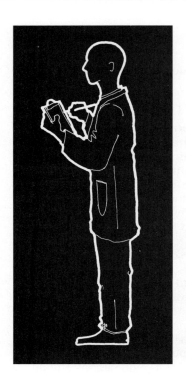

Chapter 35

Functional Evaluation of the Wrist and Hand

Jane Bear-Lehman

CONTENTS

Functional evaluation of the wrist and hand is both a quantitative and a qualitative process. The aim of functional evaluation is to help the therapist construct and then monitor the effectiveness of the treatment plan. Treatment of a patient who has sustained a musculoskeletal occupational injury of the wrist and hand focuses on helping the patient achieve maximal function of both body and limb and on restoring independence in personal and instrumental activities of daily living. Occupational musculoskeletal wrist and hand injuries can result from direct or indirect trauma in the workplace. The injury affects the musculoskeletal system, which includes the bone and its joints and their related structures: muscles, tendons, ligaments, nerves, and arteries. Direct trauma injuries are usually a medical emergency; they have a date, time, and place of injury and may result from a fall in the workplace or adverse physical contact with tools or machinery in the environment. Indirect trauma is microtrauma to the muscles, tendons, ligaments, nerves, or arteries that persists and develops over time. Evaluation and treatment of a patient with direct or indirect trauma to the wrist and hand address both the injured and adjacent body parts as is appropriate for the medical and surgical stage of recovery; results are compared with function of the uninjured limb if available.

Several quantitative measures and instruments used in the therapeutic setting to assess range of motion (ROM), muscle performance, edema, sensation, dexterity, and physical capacity are reviewed in this chapter. Attention will be brought to each instrument's stage of development and achieved reliability and validity. Although it may be perceived that the use of reliable and valid tests will increase the statistical probability for making correct clinical decisions, we are cautioned to not rely exclusively on quantitative data. Qualitative behavior, such as patient attitude, response to pain, fear, and loss of control, will often influence the quantitative wrist and hand functional evaluation results.[1,10]

Functional evaluation of a patient with a musculoskeletal disorder affecting the wrist and hand tends to follow a biomechanical frame of reference. The problems are identified by gathering and then synthesizing subjective, observational, and objective information about the patient. This information is derived from the patient, the therapist's observation of the patient visually and through touch (palpation), and the outcome performance the patient achieves on administered tests. Functional evaluation primarily relies on the voluntary cooperation of the patient to clinical stimuli, inquiries, and directives.

To begin a functional evaluation, the therapist gathers a history from the patient's perspective about the nature and the course of the injury, prior medical and therapeutic attention sought, and success of the prior interventions. This report from the patient's perspective is compared for congruity with the written history. Many questions about lifestyle adjustment are posed to the patient so that the therapist can document the alterations, but more so to appreciate the patient's ability to recognize, understand, and function within the restrictions imposed by the physical problem. Therefore patients are asked to describe how the impact of the injury has affected their lifestyle, namely, the changes in ability to perform personal and instrumental activities of daily living tasks at home, at work, and at leisure.[22] The course, location, duration and type of pain are addressed through standardized questionnaires such as the McGill Pain Profile or the Cornell Medical Index Health Questionnaire to detect patterns about the patient's pain and methods to control pain. Finally, patients are asked to describe their expectations and goals for treatment.[28] As subjective information is being gathered, the therapist visually observes how the patient moves.

The therapist observes the patient's posture and attitude of the injured wrist or hand and its adjacent structures to answer the following questions. Is the patient favoring a posture to protect the injured part from contact with the environment through upper extremity flexion and adduction? Is there biomechanical alteration in the body to compensate for the poverty of movement or increase in pain? Is there symmetry in size and shape between the injured and uninjured wrist and hand? Does the body move symmetrically? What are the preferred postures during static positions such as sitting? What are the transition patterns, that is, moving from sitting to standing, and the dynamic patterns of movement such as walking? What is the quality of movement at the injured site and in the adjacent structures? Is there a change in coloration at the injured site; does the coloration vary? Palpation of the skin gives the therapist more information about the skin's temperature, the presence of nodules, and the tightness of muscle-tendon units.

Measurement is a continuous and ongoing process; it is carefully coordinated and monitored with the stage of healing and the plan for movement during healing. Physiologic changes can and do occur quite rapidly during the acute stage.[17] Objective measures provide the treating therapist with information about the effectiveness of a given treatment, confirm the need to continue with a given treatment regimen, or signal the need for revision if the progress is not as anticipated. The data are used to justify the need for continuation of treatment, when applicable, to those who are financially supporting the treatment services.

CLINICAL ASSESSMENT OF THE MUSCULOSKELETAL SYSTEM

Range of Motion

Since the 1940s, therapists have been reporting their use of the goniometric system to obtain accurate information about patients' joint status and its movement capacity. Although technically not a standardized assessment tool, the universal goniometer is the most widely selected tool for measuring joint range of motion (ROM) as shown in **Figure 35-1**. The American Academy of Orthopaedic Surgeons (AAOS) guide is used as a reference for normative values.[3] In terms of reliability, Hamilton and Lachenbruch[19] have found no difference in the results of determining joint angles with different goniometers. The reliability of readings by the same tester over time has shown a 5 degree error. The method of recording continues to follow the guideline of the academy in which minus sign notation is used to show an extension limitation and a plus sign is used to indicate hyperextension. The American Society for the Surgery of the Hand (ASSH) has accepted the method of reporting goniometric scores in terms of the total arc of movement at a given joint or a related series of joints; scores are reported as total active movement (TAM) and total passive movement (TPM).[13,17] Use of this method for a summation of the angles of the three finger joints, metacarpophalangeal (MCP), proximal interphalangeal (PIP), and distal interphalangeal (DIP), with full ROM

yields a score approximating 260 degrees. This composite measurement does not isolate the individual joint that is creating the deficit, but it is suited for graphic representations of the patient's performance over time, particularly for a patient with a tendon or nerve repair.

Range-of-motion measurements are conducted on the adjacent joints in the acute stage of recovery; deficits in the adjacent joints that were not present before the injury are remediated in therapy. Depending on the nature of the injury and the medical or surgical protocol, measurements may be taken for active or passive ROM at the injury site immediately or may be deferred until the integrity of the joint or the surrounding tissue will allow a measurement. Range-of-motion assessment of the injured joints depends on the type of protection and stabilization used for healing. If complete rest of the injured region is required, measurements are delayed until movement is permissible. If controlled movement at the injured site is allowed, the therapist measures the type of movement allowed active or passive, within the range allowed and restricts movement beyond the prescribed arc.

Edema

Following trauma or surgery, there is frequently an abnormal accumulation of fluid in the interstitial spaces of tissues resulting in an increase in limb size. This edematous state limits ROM and ultimately function. Measurement of wrist and hand size circumferentially with a tape measure is often done at three locations: proximal to and distal from the edematous part and over the edematous part. To allow for a more valid comparison of sequential measurements, anatomic landmarks are used as reference points for placement of the tape measure. Placement and tension of the tape

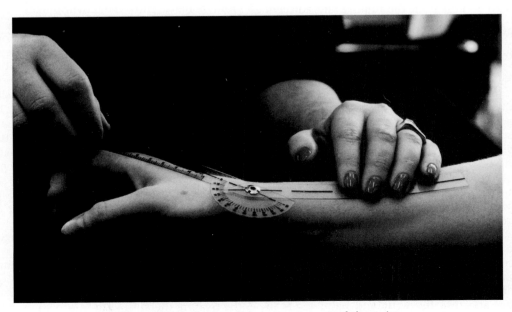

Figure 35-1 Goniometric measurement of the wrist.

measure or finger gauge affect intertester and intratester reliability. Jewelers' rings can reduce the measurement error related to tension on the tape measure (see **Fig. 35-2**). Because edema may not be localized in a digital segment but instead, more generalized over the hand and arm, a volumeter method is preferred (**Fig. 35-3**). The volumeter, based on Archimedes' principle of water displacement, is used to measure composites of hand mass. Waylett and Seibly[34] have documented 10-ml test-retest reliability when the manufacturer's guidelines are followed.[21] Normative values are not available for any of these measures, and in all cases the contralateral side is used as the approximate normal value for that patient. Hand-size changes may be attributed to factors other than edema such as normal asymmetry and muscle atrophy from disuse. Care must be taken regarding generalization and interpretation of the hand size changes. Abnormal findings using circumferential measures or the volumeter indicate the immediate need to implement edema reduction and control measures.[32]

Muscle Performance Testing

The manual muscle test designed by Lovett and Martin[24] is a screening device that relies on the external forces of gravity and resistance to assess muscle strength. The strength of muscle contractions can be measured clinically by means of spring scales, dynamometers, weights, or manual resistance. Manual resistance is added to voluntary maximal contraction once it has been established that the muscle exertion and the applied resistance will not adversely affect the healing bone, joints, and related structures. Muscle testing is used to evaluate the level of nerve injury and the regeneration of nerves. It is also used in the preoperative determination of potential donors in tendon transfer surgery.

There is no agreement regarding whether isometric or isotonic contraction should be used in muscle testing or whether testing scores are best derived from the muscles' isometric contractibility under load at the end of the range. The end of the range is often chosen as the point for applied resistance.[20] Few discrepancies are found in manual muscle testing procedures. Daniels and Worthingham[14] use a gravity-eliminated position

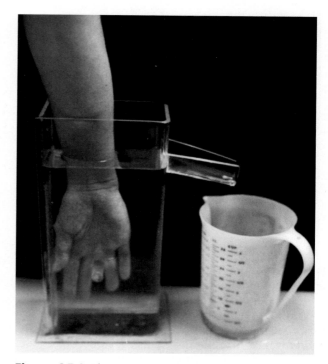

Figure 35-3 The volumeter measures upper limb size by measurement of water displaced in milliliters.

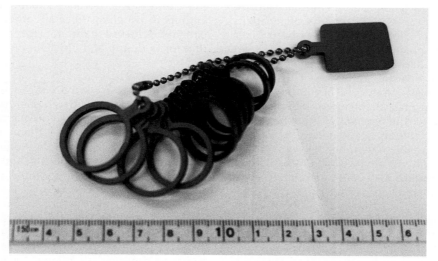

Figure 35-2 These are jewelers rings for measuring the size of the digits; scores are reported in actual ring size. The tape measure is used to measure the limb circumferentially; scores are reported in metric units.

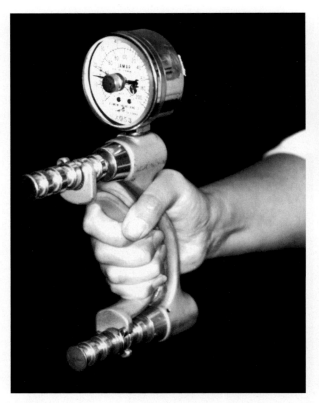

Figure 35-4 The handheld Jamar dynamometer records grip strength in kilograms-force or pounds-force.

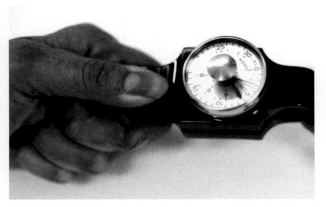

Figure 35-5 The pinch meter records pinch patterns in kilograms-force or pounds-force.

to test MCP joint extension, whereas Kendall, McCreary, and Provance[20] do not distinguish the effect of gravity in the hand. The scoring methods of Lovett[23] and Brunnstrom and Denner[12] continue to be used: 0 (zero), 1 (trace), and 2 (poor) represent test results in the gravity-eliminated posture; 3 (fair) uses the external force of gravity; and 4 (good) and 5 (normal) add the dimension of resistance. Overall, reports of reliability are descriptive. No predictive validity has been established for grip and pinch scores, although many are hypothesized, nor is hand function predictive.

Grip and pinch tests are administered to measure functional hand strength. In the case of a distal forearm, wrist, or hand fracture, measurements are deferred for at least 2 to 4 weeks after the removal of immobilization. Grip is the most common, standardized assessment using the Jamar adjustable dynamometer, as shown in **Figure 35-4**; pinch patterns are measured using a pinch meter, as shown in **Figure 35-5**. Both instruments allow for readings in kilograms-force and pounds-force. If regularly calibrated, both instruments have been shown to be reliable.[6] The literature shows a variety of test procedures that can have an impact on interrater and intrarater reliability, as well as its normative data pool.[26] The ASSH and the American Society of Hand Therapists (ASHT) accept the seated posture with humeral adduction and neutral humeral rotation, the elbow flexed to

90 degrees, and the forearm and wrist in neutral position as the desired body posture for grip testing.[25]

Norms have been established for age 5 to adulthood. Healthy adult grip strength values for the five handle positions, when providing full voluntary effort, will yield a normal bell-shaped curve.[30] The first position, the closest, is the least advantageous because it relies primarily on the ulnar nerve–innervated hand intrinsics, whereas the widest, or fifth position relies on the median nerve–innervated long finger flexors. Middle-range handle positions require the intrinsic and extrinsic musculature to work together. A patient without neural or tendon damage who has a flattened curve may be suspected of providing submaximal voluntary effort. The traditional pinch patterns of lateral (shown in **Fig. 35-5**), palmar (also known as three-jaw chuck), and tip pinch are reported as the average of three trials for each type of pinch. Swanson, Swanson, and Goran-Hagert[31] also recommend a pulp-to-pulp pinch of each digit to the thumb. The normative data described by these authors in kilograms-force are often used to determine patients' achieved status for age, gender, and occupation for both grip and pinch.

Sensation

The hand is a complex organ whose function depends on harmony between sensory and motor abilities.[15] Sensory testing can frequently identify sensorineural changes earlier than traditional motor examination can. For example, studies have shown that in median nerve entrapment at the carpal canal level, sensory changes precede motor changes, and clinical tests of vibration and Semmes-Weinstein monofilament testing show changes before electromyographic (EMG) studies do because EMG does not show the process of change.[7] Many of the tools used to test sensation clinically are being revised and improved; in addition, because of the changes offered by microsurgery, more patients now have greater potential than before to have sensory results of higher quantity and quality. Sensory

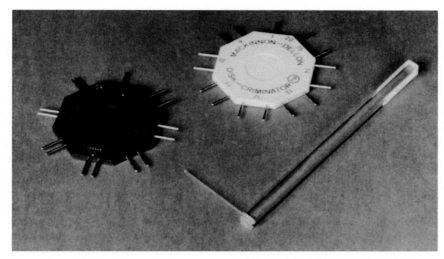

Figure 35-6 Two-point discrimination disks shown left and top; one element of the monofilament test is to the right.

testing of a patient with a wrist and hand injury addresses the ability of the patient to perceive light touch and deep pressure, to discriminate touch, and to perceive vibration. To monitor the progress of a patient's sensory status, particularly if a neural injury is suspected, it is advisable to use instruments that yield ordinal data rather than nominal data. Early methods to test light touch and deep pressure called for the use of a cotton ball or a cotton-tipped applicator. When this form of testing took place, it resulted in information that the patient perceived the touch, may not have perceived it fully, or did not perceive it; these are nominal data where 2 is normal, 1 is impaired, and 0 is absent. If abnormal or diminished results are determined during the evaluation, they need to be monitored. It is expected that sensitivity over scars and pin tracks will be heightened.

von Frey,[33] a surgeon who had a passion for learning about sensation and a love of horses, discovered that some of his patients could only detect the sensation of thicker horse hairs when applied to their skin surfaces, and as they healed, they could begin to feel the finer horse hairs. This finding led to the deep pressure–to–light touch hierarchy for sensation in the hand. The horse hairs that were first used are now 20 calibrated nylon monofilaments graded in diameter and individually attached to Plexiglass handles (see **Fig. 35-6**). The amount of force transmitted is directly related to the diameter of each filament. Each filament bends at a specific force controlling the magnitude of the touch-pressure stimulus.[8] A smaller pocket version was made by the Hansens Disease Center to screen patients in deep pressure–to–light touch responses, and Weinstein[35] has developed an even smaller, more portable version of his original test for ease of use in the clinic.[9] The larger set of 20 provides greater specificity for those patients who require it.

To test for discriminatory touch sensation, the static or stationary two-point discrimination (2PD) instrument

continues to be challenged. The Weber 2PD instrument's sliding scale allows for adjustment of the spacing between the two points; however, the adjustment may not allow the same precision as a tool with fixed points. Some practitioners open up paper clips to approximate distances, which leads to variability in spacing and uneven pressure between points. The 2PD instrument designed by Dellon, Mackinnon, and Crosby[16] controls for the precision between points and provides even application when two points are applied (see **Fig. 35-6**). However, studies show that the amount of pressure offered when two points are applied is very different than when just one is applied.

The ability to perceive vibratory stimuli is of clinical value when the patient has undergone nerve repair or when nerve compression or a peripheral neuropathy is suspected. The 30-Hz and 256-Hz tuning forks have been used to test for vibratory response. Clinical studies have proposed that both the 30-Hz and the 256-Hz tuning forks be used because it is believed that each elicits the response of an individual sensory neurite receptor. The 30-Hz fork is believed to elicit the response of the Meissner corpuscle, and the 256-Hz fork seems to evoke a response from the pacinian corpuscle.[15] Whether the prong or the stem should be applied to the skin surface is debated; in either event, the lack of control of amplitude and variability in technique make the reliability of the test inconsistent.[6] Only nominal data will be gleaned from this form of testing and will produce results that are not quantifiable. A vibrometer with a fixed frequency level provides a result measured in microns of motion at 120 c/s (see **Fig. 35-7**). The data are ordinal, and the raw score is a logarithmic function of probe displacement measured in microns. A table is provided with the instrument to convert scores into displacement. Normal expected values of the displacement for skin surface are presented in an anatomic diagram and table format.

Pain is observed during the course of the evaluation

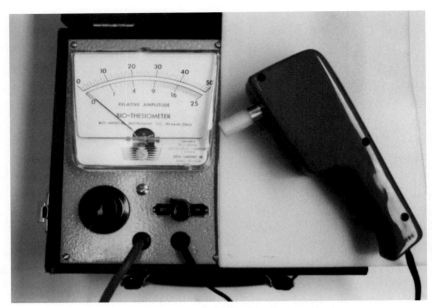

Figure 35-7 The bioesthesiometer probe is shown on the right; gauge and controls, part of the base unit, are shown on the left.

and can be monitored over time by the use of a pain analogue.[28] The patient is asked to describe the type, location, and threshold of pain perceived before, during, and after each therapy session. Perception of pain does vary from one patient to the next with the same injury and also varies for the same patient over time. The therapist must also observe and address signs that may be causing pain such as a constrictive dressing, cast, or splint or an infection. Pain may and often does occur at the onset of therapy; this form of pain is localized and should subside within 2 hours of the therapy session.

FUNCTIONAL ASSESSMENT OF THE MUSCULOSKELETAL SYSTEM

Information Processing

The patient comes to the medical setting mainly because of pain, fear, and disability.[5] A satisfactory result depends not only on the technical skills of the team but also on the team's ability to communicate, engender confidence, and fully understand and explain the problem to the patient.[11] It is necessary for the therapist to look at the process of therapy and how the patient is responding to the therapy situation. Guidelines for practice for occupational therapy rely on biological and behavioral theories.[27] The biological theories guide practice for wound healing, scar tissue management, and muscle strengthening. The process of change learned in therapy is related to the therapist's ability to teach the patient how to move again, and this process of change is based on behavioral theories, particularly theories of learning.[29]

The therapist helps the patient by designing a learning environment that emphasizes the salient traits and the characteristics of the problem to be solved or the condition to be learned. One method is to engage the patient in metacognitive experiences. Metacognitive experiences are conscious thinking and awareness of feelings that accompany and pertain to the problem-solving task. Flavell[18] defines metacognitive knowledge as information or beliefs about the course and outcome of the cognitive enterprise in three areas of cognitive awareness: person, task, and strategy. Every patient has a different level of cognitive awareness and a variety of beliefs, feelings, understanding of goals, and strategies for problem solving.

In therapy, practice or instructional programs are systematically used and the focus is on the process rather than the content.[29] Each task is analyzed relative to its repetition, imitation, and substitution. The training is assessed for the patient's need to have cues or anchors and intermodal training and for the patient's performance in a novel or new learning situation. How the patient accepts the information that has been shared and responds to it is viewed in not just a physical sense. Fear, pain, or side effects of medications often intervene in the patient's ability to orientate to the therapy situation and focus attention (alertness); this also affects the patient's ability to learn. A patient in pain may find one voice instrumental in helping learn the new way of moving the wrist. A verbal, visual, or kinesthetic voice (cue) from the therapist may be sufficient as the patient learns to move the wrist and hand again. Two voices, visual and verbal, may be needed, or the two voices may bombard the patient's ability to concentrate if given at the same time because of the high threshold of pain. The therapist observes how the patient learns to move again and how feedback is obtained and used.[2] The therapist determines whether the patient is reliant on others for direction and guidance to perform tasks or is self-directed and self-regulated in task performance.[29] It is important to know whether the patient can detect an error in movement alone, how the error is corrected, and what kind of reinforcement is required.

The therapist also observes the patient's ability to cope with the injury. After guidance in how to select and terminate activities that correspond to the patient's stage of healing, the therapist observes how the patient follows such guidelines in performing daily tasks, in participating in rehabilitation, and in assuming societal and family roles. The patient is observed for the ability to adhere to safety precautions and exhibit self-control in terms of physical limitations and pain reactions.

Activities of Daily Living

The quantity and the quality of the patient's performance of activities of daily living is ascertained by interview. For deficit areas, the therapist may observe the patient's actual performance. Early in the healing process when medical restrictions are in place as to the amount of movement or force allowed at the site of injury or whether the injured part can get wet, the patient needs to be assessed for methods of accommodation in activities of daily living.[4] For patients with a wrist or hand injury, this may require an assessment of eating, personal hygiene, dressing, bathing, and communication. Adaptive methods and devices may be indicated to temporarily facilitate one-handed methods such as a rocker knife for cutting meat or a button hook for fastening buttons.

During the course of the rehabilitation program it is important for the therapist to guide the patient as to when and how the injured wrist and hand can be safely reintegrated into the performance of activities of daily living corresponding with the clinical progress. The first reintegration will be in the performance of personal activities of daily living. When strengthening is introduced into the clinical program, the therapist needs to consider the patient's need to perform instrumental activities of daily living, which includes those tasks that are related to meal preparation, household management and shopping, and the care of others.

For many patients, the ability to work during the acute phase of recovery is not possible, whereas others may not have an interruption from their work. For those who are working, the therapist identifies the components and demands of the patient's job by interview and helps the patient assume those tasks that correspond to the achieved clinical status. For those who are unable to work, a delineation of the patient's job demands is determined to develop the requirements for return to work and the goals for therapy. As treatment progresses, the patient's performance level is viewed and compared with the levels needed for return to work. The feasibility of meeting the physical demand levels of dexterity, strength, and endurance are determined during the rehabilitation process.

Dexterity

Dexterity is commonly defined as skill and ease in using the hands. The Moberg Pick Up test can be classified as a sensory and dexterity test because it brings together the sensate and motor functions. This test is usually performed with unrestricted vision and with vision occluded, and the patient is timed as the familiar objects are scooped, handled, identified, and placed in a designated location.

To assess manual dexterity or physical functioning efficiently, the examiner must select the standardized test that suits the patient's abilities and needs. Most have a high index of reliability (greater than .75) and show good face and content validity; little has been done on concurrent validity or what is most needed for the clinical decision-making process—predictive validity.[6] Predictive validity is what is needed to answer whether the patient, based on the performance on the test, is ready to return to work.

Dexterity tests can be classified by their demand for fine to gross motor movement patterns, requirement for one hand to perform the task or the integration of both hands for task completion, whether a tool is required for their administration, and the length of time the test takes to perform. The Nine Hole Peg Test (see **Fig. 35-8**), the Purdue Pegboard (see **Fig. 35-9**), the O'Connor Tweezer Dexterity Test, the O'Connor Finger Dexterity Test, and the Crawford Small Parts Test are all examples of fine-motor dexterity movement patterns. However, the Nine Hole Peg Test and the Purdue Pegboard Test are short tests that do not provide information about endurance; the Purdue Pegboard Test does require the use of one hand as well as the use of both hands in parallel and in an integrated fashion as shown in **Figures 35-8 and 35-9**. The O'Connor Tweezer Dexterity Test and the Crawford Small Parts Test both require the use of a small tool to handle and manipulate the test parts. The former requires the use of small tweezers and testing is completed on the use of one hand at a time for all functions; the latter requires the use of tweezers or a screwdriver in one hand while the alternate hand is assistive. The Minnesota Rate of Manipulation Test and the Bennett Hand-Tool Dexterity Test assess gross motor function; the former requires the patient to handle the test items directly whereas the later requires the use of ordinary mechanics tools; both allow for the use of both hands during some of the test components.

The outcome scores for manual dexterity performance are reported as the amount of time, the speed, that the patient required to perform the task, and the increments of time are compared with normal data based on age, gender, and occupation published in the test manuals. The therapist also reports the preferred prehensile patterns used during the course of the tasks and the control the patient had over task performance.

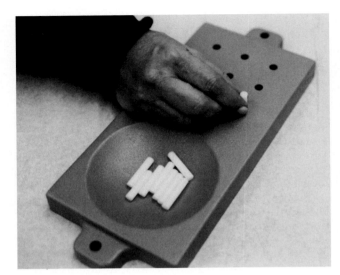

Figure 35-8 The Nine Hole Peg Test.

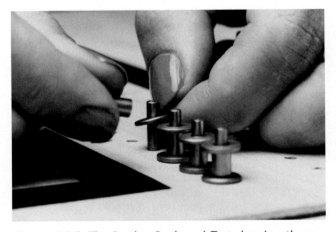

Figure 35-9 The Purdue Pegboard Test showing the assembly subtest.

Observations of motor control are discussed relative to the patient's safe use of the injured part, biomechanical alignment of the injured part relative to the body, postural accommodation of the body to the injured part, and quality of task performance. Qualities of concern include the patient's ability to spontaneously integrate the injured hand or wrist into the dexterity pattern, the ability of the two hands to work together as a dominant and subdominant pair, and the ability of the patient to spontaneously integrate the principles of joint protection into task performance. The patient is observed for safety relative to the injured part, himself, and others.

Physical Capacity Evaluation

Most physicians and therapists use a physical capacity evaluation to try to answer the question of whether a patient can safely return to work. Many sophisticated instruments are on the market; they are just beginning to have normative standards, and few are tied to motion-times-measurement standards.[6] The theoretical model that is followed is Parson's trait factor from the early 1900s in industrial engineering. The procedure is to identify the traits that the patient now has physically, behaviorally, and cognitively, to keep symptoms under control to work safely and effectively, and then to match these to the factors of the environment, including the medium at the work station.

SUMMARY

Success in rehabilitation of the wrist and the hand is measured by the patient's ability to spontaneously use the injured part in usual and customary activities. Instruments that produce reliable and valid data will assist in accountability for the assessment of upper extremity function. However, the art of practice requires awareness and documentation of the patient's qualitative wrist and hand dysfunction characteristics, not just the quantitative ones. To move effectively and efficiently, the patient needs to learn how to move again in a controlled, rhythmic way. Therefore, therapy to restore function of the upper extremity cannot rely alone on biological theories to effect change. It is the behavioral theories, the theories of learning, that guide the therapy practice for this achievement.

References

1. Abreu BC: *Evaluation.* In Abreu BC, editor: *Physical disabilities manual,* New York, 1981, Raven Press; pp 1-7.

2. Abreu BC: The quadraphonic approach: management of cognitive-perceptual and postural control dysfunction, *Occup Ther Pract* 3:12-29, 1992.

3. American Academy of Orthopedic Surgeons: *Joint motion: method of measuring and recording,* Chicago, 1965, The Academy.

4. Appelby MA, Schkade JK, Gilkeson GE: Timing of ADL education with hand surgery patients, *J Hand Ther* 5:218-225, 1992.

5. Bear-Lehman J: Factors affecting return to work after hand injury, *Am J Occup Ther* 37:189-194, 1983.

6. Bear-Lehman J, Abreu BC: Evaluating the hand: issues in reliability and validity, *Phys Ther* 69:1025-1033, 1989.

7. Bear-Lehman J, Bielawski T: The carpal tunnel syndrome: back to the source, *Rehabil Res Canada* 1:13-20, 1988.

8. Bell-Krotoski JA: *Light touch-deep pressure testing using Semmes Weinstein monofilaments.* In Hunter J et al, editors: *Rehabilitation of the hand,* ed 3, St Louis, 1990, Mosby–Year Book; pp 585-593.

9. Bell Krotoski J, Weinstein S, Weinstein C: Testing sensibility including touch pressure, two point discrimination, point localization, and vibration, *J Hand Ther* 6:114-123, 1993.

10. Brand PW: The mind and spirit in hand therapy, *J Hand Ther* 1:145-147, 1988.

11. Brown PW: The role of motivation in patient recovery, *Conn Med* 42:555-557, 1978.

12. Brunnstrom S, Denner M: *Round table on muscle testing.* Annual conference of American Physiotherapy Association, Federation of Crippled and Disabled, New York, 1931.

13. Cambridge CA: *Range of motion measurement of the hand.* In Hunter J et al, editors: *Rehabilitation of the hand,* ed 3, St Louis, 1990, Mosby–Year Book; pp 82-92.

14. Daniels I, Worthingham C: *Muscle testing techniques of manual examination,* ed 3, Philadelphia, 1972, WB Saunders.

15. Dellon AL: *Evaluation of sensibility and re-education of sensation in the hand,* Baltimore, 1981, Williams & Wilkins.

16. Dellon AL, Mackinnon SE, Crosby PM: Reliability of two point discrimination measurements, *J Hand Surg [AM]* 12A:693-696, 1987.

17. Fess EE: *Hand rehabilitation.* In Hopkins HL, and Smith HS, editors: *Willard and Spackman's occupational therapy,* ed 8, Philadelphia, 1993, JB Lippincott; pp 674-690.

18. Flavell JH: Metacognition and cognitive monitoring: a new era of cognitive developmental inquiry, *Am Psychol* 34:906-911, 1979.

19. Hamilton GF, Lachenbruch PA: Reliability of goniometers in assessing finger joint angle, *Phys Ther* 49:465-469, 1969.

20. Kendall FP, McCreary EK, Provance PG: *Muscles: testing and function,* ed 4, Baltimore, 1993, Williams & Wilkins.

21. King TI: The effect of water temperature on hand volume during volumetric measurement using water displacement method, *J Hand Ther* 6:202-204, 1993.

22. Law M: Evaluating activities of daily living: directions for the future, *Am J Occup Ther* 47:233-237, 1993.

23. Lovett RW: *The treatment of infantile paralysis,* ed 2, Philadelphia, 1917, Blakiston.

24. Lovett RW, Martin EG: Certain aspects of infantile paralysis and a description of a method of muscle testing, *JAMA* 6:729-733, 1916.

25. Mathiowetz V et al: Grip and pinch strength: normative data for adults, *Arch Phys Med Rehabil* 66:69-74, 1985.

26. Mathiowetz V et al: Reliability and validity of hand strength evaluation, *Journal of Hand Surgery [AM]* 9A:222-226, 1984.

27. Mosey AC: *Applied scientific inquiry in the health professions: an epistemiological orientation,* Rockville, Md, 1992, American Occupational Therapy Association.

28. Schultz KS: The Schultz structured interview for assessing upper extremity pain, *Occup Ther Health Care* 1:69-82, 1984.

29. Schwartz RK: *Therapy as learning,* Rockville, Md, 1985, American Occupational Therapy Association.

30. Stokes HM: The seriously injured hand: weakness of grip, *J Occup Med* 25:683-684, 1983.

31. Swanson AB, Swanson G, Goran-Hagert C: *Evaluation of impairment of hand function.* In Hunter J et al, editors: *Rehabilitation of the hand,* ed 3, St Louis, 1990, Mosby–Year Book.

32. Vasudevan SV, Melvin JL: Upper extremity edema control: rationale of the techniques, *Am J Occup Ther* 33:520-523, 1979.

33. von Frey M: Zur physiologie der juckempfindung, *Arch Neurol Physiol* 7:142, 1922.

34. Waylett J, Seibly D: A study of the accuracy of a commercially available volumeter, *J Hand Ther* 4:10-13, 1991.

35. Weinstein S: Fifty years of somotosensory research: from the Semmes-Weinstein monofilaments to the Weinstein enhanced sensory test, *J Hand Ther* 6:11-22, 1993.

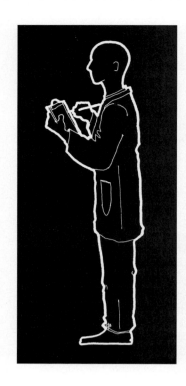

Chapter 36

Work-Related Disorders of the Arm: A Team Approach to Management

Lewis H. Millender
Beth D. Keelan
Paul J. Bonzani
Marjorie G. Mangieri

CONTENTS:

Work-related injuries to the upper extremity and hands have increased in recent years, and work-related cumulative trauma disorders (CTDs) now account for 52% of all occupational illnesses reported in the United States.[12] The incidence of work-related injuries has remained relatively stable over the past several years, but the type of injury has changed dramatically. In the upper extremity, the incidence of so-called CTDs or repetitive strain injuries (RSIs) has markedly increased. The Bureau of Labor Statistics estimates that these disorders have increased 500% in the past five years.[12] These disorders are costly in terms of time lost from work and prolonged disability.[17]

Although the incidence of CTD has increased, the etiology for the problem has been difficult to establish. Some researchers in the field disagree about the relative importance of high force and high repetition on the job versus the rising number of psychosocial complaints that accompany worker's compensation claims. On the one hand, a group of ergonomists believe that these injuries are true musculotendinous disruptions basically caused by force, repetition, abnormal postures, and vibrations.[16] Ergonomic and epidemiological studies have shown a higher incidence of these disorders in workers carrying out repetitive and forceful tasks.[13] On the other side, some researchers attribute many of these conditions to psychosocial and political factors. They attribute the increased incidence of CTD to changing work ethics, feelings of entitlement by workers, and a flawed worker's compensation system.[8,9]

Treatment of the most common disorders of the hand and fingers are discussed in this chapter. The most important part of treatment is proper classification of the disorder, particularly in the absence of objective physical findings or confirmatory radiological or laboratory data. For example, when a patient has a clear-cut musculoskeletal diagnosis such as a mild carpal tunnel syndrome or DeQuervain's tenosynovitis without ergonomic or psychosocial components, traditional nonsurgical treatment is instituted. When work station or ergonomic issues are involved, evaluations are conducted, recommendations and adjustments are made, modified duty or job enlargement is arranged, and breaks and stretches are prescribed.[5,13] When minor or major psychosocial issues are present, the therapist and surgeon are faced with a greater challenge. These underlying psychosocial issues often constitute the most limiting factor in the ability of therapists and surgeons to treat and resolve upper extremity CTDs and are a significant predictor of chronicity in this group of patients.[1,5,10] These issues become more complicated when insurers and at-torneys ask physicians to establish causal relationships between the job and the complaints.[7]

EVALUATION AND CLASSIFICATION

The following classification has been found helpful in evaluating and treating soft tissue and tendon disorders of the upper extremity. It is based on differentiating conditions with *objective* findings from those with *subjective* findings and then further separating the conditions with subjective findings into those with *reasonable subjective* findings and from those with *unreasonable subjective* findings.

The diagnosis is established by a careful history and physical examination plus an evaluation of the patient's response to treatment. Most patients with objective or reasonable subjective findings will respond to appropriate conventional conservative treatment. Laboratory tests and radiographs are usually normal. Excessive and expensive tests such as computed tomography (CT) and magnetic resonance imaging (MRI) should be discouraged.

The history begins with a description of the incident, the discomfort history, and the response to treatment. Pertinent questions include the location of pain, activities that exacerbate or improve the pain, the severity of the pain, the known events that led to the initiation of symptoms, the length of time the pain has been present, and the previous medical evaluations and results of any treatment. It is also important to inquire about the past medical history, family history, and previous injuries.

The job and nonmedical history is always important, especially for patients with subjective findings. Physicians must clearly understand the job requirements and the patient's personal job history. It is important to listen and ask questions and encourage patients to bring tools and materials that they believe are contributing to their injury; this helps physicians understand the job and shows their level of interest and commitment to the patient. It is also useful for physicians to understand the vibration, postures, and ergonomics of the job, especially the amount of force and repetition required to perform the job. Physicians should also discover whether other workers have experienced similar work-related symptoms. Are symptoms worse at the end of the day or the end of the week? Do rest breaks help with the pain and are breaks available? Are job enlargement and job rotation available? How long has the patient been at this job and how long has the patient worked at this company? How much job stress, job support, and job satisfaction are present? How frequently has the patient changed jobs and for what reasons? Is the patient a skilled or unskilled worker; what is the pay scale; and what transferable skills does the patient possess?[11]

Nonmedical issues are especially important in category 3, the patient with unreasonable subjective findings. The physician should collect information about the family as well as job stress, any drug or alcohol abuse, and other emotional issues that may be contributing to the patient's present pain. A family history of disability and the involvement of lawyers are important confounders to treatment of this category of patient.

It is very straightforward to establish the diagnosis and treatment protocol for patients with objective findings or reasonable subjective findings. In most of these cases, the diagnosis, etiology, and causal relationship to the job are established, and appropriate treatment methods can be instituted with resultant resolution of symptoms. In the third category, patients with magnified symptoms and unreasonable complaints, a diagnosis of chronic pain syndrome can be established, especially if the classic 6 *D*'s of symptom magnification are present: duration, drugs, disability, dramatization, distress, and doctor shopping. The most difficult cases are those in which a real musculotendinous pathology is present along with unreasonable subjective findings. Treatment in these cases must be delivered according to the degree of unreasonable symptoms and findings.

Objective Findings

Objective findings are determined by the physician's observation and require no patient involvement or cooperation. Objective findings include erythema; observed swelling; muscle atrophy; tendon or joint crepitation associated with motion; masses; or joint stiffness, deformity, or instability. Although these objective findings are subject to physical interpretation, they require no patient involvement for diagnosis. Radiological and laboratory tests are objective. When objective findings are present, the diagnosis is easily established.

Several work-related conditions are associated with objective findings. These include trigger fingers with locking, DeQuervain's tenosynovitis with obvious swelling or snapping, and median or ulnar nerve entrapment with muscle atrophy. Dorsal or volar wrist ganglia and dorsal tenosynovitis have objective findings. Patients may have an acute onset of joint pain associated with changed activity and radiographs will demonstrate a preexisting arthritis condition or a bony nonunion (see **Figs. 36-1; 36-2,** *B, C*).[10,11,13]

Reasonable Subjective Findings

Pain, tenderness, limited active range of motion, weakness of grip and pinch, and sensory complaints are subjective findings because they require the patient's cooperation and input. Subjective findings can be classified as reasonable or unreasonable by evaluating the entire clinical picture. Because the majority of CTDs are not associated with any objective findings, it is important to establish whether a particular patient's subjective findings are reasonable or unreasonable (see **Figs. 36-2***A,* **36-3,** and **36-4**).

Patients with reasonable subjective findings will give a reasonable history, and the physical findings will verify the history obtained. For example, a person reports symptoms of forearm pain and weakness of grip following chipping paint for 2 days. Physical examina-

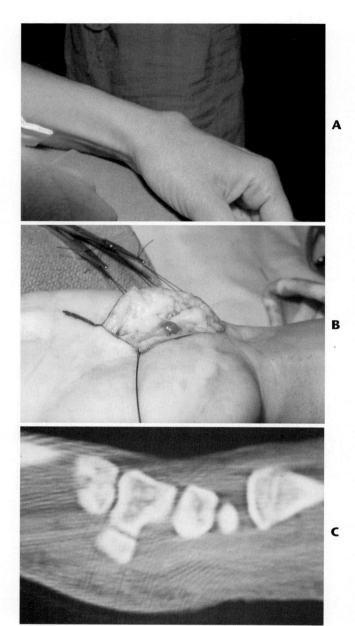

Figure 36-1 Objective findings. **A,** Dorsal wrist ganglion. **B,** Aneurysm of the ulnar artery. **C,** Fractured hook hamate seen on computed tomography.

tion demonstrates lateral epicondylar tenderness, pain on active resisted wrist extension, and pain on passive wrist flexion and elbow extension. These are reasonable subjective findings and a diagnosis of lateral epicondylitis is established.

In other cases, the clinical picture is less clear, but when the entire story follows a pattern, the patient can be categorized as having reasonable subjective findings. A patient is examined for vague mild diffuse discomfort over the dorsum of the hand, wrist, and forearm associated with excessive word processing. Physical examination may show mild discomfort on wrist extension or mild tenderness over the extensor muscle mass. Some-

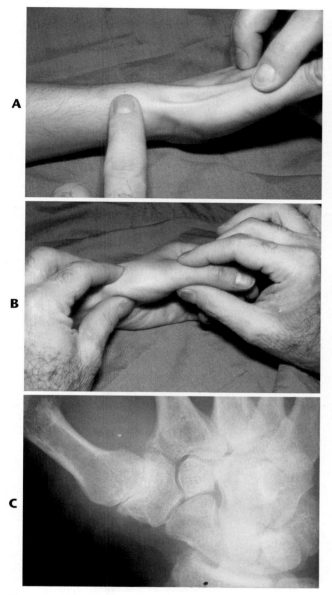

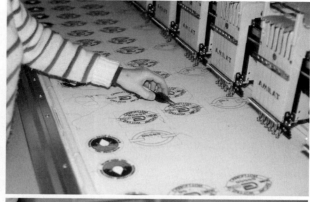

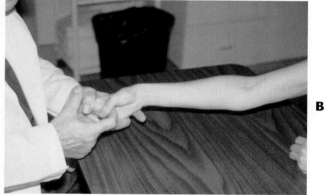

Figure 36-3 Reasonable subjective findings. **A,** Job requires repetitive and forceful pinch and patient complains of thenar muscle pain. **B,** Pain reproduced with thumb-resisted opposition.

Figure 36-2 Radial-sided wrist pain. **A,** Patient with De-Quervain's tenosynovitis manifests tenderness directly over the first extensor compartment and pain on active thumb abduction. **B,** Carpometacarpal joint degenerative arthritis: painful carpometacarpal joint grind test and painful instability of the carpometacarpal joint. **C,** Radiograph demonstrating degenerative arthritis of the carpometacarpal joint.

times the examination is completely normal; however, the work and pain history are reasonable and a diagnosis of extensor tendinitis can be made. It can be further confirmed if work station adaptation plus ergonomic issues are addressed and the condition resolves.

Several well-established musculotendinous conditions fit into this category. Although these conditions can occur spontaneously, usually a history of prolonged activity or a new or changed job will be elicited. Flexor carpi radialis tendinitis, flexor carpi ulnaris tendinitis,

extensor carpi ulnaris tendinitis, and extensor carpi radialis longus and brevis tendinitis are examples in the wrist. Extensor digitorium communis tendinitis and DeQuervain's tendinitis are examples of digital extensor tendinitis. Bicipital tendinitis, supraspinatus tendinitis, and cervicobrachial syndrome are examples in the shoulder. Lateral and medial epicondylitis are examples around the elbow (see **Fig. 36-5**).

Unreasonable Subjective Findings

Patients with unreasonable subjective findings are the most difficult to evaluate, and both experience and judgment are required by the examining physician to establish the diagnosis or nondiagnosis. The primary responsibility of the physician is to rule out organic pathology before making the diagnosis of a nonorganic cause of the patient's pain. Many patients who are classified in this category may have an organic component for their pain, but the overlying nonmedical issues confuse the picture and make it impossible to establish any secure diagnosis. A patient may have both objective findings and unreasonable subjective findings, or a patient may have subjective findings that cannot be totally characterized. Some of their findings seem reasonable, but symptom magnification and other emotional issues confuse the diagnosis.

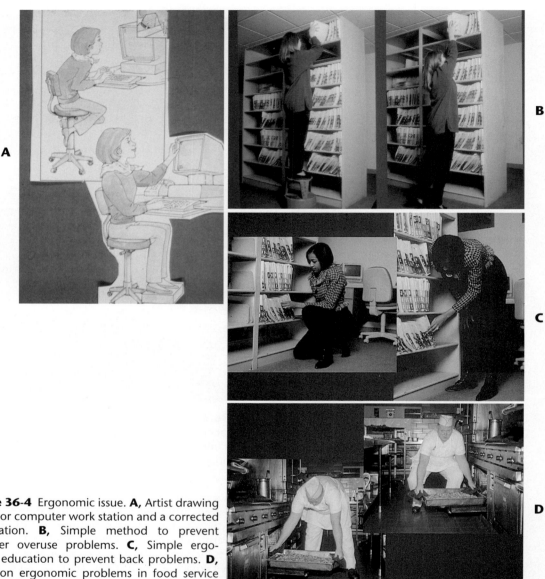

Figure 36-4 Ergonomic issue. **A,** Artist drawing of a poor computer work station and a corrected workstation. **B,** Simple method to prevent shoulder overuse problems. **C,** Simple ergonomic education to prevent back problems. **D,** Common ergonomic problems in food service departments.

Some patients are seen with completely unreasonable subjective findings.[3,5,13] These are associated with psychosocial issues often attributed to the work-related injury. A history will elicit conflicts between the worker and the employer or the worker and the insurer. Many of these patients have poor job performance evaluations or a troubled past work history and significant psychological problems. On physical examination, the findings can run a wide gamut. On one extreme is a person who seems to have DeQuervain's tenosynovitis, but the pain and tenderness is out of proportion to what should be expected and the pinch strength is 1 to 2 lb. On the other extreme is a person with truly bizarre findings of generalized pain, tenderness throughout the extremity, inability to flex the digits, and absolutely no history to substantiate these findings.

TREATMENT

In the first two categories, treatment is usually straightforward and successful. The principles are based on appropriate nonsurgical treatment, job modification when necessary, work station evaluation, and teaching ergonomic principles. Depending on the degree of symptoms, a short course of nonsteroidal antiinflammatory medications and splinting is instituted. When symptoms are mild or after the symptoms have subsided, a short course of therapy is instituted that includes education in proper work methods and developing good exercise habits. (see **Fig. 36-4**).[13,14] When patients have trigger fingers, DeQuervain's tenosynovitis, or other types of tenosynovitis, cortisone injections are helpful.

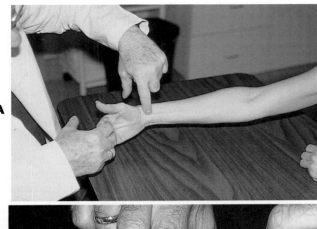

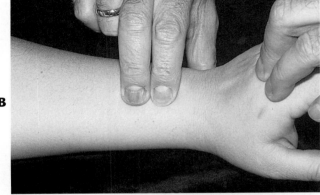

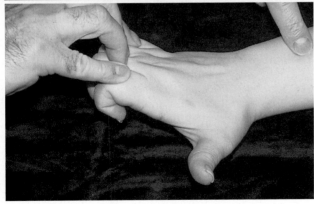

Figure 36-5 Wrist pain with reasonable subjective findings. **A,** Flexor carpi radialis tendinitis in a patient with tenderness over the flexor carpi radialis tendon and pain on resisted wrist flexion. **B,** Extensor carpi radialis longus and brevis tendinitis manifested as tenderness located over the extensor carpi radialis longus and brevis and pain on resisted wrist extension. **C,** Extensor digitorum communis tendinitis causing pain on resisted digital extension.

In more chronic cases of the first two types, the physician and therapist should have a clear understanding of the work situation of the patient. In this case, job evaluations may be performed and attempts made to modify the job or for the patient to change jobs. When employers are cooperative, the problems are more readily resolved. When accommodations are not avail-

able, conflict and long-standing disability may result. Sometimes surgery is indicated, especially for patients with objective findings, but when workers have nonmedical issues that are not addressed, recovery may not be complete and the problem may remain unresolved. It is therefore important to address nonmedical issues in all cases before treatment to ensure optimal recovery from the intervention. Occasionally surgery is necessary even when significant nonmedical issues are present, and the team should be prepared for a longer and more difficult recovery period that may include disability and pain management.

For patients with unreasonable subjective findings, it is difficult to prescribe an effective treatment plan. When significant adversarial and legal issues are present with long-standing disability, the physician can do little to alleviate the problem. These patients may be considered to have a chronic pain syndrome and should be treated in an appropriate pain program. In less severe cases where a team can assist in the resolution of some nonmedical issues, it is possible to restore the worker to productive employment. This requires the commitment of both the patient and a dedicated, multidisciplinary team that includes psychological counseling and the support of the employer.

MANAGEMENT OF CHRONIC PATIENTS

In this section, the multidisciplinary approach to the treatment and management of CTD patients who exhibit unreasonable subjective findings is discussed. The recommended configuration of an occupational hand clinic includes an expanded role for hand therapists. To successfully manage occupational CTD, physicians and therapists must broaden their traditional roles and work together in evaluating and treating patients. These new roles are discussed in the following sections.[13]

Case Management

In an occupational hand clinic, evaluation includes a detailed job history, a history of the present illness, and a description of job tasks. A member of the workplace staff is included in the coordination of care. This person may be the rehabilitation nurse, supervisor, or employer who will play a role in keeping the employee on the job throughout the rehabilitation process, either in the same job modified according to need or in another temporary position. Work site visits are an important component of performing an ergonomic analysis and making recommendations for changes in the job, work environment, or tools. This also helps the team become aware and proactive in any interpersonal issues that may be present on the job site.

Traditional medical and therapeutic treatment takes place alongside these workplace assessments to ensure that other psychosocial issues do not impede recovery of the patient from surgery or therapy. Dealing with work-related illness is different from other hand injury treatment, and the multidisciplinary team must recognize and deal with the occupational issues to facilitate recovery. The hand therapist will assume the lead role in assessment and education of the patient and coordinate the activities of all other team members, including the physician, physical therapist, and psychologist. The hand therapist, usually an occupational therapist, will coordinate the evaluation and treatment, as well as interact with the employer to understand and improve any workplace issues that exacerbate the illness.

In a large proportion of cases, the determining factor in minimizing disability revolves around nonorthopaedic issues, including job dissatisfaction, job stress, anger, resentment, or other effects of the adversarial worker's compensation system. A major predictor of disability is unresolved psychosocial issues.[1] A strong case management approach that includes therapy is effective in maintaining a patient on the job and returning patients to work after a short absence. The therapist must understand not only the physical limitations of the injury but also the job-related factors and any problems at home that contribute to the disability behavior of the patient. The trust and confidence that build between a patient and therapist are important in revealing and addressing other factors such as problems at home, drug and alcohol abuse, and work-related dissatisfaction. The team aggressively investigates the work site and encourages the employer's participation in resolving ergonomic problems as well as job dissatisfaction, negative relationships between management and the patient or between the patient and co-workers, and other work-related issues. This active role encourages patients to express their feelings and helps to facilitate improved communication between the employer and the patient. In any event, patients grow to trust the therapist as being "in their corner," and this can only improve their chances for recovery.

The Industrial Athlete

Active involvement of the patient is key to the success of recovery. Often, in traditional physical therapy programs patients are not taught to use stretching and strengthening techniques.[15] General conditioning and aerobic exercises are appropriate for all patients, who should be treated like "industrial athletes" and conditioned for their return to work. The team at the occupational hand clinic encourages active, aggressive, conservative care (stretching, strengthening, aerobic conditioning, and body mechanics training) that focuses on wellness rather than illness. The presence of minor musculoskeletal problems is more manageable by individuals who perceive themselves as healthy than by someone who feels "disabled" by an injury or pain.

Education and prevention are a big part of this approach. Patients are taught to keep themselves in good condition to recover from and prevent future injuries. Patients with upper extremity CTDs and chronic pain are often found to be weak and decondi-

tioned. Being involved and active is a source of self esteem for most individuals. Their participation in an aerobic conditioning and body strengthening program is effective in changing attitudes and behavior associated with chronic pain and decreasing upper extremity pain.[4,6] Treatment programs should educate patients about the benefits of fitness, and individually designed treatment programs should focus on the specific conditioning needs of the patient for work readiness. These exercise programs should not end when the treatment program is completed, but should be considered a part of the patient's work routine. Patients should be encouraged to continue with such programs and employers educated to support their inclusion in an injury prevention program for all their workers.[2] A simple cost-benefit comparison shows that prevention programs that include ergonomics and physical fitness are significantly less costly than medical expenses for injury, rehabilitation, worker's compensation, and possible disability.

CONCLUSIONS

Each patient with an upper extremity injury should be evaluated on three levels: musculoskeletal, ergonomic, and psychosocial. The following summarizes the important points in each category.[1]

1. **Musculoskeletal disorder**
   A. *Objective findings:* swelling, joint or tendon crepitation, limited joint motion, abnormal radiographic or electromyographic findings
   B. *Reasonable subjective findings:* pain, tenderness, sensory loss or weakness appropriate and consistent with the injury and the history
   C. *Unreasonable subjective findings:* diffuse, vague, unreproducible pain and tenderness not corresponding to anatomic distribution or inconsistent with the history of the injury

2. **Ergonomic issues**
   A. *Minor issues:* correctable work station problems or minor ergonomic instruction
   B. *Moderate issues:* high repetition, high force, or abnormal positions that are correctable
   C. *Major issues:* high repetition, high force, or abnormal positions that are not correctable

3. **Psychosocial issues**
   A. *Minor psychosocial issues:* usually administrative issues such as providing temporary modified duty or minor conflicts with the supervisor
   B. *Moderate psychosocial issues:* job frustration, job stress, management insensitivity, employee anger that is treatable
   C. *Major psychosocial issues:* long-standing and unresolved frustration, anger, job stress, plus degrees of depression that are untreatable by an occupational clinic

In a study of 50 workers, these authors found that the musculoskeletal classification is important in the diagnosis of the patients with the CTDs and in predicting their return to work.[1] In CTD, objective findings are uncommon, and this creates difficulties in evaluating the significance of subjective findings. When subjective findings of pain, tenderness, weakness, and sensory loss are reasonable and consistent with the history of the injury, patients respond to the treatment predictably. Return-to-work rates are identical for the objective group and the reasonable subjective group. The ergonomic classification does not independently determine a patient's ability to return to work. Regardless of the ergonomic classification, all patients without group B or C psychosocial issues returned to work.

Therefore, the presence of anything greater than minor psychosocial issues is the primary factor contributing to the prolonged disability of workers with CTD. Workers who have objective or reasonable subjective findings and who lack moderate or major psychosocial issues returned to work in all cases. Patients with unrea-

sonable subjective findings and moderate or major psychosocial issues do not respond to conventional treatment, and disability was prolonged in about one third of those cases. Those patients who continued to work while being treated for CTD were maintained in their jobs, even in the presence of moderate or major psychosocial issues.[1]

The presence of psychosocial stressors and the employment status of the patient at the time of CTD diagnosis are significant predictors of recovery and return to work. A multidisciplinary approach with a strong case management component is believed to be the most effective way to return a patient to work. Clinicians must be willing to interface with employers to facilitate resolution of job stresses and frustrations and to encourage modified-duty programs that permit a rapid return to work. Inclusion of the employer in the educational process is critical to the successful treatment of these patients and a reduction of similar injuries in the future.

References

1. Bonzani P et al: Factors prolonging disability in work-related cumulative trauma disorders, *J Hand Surg* (in press).

2. Bullock MI: Musculoskeletal disorders in the workplace. In Kumashiro M, Megaw ED, editors: *Towards human work: solutions to problems in occupational health and safety*, New York, 1991, Taylor & Francis.

3. Carti DJ, Burton WN: Economic impact of depression in a workplace, *J Occup Med* 36, 983-988, 1994.

4. Caudill MA: *Managing chronic pain: a behavioral medicine workbook*, Boston, 1993, Deaconess Hospital, and Nashua, NH, Hitchcock Clinic; pp 61-81.

5. Dawson DM, Hallett M, Millender, LH: *Entrapment neuropathies*, ed 2, Boston, 1990, Little, Brown.

6. Fuerstein M et al: Multidisciplinary rehabilitation of chronic work-related upper extremity disorders, *J of Occup Med* 35: 396–403, 1993.

7. Hadler NM: Cumulative trauma, carpal tunnel syndrome in the workplace: epidemiological and legal aspects. In Gelberman R, editor: *Operative nerve repair and reconstruction*, New York, 1991, JB Lippincott.

8. Hadler NM: Cumulative trauma disorders: an iatrogenic concept, *J Occup Med* 32(1):38-41, 1991.

9. Ireland DCR: Psychological and physical affects of occupational arm pain, *J Hand Surg* 13(1)B:5-10, 1988.

10. Kasdan M, editor: *Occupational hand and upper extremity injuries and diseases*, Philadelphia, 1991, Hanley & Belfus.

11. Louis DS: Evaluation and treatment of medial neuropathy associated with cumulative trauma. In Gelberman R, editor: *Operative nerve repair and reconstruction*, New York, 1991, JB Lippincott.

12. Martin T: Cumulative trauma disorder comes knocking: repetitive stress injuries on the rise, *Boston Computer Society Update*, 1992; pp 13-15.

13. Millender LH, Louis DS, Simmons, BP: *Occupational disorders of the upper extremity*, New York, 1992, Churchill Livingstone.

14. Rempel D, Harrison R, and Barnhart S: Work-related cumulative trauma disorders, *JAMA*, 267, 838-842, 1992.

15. Saunders R, Anderson M: Early treatment intervention, *Orthop Phys Ther Clin* 1(1):67-74, 1992.

16. Silverstein B, Fine LJ, Armstrong TJ: Hand and wrist cumulative trauma disorders in industry, *Br J Ind Med* 43:779-784, 1986.

17. Williams R, Westmorland M: Occupational cumulative trauma disorders of the upper extremity, *Am J Occup Ther* 48(5):411-420, 1994.

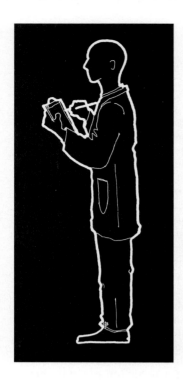

Chapter 37

Biomechanical Aspects of Hand Tools

Robert G. Radwin
Seoungyeon Oh
Christopher Carlson-Dakes

CONTENTS

The mechanical relationships between hand tools and tool operation can be used for understanding and controlling physical stress in the hands of tool operators. Hand exertions needed for many tool operations are directly affected by the selection of specific tools and accessories for the task. Many of the recommendations in this chapter are based on simple mechanical principles and reasonable assumptions about static mechanical relationships between tools and their operators. The objective is to illustrate how the characteristics of a particular tool (e.g., size, shape, output, accessories) can have a significant effect on the effort needed for performing specific tasks.

Both manual (hand-powered) and power (electric, pneumatic, or hydraulic) hand tools require that operators produce forces at varying levels. Manual tools may require exerting forces needed for squeezing together tool handles, such as with pliers and cutting tools. Other manual tools may require twisting, pulling, or pushing. Safe power tool operation requires that an operator possess the ability to adequately support the tool in a particular position and apply the necessary force while reacting against the force generated by the power tool itself. Force demands that exceed an operator's strength capabilities can cause loss of control and result in an accident or an injury. If improper selection, installation, or use of a power tool requires an operator to make substantially greater exertion than necessary, it may lead to muscle fatigue or a musculoskeletal disorder.[1,4,16,26,27] Tools that are selected for minimizing hand forces are usually the best tools for the task.

The discussion begins with simple manually operated hand tools, including screwdrivers and pliers. Then the means by which different kinds of screw fasteners can affect forces in the hands is investigated. Finally, control of static hand forces associated with power hand tool use through tool selection and installation is explored.

MANUAL SCREWDRIVERS

Screwdrivers are one of the most common hand tools used. They are available in a variety of sizes and forms suitable for different types of screws and work situations. A screw is usually tightened by grasping the screwdriver handle and simultaneously applying a torque while exerting a push force. The amount of torque T needed for tightening a screw depends on the kind of screw and the characteristics of the screw joint, such as friction, bolt diameter, thread, and clamping load. The push force is often called *feed force*. Feed force F is the axial force applied against the screwdriver shaft that is needed for threading the screw and keeping the screwdriver blade seated. Numerous task-related factors affect feed force, including thread type (i.e., whether the screw is self-tapping or threaded), material hardness, thread size, and hole diameter. The choice of a particular size screwdriver can have a great effect on the hand exertion required for a task.

Handle Length

A question often asked is *how does screwdriver length affect hand force?* Experience has found that a longer screwdriver handle generally results in less effort.[19] This can be explained by considering the motions needed for tightening a screw. When a screw is tightened, torque is transferred to the handle, usually by rotating the forearm in combination with flexion and ulnar deviation of the wrist. The asymmetry of the hand, wrist, and forearm relative to the screwdriver's radial axis produces eccentric rotation of the handle that causes perturbation of the screwdriver handle and shaft along a horizontal displacement Δ from the vertical axis (**Fig. 37-1**). The magnitude of this displacement depends on the particular action and anthropometry of the wrist. This perturbation causes the screwdriver shaft to tilt a maximum angle θ as the screwdriver rotates.

All things remaining the same (i.e., handle size, handle diameter, handle shape, screwdriver shaft diameter), hand and wrist rotation is unaffected by the screwdriver shaft length, so the handle perturbation is

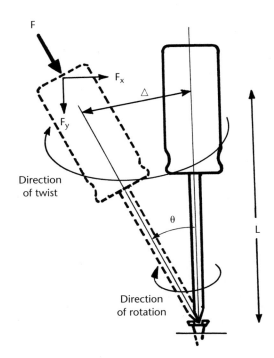

Figure 37-1 Rotation and perturbation of a manual screwdriver when the handle is twisted in the hand.

the same regardless of the screwdriver shaft length. Assuming that the handle displaces the same distance Δ from the axis of the fastener shaft (see **Fig. 37-1**), the maximum angle θ that the screwdriver shaft tilts as it is twisted can be described as

$$\theta = \sin^{-1}\left(\frac{\Delta}{L}\right) \tag{1}$$

Orthogonal feed force components (**Fig. 37-1**) can be resolved into

$$F_y = F \cos\theta \quad F_x = F \sin\theta \tag{2}$$

If a screwdriver has a length L, then the maximum component parallel to the fastener shaft is F_y:

$$F_y = F \cos\theta = F \cos\left[\sin^{-1}\left(\frac{\Delta}{L}\right)\right] \tag{3}$$

Solving for F,

$$F = \frac{F_y}{\cos\left[\sin^{-1}\left(\frac{\Delta}{L}\right)\right]} \tag{4}$$

A consequence of this relationship is that if the required axial force component F_y remains constant, F decreases as L increases. Hence the hand force exerted can be reduced by increasing L and using the longest screwdriver available. For example, if the shaft of a 6-cm screwdriver displaces $\Delta = 3$ cm, the feed force F needed to drive a screw is

$$F = \frac{F_y}{\cos\left[\sin^{-1}\left(\frac{3}{6}\right)\right]} = 1.15 \times F_y \tag{5}$$

Therefore, the maximum feed force can be as much as 15% greater than the axial force needed. If the screwdriver length is increased to 25 cm, the feed force needed to drive a screw would be

$$F = \frac{F_y}{\cos\left[\sin^{-1}\left(\frac{3}{25}\right)\right]} = 1.01 \times F_y \tag{6}$$

which decreases the force feed to only as much as 1% more force than is actually needed. Of course, a very long screwdriver may not be practical under all circumstances. Clearance and spatial constraints may limit the size of screwdriver that is practical. Furthermore, a very short screwdriver can facilitate the precision grip needed for light precise work, such as that afforded with a jeweler's screwdriver.

Another way to limit the horizontal perturbation of a screwdriver as it rotates in the hand is by supporting the screwdriver shaft, as might be done when two hands are used. If the screwdriver were held straight by supporting the shaft with the fingers of the free hand, then the tilt angle θ remains close to 0 degrees and $F_y \approx F \cos$

0 degrees $\approx F$. This action therefore aids the operator by keeping the axial feed force requirements minimum and unaffected by screwdriver length. Screwdriver shafts should be long enough to be pinched or gripped by the other hand as a guide when high feed forces are required. The hand force needed for a nutdriver, using a similar argument, should be mostly independent of the shaft length because the shaft is coupled to the nut, which permits concentric rotation with the handle despite the asymmetries of the hand and forearm.

Handle Diameter

Another common question is *how does a screwdriver handle diameter affect hand force?* Several studies have investigated the effect of handle diameter on the torque capability of the hand. A study involving volitional torque exerted for different manual screwdrivers, locking pliers, and wrenches found that the resulting torque magnitude was strongly influenced by the kind of tool and the posture assumed.[14] From a purely mechanical standpoint, a greater handle diameter should result in more torque at the screwdriver shaft for the same effort, provided that the frictional properties of the handles are similar and the handle diameter is not too large.

The diameter of a screwdriver handle plays a critical role in limiting a person's torque-generating capability. Large grip forces are often needed for sustaining a grip and coupling the hand and the tool to prevent the handle from slipping. A simplified relationship between the torque and diameter illustrates the effect of mechanical advantage on torque:

$$T = F_S D = \mu F_G D \tag{7}$$

where T is torque, F_S is the shear grip force, D is the handle diameter, μ is the coefficient of friction between the hand and the handle, and F_G is grip compression force.[19] If F_G remained constant, torque would linearly increase as the handle diameter increased. Grip strength, however, is not constant for all diameters. It is well known that grip strength is affected by handle size.[3,12,13] If a handle is too large or too small, the strength of the hand is greatly compromised. The relationship between cylindrical handle size and grip strength is summarized in **Figure 37-2**.[17] Maximum grip force occurs around 6 cm. Consequently, the optimal diameter is one in which a further increase in diameter increases the mechanical advantage while simultaneously decreasing grip force. Research has found that this optimum depends on handle design, friction, gender, and hand size.[19] Torque performance diminishes when handle diameters are greater than 5 cm.[20] A diameter of 4 cm is sometimes recommended for screwdrivers.[6,7]

Sufficient friction must be present between the handle and the hand to provide a secure grip and prevent a tool from slipping. Handle frictional characteristics affect the grip force needed to maintain control of the tool and the ability to exert force or torque.

Surfaces that do not provide adequate friction require greater grip force that may result in greater effort and even loss of control of the tool. The amount of friction depends on the coefficient of friction between the hand and the material or object grasped. Some materials have greater coefficients of friction and consequently better frictional characteristics than others.

No one handle size is practical for all tasks, and certain handles serve some objectives better than others. A panel of ergonomics experts recommend using a small-diameter handle (8 to 13 mm) for a precision grip and a large-diameter handle (50 to 60 mm) for a power grip.[15] In one study, handles between 31 and 38 mm in diameter were considered optimum for a power grip.[9] Several studies recommend 50 mm as an upper-limit diameter for handles used with a power grip.[3,20,25]

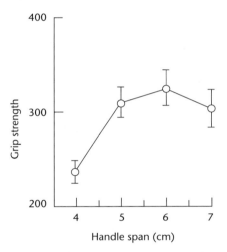

Figure 37-2 Grip strength for a population of 29 subjects (19 university students and 10 factory workers). Error bars represent one standard error of the mean.

SCREWDRIVER BLADES AND SCREW HEADS

Screwdriver feed force can be affected by the particular type of screw fastener head and screw tip needed.[5] Self-tapping screws require more feed force than do screws tightened through pretapped holes. Material hardness and friction are also important factors to consider for self-tapping screws. Feed force requirements increase as the torque level increases for cross recess screws. Allowances should be made for all these factors. The three most common threaded fastener heads are (1) slotted, (2) Phillips head, and (3) Torx head (**Fig. 37-3**). Feed force requirements differ between these three screw head types.

Slotted Screws

A slotted screw, the simplest and oldest type of screw head, has a single slot that goes across the entire diameter of the head. When a screwdriver blade is inserted inside a screw slot and rotated, contact is usually made at the two edges of the blade, as shown in **Figure 37-4**. The size of the screwdriver width w, limited by the radius of the screw head, provides a slight mechanical advantage for applying torque against the screw. Wider screw heads and screwdriver blades generally require less torque exerted at the screwdriver shaft.

We shall ignore frictional force by assuming that friction between the screw and screwdriver blade is zero (because friction in this case assists the operator by helping keep the screwdriver blade in the screw slot, an assumption of zero friction should be considered the worst-case condition). If the width of the screwdriver blade is w and the applied torque at the screwdriver shaft is T, then the normal contact force F_C between the blade and the screw head slot is

$$F_C = \frac{T}{W}$$

(8)

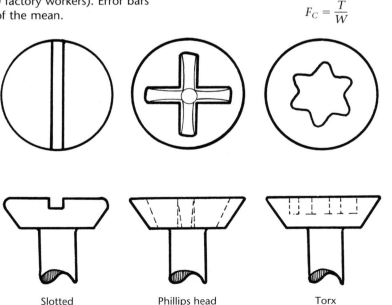

Slotted   Phillips head   Torx

Figure 37-3 Slotted head, Phillips head, and Torx head screws.

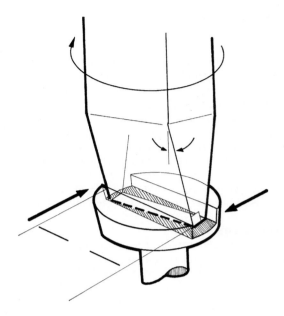

Figure 37-4 Static forces acting on a slotted screwdriver blade and shaft.

Because the blades of slotted screwdrivers are usually tapered an angle ϕ to facilitate insertion of the screwdriver blade and accommodate different-size screw slots, the normal contact force F_C is not actually perpendicular to the screwdriver shaft but rather acts at an angle perpendicular to the blade edge (see **Figure 37-4**). This results in an axial force at each contact point

$$F_y = F_C \sin\phi = \frac{T}{W} \sin\phi \tag{9}$$

that acts to push the screwdriver blade out of the slot as torque is applied to the screwdriver shaft. The hand must react against this force by exerting an equal and opposite axial force F_y that is a component of the feed force. Because there are two contact points, the total axial force is $2F_y$. Consequently, the axial force required to keep the blade from coming out of the slot is

$$F = 2F_y = 2\frac{T}{W} \sin\phi \tag{10}$$

The greater the torque T, the greater the axial force needed to keep the screwdriver blade in the slot. If the screwdriver blade taper angle ϕ is 12 degrees,

$$F = 2\frac{T}{W} \sin(12°) = 0.42\frac{T}{W} \tag{11}$$

If the screwdriver blade angle is not tapered but parallel to the slot, this force is negligible ($F_y = 0$) because no axial force acts to unseat the blade. Such a screwdriver, however, would be limited to certain size slots and it would be more difficult to insert the screwdriver into the screw slots.

Phillips Head Screws

Although slotted screws are simpler, screwdriver blades sometimes slip out of slotted heads and have the potential to damage or scratch the workpiece. The Phillips head screw (**Fig. 37-4**) gained popularity because it prevented slippage and discouraged vandals from removing screws in public places with a coin or knife edge.[18]

A Phillips head screwdriver blade contains four wedges acting on the blade. Similar to the slotted screwdriver, the axial forces acting parallel to the fastener can be described by the equation

$$F = 4F_y = 4F_C \sin\phi = 4\frac{T}{W} \sin\phi \tag{12}$$

Because ϕ is typically greater for Phillips head screws and w is much smaller, F_y is considerably more for Phillips head screwdrivers than for slotted screwdrivers. The typical taper angle for a Phillips head screw is $\phi = 40$ degrees, so

$$F = 4\frac{T}{W} \sin(40°) = 2.57\frac{T}{W} \tag{13}$$

which is more than six times the force needed for a slotted screw with an equivalent-diameter head.

Torx Head Screws

Torx screws have the advantages of *both* slotted screws and Phillips head screws. Because $\phi = 0$ for Torx head screws (**Fig. 37-3**), no other axial force component than the actual feed force is required to advance the fastener. Torx head screws are not as flexible as slotted or Phillips head screws because the screwdriver blade cannot be tapered to accommodate different-size screws. The mechanical advantage of Torx head screws may outweigh the disadvantage of requiring a large assortment of screwdrivers with corresponding blade sizes. Furthermore, they are more difficult to tamper with because Torx head screwdrivers are not as readily available as slotted and Phillips screwdrivers and an assortment of sizes are needed. The advantages and disadvantages of slotted, Phillips, and Torx head screws are summarized in **Table 37-1**.

PLIERS AND CUTTING TOOLS

The particular finger or combination of fingers used can affect grip strength.[2,23] The thumb, index, and middle fingers are the strongest fingers, and they should be used for producing the most grip force. The ring finger and small finger are capable of less strength and should be used for stabilizing handles rather than acting as primary force contributors. Sometimes tool operators handle tools in ways that take this into account.

Pliers are often used for pinching, grasping, and cutting by way of the mechanical advantage provided from squeezing together two opposing lever arms. The

Table 37-1	Summary of ergonomic advantages and disadvantages of different screw heads	
Screw Head	**Advantages**	**Disadvantages**
Slotted	Very flexible tool—one size fits all Requires little axial feed force	Difficult to keep seated in the slot Can slip and damage workpiece
Phillips	Easy to keep seated in head Flexible tool	Requires more axial feed force
Torx	No axial feed force needed Easy to keep seated in head	Inflexible—must have a specific size for an associated screw head

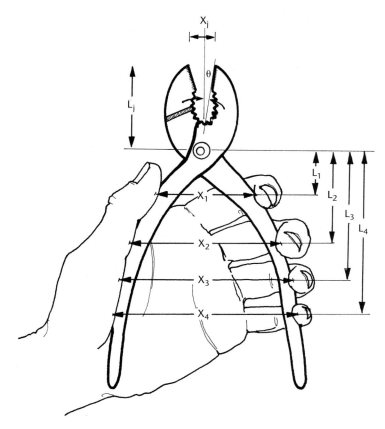

Figure 37-5 Static forces acting on the hand when a pair of pliers is grasped.

common use of pliers involves a grip depicted in **Figure 37-5**, where the pliers jaw is held on the radial side of the hand. In many instances, however, this grip does not optimize the mechanical advantage with finger strength and can result in greater exertion than necessary.

Swedish researchers observed that some sheet metal workers held metal shear blades on the ulnar side of the hand by using an inverted grip (see **Fig. 37-6**), rather than the way that conventional shears were held.[8,28] Finger strength data revealed that the inverted grip allowed a greater span between the larger index finger and thumb than between the small finger and the palm,

providing a better-suited handle size for more force in each cut.[10]

The articulation angle from the closed position to the pivot point is defined as θ. The jaw span X_j is related to the grip span X_i as

$$X_i = X_J \frac{L_i}{L_J} \tag{14}$$

where

L_i = Distance from the fulcrum to the finger i
L_j = Distance from the fulcrum to the jaw tip
X_i = Grip span available for finger i

Assuming there are no coupling effects between fingers the resultant force is the sum of all four fingers. Individual-finger normal strengths for the distal phalanx while grasping handles of different sizes are taken from Amis.[2] By summing the moments about the pivot point, the total moment is

$$M_J = F_1L_1 + F_2L_2 + F_3L_3 + F_4L_4 \qquad (15)$$

This moment is counteracted by the moment produced from reaction forces at the jaw. Consequently, the maximum jaw force is

$$F_J = \frac{M_J}{L_J} \qquad (16)$$

By using the dimensions provided in **Table 37-2**, the maximum jaw force available increases from 714 to 786 N (10%) just by inverting the handle. Because the index and middle fingers have the greatest strength, they are provided with larger moment arms for generating force with the inverted grip. Inverting the pliers in the hand provides additional mechanical advantage for the fingers with the greatest strength (the index and middle fingers). One study observed that the maximum force of one finger depended not only on its grip span but also on the grip span of the other fingers.[10]

POWER HAND TOOLS

One of the best methods for controlling applied hand exertion is to substitute a power hand tool for a manual tool. In fact, many repetitive jobs could not be performed without the use of power tools. Modern power hand tools can operate at high speeds and are capable of producing very high forces. Exertions and

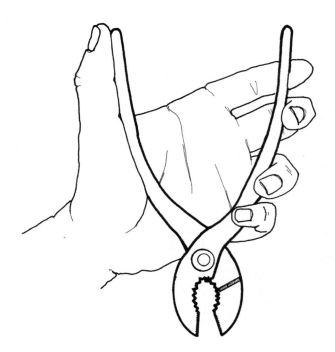

Figure 37-6 Inverted pliers grip.

Table 37-2	Pliers handle dimensions and associated finger strength for showing the mechanical advantage using an inverted grip				
Grip	**Index**	**Middle**	**Ring**	**Small**	**Total**
CONVENTIONAL					
Grip span X_i (cm)	6.0	6.6	6.4	5.4	
Grip strength F_i (N)	60	63	44	37	204
Finger distance L_i (cm)	7.0	8.3	10.2	11.4	
Torque (Nm)	420	523	449	422	1814
Jaw force F_J	165	206	177	166	714
INVERTED					
Grip span X_i (cm)	5.4	6.4	6.6	6.0	
Grip strength F_i (N)	62	64	43	35	204
Finger distance L_i (cm)	11.4	10.7	8.3	7.0	
Torque (Nm)	707	685	357	245	1994
Jaw force F_J	278	270	141	97	786

forces acting against the hand in power tool operation can be reduced by eliminating excess weight, by making the best use of the mechanical advantage, or by providing mechanical aids for holding tools, parts, and materials. Selecting a power hand tool having certain dimensions and shapes can often reduce tool reaction forces and provide mechanical advantages that assist the operator. Increasing friction between the hand and objects grasped can also reduce the forces required for gripping tools.

Power hand tools used for tightening threaded fasteners such as screwdrivers, sometimes called nutrunners, are commonly configured as (1) in-line, (2) pistol grip, and (3) right angle. A mechanical model of a power hand nutrunner was developed for static equilibrium (no movement) conditions. Hand force, reaction force from the workpiece, tool weight, and tool torque were included in this model.

The model uses a Cartesian coordinate system relative to the orientation of the handle grasped in the hand using a power grip. This coordinate system has the x-axis perpendicular to the axial direction of the handle, the y-axis passes through the long axis of the handle, and the z-axis is perpendicular to the x-axis and y-axis. The origin is located at the end of the bit or socket. Hand forces will be described in relation to these coordinate axes. To simplify the model, we will assume that orthogonal forces can be summed along the handle without producing coupling moments. This assumption allows force to be considered as having a single point of application. The resultant hand force F_H at the grip center is the vector sum of the three orthogonal force components

$$F_H = F_{H_x}i + F_{H_y}j + F_{H_z}k$$

(17)

where the hand force magnitude is

$$|F_H| = \sqrt{F_{H_x}^2 + F_{H_y}^2 + F_{H_z}^2}$$

(18)

and *i, j,* and *k* are the unit vectors.

In-line Power Drivers

The torque developed at an in-line power hand tool spindle has an equal and opposite reaction torque T_R that must be overcome by tangential shear forces between the hand and the handle. The tangential shear force F_S produces torque about the spindle axis for a moment arm D, which is the tool diameter. The shear force F_S is proportional to the compressive hand force F_G and the coefficient of friction μ between the hand and the handle, similar to a manual screwdriver except in this case the spindle is producing the torque rather than the hand. Therefore, in-line power driver operation is limited by the maximum compressive grip force an operator can produce and by tool dimensions. The forces and moments involved in operating an in-line power tool are shown in **Figure 37-7**. The relationship

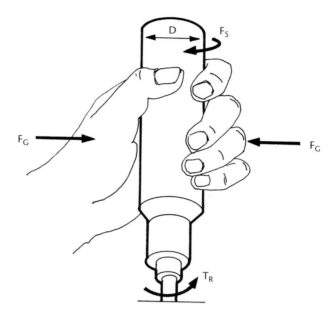

Figure 37-7 Forces acting in the hand when an in-line nutrunner is operated.

between the torque, grip force, and tool diameter is similar to manual screwdriver operation:

$$T_R = F_S D = \mu F_G D$$

(19)

Push-to-start activated power hand tools free the operator from having to squeeze a trigger or lever, but they can increase force requirements because they require more feed force to start them. A flange at the end of in-line handles helps prevent the hand from slipping during feed force exertion.[11]

Pistol-Grip and Right-Angle Power Drivers

Consider the free-body diagram of the pistol-grip nutrunner in **Figure 37-8**. The spindle torque T acts clockwise in the *xy*-plane. The tool operator has to oppose this equal and opposite reaction torque T_R in the counterclockwise direction by producing a reaction force F_{H_x} along the *x*-axis. This is not the only force that the tool operator must produce, however. A force acting along the z-axis F_{H_z} provides feed force and produces an equal and opposite reaction force F_{R_z}. In addition, the operator has to react against the tool mass to support and position the tool by producing a vertical force component F_{H_y}. The tool weight W_T and push force F_{H_z} tend to produce a clockwise rotation of the power tool about the spindle in the *yz*-plane that is countered by this vertical support force.

When a body is in static equilibrium, the sum of the external forces and the sum of the moments are equal to zero. Using this relationship, the following system of

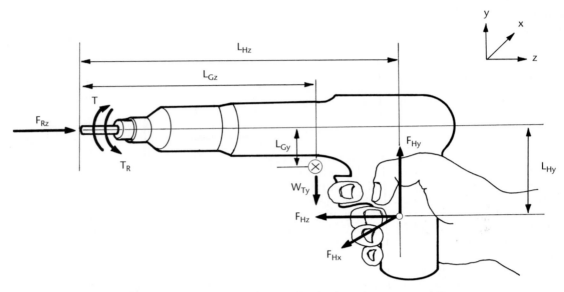

Figure 37-8 Static forces during pistol-grip nutrunner operation.

equations was developed for the pistol-grip nutrunner to describe these static forces:

$$F_{H_z} + F_{R_z} = 0 \tag{20}$$

$$F_{H_y}L_{H_z} - F_{H_z}L_{H_y} + W_{T_y}L_{G_z} = 0 \tag{21}$$

$$T_R - F_{H_x}L_{H_y} = 0 \tag{22}$$

This system of equations can be solved, and the resulting individual hand force components are

$$F_{H_x} = \frac{T_R}{L_{H_y}} \tag{23}$$

$$F_{H_y} = \frac{1}{L_{H_z}}(F_{H_z}L_{H_y} - W_{T_y}L_{G_z}) \tag{24}$$

$$F_{H_z} = -F_{R_z} \tag{25}$$

These equations reveal several relationships between tool parameters and hand force. Torque reaction force F_{H_x} is directly proportional to the reaction torque T_R and inversely proportional to the tool length L_{H_y}. Therefore, the torque reaction force is less for longer tool handles than for shorter handles. The vertical support force F_{H_y} is inversely proportional to the tool length L_{H_z} and is also dependent on tool weight, center of gravity location, handle length L_{H_y}, and push force F_{H_z}. The equations indicate that less effort is probably needed for supporting a pistol-grip power hand tool when the tool body is long than when the tool body is short. When feed force is large, supporting force decreases when the handle length is short. This is why power hand tools with handles aligned close to the tool spindle axis and with long tool bodies are advantageous for tools such as power hand drills. Power hand drills often require con-

siderable feed force, whereas torque reaction forces are relatively less than for a nutrunner. Therefore a short handle is favorable. Alternatively, when torque is large and feed force is small, a tool with a long handle is advantageous. However, when both feed force and torque are significant factors, these parameters have to be optimized. This condition can exist, for example, when drilling large holes or shooting self-tapping screws in hard wood.

The model can be used for comparing resultant hand forces associated with different tools for the same operation and for selecting the tool requiring the least exertion. Consider the four hypothetical power nutrunners shown in **Figure 37-9**. All four tools weigh the same (30 N) and have the same torque output. The difference is their dimensions and mass distribution. Comparisons between the four tool dimensions are provided in **Table 37-3**.

Assuming one-hand operation, resultant hand force was predicted by using the model for the four different tools and plotted as a function of torque in **Figure 37-9**. Hand force was determined for both low–feed force (1 N) and high–feed force (100 N) conditions when the tools were operated against a vertical surface. When feed force was small, the resultant hand force was mostly affected by the torque reaction force, which increased as torque increased for all four tools. Because the greatest force component in this case was the torque reaction force, tools 3 and 4 resulted in the least resultant hand force because they had the longest handles (See **Table 37-3**). Tool 3, however, had a considerably greater resultant hand force when feed force was high because the hand was located farthest from the spindle for that tool. This effect was not observed for tool 4, which also had a long handle, because of its greater tool body length.

Tool types

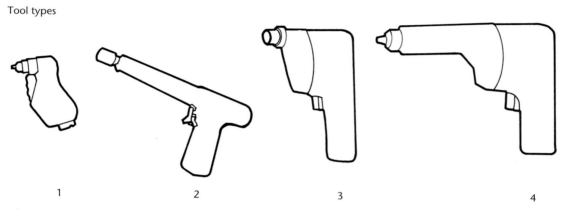

| 1 | 2 | 3 | 4 |

Figure 37-9 Comparison of resultant hand forces acting on the hand for four equivalent power screwdrivers plotted against reaction torque.

Table 37-3	Pistol-grip nutrunner dimensions, load, and center of gravity location			
Tool	**Weight (N)**	L_{H_z} (m)	L_{H_y} (m)	L_{G_z} (m)
1	30	0.09	0.06	0.07
2	30	0.40	0.09	0.26
3	30	0.11	0.50	0.07
4	30	0.40	0.50	0.32

Although tool 4 had the least resultant hand force when both feed force and torque levels were high, tools 1 and 2 had less resultant hand force for high feed force and low torque because these tools permitted the hands to grasp the tool close to the spindle axis. Consequently, the best tool depended on both feed force and the torque requirements for the task.

All tools were assumed to weigh the same. Of course, if these tools had different weights, the differences might have been even greater. Additional factors the model can consider include relative tool weight, mass distribution, and tool orientation. This analysis does not take into account the relative strength capabilities of the hand in the three component directions, although use of such a model does not exclude strength comparisons.

The reaction force transmitted to the hand for right-angle power drivers is also affected by the magnitude of spindle torque and the tool dimensions. Right-angle nutrunner spindle torque can range from less than 0.8 Nm to more than 700 Nm. A tool operator opposes these forces while supporting the tool and preventing it from losing control. This torque is transmitted to the operator as a reaction force and opposed by the great mechanical advantage provided by the long reaction arm created by the tool handle.[23]

Right-angle nutrunners are functionally nothing more than pistol-grip nutrunners with a very short body and a very long handle. The model for a right-angle nutrunner is shown in **Figure 37-10**. Because right-angle nutrunners are usually operated with two hands, two hand forces are now in the z-axis; $F_{H_{z1}}$ is applied at the handle for supporting the tool, and $F_{H_{z2}}$ is applied over the tool spindle to help provide feed force. When a right-angle nutrunner is operated on a horizontal surface, it is assumed that

$$F_{H_y} = W_{T_y} = W_{T_x} = 0 \tag{26}$$

The system of equations for a right-angle nutrunner is

$$F_{R_z} + F_{H_{z1}} + F_{H_{z2}} + W_{T_z} = 0 \tag{27}$$

$$F_{H_{z1}}L_{H_{z2}} + F_{H_{z2}}L_{H_{y2}} + W_{T_z}L_{G_y} = 0 \tag{28}$$

$$T_R - F_{H_x}L_{H_{y1}} = 0 \tag{29}$$

The solution for this system of equations results in the following hand force components:

$$F_{H_x} = \frac{T_R}{L_{H_{y1}}} \tag{30}$$

$$F_{H_y} = 0 \tag{31}$$

$$F_{H_{z1}} = \frac{L_{H_{y2}}(W_{T_z} + F_{R_z}) - L_{G_y}W_{T_z}}{L_{H_{y1}} - L_{H_{y2}}} \tag{32}$$

$$F_{H_{z2}} = \frac{-L_{H_{y1}}(W_{T_z} + F_{R_z}) + L_{G_y}W_{T_z}}{L_{H_{y1}} - L_{H_{y2}}} \tag{33}$$

These equations can be used for comparing hand forces between a right-angle and a pistol-grip power nutrunner used on a horizontal surface (see **Fig. 37-11**). The right-angle nutrunner in this example weighs 20 N, whereas the pistol-grip nutrunner weighs 50 N. A graph of torque reaction force plotted against torque shows that the mechanical advantage of the right-angle nut-

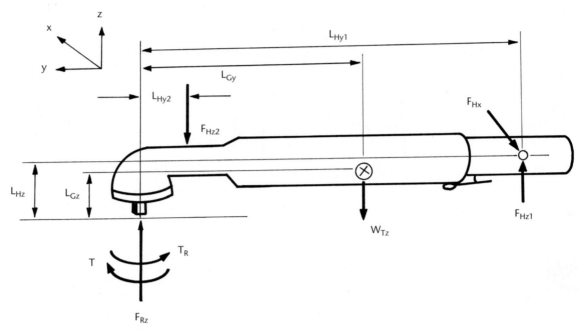

Figure 37-10 Static forces for right-angle nutrunner operation.

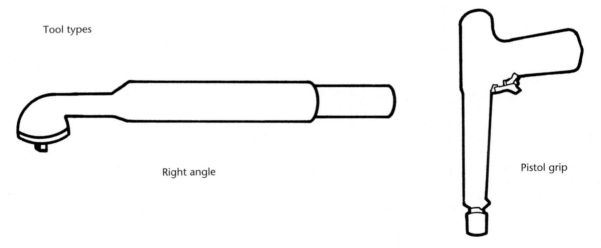

Figure 37-11 Comparison of hand forces between a right-angle nutrunner and a pistol-grip nutrunner operated on a horizontal surface.

runner for high torque levels is considerable. The other hand, however, exerts greater feed force for the right-angle nutrunner than for the pistol-grip nutrunner. Because the pistol-grip nutrunner weighs more and has its center of gravity closer to the tool spindle, it requires less support force for $F_{H_{z1}}$ and $F_{H_{z2}}$ than for the right-angle nutrunner (see **Fig. 37-11**).

ACCESSORY HANDLES AND TORQUE REACTION ARMS

Accessory handles can assist a pistol-grip power tool operator by providing an additional handle for two-handed operation. A torque reaction bar can sometimes be used to transfer loads back to the workpiece. Tools that can be equipped with a stationary reaction bar adapted to a specific operation so that reaction force can be absorbed by a convenient solid object can completely eliminate reaction torque from the operator's hand. These bars can be installed on in-line, pistol grip, and angled tools. The advantages of tool-mounted reaction devices are that (1) all reaction forces are removed from the operator; (2) one-hand–operated pistol-grip and in-line reaction bar tools can be used rather than right-angle nutrunners, which usually require two hands; (3) reaction bar tools can be less restricting on the operator's posture; (4) tool speed and weight are

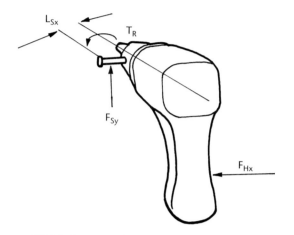

Figure 37-12 Force and moment arm for a pistol-grip nutrunner equipped with a torque reaction bar.

improved over right-angle nutrunners in most tool sizes; and (5) the use of reaction bars can improve tool performance.

The limitations are that reaction bars must be custom-made for each operation, and the combination of several attachments for one tool can be difficult. Torque reaction bars also add weight to the tool and can make the tool more cumbersome to handle. Providing tools with torque reaction bars or using torque-absorbing suspension systems can eliminate torque reaction effects completely, although these interventions are not always practical, especially when accessibility is limited, manipulation is restricted, or the reaction bars have no surfaces to contact. However, a shorter tool can be used if a reaction bar is provided.

When an accessory handle or torque reaction bar is used with a pistol-grip nutrunner, the horizontal hand force F_{H_x} is reduced. If a vertical force is applied to a torque reaction bar, as depicted in **Figure 37-12**, an additional term is needed for the sum of the moments in the z-axis:

$$T_R - F_{H_x}L_{H_y} + F_{S_y}L_{S_x} = 0 \tag{34}$$

As a result, F_{H_x} becomes

$$F_{H_x} = \frac{-F_{S_y}L_{S_x} + T_R}{L_{H_y}} \tag{35}$$

If a torque reaction bar is used and all the torque reaction force acts against a stationary object, then

$$T_R = -F_{S_y}L_{S_x} \tag{36}$$

Consequently,

$$F_{H_x} = 0 \tag{37}$$

TOOL COUNTERBALANCERS

The force requirements for a job are often related to the weight of the tools being handled. The effort needed

for holding an object in the hands is usually associated with its mass.[21,22] Consequently, heavier tools generally require greater exertion. There is a trade-off between selecting a lightweight tool and the benefit of the added weight for performing operations that require high feed force. A counterbalance can help reduce the load from heavy tools that are operated frequently.

When a counterbalance is used to support the tool, the counterbalance produces a force that opposes gravitational force. This is illustrated with a pistol-grip power tool in **Figure 37-13**. When the tool is freely held in the hand, there is no torque to react against ($T_R = 0$) and consequently no reaction force ($F_{H_x} = 0$). The counterbalance force F_{C_y} can create a moment in the yz-plane and also influences F_{H_y}. This moment is counteracted by a coupling moment C from the hand, as described in the following equations:

$$F_{H_y} + W_{T_y} + F_{C_y} = 0 \tag{38}$$

$$F_{H_y}L_{H_z} + W_{T_y}L_{G_z} + F_{C_y}L_{C_z} + C = 0 \tag{39}$$

If the counterbalance force F_{C_y} is set to counteract the tool weight W_{T_y}, then

$$F_{C_y} = -W_{T_y} \tag{40}$$

Consequently, the y-axis component of the hand force becomes $F_{H_y} = 0$. The location that the counterbalance force acts against the tool can also affect operator exertion when holding the tool. Solving for the coupling moment C,

$$C = F_{C_y}(L_{G_z} - L_{C_z}) \tag{41}$$

The equation shows that the coupling moment can be eliminated ($C = 0$), if

$$L_{G_z} = L_{C_z} \tag{42}$$

Therefore, balancers should be attached to tools at or near their centers of gravity. Tool balancers attached away from the center of gravity require additional effort by the tool operator to counteract the handle moment.

Spring counterbalances or air balancers are available for counteracting tool loads in the hands. Special attention may be required when balancers are installed so that minimal effort is needed when holding and using the tools in the desired work location. Spring counterbalances produce a force that opposes gravitational force so the tool weight is reduced. If these balancers are installed incorrectly, however, they can actually have the reverse effect of increasing force. Spring tension should be adjusted so that the operator does not have to counter more force than necessary. Balancers should be adjusted so that the tool aligns as close to the work area as possible to prevent unnecessary reaching. The counterbalance should not lift the tool when it is released so that the operator must elevate the shoulder to reach the tool. The tool should remain suspended at the same

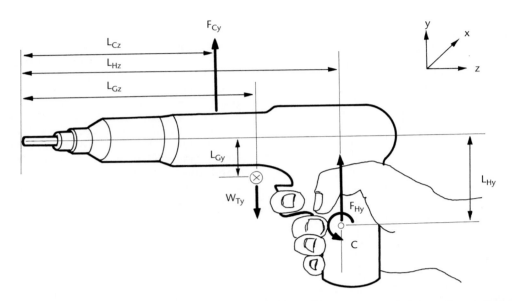

Figure 37-13 Static forces when handling a pistol-grip power hand tool with a counterbalance. Counterbalance force F_{C_y} creates a moment in the *yz*-plane that is counteracted by a coupling moment *C*.

height at which it was released. Also, situations where operators tend to work ahead or behind the assembly line should be avoided. A trolley and rail system should be installed if a tool is moved horizontally. Special attention may be required to be sure that the balancer is attached directly above the work.

CONCLUSIONS AND RECOMMENDATIONS

Tool operator exertion can be minimized by considering the forces acting on the tools and the way the tools are used for a specific task. The selection of alternative hand tools for different work situations can be assisted by comparing the mechanical relationships between the task and tool parameters. Other aspects that should be considered that are not covered in this chapter include repetitive use, postures assumed, vibration exposure, and contact stress.

The following recommendations can be made:

1. When large feed forces are necessary, use the longest manual screwdriver available and provide a screwdriver shaft long enough so that it can be gripped by the other hand as a guide. Nutdrivers and socket drivers also help reduce hand forces by providing concentric handle rotation and additional mechanical advantage at the screw head.
2. Large-diameter manual screwdriver handles with high frictional characteristics are recommended; however, if the handle diameter is too large, the

mechanical advantage may be counteracted by reduced grip strength.
3. Avoid using Phillips head screws because they require greater axial push force as torque increases. Torx head screws provide the least axial reaction force.
4. Pliers and shears can sometimes be used to a greater mechanical advantage by gripping them so that the pivot is on the ulnar rather than the radial side of the hand.
5. Torque reaction force is less for longer pistol-grip and right-angle nutrunners than for equivalent tools with shorter handles.
6. When pistol-grip power hand tools that have longer tool bodies are used, less vertical support force is required than for equivalent tools with shorter tool bodies, provided that their mass distribution is similar.
7. All other factors being equivalent, when feed force is large and torque is small, a pistol-grip power tool with a shorter handle should be used. When feed force is small and torque is large, a pistol grip power hand tool with a longer handle is more advantageous.
8. Torque reaction bars help eliminate torque reaction forces and accessory handles help distribute torque reaction forces among the two hands.
9. A tool counterbalance can help reduce the force needed to support a power hand tool. The optimal location for attaching a balancer is at the tool center of gravity.

References

1. Aghazadeh F, Mital A: Injuries due to hand tools, *Appl Ergonom* 18(4):273-278, 1987.

2. Amis AA: Variation of finger forces in maximal isometric grasp tests on a range of cylinder diameters. *J Biomed Eng* 9:313-320, 1987.

3. Ayoub MM, LoPresti PL: The determination of an optimum size cylindrical handle by the use of electromyography, *Ergonomics* 14(4):509-518, 1971.

4. Cannon LJ, Bernacki EJ, Walter SD: Personal and occupational factors associated with carpal tunnel syndrome, *J Occup Med* 23:255-258, 1981.

5. Cederqvist T, Lindberg M: Screwdrivers and their use from a Swedish construction industry perspective, *Appl Ergonom* 24(3):148-157, 1993.

6. Cochran DJ, Riley MW: *An evaluation of handle shapes and sizes.* Proceedings of the 26th Annual meeting of the Human Factors Society, Seattle, Wash., 1982; pp 408-412.

7. Cochran DJ, Riley MW: The effect of handle shape and size on exerted forces, *Hum Factors* 27:253-265, 1986.

8. Dahlman S, et al: Tools and hand function: requirements of the users and the use situation. In Quéinnec Y, Daniellou F, editors: *Designing for everyone*, London, 1991, Taylor & Francis.

9. Drury CG: Handles for manual materials handling, *Appl Ergonom* 11(1):35-42, 1980.

10. Fransson C, Winkel J: Hand strength: the influence of grip span and grip type, *Ergonomics* 24(7):881-892, 1991.

11. Grant KA, Habes DJ: Effectiveness of a handle flange for reducing manual effort during hand tool use, *Int J Ind Ergonom* 12:199-207, 1993.

12. Greenberg L, Chaffin DB: *Workers and their tools*, Midland, Mich, 1977: Pendell.

13. Hertzberg T: Some contributions of applied physical anthropology to human engineering, *Ann NY Acad Sci* 63(4):616-629, 1955.

14. Mital A: Effect of body posture and common hand tools on peak torque exertion capabilities, *Appl Ergonom* 17(2):87-96, 1986.

15. Mital A, Kilbom A: Design selection and use of hand tools to alleviate trauma of the upper extremities. Part I — Guidelines for the practitioner, *Int J Ind Ergonom* 10:1-5, 1992.

16. Myers JR, Trent RB: Hand tool injuries at work: a surveillance perspective, *J Saf Res* 19:165-176, 1988.

17. Oh S, Radwin RG: Pistol grip power tool handle and trigger size effects on grip exertions and operator preference, *Hum Factors* 35(3):551-569, 1993.

18. Petroski H: *The evolution of useful things,* New York, 1992, Alfred A Knopf.

19. Pheasant S: *Body space: anthropometry, ergonomics and design,* London, 1988, Taylor & Francis; pp 227-233.

20. Pheasant S, O'Neill D: Performance in gripping and turning—a study in hand/handle effectiveness, *Appl Ergonom* 6(4):205-208, 1975.

21. Radwin RG, Armstrong TJ: Assessment of hand vibration exposure on an assembly line,. *Am Ind Hyg Assoc* 46(4):211-219, 1985.

22. Radwin RG, Armstrong TJ, Chaffin DB: Power hand tool vibration effects on grip exertions. *Ergonomics* 30(5):833-855, 1987.

23. Radwin RG, VanBergeijk E, Armstrong TJ: Muscle response to pneumatic hand tool reaction forces, *Ergonomics* 32(6):655-673, 1989.

24. Radwin RG et al: External finger forces in submaximal static prehension, *Ergonomics* 35(3):275-288, 1992.

25. Replogle JO: Hand torque strength with cylindrical handles. Proceedings of the 27th annual meeting of the Human Factors Society, Norfolk, Va., 1983; pp 412-416.

26. Rothfleish S, Sherman D: Carpal tunnel syndrome: biomechanical aspects of occupational occurrence and implications regarding surgical management, *Orthop Rev* 7:107-109, 1978.

27. Silverstein BA, Fine LJ, Armstrong TJ: Occupational factors and carpal tunnel syndrome, *Am J Ind Med* 11:343-358, 1987.

28. Swedish National Institute of Occupational Health: *Forskning & Praktik*, vol 2, 1993, The Institute; pp 14-17 (English edition).

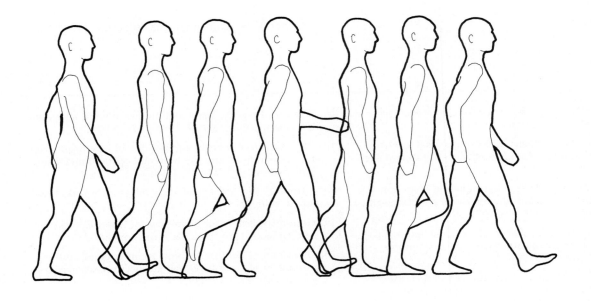

SECTION 4

Hip and Knee

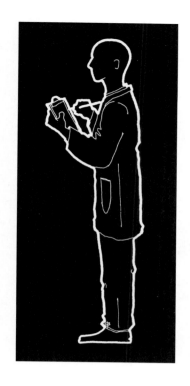

Chapter 38

Epidemiology of the Lower Extremity

Carl Zetterberg

CONTENTS

Musculoskeletal impairments increase linearly with age. In a study by Praemer, Furner, and Rice,[22] 2% of teenagers in the United States to 7% of 75-year-olds are disabled, and many more have pain. Daily joint pain during the previous 2 weeks was experienced by 19% of persons 25 to 74 years of age and 12% of persons 25 to 44 years of age. The sites of joint pain for persons 25 to 74 years of age were the knee in 46%, the shoulder in 35%, the fingers in 32%, the hip in 7%, and the ankle in 4%. Knee pain was equally common among males and females, whereas hip pain was more common among women. In the first National Health and Nutrition Examination Survey (NHANES I),[1] a prevalence of knee pain of 5% to 20% in persons 25 to 74 years of age was recorded.

In a population-based study of 55-year-olds (575 subjects), Bergenudd[4] showed that 11% had femoropatellar pain and 10% had knee joint pain. The prevalence was higher in women than in men. In a study correlating knee pain and low IQ measured 40 years earlier, low job satisfaction, obesity, and increased s-glutamyltransferase were found in men, whereas low education level, low income, low life success, and sleeping disturbances were found in women. For the entire group, knee pain and high occupational workload were also correlated. Similar results were found for hip pain. Occupational workload correlated with hip pain in men but not in women. Increased body weight correlated with knee pain in men and hip pain in women.

Therefore, as with back pain, the background for symptoms from the knee and hip is multifactorial. Age, sex, and social life are of importance along with occupational factors. When compared with the upper extremities, neck, and lower back, diseases and disorders of the lower extremities have less relation to work.[10] Worker's compensation claims for disorders of the lower extremities account for fewer than 10% of all the musculoskeletal claims in Sweden.

DEFINITIONS

From an etiological point of view, occupational musculoskeletal disorders can be classified as work related (worsened) or caused by the work. To use the etiological diagnoses cumulative trauma disorder (CTD) or occupational cervicobrachial disorder (OCD), for example, is not meaningful because the cause of any musculoskeletal disorder is multifactorial, and the same clinical entity can occur unrelated to the work. The clinical diagnosis is often either a symptom diagnosis or a pathophysiologic diagnosis.

An *occupational injury* is defined as any injury that results from a work-related accident or exposure involving a sudden event in the work environment.[22]

An *occupational illness* is any abnormal condition or disorder other than that resulting from occupational injury that is caused by exposure to factors associated with employment.[22]

OCCUPATIONAL INJURIES

In the United States, injuries to the musculoskeletal system have an annual incidence rate of 14%.[22] Injuries among men are most common between 18 and 44 years of age. Of all injuries that led to medical attention or at least half a day of restricted activity, 14% were industrial injuries. Thirteen percent of all fractures occur in industry, along with 16% of all sprains or strains.[22] Back pain accounts for 48% of all occupational injuries involving work loss. Among fractures, finger fractures account for 19%. **Table 38-1** shows the corresponding figures for the lower extremities.

Rupture of tendons and muscles is not often caused by occupational loading. The strength of tissues decreases with age, but ruptures are most often seen in sports activities and as a result of rather high-loading injuries.

OCCUPATIONAL ILLNESS

Joints are made for loading and movement. Nutrition of the cartilage is partly provided by compression from loading. The cartilage of the joints is well designed to withstand compression, translation, and shear forces. Deleterious types of loading are loads in extreme positions (nutcracker effect) and axial impact loads at high speed.[20] Low-frequency vibrational loading may be deleterious to the joints and the joint cartilage. High-frequency vibration may induce other problems, for example, the white-finger syndrome. Highly repetitive, monotonous work can cause a variety of problems in

Table 38-1	Occupational injuries of the lower extremities as a percentage of all injuries. US Data.			
Diagnosis	**Hip**	**Knee**	**Lower Leg**	**Multiple**
Fracture	0.3	2.6	2.0	1.2
Sprain and strain	0.3	7.9	0.3	0.8

From Praemer A, Furner S, Rice DP: Musculoskeletal conditions in the United States, Park Ridge, Ill., 1992, AAOS.

the joints, tendons, and peripheral nerves. These are not often seen in the lower extremities in relation to occupation, but rather are more common in sports activities.

Tendinitis

Tendinitis, tenosynovitis, myalgia, and other conditions of muscles and tendons are not as common in the lower extremities as in the upper.

Bursitis

Eighteen bursae surround the hip joint, and approximately 10 surround the knee joint. Specific diagnoses are often difficult to make. Bursitis caused by sports overuse is not uncommon, but bursitis around the hip as an occupational illness is more rarely seen. Bursitis of the knee, especially prepatellar or infrapatellar, is often seen in jobs that require kneeling, for example, floor layers, fishermen, and plumbers.[24-26] Bursitis most often leads to minor disability.

Nerve Entrapments

Only occasionally is nerve entrapment seen in the lower extremities. Ischial neuralgia, or "wallet-sciatica," a sensation along the ischial nerve caused by compression at the infrapiriform foramen, may be encountered by sitting. Peroneal nerve compression at the side of the knee may cause palsy. This may happen to tractor drivers during prolonged sitting in a twisted position and from accidents. Ilioinguinal neuralgia and lateral cutaneous nerve neuralgia are seen as occupational illnesses. The mechanism is often some sort of pressure on the anterior part of the iliac crest from belts or other equipment, especially if loaded with tools or other weights. Edema, tiredness, and dull pain in the legs are more common in those with static sitting or standing occupations than in those who work in a more varied posture.[33] Compartmental syndromes are rarely due to occupational loading of the lower extremities. This syndrome is more often seen as a result of sports activities and as a complication of fractures and other traumatic injuries.

Rheumatic Diseases

Arthritis and rheumatism account for 66% of the musculoskeletal conditions among women and 51% among men. Osteoporosis accounts for an additional 11% of musculoskeletal disease, predominantly in females.[22] Rheumatic diseases are not caused by occupational loading but may be worsened by it.

Osteoarthritis

The prevalence of osteoarthritis (OA) is greater in women than in men. Physical examination more often results in a diagnosis of OA, as compared with radiographic examination, when narrowing of the joint space is used as the criterion. If osteophytosis is included as a sign of OA, the prevalence is much higher. Around 12% of the U.S. population have OA in any joint.[6,10,15] **Table 38-2** shows the prevalence of OA diagnosed by radiographic examination in different age groups.[15,22] Diagnosis by examination revealed more OA than diagnosis by history. The explanation is that many individuals are symptom free.

In the NHANES I study,[1] the prevalence of OA of the knee was 2.3% to 18% in 45- to 74-year-olds, with a larger prevalence in the elderly and in women. Hip OA was found in 0.2% to 6.6% of 25-year-olds to 74-year-olds, more in the elderly but with less sex difference than OA in the knee. Osteoarthritis of the hip and knee has been studied in relation to occupational as well as other factors. *Secondary OA* is due to previous, known trauma (e.g., fracture, surgery) or disease (e.g., hip dysplasia, osteochondritis, Perthes' disease). *Primary OA* has been shown to have a multifactorial background. Bilateral hip and knee OA has been suggested to have an etiology different from that of unilateral OA.

HEREDITY

In a comparative population study in San Francisco, standardized rates of primary hip OA, expressed as numbers per 100,000 population per year, were 1.5 in Japanese, 1.5 in Chinese, 1.6 in Filipinos, 5.1 in Hispan-

| **Table 38-2** | Prevalence of osteoarthritis as diagnosed by history or examination by gender and age group. |

	Rate per 100 persons			
	Diagnosis by History		Diagnosis by Examination	
Age	Males	Females	Males	Females
Less than 20 years	—	—	—	—
20–39 years	0.2	0.4	—	0.2
40–59 years	3.4	8.4	4.0	8.9
Over 60 years	17.0	29.6	20.3	40.8
All ages	1.9	4.0	2.2	5.0
All ages over 20 years	4.5	7.3	4.2	9.0

ics, 8.3 in blacks, and 29.4 in Caucasians. The hereditary factor often results in a more generalized OA in different locations of the body.[18]

The percentage of hip OA, defined as lowered height of the joint cartilage, at 70 years of age in Sweden is about 2% in both sexes. Knee OA has a prevalence of 2% in men and 3% in women at 70 years of age in Sweden. However, a relation to occupational loading or sports is more clearly shown in men, whereas obesity correlates more with knee OA in women. Consequently, a hereditary factor increasing the risk for females to contract OA of the knee is likely.[18] Obesity correlates with symptomatic OA in the hip[27] and also in the knee, which is clearly shown in females, and has a relative risk (RR) of about 4.[8,18]

HIP OSTEOARTHRITIS

Sports Lindberg and Montgomery[17] found a 2.8% prevalence of hip OA in controls as compared with 5.6% in athletes and 14% in elite athletes (soccer players). Similar results have been shown by Klunder, Rud, and Hansen.[13] Among those undergoing a total hip procedure because of OA, Vingård et al[18,28,30,32] found an RR of 4.5 for athletes. Those athletes who also had a physically demanding job had an RR of 8.5. Different results have been shown in studies of long-distance runners.[7]

Occupation Vingård et al[28-34] found more symptoms caused by hip OA in men exposed to greater physically demanding jobs. Farmers, construction workers, firefighters, and food processing workers had significantly more OA than expected (RR, 2.4). For those exposed to both occupational loading and sports activities, the RR was 8.5, and for sports alone, the RR was 2.5. Disability pension for hip OA was more often received by those with high occupational load exposure than by those with low exposure (RR, 12.4).[30] The risk occupations were construction workers, metal workers, farmers, and forestry workers. An increased risk for hip OA has been shown in farmers, with RRs of 9.7 to 12 in several studies.* In female farmers, no difference from controls was found.[3]

*References 3, 5, 9, 12, 16, 23.

KNEE OSTEOARTHRITIS

Sports A Swedish study[18] found a knee OA prevalence of 7% in soccer players as compared with 1.6% in controls. The prevalence was higher in those with known meniscal tears or anterior cruciate ligament ruptures.

Occupation The Framingham study showed an odds ratio (OR) of 2.2 for OA of the knee in jobs requiring knee bending and at a least a medium level of physical activity.[8] The etiological fraction or attributable proportion of knee OA to occupational physical loading was 15%. Obesity accounted for 10%. Only a few females had physically demanding jobs in the study, and no gender association was found.[8] In the NHANES study, knee OA was increased among men and women with physically demanding jobs: an OR of 1.88 in women (not significant) and 3.13 in men in younger ages; in higher ages, ORs of 3.49 and 2.45, respectively. The occupational etiologic fraction was estimated to be 32%.[1]

Dock workers have been shown to have more knee OA than office workers.[21] Lindberg and Montgomery[17] found an increasing risk for knee OA in shipyard workers as compared with office workers and teachers. Vingård et al[18,28,29,30,32] found an increased risk for knee OA among farmers, construction workers, and firefighters. That study also showed an increased risk of knee OA symptoms in female janitors and letter carriers. Therefore, a moderately increased risk of symptomgiving knee OA has been shown in physically demanding occupations.[11,14,19] Overweight and some sports activities seem to increase the risk of symptom-giving knee OA more than any occupation.

A consensus discussion in 1992 in Malmö on the etiology of OA concluded that unfavorable weight bearing and repeated minor trauma may contribute to OA.[18] This is in agreement with the current etiologic hypotheses. Static load, repeated trauma over long periods, and an unnatural use of joints are likely to contribute to OA. Regarding occupation, farmers, professional ballet dancers,[2] and professional soccer players have a much higher frequency of OA than expected and are therefore considered to carry an increased risk for OA. Other physically demanding jobs have less of an increase in RR for OA, around 2 to 3, similar to the RR for obesity and lower than the increased risk in some elite athletes.[18]

References

1. Andersson JJ, Felson DT: Factors associated with osteoarthritis of the knee in the first National Health and Nutrition Examination Survey (NHANES I): evidence for an association with overweight, race, and physical demands of work, *Am J Epidemiol* 128(179):89, 1988.

2. Andersson S et al: Degenerative joint disease in ballet dancers, *Clin Orthop* (in press).

3. Axmacher B, Lindberg H: Coxarthrosis in farmers, *Clin Orthop* 287:82-86, 1993.

4. Bergenudd H: *Talent, occupation, and locomotor discomfort,* doctoral thesis, Malmö, Sweden, 1989, Lund University.

5. Croft P et al: Osteoarthritis of the hip: an occupational disease in farmers, *BMJ* 304:1269-1272, 1992.

6. Cunningham LS, Kelsey JL: Epidemiology of musculoskeletal impairments and associated disability, *Am J Public Health* 74:574-579, 1984.

7. Ernst E: Jogging—for a healthy heart and worn out hips? *J Intern Med* 228:295-297, 1990.

8. Felson D et al: Occupational physical demands, knee bending and knee osteoarthritis: results from the Framingham study, *J Rheumatol* 18:1587-1592, 1991.

9. Forsberg K, Nilsson B: Coxarthritis on the island of Gotland. Increased prevalence in a rural population, *Acta Orthop Scand* 63:1-3, 1992.

10. Hadler NM: *Occupational musculoskeletal disorders*, New York, 1993, Raven Press.

11. Hult L: The Monkfors investigation, *Acta Orthop Scand Suppl* 16, 1954; pp 1-76.

12. Jacobsson B, Dalén N, Tjörnstrand B: Coxarthrosis and labour, *Int Orthop* 11:311-313, 1987.

13. Klunder KB, Rud B, Hansen J: Osteoarthritis of the hip and knee joint in retired football players, *Acta Orthop Scand* 51:925-927, 1980.

14. Kohatsu N, Schurman D: Risk factors for the development of osteoarthritis of the knee, *Clin Orthop 261:242-246, 1990.*

15. Lawrence RC et al: Estimates of selected arthritic and musculoskeletal diseases in the U.S., *J Rheumatol* 16(4):427-441, 1989.

16. Lindberg H, Axmacher B: Coxarthrosis in farmers, *Acta Orthop Scand* 59:607, 1988.

17. Lindberg H, Montgomery F: Heavy labor and the occurrence of gonarthrosis, *Clin Orthop* 214:235-236, 1987.

18. Nilsson BE: The Tore Nilson Symposium on the etiology of degenerative joint disease, *Acta Orthop Scand Suppl* 64(suppl 253): 54-61, 1993.

19. Nicolaisen T: *Health among postmen*, 1983, General Directorate for Post and Telegraph, Copenhagen (in Danish).

20. Nordin M, Frankel VH: *Basic biomechanics of the musculoskeletal system*, ed 2, Philadelphia, 1989, Lea & Febiger.

21. Partridge REH, Dulthie JJR: Rheumatism in dockers and civil servants, *Ann Rheum Dis* 27:559-568, 1968.

22. Praemer A, Furner S, Rice DP: *Musculoskeletal conditions in the United States*. Park Ridge, Ill., 1992, AAOS.

23. Thelin A: Hip joint arthrosis: an occupational disorder among farmers, *Am J Ind Med* 18:339-343, 1990.

24. Törner M: *Musculoskeletal stress in fishery: causes, effects, and preventive measures*, doctoral thesis, University of Göteborg, Sweden, 1991.

25. Törner M et al: Musculoskeletal symptoms and signs and isometric strength among fishermen, *Ergonomics* 33:1155-1170, 1990.

26. Törner M et al: Workload and musculoskeletal problems: a comparison between welders and office clerks, *Ergonomics* 34:1179-1196, 1991.

27. Vingård E: Overweight predisposes to coxarthrosis. Body mass studied in 239 males with hip arthroplasty, *Acta Orthop Scand* 62:106-109, 1991.

28. Vingård E: *Work, sports, overweight and osteoarthrosis of the hip*, Arbete och Hälsa 25, doctoral thesis, 1991, Karolinska Institute.

29. Vingård E et al: Coxarthrosis and physical load from occupation, *Scand J Environ Health* 17:104-109, 1991.

30. Vingård E et al: Disability pensions due to musculoskeletal disorders among men in heavy occupations, *Scand J Soc Med* 20:31-36, 1992.

31. Vingård E et al: Ökad risk för arthros i knän och höfter för arbetare i yrken med hög belastning på benen, *Läkartidningen*:4413-4416.

32. Vingård E et al: Sports and osteoarthrosis of the hip, *Am J Sports Med* 21(2):195-200, 1993.

33. Winkel J: *On fast swelling during prolonged sedentary work and the significance of leg activity*, Arbete och Hälsa, doctoral thesis, Stockholm, 1985, National Institute of Occupational Health.

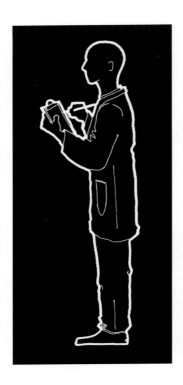

Chapter 39

Biomechanics of the Hip and the Knee

Debra E. Hurwitz
Thomas P. Andriacchi

CONTENTS

$\mathbf{I}$nformation on loading at the hip and knee joints during daily activities that occur in the home and work environment is helpful in determining the influence of work and the work environment on the lower extremity joints. Loads at joints have primarily been determined in two manners. In a few instances, forces at the hip have been measured directly in subjects by using implants with transducers. For example, during gait, average peak forces were measured in the range of 3 to 4 body weights (BWs),[4,8] whereas during ascending and descending stairs they ranged from 3 to 5 BWs.[5]

Loads at the hip and knee have also been calculated using analytical methods. Because the number of unknown muscle forces far exceeds the number of equilibrium equations, the problem is statically indeterminate. This means that a single unique solution of hip or knee loads cannot be directly solved. To solve this type of problem, several analytical approaches have been developed.

The reduction approach reformulates the statically indeterminate problem into a statically determinate one by combining muscles into functionally similar groups. This reduces the number of unknowns until the number of unknowns no longer exceeds the number of equations. The statically indeterminate problem is thus reformulated as a statically determinate one. With this approach, estimates of peak hip forces during gait have ranged from 4 to 7 BW[13] and peak knee forces from 2 to 4 BW.[12]

Another analytical method uses optimization methods to determine muscle forces. In this formulation the forces are distributed among the muscles acting across a joint in such a manner to optimize a "cost function" like muscle endurance, fatigue, or effort. With this approach, peak hip forces calculated during gait have ranged from 2 to 6 BW[6,15] and peak knee forces from 3 to 7 BW.[15] During stair climbing, forces at the hip were calculated to be as high as 7 BW.[7]

The relationship between the muscle and joint forces that occur during activities of daily living and the kinematics and kinetics of the hip and knee joints are the focus of this chapter. The relationship between the measured kinematics and kinetics of the lower extremity and the calculated external forces and moments at the hip and knee joints are first derived. Subsequently, the relationship between these external forces and moments and the muscle forces and resulting loads on the hip and knee is examined for a variety of activities. The activities discussed are gait, stair climbing, rising from a chair, and lifting weights.

KINEMATICS AND KINETICS OF THE LOWER EXTREMITY DURING FUNCTIONAL ACTIVITIES

Understanding the kinetics (forces and moments) of human movement is fundamental to understanding the musculoskeletal system inasmuch as the kinematics (motion) of the musculoskeletal system result from a balance between the external and internal forces. External forces represent the action of other bodies on the rigid body of interest. In the musculoskeletal system, external forces frequently include the ground reaction force, the weight of the limb segment, and the force of one segment on another. Internal forces are responsible for holding together the individual components of the rigid body of interest. In the musculoskeletal system, internal forces are primarily generated by muscle contractions, passive soft tissue stretch, and articular reaction forces.

The determination of forces and motion relies on Newton's second law of motion: if the resultant force acting on a body is not zero, the body will have an acceleration proportional to the magnitude of the resultant force and in the direction of this resultant force. For a three-dimensional analysis, Newton's second law results in six equilibrium equations (three force and three moment equations). A two-dimensional analysis has only three equilibrium equations. The governing equations for a two-dimensional example are

$$\Sigma \; F_v = ma_v$$
$$\Sigma \; F_h = ma_h$$
$$\Sigma \; M_o = I\alpha$$

where

$\Sigma \; F_v, \Sigma \; F_h$ = Sum of the forces in the vertical and horizontal directions
$\Sigma \; M_o$ = Sum of the moments about point **o**
I = Mass moment of inertia of the body
α = Angular acceleration of the body
a_v, a_h = Linear acceleration in the vertical and horizontal directions
m = Mass of the body

Newton's second law allows the forces and moments acting on the musculoskeletal system to be calculated from measurements of segmental motion and mass. The relative segmental angles at the hip and knee for many activities have been extensively characterized with either goniometers or optoelectronic systems.[2,3,11,14] Foot-ground reaction forces have frequently been measured with multicomponent force plates.

In the following example, the equilibrium equations just presented are used to determine the unknown forces (F^r_v, F^r_h) and moment (M_o) at the knee joint during gait from measurements of the limb segment displacement, body mass, and ground reaction force[1] (**Fig. 39-1**). The weight and inertial forces are obtained

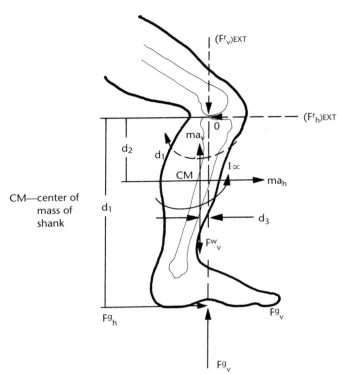

CM—center of mass of shank

Figure 39-1 External forces acting on the shank. *(From Andriacchi TP, Mikosz RP: Musculoskeletal dynamics, locomotion and clinical applications. In Mow VC, Hayes WC, editors: Basic orthopaedic biomechanics, New York, 1991, Raven Press; pp. 51-92.)*

by modeling the leg as a collection of segmental masses. The entire mass of each segment is modeled at the center of each segment. It is assumed that the ankle has negligible mass as compared with the shank.

$$(F^r_v)_{external} = -F^w_v + F^g_v + -ma_v$$
$$(F^r_h)_{external} = F^g_h + -ma_h$$
$$(M_o)_{external} = F^g_h \, (d_1) + F^w_v(d_3) - ma_v \, (d_3)$$
$$+ ma_h \, (d_2) - I\alpha$$

where

$$(F^r_v, F^r_h)_{external} = \text{Unknown external vertical and}$$
$$\text{horizontal forces at the knee}$$
$$(M_o)_{external} = \text{Unknown external moment at}$$
$$\text{the center of the knee joint}$$
$$F^w_v = \text{Weight of the segment}$$
$$F^g_v, F^g_h = \text{Vertical and horizontal ground}$$
$$\text{reaction forces}$$
$$d_1, d_2, d_3 = \text{Moment arms of the forces}$$

Typical values for the external forces acting on the lower limb for level walking at a normal speed (1 m/sec) at the instance just before toe-off during stance phase are given in **Table 39-1**. The relationship between these external reaction forces and the internal forces are covered in the next section.

RELATIONSHIP BETWEEN INTERNAL (MUSCLE FORCES) AND EXTERNAL FORCES

To maintain equilibrium, the external forces and moments must be balanced by a set of forces and moments equal in magnitude but opposite in direction that act internally. These internal moments are predominately generated from muscle forces. Therefore, large joint reaction forces result primarily from muscle contractions.

Because three-dimensional space analysis involves only six equilibrium equations, it is possible to solve for at most six unknown values. However, in general there are more than six internal or muscle forces. Therefore, in solving one of the analytical methods mentioned in the beginning of the chapter must be used or additional information about the muscle force relations must be obtained.

INTERNAL FORCES AT THE KNEE JOINT IN STATICALLY INDETERMINATE CASES

Muscle forces about the knee joint can be estimated by using the external forces and moments shown by the simplified free-body diagram of the knee joint (**Figure 39-2**). In this simplified case, the horizontal components of the forces are usually small in relation to the vertical ones and will not be considered. This reduces the number of equilibrium equations from three to only two. The unknowns are the vertical forces of the quadriceps and hamstring muscles (F^q_v, F^h_v) and the tibial femoral contact force (F^c_v). The external vertical reaction force and moment (F^r_v, M_o)$_{external}$ were solved for using the methods presented in the previous section. These two equations are as follows:

$$F^h_v + F^q_v - F^c_v + (F^r_v)_{external} = 0$$
$$(F^q_v - F^h_v)d + (M_o)_{external} = 0$$

where

$$F^h_v = \text{Vertical force in the hamstrings muscles}$$
$$F^q_v = \text{Vertical force in the quadriceps muscles}$$
$$F^c_v = \text{Vertical tibial-femoral contact force}$$
$$d = \text{Moment arm of quadriceps and}$$
$$\text{hamstrings force}$$

Even this simplified case has one more unknown than equations. An additional relationship is still needed to directly solve these equations. The additional relationship is obtained from experimental results of the external moment acting at the knee joint and an assumed relationship between the relative quadriceps and hamstring forces.

The external sagittal-plane moment acting at the knee joint for normal level walking at a speed of 1 m/sec is shown in **Figure 39-3**. Above the moment graph are the electromyographic (EMG)[17] activities of the gastroc-

Table 39-1	Numerical values for example 1: application of kinetics in gait analysis	
Description	**Symbol**	**Value**
KNOWNS		
Ground Reaction		
Vertical	F^g_v	700 N
Horizontal	F^g_h	150 N
Shank Weight		
Vertical	F^w_v	28 N
Inertial Forces		
Shank mass (m) × Vertical acceleration (a_v)	ma_v	3.3 N
Shank mass (m) × Horizontal acceleration (a_h)	ma_h	0.7 N
Inertia (I) × Angular acceleration (α)	$I\alpha$	0.06 Nm
Lever Arms		
Floor to knee center	d_1	0.4 m
Shank mass center to knee center	d_2	0.1 m
Horizontal distance, shank mass center to point 0	d_3	0.03 m
UNKNOWNS		
External Reaction		
Vertical	$(F^r_v)_{ext}$	668 N
Horizontal	$(F^r_h)_{ext}$	149 N
Moment	$(M_O)_{ext}$	61 Nm

From Andriacchi TP, Mikosz RP: Musculoskeletal dynamics, locomotion and clinical applications. In Mow VC, Hayes WC, editors: Basic orthopaedic biomechanics, *New York, 1991, Raven Press; pp. 51-92.*

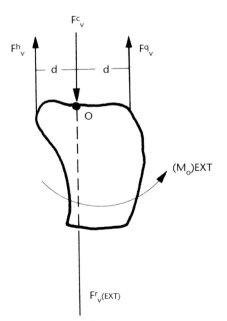

Figure 39-2 Free-body diagram of external and internal forces acting at the center of the knee on the tibial plateau, statically indeterminate. *(From Andriacchi TP, Mikosz RP: Musculoskeletal dynamics, locomotion and clinical applications. In Mow VC and Hayes WC, editors:* Basic orthopaedic biomechanics, *New York, 1991, Raven Press; pp 51-92.)*

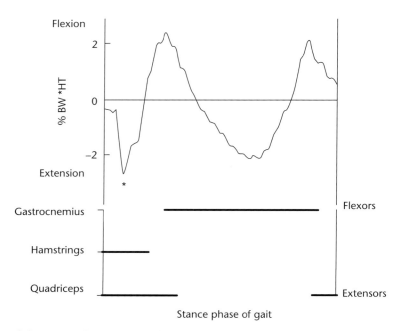

Figure 39-3 Illustration of the external moment at the knee joint during level walking along with the electromyographic activity of various muscle groups. *(From University of California:* Univ Cal Prosthet Dev Res Rep, *2(25): 1-41, 1953.)*

nemius, hamstring, and quadriceps muscles presented as either "on" (solid line) or "off." The external moment at the knee joint at the instant just after heel-strike is one that tends to extend the joint. The hamstring muscles, which are active at this point in the gait cycle, generate a moment that balances this external extension moment. At this point the quadriceps muscles are also active and provide antagonistic muscle activity. The external moment therefore represents the balance between the moment from the agonist muscles (hamstring muscles) and the antagonist muscles (quadriceps muscles). Because the net internal moment must balance the external extension moment, it will arbitrarily be assumed that the vertical force in the hamstring muscles (knee flexors) is twice that of the quadriceps muscles (knee extensors) ($F^h_v = 2F^q_v$).

Solving the moment equilibrium equation (**Table 39-2**) for the vertical force in the hamstrings, we determine that $F^h_v = 1667$ N. This yields a vertical contact force of 3200 N, or approximately 4.6 BW.

In this example the external moment acting at the joint was indicative of the net muscle activity. If the externally applied moment $(M_O)_{external}$ increases and the ratio of antagonist to agonist muscle force remains constant, the forces in both the quadriceps and hamstring muscles would have to increase proportionately. This would increase the contact force at the knee joint. In relative studies of muscle and joint forces, the moments are extremely useful. The external moment direc-

tions and the EMG data can be used to simplify a statically indeterminate problem into one that is statically determinate.

A PARAMETRIC APPROACH FOR DETERMINING HIP MUSCLE FORCES IN STATICALLY INDETERMINATE CASES

Expanding on this previous approach leads to a parametric determination of the muscle force distributions needed to balance the external moments and maintain equilibrium.[9] To apply this to the hip joint, the muscles crossing the hip joint are divided into agonists or antagonists based on either their sagittal-plane or frontal-plane moment. The agonist muscle force distributions are then evaluated at incremental levels of antagonistic muscle activity that range from 0%, no antagonistic activity, to 100%, where the antagonist muscle forces are at their maximum isometric force.

At each level of antagonistic muscle activity, the agonist muscles are further subdivided according to their moment in the other plane. The forces are determined such that the moment from the two groups of agonist muscles balances the external moment present along with the moment from the selected level of antagonistic activity. To maintain mechanical equilibrium, the moment from the agonist muscles must there-

Table 39-2	Numerical values for example 2: practical use of moments	
Description	**Symbol**	**Value**
KNOWNS		
External Reaction		
Vertical	$(F^r_v)_{ext}$	668 N
Moment	$(M_o)_{ext}$	25 Nm
Lever Arms		
Point 0 to vertical force in quadriceps muscle	d	0.03 m
Point 0 to vertical force in hamstring muscle	d	0.03 m
UNKNOWNS		
Hamstring Force		
vertical	F^h_v	1667 N
Quadriceps Force		
vertical	$F^q_v = \frac{1}{2}F^h_v$	833 N
Tibial-Femoral Contact Force		
vertical	F^c_v	3168 N

From Andriacchi TP, Mikosz RP: Musculoskeletal dynamics, locomotion and clinical applications. In Mow VC, Hayes WC, editors: Basic orthopaedic biomechanics, New York, 1991, Raven Press; pp 51-92.

fore be equal in magnitude but opposite in direction to the external moment and the moment from the antagonistic muscle forces. This results in two linear equations, one for sagittal-plane moment (given below) and one for frontal-plane moment.

$A *$ Total maximum flexion moment of agonist
muscle group A
+
$B *$ Total maximum flexion moment of agonist
muscle group B
=
$-1 *$ (External flexion moment during gait)
+
$-1 *$ (Total flexion moment of antagonist muscles)

The two unknowns, A and B, represent the activation levels or the required percentage of maximum isometric force of each agonist muscle in group A and group B needed to maintain mechanical equilibrium.

The range of agonist muscle force that maintains mechanical equilibrium is obtained by iteratively solving these equations with the following modification. The maximum isometric force or moment of each agonist muscle is incrementally decreased from 100%, indicating full activation, to 0%, indicating that the muscle is inactive. This is done in increments of 20% for each agonist muscle as well as for selected subgroups of agonist muscles. In this manner the range of agonist

muscle forces that satisfy the external moments is determined for each selected level of antagonistic muscle activity.

Figure 39-4 shows the external sagittal-plane and frontal-plane moments during gait for the hip joint along with the corresponding EMG data. When this parametric approach is used, the contact force during the initial hip peak adduction moment ranges from 2 to 4 BWs (**Fig. 39-5**). At this instance in the gait cycle the contact force is mainly influenced by the level of antagonistic muscle activity rather than by the distribution of agonistic muscle forces.

RELATIONSHIP BETWEEN NET JOINT REACTION MOMENTS AND MUSCLE ACTIVITY

The same relationship between the moments and the muscle forces seen during gait also applies to more stressful activities of daily living. **Figure 39-6** shows the relationship between EMG muscle activity at the hip and knee[3,10] and the corresponding external sagittal-plane moment patterns during stair climbing. During stair climbing, the net external moments at the hip and knee are primarily flexion moments. At the hip, the gluteus maximus and hamstring muscles provide the necessary extensor moment to balance the external

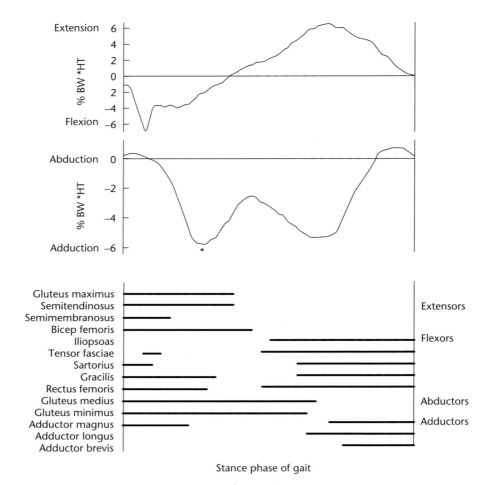

Figure 39-4 Illustration of the external moment at the hip joint during level walking along with the electromyographic activity of various muscle groups. *(From University of California:* Univ Cal Prosthet Dev Res Rep *2(25): 1-41, 1953.)*

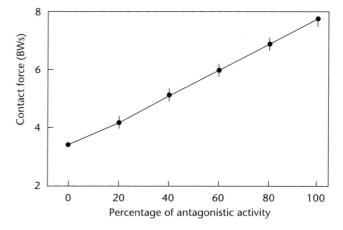

Figure 39-5 Parametric evaluation of the contact force at the hip for an instance during the gait cycle. The agonist muscles are the hip extensors. Agonist muscle group A consists of the gluteus medius and minimus, and agonist muscle group B consists of the gluteus maximus and the hamstring muscles. The antagonist muscles are the hip flexors and consist of the rectus femoris, tensor fasciae latae, and gracilis.

flexion moment and any moment resulting from the antagonistic muscle activity of the rectus femoris, tensor fasciae latae, and gracilis. At the knee, the quadriceps muscles provide the necessary extensor moment to balance the external knee flexion moment and any

moment resulting from the antagonistic muscle activity. The hamstring muscles that acted as agonists at the hip are providing antagonistic muscle activity at the knee joint.

As seen in this example, some muscles cross both

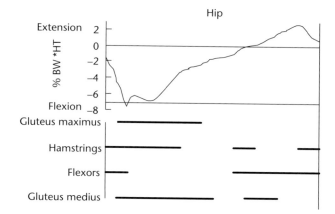

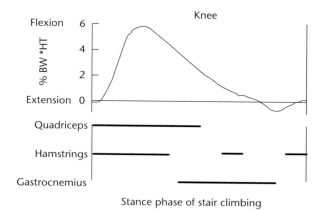

Stance phase of stair climbing

Figure 39-6 Illustration of the external sagittal-plane moments at the hip and knee joints during the stance phase of stair climbing along with the electromyographic activity of various muscle groups. *(From Andriacchi TP et al: J Bone Joint Surg Am 62:749-757, 1980; and University of California: Univ Cal Prosthet Dev Res Rep 2(25): 1-41, 1953.*

the hip and knee joint. These muscles frequently generate agonist muscle activity at one joint and antagonistic muscle activity at the other joint. For example, the rectus femoris, one of the quadriceps muscles active during stair climbing, acts as an agonist at the knee joint by balancing the knee extension moment. The rectus femoris is also a hip flexor and therefore provides antagonistic muscle activity with respect to the external hip flexion moment.

RELATIONSHIP BETWEEN JOINT LOADING AND THE INTENSITY OF THE TASK

The magnitude of the net external moment relates to the magnitudes of the muscle forces and internal joint reaction forces. As the intensity or physical demands of a task increase, the external moments and therefore muscle and joint forces increase.

This is clearly seen during gait. As walking speed increases, the flexion-extension moments increase (**Fig. 39-7**). Because the internal forces are related to the joint moments, the internal forces acting on the joints also increase with walking speed. A similar effect can be seen when rising from a chair. As the chair-rising task becomes more difficult by lowering the chair height, the knee flexion moment increases (**Fig. 39-8**). This reflects the increased demand on the quadriceps muscles needed to rise from chairs with lower heights.

In a similar manner, the loads at both the hip and L5/S1 increase substantially as a lifting task becomes more difficult.[16] Increases in both the speed of lifting and the weight of the object being lifted result in increased peak hip moments. At a normal lifting speed, the hip moment increases from 12% to 15% BW*HT as the load lifted increases from 50 to 150 N.

The relative magnitudes of the moments during various activities serve as indicators of the relative forces acting on the joint. Comparing the relative peak moments of different activities helps identify those activities that place the greatest demands on the muscles and joints. The largest moment magnitudes during most activities of daily living are in directions tending to flex the joints, which places demands on the extensor muscles. A comparison of the maximum flexion moments during walking, ascending stairs, descending stairs, rising from a seated position, and lifting a weight indicates a substantial variation in the peak values at the joint (**Fig. 39-9**). Lifting weights places relatively large demands on the hip extensor muscles whereas descending stairs places relatively large demands on the quadriceps muscles. Although the range of motion and the moment magnitudes may vary between tasks, the moment–muscle activity relationships remain consistent.

ANTAGONIST-AGONIST MUSCLE FORCES

The external moment patterns reflect the net activity of the muscle groups. As antagonistic muscle activity increases, the forces in the agonist muscles must also increase to counteract the contribution of the antagonistic muscle activity to the internal moment. This increases the load at the joint. Therefore, if no antagonistic muscle activity is present, the moment magnitude and direction reflect a lower bound for muscle and joint forces. Increasing antagonistic activity increases both muscle and joint forces.

During normal walking, the net sagittal-plane moment at the knee just after heel-strike tends to extend the knee (**Fig. 39-3**). Measurements of EMG activity consistently show both agonist flexor and antagonistic extensor muscle activity. If the muscles were acting solely to balance the external extension moment, only the flexors would be needed. The antagonistic muscle activity appears to be contraindicated with many of the

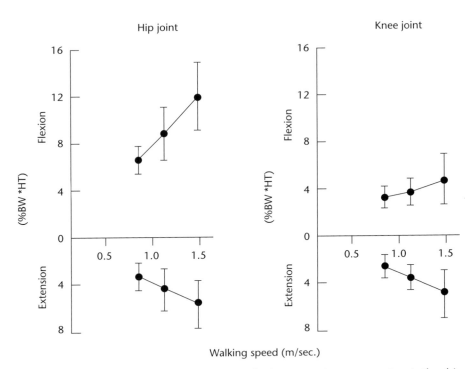

Figure 39-7 Illustration of walking speed dependence on flexion-extension moments at the hip and knee. *(From Andriacchi TP, Strickland AB: Lower limb kinetics applied to the study of normal and abnormal walking. In Berme N, Engin AE, Correia Da Silva KM editors:* Biomechanics of normal and pathological human articulating joints, *NATO ASI Series E, No 93, Dordrecht, The Netherlands, 1985, Martinus Nijhoff; pp. 83-102.)*

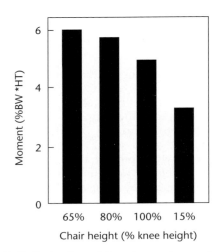

Figure 39-8 Illustration of the change in maximum flexion moment with chair height at the knee. At the knee joint a greater than 50% reduction in flexion moment resulted from the difference between the lowest and highest chair height. *(From Rodosky MW, Andriacchi TP, Andersson GBJ:* J Orthop Res *7:266-271, 1989.)*

optimal theories related to the energy efficiency of normal gait.

As mentioned earlier, antagonistic muscle activity frequently results from muscles that span two joints. Muscle activity during stair climbing involves muscles that cross both the hip and knee joints and often results in antagonistic activity at one of the two joints. This is also seen when rising from a chair, where the hamstring muscles act as agonists with respect to the hip flexion moment but as antagonist muscles with respect to the knee flexion moment.

Muscles also have multiple roles by generating moments in more than one plane. A muscle may act as an agonist in one plane and as an antagonist in another plane. This frequently occurs during gait at the hip joint. The gluteus medius acts as both an abductor and extensor. During the second half of stance, the external hip moments are ones of extension and adduction. The gluteus medius therefore provides not only agonistic activity with respect to the frontal-plane moment but also antagonistic activity with respect to the sagittal-plane moment.

When the total mechanics of the joint and its complex three-dimensional loading are considered, it becomes apparent that antagonistic muscle action can also provide increased stability for other types of load-

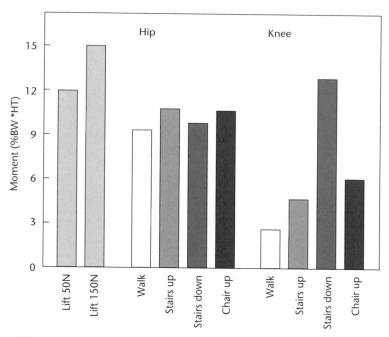

Figure 39-9 Comparison of the magnitude of flexion moments during various activities of daily living. *(From Andriacchi TP, Mikosz RP: Musculoskeletal dynamics, locomotion and clinical applications. In Mow VC, Hayes WC, editors:* Basic orthopaedic biomechanics, *New York, 1991, Raven Press; pp 51-92; and Tsuang YH et al:* Ergonomics *(4): 437-444, 1992.)*

ing. This increased need for stability is apparent at the knee joint where in addition to flexion-extension moments, other large moments tend to adduct the knee during activities of daily living. The cocontraction of agonist-antagonist muscle groups may stabilize the joint to large out-of-plane loading like the adduction moment that normally occurs during gait.

SUMMARY

Relevance of Joint Mechanics to the Analysis of Activities of Daily Living

The fundamental theory presented in this chapter provides a basis for the analysis and interpretation of joint forces and muscle loading during various activities of daily living. Clearly, the muscular demand is related to both the direction and magnitude of the external moments that tend to flex and extend the joints during various activities. As moment magnitudes increase, the net demand for flexor or extensor muscle forces increases. Therefore, the effect of parameters such as walking speed on hip and knee joint loads and muscular effort can be analyzed. For example, the magnitude of the flexion moment at the hip tends to increase substantially with increased walking speed (**Fig. 39-7**). This suggests that the demand on hip extensor muscles to balance this external flexion moment will increase substantially with increased walking speed. Similarly, the influence of chair height on knee extensor muscle demand can be evaluated by looking at the relative change in knee joint moments with changes in chair height (**Fig. 39-8**). A substantial reduction in extensor muscle demand at the knee can be achieved by increasing chair height from 80% to 100% of knee height.

Moments at the joints can be used to study muscle function, forces on the joints, and stresses in the soft tissues surrounding the joints. A knowledge and understanding of the factors influencing joint moments and loads can be extremely valuable for assessing the effects of activities that routinely occur in the home and work environment on the loads at the hip and knee joints. Activities that may potentially overload healthy and injured joints can be analyzed with this information.

References

1. Andriacchi TP, Mikosz RP: Musculoskeletal dynamics, locomotion and clinical applications. In Mow VC, Hayes EC, editors: *Basic orthopaedic biomechanics,* New York, 1991, Raven Press; pp 51-92.

2. Andriacchi TP, Strickland AB: Lower limb kinetics applied to the study of normal and abnormal walking. In Berme N, et al, editors: *Biomechanics of normal and pathological human articulating joints,* NATO ASI Series E, No 93, Dordrecht, The Netherlands, 1985, Martinus Nijhoff; pp. 83-102.

3. Andriacchi TP et al: A study of lower-limb mechanics during stair-climbing, *J Bone Joint Surg* 62A(5): 749-57, 1980.

4. Bergmann G, Graichen F, Rohlmann A: Hip joint loading during walking and running measured in two patients, *J Biomech* 26(8): 969-990, 1993.

5. Bergmann G, Graichen F, Rohlmann A: Load directions at hip prostheses measured in vivo. Abstracts International Society of Biomechanics XII Congress 1989, *J Biomech* 22(8/9): 986, 1989.

6. Brand RA et al: Comparison of hip force calculations and measurements in the same patient, *J Arthro* 9(1): 45-51, 1994.

7. Crowninshield RD, Brand RA: A physiologically based criterion of muscle force prediction in locomotion, *J Biomech* 14(11): 793-801, 1981.

8. Davy DT et al: Telemetric force measurements across the hip after total hip arthroplasty, *J Bone Joint Surg* 70A(1): 45-50, 1988.

9. Hurwitz D: *Biomechanics of the hip as related to total hip replacements*, PhD dissertation, 1994, University of Illinois at Chicago.

10. Joseph J, Watson R: Telemetering electromyography of muscles used in walking up and down stairs, *J Bone Joint Surg* 49B(4): 774-780, 1967.

11. Lamourex L: Kinematic measurements in the study of human walking, *Bull Prosthet Res* Spring: 3-84, 1971.

12. Morrison JB: The mechanics of the knee joint in relation to normal walking, *J Biomech* 3:51-61, 1970.

13. Paul JP: Loading on normal hip and knee joints and on joint replacements. In Schaldach M et al, editors: *Engineering and medicine 2: advances in artificial hip and knee joint technology*, New York, 1976, Springer-Verlag; pp. 53-70.

14. Rodosky MW, Andriacchi TP, Andersson GBJ: The influence of chair height on lower limb mechanics during rising, *J Orthop Res* 7:266-271, 1989.

15. Seireg A, Arvikar RJ: The prediction of muscular load sharing and joint forces in the lower extremities during walking, *J Biomech* 8:89-102, 1975.

16. Tsuang YH et al: Influence of body segment dynamics on loads at the lumbar spine during lifting, *Ergonomics* 35(4): 437-444, 1992.

17. University of California: The pattern of muscular activity in the lower extremity during walking, *Univ Cal Prosthet Dev Res Rep* 2(25): 1-41, 1953.

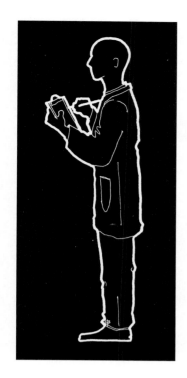

Chapter 40

Clinical Evaluation of the Hip and Knee

Gunnar B. J. Andersson

CONTENTS

Acareful clinical evaluation of the hip and knee is important to determine the presence of disease or injury, that is, for the purposes of establishing the nature of a complaint. Only by means of an accurate diagnosis is it possible to select appropriate treatment. This is true in occupationally injured patients as well as any other patients. Because of the importance of the clinical evaluation, textbooks are available that deal with this topic in great detail.[2,4] It is beyond the scope of this chapter to provide a complete description of how to obtain the history and perform a physical examination of patients with hip and knee problems, nor is it the purpose to completely describe all other techniques used for diagnostic purposes in patients with hip and knee complaints. Rather, the focus is on providing the clinician with the basic skills needed to make an accurate diagnosis in most patients with occupationally related complaints about the hip and knee.

HISTORY AND PHYSICAL EXAMINATION

The patient history and the physical examination are the mainstays of clinical medicine. Although modern technology and advanced imaging methods have added tremendously to our diagnostic ability, it is still the history and physical examination that provide the basis on which technology can build. Indeed, it is extremely inefficient and costly to simply apply a variety of technical tests without appropriate guidance from a thorough history and physical examination.

Obtaining a patient history is slightly different in a patient with an occupationally related disorder than it is in a patient with a general complaint, not only because occupational factors may provide additional information useful to obtain a correct diagnosis but also because any relationship between the patient's complaint and the job must be more carefully documented for legal, medical, and rehabilitation purposes. In general, a structured history and physical examination should follow the guidelines provided in the box opposite. The order in which the history is obtained may vary, but the table outlines an order that is useful. Clearly, if the patient's complaints are few and specific, a more thorough review of previous illnesses is not as necessary. In general, previous illnesses are of less importance in an occupational orthopaedic practice than they may be in an orthopaedic practice of a different nature because often but not always the complaint can

---

Example of structured history
Main current symptoms (present illness) Description of symptoms When did they start? How did they start? What do you think caused the symptoms? Previous evaluation and treatment Relationship between symptoms and activities Previous history (joint specific) Organ systems review Occupational history Personal and social history

---

be attributed to a triggering event (accident). For the purposes of determining whether this event caused an initial injury or is an aggravation of a preexisting condition, information about previous illnesses and injuries must be obtained, however.

The history should start with questions regarding the main current complaints and present illness, and they should be documented in chronological order. It is important to determine what the patient's principal complaints are, when the symptoms started, how they started, what the patient believes caused the symptoms, what evaluation and treatment has occurred, and how the symptoms have responded to any previous treatment. The physician also needs to know whether the symptoms are increased by specific activities and decreased by others. Typically, this would cover basic functional activities such as sitting, standing, walking, bending, twisting, lifting, and sleeping. The biomechanical influences of different activities on the hips and knees are described in Chapter 39. It becomes apparent that hip and knee problems greatly influence the ability to walk, climb stairs, get in and out of a chair, use public transportation, and so on.

The next part of the history deals with whether the patient has had previous problems from the hip or knee. This is obviously important and should include information about problems dating as far back as childhood because many injuries and diseases in childhood may affect the hip and knee in adult life. For the same reason, previous or present major diseases involving other organ systems must be ascertained. As outlined elsewhere in this book, it is also necessary to obtain a good personal and social history, including an occupational history, and information about recreational habits, smoking, alcohol use, and family life.

PHYSICAL EXAMINATION OF THE HIP

The physical examination of a patient with a hip problem begins by observing the patient's gait. For the purpose of the examination, the patient needs to be sufficiently undressed so that movements of the hip and

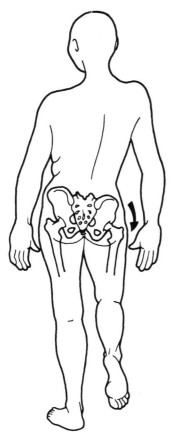

Figure 40-1 Trendelenburg test. The unaffected hip drops when standing on the affected leg.

knees can be observed appropriately, in other words, so that the lower extremities are exposed. Gait observation will allow detection of limp, deformity, and leg-length discrepancy. It is important to understand a few basic elements of gait to make useful observations. It is also important to be able to identify certain specific pathologic gait patterns.

An antalgic gait is commonly seen in painful conditions of the hip. It results from the patient's attempt to reduce pain in the hip caused by weight bearing during stance phase. By shortening the stance phase as much as possible, the hip is loaded for a short period of time only. A different type of gait is the gluteus medius or abductor gait. This gait is the result of a weakness of the hip abductors that causes the affected hip to list downward when the leg is in swing phase. The patient will compensate by shifting the trunk in the opposite direction in an attempt to maintain the center of gravity closer to the stance leg.

A Trendelenburg test involves asking the patient to stand on one leg and then observing the pelvis (**Fig. 40-1**). Normally, when the patient stands on the right leg, the right gluteus medius will contract and elevate the pelvis on the left side. In the case of weakness or paralysis of that muscle, the pelvis on the left side, in

this example, will sink, and the patient will shift the trunk to the right. The Trendelenburg sign is not specific to a disease entity of the hip but occurs in a number of different hip conditions such as fractures, hip deformities, neurologic diseases, and arthritic conditions. The test is typically recorded as positive (abnormal) or negative.

Further observation of the patient's hip should include the skin surface to note abrasions, discolorations, swelling, and any deformity. Observation is followed by palpation. This should first be done in the standing position, where the presence or absence of pelvic obliquities is determined by identification of the anterior superior iliac spines and the iliac crests and the greater trochanteric area is palpated. Normally, the trochanter should be at the same level on both legs and should not be tender. Tenderness sometimes occurs with bursitis and other hip conditions. Not only is it important to palpate the bony structures, but the soft tissue structures should be palpated as well. This includes the femoral triangle area anteriorly, the sciatic notch posteriorly, and the individual muscles. Tenderness may result from tendinitis, bursitis, or sprain and strain injuries.

Range of motion is normally measured with the patient supine on the examination table. A complete examination includes flexion, extension, rotation, and abduction, and adduction. To determine the presence or absence of a flexion contracture, it is useful to know the Thomas test, in which one hip is flexed to eliminate the lumbar lordosis and then the residual flexion, if any, of the opposite hip is observed (**Fig. 40-2**). Normal range of hip flexion is about 120 to 135 degrees (**Fig. 40-3**). Extension is easiest to measure with the patient prone and should normally be about 30 degrees (**Fig. 40-4**). Abduction, adduction, and rotation are usually measured with the patient supine (**Fig. 40-5**). It is important to place one hand on the iliac crest when performing abduction and adduction tests so that any associated pelvic movement can be detected. Typically, abduction should be about 45 to 50 degrees and adduction about 20 to 30 degrees. Rotation can be measured with the hip in extension or 90 degrees of flexion (**Fig. 40-6**). Internal rotation is normally 30 to 35 degrees and external rotation about 45 degrees.

In cases of hip disease it is also sometimes important to ascertain whether muscle strength is impaired. A full examination of strength should include testing of the flexors, extensors, abductors, and adductors. Hip flexion strength can be tested by having the patient in the sitting posture and flexing the hip against manual resistance. Hip extensors are more easily tested in the prone position and asking the patient to extend the hip against the examiner's hand. Hip adductors are partly tested through the Trendelenburg test, but they can be additionally tested by abduction against manual receivers with the patient in a lateral position on the examination table. To test the adductors, the patient is first asked to abduct the legs and then adduct against resis-

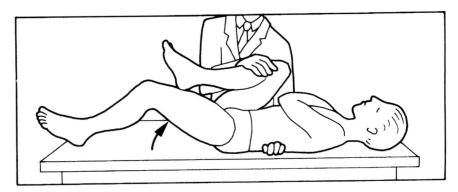

Figure 40-2 Thomas test. The test is used to detect flexion contractures of the hip and evaluate the range of hip flexion.

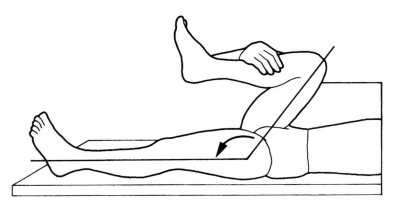

Figure 40-3 Hip flexion, normally 120 to 135 degrees.

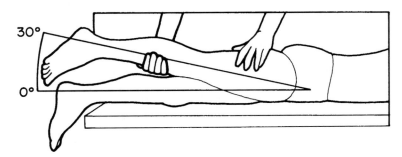

Figure 40-4 Hip extension, normally 30 degrees.

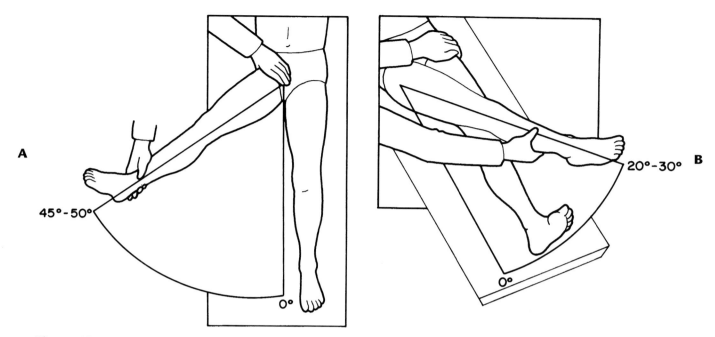

Figure 40-5 A, Abduction and **B,** Adduction. Abduction is normally 45 to 50 degrees, and adduction is normally 20 to 30 degrees.

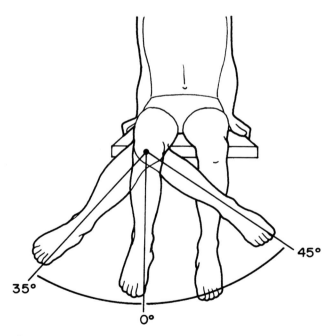

Figure 40-6 Rotation tested in the flexed position, normally 30 to 35 degrees internal and 40 to 45 degrees external.

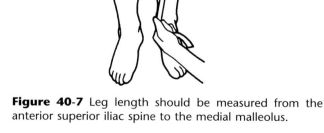

Figure 40-7 Leg length should be measured from the anterior superior iliac spine to the medial malleolus.

tance. Sensory changes are rarely critical parts of a hip examination, nor are they reflex changes.

A complete examination of a hip should also include length measurements. Actual leg length is measured with a tape measure as the distance between the anterior superior iliac spine and the medial malleolus (**Fig. 40-7**). Apparent leg length inequality may result from pelvic obliquity, in which case the distance between the umbilicus and medial malleolus will be different from one leg to the other.

PHYSICAL EXAMINATION OF THE KNEE

In general, physical examination of the knee follows the same pattern as physical examination of the hip. When the patient's gait is examined, special attention should be placed on the presence or absence of deformities such as varus or valgus deformity and whether those deformities increase with weight bearing (**Fig. 40-8**). Normally, there is about 7 degrees of valgus of the knee during weight bearing. Often it is also possible to detect atrophy by inspection. Because hip diseases sometimes result in pain about the knee, it is important to study the gait pattern as discussed previously. A positive Trendelenburg sign, for example, may be important in arriving at a differential diagnosis. Patients with severe arthritic changes of the knees are sometimes observed as having sudden gait instability, where there is an apparent thrust laterally or medially of the knee upon weight bearing.

Inspection of the area of the knee follows next to determine any skin changes and any deformity, swelling, or obvious atrophy. Swelling is not infrequently part of a knee injury, and its size, shape, and location should be noted. Localized swelling over the patella may be caused by bursitis or an infection of the prepatellar bursa. More general swelling about the knee may be due to an interior knee disarrangement. Localized swelling in the popliteal fossa may be a Baker's cyst.

Palpation about the knee requires some basic understanding of the underlying potential conditions described in a subsequent chapter. Tenderness at the inferior pole of the patella may occur from tendon insertion disorders, and tenderness over the tibial tubercle with or without swelling may indicate the presence of Osgood-

Schlatter disease. In evaluating patella problems, the patella needs to be moved from side to side while noting how much it moves, how easily it moves, whether movement is painful, and whether crepitations are present. This is necessary to determine the possible presence of such problems as recurrent patella dislocation, chondromalacia patellae, and general osteoarthritis of the knee. Normally the patella is fixed in flexion and mobile in extension. Movement should be pain free and without crepitus. When the patient's patella is observed, it is useful to measure the so-called Q angle. The Q angle is the angle formed by a line drawn along the axis of the quadriceps tendon to the anterior superior iliac spine and a second line drawn from the tibial tubercle across the patella. A normal Q angle should be 15 to 20 degrees as measured with the patient supine and the knee extended. Patella dislocations may result in a reduced Q angle. Palpation of the anterior aspect of the patella is done to determine tenderness or swelling resulting from chronic irritation, trauma, or infection in the prepatellar bursa. Palpation of the joint will allow detection of joint effusion that may be visually undetected if the effusion is small. The knee joint should also be palpated for tenderness and swelling along the joint margins. This is easier to do if the knee is flexed to 90 degrees. Tender sites should be noted and may indicate meniscus tears. Other causes of joint line tenderness include patella problems and inflammatory or bursa conditions. Palpation along the attachment sites of the collateral ligaments is important because this may allow a diagnosis of acute sprains that typically result in well-localized tenderness. This palpation should include the fibular head where the lateral collateral ligament inserts and where evulsion injuries can occur.

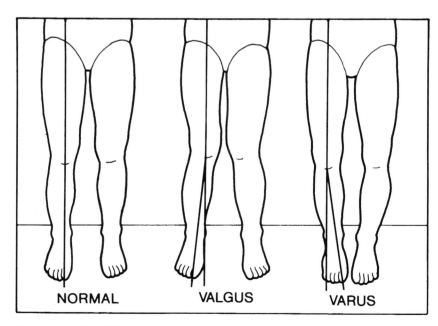

Figure 40-8 Varus/valgus deformity of the knee.

Range-of-motion measurements of the knee include flexion and extension. Normal values are full extension and 135 to 150 degrees of flexion (**Fig. 40-9**). Active knee extension is best tested with the patient sitting, whereas passive knee extension can be tested in both the sitting and lying positions. Inability or difficulty in actively extending the knee may be indicative of an extensor injury to either the quadriceps tendon or the patella itself or simply quadriceps weakness. It is referred to as an extension lag (**Fig. 40-10**). Flexion deficits may be due to a variety of knee conditions and will occur with any swelling of the knee. An inability to move the knee into full extension is called a locked knee. This can be caused by, for example, a meniscus tear. Extension beyond the straight line into a position of recurvatum is normal up to 20 degrees if similar for both knees. If this occurs on one side only, however, it may indicate a cruciate ligament injury.

A variety of special tests have been developed to determine the presence of a meniscus tear. Such tears are important not only in an acute injury situation but also as part of a degenerative process of the knee. Not

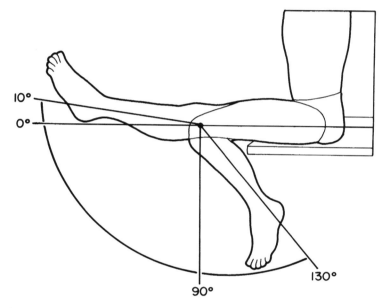

Figure 40-9 Flexion-extension of the knee—normal extension, 10 degrees; flexion, 135 to 150 degrees.

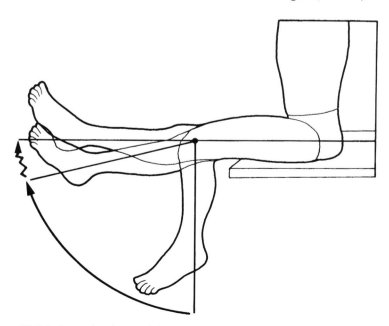

Figure 40-10 Extension lag is defined as an inability to actively extend the knee.

infrequently the patient has a history of joint pain with rotation. Periodic swelling and relief of pain with rest are also often noted. As discussed previously, it is always possible that a locked knee is a meniscus tear, but a truly locked knee is uncommon. Among the special clinical tests used to detect meniscus injuries, some are more popular than others. The McMurray test is a rotational test in which the knee is first rotated in full flexion, either internally or externally, and then the knee is extended (**Fig. 40-11**). Usually this is done with the patient lying supine and the examiner palpating the joint margin with one hand while keeping the patient's foot rotated with the other. Snaps or clicks should be noted as well as pain. The Steinmann test is a test in which the patient is sitting with the knees in 90 degrees of flexion and then the tibia is vigorously rotated, externally or internally. Although this is a fairly sensi-

tive test for a meniscus tear, it is unfortunately nonspecific.

The Apley test is done with the patient prone and is an extension of the McMurray test. In the Apley test the knee is flexed to 90 degrees and the foot internally or externally rotated (**Fig. 40-12**). This rotation is done while compressing the knee joint either manually or with distraction by pulling at the foot while keeping the patient's thigh on the couch by pressure from the examiner's knee. If compression produces increased pain, the test is considered positive. Unfortunately, again, this test, although sensitive, is not entirely specific, even though it is probably a better test than the two previously mentioned.

The stability of the ligaments is important to establish. Lateral stability is typically tested by applying a lateral or medial moment to the knee joint (**Fig. 40-13**).

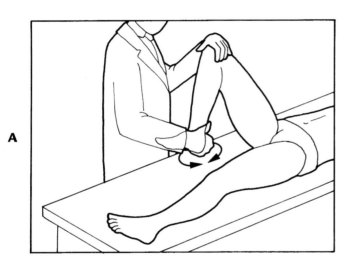
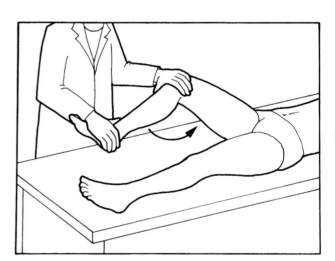

Figure 40-11 McMurray test. The knee is first rotated in full extension **A** and then extended **B**.

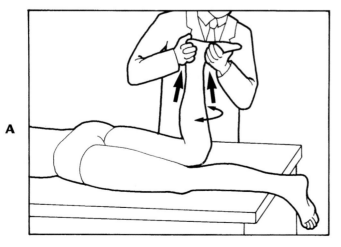
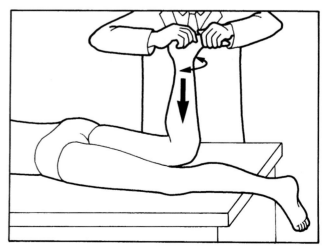

Figure 40-12 Apley test. With the patient prone, the knee is flexed and the foot internally and externally rotated **A** with distraction and **B** with compression.

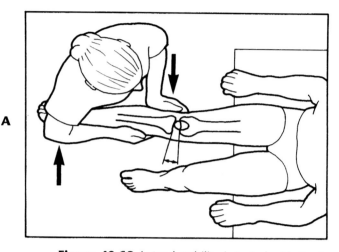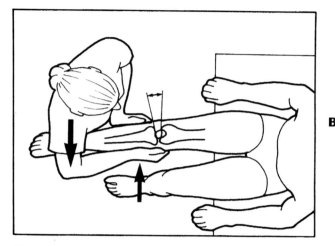

Figure 40-13 Lateral stability is tested with the knee in 15 to 20 degrees of flexion (**A,** medial; **B,** lateral).

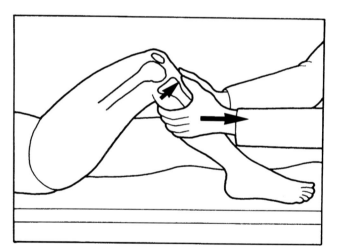

Figure 40-14 Anterior drawer test to detect cruciate ligament injury.

This is ideally done with the knee in 15 to 20 degrees of flexion to prevent false-negative results from occurring in extension because of the geometry of the joint itself, which is more static in extension. Injuries to the anterior and posterior cruciate ligaments are measured through a variety of tests. Tests of the anterior cruciate ligament (ACL) include the anterior drawer sign, the Lachman test, and the pivot/shift test. The anterior drawer test is historically used by almost all examiners (**Fig. 40-14**). It is typically performed with the knee in 90 degrees of flexion. Although it is a good test to detect chronic ACL deficiency, the anterior drawer test is not a good test in the acute stage when other secondary restraints about the knee can compensate for an ACL deficiency. The Lachman test is superior in that respect. This test is also, in a way, an anterior drawer test and is performed with the knee in 20 to 30 degrees of flexion. The femur is firmly held by one hand and an anterior

force is applied to the tibia with the other hand while noting how far the tibia moves on the femur and whether the movement has a clear end point. The pivot shift test is also an excellent test for ACL injuries, but it is less frequently used because it can be quite painful. It is important that the patient be completely relaxed when this test is performed. Typically, the patient is in a supine position and the knee is flexed to about 30 degrees. The foot is held in a midinternal position and a valgus force is then created on the knees by placing the opposite hand on the tibia. The knee is now extended, and if the valgus forces are continued and an ACL rupture is present, a "jump" would be noted at about 20 to 30 degrees. This shift is the result of the tibia suddenly subluxating forward on the femur.

The posterior cruciate ligament is also tested clinically. A posterior drawer test is performed by applying a posterior force to the tibia with the knee flexed at about 90 degrees. A variety of other tests have been developed for the purpose of determining posterolateral stability and can be reviewed in textbooks specifically dealing with this problem. These injuries are not common in the industrial setting.

IMAGING DIAGNOSIS

The Hip

Radiographic examination of the hip should include at least an anteroposterior (AP) and a lateral view. Other views may be necessary under certain conditions, such as oblique views for suspected acetabular fractures. An AP pelvic overview is helpful in that both hips can be compared. Plain-film radiography is the standard technique for evaluation of trauma and arthritis.[1] Osteoarthritis (OA) is characterized by joint narrowing, particularly in the superolateral position of the joint. Subchondral sclerosis and osteophyte formation are often present, and subchondral cysts may occur. In the early stages the joint narrowing in OA may be visible on weight-bearing views only.

Rheumatoid arthritis is characterized by a more symmetric narrowing of the joint space. Osteophyte formation is rarely present in the early stages but later may be present as secondary OA develops. Seronegative arthritides usually affect the sacroiliac joints before the hip joints. Tomography is sometimes used to detect fractures and special evaluations, whereas arthrography is mainly used in pediatric orthopaedics and sometimes in adult patients with painful hip implants. Radionuclide imaging is mainly used to screen for metastatic lesions or suspected fractures. In an occupational injury, a bone scan may help distinguish between an old and a new lesion (fracture). Unfortunately, bone scans are extremely sensitive but very nonspecific.

Computed tomography (CT) permits radiographic reconstruction of the hip joint. Acetabular fractures can be precisely evaluated and complex reconstructive procedures better planned. In addition, CT is used to evaluate tumors, although magnetic resonance imaging (MRI) has many advantages. Magnetic resonance imaging is the most sensitive test to diagnose ischemic necrosis, a painful hip disorder sometimes undetected by other techniques.

Knee

Routine radiographic examination of the knee includes a minimum of two views: AP and lateral. In addition, a tunnel view and a patellofemoral view are often included.[3] The AP view should preferably be taken with the patient standing to evaluate the joint space and alignment. The lateral view is typically taken in 30 degrees of flexion with the patient lying on the affected limb. The tunnel view, which is a frontal view with the knee in 60 degrees of flexion, provides additional information about the posterior condyles, the intercondylar notch, and the tibial plateau. Patellofemoral views are useful to determine patellar alignment and demonstrate the patellofemoral joint.

Femorotibial alignment is measured from the standing AP view. It should normally be about 7 degrees of valgus.

Radiographs are important in trauma and to determine degenerative joint conditions. Soft bone abnormalities such as joint effusion or ruptures of the quadriceps and patella tendons can often be detected on plain radiographs, as can the calcification of articular and meniscal cartilage often referred to as chondrocalcinosis.

Degenerative arthritis is characterized by joint space narrowing (often requires standing films), subchondral sclerosis, subchondral cysts, and osteophytes. One, two, or all three compartments may be involved, usually one more than the other. In rheumatoid arthritis, the joint space may be more uniformly narrowed and osteopenia is often present. Tomography and CT scanning are primarily used to evaluate trauma. Bone scans are helpful in patients with pain after trauma when radiographs are uncertain and pain persists. Arthrograms were often used in the past to evaluate internal knee derangements such as ligament or cartilage tears.

To some degree MRI has replaced arthrography, but it is more expensive. Arthroscopy has also reduced the use of arthrograms. Magnetic resonance imaging is highly sensitive to ACL injuries, and its specificity is also acceptable. It is also an excellent method to detect posterior cruciate ligament injuries, but it has little to offer over physical examination in an evaluation of the more common medial collateral ligament injuries. Magnetic resonance imaging has good sensitivity and specificity for meniscal tears and also detects meniscal cysts.

Arthroscopy

Arthroscopic examination of the knee joint is commonly done for diagnostic purposes. Because of the invasive nature of arthroscopy, it should only be used when other diagnostic procedures fail and when treatment can also be provided. The greatest advantage of arthroscopy lies in the ability to diagnose and treat in one setting.

SUMMARY

Clinical evaluation of the hip and knee often allows the physician to make a diagnosis and plan for treatment. Imaging is sometimes a necessary complement but should always be evaluated in light of the clinical findings.

References

1. Dalinka MK, Neustadler LM: Radiology of the hip. In Steinberg ME, editor: *The hip and its disorders*, Philadelphia, 1991, WB Saunders; pp. 56-71.

2. Hoppenfeld S: *Physical examination of the spine and extremities*, New York, 1976, Appleton-Century-Crofts.

3. Pavlov H: Radiographic examination of the knee. In Insall JN, editor: *Surgery of the knee*, New York, 1984, Churchill Livingstone; pp. 73-98.

4. Post M: *Physical examination of the musculoskeletal system*, Chicago, 1987, Mosby–Year Book.

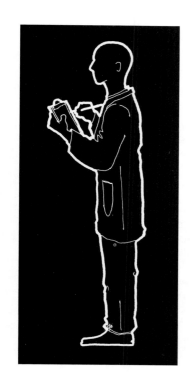

Chapter 41

Treatment of the Common Disorders of the Knee and Hip

Craig D. Silverton

CONTENTS

Because a comprehensive, detailed review of treatment of hip and knee disorders is difficult in a limited format, a moderately detailed review is offered that will leave some readers with a wish to further pursue the subject matter. For that purpose, a few textbooks are recommended in the list of references.[1,7-12] For those who do not specifically treat hip and knee disorders but are still exposed to patients with hip and knee complaints or to patients with sequelae from these disorders, this review, together with Chapter 40, aims to provide the basis for a better understanding of hip and knee pathology as it relates to symptoms, diagnosis, and treatment.

TREATMENT OF KNEE DISORDERS

Fractures About the Knee

Fractures about the knee can be divided into three areas: (1) supracondylar and intercondylar distal femur fractures, (2) tibial plateau fractures, and (3) patella fractures. All these fractures, whether intraarticular or extraarticular, have in common the potential sequelae of posttraumatic knee arthritis with accompanying pain if axial malalignment and articular incongruities are not corrected.

In the past 30 years, there has been an evolution from nonoperative to operative treatment for many fractures.[8] The Swiss group of surgeons who formed the Association for Osteosynthesis/Association for the Study of Problems of Internal Fixation (AO/ASIF) in the late 1950s believed in stable fixation of fractures and early motion to prevent what they termed "fracture disease." This was a term used to describe the osteoporosis, soft tissue atrophy, chronic edema, and joint stiffness manifested after traditional immobilization for the treatment of fractures. Their principles of internal fixation stressed (1) anatomic restoration of joint surfaces, (2) stable internal fixation, (3) preservation of blood supply to the bone fragments and soft tissue, and (4) early active joint motion based on obtaining stability of the fracture at the time of surgery. Fulfillment of these principles in the operative treatment of fractures about the knee will give the patient the best chance of avoiding a posttraumatic painful, stiff arthritic knee.

Supracondylar and intercondylar femur fractures are complex injuries that are difficult to treat. Many of these injuries involve young patients in high-energy accidents. The elderly population with osteoporosis also seems to be susceptible to these fractures. Initial examination will show marked swelling at the fracture site. It is important to check the distal circulation to determine the presence of a vascular injury to the femoral artery,

which lies adjacent to the shaft of the femur. Standard anteroposterior and lateral films will usually give adequate information to determine the treatment protocol.

The relative roles of nonoperative and operative treatment of distal femur fractures continue to be debated. Factors affecting the decision include the patient's age, activity level, other associated injuries, and the ability to tolerate traction, casting, or surgery.[2,8] Most nonoperative treatment uses either skeletal traction or a cast brace that allows some motion at the knee joint. The majority of supracondylar and intercondylar femur fractures require open reduction and internal fixation (ORIF). This is done by using screws either alone or in combination with various buttress, condylar, or blade plates, antegrade or retrograde intramedullary nails, or external fixation devices. Three millimeters of intraarticular displacement is a widely accepted indication for operative treatment.

Supracondylar femur fractures above total knee replacements are occasionally seen in the elderly. Most of these injuries are caused by a low-energy fall, with the fracture occurring at the weak area of the metaphyseal-diaphyseal junction. The decision between nonoperative and operative treatment is determined by the ability of the cast to maintain acceptable alignment and by the stability of the knee prosthesis before and after the fracture. A revision total knee arthroplasty may be the only way to salvage this difficult problem. Recently, reports show that the use of retrograde locked intramedullary nails has been effective in selected cases of supracondylar femur fractures above a total knee replacement.

The tibial plateau is one of the most critical weight-bearing areas in the body. Plateau fractures are caused by either high- or low-energy trauma and tend to occur later in life. Ligamentous injuries (medial collateral ligament [MCL]) are commonly associated with lateral plateau fractures. Patients initially have a large hemarthrosis unless a tear in the joint capsule allows blood to extravasate. Tenderness over the fracture site and limited range of motion are seen. Assessment of the collateral ligaments is important; however, unless the joint is aspirated and filled with lidocaine (Xylocaine), most patients are too uncomfortable to undergo stress radiographs. Routine anteroposterior and lateral views of the knee will document most tibial plateau fractures. The tibial plateau angle view (obtained by tilting the x-ray tube 15 degrees caudad) will more accurately determine the amount of plateau depression present. Computed tomography (CT), conventional tomograms, and magnetic resonance imaging (MRI) all give additional information concerning the fracture pattern and degree of displacement. Stress films in varus and valgus rarely give additional information that cannot be obtained on physical examination.

Traditional management has used closed methods in the past. This included skeletal traction, casting, cast-bracing, and early mobilization with active range of motion. Operative treatment of displaced or depressed tibial plateau fractures remains the current treatment of choice.[4,5] Opinion varies as to what constitutes significant depression, with numbers ranging from 0 to 10 mm. Surgical repair using various screws, plates, and external fixation devices is standard. The use of arthroscopy to guide the intraarticular reduction of fracture fragments together with cannulated screw fixation has provided another treatment modality to those skilled in this technique. Regardless of the specific method of fracture fixation, the following principles must be followed: (1) anatomic reduction, (2) restoration of articular surfaces, (3) stable fixation, (4) bone grafting of defects, (5) treatment of ligament injuries, (6) preservation of the meniscus, (7) early range of motion, and (8) non–weight bearing until healing occurs. All these goals should be met while keeping in mind the words of two of the leading fracture surgeons, Drs Schatzker and Tile: "the result of a failed open reduction and internal fixation is always worse than the result of a failed closed treatment." Following these principles will minimize the chance of development of a post-traumatic stiff, painful, and arthritic knee joint.

Tibial fractures in association with a total knee arthroplasty are rare. The majority of these fractures can be managed nonoperatively by ensuring that correct limb alignment is maintained and that tibial components have not loosend. Revision of the tibial component with a long stem may be necessary in selected cases.

Fractures of the patella are common in the 20- to 45-year-old age group. The subcutaneous location of this bone directly anterior to the knee joint makes it susceptible to direct injuries. Diagnosis of this injury is easy because patients have a large effusion, pain with passive movement of the patella, and a palpable defect. Inability to extend the knee may indicate major disruption of the extensor retinaculum in association with a patella fracture. Standard anteroposterior and lateral radiographs suffice for the diagnosis of patella fracture.

The goals of treatment are similar to those already discussed. Nonoperative treatment consists of immobilization in a long leg cylinder cast in full extension for at least 6 weeks. Operative treatment is indicated if the articular step-off is greater than 3 mm or the extensor mechanism is directly disrupted. Internal fixation is performed with a variety of cerclage and tension band wires, pins, and screws. Repair of the extensor retinaculum is essential for a good result. Active knee motion is begun soon after surgery. Posttraumatic patellofemoral arthritis is the most common major sequela of this injury. This may be in part due to the direct insult to the cartilage at the time of injury; however, attention to anatomic reduction of the articular surfaces may lessen the likelihood of posttraumatic arthritis developing.

Ligamentous Injuries

Knee ligament injuries revolve around the so-called crucial ligaments of the knee—the anterior and posterior cruciate ligaments (ACL and PCL). These two strong intraarticular ligaments form an "x" as they cross through the middle of the knee. The MCL and lateral collateral ligament (LCL) provide extra-articular ligamentous support to the knee joint.

Ligamentous injury to the knee joint is basically caused by four primary mechanisms. Valgus stress with the knee in slight flexion is the most common. This usually results in tearing of the MCL and ACL. O'Donoghue described a triad of these two ligamentous injuries in association with a medial meniscus tear. This injury complex is commonly referred to as the "terrible triad of O'Donoghue." The next most common injury is hyperextension of the knee. This initially tears the ACL and then proceeds onward to the PCL and posterior of the capsule and ultimately into the neurovascular bundle. Meniscus injuries are common with this injury complex. The third most common injury pattern is a posteriorly directed force into the flexed knee. This is a common occurrence in an automobile accident when the knee strikes the dashboard and drives the tibia posterior on the femur thereby tearing the PCL from its tibial insertion. The fourth pattern is a varus stress from a direct blow on the medial side of the knee. This initially leads to disruption of the LCL, then the posterolateral capsule, and ultimately the PCL. Not all injury patterns follow these mechanisms exactly. A combination of any of these patterns can lead to additional ligamentous injuries and possible knee dislocation.

Patients may give a history of hearing a "pop" following their injury; this corresponds to a torn ACL in 85% of patients. Examination of the knee reveals a tense effusion and limited range of motion. The presence of swelling will tend to position the knee in 30 degrees of flexion, a position in which intraarticular pressure is the lowest. The absence of swelling may be significant and indicate a severe knee injury with disruption of the joint capsule leading to extravasation of blood outside the knee joint. The collateral ligaments are examined with a valgus stress for the MCL and a varus stress for the LCL. The stress test is performed in both full extension and then in 30 degrees of flexion allowing the posterior capsule and PCL to relax. Grading of the laxity is from I through III, with grade I being a partial tear and grade III a complete tear. A multitude of tests are available to check the integrity of the ACL but are beyond the scope of this chapter.[6] The Lachman test is the most sensitive ACL test and is performed with the knee flexed 30 degrees and anterior pressure applied to the proximal tibia. The degree of anterior subluxation of the tibia in relation to the femur is noted and compared with the uninjured knee. The anterior drawer test is performed with the knee joint flexed to 90 degrees and an anteriorly directed force applied to the proximal tibia. This test is said to emphasize the anteromedial bundle of the ACL, and the Lachman test is said to emphasize the posterolateral bundle. Similar tests can be performed for evaluation of the PCL, that is a posteriorly directed force placed on the proximal end of the tibia at both 30 and 90 degrees of knee flexion.

Radiographic evaluation should always be performed on an acutely injured knee to rule out a fracture.

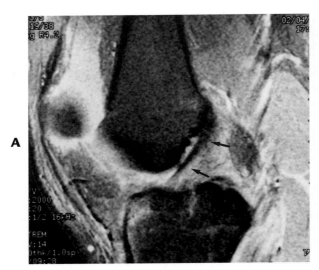 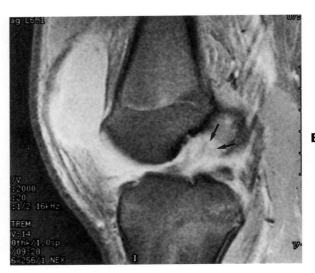

Figure 41-1 A, T2-weighted MRI of a normal anterior cruciate ligament (ACL) that has a low-intensity (*black edge*), straight anterior margin (*arrow*). The posteroinferior edge of a normal ACL is variable in appearance; it is high in intensity in this case. **B**, T2-weighted MRI of a torn ACL. Tissue in the expected region of the ACL is high in signal and disorganized, indicating a tear. Note the frayed ends of the torn ligament (*arrow*).

A depressed tibial plateau fracture may mimic a ligamentous injury to the knee until radiographs demonstrate the actual pathology. A minimum of three views, including an anteroposterior, lateral, and notch view, should be obtained. Magnetic resonance imaging may be helpful for further evaluation of the ligaments (**Fig. 41-1, A** and **B**), menisci, articular cartilage surface, and subchondral bone; however, physical examination is usually sufficient to diagnose the majority of ligamentous injuries to the knee.

Treatment recommendations for ligamentous injuries to the knee are quite complex because it is only a rare patient who has an isolated ligament injury. In those acute knee injuries involving only the MCL or LCL, nonoperative management is recommended. This consists of a short period of immobilization followed by an aggressive physical therapy program. Recovery time is based on the severity of the injury, and most patients are able to return to full function within 6 to 8 weeks. Management of MCL or LCL injuries in association with a cruciate injury requires a more aggressive approach to treatment. In the athletic population this usually requires operative intervention with reconstruction of the torn ACL or PCL, by using either a portion of the patellar tendon or hamstring tendons for substitution of the torn ligament.[2] Primary repair of torn cruciate ligaments has not had a successful track record to date. Cruciate ligament surgery is usually performed 3 to 4 weeks after the initial injury, during which time aggressive physical therapy is instituted to minimize muscle atrophy and maintain full range of motion. Knee arthroscopy precedes the knee reconstruction, at which time the menisci are evaluated and treated, with repair of the meniscus emphasized when possible. The knee reconstruction is done either arthroscopically or open

(through the patellar tendon defect). Following surgery, an aggressive therapy program continues, and most patients are able to return to sporting activities in 6 to 8 months. Use of a brace following surgery has not been proven to prevent reinjury to the knee. The majority of knee reconstructions involve a torn ACL, but newer arthroscopic techniques have made reconstruction of a PCL-injured knee a reasonable alternative.

Treatment for an isolated ACL injury is not clear-cut. The natural history of an ACL-deficient knee would lead us to believe that all patients should have a reconstruction to prevent further injury to the menisci and subsequent degenerative changes. Patient selection for treatment recommendations should be based on the following: lifestyle, age, degree of functional instability, and patient cooperation. The primary determinant in making the decision for nonoperative treatment should be based on the preinjury level of activity and the patient's desire to return to this level. Those patients who want to maintain an active lifestyle, including sports, will probably experience episodes of "giving way," pain, and swelling. The degree of instability on physical examination may be related to the integrity of the secondary stabilizers and should be considered in treatment recommendations. If nonoperative treatment is elected, low-risk activities such as swimming and bicycling are reasonable. Functional bracing alone is not adequate to prevent reinjury to the knee, and some patients may benefit from improved proprioception to reduce episodes of "giving way."

Isolated PCL injuries are much less common than isolated ACL injuries, and their natural history is much more obscure. The majority of PCL injuries are complex and involve other ligaments around the knee (**Fig. 41-2, A,B**). Management of isolated PCL-injured knees is

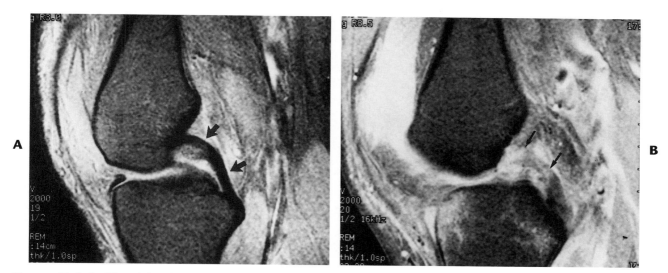

Figure 41-2 A, T2-weighted MRI of a normal posterior cruciate ligament (PCL) in a 25-year-old male. The ligament (*arrow*) is normally black, as it is in this case. **B**, MRI, torn PCL. The bright appearance of the proximal end of the ligament and its discontinuity (*arrow*) indicates a tear at its attachment to the femur.

controversial, with enthusiastic reports of good results with both operative and nonoperative treatment. Until better follow-up studies are available, nonoperative management is probably the treatment of choice in isolated PCL injured knees.

Meniscal Injuries

Tears of the semilunar cartilage, or menisci, are the most common cause of mechanical knee symptoms such as locking, catching, and giving way of the knee. The medial and lateral menisci function to distribute loads across the knee joint. Any tears of the menisci may cause a portion of the meniscus to become abnormally mobile and lead to pain, locking, and local synovitis. The type of tear, location, and extent will determine the symptomatology. Patients typically give a history of a twisting-type knee injury followed by localized tenderness and swelling. Signs and symptoms of a meniscal tear include an effusion, joint line tenderness, inability to fully extend the knee, and a positive Apley or McMurray test.

Standard anteroposterior and lateral radiographs are seldom of benefit in evaluating a patient in whom a meniscal tear is suspected. Standing radiographs (weight bearing) in full extension and 45 degrees of flexion (skier's view) can be helpful in evaluating joint space loss and early degenerative changes. Although arthrography was the gold standard for diagnosis of a meniscal tear, MRI has emerged as the diagnostic modality of choice for imaging the menisci of the knee. Magnetic resonance imaging is very sensitive and enables the diagnostician to accurately delineate the type of tear as well as the extent and size (**Fig. 41-3, A, B**). The remainder of the soft tissues in and around the knee are also seen with outstanding accuracy. Subchondral bone edema, articular surface damage, and areas of avascular

necrosis (AVN) that can mimic a meniscal lesion on physical examination are easily detected with MRI. Unfortunately, this test has replaced good physical examination and is commonly used as a diagnostic screening test for routine patients with knee pain. In a patient with a history of a twisting-type knee injury, effusion, joint line tenderness, and a positive McMurray test, MRI is unnecessary. The MRI should be reserved for those patients in whom a good physical examination has been performed and an appropriate trial of conservative treatment has been instituted for at least 4 weeks. If questionable symptoms of a meniscal lesion persist and operative intervention is contemplated, then an MRI may be indicated. However, it is most important to correlate the patient's subjective complaints and objective examination results with the MRI findings because the frequency of asymptomatic meniscal lesions is high in the normal population, especially in patients over the age of 50. A positive MRI report should not be used as an indication for surgery in as much as many small interstitial, cleavage, and degenerative tears may be managed appropriately with nonoperative treatment. Furthermore, the menisci in these situations are frequently functioning properly and early removal may well be more deleterious than beneficial to the long-term survival of the knee joint. The introduction of MRI has given us information about the menisci, cartilage, subchondral bone, and soft tissues around the knee not previously available. However, if this information is not properly correlated with the clinical picture, many unhappy patients will return to their care provider after operative arthroscopy with no change in their subjective complaints.

In the past, meniscal tears were treated with an arthrotomy and total meniscectomy. Long-term studies of open total meniscectomy reveal a high incidence of

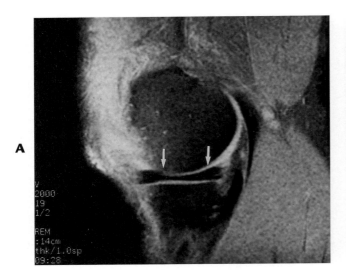 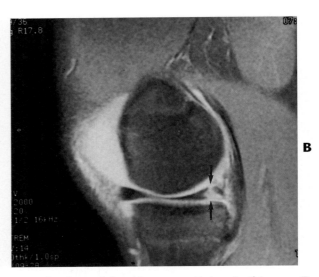

Figure 41-3 A, MRI of a normal meniscus appears black in a proton-density–weighted image, as it does in this case. **B**, MRI of a torn meniscus. The posterior horn tear (*arrow*) appears as a high-intensity white line or band (*arrows*).

progressive degenerative changes in the knee. With the introduction of arthroscopy in the 1970s, meniscal lesions were better visualized and subtotal or partial meniscectomy emerged as the treatment of choice, the thought being that retaining a portion of the menisci would decrease the incidence of degenerative arthritis. However, as the physiology of the meniscus was better understood, preservation of this important stabilizer and load-sharing device has become increasingly important. Preservation of the menisci by arthroscopic or open repair is an attainable goal when the tear is near the vascular periphery and does not have a complex pattern. Other criteria for successful meniscal repair include an acute (less than 6 weeks since injury) longitudinal tear in a stable knee with the remainder of the menisci and articular cartilage normal. Unfortunately, repairable tears are relatively infrequent, and when the indications are extended to include complex tears and tears in the avascular portion of the menisci, failures are common. Young patients with an associated ACL tear have benefited from this technically difficult procedure because the stability afforded by the medial meniscus is crucial to having a successful long-term result following cruciate ligament reconstruction. Arthroscopic meniscectomy remains the procedure of choice for most symptomatic meniscal tears. Current techniques continue to emphasize retaining an intact ring of the meniscus to act as a stabilizer and load-sharing device, although no long-term reports have demonstrated a decreased incidence of degenerative arthritis with this technique.

In an attempt to minimize degenerative arthritis of the knee in young patients following meniscectomy, replacement of the meniscus with an allograft has recently gained popularity. These meniscal transplants have shown some promise at short-term follow-up, but the data are currently insufficient to support this proce-

dure as an alternative salvage procedure in a postmeniscectomy patient.

Patellofemoral Pain

One of the most common complaints referable to the knee is patellofemoral pain.[3] There is still confusion as to the exact causes of patellofemoral pain. Chondromalacia patellae, plicas, osteoarthritis, subluxation, patellar tilt, and reflex sympathetic dystrophy have all been implicated as causes of patellofemoral pain. Most patients have no history of trauma and complain of a dull, aching discomfort in the anterior aspect of the knee that may be aggravated by going up and down stairs, squatting, kneeling, or prolonged sitting with the knee flexed. It is most commonly seen in young females and many times interferes with their sports activities.

Physical examination of a patient with patellofemoral pain may show an increase in the quadriceps (Q) angle, which is formed by the line of the quadriceps muscle and the patellar ligament. The average Q angle is about 15 degrees, and any angle greater than 20 degrees has been associated with recurrent patellar subluxation and chondromalacia patellae. Other physical findings include atrophy of the vastus medialis muscle (VMM) and a positive apprehension sign (the patella is forced laterally while the knee is flexed). Palpable and audible crepitus may be detected, but this is not pathognomonic of patellofemoral pain syndrome and may commonly be present in an asymptomatic individual. Effusion is sometimes present along with peripatellar tenderness.

Routine radiographs should include a skyline or Merchant view which will show both the medial and lateral patellar facets and provide an evaluation of the patellofemoral joint. The presence of patellar tilt, joint space loss, and osteoarthritic spur formation may be seen on the skyline view. In those rare cases of patellofemoral pain where nonoperative treatment has not benefited the patient, additional studies may be indicated. Computed tomography in association with an arthrogram has gained popularity in evaluating the patellar cartilage. Computed tomography of the patellofemoral joint in full extension and various degrees of flexion is an excellent modality for evaluating patellar tracking and malalignment problems. Magnetic resonance imaging of the patellofemoral joint is best for evaluating the soft tissues surrounding the patella, although posttraumatic osseous changes of the patella can also be visualized.

Chondromalacia patellae is the term most commonly associated with patellofemoral pain. This term is a pathologic diagnosis and refers to softening and progressive breakdown of the articular cartilage. It is usually secondary to either a single episode of trauma or repetitive microtrauma secondary to a malalignment problem. Chondromalacia patellae is a distinct clinical entity and is not synonymous with patellofemoral syndrome. Arthroscopy has helped in the grading of this lesion (grades 0 to IV), with grade I representing softening of the cartilage and grade IV indistinguishable from osteoarthritis with exposed subchondral bone. It is not well understood why breakdown of the articular surface causes pain because nerve endings are not present within the cartilage. The source of pain is probably from both the subchondral bone itself and the severity of synovitis present. It should be emphasized that chondromalacia patellae is common in asymptomatic patients and the coexistence of pain and this lesion can be unrelated. The presence of chondromalacia does not imply symptoms.

Osteoarthritis of the patellofemoral joint is common in the older population. These patients frequently complain of pain when climbing stairs or rising from a sitting position. Stiffness and swelling of the knee are common. Most of these patients have disease of either their medial or lateral knee compartments or both. Lateral and skyline radiographs demonstrate joint space narrowing, subchondral sclerosis, and osteophytes; these are typical findings in osteoarthritis.

Dislocation or subluxation of the patella is a traumatic event. However, the presence of a shallow trochlea, patellar malalignment, weak VMO, or a tight lateral retinaculum has been shown to predispose patients to this entity. The patella usually reduces on its own, and patients complain of pain along the medial border of the patella. For many patients, this becomes a chronic problem and surgical intervention becomes necessary.

The presence of synovial folds (plicas) in the suprapatellar pouch represents embryonic remnants that have no known physiologic function. These plicas are a normal finding during routine arthroscopy. Occasionally plicas become inflamed or thickened and impinge as the knee flexes and the plica glides over the femoral condyle. The plica is such an easy structure to locate and cut during routine arthroscopy that it has become

the "fall guy" for unexplained knee pain. The plica syndrome is overdiagnosed and only occasionally is the cause of patellofemoral pain.

Other causes of peripatellar knee pain include patella tendinitis (jumper's knee), prepatellar bursitis (housemaid's knee), inflammation of the infrapatellar fat pad (Hoffa's syndrome), and iliotibial band friction syndrome.

Initial treatment for the majority of patellofemoral problems is nonoperative. Ice, rest, nonsteriodal antiinflammatory drugs (NSAIDs) and physical therapy will be successful in minimizing symptoms in up to 90% of cases. A minimum of 6 to 12 months of conservative therapy is usually recommended before surgical options are considered. Surgery is more likely to be successful in a patient with a specific patellar tracking malalignment than in a patient with symptoms of chondromalacia patellae not associated with malalignment. Tibial tubercle osteotomies, transfers, and anterior elevation have been performed for a variety of patellofemoral complaints, with good results in those patients whose complaints were secondary to a malalignment problem. Again, patients with chondromalacia patellae and no specific malalignment pathology do not consistently achieve reproducibly good results with transfer of the tibial tubercle.

No surgical procedure can replace or repair damaged articular cartilage. Although arthroscopy is an excellent tool for the diagnosis of articular surface damage, debridement of the diseased cartilage has not proved to be beneficial. Arthroscopic release of the lateral retinaculum was extensively used in the past for the treatment of generalized patellofemoral pain and for patients with lateral subluxation of the patella. Good short-term results were reported. The enthusiasm for this procedure has waned recently, and currently, specific indications for lateral retinacular release include both physical examination and CT evidence of patellar tilt, with arthroscopic evidence of minimal degenerative changes of the patellofemoral joint. Isolated patellofemoral arthroplasty was developed for the treatment of degenerative changes of the patellofemoral joint, but results were poor and this procedure is no longer recommended. Patellar excision or patellectomy is a salvage procedure and can only be recommended as a last resort in the treatment of patients with patellofemoral arthrosis. Patients may lose up to 50% of their knee extension power following complete patellectomy. Many of these patients have disease involving either their medial or lateral compartments and will require a total joint arthroplasty in the future. These patients are better served with a total joint arthroplasty and resurfacing of the patella to maintain extension power.

Arthritis

Osteoarthritis is the most common type of arthritis seen at the knee and is most commonly reported in the elderly population. Classic osteoarthritis involves the medial compartment and patellofemoral joint but spares the lateral compartment. Patients complain of pain with ambulation, swelling, crepitance, and stiffness, and as the disease progresses, patients may even awaken at night with severe discomfort. Physical examination will demonstrate effusion in over 50% of patients, limited range of motion, and marked crepitance. Standing or weight-bearing anteroposterior radiographs of the involved knee are necessary to evaluate joint space collapse because standard radiographs will frequently falsely demonstrate joint space integrity. Complete loss of joint space, marginal osteophytes, and subchondral cyst formation are the classic radiographic findings in osteo- arthritis of the knee. Weight-bearing mechanical axis views are advantageous in evaluating the axial alignment of the lower extremity. Many patients with medial joint arthrosis will lose the normal 5 to 7 degrees of valgus alignment of the lower extremity and drift into a varus attitude (bowlegged) as the disease progresses (**Fig. 41-4, A, B**). Conversely, patients with lateral joint arthrosis may have a more severe valgus deformity (knock knee).

The first line of treatment in osteoarthritis of the knee is conservative: NSAIDs, activity modification, and weight reduction if needed. The efficacy of the NSAID may be short-lived, and either dosage modification or changing to another drug may be necessary. Physical therapy may be beneficial in maintaining range of motion and temporarily alleviating symptoms. An intraarticular injection of a steroid preparation may occasionally provide long-lasting pain relief. However, none of these conservative measures will alter the course of the disease, and in many patients sufficient symptoms will develop to warrant operative intervention.

The success of total-knee replacements in the past 20 years in relieving pain and increasing function has led many patients and physicians to regard this as the only procedure available for the treatment of knee osteoarthritis. No currently available synthetic materials can replace the ability of the articular surface to provide a painless, gliding surface that is nearly wear free. Despite the design improvements and better operative techniques, the mechanical nature of knee replacements limits their life span. Infection, aseptic loosening, and excessive component wear will eventually lead to failure over time. In the elderly population with tricompartmental degenerative joint disease, total knee replacement may be the only option. However, in the younger patient population when only one compartment is diseased (unicompartmental), other surgical options that preserve articular surfaces are available and may slow the progression of osteoarthrosis.

Osteotomy, either proximal tibial or distal femoral, changes the axial alignment of the lower extremity and alters the loads applied to the knee joint, with a subsequent decrease in stress on the diseased compartment. Frequently, a radiographically visible joint space may be created where previously bone-on-bone contact was seen. A fibrocartilaginous articular surface forms over the previously diseased segment. Patients can expect a

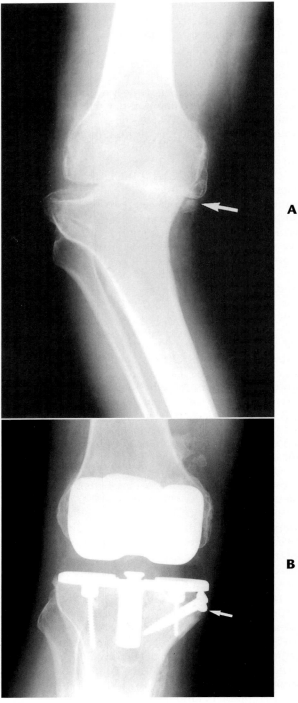

Figure 41-4 A A severe varus deformity in an 8-year-old female with partial loss of the medial tibial plateau. **B,** Total knee arthroplasty required a bone graft fixed with screws on the medial side to support the tibial plate (*arrows*).

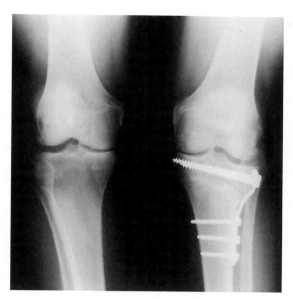

Figure 41-5 Bilateral varus deformities with medial joint arthritis in a 41-year-old female treated with a high tibial osteotomy on the left side to correct her varus alignment.

decrease in their symptoms and improved function, although the results of this procedure are variable and generally decline with time. The ideal candidate for an osteotomy is a young, active male (less than 50 years old) with disease limited to either the medial or lateral compartment and no patellofemoral symptomatology. With proper preoperative planning, patient selection, and an adequate amount of axial correction, high tibial or distal femoral osteotomy has the potential of providing good results in the young active patient population (**Fig. 41-5**).

Arthroscopic debridement of the arthritic joint was a popular procedure in the past, although no evidence suggests that procedure changes the natural course of the disease. Patients do report a decrease in their symptoms after arthroscopic lavage, and theoretically this may be due to removal of cartilage debris and associated synovial inflammatory mediators with a subsequent decrease in synovial irritation. Combining this procedure with abrasion of the damaged articular surface is thought by some authors to stimulate the formation of a new articular surface. The quality of this fibrocartilaginous articular surface is in question because it lacks the composition, mechanical properties, and durability of host articular cartilage. The results of this procedure are once again variable, with some patients reporting a decrease in their symptoms and others reporting no change or worsening of their symptoms. Although success rates for arthroscopic debridement of the knee joint vary between 50% and 65%, this procedure may have a place in the treatment of young patients with limited disease and in those older patients who are unwilling or unable to undergo a total joint arthroplasty.

The evolution of total knee replacement over the past 25 years has resulted in current knee designs that have a survival rate of up to 95% at 15-year follow-up. The ability of this operation to consistently relieve pain is unsurpassed by any previous surgical procedure. Although design changes are still being debated, the basic total knee arthroplasty (tricompartmental) consists of either a cobalt chrome or titanium femoral component, a polyethylene tibial articulating surface that is locked in place onto a tibial base plate, and a polyethylene patella. Either components are cemented in place, or in some designs (cementless), biological ingrowth into the porous surfaces of the femoral and tibial components provides long-term fixation. Cement was originally thought to be the culprit in early failures of some total knee designs; therefore, cementless components were developed as an alternative for younger, more active patients. Both cemented and cementless total knee arthroplasty designs have now shown consistently good results at long-term follow-up in all age groups. Candidates for total knee arthroplasty should have been through a complete trial of conservative treatment options and failed. Most patients will complain of pain at rest, night pain, and an inability to ambulate more than one or two blocks without significant pain. Weight-bearing radiographs will show joint space collapse, subchondral cyst formation, and angular deformities.

In those select patients who have osteoarthritis limited to only one compartment, another surgical option is unicompartmental knee arthroplasty. This involves replacement of only one compartment (usually medial) with the advantage of preserving normal knee kinematics. Patients enjoy an increased range of motion and earlier rehabilitation as compared with tricompartmental knee replacement. The ideal candidate for unicompartmental replacement is 60 years of age or older with disease limited to either the medial or lateral compartments, an intact ACL, range of motion greater than 90 degrees, and minimal angular deformity. If these criteria are met, the clinical results of unicompartmental knee replacement can be even better than those of tricompartmental knee arthroplasty.

Knee fusion, or arthrodesis, is a good surgical option in a young patient who has posttraumatic tricompartmental knee arthritis. However, this procedure is now rarely performed because the results of total knee arthroplasty continue to be promising even in the younger patient population. Although the option of total knee arthroplasty in a young patient is inviting to both the physician and patient, failure of the total knee and a lifetime of revision surgery may await these patients. Knee arthrodesis is a one-time operation with a high rate of success but unfortunately enjoys low patient acceptance. Consequently, the most common indication for knee arthrodesis today is failed total knee arthroplasty secondary to sepsis (**Fig. 41-6**).

Other systemic inflammatory arthritic conditions can also affect the knee joint, including rheumatoid arthritis, gout, pseudogout (calcium pyrophosphate dihydrate deposition disease [CPDD]), psoriatic arthropa-

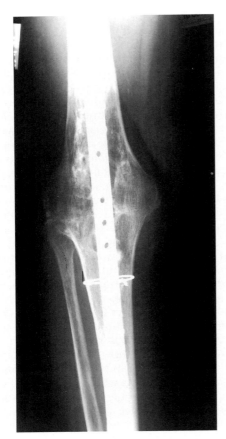

Figure 41-6 A healed knee fusion using an intramedullary rod in a 62-year-old female who underwent multiple surgeries after her primary total knee arthroplasty became infected.

thy, and Lyme disease. Some HIV-positive patients also may demonstrate an inflammatory-type arthritis of the knee before the onset of AIDS. Neuropathic arthropathies (Charcot joint) may affect the knee and are most commonly caused by diabetes and syphilis. Diagnosis of these various disease processes has been previously described, and in the case of gout and pseudogout, the diagnosis may depend on the demonstration of characteristic crystals in the synovial fluid.

Medical management is the cornerstone of treatment for these systemic diseases. The use of intraarticular steroids such as methylprednisolone (20 to 40 mg) may induce some improvement in symptoms, and relief typically lasts from several weeks to months. If symptoms worsen despite a reasonable trial of conservative medical therapy, surgical intervention may be necessary. Early prophylactic synovectomy (either open or arthroscopically) may be appropriate in some patients, although this procedure is performed less frequently since the introduction of total knee arthroplasty. Ultimately, most patients will eventually require total knee arthroplasty (**Fig. 41-7**).

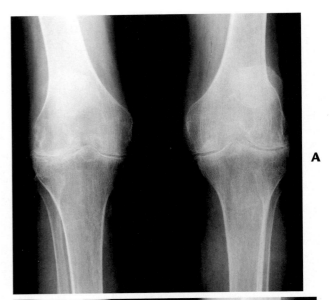

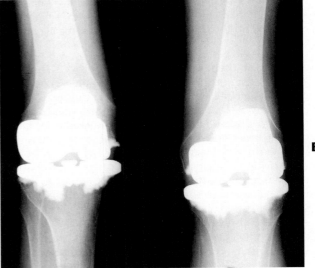

Figure 41-7 A, Bilateral degenerative joint disease in a 56-year-old female rheumatoid patient. Note the complete loss of joint space, severe osteopenia, and lack of osteophytes typical of rheumatoid arthritis. **B**, Bilateral total knee arthroplasties were cemented in place because of poor bone quality in this patient.

Osteonecrosis of the Knee

Spontaneous osteonecrosis of the knee is a relatively common knee disorder primarily seen in women over 60 years of age. The exact etiology is unknown, and patients relate a history of sudden pain on the medial aspect of the knee that may or may not have been precipitated by an injury. The pain can be quite severe and is frequently worse at night. Physical examination shows an area of localized tenderness over the medial femoral condyle, which may be confused with a torn medial meniscus. Plain radiographs may appear normal. Consequently, early in the course of the disease bone scan has been used to make the diagnosis. However, MRI frequently yields more specific diagnostic information and is currently the easiest way to make the diagnosis of osteonecrosis of the knee.

Treatment options vary as to the size and extent of the lesion. Small lesions may do well with protected weight bearing and nonoperative treatment; however, with progressive collapse and severe symptoms, joint arthroplasty (either unicompartmental or tricompartmental) produces the most predictable results.

TREATMENT OF HIP DISORDERS

Fractures

Fractures around the hip are the most common orthopaedic diagnosis, constituting an average of 30% of orthopaedic hospital admissions. Hip fractures are usually traumatic in origin and involve either the femoral neck or intertrochanteric regions of the proximal femur. Patients give a history of falling and are unable to ambulate following their injury. In those patients who sustain only a nondisplaced crack of the femoral neck, many will complain of only groin discomfort and continue to ambulate. This picture is also common in stress fractures of the femoral neck that are occasionally seen in younger patients pursuing vigorous athletic endeavors. High-speed motor vehicle accidents also can cause fractures around the hip; fracture-dislocations of the hip joint are more likely to occur when the patient's knee strikes the dashboard, the femoral head is driven posteriorly, and the femoral head or acetabulum is fractured and dislocated. Thus fractures of the pelvis and acetabulum are also common following high speed accidents.

Radiographic analysis of the hip joint is the only reliable way to diagnose a hip fracture. Routine films should include an anteroposterior and lateral projection of the hip joint. A frog-leg lateral view may be substituted for a true lateral projection. In those patients who sustain a nondisplaced fracture or a stress fracture, a bone scan may be necessary for a definite diagnosis (**Fig. 41-8, C**). If the initial radiographs fail to reveal a fracture and the patient continues to complain of pain, repeat films are indicated in 2 to 3 weeks or sooner if the symptoms worsen because some nondisplaced fractures are often not visible on the initial radiographs (**Fig. 41-8, A, B**). Fractures that involve the acetabulum may require oblique (Judet) views of the pelvis or CT to better delineate the fracture pattern (**Fig. 41-9, A, B**).

The treatment for most fractures around the hip is ORIF (**Fig. 41-9, C**). Intertrochanteric fractures nearly always require ORIF. Only those femoral neck fractures that are not displaced may be considered for nonoperative treatment, and even these are typically treated surgically to prevent displacement. Nonoperative treatment requires non–weight bearing on the side of the injury for a period of at least 6 to 8 weeks. Repeat radiographs are indicated every 3 weeks to evaluate fracture alignment and radiographic evidence of healing (callus formation). Many of these nondisplaced femoral neck and stress fractures go on to displacement despite conservative treatment and then require ORIF. For this reason, many of these fractures are operated prophylactically to prevent further displacement. Displaced femoral neck fractures that disrupt the blood supply to the femoral head are not amenable to fixation and will usually require hemiarthroplasty or total joint arthroplasty. A bone scan may be indicated to assess the viability of the femoral head.

Avascular Necrosis

Avascular necrosis is a debilitating disease of the hip joint frequently seen in patients who are in their third, fourth, or fifth decade of life. It is characterized by areas of dead trabecular bone within the femoral head. The femoral head gradually progresses to collapse around areas of dead bone, thereby leading to mechanical incongruity of the joint. Secondary osteoarthritis will develop in most patients, and eventually total hip replacement is required. Patients most often have a history of intermittent groin pain that may radiate to the knees or buttocks. The pain is exacerbated by weight bearing, and although range of motion of the hip may be normal, pain with forced internal rotation and abduction is often present. A limp frequently develops and gets worse with advancing disease. The opposite hip must always be examined because the prevalence of bilaterality is over 60% in most series.

The etiology of AVN may be secondary to a previous fracture with subsequent compromise of the blood supply to the femoral head. Other causes of AVN are not as well understood. The most common risk factors include the use of alcohol, use of corticosteroids, sickle-cell disease and other hemoglobinopathies, coagulation deficiencies, caisson disease, and a history of radiation to the hip joint. Exposure to corticosteroids and excessive alcohol intake account for approximately 90% of all reported causes of AVN.

Treatment success of AVN of the femoral head is related to the diagnostic stage at which care is initiated. Diagnostic techniques include plain radiographs, bone scanning, MRI, and CT. In the earliest stages of the disease, plain radiographs may be negative. It is imperative to obtain a good frog-leg lateral radiograph, however, because subtle evidence of cystic changes may not be seen on the anteroposterior film (**Fig. 41-10, A, B**). Magnetic resonance imaging is regarded as the most accurate imaging modality for the early stages of AVN (**Fig. 41-10, C**). Intraoperative diagnostic testing includes venography and bone marrow pressure, but these invasive tests are rarely needed since the introduction of MRI. Core biopsy still remains the definitive test for AVN.

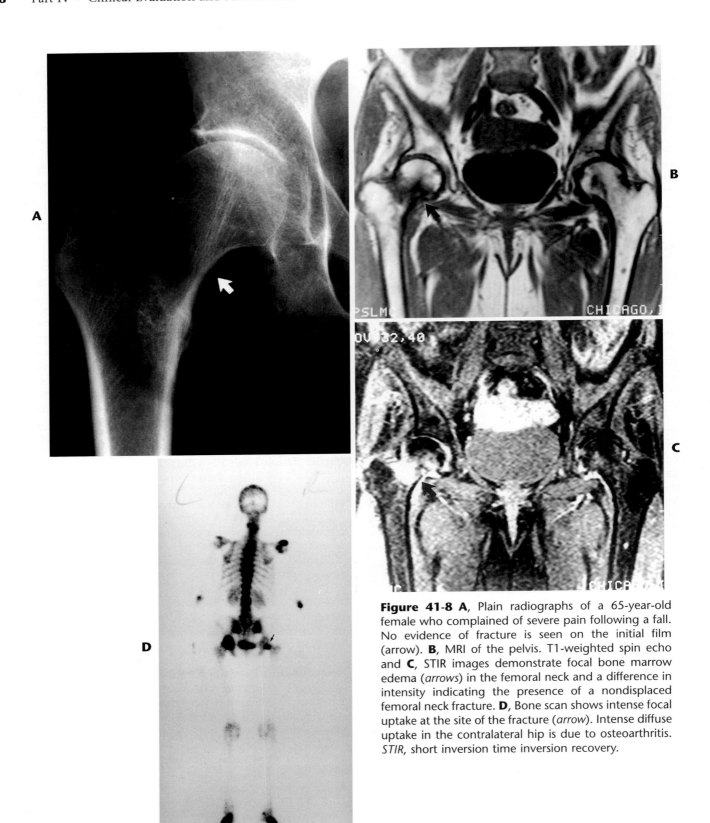

Figure 41-8 A, Plain radiographs of a 65-year-old female who complained of severe pain following a fall. No evidence of fracture is seen on the initial film (arrow). **B**, MRI of the pelvis. T1-weighted spin echo and **C**, STIR images demonstrate focal bone marrow edema (*arrows*) in the femoral neck and a difference in intensity indicating the presence of a nondisplaced femoral neck fracture. **D**, Bone scan shows intense focal uptake at the site of the fracture (*arrow*). Intense diffuse uptake in the contralateral hip is due to osteoarthritis. *STIR*, short inversion time inversion recovery.

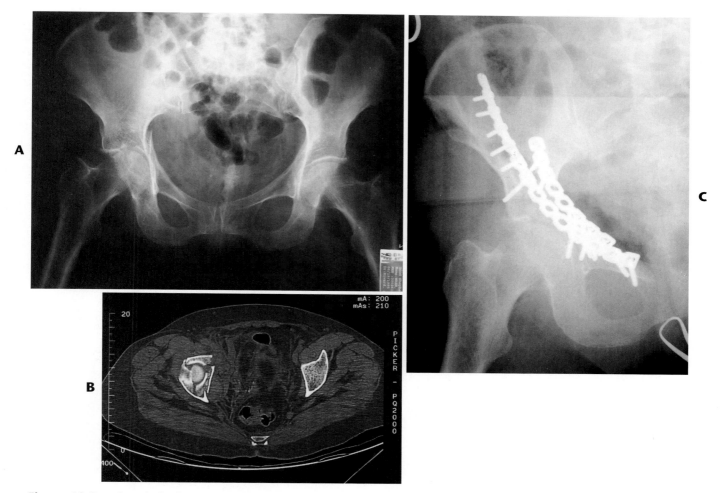

Figure 41-9 a, Acetabular fracture in a 61-year-old female who slipped and fell on her hip after exiting a swimming pool. Note the protrusion of the femoral head into the pelvis, loss of continuity of the articular surface, and disruption of the medial wall (*arrows*). This injury is not usually seen in a low-velocity setting. **B**, Computed tomography shows the dome of the acetabulum blown out as the femoral head protrudes (*arrows*). **C**, Restoration of the articular surface and medial wall required open reduction/internal fixation with long plates and screws applied to the inner surface of the pelvis.

Treatment of AVN encompasses a large variety of treatment modalities from conservative methods that strive to decrease pressure across the hip joint to replacement of the diseased femoral head. Because the natural history of this disease is unclear, evaluating the different treatment methods is difficult. However, if no treatment is instituted, up to an 85% rate of further collapse of the femoral head may be seen at 2 years. Most nonoperative treatment has had poor results, although the use of electrical stimulation has shown promising results in the early stages of the disease (electrical stimulation has not been approved for the treatment of AVN by the Food and Drug Administration and is currently undergoing investigation). Operative treatment may be as simple as a core decompression that involves removing an 8 to 10 mm-diameter core of bone from the femoral neck and head or as complex as

a total hip arthroplasty. Other options include nonvascularized or vascularized bone grafting, angular or rotational osteotomies of the femur, and surface replacement of the femoral head. Hip fusion may be indicated for a young patient with unilateral disease; however, with the high incidence of bilaterality, this is rarely performed except in the post-traumatic patients with AVN. In general, core decompression is indicated for the early stages of the disease, total hip arthroplasty for the most advanced stages, and bone grafting and osteotomy for the intermediate stages.

Transient Osteoporosis of the Hip

Transient osteoporosis of the hip is often confused with early AVN of the femoral head. The exact etiology is unknown; however, there may be some correlation to reflex sympathetic dystrophy. The pain begins without a

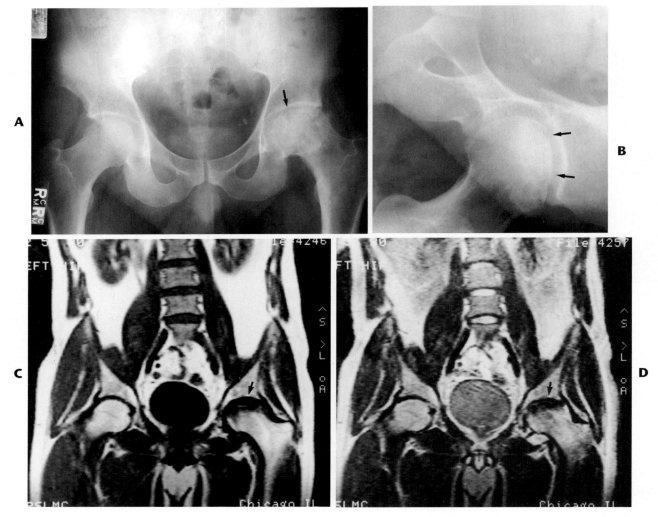

Figure 41-10 A, Severe avascular necrosis of the femoral head in a 35-year-old alcohol abuser. Note the incongruity of the femoral head with collapse (*arrow*). **B,** Frog-leg lateral demonstrates severe collapse of the superior portion of the femoral head. **C,** MRI of the pelvis. T1-weighted and T2-weighted **(D)** spin-echo images demonstrate the extent of osteonecrosis in the femoral head.

history of significant trauma and may become so severe as to require narcotics for pain control. Typically this is a self-limiting disease resolving on its own in 6 to 12 months. Conventional radiographs are negative early in the course of the disease. Bone scanning will show increased uptake in the femoral head and neck, and MRI findings of diffuse bone marrow edema are observed in the femoral head and neck. These findings tend to regress with the clinical symptoms, unlike those of AVN, where progressive collapse of the femoral head is noted.

Treatment of transient osteoporosis of the hip is symptomatic and nonoperative inasmuch as the disease is self-limiting. Patients do well with NSAIDs and protected weight bearing. It is important, however, to differentiate this disease process from the early stages of AVN because the treatment of these two entities is distinctly different.

Osteoarthritis

Osteoarthrosis of the hip is one of the most common causes of disability in our society. Primary osteoarthritis (OA) is the term used for those cases in which no etiology can be identified. Secondary OA, which is the most common type of osteoarthritis of the hip, has one or more predisposing factors that lead to destruction of the hip joint. These include congenital anatomical deformities (acetabular dysplasia, Perthes' disease, slipped capital femoral epiphysis [SCFE]), sepsis (old tuberculosis of the hip, childhood infection), trauma (femoral head and neck fractures), and various metabolic disorders (rheumatoid arthritis, gout, pseudogout).[9,12]

Patients seen in early stages of the disease have a history of dull, aching pain poorly localized to the groin and buttock region. As the osteoarthritis progresses, patients frequently complain of awakening at night

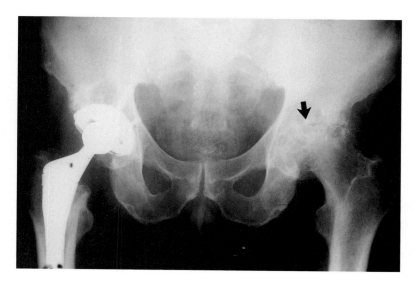

Figure 41-11 Severe osteoarthritis of the left hip with cystic changes in both the acetabulum and femoral head (*arrows*) in a 59-year-old school teacher. The contralateral hip was treated with a cementless total hip arthroplasty.

with pain and also begin to limp. Patients with OA of the hip have an increased incidence of spinal stenosis, and it is important to differentiate these two separate disease processes during the physical examination. The pain with OA of the hip is worse with ambulation and relieved with rest. Range of motion of the hip is decreased and ambulation becomes more difficult. Radiographs in the anteroposterior and lateral planes (weight bearing) show collapse of the joint space with sclerosis and arthritic spur formation (osteophytes) as well as subchondral cyst formation (**Fig. 41-11**).

Initial management of OA of the hip consists of NSAIDs, physical therapy, weight reduction if needed, and activity modification, including the use of a cane. Although none of these conservative measures have any impact on natural progression of the disease, they do form the first line of treatment in the early and intermediate stages. Empiric trials with various different NSAIDs may be necessary. The efficacy of a specific drug may be short-lived, and either dosage modification or changing to a different type of NSAID is frequently necessary. Injection into the hip joint with Xylocaine and a steroid preparation may be beneficial as a diagnostic tool but rarely provides sufficient duration of relief to be considered as therapeutic modality.

Patients with progressively severe symptoms of osteoarthritis of the hip will eventually require surgery. In many of these patients the cause of the osteoarthrosis is mechanical and secondary to residual deformity from developmental hip disease. The role of reconstructive osteotomy in the prevention of hip osteoarthrosis is a surgical option for a young patient (less than 45 years of age) with early disease and evidence of developmental hip deformity (acetabular dysplasia, Perthes' disease). The osteotomy is performed on either the femoral or acetabular side of the hip joint (and sometimes both) and changes the direction of the forces across the joint by realigning the bony architecture. A preventive realignment osteotomy is called a reconstructive os-

teotomy; once osteoathrosis has been established, this is called a salvage osteotomy. A salvage osteotomy is an option for those patients with intermediate disease who are considered to be poor candidates for a total hip arthroplasty.

Hip fusion (arthrodesis) is a good alternative for a young patient with unilateral hip disease who is not a candidate for osteotomy. The contralateral hip, ipsilateral knee, and lumbar spine must be normal for a successful hip arthrodesis. Patients with a history of back pain are not good candidates for this procedure. Although enthusiasm for this procedure has diminished since the introduction of hip arthroplasty, hip arthrodesis is still a viable surgical treatment option in selected patients (**Fig. 41-12**).

Hip arthroscopy has recently emerged as a diagnostic and therapeutic tool in the treatment of specific hip pathology. Removal of a torn labrum, loose bodies, and synovial biopsies are performed on a limited basis. The use of arthroscopy for the diagnosis and treatment of osteoarthritis of the hip is rarely indicated.

Resection arthroplasty (also known as the Girdlestone procedure) involves complete resection of the femoral head and neck of the femur as well as the protruding margins of the acetabulum. Originally used for the treatment of tuberculosis and pyogenic arthritisof the hip, resection arthroplasty is now most often used for salvage of a failed or infected total hip arthroplasty. This procedure may still have a role in the primary setting under special circumstances. Relative indications for primary resection arthroplasty include (1) a septic hip with bone loss, (2) fractures in a nonambulatory patient, (3) dislocation with spasticity, (4) severe contractures, and (5) bone stock that will not support a prosthesis.

The role of total hip replacement in the past 25 years has changed the prognosis for thousands of arthritic patients around the world. Approximately 125,000 total hip replacements are performed annually in the United

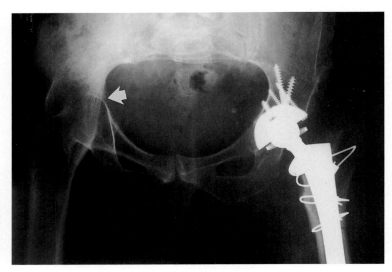

Figure 41-12 A solid hip fusion performed over 30 years ago in a 58-year-old male. The patient has done well with his fusion; however, the total hip arthroplasty performed on his contralateral hip required revision after 6 years and a constrained cup was necessary to prevent recurrent dislocations.

States for OA of the hip. The ability of this operation to consistently relieve pain has been outstanding. Indications for total hip arthroplasty include (1) severe pain not controlled by medication, (2) night pain and pain at rest, and (3) radiographic evidence of degenerative changes in the hip. Over the past 25 years, refinements in implant materials, design, and surgical instrumentation have resulted in our current generation of total hip replacement implants. The femoral and acetabular components are either of the cementless design, which requires press fitting for initial stability and biological ingrowth for long-term stability, or the cemented design, which uses polymethylmethacrylate (bone cement) for initial and long-term stability. The socket or acetabulum is lined with a high-density polyethylene material that articulates with the femoral head. Titanium and cobalt chrome are the standard materials used for manufacturing the femoral components and the acetabular shell. Titanium is generally restricted for use with the cementless designs because of its biocompatibility and elastic modulus, which more closely resembles bone (as compared with cobalt chrome). Cemented titanium components have not enjoyed the same success as their cobalt chrome counterparts. Femoral heads are modular and have been made from cobalt chrome or ceramic since discontinuation of the use of titanium femoral heads because of poor wear characteristics.

Excellent results can be expected with both cemented and cementless designs. In an occasional young patient who has disease limited to the femoral side of the hip joint, replacement of only the femoral head with a cup arthroplasty or bipolar prosthesis can be done. This procedure has not yielded results comparable to those of total hip arthroplasty.

Despite improvements in total hip replacement designs and materials, the longevity of these systems is still limited by their mechanical nature. As younger (less than 50 years old) and more active patients have been

treated by total hip arthroplasty, the longevity of these devices has decreased markedly. Whereas at one time we could count on a 15 to 20-year service life for total hip replacements in elderly patients, many young patients are now having their replacement revised as early as 5 to 10 years postoperatively for either mechanical loosening or component wear. Microscopic polyethylene debris generated by wear is known to be responsible for areas of lysis that surround both cemented and cementless femoral components. This lysis leads to the loss of bone stock, which makes future reconstruction more difficult. Because the results of revision hip replacement are not nearly as successful or long-lived as primary hip replacement, renewed interest in the prevention of OA with reconstructive osteotomy has recently gained popularity.

Inflammatory Arthropathies

The inflammatory arthropathies that involve the hip joint include rheumatoid arthritis, seronegative spondyloarthropathies (e.g., ankylosing spondylitis), crystal-induced arthritis (e.g., gout), and other inflammatory disorders (e.g., Lyme disease).

Rheumatoid arthritis, a systemic disease that attacks the synovial lining of the joints, causes inflammation and proliferation of the synovium, which eventually destroys the joint cartilage. Despite many years of exhaustive investigative work, the etiology of rheumatoid arthritis remains obscure, but it is known to be autoimmune in nature. A patient is said to have rheumatoid arthritis according to the *Primer on the Rheumatic Diseases* if they have at least four of the following seven criteria: (1) morning stiffness, (2) arthritis of three or more joints, (3) arthritis of hand joints, (4) systemic arthritis, (5) rheumatoid nodules, (6) positive serum rheumatoid factor, and (7) radiographic changes typical of rheumatoid arthritis of the hand and wrist.[10]

Radiographic evaluation of both hips shows a symmetrical loss of joint space, medial migration of the femoral head (protrusio acetabuli), and subchondral erosions with localized bone resorption. Little or no osteophyte formation may be present. Initially, these findings may appear similar to those of primary osteoarthritis; however, the presence of symmetric loss of the joint space in both hips with localized osteopenia, lack of osteophytes, and femoral head protrusion are more typically seen in rheumatoid arthritis.

Because rheumatoid arthritis is a systemic disease, drug therapy is the mainstay of treatment. Initially, patients are placed on a regimen of aspirin or an NSAID. Should the disease not be controlled by one of these agents, use of the so-called disease-modifying antirheumatic drugs (DMARDs) such as gold salts, methotrexate, azathioprine, and cyclophosphamide may be tried.

Once a patient fails all forms of nonoperative treatment, surgical intervention may be necessary. Although the disease attacks the synovium initially, the results of synovectomy alone are not gratifying. Indications for total hip replacement in a rheumatoid patient are similar to those seen with degenerative arthritis of the hip, that is, pain and loss of function. Total hip replacement is the treatment of choice, and it is not uncommon to have rheumatoid patients in their fifth decade of life with bilateral hip and knee prostheses. The incidence of both wound complications and deep infections following hip replacement appears to be higher in rheumatoid patients.

Seronegative spondyloarthropathies encompass those diseases that are characterized by inflammation at the ligamentous insertion into the bone (enthesopathic). This is in contrast to rheumatoid arthritis, where the synovium is the site of predilection. Ankylosing spondylitis, Reiter's syndrome, psoriatic arthritis, reactive arthropathy, and intestinal arthropathy all fall into this category. Typically, most of these patients are HLA-B27 positive and rheumatoid factor negative. Whereas 90% of Caucasian patients with ankylosing spondylitis will be HLA-B27 positive, only about 60% of African Americans with the disease are HLA-B27 positive. Approximately 5% of the normal Caucasian population is HLA-B27 positive, and presence of the HLA-B27 antigen alone is not diagnostic for a seronegative spondyloarthropathy.

Hip involvement is seen in approximately 10 to 30% of patients with seronegative arthropathy. It is more commonly seen in patients with ankylosing spondylitis and is frequently manifested as morning stiffness. However, the hip is the second most common site of joint involvement after the knee in ankylosing spondylitis. Range of motion of the hip becomes limited as the disease progresses, and bilateral hip involvement is frequent.

The sine qua non for radiographic diagnosis of ankylosing spondylitis is involvement of the sacroiliac joints. This sacroiliitis must be differentiated from Paget's disease, metastatic disease, and osteitis condensans ilii. The classic "bamboo spine" may be seen on thoracolumbar radiographs; however, relatively few patients actually progress to this stage of the disease. Hip radiographs of patients with ankylosing spondylitis demonstrate the usual destructive changes of a degenerative process of a large joint with loss of joint space, osteophyte formation, subchondral cysts, and mild protrusio acetabuli. In those patients with psoriatic arthritis, enteropathic arthritis, Reiter's syndrome, and concomitant hip involvement, similar radiographic findings are seen.

Both nonoperative and operative management of patients with a seronegative spondyloarthropathy and hip joint involvement is similar to that of patients with rheumatoid arthritis. Radiation therapy alone was once used to treat those patients with ankylosing spondylitis; however, its use is now limited to prophylaxis against heterotopic bone formation after total hip replacement. Because many patients with ankylosing spondylitis have restricted motion of the hip, total joint replacement has the added benefit of significantly improving joint motion.

Gout, pseudogout (CPPD), and apatite deposition encompass those systemic arthritic disease processes that are crystal induced. Gout results from the articular deposition of monosodium urate crystals in the joint, in contrast to pseudogout, which results from the deposition of calcium pyrophosphate crystals and apatite, a form of calcium. Examination of the synovial fluid under polarized light microscopy is diagnostic for gout and pseudogout. Individual apatite crystals are only visible with electron microscopy.

Hip joint involvement is not common in gout or apatite deposition; however, the hip is involved in approximately 30% of patients with pseudogout at some time during the course of their illness. Radiographic studies frequently reveal rapidly destructive arthritis of the hip.

Treatment of the crystal-induced arthritic diseases involves the use of NSAIDs and colchicine to control acute attacks. Total hip replacement is reserved for those patients who do not improve with conservative measures, demonstrate severe pain, and have radiographic evidence of destructive arthritis.

Other miscellaneous inflammatory disorders include Lyme disease, which is caused by a spirochete transmitted by the tick *Ixodes dammini*, and acute febrile juvenile rheumatoid arthritis in adults (Still's disease). Both of these diseases may have hip joint involvement. Radiographic diagnosis and treatment of their hip involvement are similar to that of the other inflammatory disorders previously discussed.

Developmental deformities about the hip

The three major developmental diseases of the hip are SCFE, Perthes' disease, and dysplasia resulting from congenital hip dislocation (subluxation).

Slipped capital femoral epiphysis is characterized by gradual displacement of the epiphysis (growth plate) of the femoral head. This separation is through the growth plate of the femoral head and resembles a fracture

(Salter-Harris type I). The difference is in the abnormal growth plate of patients with SCFE; normal physiological shear stresses are not tolerated, and a resulting slip occurs. In contrast, patients with a fracture through the growth plate (Salter type I), have a normal epiphysis before injury. Slipped capital femoral epiphysis is seen in the pubertal years, with a 2:1 predominance of occurrence in males, and typically involves both hips. Definitive diagnosis is made only by radiographs. Because the predominant direction of slip occurs posteriorly, it is imperative to obtain a frog-leg lateral view (Lauenstein's view). Computed tomography and MRI may be beneficial in providing three-dimensional views of the proximal femur. A bone scan is beneficial to assess preoperative vascularity of the femoral head. Slipped capital femoral epiphysis is an orthopaedic emergency, and operative pinning of the slip is the current standard treatment to prevent further displacement. Other options include traction, plaster immobilization, epiphysiodesis, closed and open reduction with pinning, and various proximal femoral osteotomies.

Avascular necrosis of the femoral head is a serious complication of SCFE and may follow closed or open reduction of a slip, proximal femoral osteotomy, or pinning in situ (which disturbs the intraosseous blood supply). Depending on the amount of femoral head displacement or collapse, a rotational osteotomy of the proximal femur may be beneficial. If the collapse is total, osteotomy is not indicated. Surface replacement of the diseased femoral head has had poor results, and because most patients are too young for a total hip replacement, hip fusion may be the best option.

Progression to osteoarthritis of the hip, which is the ultimate poor outcome, results from malalignment of the proximal epiphysis on the metaphysis of the femur. Depending on the severity of the slip, proximal femoral osteotomy may improve this malalignment in adult patients; however, long-term data are insufficient to determine whether osteotomy will prolong the useful life of the hip. Once the degenerative process begins, treatment protocols are similar to those of OA, and many patients will ultimately require total hip replacement.

Perthes' Disease

Legg-Calvé-Perthes disease is a self-limited disease of the hip produced by femoral head ischemia with various degrees of necrosis of the femoral head. Although the disease is produced by avascularity of the femoral head, the exact etiology is unknown. The clinical onset is between the ages 4 and 9 years, with a 4:1 predilection for males. The initial complaints are a limp and pain of several weeks' duration. Pain referral to the knee in many cases follows the sensory distribution of the obturator nerve. Hip motion may be limited. Radiographic evaluation shows a widened articular cartilage space with a small ossific nucleus. Subchondral fracture and collapse of the femoral head may be present. Bone scans show decreased uptake in the avascular femoral head.

The prognosis of Perthes' disease is proportional to the extent of involvement of the femoral head: the greater the involvement and the younger the patient at the time of diagnosis, the poorer the prognosis. Treatment protocols depend on the severity of involvement. The goals of treatment are to maintain full range of motion of the hip while keeping the femoral head contained within the acetabulum. This may involve wearing a brace (hip orthosis; **Fig. 41-13A**) until the reparative stage of the disease is established. Patients with femoral heads that are not able to be contained within the acetabulum with a brace may need a femoral or acetabular osteotomy for coverage to be acceptable (**Fig. 41-13B**).

Although the etiology of the disease is unclear, the long-term prognosis is. Significant arthritis will develop in over 50% of patients by the age of 50. Ten percent of patients will require reconstructive surgery by the age of 35. Many of these patients will progress to total joint replacement surgery. Reconstructive osteotomy may have a role in the prevention of secondary osteoarthritis caused by a malformed femoral head. Once secondary osteoarthritis develops, the surgical options for Perthes' disease are similar to those for primary osteoarthrosis of the hip.

Developmental Dysplasia of the Hip

Developmental dysplasia of the hip in a newborn encompasses a wide range of abnormalities ranging from simple hip instability on manual testing to complete dislocation of the femoral head out of the socket (congenital dislocation of the hip [CDH]). This dislocation of the femoral head results in concomitant dysplasia of the acetabulum. Many factors are involved in the etiology of CDH, including ligamentous and capsular hyperlaxity, intrauterine malposition, genetic influences, and postnatal environmental factors. The diagnosis of CDH is made by physical examination of the newborn and use of the Ortolani and Barlow tests. Because the femoral head is cartilaginous and not visualized radiographically, radiographs are frequently normal in newborns with unstable hips. Subsequently, ultrasound has recently become the primary imaging tool in evaluating the hip of a neonate.

Reduction and maintenance of the subluxated or dislocated hip is the first step in the treatment of CDH. Various splints and harnesses have been designed for this purpose. Early diagnosis is the key to a successful outcome of a normal hip. If the diagnosis is missed in the newborn, reduction becomes progressively more difficult over the next year, and traction, closed or possibly open, reduction of the dislocated hip will be required. Femoral and acetabular osteotomies may be indicated for those cases in which closed treatment has failed and an incongruity of the hip joint remains. Development of the acetabulum may be delayed in

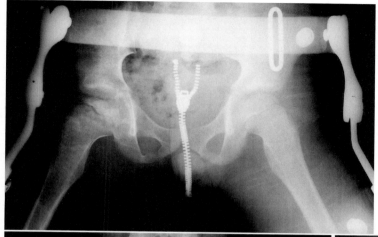

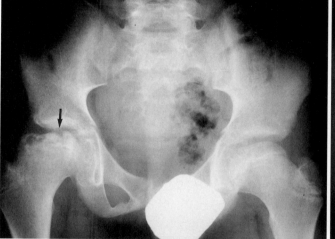

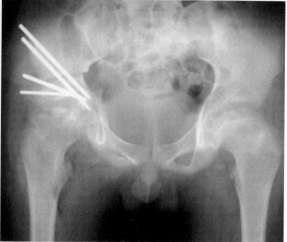

Figure 41-13 A, Avascular necrosis of the femoral head (Perthes' disease) in a 7-year-old boy treated with an abduction brace. **B**, Despite treatment, the disease progressed and the boy needed an acetabular osteotomy **(C)**.

many cases, with resultant acetabular dysplasia.

Once acetabular dysplasia develops, the chance of secondary OA developing by the age of 50 years is 50% (**Fig. 41-14, A, B**). In acetabular dysplasia as well as other developmental disorders about the hip (SCFE, Perthes' disease), the age at the onset and the severity of the secondary osteoarthrosis appear to be related to the degree of deformity at the end of growth. A reconstructive osteotomy of the pelvis is the best way to limit the amount of osteoarthrosis that will develop secondary to the acetabular deformity (**Fig. 41-14, C, D**). Reconstructive osteotomy should be undertaken at a stage when the hip has full range of motion and minimal radiographic evidence of OA. This will give the patient the best chance of avoiding degeneration in a hip in which osteoarthrosis is otherwise destined to develop. Once secondary OA develops, treatment modalities similar to those for primary OA are indicated.

Tumors Around the Hip

The diagnosis of bone and soft tissue tumors around the hip revolves around the use of specialized radio-

graphic studies, as well as biopsy of the lesion. The key to a successful outcome of many of these lesions is prompt diagnosis and treatment.

Routine anteroposterior and lateral films of the hip should initially be obtained. Computer tomography is excellent at delineating bone abnormalities, but soft tissue visualization is not as good. Magnetic resonance imaging is the study of choice for imaging soft tissue tumors and bone tumors with a soft tissue extension. It will also locate neurovascular structures and can aid in evaluating bone marrow involvement representing tumor extension. The bone scan gives additional information concerning the biological activity of the tumor. "Blood pool" images (the second phase of the scan taken 5 to 10 minutes postinjection) will be positive in those tumors that are highly vascular such as giant cell tumors and Ewing's sarcoma. Arteriograms may be necessary for surgical planning, but they do not aid in the diagnosis.

The most critical aspect of the diagnostic regimen is the biopsy. This should be performed by the surgeon who will be planning the definite procedure. In a ma-

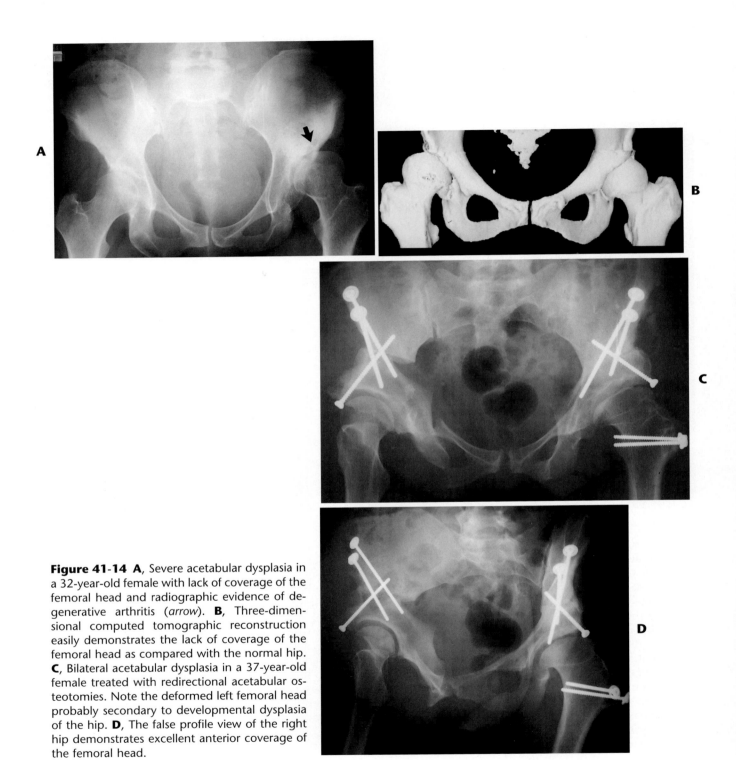

Figure 41-14 A, Severe acetabular dysplasia in a 32-year-old female with lack of coverage of the femoral head and radiographic evidence of degenerative arthritis (*arrow*). **B**, Three-dimensional computed tomographic reconstruction easily demonstrates the lack of coverage of the femoral head as compared with the normal hip. **C**, Bilateral acetabular dysplasia in a 37-year-old female treated with redirectional acetabular osteotomies. Note the deformed left femoral head probably secondary to developmental dysplasia of the hip. **D**, The false profile view of the right hip demonstrates excellent anterior coverage of the femoral head.

lignancy, the biopsy specimen contaminates the tract and needs to be harvested during the definitive procedure. Whether the biopsy is performed open or with a fine needle depends on the surgeon's preference, the pathologist's experience, and the accessibility of the lesion.

Treatment of tumors around the hip is based on obtaining adequate margins for the biological behavior of the lesion. A simple benign cyst may be treated by curettage and packed with bone graft, whereas an aggressive, malignant tumor may require a large en bloc resection. Frequently, the functional deficit following tumor surgery around the hip requires additional reconstructive surgery to maintain ambulation. Preoperative radiation and chemotherapy have had a positive impact in shrinking tumor bulk and increasing disease-free survival in certain high-grade malignant lesions.

Bursitis and Inflammatory Syndromes

At least 13 bursae are present around the hip joint, and each is subject to inflammation. Bursitis in the region of the hip joint can mimic other pathology, including OA and AVN of the hip joint as well as radicular pain secondary to nerve root irritation. Radiographs are usually negative, although occasionally calcification may be found in the bursa.

Trochanteric bursitis is the most common site of inflammation around the hip joint and is also the most overlooked. Patients complain of a dull, deep, aching pain with burning and tingling that radiates down the lateral aspect of the leg. The pain is worse with activity and when sitting on the affected side for an extended period of time (e.g., driving a car). Palpation along the posterior edge of the trochanter elicits pain, and in the acute stages, internal and external rotation of the hip may be painful. The two most common diagnoses to be excluded are osteoarthritis of the hip and acute low back pain with radiation to the posterolateral buttock.

Treatment consists of physical therapy and NSAIDs. Those patients who do not respond to physical therapy may be helped with an intrabursal injection of local anesthetic and steroid. The use of a local anesthetic confirms the diagnosis and rules out other disease processes. The biggest problem in the treatment of trochanteric bursitis is establishing the diagnosis. Once this is confirmed, the prognosis is generally favorable.

Other areas of bursitis around the hip include the iliopectineal bursa and the ischiogluteal bursa, which are much rarer. Treatment of these areas is similar to treatment of the aforementioned trochanteric bursitis.

Some patients complain of a snapping sensation on the lateral aspect of the thigh. This involves the posterior border of the iliotibial band snapping as it roles over the greater trochanter. On physical examination, the patient may be able to flex the thigh and internally rotate the hip to reproduce the snap. Some patients make this a nervous habit and cause a chronic trochanteric bursitis. Treatment consists of NSAIDs, physical therapy, and recognition of the problem. Surgical treatment is rarely indicated.

References

1. Browner BD, Jupiter JB, Levine AM, Grafton PG: *Skeletal trauma*, Philadelphia, 1992, WB Saunders.

2. Delee, JC, Drez, D: *Orthopaedic sports medicine: principles and practice*, Philadelphia, 1994, WB Saunders.

3. Fox, JM: *The patellofemoral joint*, New York, 1993, McGraw-Hill.

4. Fu FH, Harner CD, Vince KG: *Knee Surgery*, Baltimore, 1994, Williams & Wilkins.

5. Insall JN: *Surgery of the knee*, New York, 1993, Churchill Livingstone.

6. Jackson DW: *The anterior cruciate ligament*, New York, 1993, Raven Press.

7. Kelly WN, Harris ED: *Textbook of rheumatology*, ed 4, Philadelphia, 1993, WB Saunders.

8. Rockwood C, Green DP, Bucholz RW: *Fractures in adults and children*, ed 3, Philadelphia, 1991, JB Lippincott.

9. Rothman RH, Balderston RA, Booth, RE, Hozack WJ: *The hip*, Philadelphia, 1992, Lea & Febiger.

10. Schumacher, HR: *Primer on the rheumatic diseases*, ed 10, Atlanta, 1993, Arthritis Foundation.

11. Scott WN: *The knee*, St. Louis, 1994, Mosby–Year Book.

12. Steinberg, ME: *The hip and its disorders*, Philadelphia, 1982, WB Saunders.

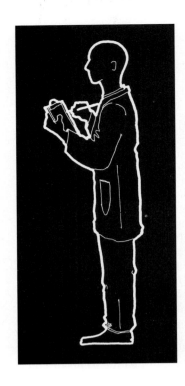

Chapter 42

Job Accommodation with Respect to the Lower Extremity

Steve A. Lavender
Gunnar B. J. Andersson

CONTENTS

Some of the most frequent and severe musculoskeletal disorders in the workplace are localized to the upper extremity and the back. As a result, much of the ergonomic literature has focused on the prevention and accommodation of disorders in these body segments through engineering and administrative controls. Comparatively little attention has been given to the prevention and accommodation of occupational lower extremity musculoskeletal disorders. The first question that most readers will ask concerns the significance of the problem. The second question, once convinced that the problem is significant, has to do with the types of control measures available for lower extremity injury prevention and accommodation. These two issues are addressed in this chapter.

DOES AN OCCUPATIONAL LOWER EXTREMITY PROBLEM EXIST?

Most of the lower extremity disorder literature has focused on both acute and cumulative trauma stemming from athletic and recreational activities. However, recent studies have begun to report a relationship between knee trauma and, to a lesser extent, hip trauma and occupational factors. Lindberg and Axmacher[23] reported the prevalence of coxarthrosis in the hip to be greater in male farmers than in an age-matched group of urban dwellers. Vingard et al[54] classified blue-collar occupations as to whether static or dynamic forces could be expected to act on the lower extremity. The authors found that those employed in occupations that experienced greater loads on the lower extremity, namely, farmers, construction workers, firefighters, grain mill workers, butchers, and meat-preparation workers, had an increased risk of osteoarthrosis of the hip. Similarly, Vingard et al[53] found that disability pensions for hip osteoarthrosis were significantly more likely to be received by males employed as farmers, forest workers, and construction workers.

Lindberg and Montgomery[24] reported that knee gonarthrosis (osteoarthritis [OA]), defined by them as a "narrowing of the joint space with a loss of distance between the tibia and the femur in one compartment, of one-half or more of the distance in the other compartment of the same knee joint or the same compartment of the other knee, or less than 3 mm," was more common in those who had performed jobs that required heavy physical labor for a long time. Kohatsu and Schurman[18] found that relative to controls, indi-

viduals with severe OA were two to three times more likely to have worked in occupations requiring moderate to heavy physical work. Personal risk factors for osteoarthrosis of the knee include obesity and significant knee injury. These authors found no relationship between leisure activities and knee OA. Anderson and Felson[2] reported a relationship between the frequency of knee bending required in a respondent's occupation and OA in the older working population (55 to 64 years old). Moreover, these same authors have shown that the strength demands of the job were predictive of knee OA in women from this older age group. The authors suggest that the increased OA in those with long exposure to occupational tasks is indicative of the role of repetitive occupational exposure.[2]

When concrete reinforcement workers were compared with painters, no differences were found with regard to the occurrence of knee accidents, knee stiffness, or sick leave taken for knee trouble.[55] However, the work for concrete reinforcement workers required heavier lifting and often slippery work surfaces. In fact, these authors report that slipping and stumbling accounted for 70% of the minor injuries in concrete reinforcement workers whereas in painters, slipping and stumbling accounted for only 8% of the minor injuries.

Cumulative trauma injuries can take the form of stress or fatigue fractures. Linenger and Shwayhat[25] reported that training-related injuries to the foot occurred in military personnel undergoing basic training at a rate of three new injuries per 1,000 recruit days. These authors found that stress fractures to the foot, ankle sprains, and Achilles tendinitis accounted for the bulk of the injuries. Anderson[1] found that stress fractures were most common in the distal second and third metatarsal bones but could occur in any of the bones in the foot. Giladi and coworkers' findings[13] indicated that 71% of the stress fractures in their sample of military recruits occurred in the tibia and 25% in the femoral shaft. Moreover, they found the fractures to occur later in the training process than reported by others. Giladi et al[12] also reported the influence of individual factors on the incidence of fatigue fractures. Specifically, they found that individuals with narrow tibias and/or greater external rotation of the hip were more likely to experience fatigue fractures. The effectiveness of shoe insoles and variations in shoe design as preventive measures will be reviewed later in this chapter.

Törner et al[51] reported that chronic prepatellar bursitis was the predominant knee disorder in 120 fishermen who underwent an orthopaedic physical examination. Forty-eight percent of the men examined showed this disorder. Interestingly, the finding was as common among the younger men as the older men. The authors believe that this disorder is a secondary effect of the boat's motion. The knees are used to stabilize the body by pressing against gunwales or machinery as tasks are performed with the upper extremities. Furthermore, just standing in mild sea conditions (maximum roll angles of 8 degrees) has been shown to considerably elevate moments at the knees because motion in the lower extremities and the trunk is the primary means for counteracting a ship's motions.[50]

The etiology of "beat knee" was described by Sharrard.[43] He reported on the examination of 579 coal miners, 40% of whom were symptomatic or had previously experienced symptoms. Most of the injuries could be characterized as acute simple bursitis or chronic simple bursitis. The majority of the affected miners were colliers whose job requires constant kneeling at the mine face. They found a strong relationship between the coal seam height (directly related to roof height in a mine) and the incidence of beat knee. The incidence rates were much higher in mines with a roof height under 4 feet as compared with those with greater roof heights. Obviously, this factor greatly affects the work posture of the miners. With higher roof heights, miners can alternate between stooped and kneeling postures, but when the seams are 1 m or less, the stooped posture is no longer an alternative. Gallagher and Unger,[10] for example, present recommendations for weight limits of handled materials in underground mines. Below 1.02 m, these are based on miners in kneeling postures. Sharrard[43] also speculated on the individual factors attributable to the disorder and found a higher incidence among younger men. However, this may be due to a "healthy worker effect"[3] in which older miners with severe "beat knee" have left the mining occupation.

Tanaka et al[46] reported that the occupational morbidity ratios for worker's compensation claims of knee joint inflammation among carpet installers was twice that found in tile setters and floor layers and was over 13 times greater than that of carpenters, sheet metal workers, and tinsmiths. Others have shown that the knees of those involved in carpet and flooring installation are more likely to have fluid collections in the superficial infrapatellar bursa, a subcutaneous thickening in the anterior wall of the superficial infrapatellar bursa, and an increased thickness in the subcutaneous prepatellar region.[31]

Thun et al[48] determined the incidence of repetitive knee trauma in the flooring installation professions. Although all flooring installers spend a large amount of time kneeling, the authors divided the 154 survey respondents into two groups, tile setters and floor layers, based on their use of a "knee kicker." This device is used to stretch the carpet during the installation process. These respondents were compared with a group of millwrights and brick layers whose jobs did not require extended kneeling and/or the use of a knee kicker. Of the 112 floor layers (those who used the knee kicker), the prevalence rate of bursitis was approximately twice that found in the 42 tile setters, and over three times that found in the 243 millwrights and brick layers. However, the prevalence in both groups of flooring workers of having required needle aspiration of the knee was almost five times that of millwrights and bricklayers. These results suggest that long durations of occupational kneeling are related to fluid accumulation, yet the

bursitis is due to the repetitive trauma endured by the floor layers using the knee kicker. Village, Morrison, and Leyland[52] found that the peak impulse forces generated in the knees of carpet layers when using the knee kicker were on the order of 3000 N. The opposite knee that was supporting the body during this action had an average peak force of 893 N. Bhattacharya, Mueller, and Putz-Anderson[6] reported knee impact forces of 2469 N (about three times body weight) for a light kick and 3019 N (or about four times body weight) for a hard kick. These light and hard kicks resulted in impact decelerations of 12.3 and 20 g, respectively. The authors observed that the knee kicking action during flooring installation occurred at a rate of 141 kicks per hour. However, to put the knee injuries in perspective, pain was reported by 22% of questionnaire respondents in a tufting job in a carpet manufacturer, but knees were only listed in 2.4% of the accident records. Theoretically, the knee is frequently the site of discomfort, although there may be few lost days associated with knee pain.[47]

In summary, several occupational risk factors have been identified that place an employee at increased risk for disorders in the lower extremity. The literature has shown that heavy physical labor and frequent knee bending are factors, especially in the older component of the workforce, thereby suggesting an interaction between the age degenerative processes and cumulative work experience. In other occupations, the risk of lower extremity disorders is increased through poor footing conditions. Clearly, the role of direct cumulative trauma in those employees who must maintain kneeling postures and use their the knees to strike objects (knee kicker) cannot be overlooked when preventive measures are considered.

PREVENTING INJURY AND REINJURY: TYPES OF ERGONOMIC CONTROLS

Several types of control mechanisms to prevent or accommodate lower extremity disorders are available. This section will focus on techniques whereby the foot-floor interface can be optimized. This includes measures to prevent slips, falls, and stress fractures, as well as measures to improve circulation and comfort in the lower extremities for those who remain in relatively static work postures throughout the day.

Floor Mats

Floor mats are often used for local slip protection. Although inexpensive, they create a possible trip hazard, interfere with operations or cleanliness, and wear excessively.[4] Several investigators have looked into the use of floor mats to reduce the fatigue effects observed in jobs that require prolonged standing. The subjects tested by Kuorinka et al[19] indicated through subjective ratings that they preferred to work on softer surfaces as opposed to harder surfaces. A foam plastic surface was rated the best and concrete the worst. These authors reported a moderate correlation between the subjective comfort ratings of the five surfaces tested and the order of surface hardness. However, integrated electromyographic (EMG) signals, median frequency of the EMG, measures of postural sway, and measures of calf circumference did not show any significant differences between floor coverings. Hinnen and Konz[16] asked employees in a distribution center to stand for two 8-hour shifts on each of five mats tested in the study. Approximately every hour, the employees rated their comfort in several body regions, including the upper leg, lower leg, ankle, and back. A scale of 0 (no discomfort at all) to 10 (extreme discomfort) was used. Although these workers experienced relatively little discomfort, mats with compressibility between 3% and 4% did best in the upper leg discomfort rankings as well as in subject preference rankings. Marginally significant changes in discomfort ratings were reported for the ankle. The ratings of lower leg and back discomfort showed no significant differences.

Rys and Konz[39,40] reported on several anthropometric and physiological measures, including changes in foot size and skin temperature at the instep and the calf. In general, the mats included in this study were significantly different from concrete in that skin temperature was greater at both measured locations and comfort ratings were greater. These authors report that comfort was inversely related to mat compressibility.

Cook et al[8] used surface EMG to study recruitment of the anterior tibialis and paraspinal muscles when standing on linoleum-covered concrete versus an expanded vinyl, 9.5-mm-thick surgical mat. After the subjects stood for two sessions of 2 hours' duration on the mat and on the linoleum, it was concluded that the mats caused no significant changes in the mean of the rectified EMG signals in either muscle. As in the aforementioned studies, subjective data support use of the mat.

Kim, Stuart-Buttle, and Marros[17] tested two types of floor mats and a control condition in which subjects stood on concrete. Although these authors observed muscular fatigue, as determined by a shift in the EMG median frequencies in the gastrocnemius and anterior tibialis muscle, the EMG median frequencies in these muscles were not affected by the use of floor mats. The median frequency shift in the erector spinae was reduced when subjects stood on the thinner and more compressible mat. The authors hypothesized that greater compressibility would have made for a less stable base of support, thereby requiring more frequent postural changes in the trunk to overcome the destabilization associated with postural sway. Therefore the dynamic use of erector spinae muscles to correct for postural sway would facilitate oxygen delivery and removal of contractile by-products through increased blood flow. A further test of this hypothesis would evaluate whether this motion occurred only in the trunk or whether it occurred in the lower extremities, which did not show the spectral shift caused by the floor condition.

Shoe Insoles

The critical role that shoe design plays in the development of overuse syndromes in runners is widely recognized.[22,28,33] Moreover, the role of the shoe in controlling lower extremity kinematics has been reviewed by Frederick[9] and discussed by McKenzie Clement, and Taunton.[28] Similarly, the use of wedged insoles has been shown to alter the static posture of the lower extremity.[56] Sasaki and Yasuda[42] have shown the use of wedged insoles to be a good conservative treatment for medial OA of the knee in the early stages. These authors reported that patients with early radiographic stages of OA who were provided with a wedged insole had reduced pain and improved walking ability relative to controls without the insole.

Clearly, the lower extremity disorders reported by runners represent extreme overuse; however, the treatment and prevention mechanisms may be applicable to occupational settings where employees must stand, walk, run, or even jump during their normal work activities. Padded insoles have been investigated for their shock-abating effects on the skeletal system. Loy and Voloshin[26] used lightweight accelerometers for measuring the shock waves as subjects walked, ascended and descended stairs, and jumped off platforms of a fixed height. The peak magnitude of the shock waves during jumping activities was approximately eight times that seen during normal walking. The results indicated that the insoles reduced the amplitude of the shock wave by between 9% and 41% depending on the activity performed. The insoles were most effective at reducing heel-strike impacts and had the largest effect with jumping activities.

Milgrom et al[30] tested the effects of shock attenuation on the incidence of overuse injuries in infantry recruits. Earlier studies conducted by fixing accelerometers to the tibial tubercle showed that soldiers wearing modified basketball shoes had mean accelerations that were 19% less than those of soldiers wearing lightweight infantry boots. These authors also found that over the 14 weeks of basic training, the modified basketball shoes reduced the incidence of metatarsal stress fractures; however, tibial and femoral stress fractures were not affected by the shoes worn. Gardner et al[11] compared a viscoelastic polymer insole and a standard mesh insole that were issued to a platoon of over 3000 marine recruits. Although the polymer insole had good shock-absorbing properties, the incidence of lower extremity stress injuries over the 12-week basic training program was unaffected by the insole used.

Several studies have been conducted to evaluate variations in insole materials. Leber and Evanski[20] describe the characteristics of the following seven insole materials: Plastazote, latex foam, Dynafoam, Ortho felt, Spenco, Molo, and PPT. These authors measured plantar pressures in 26 patients with forefoot pain. All insole materials reduced plantar pressure by between 28% and 53% relative to a control condition; however, PPT, Plastazote, and Spenco were the superior products. Viscolas and Poron[35] were found to have the best shock absorbency of the five insole materials tested by Pratt, Rees, and Rodgers.[36] Maximum plantar pressures were found to be significantly reduced in the forefoot region with PPT, Spenco, and Viscolas, although the three materials were not significantly different.[29] In the rearfoot region, however, McPoil and Cornwall[29] report that only the PPT and the Spenco insole materials reduced the maximum plantar pressure relative to the barefoot condition. The plantar pressure in the rearfoot region was not significantly reduced with the Viscolas. Interestingly, based on the shock absorbency data from Pratt's 30-day durability test,[34] the resilience of Viscolas, PPT, and Plastazote could be described as excellent, good, and poor, respectively. Sanfilippo, Stess, and Moss[41] also reported the change in foot-to-ground contact area as a function of insole material. Plastazote, Spenco, and PPT led to a significantly greater contact area than did the other materials tested.

In summary, insoles appear to be effective at modifying lower extremity kinematics and reducing peak plantar pressures, although their effectiveness is dependent on the material used. Additional research is needed to clarify the effectiveness of insoles in controlling lower extremity stress injuries. From the previous discussion it should be clear that the effectiveness of this control strategy will be dependent on shock-absorbing capacity, pressure dispersion, and the durability properties of the insole materials selected.

The Foot-Floor Interface

Controlling slip and fall injuries requires a multifaceted approach. The foot-floor interface is analogous to the four-legged stool shown in **Figure 42-1**. To optimize postural stability, all four legs need to be in place and of equal length. The obvious legs are the flooring material and the shoe tread material and design. Environmental conditions represent the third leg because these affect the coefficient of friction (COF) between the shoe and the floor. The fourth leg of the stool pertains to the behavior of the individual wearing the shoe. This behavioral component includes an individual's locomotion pattern, perception of environmental conditions,

and allocation of the attentional resources necessary for adaptive behavior. If any of the four primary components are missing, at least to some degree, a leg of the stool is cut off by some random amount. For example, if the environmental conditions result in an oil film on the floor surface, the stool may still stand on the three remaining legs, provided that the shoe design and floor material are adequate and that the individual perceives the environmental conditions and adapts accordingly. Thus the stool remains standing, although precariously, in spite of a shortened leg. If the individual did not attend to the environmental conditions, the psychomotor leg would have been shortened, thereby making it unlikely that the stool would remain standing. In summary, the prevention of lower extremity injuries caused by slips and falls requires that attention be paid to each component or leg of the stool responsible for maintaining the body's stability.

In considering slip and trip prevention, it is the dynamic friction of the interface, as opposed to static friction, that is considered more critical in determining slip potential inasmuch as most slips occur when the heel initially contacts the ground.[36,44] Gronqvist, Hirvonen, and Skytta[15] have quantified slip resistance by determining the COF between the interacting surfaces and possible contaminants. These authors reported that the important countermeasures against floor slipperiness are the microscopic porosity and roughness of floor coverings. Flooring materials that have rough, unglazed, raised patterns or those made from porous ceramic tiles are best for reducing slipping hazards in areas that must maintain very high standards for hygiene. In environments where the hygiene standards can be relaxed, very rough epoxy or acrylic resin floor materials should be used. Floor surface issues become even more critical on ramps and other inclined work surfaces. Redfern and McVay[37] reported that when walking down ramps, the *required* COF increased in a nearly linear fashion as the ramp angle increased. This was due to the high shear forces encountered during heel-strike as an individual walks down a ramp.

Gronqvist and Hirvonen[14] studied the slip resis-

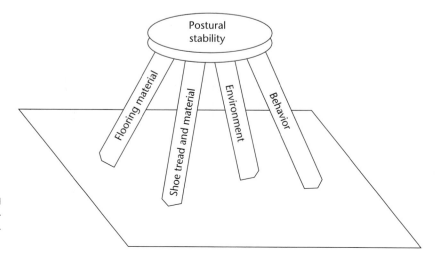

Figure 42-1 Four-legged stool showing the interdependence of the factors affecting postural stability at the foot-floor interface.

tance properties of footwear on iced surfaces. They found that the shoe material significantly affected slip resistance. Shoe heels and soles constructed from thermoplastic rubber with a large cleated area were best for dry ice conditions (-10° C). Very few of the shoes tested functioned well on wet ice (0° C), where there is a boundary layer of water on top of the ice. In fact, the shoes that worked best in a dry ice condition were among the worst when tested in the wet ice condition. Shoes with the sharpest cleats yielded the greatest friction readings under this condition. The hardness of the heel and sole material was not a significant factor on wet ice.

Little consensus is found in sole hardness data, and what differences exist are not of practical significance.[21] In general, microcellular polyurethane heels and soles are recommended, although footwear showed less of an effect on the kinetic COF than did variations in floor surface.[15] Relative to rubber soles and heels, Manning, Jones, and Bruce[27] reported that boots with microcellular polyurethane soles and heels better resisted polishing caused by smooth, wet, or oily floors; had a longer life; and had a greater average COF. The COF of the polyurethane improved over time, thus indicating that the initial smooth surface of the boots should be roughened before use. Tisserand[49] recommends avoiding the use of "microtreads" or small bumps. However, tread design and material are not independent factors when it comes to the coefficient of dynamic friction. Leclercq, Tisserand, and Saulnier[21] stress that the ridges in the tread need to be as sharp as possible to wipe away contaminants on the surface. In addition, these authors point out that the tread design needs to provide channels for the surface contaminants to flow through. Slipping risk is greatest at heel-strike, and therefore the heel of the shoe requires considerable attention. A controversial issue is whether the use of a beveled heel to increase contact surface area is superior to the use of a small contact surface that would result in high contact pressure.[21]

Tisserand[49] has promoted the concept of a mental model whereby an individual has constant input as to the friction available from the surface being walked on. The model is updated as new information indicating a change in surface conditions is received. Slips occur when a discrepancy exists between the mental model of the surface and the actual conditions. Therefore, as Tisserand points out: "The risk of slipping lies more in the gradient of the friction coefficient of the surface than in its absolute value: such as when in a car, a small patch of ground with a low coefficient (an isolated patch of ice, for example, on a large surface with a high coefficient of friction) is more dangerous than a surface with a medium but constant coefficient of friction."

Swensen et al[45] assessed the subjective judgments of surface slipperiness by having groups of iron workers and students walk across steel beams. The subjects were asked to rank the slipperiness of four types of steel coatings and four levels of surface contamination: none,

water, clay, and plastic covering oil. The static COF values ranged between .98 and .20. For experienced and inexperienced subjects, the correlation between the subjective surface ratings and the actual COF measured following the test were .75 and .90, respectively. The subjects exposed to the very slippery conditions created by the oil and plastic (COF = .20) compensated by shortening their stride length, thereby lessening foot velocity and shear forces, and maintained the body's center of gravity within the smaller region of stability. Thus people can detect the COF and adapt their gait accordingly. When this adaptation fails to take place, an individual is much more likely to slip and possibly fall.

Ideally, with the perfect shoe-floor interface—one with no environmental contaminants—the individual's behavior would be not be a factor. However, this exists in few cases, and then even a small fluctuation in the environment would be enough to disrupt the balance of the now three-legged stool. Therefore administrative control measures need to be considered as a means for maintaining the behavior necessary for stable work postures. Employees should be trained to recognize where slippery conditions are likely within a facility and be alert to changing environmental conditions. Further, employees should be encouraged to report maintenance problems with machines that affect the flooring conditions.

Stair Design

Pauls[32] reports that only 6% of stair accidents entail slips and more often accidents are due to "overstepping." This author suggests that the overstepping occurs because the individual descending the stairs does not accurately perceive the stair width (also known as tread length). Therefore, the foot is placed too far forward on the step. This scenario accounts for 19% of all stair accidents. This work highlights the interplay between engineering design factors (stair size) and behavioral factors. Research has suggested that stairs should have risers no higher than 178 mm (7 in) and treads no shorter than 279 mm (11 in).

A secondary issue in stair design is the complex effect of visual distractions. Pauls[32] reported that when visual distractions were present, people actually focused harder on descending the stairs. When no distractions were present, people exhibited less caution. Similarly, patients commonly reported that falls leading to femoral neck fractures were initiated with missing a step down, for example, unexpectedly stepping off a curb.[7] This suggests that when the brain recognizes the potential distractions, attention resources are allocated to the task at hand, whereas without some overt distraction, the brain may allocate adequate attentional resources or it may not. Archea[5] has stressed that an older population that may not have the perceptual and motor capabilities found in younger individuals is more vulnerable to accidents on stairs. These findings suggest that the effects of distractions around stairs change through the aging process.

Help for Those in Kneeling Postures

Sharrard[43] reported that the type of knee pads used was not related to the incidence of beat knee in miners. This author recorded peak pressures on the order of 35.7 kg/cm² as simulated mining tasks were performed. These compression forces were shown to vary widely throughout the 2.5-second cycle time for a shoveling task. Unfortunately, the author had no instrumentation capable of determining the shear forces and the torsional moments placed on the knee during the simulated tasks. At the time of Sharrard's paper, a "bursa pad" had been designed that allowed perspiration to escape, pushed coal particles away from the skin, and provided satisfactory cushioning. Although no control group was used, the author reported that of the 24 previously affected men selected to test the pad under working conditions, only 2 reported a recurrence of beat knee after a 12-month period.

Ringen, Englund, and Seegal[38] reported on a new tool to reduce knee and back trauma in those who tie rebar rods together in preparation for pouring concrete. No longer will concrete workers need to kneel or stoop for extended periods to interconnect the iron rods because this tool allows the operator to work in a standing posture.

Powered carpet stretching tools are available to remove the repeated trauma experienced by carpet layers. However, their widespread implementation depends on educating flooring workers on the trade-offs between the additional time necessary to operate the tool and the knee disorders associated with the conventional technique.

SUMMARY

Ergonomic texts have historically focused relatively little attention on the prevention of lower extremity disorders or the accommodation of individuals returning to work who have experienced a lower extremity disorder. In part, this may be due to an underappreciation of the frequency and severity of occupational lower extremity disorders. Unlike many back or upper extremity disorders that have their origins in the repeated stresses placed on muscular, tendinous, and ligamentous tissues, many of the occupational lower extremity disorders occur through direct compression of body tissues by a surface in the environment. As a result, occupational lower extremity disorders often involve cartilaginous tissue and bone. Therefore, accommodation and prevention of these disorders occur primarily by optimizing the body's contact with surfaces in the environment. This chapter has illustrated some of the key ways in which this can be accomplished.

References

1. Anderson EG: Fatigue fractures of the foot, *Injury* 21:275-279, 1990.

2. Anderson JJ, Felson DT: Factors associated with osteoarthritis of the knee in the first National Health and Nutrition Examination Survey (HANES I), *Am J Epidemiol* 128:179-189, 1988.

3. Andersson GBJ: The epidemiology of spinal disorders. In Frymoyer JW, editors: *The adult spine: principles and practice,* New York, 1991, Raven; pp. 107-146.

4. Andres RO, O'Conner D, Eng T: A practical synthesis of biomechanical results to prevent slips and falls in the workplace. In Kumar S, editor: *Advances in industrial ergonomics and safety IV,* London, 1992, Taylor & Francis; pp. 1001-1006.

5. Archea JC: Environmental factors associated with stair accidents by the elderly, *Clin Geriat Med* 1:555-569, 1985.

6. Bhattacharya A, Mueller M, Putz-Anderson V: Traumatogenic factors affecting the knees of carpet installers, *Appl Ergonom* 16:243-250, 1985.

7. Citron N: Femoral neck fractures: are some preventable? *Ergonomics* 28:993-997, 1985.

8. Cook J, Branch TP, Baranowski TJ, Hutton WC: The effect of surgical floor mats in prolonged standing: an EMG study of the lumbar paraspinal and anterior tibialis muscles, *J Biomed Eng* 15:247-250, 1993.

9. Frederick EC: Kinematically mediated effects of sport shoe design: a review, *Sports Sci* 4:169-184, 1986.

10. Gallagher S, Unger RL: Lifting in four restricted lifting conditions, *Appl Ergonom* 21:237-245, 1990.

11. Gardner LI, Dziados JE, Jones BH, Brundage JF: Prevention of lower extremity stress fractures: a controlled trial of a shock absorbent insole, *Am J Public Health* 78:1663-1667, 1988.

12. Giladi M, Ahronson Z, Stein M, Danon YL, Milgrom C: Unusual distribution and onset of stress fractures in soldiers, *Clin Orthop Related Research* 192:142-146, 1985.

13. Giladi M, Milgrom C, Simkin A, Danon Y: Stress fractures: identifiable risk factors, *Am J Sports Med* 19:647-652, 1991.

14. Grönqvist R, Hirvonen M: Pedestrian safety on icy surfaces: anti-slip properties of footwear. In Aghazadeh F: *Advances in industrial ergonomics and safety VI,* London, 1994, Taylor & Francis; pp. 315-322.

15. Grönqvist R, Hirvonen M, Skytta E: Countermeasures against floor slipperiness in the food industry. In Kumar S, editor: *Advances in industrial ergonomics and safety IV,* London, 1992, Taylor & Francis; pp. 989-996.

16. Hinnen P, Konz S: Fatigue mats. In Aghazadeh F, editor: *Advances in industrial ergonomics and safety VI,* London, 1994, Taylor & Francis; pp. 323-327.

17. Kim JY, Stuart-Buttle C, Marras WS: The effects of mats on back and leg fatigue, *Appl Ergonom* 25:29-34, 1994.

18. Kohatsu ND, Schurman DJ: Risk factors for the development of osteoarthrosis of the knee, *Clin Orthop* 261:242-246, 1990.

19. Kuorinka I, Hakkanen S, Nieminen K, Saari J: Comparison of floor surfaces for standing work. In Asmussen E, Jorgensen K, editors: *Biomechanics VI-B*, Proceedings of the Sixth International Congress of Biomechanics, Baltimore, 1978, University Park Press; pp. 207-211.

20. Leber C, Evanski PM: A comparison of shoe insole materials in plantar pressure relief, *Prosthetics and Orthotics International* 10:135-138, 1986.

21. Leclercq S, Tisserand M, Saulnier H: Slip resistant footwear: a means for the prevention of slipping. In Aghazadeh F, editor: *Advances in industrial ergonomics and safety VI*, London, 1994, Taylor & Francis; pp. 329-337.

22. Lehman WL: Overuse syndromes in runners, *American Family Physician* 29:157-161, 1984.

23. Lindberg H, Axmacher B: Coxarthrosis in farmers, *Acta Orthop Scand* 59:607, 1988.

24. Lindberg H, Montgomery F: Heavy labor and the occurrence of gonarthrosis, *Clin Orthop* 214:235-236, 1987.

25. Linenger JM, Shwayhat AF: Epidemiology of podiatric injuries in US Marine recruits undergoing basic training, *J Am Podiat Med Assoc* 82:269-271, 1992.

26. Loy DJ, Voloshin AS: Biomechanics of stair walking and jumping, *J Sports Sci* 9:136-149, 1991.

27. Manning D, Jones C, Bruce M: Boots for oily surfaces, *Ergonom* 28:1011-1019, 1985.

28. McKenzie DC, Clement DB, Taunton JE: Running shoes, orthotics, and injuries, *Sports Med* 2:334-347, 1985.

29. McPoil TG, Cornwall MW: Effect of insole material on force and plantar pressures during walking, *J Am Podiatr Med Assoc* 82:412-416, 1992.

30. Milgrom C, Finestone A, Shlamkovitch N, Wosk J, Laor A, Voloshin A, Eldad A: Prevention of overuse injuries of the foot by improved shoe shock attenuation: a randomized prospective study, *Clin Orthop* 281:189-192, 1992.

31. Myllymaki T, Tikkakoski T, Typpo T, Kivimaki J, Suramo I: Carpet-layer's knee: an ultrasonographic study, *Acta Radiol* 34:496-499, 1993.

32. Pauls JL: Review of stair safety research with an emphasis on Canadian studies, *Ergonomics* 28:999-1010, 1985.

33. Pinshaw R, Atlas V, Noakes TD: The nature and response to therapy of 196 consecutive injuries seen at a runners' clinic, *S Afr Med J* 65:291-298, 1984.

34. Pratt DJ: Medium term comparison of shock attenuating insoles using a spectral analysis technique, *J Biomed Eng* 10:426-429, 1988.

35. Pratt DJ, Rees PH, Rodgers C: Assessment of some shock absorbing insoles, *Prosthet Orthot Int* 19:43-45, 1986.

36. Redfern MS, Bidanda B: The effects of shoe angle, velocity, and vertical force on shoe/floor slip resistance. In Kumar S, editor: *Advances in industrial ergonomics and safety IV*, London, 1992, Taylor & Francis; pp. 997-1000.

37. Redfern MS, McVay EJ: Slip potentials on ramps. Proceedings of the Human Factors and Ergonomics Society 37th Annual Meeting 2:701-703, 1993.

38. Ringen K, Englund A, Seegal J: Construction workers. In Levey BS, Wegman DH, editors: *Occupational health: recog-*

nizing and preventing work-related disease, Boston, 1995, Little, Brown; pp. 685-701.

39. Rys M, Konz S: An evaluation of floor surfaces. Proceedings of the Human Factors Society 33th Annual Meeting 1:517-520, 1989, Denver, Colo.

40. Rys M, Konz S: Floor mats. Proceedings of the Human Factors Society 34th Annual Meeting 1:575-579, 1990, Orlando, Fla.

41. Sanfilippo PB, Stess RM, Moss KM: Dynamic plantar pressure analysis. Comparing common insole materials, *J American Podiatric Medical Association* 82:502-513, 1992.

42. Sasaki T, Yasuda K: Clinical evaluation of the treatment of osteoarthritic knees using a newly designed wedged insole, *Clin Orthop* 221:181-187, 1987.

43. Sharrard WJW: Aetiology and pathology of beat knee, *Br J Ind Med* 20:24-31, 1963.

44. Strandberg L: On accident analysis and slip-resistance measurement, *Ergonomics* 26:1983.

45. Swensen EE, Purswell JL, Schlegel RE, Stanevich RL: Coefficient of friction and subjective assessment of slippery work surfaces, *Hum Factors* 34:67-77, 1992.

46. Tanaka S, Smith AB, Halperin W, Jensen R: Carpet-layers knee, *N Engl J Med* 307:1276-1277, 1982.

47. Tellier C, Montreuil S: Pain felt by workers and musculoskeletal injuries: assessment relating to tufting shops in the carpet industry. In Queinnec Y, Daniellou F, editors: *Designing for everyone* 1:287-289, 1991.

48. Thun M, Tanaka S, Smith AB, Haperin WE, Lee ST, Luggen ME, Hess EV: Morbidity from repetitive knee trauma in carpet and floor layers, *BMJ* 44:611-620, 1987.

49. Tisserand M: Progress in the prevention of falls caused by slipping, *Ergonomics* 28:1027-1042, 1985; p. 1039.

50. Törner M, Almström C, Karlsson R, Kadefors R: Biomechanical calculations of musculoskeletal load caused by ship motions, in combination with work, on board a fishing vessel. In Queinnec Y, Daniellou F, editors: *Designing for everyone*, 1991, London, Taylor & Francis; pp 293-295.

51. Törner M, Zetterberg C, Hansson T, Lindell V: Musculoskeletal symptoms and signs and isometric strength among fishermen, *Ergonomics* 33:1155-1170, 1990.

52. Village J, Morrison JB, Leyland A: Carpetlayers and typesetters: ergonomic analysis of work procedures and equipment. In Queinnec Y, Daniellou F, editors: *Designing for everyone*, 1991, London, Taylor & Francis; pp. 320-322.

53. Vingard E, Alfredsson L, Fellenius E, Christer H: Disability pensions due to musculo-skeletal disorders among men in heavy occupations, *Scand J Soc Med* 20:31-36, 1992.

54. Vingard E, Alfredsson L, Goldie I, Hogstedt C: Occupation and osteoarthrosis of the hip and knee: a register-based cohort study, *Int J Epidemiol* 20:1025-1031, 1991.

55. Wickström G, Hanninen K, Mattsson T, Niskanen T, Riihimaki H, Waris P, Zitting A: Knee degeneration in concrete reinforcement workers, *Br J Ind Med* 40:216-219, 1983.

56. Yasuda K, Sasaki T: The mechanics of treatment of the osteoarthritic knee with a wedged insole, *Clin Orthop* 215:162-172, 1987.

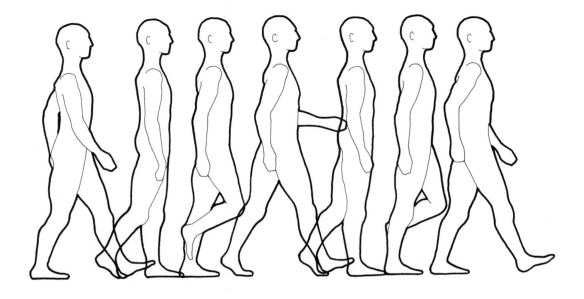

SECTION 5

Foot and Ankle

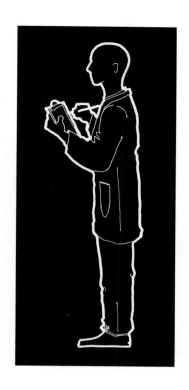

Chapter 43

Epidemiology of Foot and Ankle Disorders

Beat Hintermann
Benno M. Nigg

CONTENTS

Acute and overuse injuries of the foot and ankle are among the most common injuries in the musculoskeletal system. It has been reported that for every 300 men working in heavy industry, 15 working days per month are lost as a result of foot problems, 65% of which are the result of trauma.[28] Based on 15,000 completed questionnaires by family shoe store customers, it was determined that 40% of the population in the United States has foot problems, 12% of which had surgery and 7% have been left untreated.[54]

Given the emphasis that our society places on sports and recreation, it is not surprising that the number of athletically related injuries has increased. Professional sport activities have also markedly increased in the last 20 to 30 years. In sports practice, however, it is often not easy to distinguish between professional and recreational activities, and therefore it is difficult to strictly separate work-related from recreation-related sport injuries.

The following general comments on the epidemiological assessment of disorders and injuries to the foot and ankle are meant to show the general problems and difficulties in attempting to reveal and compare data from a literature review. More detailed considerations about epidemiology are separately made for work-related, military-related, and sport-related injuries, although as mentioned earlier, strict differentiation between these activities is often not possible. There has been a growth in the number of athletically related injuries coincident with an enlarging search by the public for specialists to provide the necessary treatment. Hence it is not surprising that athletic-related injuries are at this time among the best-investigated injuries. The knowledge gleaned from such specific studies, however, has contributed to a better understanding of injuries occurring during work and military service and has led to improvements in equipment. As an example, shoe construction and design have markedly profited by the research activities of sport shoe companies.

EPIDEMIOLOGICAL STUDIES—CRITICAL ASPECTS IN METHODOLOGY

One of the goals of preventive medicine is to reduce the health risk of both occupational exposure and athletic participation through recognition and control of the risk factors. From the vantage point of careful epidemiological study, it is possible to identify and quantify risk along with the incidence and prevalence of injury for a given set of conditions.[78,125]

To properly analyze epidemiological data, it is critical that the population being analyzed is assiduously defined. Many studies of athletic injuries that have engendered prejudicial thinking about the causes of injuries are flawed because of their methodology.[22] Most of the existing information on observed causes of athletic injuries comes from reports of case studies. Many of these studies report an injury rate, although they have often failed to accurately define the population at risk for injury. For instance, the prevalent idea that runners who overpronate are at a greater risk for injury, as reported by James, Bates, and Osternig,[73] was fostered by noting that 58% of their 180 patients had a pronated foot configuration. This study does not take into consideration the total number of people in the running population from whom this select group was derived who also pronate but do not have an injury problem.

Another aspect in epidemiological studies is the failure to provide an accurate definition of the factor to be analyzed. In sport injury studies, significant variations are seen in the definition of what constitutes an injury. As an example, it is difficult to compare studies where an injury is anything that causes an athlete to require medical attention and lose time from participation[12,133] with studies that have much stricter definitions and classifications.[60,157] The comparison difficulties are further increased when different sports and participation levels are compared. There may be significant differences in considering the injury of a recreational runner as opposed to that of a professional rugby player.[25] In addition, pain recognition and processing by the central nervous system may change during the years of hard training.[139]

Finally, the homogeneity of the population being studied is important. This relates to such considerations as exposure to injury, age differences, gender differences, preexisting injury, and other confounding variables that may significantly influence injuries.[22] For instance, it has been demonstrated in several studies that weekly running mileage is the single most critical factor in the risk of injury in the running population.[13,90,96,122,160] At distances of over 64 km (40 miles) per week, the injury rate seems to increase exponentially. Other risk factors have not been confirmed through all these studies.

WORK-RELATED INJURIES

Epidemiology

Attempts to characterize and quantify work-related injuries to the foot and ankle are few. Jobs involving extensive manual material handling or vehicular operations were the occupations most often listed by those with foot-related injuries.

Etiology

Specifically, foot injuries were found to be associated with being struck by boxes, metal objects, or vehicles, or to being caught in, under, or between vehicles or machinery. From a total of 990 work-related injuries to the foot, being struck accounted for 58.4% across occupational groups.[114] Regardless of the industry group, metal items and vehicles were related to 50.7% of all work-related foot injuries.

Prevention

To reduce the incidence of foot injuries, workers in many industries are required to wear safety footwear incorporating a steel toe cap. In Australia, an investigation of 321 workers employed in a broad range of work activities and required to wear safety footwear revealed an extremely high percentage (91%) of subjects reporting one or more foot problems that were verified by a professionally trained podiatrist.[95] Most of these subjects believed that the safety footwear either caused the problem or adversely affected an existing foot condition. The main shoe concerns were excessive heat (65%), inflexible soles (52%), weight (48%), and pressure from the steel toe cap (47%). Whether the priority is safety or comfort may obviously create a conflict. Ideally, there is a compromise between knowledge and experience in choosing shoes for industry workers to allow the best possible supply of safety footwear.

MILITARY-RELATED INJURIES

Epidemiology

Among the U.S. Marine Corps, training-related initial injuries to the foot were found at a rate of 3.0 new injuries per 1000 recruit days.[88] The highest specific rates of injuries occurred with stress fractures to the foot (0.56 per 1,000 recruit days), ankle sprains (0.53), and Achilles tendinitis (0.39). Among an air assault division, foot and ankle injuries were the most prevalent and severe category of injury for combat unit soldiers.[40] In a 1-year period, the average combat unit soldier sustained 0.16 foot injuries with an estimated 3.2 effective duty days lost. A prospective study of 295 male Israeli military recruits reported a 31% incidence of stress fractures.[107] Most of the fractures (80%) were in the tibial or femoral shaft, whereas only 8% occurred in the tarsus and metatarsus. Excessive rates of stress fractures were also found by other authors.[10,11,135]

Etiology

Stress fractures are common injuries sustained during military training. Excessive physical demands in military service may cause the majority of these injuries to the foot and ankle.[10,11,79,107] Typically, fatigue fractures were seen mostly in the first months of enlistment, indicating an acute overuse of bones.[135]

Flatfeet have been a disqualifying factor for military service in the past. Specific studies, however, have shown that those recruits with flat or pronated feet had no greater incidence of stress fracture than the normal population.[29,52] In contrast, a more recent study of Israeli military recruits showed that those recruits with a

low arch had a higher incidence of metatarsal stress fractures than did those who had a higher arch, whereas the number of stress fractures of the tibia and femur was lower in low-arch than in high-arch feet.[143] Other causes are cold weather injuries[152] and inflammatory foot lesions.[67]

Prevention

To determine the effect of the appropriateness of foot-shoe fit and training shoe type on the incidence of overuse injuries, the Israeli Defense Forces Medical Corps conducted a prospective study.[39] Among infantry recruits, they found that three shoe widths for each shoe length size were necessary to adequately accommodate the recruit population's foot anatomy. Recruits compensated for the lack of available shoe widths by choosing larger shoe sizes, which did not result in a higher incidence of overuse injuries. Switching to tennis shoes substantially reduced calcaneal stress fractures in military recruits.[56] A study of South African military recruits reported a reduction in overuse injuries by incorporating a neoprene insole into the shoe used in training.[140] However, surprisingly, no mid-term to long-term studies have systematically assessed the effectiveness of footwear improvements on the fitness for action of soldiers, although such knowledge should be of highest interest.

SPORT-RELATED INJURIES

Epidemiology

Injuries to the lower extremities constitute the majority of injuries in most sports, especially in the running, jumping, and kicking sports. Twenty-five percent of 12,681 injuries in the top 19 sports injuries seen in a multispeciality sports medicine clinic occurred at the ankle and foot. The percentages of foot and ankle injuries varied substantially from sport to sport, as did the proportion of sprains versus overuse injuries at each location.[49] If injury rates for the foot and ankle are determined from studies performed for various sports (**Table 43-1**), the magnitude of the athletic injury problem can be estimated by multiplying these rates by the number of participants in the given sport. Obviously, some sports have an extremely high risk for injuries to the ankle or foot, whereas the injury rate is minimal in other sports.

Etiology

The risk of sustaining an injury in a given sport may depend on different factors such as velocity, exposure to other players or obstacles, playing environment, training techniques, and equipment. These factors are among some of the extrinsic factors, whereas the individual's physical and personality traits constitute the intrinsic factors.[22] The factors most associated with injuries to the foot and ankle in sports include anatomical or biomechanical abnormalities, lack of flexibility,

Table 43-1 Injury rates calculated for the foot and ankle in various sports from a review of the literature.

Sport	First Author	Year	Skill Level	Ankle Injury (%)	Foot Injury (%)
Aerobics	Garrick[47]	1986	Recreational	11	18
	Rothenberger[131]	1988	Recreational	12	5
Ballet	Garrick[45]	1986	Various	17	22
	Sohl[148]	1990	Review of literature	14	15
	Garrick[48]	1993	Various	12	22
Baseball	Garfinkle[44]	1981	Professional	10	4
Basketball	Moretz[108]	1978	High school	31	8
	Henry[59]	1982	Professional	18	6
	Zelisko[164]	1982	Professional	19	4
Cycling	Davis[27]	1980	NA*	F&A	8
	Kiburz[82]	1986	Club	F&A	14
Dance (general)	Washington[161]	1978	Various levels	17	15
	Rovere[132]	1983	Students	22	15
Equestrian	Bernhang[6]	1983	Top class	F&A	13
	Bixby-Hammett[9]	1985	Top class	F&A	6
Football	Blyth[15]	1974	High school	15	2
	Canale[20]	1981	College	11	2
	Culpepper[26]	1983	High school	11	4
	Zemper[165]	1989	College	16	4
Golf	McCarrol[98]	1982	Professional	2	3
	McCarrol[99]	1990	Amateur	3	2
Gymnastics	Garrick[50]	1980	High school	10	8
	Caine[19]	1989	Club	21	3
Handball	Lindblad[87]	1992	Various	21	5
Ice hockey	Sutherland[151]	1976	Amateur	0	0
			High school	0	0
			College	7	10
			Professional	0	0
	Park[115]	1980	Junior	4	1
Lacrosse	Nelson[111]	1981	College	14	4
	Müller[110]	1982	College	15	4
Mountaineering	McLennan[100]	1983	NA	41	8
	Tomczak[154]	1989	NA	40	35
Netball	Hopper[69]	1993	Australian elite	14	NA

Adapted from Clanton TO: Etiology of injury to the foot and ankle. In Drez D Jr, DeLee JC, editors: Orthopaedic sports medicine, *Philadelphia, 1992, WB Saunders.*

*NA, not available; F&A, foot and ankle; USSA, U.S. Skiing Association.

Table 43-1 Injury rates calculated for the foot and ankle in various sports from a review of the literature—cont'd.

Sport	First Author	Year	Skill Level	Ankle Injury (%)	Foot Injury (%)
Orienteering	Johansson[76]	1986	Elite	26	13
	Hintermann[63]	1992	Various	24	11
Parachuting	Petras[120]	1983	Military	7	0.3
Rodeo	Meyers[103]	1990	College	6	1
Roller skating	Ferkel[38]	1981	College	10	NA
	Perlik[116]	1982	NA	8	2
Rugby	Micheli[104]	1974	College/club	8	2
	Gibbs[51]	1993	Professional	F&A	4
Running	Gottlieb[53]	1980	Recreational	19	11
	Temple[153]	1983	NA	26	26
	Marti[96]	1988	NA	30	10
	Walter[160]	1989	Recreational	15	16
Ice skating	Smith[145]	1982	Ages 11-19 yr	29	8
	Brown[17]	1987	National males	8	8
Skiing (downhill)	Johnson[77]	1980	Various	9	NA
	Blitzer[14]	1984	Youth	F&A	8
	Bladin[12]	1993	Various	F&A	6
Skiing (freestyle)	Dowling[30]	1982	USSA	8	NA
Skiing (snow boarding)	Pino[121]	1989	Recreational	26	3
	Bladin[12]	1993	Various	F&A	23
Skiing (jumping)	Wright[163]	1991	Various	5	1
Skiing (cross-country)	Hintermann[60]	1992	Youth elite	8	18
Soccer	Ekstrand[33]	1983	Swedish senior division	17	12
	Nielson[112]	1989	Various	36	8
	Berger-Vachon[5]	1986	French amateur leagues	20	NA
Squash/racquetball	Berson[7]	1978	Recreational	21	2
	Soderstrom[147]	1982	NA	20	7
Tennis	Winge[162]	1989	Elite	11	9
Volleyball	Schafle[137]	1990	National amateur	18	6
Water skiing	Hummel[73]	1982	NA	4	15
Weight training	Kulund[84]	1978	Elite/Olympic	2	0
Wind surfing	Mettler[102]	1991	Various	NA	1
Wrestling	Lok[89]	1975	Olympic	10	0
	Roy[134]	1979	College	10	3
	Requa[124]	1981	High school	4	NA
	Snook[146]	1982	College	4	0

poor strength or muscle imbalance, the type of shoe and/or use of orthoses, and the type of playing surface.[22,25]

ANATOMIC/BIOMECHANICAL ABNORMALITIES

Various anatomical conditions have been frequently associated with athletic injuries: alignment of the lower extremity and/or overpronation has been associated with injuries to the knee, ankle, and foot, and foot configuration has been associated with stress fractures of the lower extremity. The belief that runners who overpronate initially have a higher risk of sustaining a running-related injury is still held by most runners and their coaches, although no reliable study has supported this. Probably the most comprehensive study of running-related injuries, the Ontario cohort study, showed that none of the anthropometric variables such as femoral neck anteversion, knee and patella alignment, rearfoot valgus, pes cavus/planus, and running shoe wear pattern were significantly related to risk.[160] Similarly, although lower-extremity injuries in dancing have been related to poor technique and malalignment,[58,71,97] two independent studies failed to confirm such an association.[101,149]

Indeed, anatomical/biomechanical alterations appear to be casually related to injury. In running, for instance, overpronation may result in running-related overuse injuries,[60,73] but probably in fewer than 10%.[25] Nevertheless, approximately 70% of injured runners who are treated with orthotic devices will improve.[23,60,73]

FLEXIBILITY

A lack of flexibility as a result of limited joint motion is a common cause of injuries to the foot and ankle. Restricted dorsiflexion at the ankle joint is a factor in the anterior ankle pain often seen in soccer players associated with anterior tibial osteophytes (**Fig. 43-1**)[42] and/or a meniscoid lesion.[37] Also, other problems around the foot and ankle are believed to be due to restricted ankle dorsiflexion, including turf toe,[130] bunions,[94] midfoot strain and plantar fasciitis,[81,85] ankle sprains,[159] Achilles tendinitis,[21,141] calf strains,[32,33] and hyperpronation.[16,22,92] However, although these conditions have been related to a tight Achilles tendon, no study has yet confirmed such an association.

A deficit of dorsiflexion at the first metatarsophalangeal joint, as is typically the case in hallux rigidus,[66,93] has been related to turf toe injuries (**Fig. 43-2**). However, more recent work did not confirm this.[24] Limitation of motion at the interphalangeal joint is often connected to deformities such as hammer toe or mallet toe and thus creates a problem (**Fig. 43-3**).

On the other hand, hypermobility can also cause injury problems at the foot and ankle. The hypermobility syndrome has been described as a potential source of musculoskeletal symptoms.[22] In most cases this syndrome has no association with connective tissue disorders, including Down syndrome, Marfan syndrome,

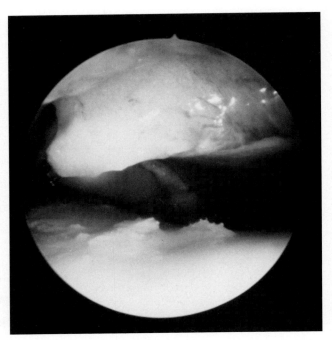

Figure 43-1 Anterior osteophytes on the distal end of the tibia in a 28-year-old soccer player (arthroscopic view in the medial plane) can cause restriction of dorsiflexion and cartilage degeneration on the talus.

Ehlers-Danlos syndrome, and osteogenesis imperfecta.[55,70,150] In certain sports, however, high flexibility is needed. Ballet dancers, divers, and gymnasts are particularly noted for the tremendous mobility in their feet and ankles that allows them to achieve maximum plantar flexion so that the foot is parallel to the lower leg. Although such increased mobility has obvious advantages, an increased incidence of injury was noted in those ballet dancers who have greater mobility.[83] At the opposite side, this can create posterior ankle pain from impingement.

A pathologic increase in joint laxity is termed *instability*.[22] Instability in the ankle joint, whether the result of a proprioceptive deficit, loss of ligamentous integrity, or some other factor, is a major factor in recurrent injuries to the ankle. Studies in Norway and Finland reported that acute ankle sprains accounted for 16% and 21% of all athletic injuries, respectively, in those countries.[91,136] In basketball, ankle sprains accounted for 45% of all injuries, and in soccer, 17% to 31% of all injuries are ankle sprains.[35,46,136] A history of a previous ankle sprain makes a soccer player twice as likely to have a new ankle sprain as a player without prior injury.[33] The same observation was made in orienteers.[62,76]

STRENGTH

The belief that weak musculature predisposes an individual to injury in sports has been supported by various studies. Soccer players who sustained a minor

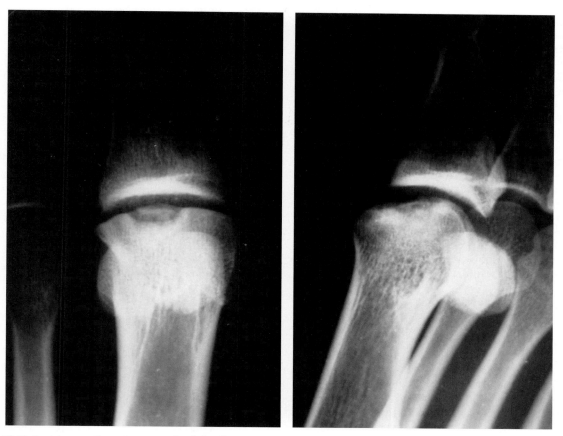

Figure 43-2 Post traumatic osteonecrosis of the first metatarsal head following a turf toe injury in a 19-year-old orienteer. As the apex of the head breaks, the phalanx starts to impinge on the dorsal aspect, which results in dorsal capsulitis and osteophyte formation limiting dorsiflexion. *(From Hintermann B et al:* Unfallchirurg 230 (suppl): *425-432, 1993.)*

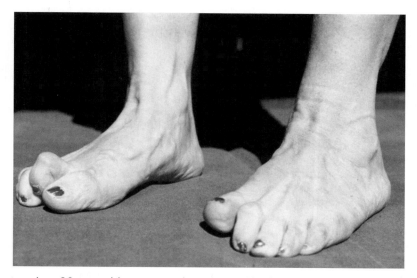

Figure 43-3 Hammer toes in a 39-year-old runner as the source of both pain and shoe-fitting problems.

injury during the preceding 2 months and subsequently had inadequate rehabilitation and poor muscle strength had a 20% increase in risk for a more serious subsequent injury.[31,33] Among 1139 young soccer players, 216 injuries were observed during a summer training camp.[3] Most of these injuries involved the ankle joint. The highest incidence of injury occurred in boys who were tall and had a weak grip strength, which suggests that skeletally mature but muscularly weak boys were at increased risk for injury as compared with their peers. Other studies have concluded that strength differences of more than 10% between the right and left legs increased the risk for injury.[4,18] This corresponds to the observation that the institution of a prophylactic program, including rehabilitation to the point that 90% of muscle strength had been regained, reduces the incidence of injury in soccer players by 75%.[34] Other studies have also shown that improving strength can reduce the risk for reinjury.[1,33]

SHOE WEAR AND ORTHOSES

Foot fixation on a playing surface resulting in abnormal torque is the most commonly cited etiological factor for noncontact injuries to the knee and ankle.[25] These injuries obviously depend on the playing surface and are often attributed to the shoe-surface interface. This aspect will be discussed in a later section.

When the shoe is improperly fitted, an overly high shoe causes pressure-related pain at the site of bunions and bunionettes. As an example, one can see aggravation of a bunion in a metatarsus primus varus or an accessory navicular from an ice skating boot and irritation of the Achilles tendon from many varieties of shoe wear. It could be that local pressure at the heel may in some cases produce retrocalcaneal bursitis.[57] The painful irritation of the retrocalcaneal bursa (**Fig. 43-4**) often seen in runners and cross-country skiers,[60,61] however, is more likely to be caused by the friction resulting from gliding of the tendon over the posterior calcaneal bone due to eversion-inversion movement of the calcaneus than by an improperly fitted shoe heel.[64] When the shoe is too short, the toes jam into the end, and nail problems occur. When the shoe is too loose, it allows the foot to slide, and blisters result.

A lack of cushioning and/or support by the shoe has also been implicated as a specific factor in overuse injuries.[113] Whereas some reports showed beneficial effects of cushioned shoes in reducing injuries,[56,126,140] other studies have been less conclusive or have shown no benefit from increased shock absorption in either shoes or insoles.[43,79,105,106] There is even an interesting counterproposal to the idea that improved cushioning in the shoe is protective to the body.[129] The authors hypothesize that increased cushioning can actually be an etiological factor in injury by dampening the body's own sensory feedback mechanism coming from the plantar surface of the foot.[127,128]

Torque is one of the most dangerous forces to which the body is subjected in sports.[25] Cleating of the athletic

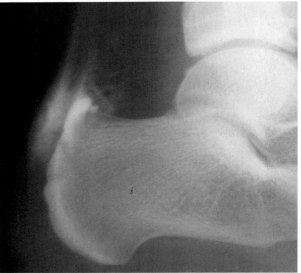

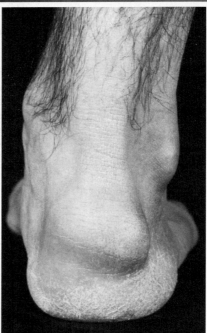

Figure 43-4 Retrocalcaneal bursitis in a 26-year-old orienteer as the source of pain, restriction of dorsiflexion at the ankle, and shoe-fitting problems.

shoe is designed to improve traction for more efficient performance but can significantly contribute to rotational load.[2,138,158] The number, length, and pattern of the cleats[156] as well as the outsole material and sole pattern[123] have been shown to substantially influence traction. In high school football, the number of ankle injuries was halved by changing from the traditional seven-cleated grass shoe to a soccer-style shoe.[133] The same result was found in another study, where the rate of ankle injuries decreased from 0.45 to 0.23 per team per game when soccer-style shoes were used.[155] On the other hand, a lack of traction can potentially cause injury by increasing the frequency of slips and falls.[25] As an example, slipping on wet tennis surfaces was a factor in 21% of injuries.[8] Obviously, superior performance demands maximum traction, but at some point this can exceed the body's ability to handle the load.

PLAYING SURFACES

Resurfacing and maintaining the grass practice and game fields can reduce injury rates about 30%.[110] Several studies of soccer,[68] dance,[47,58] and ice hockey[36,142] also indicated the playing surface as a relevant factor in injury. Janda and coworkers[74] found that 70% of recreational softball injuries were related to sliding into fixed bases. Follow-up to this study showed a 98% reduction in serious injuries when breakaway bases were used, which demonstrates a potential for significant savings in medical care costs.[75] In running, however, although the opinion that hard surfaces and hills are big factors in injuries is widely held, several studies did not prove a relationship between surface and injury.[90,122,160]

PREVENTION

By analysis of the risk factors, as mentioned in the preceding section, it is sometimes possible to intervene in a way to reduce or eliminate the risk factor and thereby lower the risk for injury. This is indeed the aim of preventive sports medicine. Examples of such intervention include rule changes in football to eliminate the crackback block[117-119] and improved generations of synthetic grass and underpadding brought about by research into the relationship between artificial turf and injury.[86,144] In softball, a reduction in injuries of about a factor of 23 was shown when breakaway bases were used instead of stationary bases.[75] During a 3-year follow-up in junior elite cross-country skiers, the prevalence of overuse injuries to the lower extremity decreased from 62% to 22% when individual shoe adaptations and/or orthotic devices were made (**Fig. 43-5**).[60] Supervision by a doctor and physiotherapist,[34] a reduction in muscle tightness,[1,33] the use of shock-absorbent insoles,[43,105,106,140] orthotic devices,[143] external support (**Fig. 43-6**),[65,80] or ankle taping,[41] and injury prevention through barefoot adaptations[129] are among some of the preventive means to reduce injuries to the foot and ankle.

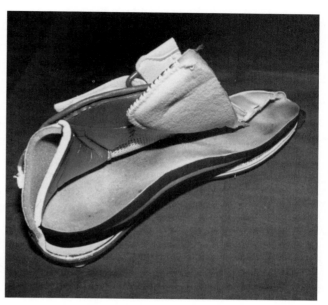

Figure 43-5 Individual corrections by an orthotic device that replaces the custom-made insole may prevent injury, as our study in youth cross-country skiers showed. *(From Hintermann B: Swiss Praxis 81:389-393, 1992.)*

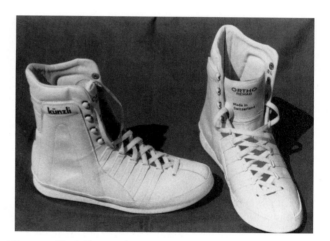

Figure 43-6 External support of the ankle joint, on the medial and lateral side, as in these shoes, may prevent injury. In addition, these shoes allow the injured individual to start working and training early.

References

1. Agre JC: Hamstring injuries: proposed etiologic factors, prevention, and treatment, *Sports Med* 2:21-33, 1985.

2. Andreasson G, Lindenberger U, Renström P, et al: Torque developed at simulated sliding between sport shoes and an artificial turf, *Am J Sports Med* 14:225-230, 1986.

3. Backous DD, Friedl KE, Smith, NJ, et al: Soccer injuries and their relation to physical maturity, *Am J Dis Child* 142:839-842, 1988.

4. Bender JA, Pierson JK, Kaplan HM, et al: Factors affecting the occurrence of knee injuries, *J Assoc Phys Ment Rehabil* 18:130-134, 1964.

5. Berger-Vachon C, Gabard G, Moyen B: Soccer accidents in the French Rhone-Alps Soccer Association, *Sports Med* 3:69-77, 1986.

6. Bernhang AM, Winslett G: Equestrian injuries, *Phys Sports Med* 11:90-97, 1983.

7. Berson BL, Passoff TL, Nagelberg S, et al: Injury patterns in squash players, *Am J Sports Med* 6:323-325, 1978.

8. Biener K, Caluori P: Sports accidents in tennis players, *Med Klin* 72:754-757, 1977.

9. Bixby-Hammett DM: Youth accidents with horses, *Phys Sports Med* 13:105-117, 1985.

10. Black JR: Stress fractures of the foot in female soldiers: a two-year survey, *Mil Med* 146:694-695, 1982.

11. Black JR: Stress fractures of the foot in male soldiers: a two-year survey, *J Am Podiatr Assoc* 73:633-634, 1983.

12. Bladin C, Giddings G, Robinson M: Australian snowboard injury data base study: a four-year prospective study, *Am J Sports Med* 21:701-704, 1993.

13. Blair SN, Kohl HW, Goodyear NN: Rates and risks for running and exercise injuries: studies in three populations, *Res Q* 58:221-228, 1987.

14. Blitzer CM, Johnson RJ, Ettlinger CF, et al: Downhill skiing injuries in children, *Am J Sports Med* 12:142-147, 1984.

15. Blyth CS, Müller FO: Football injury survey: Part 1. when and where players get hurt, *Phys Sports Med* 2:45-52, 1974.

16. Brody DM: Running injuries—prevention and management, *Clin Symp* 39:1-36, 1987.

17. Brown EW, McKeag DB: Training experience, and medical history of pairs skaters, *Phys Sports Med* 15:101-114, 1987.

18. Burkett LH: Causative factors in hamstring strains, *Med Sci Sports Exerc* 2:39-42, 1970.

19. Caine D, Cochrane B, Caine C, et al: An epidemiological investigation of injuries affecting young competitive male gymnasts, *Am J Sports Med* 17:811-820, 1989.

20. Canale ST, Cantler ED, Sisk TD, et al: A chronicle of injuries of an American intercollegiate football team, *Am J Sports Med* 9:384-389, 1981.

21. Clancy WG Jr: Tendinitis and plantar fasciitis in runners. In D'Ambrosia RD, Drez D Jr, editors: *Prevention and treatment of running injuries,* ed 2, Thorofare, N.J., 1989, Charles B. Slack.

22. Clanton TO: Etiology of injury to the foot and ankle. In Drez D Jr, DeLee JC, editors: *Orthopaedic sports medicine,* Philadelphia, 1992, WB Saunders.

23. Clanton TO: Sport shoes, insoles and orthoses. In Drez D Jr, DeLee JC, editors: *Orthopaedic sports medicine,* Philadelphia, 1992, WB Saunders.

24. Clanton TO, Eggert KE, Pivarnik JM, et al: First metatarsophalangeal joint range of motion as a factor in turf toe injuries, *Am J Sports Med,* (in press).

25. Clanton TO, Schon LC: Athletic injuries to the soft tissues of the foot and ankle. In Mann RA, Coughlin NJ, editors: *Surgery of the foot and ankle,* St. Louis, 1993, Mosby–Year Book; pp. 1095-1224.

26. Culpepper MI, Niemann KMW: High school football injuries in Birmingham, Alabama, *South Med J* 76:873-878, 1983.

27. Davis MW, Litman T, Crenshaw RW: Bicycling injuries, *Phys Sports Med* 8:88-96, 1980.

28. DeLee JC: Fractures and dislocations. In Mann RA, Coughlin MJ, editors: *Surgery of the foot and ankle,* St. Louis, 1993, Mosby–Year Book; pp. 1465-1467

29. DeVan WT, Carlton DC: The march fracture persists: a report on 143 cases during a fifteen-month period at an infantry basic center, *Am J Surg* 87:227-231, 1954.

30. Dowling PA: Prospective study of injuries in United States Ski Association freestyle skiing: 1976-77 to 1989-80, *Am J Sports Med* 10:268-275, 1982.

31. Ekstrand J, Gillquist J: The avoidability of soccer injuries, *Int J Sports Med* 4:124-128, 1983.

32. Ekstrand J, Gillquist J: The frequency of muscle tightness and injuries in soccer players, *Am J Sports Med* 10:75-78, 1982.

33. Ekstrand J, Gillquist J: Soccer injuries and their mechanisms: a prospective study, *Med Sci Sports Exerc* 15:267-270, 1983.

34. Ekstrand J, Gillquist J, Liljedahl SO: Prevention of soccer injuries: supervision by doctor and physiotherapist, *Am J Sports Med* 11:116-120, 1983.

35. Ekstrand J, Tropp H: The incidence of ankle sprains in soccer, *Foot Ankle* 11:41-44, 1990.

36. Feriencik K: Trends in ice hockey injuries: 1965-1977, *Phys Sports Med* 7:81-84, 1979.

37. Ferkel RD, Karzel RP, Pizzo WD, et al: Arthroscopic treatment of anterolateral impingement of the ankle, *Am J Sports Med* 19:440-446, 1991.

38. Ferkel RD, Mai LL, Ullis KC, et al: An analysis of roller skating injuries, *Am J Sports Med* 9:24-30, 1981.

39. Finestone A, Shlamkovitch N, Eldad A, et al: A prospective study of the effect of the appropriateness of foot-shoe fit and training shoe type on the incidence of overuse injuries among infantry recruits, *Mil Med* 157:489-490, 1992.

40. Fleming JL: One-year prevelance of lower extremity injuries among active duty military soldiers, *Mil Med* 153:476-478, 1988.

41. Fumich RM, Ellison AE, Guerin GJ, et al: The measured effect of taping on combined foot and ankle motion before and after exercise, *Am J Sports Med* 9:165-190, 1981.

42. Gächter A, Hintermann B: *Post-traumatic changes of the ankle joint: alterations of the ventral tibial lip* (unpublished study).

43. Gardner L, Dziados JE, Jones BH, et al: Prevention of lower extremity stress fractures: a controlled trial of a shock absorbent insole, *Am J Publ Health* 78:1563-1567, 1988.

44. Garfinkle D, Talbot AA, Clarizio M, et al: Medical problems on a professional baseball team, *Phys Sports Med* 9:85-93, 1981.

45. Garrick JG: Ballet injuries, *Med Probl Perform Arts* 1:123-127, 1988.

46. Garrick JG: The frequency of injury, mechanism of injury, and epidemiology of ankle sprains, *Am J Sports Med* 5:241-242, 1977.

47. Garrick JG, Gillien DM, Whiteside P: The epidemiology of aerobic dance injuries *Am J Sports Med* 14:67-72, 1986.

48. Garrick JG, Requa RK: Ballet injuries: an analysis of epidemiology and financial outcome, *Am J Sports Med* 21:586-590, 1993.

49. Garrick JG, Requa RK: The epidemiology of foot and ankle injuries in sports, *Clin Podiatr Med Surg* 6:629-637, 1989.

50. Garrick JG, Requa RK: Epidemiology of women's gymnastics injuries, *Am J Sports Med* 8:261-262, 1980.

51. Gibbs N, Dip G: Injuries in professional rugby league: a three-year prospective study of the South Sydney Professional Rugby League Football Club, *Am J Sports Med* 21:696-700, 1993.

52. Gilbert RS, Johnson HA: Stress fractures in military recruits—a review of twelve years' experience, *Mil Med* 131:716-721, 1966.

53. Gottlieb G, White JR: Responses of recreational runners to their injuries, *Phys Sports Med* 8:145-149, 1980.

54. Gould N, Schneider W, Ashikaga T: Epidemiological survey of foot problems in the continental United States, *Foot Ankle* 1:8-10, 1980.

55. Grahame R: Joint hypermobility—clinical aspects, *Proc R Soc Med* 64:692-694, 1971.

56. Greaney RB, Gerber FH, Laughlin RL, et al: Distribution and natural history of stress fractures in US Marine recruits, *Radiology* 146:339-346, 1983.

57. Haglund P: Contribution to the clinic of the Achilles tendon, *Orthop Chir* 49:49-58, 1928.

58. Hamilton WG: Foot and ankle injuries in dancers, *Clin Sports Med* 7:143-173, 1988.

59. Henry JH, Lareau B, Neigut D: The injury rate in professional basketball, *Am J Sports Med* 10:16-18, 1982.

60. Hintermann B: Long-term results after static correction of the lower extremity in young cross-country skiers, *Swiss Praxis* 81:389-393, 1992.

61. Hintermann B: Overuse injuries in cross-country skiing. In Matter P, Holzach P, Heim D, editors: *Winter sports accidents in Davos during the last 20 years,* Bern, Switzerland, 1993, Haupt.

62. Hintermann B, Hintermann M: Ankle sprains in orienteering—a simple injury? *Sci J Orienteering* 2:79-86, 1992.

63. Hintermann B, Hintermann M: A study of the 1991 Swiss 6-days orienteering event, *Sci J Orienteering* 2:72-78, 1992.

64. Hintermann B, Holzach P: The retrocalcaneal bursitis—a biomechanical analyzis and clinical study, *Z Orthop* 130:114-119, 1992.

65. Hintermann B, Holzach P, Matter P: The treatment of the lateral ankle ligament injury using the Ortho-Rehab-Shoe, *Schweiz Z Sportmed* 38:87-93, 1990.

66. Hintermann B, Weber M, Dick W, Feinstein R: Hallux rigidus—a post-traumatic osteonecrosis? *Unfallchirurg* 230(suppl.):425-432, 1993.

67. Hodges GR, DuClos TW, Schnitzer JS: Inflammatory foot lesions in naval recruits: significance and lack of response to antibiotic therapy, *Mil Med* 140:94-97, 1975.

68. Hoff GL, Martin TA: Outdoor and indoor soccer: injuries among youth players, *Am J Sports Med* 14:231-233, 1986.

69. Hopper D, Elliott B: Lower limb and back injury patterns of elite netball players, *Sports Med* 16:148-162, 1993.

70. Horan FT, Beighton PH: Recessive inheritance of generalized joint hypermobility, *Rheum Rehab* 12:47-49, 1973.

71. Howse J: Disorders of the great toe in dancers, *Clin Sports Med* 2:499-505, 1983.

72. Hummel G, Gainor BJ: Waterskiing-related injuries, *Am J Sports Med* 10:215-218, 1982.

73. James SL, Bates BT, Osternig LR: Injuries to runners, *Am J Sports Med* 6:40-50, 1978.

74. Janda DH, Wojtys EM, Hankin FM, et al: Softball sliding injuries: a prospective study comparing standard and modified bases, *JAMA* 259:1848-1850, 1988.

75. Janda DH, Wojtys EM, Hankin FM, et al: A three-phase analysis of the prevention of recreational softball injuries, *Am J Sports Med* 18:632-635, 1990.

76. Johansson C: Injuries in elite orienteers, *Am J Sports Med* 14:410-415, 1986.

77. Johnson RJ, Ettlinger CF, Campbell RJ, et al: Trends in skiing injuries: analysis of a 6-year study (1972-1978), *Am J Sports Med* 8:106-113, 1980.

78. Jones BH, Haris JM, Vinh TN, et al: Exercise-induced stress fractures and stress reactions of bone: epidemiology, etiology, and classification, *Exerc Sport Sci Rev* 17:379-422, 1989.

79. Jones RO, Christenson CJ, Lednar WM: Podiatric utilization referral patterns at an Army medical center, *Mil Med* 157:7-11, 1992.

80. Karlsson J, Andreasson GO: The effect of external ankle support in chronic lateral ankle joint instability: an electromyographic study, *Am J Sports Med* 20:257-261, 1992.

81. Kibler WB, Goldberg C, Chandler TJ: Functional biomechanical deficits in running athletes with plantar fasciitis, *Am Sports Med* 19:66-71, 1991.

82. Kiburz D, Jacobs R, Reckling F, et al: Bicycle accidents and injuries among adult cyclists, *Am J Sports Med* 14:416-419, 1986.

83. Klemp P, Chalton D: Articular mobility in ballet dancers: a follow-up study after four years, *Am J Sports Med* 17:72-75, 1989.

84. Kulund DN, Dewey JB, Brubaker CE, et al: Olympic weight lifting injuries, *Phys Sports Med* 6:111-119, 1978.

85. Kwong PK, Kay D, Voner RT, et al: Plantar fasciitis: mechanics and pathomechanics of treatment, *Clin Sports Med* 7:119-127, 1988.

86. Levy IM, Skovron ML, Agel J: Living with artificial grass: a knowledge update. Part 1: Basic science, *Am J Sports Med* 18:406-412, 1990.

87. Lindblad BE, Hoy K, Terkelsen CJ: Handball injuries: an epidemiologic and socioeconomic study, *Am J Sports Med* 20:441-444, 1992.

88. Linenger JM, Shwayhat AF: Epidemiology of podiatric injuries in US Marine recruits undergoing basic training, *J Am Podiatr Med Assoc* 82:269-271, 1992.

89. Lok V, Yuceturk G: Injuries of wrestling, *J Sports Med* 2:324-328, 1975.

90. Macera CA, Pate RR, Powell KE, et al: Predicting lower-extremity injuries among habitual runners, *Arch Intern Med* 149:2565-2568, 1989.

91. Maehlum S, Daljord OA: Acute sports injuries in Oslo: a one-year study, *Br J Sports Med* 18:181-185, 1984.

92. Mann RA, Baxter DE, Lutter LD: Running symposium, *Foot Ankle* 1:190-224, 1981.

93. Mann RA, Clanton TO: Hallux rigidus: treatment by cheilectomy, *J Bone Joint Surg* 70A:400-406, 1988.

94. Mann RA, Coughlin MJ: Hallux valgus and complications of hallux valgus. In Mann RA, editors, *Surgery of the foot,* ed 5, St. Louis, 1986, Mosby–Year Book; pp. 70-71.

95. Marr SJ, Quine S: Shoe concerns and foot problems of wearers of safety footwear, *Occup Med* 43:73-77, 1993.

96. Marti B, Vader JP, Minder CE, et al: On the epidemiology of running injuries. The 1984 Bern Grand-Prix study, *Am J Sports Med* 16:285-294, 1988.

97. Marshall P: The rehabilitation of overuse foot injuries in athletes and dancers, *Clin Sports Med* 7:175-191, 1988.

98. McCarroll JR, Gioe TJ: Professional golfers and the price they pay, *Phys Sports Med* 10:64-70, 1982.

99. McCarroll JR, Rettig AC, Shelbourne KD: Injuries in the amateur golfer, *Phys Sports Med* 18:122-126, 1990.

100. McLennan JG, Ungersma J: Mountaineering accidents in the Sierra Nevada, *Am J Sports Med* 11:160-163, 1983.

101. McNeal AP, Watkins A, Clarkson PM, et al: Lower extremity alignment and injury in young, preprofessional, college and professional ballet dancers. Part II: Dancer-reported injuries, *Med Probl Perform Arts* 5:83-88, 1990.

102. Mettler R, Biener K: Athletic injuries in wind surfing, *Schweiz Z Sportmed* 39:161-166, 1991.

103. Meyers MC, Elledge JR, Sterling JC, et al: Injuries in interscolastic rodeo athletes, *Am J Sports Med* 18:87-91, 1990.

104. Micheli LJ, Riseborough EM: The incidence of injuries in rugby football, *J Sports Med* 2:93-98, 1974.

105. Milgrom C, Burr DB, Boyd RD, et al: The effect of a viscoelastic orthotic on the incidence of tibial stress fractures in an animal model, *Foot Ankle* 10:276-279, 1990.

106. Milgrom C, Giladi M, Kasthan H, et al: A prospective study of the effect of a shock-absorbing orthotic device on the incidence of stress fractures in military recruits, *Foot Ankle* 6:101-104, 1985.

107. Milgrom C, Giladi M, Stein M, et al: Stress fractures in military recruits: a prospective study showing an unusually high incidence, *J Bone Joint Surg* 67B:732-735, 1985.

108. Moretz A. III, Grana WA: High school injuries. *Phys Sports Med* 6:92-95, 1978.

109. Müller FO, Blyth CS: North Carolina high school football injury study: equipment and prevention, *Am J Sports Med* 2:1-10, 1974.

110. Müller FO, Blyth CS: A survey of 1981 college lacrosse injuries, *Phys Sports Med* 10:87-93, 1982.

111. Nelson WE, DePalma B, Gieck JH, et al: Intercollegiate lacrosse injuries, *Phys Sports Med* 9:86-92, 1981.

112. Nielson AB, Yde J: Epidemiology and traumatology of injuries in soccer, *Am J Sports Med* 17:803-807, 1989.

113. Nigg BM: Biomechanical aspects of running. In Nigg BM, editor: *Biomechanics of running shoes,* Champaign, Ill., 1986, Human Kinetics; pp. 1-25.

114. Oleske DM, Hahn JJ, Leibold M: Work-related injuries to the foot: data from an occupational injury/illness surveillance system, *J Occup Med* 34:650-655, 1992.

115. Park RD, Castaldi CR: Injuries in junior ice hockey, *Phys Sports Med* 8:81-90, 1980.

116. Perlik PC, Kalvoda DD, Wellman AS, et al: Rollerskating injuries, *Phys Sports Med* 10:76-80, 1982.

117. Peterson TR: Blocking at the knee, dangerous and unnecessary, *Phys Sports Med* 1:46-50, 1973.

118. Peterson TR: The cross-body block, the major cause of knee injuries, *JAMA* 211:449-452, 1970.

119. Peterson TR: Knee injuries due to blocking: a continuing problem, *Phys Sports Med* 7:99-104, 1979.

120. Petras AF, Hoffman EP: Roentgenographic skeletal injury patterns in parachute jumping, *Am J Sports Med* 11:325-328, 1983.

121. Pino EC, Colville MR: Snowboard injuries, *Am J Sports Med* 17:778-781, 1989.

122. Powell KE, Kohl HW, Caspersen CJ, et al: An epidemiological perspective on the causes of running injuries, *Phys Sports Med* 14:100-114, 1986.

123. Rheinstein DJ, Morehouse CA, Niebel BW: Effects on traction of outsole composition and hardnesses of basketball shoes and three types of playing surfaces, *Med Sci Sports Exerc* 10:282-288, 1978.

124. Requa R, Garrick JG: Injuries in interscholastic wrestling, *Phys Sports Med* 9:44-51, 1981.

125. Rice SG: Epidemiology and mechanisms of sports injuries. In Teitz CC, editor: *Scientific foundations of sports medicine,* St. Louis, 1989, Mosby–Year Book; pp. 3-23.

126. Richie DH Jr, Delso SF, Belluci PA: Aerobic dance injuries: a retrospective study of instructors and participants, *Phys Sports Med* 13:130-140, 1985.

127. Robbins SE, Gouw GJ: Athletic footwear and chronic overloading: a brief review, *Sports Med* 9:76-85, 1990.

128. Robbins SE, Gouw GJ: Athletic footwear: unsafe due to perceptual illusions, *Med Sci Sports Exerc* 23:217-224, 1991.

129. Robbins SE, Hanna AM: Running-related injury prevention through barefoot adaptations, *Med Sci Sports Exerc* 19:148-156, 1987.

130. Rodeo SA, O'Brian S, Warren RF, et al: Turf-toe: an analysis of metatarsophalangeal joint sprains in professional football players, *Am J Sports Med* 18:280-285, 1990.

131. Rothenberger LA, Chang JI, Cable TA: Prevalence and types of injuries in aerobic dancers, *Am J Sports Med* 16:403-407, 1988.

132. Rovere GD, Webb LX, Gristina AG, et al: Musculoskeletal injuries in theatrical dance students, *Am J Sports Med* 11:195-198, 1983.

133. Rowe ML: Varsity football: knee and ankle injury, *NY State J Med* 69:3000-3003, 1969.

134. Roy SP: Intercollegiate wrestling injuries, *Phys Sports Med* 7:83-91, 1979.

135. Ruckert KF, Brinkmann ER: Fatigue fractures of the calcaneus in soldiers of the Federal Forces, *Munch Med Wochenschr* 117:681-684, 1975.

136. Sandelin J: *Acute sports injuries: a clinical and epidemiological study*, thesis, Helsinki, 1988, University of Helsinki; pp. 1-66.

137. Schafle MD, Requa RK, Patton WL, et al: Injuries in the 1987 National Amateur Volleyball Tournament, *Am J Sports Med* 18:624-631, 1990.

138. Schläpfer F, Unold E, Nigg BM: The frictional characteristics of tennis shoes. In Nigg BM, Kerr BA, editors: *Biomechanical aspects of sport shoes and playing surfaces,* Calgary, 1983, University of Calgary Press; pp. 153-160.

139. Schrode N, Larbig W, Heitkamp H, et al: Psychophysiological changes in marathon runners, *Sportwiss* 16:303-315, 1986.

140. Schwellnus MP, Jordaan G, Noakes TD: Prevention of common overuse injuries by the use of shock absorbing insoles: a prospective study, *Am J Sports Med* 18:636-641, 1990.

141. Segesser B, Nigg BM: Insertion tendinitis on the tibia, Achilles tendinitis and overuse injuries of the foot—etiology, biomechanics, and treatment, *Der Orthopäde* 9:207-214, 1980.

142. Sim FH, Simonet WT, Melton LJ, et al: Ice hockey injuries, *Am J Sports Med* 15:30-40, 1987.

143. Simkin A, Leichter I, Giladi M, et al: Combined effect of foot arch structure and an orthotic device on stress fractures, *Foot Ankle* 10:25-29, 1989.

144. Skovron ML, Levy IM, Agel J, et al: Living with artificial grass: a knowledge update. Part 2: Epidemiology, *Am J Sports Med* 18:510-523, 1990.

145. Smith AD, Micheli LJ: Injuries in competitive figure skaters, *Phys Sports Med* 10:36-47, 1982.

146. Snook GA: Injuries in intercollegiate wrestling: a five year study, *Am J Sports Med* 6:128-131, 1978.

147. Soderstrom CA, Doxanas MT: Raquetball: a game with preventable injuries, *Am J Sports Med* 10:180-183, 1982.

148. Sohl P, Bowling A: Injuries to dancers, *Sports Med* 9:317-322, 1990.

149. Solomon RL, Trepman E, Micheli LJ: Foot morphology and injury patterns in ballet and modern dancers, *Kinesiol Med Dance* 12:20-40, 1989.

150. Steiner ME: Hypermobility and knee injuries, *Phys Sports Med* 15:159-165, 1987.

151. Sutherland GW: Fire on ice, *Am J Sports Med* 4:264-269, 1976.

152. Taylor MS: Cold weather injuries during peacetime military training, *Mil Med* 157:602-604, 1992.

153. Temple C: Hazards of jogging and marathon running, *Br J Hosp Med* 29:237-239, 1983.

154. Tomczak RL, Wilshire WM, Lane JW, et al: Injury patterns in rock climbers, *J Osteopath Sports Med* 3:11-16, 1989.

155. Torg JS, Quedenfeld T: Effect of shoe type and cleat length on incidence and severity of knee injuries among high school football players, *Res Q* 42:203-211, 1971.

156. Torg JS, Quedenfeld T: Knee and ankle injuries traced to shoes and cleats, *Phys Sports Med* 1:39-43, 1973.

157. Torg JS, Quedenfeld TC, Landau S: The shoe-surface interface and its relationship to football knee injuries, *Am J Sports Med* 2:261-269, 1974.

158. Van Gheluwe B, Deporte E, Hebbelinck M: Frictional forces and torques of soccer shoes on artificial turf. In Nigg BM, Kerr BA, editors: *Biomechanical aspects of sport shoes and playing surfaces,* Calgary, 1983, University of Calgary Press; pp. 161-168.

159. Walsh WM, Blackburn T: Prevention of ankle sprains, *Am J Sports Med* 5:243-245, 1977.

160. Walter SD, Hart LE, McIntosh JM, et al: The Ontario cohort study of running-related injuries, *Arch Intern Med* 149:2561-2564, 1989.

161. Washington EL: Musculoskeletal injuries in theatrical dancers: site, frequency, and severity, *Am J Sports Med* 6:75-98, 1978.

162. Winge S, Jorgensen U, Nielsen AL: Epidemiology of injuries in Danish championship tennis, *Int J Sports Med* 10:368-371, 1989.

163. Wright JR, McIntyre L, Rands JJ, et al: Nordic ski jumping injuries: a survey of active American jumpers, *Am J Sport Med* 19:615-619, 1991.

164. Zelisko JA, Noble HB, Porter M: A comparison of men's and women's professional basketball injuries, *Am J Sports Med* 10:297-299, 1982.

165. Zemper ED: Injury rates in a national sample of college football teams: a 2-year prospective study, *Phys Sports Med* 17:100-113, 1989.

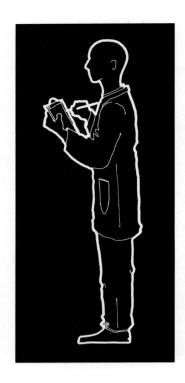

Chapter 44

Anthropometry of the Human Foot

Michael R. Hawes
Benno M. Nigg

CONTENTS

A brief description of the anatomy of the foot is presented to ensure standard nomenclature. A detailed description of the morphology of the foot will not be presented, however, because it is widely available from other excellent sources.[20,21,35]

DESCRIPTIVE ANATOMY

The foot (pes) consists of 26 bones, 12 extrinsic muscles, many more intrinsic muscles, and over 100 ligaments. It is described as having dorsal and plantar surfaces (upper and lower, respectively, in the anatomical position) and anterior, medial, and lateral borders. The hallux (great toe) and digitus minimus (little toe) are individually named, whereas the other toes are numbered from 1 to 5 medial to lateral.

Skeletal Structures

The skeletal framework of the foot is divided into the tarsus (seven irregular bones) constituting the midfoot (navicular, cuboid, and three cuneiform bones) and hindfoot (calcaneus and talus); metatarsals (five long bones in the forefoot between the tarsus and toes); and the phalangeals, which make up the toes (two in the hallux and three each in the remaining lateral toes).

Hindfoot
CALCANEUS
The heel bone projects posteriorly to the ankle joint to provide leverage for the triceps surae muscle group. The lower surface of the posterior end of the bone (the tuber) has rounded medial and lateral processes that provide contact surfaces during locomotion. Anteriorly, the calcaneus articulates with the cuboid, and superiorly and medially the sustentaculum tali supports the talus at the subtalar (talocalcaneal) joint.

TALUS
The talus is a unique bone that has no muscular attachments. Superiorly, the talus forms the ankle joint (talocrural) with the tibia and medially and laterally with the malleoli of the tibia and fibula. The inferior surface of the talus rests on the sustentaculum tali of the calcaneus, whereas anteriorly the bone articulates with the navicular.

Midfoot
NAVICULAR
The navicular lies anterior to the talus on the medial side of the foot and posterior to the cuneiform bones. On the lateral side, the navicular articulates with the cuboid.

CUNEIFORM BONES (MEDIAL, INTERMEDIATE, AND LATERAL)
The cuneiform bones lie in a series across the anterior surface of the navicular, and the lateral cuneiform articulates with the cuboid. Anteriorly, the three cuneiform bones articulate with the first three metatarsal bones.

CUBOID
The cuboid articulates posteriorly and anteriorly with the calcaneus and two lateral metatarsal bones, respectively. On the medial side, the cuboid articulates with the lateral cuneiform and the navicular.

Forefoot
The metatarsal bones are long bones with a distinct base, body, and head giving rise to five discrete rays. Each ray culminates in a digit consisting of a series of short phalangeal bones, proximal, middle, and distal in the four lateral toes and proximal and distal in the hallux.

FUNCTIONAL ANATOMY

The foot is a specialized organ that has the contrasting characteristics of providing the following:

- *Support* of body mass
- Static and dynamic *balance*
- Facilitation of *locomotion*

These characteristics are achieved by large muscles located in the shank, smaller intrinsic muscles of the foot, bony levers, and various degrees of joint mobility within the foot and ankle. Adequate muscular development and joint function are essential for normal gait and foot mechanics.

Foot Arches
Morphologically, the foot may be described as having three arches or trusses. Longitudinally, the arch of the foot is higher on the medial side than on its lateral side. The former involves the calcaneus, talus, navicular, cuneiforms, and three medial digits; the latter, although also arising from the calcaneus, proceeds through the cuboid and two lateral digits. In the midfoot region, the arch in the transverse plane is observed passing through the talus and navicular on the medial side to the calcaneus and cuboid on the lateral side. This arch gradually flattens anteriorly so that the heads of the metatarsal bones are all in the same plane. The arches are dynamically maintained by

- The keystone effect of the talus, cuboid, and middle cuneiform within the medial, lateral, and transverse arches respectively. The articular surfaces of these bones form a wedge that drops into place between adjacent bones.

- The bowstring effect of the plantar ligaments. The plantar calcaneonavicular (spring) ligament maintains the medial arch, whereas the short and long plantar ligaments maintain the lateral arch.
- The intrinsic and extrinsic muscles of the foot, which assist in maintaining the arches.

Morphologically, it is convenient to describe the foot in terms of three discrete arches; however, when forces distributed throughout the foot are considered, there is a complex interplay of stresses that acts among all the components of a single dynamic structure.

ASSESSMENT OF FOOT SHAPE AND DIMENSIONS

The dimensions and shape of the human foot are of interest for many reasons, including assessment of medical conditions, changes with growth, adaptation to functional stresses, and ergonomic considerations for the fitting of footwear. Many techniques are described in the literature, but the results may not be comparable because of differences in measurement protocol. These include different degrees of weight bearing in the measuring position,[5] nonstandard measuring devices such as cloth tape and a Brannock scale,[32] and indirect measurement from photographic images[31] that fail to account for the outward curvature of the foot from the sole to the maximum projection of bony and soft tissue. A technique[16] that consolidates many of the previously described techniques into a geometric model permitting accurate reconstruction of single or mean foot shapes for a variety of purposes (**Fig. 44-1**) will be discussed further.

Measurement Technique

Measurements are taken on one foot in a full weight-bearing position with the other foot resting lightly on a raised (25 cm) platform. The ankle joint is placed in a neutral position with the shank vertical and the body in a normal upright posture. Measurements of height (**Figs. 44-1 and 44-3**) are all taken in a vertical plane from the standing surface to the defined landmark. A vertical caliper is used to take measurements to the nearest 1 mm. Height measurements include hallux height, measured to the superior surface of the hallux. Medial and lateral metatarsal-phalangeal joint (MPJ) heights are measured to the superior points of the first and fifth joints; dorsum height is measured to the superior surface of the head of the talus; sphyrion fibulare height, pterion height, and maximum arch height are measured at the intersection of a vertical plane passing through the dorsum height on the margin of the medial plantar curvature.

LENGTH MEASUREMENTS

Length measurements (**Fig. 44-2**) are taken parallel to the long axis of the foot using a sliding caliper with adjustable branches. Measurements are recorded to the nearest 1 mm. Foot lengths to the most prominent point on the first, second, third, fourth, and fifth digits, to the metatarsal tibiale, and to the metatarsal fibulare are all measured from the most posteriorly projecting point on the heel, the pterion. Two additional length variables are measured to locate the position of the superior surface of the head of the talus (dorsum). The measurements are made from the dorsum to the akropodion and to the point of distal heel contact with the bearing surface.

BREADTH MEASUREMENTS

Breadth measurements (**Figs. 44-2 and 44-3**) are taken with a small sliding caliper to the nearest 1 mm in a horizontal plane perpendicular to the long axis of the foot. Foot breadth is measured between the metatarsal tibiale and fibulare, and maximum heel breadth is measured with compression to the bony surface at the point of maximum heel width, 2 to 3 mm above the standing surface and approximately 3 cm anterior to the

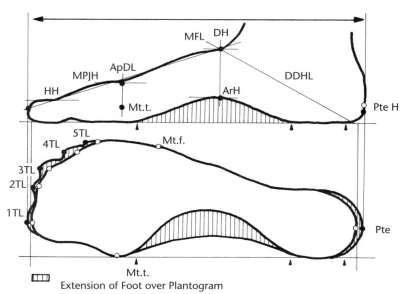

Figure 44-1 Foot model reconstructed from data points and a digitized plantogram.

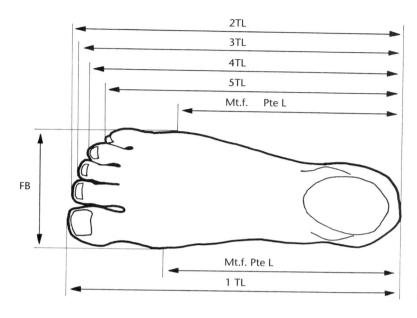

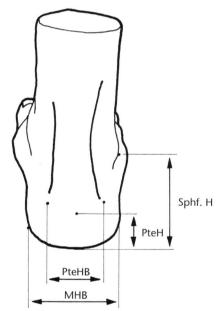

Figure 44-2 Measurement sites for length and breadth.

Figure 44-3 Measurement sites for breadths and heights and the heel.

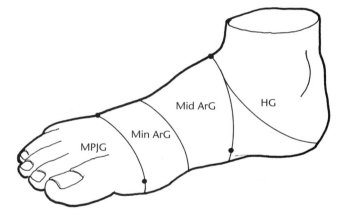

Figure 44-4 Measurement sites for girths.

pterion. Pterion heel breadth is measured by compression to the bony surface at the point of maximum width of the calcaneus at the level of the pterion.

GIRTH MEASUREMENTS

Girth measurements (**Fig. 44-4**) are taken with a narrow steel tape to the nearest 1 mm. The MPJ girth encompasses the metatarsal tibiale and fibulare. Minimum arch girth is measured with the subject elevating the heel, and minimum circumference is determined by serial measurements through the arch. Midarch girth is measured in the frontal plane passing through the

dorsum, and heel girth measurement encompasses the dorsum and the point of distal heel contact on the standing surface.

SHAPE

A basic two-dimensional shape of the foot is provided by a plantagram obtained with the subject momentarily standing with full body weight on the right foot on an ink tablet. The subject carefully transfers weight to the left foot and lifts the right foot from the ink pad. The plantagram is processed by tracing the outer contour of the print and subsequently digitizing the curve. Curves may be averaged by using a technique described by Hawes et al.[16]

Three-dimensional laser digitizing may appear to offer even more information about foot shape and dimension; however, it is limited to portrayal of the soft tissue margins and should include the more important measures associated with the underlying bony landmarks.

POPULATION DATABASES

Comprehensive descriptions of civilian populations are quite limited and often pertain to previous generations. The significance of the latter point may be debated, but genetically, a secular trend toward increased stature and mass is commonly observed in Western nations that would influence population means for foot variables from generation to generation. Additionally, the environmental influences acting on the foot, such as the shape and materials of footwear and the load-bearing characteristics of daily activity, have changed substantially in recent generations and are potential influences on the plastic elements of foot shape. Comprehensive descriptions of civilian populations include Spanish-American War veterans,[8] U.S. male veterans,[7] air-traffic controller trainees,[33] and Caucasian Canadian subjects aged 16 to 80 years.[17] Military studies include the work of Freedman and coworkers[11], who studied a large population of U.S. army inductees, and Dahlberg and Lander,[6] who reported on a Swedish population of military conscripts. **Table 44-1** compares the mean data from the latter three studies.

VARIABILITY IN FOOT SHAPE AND DIMENSION

Within the human species, variations in foot shape and proportion may appear to be relatively small, but differences are noted in the pattern of toe length (digital patterning), the height of the arch and instep (dorsum), the relationship between foot length and ball and heel breadth, the shape of the heel, and the angle across the anterior margin of the foot. Examination of the pattern and degree of variation in foot shape has significant implications within the realm of ergonomics, anthropology, and medical science.

Several factors may account for the variability in foot shape and dimension. In normal growth, the human foot changes shape and proportion as a result of the functional stresses of bipedal locomotion. The foot of an infant changes from a flat, highly mobile organ to a specialized structure that is characterized by greater rigidity and longitudinal and transverse arches.[36] Even in adulthood, the foot remains plastic. Robinson, Frederick, and Cooper[31] reported that the chronic stresses of habitual long-distance running are associated with elongation of the foot and lowering of the dorsum and the medial aspect of the MPJ. Similar results may be expected for specific jobs where foot loading is excessive. The type of footwear habitually worn may also be responsible for modifying the shape of the foot. Japanese forestry workers wearing a modified version of the traditional tabi footwear (glovelike footwear with a separate pocket for the great toe) have been shown by Morioka, Miura, and Kimura[24] to have substantially different-shaped feet when compared with city dwellers habitually wearing dress shoes. The tabi-wearing forestry workers had relatively larger and broader toes and

Table 44-1	Mean and standard deviation for foot variables with comparable values from American and Swedish military studies.				
	Current (Mean ± SD)	American	Effect Size Index (d1)	Swedish	Effect Size Index (d2)
Age (yr)	35.47 ± 11.85	22.80#		21.00‡	
N	1197	5575		8232	
Stature (cm)	176.71 ± 6.54			175.60‡	
Mass (kg)	77.31 ± 10.44			69.10‡	
HEIGHT (CM)					
HH	1.9 ± 0.40§	2.74#			
MPJH	3.55 ± 0.42§	3.88 ± 0.21	0.99		
DH	6.53 ± 0.61§	7.82 ± 0.49	2.33		
Sph f. H	5.98 ± 0.66				
Pte H	2.00 ± 0.47				
Ar H	2.12 ± 0.67§	2.83 ± 0.44	1.25		
LENGTH (CM)					
1TL	26.32 ± 1.23§‖	26.84 ± 1.16*†	0.43	26.63 ± 1.25	0.25

Table 44-1 Mean and standard deviation for foot variables with comparable values from American and Swedish military studies—cont'd

	Current (Mean ± SD)	American	Effect Size Index (d1)	Swedish	Effect Size Index (d2)
LENGTH (CM)—cont'd					
2TL	26.01 ± 1.22				
3TL	25.05 ± 1.20				
4TL	23.60 ± 1.12				
5TL	21.69 ± 1.05§	20.95 ± 0.98†	0.73		
Mt.f. Pte L	16.90 ± 0.93§	15.94 ± 0.90†	1.05		
Mt.t. Pte L	19.29 ± 0.96‖‡	19.26 ± 0.90†	0.03	19.98 ± 0.95	0.72
ApDL	14.73 ± 0.85				
DDHL	13.82 ± 0.79				
BREADTH (CM)					
FB	9.91 ± 0.57§	9.80 ± 0.52†	0.20		
MHB	6.30 ± 0.40§	6.96 ± 0.34†	1.78		
Pte HB	5.43 ± 0.53				
GIRTH (CM)					
MPJG	25.34 ± 1.30§‖	25.18 ± 1.16	0.13	25.62 ± 1.24	0.22
Min Ar G	25.43 ± 1.14‖			24.52 ± 1.16	0.95
Mid Ar G	25.38 ± 1.16‖	25.83 ± 1.14	0.39	26.12 ± 1.36	0.59
HG	35.89 ± 1.72§‖	4.41 ± 1.55	0.90	34.01 ± 1.50	1.16

Data on American studies from Freedman A, et al.: Foot dimensions of soldiers, Project No. T-13, Fort Knox, KY, 1946, Armored Medical Research Laboratory; data on Swedish military studies from Dahlberg G, Lander E: Acta Genet 1:115-161, 1948.

ApDL, *akropodion-to-dorsum length;* Ar H, *arch height;* DDHL, *dorsum-to-distal heel length;* DH, *dorsum height;* FB, *foot breadth;* HG, *heel girth;* HH, *hallux height;* MHB, *maximum heel breadth;* Mid Ar G, *midarch girth;* Min Ar G, *maximum arch girth;* MPJG, *metatarsal-phalangeal joint girth;* MPJH, *medial metatarsal-phalangeal height;* Mt. f., *metatarsale fibulare;* Mt. t., *metatarsale tibiale;* Pte H, *pterion height;* Pte HB, *pterion heel breadth;* Pte L, *pterion length;* Sph f. H, *sphyrion fibulare height;* 1TL, *foot length to the most prominent point on the first digit.*

d1, *effect size index between current and American studies;* d2, *effect size index between current and Swedish studies.*

*Correction factor applied.

†Measured from photograph

‡No significant difference reported

§Significant difference (p<0.001) between current and American studies

‖Significant difference (p<0.001) between current and Swedish studies

a reduced outward inclination of the great toe. The cleft between the first and second toe was substantially greater in the forestry workers than in the city workers. Perhaps the most dramatic example of foot adaptation to stress comes from the ancient Chinese practice of foot binding. This practice involved tight binding of the foot from a young age to reduce the length of the foot to approximately one third of the normal dimension.[25]

Ethnic Differences

Although the foot is clearly plastic in some of its elements, it has been suggested that different shape characteristics are typical of ethnic or racial populations. Cheskin[4] described foot shapes that are characteristic of the African American, Asian, and Caucasian races and asserted that "the classic Negro foot is broad in the forepart and narrow in the heel. . . . The classic

Asian foot is short and broad in the forepart and heel. The toes are straight with a large space between the big and second toe. . . . The Caucasian foot type is an equal mix of high, normal, and low arches." Freedman and coworkers[11] in a study of 6775 U.S. army personnel, draws attention to differences in foot dimensions of African American and Caucasian recruits and reports that in general, all length, breadth, and girth measurements and the dorsal toe elevation of African Americans tend to be larger than those of Caucasian subjects. On the other hand, toe length and breadth and all height measurements of the ball and arch appear to be smaller among the African American population. These statements refer to absolute differences and are not proportionate to foot length. When normalized to foot length, all height measurements of the African American sample are between −3.0% and −8.7% of the Caucasian sample, MPJ girth and instep girth are −2.1% and −1.7%, respectively, and ball breadth is −1.4% and heel breadth is +1.7% of the Caucasian sample. Therefore, in contrast to the perception of Cheskin,[4] the African American foot may be slightly narrower in the ball and wider in the heel when compared with a Caucasian foot of similar length.

Baba[1] measured the feet of a group of 826 Japanese male factory workers and compared various ratios with data published by Bernard and Hueber[3] of 5136 male French subjects. The analysis suggested that the Japanese subjects had consistently larger foot breadth and ball girth–to–foot length ratios than the French subjects did. This study tends to confirm the perception of Cheskin with respect to differences between Asian and Caucasian feet.

Hawes and coworkers[18] in a study of Japanese and Korean factory and white-collar workers, showed no practical difference in foot breadth between adult male Asian and North American Caucasian populations, although there were ergonomically significant differences between the populations in the height of the hallux, the location and angle of the MPJ axis, and the angle across the anterior margin of the foot.

Gender Differences

Although gender dimorphism has been studied extensively, the evidence in the literature about foot structure is confusing. The variable most frequently considered is foot breadth in relation to foot length. The American Standard Measurement book suggests that men's shoes should be wider than women's at any given length.[9] In contrast, Oliver[27] stated that women have proportionally wider feet than men. The Nike Laboratory reported a study using previously published data[11,23,26,28] that suggests that men and women have proportionately similar foot breadth relative to foot length. Robinson[30] reported some differences between the male and female foot, in particular, that foot breadth and dorsum height are greater in males than females at any given foot length.

Hawes[15] reported a study of 2132 subjects (1031 males and 1091 females) from three databases—North American adults, Asian adults, and North American children. A consistent dimorphic pattern was found in each of the three populations. The adult female foot appears to be proportionately narrower at both the ball and heel and to exhibit less volume throughout the ball, arch, and heel. The specific variables found to be significantly different between the two adult samples were the same in 8 of 11 variables. By contrast, children showed no evidence of dimorphism until 8 years of age, at which time the consistent adult pattern begins to emerge.

Growth

The foot assumes adult shape and dimension in a progressive manner throughout childhood as a result of genetically determined growth factors, the assumption of erect posture, and the adoption of bipedal locomotion. Throughout childhood, major changes take place in the shape, proportion, and dimension of the foot.

Although a comprehensive study of changing dimensions and proportions in children's feet does not appear to be available in the literature, some studies deal with discrete aspects of foot shape. Forriol and Pascual[10] discussed the high frequency of morphologically flat feet in young children aged 3 to 4 years. Over a period of time (up to 9 years), the authors noted a change in the footprint angle and the Chippaux-Smirak index. Beauchamp[2] noted that the normal longitudinal arch develops with correction of the physiological genu valgum by ages 5 to 6 years. Jaworski and Puch[19] noted an increase in footprint angle up to age 13 in girls and age 15 in boys. Staheli, Chew, and Corbett[34] recorded different arch index values between children and adults. Gould et al.[12] investigated the effect of different footwear on arch development from age 11 months to 5 years in 125 toddlers. Initially, all the children displayed pes planus, but the longitudinal arch developed more quickly in those subjects wearing arch support footwear. Gould and associates reported that genu valgum was present in 92.5% and hyperpronation in 77.9% of a population of 5-year-olds and that the sustentaculum tali (necessary for support of the talus) was only just showing signs of developing. Kleiger and Mankin[22] had previously reported that this structure was fully ossified by 4.5 to 5 years. In a later paper, Gould et al.[13] indicated that boys' feet are consistently one size larger than girls' feet at the same age and, in addition, are one size wider than girls'. Robinow, Johnston, and Anderson,[29] in an radiograph study of children aged 2.5 to 13 years, suggested that the changes with age in the development of the bony arch are remarkably small. The authors suggested that the arch is well developed from a very early age and also commented that differences in children's arches are largely determined by genetics. Hawes[14] described the increasingly acute angle across the anterior margin of the foot as foot length (and age) increases. In addition, the location and angle of the MPJ axis also changes with foot length, moving posteriorly and becoming more acute. The changing proportions of the many variables that describe the foot suggest that lasts for children's shoes cannot be linearly scaled from one midrange size. Although most of the length parameters are directly proportional to maximum foot length, breadth, girth, and height measurement show a diminishing relationship to maximum foot length.

References

1. Baba K: Foot measurement for shoe construction with reference to the relationship between foot length, foot breadth, and ball girth, *J Human Ergol* 3:149-156, 1975.

2. Beauchamp R: Pediatric foot and ankle problems, *Med Sport Sci* 23:128-144, 1987.

3. Bernard M, Hueber A: Connaissance du Pied Masculin Adulte, *Technicuir* 2(7):135-158, 1968.

4. Cheskin MP: *The complete handbook of athletic footwear,* New York, 1987, Fairchild Publications.

5. Cobey JC, Sella E: Standardizing methods of measurement of foot shape by including the effects of subtalar rotation, *Foot Ankle* 2(1):30-36, 1981.

6. Dahlberg G, Lander E: Size and form of the foot in men, *Acta Genet* 1(2):115-161, 1948.

7. Damon A, Seltzer CC, Stoudt HW, et al: Age and physique in healthy white veterans at Boston, *J Gerontol* 27(2):202-208, 1972.

8. Damon A, Stoudt HW: The functional anthropometry of old men, *Hum Factors* 5(5):485-491, 1963.

9. Dayton Last Works: *Standard measurements of lasts: standard margins of sole patterns,* Dayton, Ohio, 1924, Dayton Last Works.

10. Forriol F, Pascual J: Footprint analysis between three and seventeen years of age, *Foot Ankle* 11(2):101-104, 1990.

11. Freedman A, Huntington EC, Davis GC, et al: *Foot dimensions of soldiers:* Project No. T-13, Fort Knox, 1946, Armored Medical Research Laboratory.

12. Gould N, Moreland M, Alvarez R, et al: Development of the child's arch, *Foot Ankle* 9(5):241-245, 1989.

13. Gould N, Moreland M, Trevino S, et al: Foot growth in children age one to five years, *Foot Ankle,* 10(4):211-213, 1990.

14. Hawes MR: *Adidas anthropometric research report #7: changing morphometry of the human foot during growth, 2-12 years,* Calgary: Sport Anthropology Group, Human Performance Laboratory, 1991, The University of Calgary.

15. Hawes MR: *Adidas anthropometric research report #8— gender dimorphism of the human foot,* Calgary, Sport Anthropology Group, Human Performance Laboratory, 1992, University of Calgary.

16. Hawes MR, Heinemeyer R, Sovak D, et al: An approach to averaging digitized plantagram curves, *Ergonomics* 37(7):1227-1230, 1994.

17. Hawes MR, Sovak D: Quantitative morphology of the human foot in a North American population, *Ergonomics* 37(7):1213-1226, 1994.

18. Hawes MR, Sovak D, Miyashita M, et al: Ethnic differences in forefoot shape and the determination of shoe comfort, *Ergonomics* 37(1):187-197, 1994.

19. Jaworski JM, Puch EA: Morphology of overweighted children foot. In *Versammlung der anatomischen gesellschaft,* Leipzig, Germany, 1987; p. 89.

20. Jenkins DB: *Hollinshead's functional anatomy of the limbs and back,* Philadelphia, 1991, WB Saunders.

21. Kapandji IA: *The physiology of the joints,* Edinburgh, 1987, Churchill Livingstone.

22. Kleiger B, Mankin HJ: A roentgenological study of the development of the calcaneus by means of a posterior tangential view, *J Bone Joint Surg Am* 43A:961, 1961.

23. McConville JT, Churchill E, Churchill T, et al: *Anthropometry of women of the U.S. army comparative data for U.S. army men* (Report No 5), Natick, Mass, 1977, U.S. Army Research & Development.

24. Morioka M, Miura T, Kimura K: Morphological and functional changes of feet and toes of Japanese forestry workers, *J Human Ergol* 3:87-94, 1974.

25. Morris D: *Bodywatching,* London, 1987, Grafton Books.

26. Newman RW, White RM: *Reference anthropometry of army men* (Report No. 180), Lawrence, Kansas, 1951, Environmental Protection Section Quartermaster Climactic Research Laboratory.

27. Olivier G: Measurements of the lower limb. In *Practical anthropology,* Springfield, Illinois, 1969, Charles C. Thomas, pp. 29-38.

28. Randall FE, Munro EH, White RM: *Anthropometry of the foot (U.S. army white male),* Lawrence, Kansas, 1951, Department of the Army.

29. Robinow M, Johnston M, Anderson M: Feet of normal children, *J Pediatr* 23(2):141-149, 1943.

30. Robinson JR: Human sexual dimorphism of feet, *Am J Human Biol* 2:199-200, 1990.

31. Robinson JR, Frederick EC, Cooper LB: Running participation and foot dimensions, *Med Sci Sports Exerc* 16(2):200, 1984.

32. Rossi WA: The high incidence of mismated feet in the population, *Foot Ankle* 4(2):105-112, 1983.

33. Snow CC, Schneider RG: *Anthropometry of air traffic control trainees* (Report No. AM 65-26), Oklahoma, 1965, Federal Aviation Agency, Civil Aeromedical Research Institute.

34. Staheli LT, Chew DE, Corbett M: The longitudinal arch, *J Bone Joint Surg* 69A(3):426-428, 1987.

35. Stiehl JB: *Inman's joints of the ankle,* Baltimore, 1991, Williams & Wilkins.

36. Straus WL Jr: The development of the human foot and its phylogenetic significance, *Am J Phys Anthrop* IX(4):427-438, 1926.

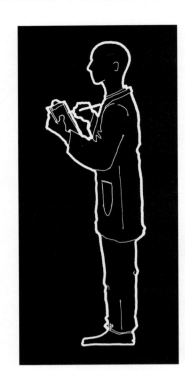

Chapter 45

Biomechanics of the Ankle Joint Complex and the Shoe

Benno M. Nigg
Beat Hintermann

CONTENTS

Shoes are used by humans to protect the foot during various activities and to support foot function and mobility. To understand foot function and the effects shoes can have on it, it is important to analyze:

- Movement of the foot and leg during typical activities
- The coupling mechanism between the foot and leg
- The forces acting on and in the human foot and ankle joint

These three aspects of foot and shoe biomechanics are discussed in this chapter, as well as how shoes may affect movement, movement transfer, and forces.

DEFINITIONS

Kinematics

The *abduction-adduction* angle of the foot is the angular position of the foot relative to the leg about an axis determined by the intersection of the frontal and the sagittal planes of the leg. The terms *abduction* and *adduction* are used to describe an angular position or a rotation of the foot with respect to the leg. Abduction represents rotation in which the tip of the foot points or moves toward the outside, and adduction is rotation toward the inside of the foot.

The *ankle joint inversion-eversion* angle is the angular position of the foot relative to the leg about an axis determined by the intersection of the transverse and sagittal planes of the foot. The terms *inversion* and *eversion* are used to describe an angular position or movement of the foot with respect to the leg. Inversion represents an angular position or a rotation of the foot sole toward the inside, and eversion is an angular position or rotation toward the outside. The terms inversion and eversion are sometimes defined with respect to the ground. To distinguish between these two definitions, the following terms are used: *foot inversion-eversion* is movement of the foot with respect to the ground, and *ankle joint inversion-eversion* is movement of the foot with respect to the leg.

The *dorsal extension–plantar flexion* angle is the angular position of the foot relative to the leg about an axis determined by the intersection of the frontal and transverse planes of the leg. The terms *dorsal extension* and *plantar flexion* are used to describe an angular position or movement of the foot with respect to the leg. *Dorsal extension* represents an extension position or movement of the foot-leg segments, whereas *plantar flexion* represents a flexion position or movement of the foot-leg segments. The term "dorsiflexion," often used in the literature, is inappropriate because the movement corresponds to extension and not to flexion. Consequently, the term *dorsal extension* will be used in this text.[35]

The *tibial rotation* angle is the angular position of the tibia relative to the foot about a longitudinal axis of the tibia. *Tibial rotation* is used to describe an angular position or movement of the leg with respect to the foot. *Internal tibial rotation* represents an angular position or rotation of the anterior part of the tibia toward the inside, and *external tibial rotation* is an angular position or rotation toward the outside.

The *pronation-supination* angle is the angular position of the foot relative to the talus about the talocalcaneal axis (subtalar joint axis). The terms *pronation* and *supination* are used to describe an angular position or movement of the calcaneus with respect to the talus. *Pronation* represents an angular position or rotation in which the foot sole moves toward the outside, and supination is used in cases in which the foot sole moves toward the inside. Pronation and supination are a combination of abduction-adduction, inversion-eversion, and plantar flexion–dorsal extension.[15]

The *ankle joint complex* is a combination of the talocrural and the talocalcaneal joints (ankle and subtalar joints) that provides the angular rotation between the leg and the foot.

The *clinical axes* are axes that are typically used in clinical assessment. For the foot, the clinical axes are the anteroposterior axis, the mediolateral axis, and the inferosuperior axis.

The *functional axes* are axes about which the actual rotation between two segments occurs. For the ankle joint complex, the two functional axes are the talocrural and the talocalcaneal joint axes (the ankle joint and the subtalar joint axes).

Kinetics

Ground reaction forces are forces acting from the ground onto an object that is in contact with the ground. Ground reaction forces are typically subdivided into three orthogonal components: a vertical, an anteroposterior, and a mediolateral component.

Impact forces in human locomotion are forces that result from a collision of two objects reaching their maximum earlier than 50 ms after the first contact of the two objects.[29]

Active forces in human locomotion are forces generated by movement that is entirely controlled by muscular activity.[29]

MOVEMENT

The ankle joint complex allows for relative movement between the foot and the leg. The following paragraphs concern possibilities to assess this movement, specifically addressing the following aspects:

- Clinical and functional variables
- Three-dimensional assessment
- Examples of foot movement variables for one specific case

Clinical and Functional Variables

Rotational movement between two segments occurs around a momentary axis of rotation that is determined primarily by the shape, the ligamentous structures, and the muscle-tendon units of the joint. Rotations describing the functional movement of two adjacent segments are rotations about *functional axes*. The ankle joint complex is a peculiar joint in the sense that during locomotion one can estimate the location of two of the three bones that make up the joint, the tibia and the calcaneus. However, it is practically impossible to estimate the location of the talus during locomotion. Additionally, it is extremely difficult to determine the ankle joint axes[6] around which the actual rotational movements occur. Consequently, it is difficult to describe the movement of the ankle joint complex by using functional axes. Movement of the foot, however, can be determined much more easily in a clinical environment by defining *foot axes* such as the anteroposterior, the mediolateral, and the inferosuperior axes.

Movement of the foot can be defined with respect to the direction of locomotion,[35] the position of the foot with respect to a laboratory coordinate system, or the position of the foot with respect to the leg. Specific descriptions of foot movement may be advantageous for specific questions. Foot movement with respect to the direction of movement of the center of mass may be appropriate for energy considerations. Foot movement relative to the leg may be appropriate for local loading aspects. In any case, it is crucial to define the system of reference clearly because depending on the system of reference, the results are different. The following discussions use variables that have been defined as movement between the foot and the leg (see definitions).

It is obvious that functional variables would be ideal in discussing functional aspects of the foot-leg complex. However, because of practical reasons, functional variables are rarely available for research and/or clinical application. Expressions such as "pronation" or "supination" are often used incorrectly when they are meant to represent "eversion" or "inversion," respectively. Clinical variables are used in the majority of clinical and research applications.

Three-Dimensional Assessment

The rapid development of technology has provided gait analysis systems that offer the possibility for three-dimensional movement analysis. This development is not without concern. Two such concerns will be discussed shortly: the use of two-dimensional analysis and the sequence of angle determination.

For many questions, a two-dimensional approach is appropriate and errors resulting from these restrictions are minimal. It is therefore appropriate to first check whether three-dimensional analysis is really necessary and what errors occur by changing to two-dimensional analysis.

A three-dimensional rotational movement subdivided into its three rotational components will provide different results depending on the sequence of the rotations chosen.[2,13] One can easily verify this by moving the arm from an "initial position," where the arms are alongside the body with the palms facing the side of the body, to a "final position," where the arm points horizontally at a 45-degree angle from the sagittal plane and the palms face the side. The angular components used are extension (EX), abduction (AB), and axial rotation (AR). One may reach the final position by first moving the arm upward and second by abducting it 45 degrees. This would correspond to an FL-AB-AR sequence with the values 90-45-0 degrees. However, one may reach the same final position by first axially rotating the arm 45 degrees and, second, by extending the arm 90 degrees. This corresponds to an AR-FL-AB sequence with the values 45-90-0 degrees. Both movement sequences include 90 degrees of extension. However, the first movement sequence includes 45 degrees of abduction and no axial rotation, whereas the second movement sequence includes no abduction but 45 degrees of axial rotation. It is therefore important to understand for which movement analyses the sequence of the angular components is crucial. This aspect is illustrated for the foot in **Table 45-1**.

Many authors have argued about the appropriateness of some of the sequences.[2,5,17] However, logical arguments described earlier[32] that have used anatomical definitions of flexion-extension, abduction-adduction, and axial rotation[26,37] indicate that the appropriate sequence that agrees with the definition of these movements for all human joints is as follows:

In general	For the ankle joint complex
• Flexion-extension	• Plantar flexion–dorsal extension (PD)
• Abduction-adduction	• Abduction-adduction (AA)
• Axial rotation	• Inversion-eversion (IE)

In any case, the results in **Table 45-1** indicate that caution is necessary when three-dimensional analysis is used to analyze mediolateral movements and to assess range of motion. However, the sequence of angular component determination is not critical for movements such as walking and running.

Examples of Foot Movement Variables

Foot movement variables have been quantified for walking and/or running by several authors.[14,25,27,35,41] Lower extremity locomotion has been subdivided into many different phases. For the purpose of a functional analysis of foot movement in this section, the gait cycle is subdivided into two phases, a stance and a swing phase. The forces acting on and in the various structures of the ankle joint complex are typically much higher in

Table 45-1	Comparison of the three components of angular position of the ankle joint complex for running, side-shuffle, and range of motion for two different sequences of Cardan angles for which these angular components were determined.		
Activity	**Component of Rotation**	**Sequence of Determination**	
		PL-DO	PL-DO
		AD-AB	IN-EV
		IN-EV	AD-AB
Running	Dorsal extension	25.0	21.4
	Abduction	10.0	10.6
	Eversion	20.0	19.7
Side shuffle	Dorsal Extension	20.0	30.3
	Abduction	15.0	18.1
	Inversion	35.0	33.6
ROM	Plantar Flexion	40.0	26.8
	Abduction	40.0	41.8
	Inversion	20.0	15.2

AB, *abduction*; AD, *adduction*; DO, *dorsal extension*; EV, *eversion*; IN, *inversion*; PL, *plantar flexion*; ROM, *range of motion*. From Nigg BM, Cole GK: Optical methods. In Nigg BM, Herzog W, editors: Biomechanics of the musculoskeletal system, Chichester, England, 1994, John Wiley & Sons; pp 254-286.

the stance phase than in the swing phase. Consequently, the following illustrations and discussions concentrate on the stance phase.

The stance phase is functionally subdivided into two parts, an impact phase and an active phase. The impact phase includes approximately the initial 50 ms of ground contact. The active phase includes the rest of the ground contact, but the boundary between these phases is fuzzy.

During the *impact phase*, the subject cannot react to sudden changes and switch strategies in muscle response. Typically, the system is preprogrammed for a given situation. However, if sudden changes occur, the system reacts with the "old" response pattern. During the impact phase, the human leg behaves like a *passive structure* with certain mechanical properties. In contrast, movement during the *active phase* is fully controlled by muscular activation and the system acts as an *active structure*.

The variables abduction-adduction, plantar flexion–dorsal extension, ankle joint inversion-eversion, and tibial rotation are illustrated in **Figure 45-1** for 10 subjects running heel-toe. The angular variables were determined using the sequence PD-AA-IE (plantar-flexion–dorsal extension, abduction-adduction, inversion-eversion).

Even though such mean curves are published in many textbooks, they may not be typical of the loading situation in a subject-specific case. The right side of **Figure 45-1** shows a subject who has movement variables for the ankle joint complex that are substantially different from the mean curves. Careful study of such graphs may provide insight into subject-specific problems or advantages.

MOVEMENT TRANSFER BETWEEN FOOT AND LEG

Let us consider the calcaneus, tibia, femur, and pelvis during one ground contact in running. The calcaneus touches the ground and everts until about midstance (at about 150 to 250 ms). The calcaneus eversion movement is associated (through the talus) with internal rotation of the tibia. At the same time (from initial contact to midstance), the pelvis rotates externally with respect to the supporting leg, which is initiating an external rotation of the femur. The two movements are, however, in opposite directions, and somewhere between the calcaneus and the pelvis, movement transfer between the neighboring segments cannot be direct.[1] Substantial transfer of the eversion movement of the calcaneus to the tibia may, however, be associated with potential overloading problems at the knee level. It is

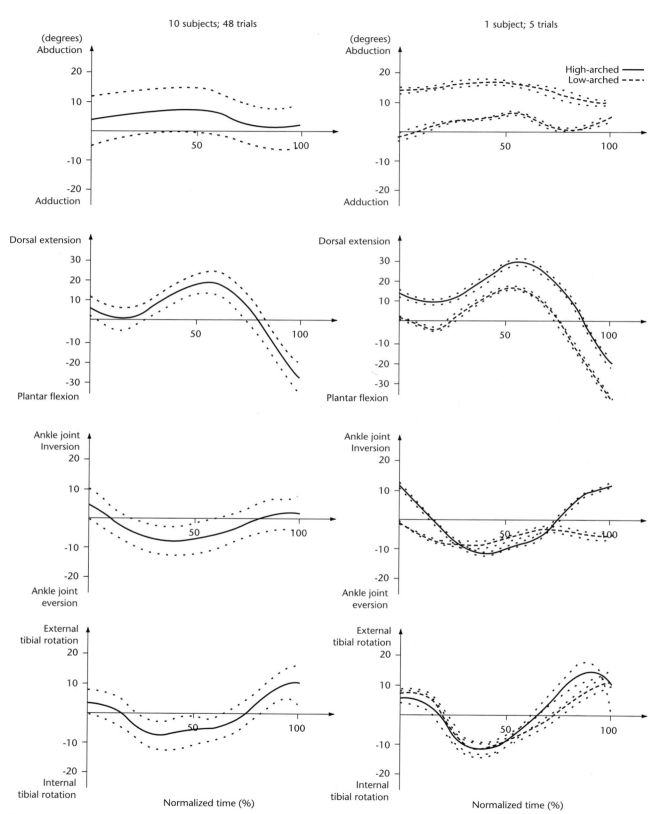

Figure 45-1 Illustration of the variables abduction-adduction, plantar flexion–dorsal extension, ankle joint inversion-eversion, and tibial rotation during ground contact for running heel-toe at a running speed of 4 m/sec. Mean and standard deviation are presented for 10 subjects (48 trials) on the left and for 1 subject (5 trials) on the right. The illustration for 1 subject (right) indicates the rather substantial variability 6–degree of freedom a single subject-shoe combination may produce.

therefore important to understand the transfer mechanism between the calcaneus and tibia. The following paragraphs address this transfer mechanism by discussing in vitro and in vivo experiments.

Movement Transfer In Vitro

Mechanical coupling between calcaneal and tibial movement can be studied by mounting a foot-leg specimen in a 6–degree of freedom fixture,[1,20] inserting bone pins with markers into the calcaneus and the tibia, and quantifying movement of the calcaneus and tibia kinematically. The relationship between calcaneal and tibial movement is illustrated in **Figure 45-2**, with movement of the calcaneus used as input and movement of the tibia used as output.

The initial calcaneal inversion of about 20 degrees results in external tibial rotation of about 5 degrees. The maximal calcaneal inversion of about 32 degrees results in external tibial rotation of about 14 degrees. Transfer in the initial phase corresponds to a transfer of about 25%, and transfer in the final inversion movement (27 to 32 degrees) corresponds to a transfer of about 100%. Return of the foot to the neutral position follows a different tibial rotation-inversion path than does onset of the inversion movement. The subsequent eversion movement of the calcaneus produces an internal rotation of the tibia. Transfer for this part of the movement corresponds to about 18%. Cutting of the anteriortalofibular and the calcaneofibular ligaments changes the transfer mechanism.

Based on these (**Fig. 45-2**) and other previously published results,[20-22] one must conclude that transfer of movement from the calcaneus to the tibia is not constant. It depends on various factors such as the type of input movement, the plantar flexion–dorsal extension position of the foot,[20,22] loading of the ankle joint complex,[28] the fusion of selected joints,[21] and the integrity of the ligaments.[20,22] Consequently, the talocrural (ankle) and the talocalcaneal (subtalar) joints are not universal joints, as had been suggested earlier.[23,39]

Movement Transfer In Vivo

Quantification of the mechanical coupling of the calcaneus and tibia is technically much more difficult in vivo than in vitro. Markers must be placed at the skin of the heel or at the heel of the shoe and on the skin of the leg, and movement of the skin markers relative to the bone is possible. Several techniques have recently been developed and should be available clinically in the near future. The following examples stress the basic possibilities, not the measuring technique. An illustration of a movement transfer characteristic (inversion-eversion versus tibial rotation) is illustrated in **Figure 45-3**.

The illustrated curve is typical for the movement analyzed, the footwear, and the anatomical specifics of the tested subject. Changes in one of these parameters, for instance, changes in footwear, will change the characteristics of the curve. Such analyses therefore have the potential to assess the appropriateness of an intervention. For example, it is possible to assess whether a foot orthotic changes the maximal eversion of the rearfoot

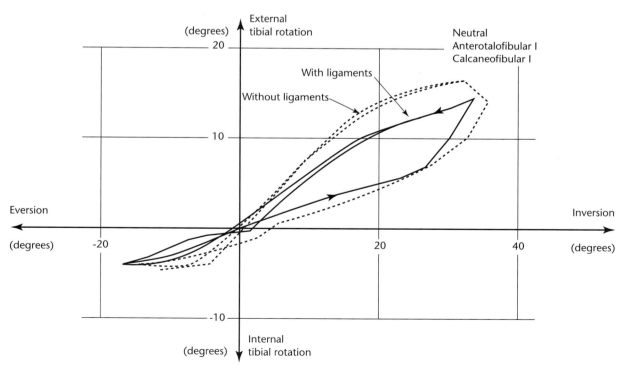

Figure 45-2 Movement transfer between the calcaneus and tibia for one cadaveric foot-leg specimen with and without intact ligaments mounted in a 6–degree of freedom fixture with calcaneal inversion-eversion as input and tibial rotation as output. The curve without ligaments illustrates the increased laxity of the ankle joint complex.

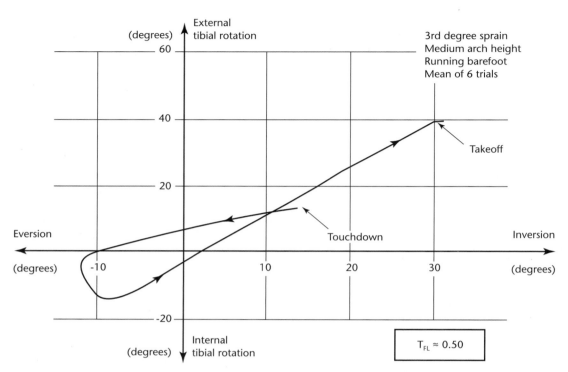

Figure 45-3 Illustration of an ankle joint movement transfer characteristic for one subject running heel-toe barefoot (mean of six trials).

or the transfer of movement from the calcaneus to the tibia. Depending on the problem at hand, interventions can be assessed and accepted or rejected. Consequently, this approach allows an understanding of functional connections in the lower extremities.

FORCES

Whenever the foot is in contact with the ground, forces act from the ground onto the foot and vice versa. These forces, called *ground reaction forces,* are resultant forces that correspond to the movement of the center of mass and gravity. Ground reaction forces are typically subdivided into *impact* and *active forces.* Examples of the magnitude of external forces, summarized in **Table 45-2,** illustrate that ground reaction forces are different for various activities and can easily exceed body weight several times. Typical ground reaction force components for heel-toe running are illustrated in **Figure 45-4** for a group of subjects and for one individual.

External forces acting on the human foot, the geometric alignment of the foot and the leg, muscle forces, and segmental inertia forces are responsible for the internal forces acting in joints and on ligaments and tendons. Mathematical models are used to estimate the magnitude of forces in internal structures such as joints, tendons, and ligaments. These estimations use several (sometimes different) assumptions that are still being discussed.[19] However, the order of magnitude of the estimated forces is assumed to be correct.

Typically, the geometry of the acting forces (i.e., the distance of the line of action of an acting force to a joint of interest) is the most important factor that determines the internal forces.

Ground reaction forces are resultant forces that are determined by movement of the various segments involved in the locomotion process. They are integral quantities and are limited in providing information on local phenomena, especially on phenomena specific for the foot. Ground reaction forces for people with high arches and flatfeet can easily look similar. Pressure distribution sensors are better suited to provide more local information. A pressure distribution sensor is a summation of many hundreds of small force plates that measure the force perpendicular to the surface.[7,18,28] Pressure distribution sensors are often used in the form of insoles to assess foot specific problems. **Figure 45-5** illustrates results from pressure distribution sensors. The example shown illustrates the maximum pressure images for a subject experiencing pain under the head of the second metatarsal while using a regular and an orthotic insole. Data were collected for the subject running on a treadmill at a speed of 5.2 m/sec in a standard running shoe.

The first illustration at 20 ms of ground contact indicates that impact loading beneath the heel is reduced by the orthotic insole. In the next picture at 80 ms, loading under the midfoot is greater and more evenly distributed to the medial side with the orthotic insole. This is the result of substantially increased arch support in the orthotic in comparison to the normal

Table 45-2	Summary of the magnitude of external and internal forces of the ankle joint complex in the unit body weight.		
Type	**Location**	**Magnitude**	**Description of Activity**
EXTERNAL	Heel	0.55	Impact forces during heel-strike while walking barefoot[9]
	Heel	0.37	Impact forces during heel-strike while walking in army boots[9]
	Heel	0.27	Impact forces during heel-strike while walking in street shoes[9]
	Forefoot	≑1	Active forces during take-off in walking
	Heel	1-4	Impact forces during heel-strike in heel-toe running for speeds between 3 and 6 m/s[8,16,31,34]
	Forefoot	3	Active forces during take-off in running at about 3 to 6 m/s[31]
INTERNAL	Ankle joint	1	Standing on one leg
	Ankle joint	0	Heel-strike for walking and heel-toe running
	Ankle joint	2-5	Stand phase and take-off in walking
	Ankle joint	3-8	Stand phase and take-off for jogging[12]
	Ankle joint	5-10	Take-off in sprinting[4]

Data from references 4, 8, 9, 12, 16, 31, 34.

insole. Finally, the illustration at 140 ms indicates that the high pressure under the first and second metatarsal heads is substantially reduced with the orthotic insole. These results show that in general, pressure distribution measurements can provide fast information about the local effect of changes in footwear. Pressure distribution insoles therefore have a wide potential field of application in occupational health assessment.

In addition to direct measurement of pressure distribution in footwear, pressure distribution sensors have been used to estimate internal forces in the anatomical structures of the human foot.[6,12] The results of pressure distribution measurements were used as localized input into the different foot structures to provide a possible means of quantifying internal forces in joints, ligaments, and tendons of the foot, an estimation that cannot be performed using the ground reaction force as force input.

SHOES

The literature on the biomechanics of shoes includes a substantial majority of reports concentrating primarily on sport shoes, specifically running shoes. However, some of the general findings may find application in everyday situations. The most important findings that have—in the view of the authors—general significance are summarized in the following paragraphs.

Impact Forces

Impact forces in structures of the lower extremities (internal impact forces) during activities such as walking and running are much smaller than internal active forces.[28,36]

Epidemiological evidence of a possible association between external or internal impact forces during walking and running and related injuries is not conclusive. Some sources speculate that impact forces are associated with the development of injuries, whereas others speculate that they are not.

It has been proposed that impact forces may be related more to comfort than to injuries.[20] It may be possible that "good cushioning" influences energy aspects and fatigue in locomotion.

Ankle Joint Eversion

Excessive ankle joint eversion has been typically associated with the development of overuse injuries in locomotion.[10,11,24] Subjects with injuries typically have foot eversion movement that is about 2 to 4 degrees greater than that of subjects with no injuries. However, between 40% and 50% of runners with excessive ankle joint eversion do not have overuse injuries.

It has been suggested that a combination of excessive ankle joint eversion and substantial movement transfer of foot eversion into internal tibial rotation is a better predictor of the development of (especially knee) overuse injuries.[3,20,30]

It has been proposed that movement transfer between foot eversion and tibial rotation is small for subjects with low arches and high for subjects with high arches.[33] Consequently, subjects with high arches are more susceptible to overuse injuries than subjects with low arches if they show excessive ankle joint eversion.

Ankle joint eversion is substantially influenced by

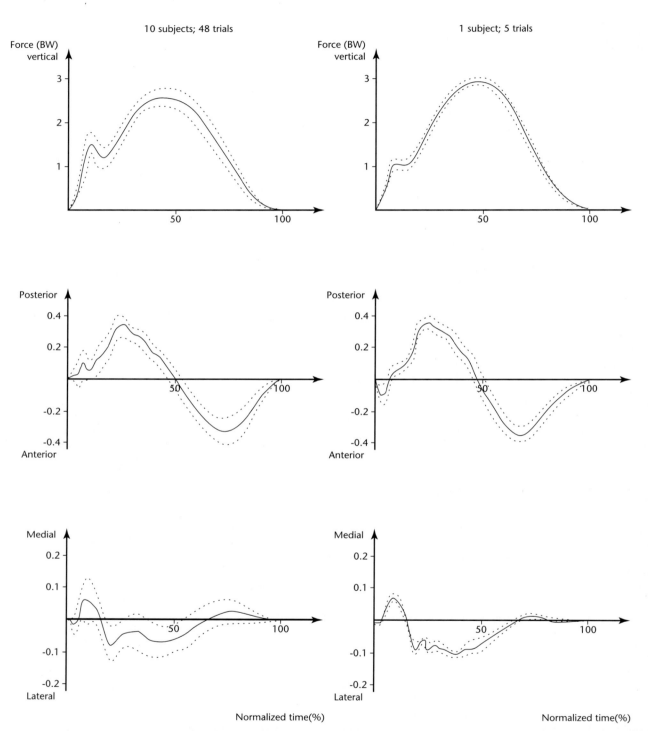

Figure 45-4 Mean and standard deviation of ground reaction force components of heel-toe running for 10 subjects (left) and 1 subject (right) illustrating the typical mean values and also possibilities substantially deviating from the "typical" mean curves.

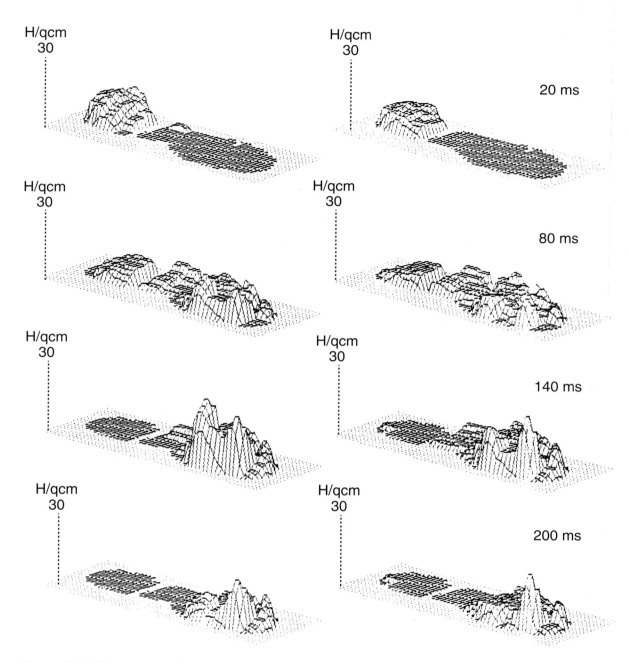

Figure 45-5 Time-sequenced pressure distribution images for a subject running with an orthotic insole (*right*) and with a normal insole (*left*) on a treadmill at a running speed of 5.2 m/sec. A time of 0 ms represents the time of initial heel contact, and the total duration of ground contact is 260 ms for both insoles.

the shoe. Differences in ankle joint eversion for a subject using different running shoes are considerable. It is easily possible that the maximal ankle joint eversion movement is 31 degrees for one and 12 degrees for another running shoe (**Fig. 45-6**).[30]

Medial support in a shoe may provide increased stability to the foot and leg and may reduce maximal ankle joint eversion. However, at the same time, medial support may increase internal rotation of the tibia. It is

assumed that this change is associated with an increased inclination of the subtalar joint axis.[33]

Torsion

Without shoes, the foot has a natural ability to allow for torsional motion between the rearfoot and forefoot. Shoes often have torsional stiffness that is too high and do not allow this movement. It is proposed that low torsional stiffness is advantageous, especially for move-

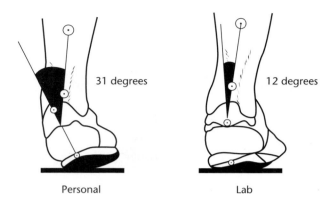

Figure 45-6 Illustration of a shoe-induced difference in maximal ankle joint eversion for two subjects running heel-toe at 4 m/sec with two different pairs of running shoes, a "personal shoe" and a "lab shoe."

ment involving landing on the forefoot, as is typical in volleyball or basketball.[38,40]

Shoe Inserts and Arch Supports

Shoe inserts and foot arch supports are often used successfully in the treatment and prevention of occupational and sports injuries. They are used to limit overuse of the foot structures, increase foot-leg stability, and/or change foot function. The application of these aids is typically based on the expertise of the orthotist and podiatrist, and many problems are successfully treated with these strategies. However, in most applications, the mechanical functioning of such orthoses is not well understood, so further research is needed to improve the functional-mechanical understanding of such orthoses.

References

1. Allinger TL, Engsberg JR: A method to determine the range of motion of the ankle joint complex in vivo, *J Biomechanics* 26:69-76, 1993.

2. Areblad M, Nigg BM, Ekstrand J, Olsson KO, Ekström H: Three-dimensional measurement of rearfoot motion during running, *J Biomechanics* 23:933-940, 1990.

3. Bahlsen A: *The etiology of running injuries: a longitudinal prospective study,* (unpublished doctoral thesis), Calgary, Canada, 1988, The University of Calgary.

4. Baumann W, Stucke H: Sportspezifische Belastung aus der Sicht der Biomechanik (Sport specific loading from a biomechanical point of view). In Cotta H, Krahl H, Steinbrück K, editors: *Die belastungstoleranz des bewegungsapparates,* Stuttgart, Germany; 1980, Georg Thieme Verlag; pp. 55-64.

5. Blankevoort L, Huiskes R, de Lange A: The envelope of passive knee joint motion, *J Biomech* 21:705-720, 1988.

6. Bogert van den AJ, Smith GD, Nigg BM: In vivo determination of the anatomical axes of the ankle joint complex: an optimization approach, *J Biomech* 27(12):1477-1488, 1994.

7. Cavanagh PR, Hennig EM, Bunch RP, Macmillan NH: A new device for the measurement of pressure distribution inside the shoe. In Morecki A, Fidelus K, Kedzior K, Wit A, editors: *Biomechanics, VII-B,* Baltimore, Md., 1983, University Park Press; pp. 1089-1096.

8. Cavanagh PR, Lafortune MA: Ground reaction forces in distance running, *J Biomech* 13:397-406, 1980.

9. Cavanagh PR, Williams KR, Clarke TE: A comparison of ground reaction forces during walking barefoot and in shoes. In Morecki A, Fidelus K, Kedzior K, Wit A, editors: *Biomechanics, VII-B,* Baltimore, Md., 1981, University Park Press; pp. 151-156.

10. Clancy WG: Tendonitis and plantar fascitis in runners. In d'Ambrosia R, Drez D, editors: *Prevention and treatment of running injuries,* Thorofare, NJ, 1982, Slade; pp. 77-87.

11. Clement DB, Taunton JE, Smart GW, McNicol KL: A survey of overuse injuries, *Phys Sports Med* 9:47-58, 1981.

12. Cole GK, Nigg BM, Fick GH, Morlock MM: Internal loading of the foot and ankle during impact in running, *J Appl Biomech* 11:25-46, 1995.

13. Cole GK, Nigg BM, Ronsky JL, Yeadon MR: Application of the joint coordinate system to three-dimensional joint attitude and movement representation: a standardization proposal, *J Biomech Eng* 115:344-349, 1993.

14. Eberhart HD, Inman VT, Bressler B: The principle elements in human locomotion. In Klopsteg PE, Wilson PD, editors: *Human limbs and their substitutes,* New York, 1968, Hafner Publishing Company; pp. 437-471.

15. Engsberg JR: A biomechanical analysis of the talocalcaneal joint in vitro, *J Biomech* 20:429-442, 1987.

16. Frederick EC, Hagy JL, Mann RA: Prediction of vertical impact forces during running, *J Biomech* 14:498, 1981.

17. Grood ES, Suntay WJ: A joint coordinate system for the clinical description of three-dimensional motions: application to the knee, *J Biomech Eng* 105:136-144, 1983.

18. Hennig EM, Cavanagh PR, Albert HT, Macmillan NH: A piezoelectric method of measuring the vertical contact stress beneath the human foot, *J Biomed Eng* 4:213-222, 1981.

19. Herzog W, Binding P: Mathematically indeterminate systems. In Nigg BM, Herzog W, editors: *Biomechanics of the musculo-skeletal system,* Chichester, U.K., 1994, Wiley and Sons; pp. 472-491.

20. Hintermann B, Nigg BM: Die Bewegungsübertragung zwischen Fuss und Unterschenkel in vitro (movement transfer between foot and leg in vitro), *Sportverletz Sportschaden* 2:60-66, 1994.

21. Hintermann B, Nigg BM, Cole GK: Influence of selective arthrodesis on the movement transfer between calcaneus and tibia in vitro, *Clin Biomech* 9(6):349-355, 1994.

22. Hintermann B, Nigg BM, Sommer C, Cole GK: Transfer of movement between calcaneus and tibia in vitro, *Clin Biomech* 9(6):349-355, 1994.

23. Inman VT: *The joints of the ankle,* Baltimore, Md., 1976, Williams & Wilkins.

24. Leach R: Running injuries of the knee. In d'Ambrosia R, Drez D, editors: *Prevention and treatment of running injuries,* Thorofare, N.J., 1982, Slade; pp. 55-75.

25. Mann RA: Biomechanics of running. In Mack RP, editor: *Symposium on the foot and leg in running sports,* St. Louis, 1982, Mosby–Year Book; pp. 1-29.

26. Moore KL: *Clinically oriented anatomy,* ed 1, Baltimore, 1980, Williams & Wilkins; pp. 403-475.

27. Murray MP, Drought AB, Kory RC: Walking pattern of normal men, *J Bone Joint Surg* 46A:335-360, 1964.

28. Nicol K, Hennig EM: Time dependent method for measuring force distribution using a flexible mat as a capacitor. In Komi PV, editor: *Biomechanics, V-B,* Baltimore, Md., 1976, University Park Press; pp. 433-440.

29. Nigg BM: Force. In Nigg BM, Herzog W, editor: *Biomechanics of the musculo-skeletal system,* Chichester, U.K., 1994, Wiley and Sons; pp. 200-224.

30. Nigg BM, Bahlsen AH, Denoth J, Lüthi SM, Stacoff A: Factors influencing kinetic and kinematic variables in running. In Nigg BM, editor: *Biomechanics of running shoes,* Champaign, Ill., 1986, Human Kinetics; pp. 139-159.

31. Nigg BM, Bahlsen HA, Lüthi SM, Stokes S: The influence of running velocity and midsole hardness on external impact forces in heel-toe running, *J Biomech* 20:951-959, 1987.

32. Nigg BM, Cole GK: Optical methods. In Nigg BM, Herzog W, editors: *Biomechanics of the musculo-skeletal system,* Chichester, U.K., 1994, Wiley & Sons; pp. 254-286.

33. Nigg BM, Cole GK, Nachbauer W: Effects of arch height of the foot on angular motion of the lower extremities in running, *J Biomech* 26:909-916, 1993.

34. Nigg BM, Denoth J: *Sportplatzbeläge (playing surfaces),* Zürich, Switzerland, 1980, Juris Verlag.

35. Perry J: *Gait analysis: normal and pathological function,* Thorofare, N.J., 1992, Slack.

36. Scott SH, Winter DA: Internal forces at chronic running sites, *Med Sci Sports Exerc* 22:357-369, 1990.

37. Snell RS: *Clinical anatomy for medical students,* ed 4, Boston, 1992, Little Brown; pp. 1-5.

38. Stacoff A, Kälin X, Stüssi E, Segesser B: The torsion of the foot in running, *Int J Sports Biomech* 5:375-389, 1989.

39. Stauffer JE, Chao EY, Brewster RC: Force and motion analysis of the normal, diseased and prosthetic ankle joint, *Clinical Orthop* 127:189-196, 1977.

40. Stüssi E, Stacoff A: Biomechanische und orthopädische Probleme des Tennis- und Hallenschuh (biomechanical and orthopaedic problems in tennis and indoor shoes), *Sportverletz-Sportschaden* 7:187-190, 1993.

41. Winter DA, Quanbury AO, Hobson DA, Sidwall HG, Reimer G, Trenholm BG, Steinkle T, Shlosser H: Kinematics of normal locomotion—a statistical study based on TV data, *J Biomech* 6:479-486, 1974.

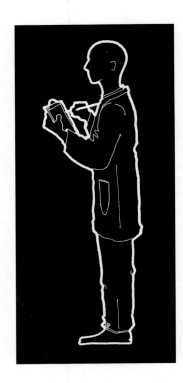

Chapter 46

Clinical and Functional Evaluation of the Foot and Ankle

Paul S. Cooper
G. James Sammarco

CONTENTS

Successful treatment of disorders related to the foot and ankle requires a meticulous history and physical examination to achieve an accurate diagnosis. The course and proximity of the various anatomic structures in the foot and ankle therefore demand a thorough knowledge of the bony and soft tissue anatomy involving the foot and ankle. Conditions of the foot and ankle often do not exist or are not manifested in isolation; therefore, a thorough examination of the relationship to the entire lower extremity is essential if successful treatment is to be obtained. Examples of this would include a rotational deformity in the lower extremity manifested as symptoms resulting from compensation by the foot and ankle. Conversely, a malalignment condition in the foot may initially be manifested as symptoms related to medial knee pain. Often, afflictions involving the foot may be the first sign of a systemic disorder; thus the clinician is obligated to extend the history and physical examination to exclude more generalized conditions.

The purpose of this chapter is to give the practicing clinician a systematic approach to the history and physical examination of the foot and ankle. The physical examination section of this chapter is grouped by sites of patient symptoms. Through this group approach it will be easier to form a differential diagnosis by patient complaint so as to devise an appropriate treatment plan.

OBTAINING THE HISTORY

The objective of the history is to narrow and direct attention toward the physical examination and the ultimate differential diagnosis. The examiner may use a questionnaire or personally record the responses for an accurate, complete documentation of the history. Standardized history and physical examination forms save time and ensure completeness and consistency, but allowances should be made for supplemental questions from the examiner. Much information is gathered in the first few minutes of the interview.[3] The patient's occupation, level of education, socioeconomic status, and level of activity help to assess the degree to which patients will be able to participate in their care. The ability of a patient to report a past medical and surgical history allows the physician to determine the level of understanding about the seriousness of the injury and subsequent treatment. The mechanism of injury and duration of symptoms should be elicited from the patient. In addition, the nature of the pain—its occurrence throughout the day and association with which activities, as well as limitations of activities—should be documented. Other symptoms should be included, such as the timing and duration of swelling and giving way. Prior procedures and previous treatments by physicians or practitioners, including injections and surgery, should be accurately documented with regard to number and occurrence. A family history to determine a hereditary predisposition for a disorder of the foot and ankle should be included because both congenital and some acquired foot disorders as well as various inflammatory and metabolic conditions may have a familial predisposition. A detailed review of symptoms should be made that includes inflammatory conditions (e.g., gout and seropositive arthropathies), metabolic conditions (e.g., diabetes mellitus), and vascular conditions (e.g., peripheral vascular disease and venous insufficiency).

EXAMINATION

Patients with lower extremity disorders should be evaluated agown with both stockings and shoes removed. Often, a symptomatic foot or ankle is shown to the examiner, and impending or copathology is overlooked on the contralateral foot. The feet should be examined, both from the front, the back, and the sides, with asymmetry noted between the legs with regard to muscular atrophy, swelling, and effusions and position of the foot. Next, the gait pattern should be assessed while the patient walks both toward and away from the examiner. The style and pattern of the gait and foot position, including rotation and arch configuration, should be recorded. Similarly, an antalgic gait, a pelvic tilt, alterations in cadence, arm swing, and foot and leg position, in both stance and swing phases, are noted. During stance, emphasis is placed on forefoot and hindfoot position and configuration of the medial longitudinal arch. Examination in the frontal plane with the patient on single and double toe rise and heel rise can give valuable information.

The examiner should inspect the shoes, both inside and out, for abnormal wear patterns and supplemental orthotics or orthoses. Asymmetry in shoe wear and asymmetry in the wear of the sole should be noted; asymmetrical wear of the outer border of the sole is often associated with a cavus or cavovarus foot, or a more symmetrical or medial wear can be associated with a plantar valgus foot. Orthotics should be evaluated for both durability and repair. Often a patient will complain of developing foot pain after wearing a semirigid orthotic for many years. On further examination, the orthosis is noted to be completely broken down and thus nonfunctioning.

Examination by Specific Systems

Once the inspection has been completed, localized examination of the bony and soft tissue–injured areas follows. It can be very helpful to have the patient first indicate, with an index finger, the specific symptomatic site. In general, in all systems to be examined, swelling from edema or effusion, skin temperature changes, and the condition of the skin should be noted, as well as previous sites of surgery or trauma. Systematic examination consists of examination of the ankle, hindfoot, midfoot, and forefoot groups based on symptoms.

The ankle joint should first be assessed for evidence of effusion versus local soft tissue swelling. The effusion can best be assessed by ballottement along the anterior ankle joint either to the medial aspect of the tibialis anterior tendon or just lateral to the extensor digitorum communis tendon (**Fig. 46-1**). This is not to be confused with inflammation and swelling of an associated bursitis as seen in the retrocalcaneal area of the Achilles tendon or with a tenosynovitis such as seen in the flexor tendon groups. Motion of the ankle is similar to a hinge and consists primarily of dorsiflexion and plantar flexion. The average arc of ankle motion consists of 20 degrees dorsiflexion to 50 degrees plantar flexion. It is

essential to measure both active and passive arcs of motion because an average difference of 14 degrees has been noted between inactive and passive motion.[2] Ankle motion is also restricted by age, with older males having an increased arch of plantar flexion and older females losing maximum dorsiflexion. Specific attention should be directed to a restricted dorsiflexion or *equinus* deformity that may create significant mechanical and functional disability if the ankle restricts the foot from becoming plantigrade during the midstance phase of gait. A restriction in ankle dorsiflexion may be attributed to a tight heel cord, posterior capsular contracture of the ankle, or bony impingement along the anterior ankle line. Passive dorsiflexion should be assessed with the knee in full extension and at 90 degrees of flexion; an increase with the knee flexed indicates a tight gastrocnemius muscle.

Pathology localized to the posterior of the ankle and hindfoot consists of Achilles tendinosis or rupture, insertional calcific tendonitis, retrocalcaneal bursitis, Haglund's deformity, and posterior impingement or os trigonum syndrome. *Achilles tendon rupture* often consists of a palpable gap and swelling approximately 2 to 4 cm above the insertion site of the Achilles tendon. With the patient lying in a prone position, the Thompson test is a reliable indicator of incompetency of the Achilles tendon unit. With the patient's legs hanging over the edge of the examining table, the clinician squeezes both gastrocnemius and soleus muscle bellies proximally. The lack of passive plantar flexion elicited by the squeeze is compatible with a rupture of the tendon. Another

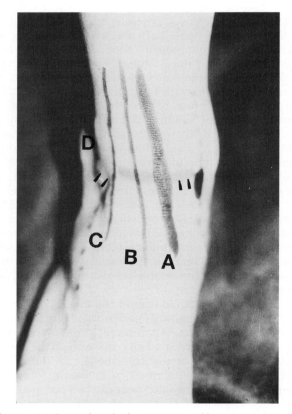

Figure 46-1 Landmarks for anterior ankle pain: *A,* anterior tibial tendon; *B,* extensor hallucis, longus; *C,* extensor digitorum communis; *D,* distal anterior tibiofibular joint (*arrows* indicate sites for ballottement of the ankle joint margin).

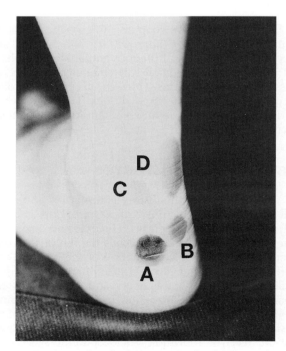

Figure 46-2 Landmarks for posterior heel pain and ankle pain: *A,* pump; *B,* insertion of the Achilles tendon; *C,* retrocalcaneal bursae; *D,* Achilles tendon.

indicator is a loss of the resting plantar flexion tension of the foot. *Achilles tendinosis* consists of an intact Achilles tendon with either fusiform or localized thickening in the Achilles tendon or paratendon that is painful on palpation. This may exist in isolation or be associated with a *retrocalcaneal bursitis* consisting of a thickening above the insertion site of the Achilles anterior to the tendon (**Fig. 46-2**). Normally, the soft tissues in this area are hollow on both the medial and lateral sides but swell and may outpouch with inflammation of the bursa. Tenderness elicited by squeezing from the medial lateral side of this bursa elicits pain. *Insertional calcific tendonitis* is noted by extreme hypersensitivity to palpation and localized swelling at the insertion site of the Achilles tendon on the os calcis. A *posterior impingement syndrome* or *os trigonum syndrome* may or may not have associated swelling in the posterior ankle joint. Palpation deep in the retrocalcaneal area on the os trigonum laterally and pain elicited with passive hyper plantar flexion of the ankle joint are characteristic of this syndrome (**Fig. 46-3**).

The lateral ankle joint is one of the most common sites for pathology frequently associated with an ankle "sprain." Because of the many anatomic sites in a limited area, orderly and specific local palpation is essential (**Fig. 46-4**). Tenderness overlying the anterior talar fibular ligament with or without associated pain along the calcaneofibular ligament is characteristic of a lateral ankle sprain. Stability testing includes the anterior drawer test and inversion stress test. The anterior drawer test should be performed with the patient relaxed and knee bent over the side of the table. One hand of the examiner is cupped around the posterior of

the heel, and with the opposite hand stabilizing the anterior tibia, an anterior drawer is applied with the ankle in approximately 10 degrees of plantar flexion (**Fig. 46-3**). Similarly, the patient is placed in the same position and inversion stress is applied to the lateral aspect of the heel while stabilizing the medial tibia. The inversion test should be applied in both dorsiflexion and plantar flexion positions to stress both calcaneofibular and anterior talofibular competency, respectively. Any laxity should be noted in the context of the contralateral ankle joint or generalized body ligamentous laxity. *Peroneus brevis* tendonitis/tears may consist of a fusiform swelling just posterior and proximal to the tip of the fibula that is associated with tenderness on palpation of the tendons in their sheath (**Fig. 46-5**).[4] Pain and weakness associated with resisted foot eversion with the ankle plantar-flexed is associated with this tendon injury. *Subtalar synovitis* resulting from a variety of causes, including arthrosis and inflammatory conditions, may be isolated by palpating the sinus tarsi region. Additionally, painful or restricted range of motion of the subtalar joint in inversion and eversion is characteristic. Measurement of subtalar motion for in-

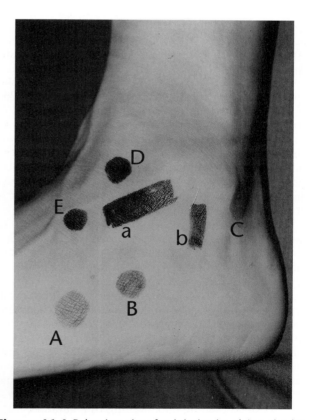

Figure 46-4 Palpation sites for injuries involving the lateral ankle. Often these sites must be differentiated on examination for a common ankle "sprain." *A,* anterotalofibular ligament; *B,* calcaneofibular ligament. *a,* Base of the fifth metatarsal styloid process; *b,* site of peroneus longus tears; *C,* site of peroneus brevis tears; *D,* site of distal tibiofibular sprains; *E,* sinus tarsi.

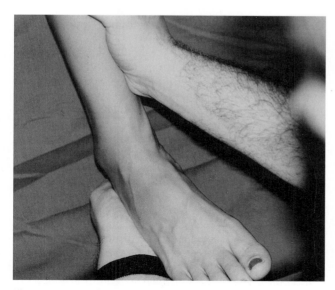

Figure 46-3 Clinical testing for anterior talofibular ligament laxity with the anterior drawer test. The ankle is held in 10 degrees of plantar flexion as an anterior drawer is applied with one hand cupped around the posterior of the heel and the other hand stabilizing the tibia.

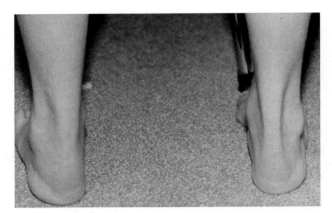

Figure 46-5 Example of swelling in the posterior lateral ankle caused by a peroneus brevis chronic tendon tear with associated tenosynovitis.

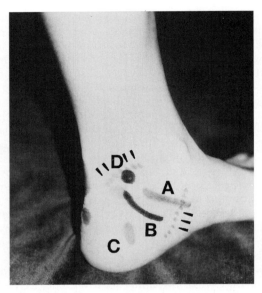

Figure 46-6 Sites of pain in the medial ankle and hindfoot. Sites for medial and ankle pathology: *A,* posterior tibial tendon; *B,* flexor hallucis longus tendon; *C,* course of the medial calcaneal nerve; *D,* posterior ankle joint (*arrows* outline the boundaries of the tarsal tunnel).

version and eversion should be done with the ankle positioned in a few degrees of dorsiflexion to restrict tibial talar joint motion while ranging the subtalar joint.[2] Inversion motion is generally greater than eversion motion by a ratio of 2:1; an individual with a cavus foot will have a decreased arc of motion through the subtalar joint whereas the arc of motion of a hypermobile planovalgus foot will be increased. *Peroneal spastic flatfoot* will be pes planus associated with a rigid subtalar joint, pain in the sinus tarsi region, and spasms involving the peroneal tendon groups posterior to the ankle joint. *Peroneus longus tendon injuries* and the *painful os peroneus syndrome* are associated with tenderness inferior and distal to the tip of the fibula when the peroneus longus tendon is palpated as it courses through the cuboid sulcus. A painful palpable os peroneum may also be encountered. Resisted plantar flexion of the first ray during palpaton of the tendon in the cuboid sulcus helps confirm the diagnosis.

Anterior ankle joint symptoms may be related to sprains of the distal tibiofibular joint, anterior impingement syndrome or arthrosis of the ankle joint, entrapment neuropathies, or tendon injuries. The *distal tibiofibular* or *"high ankle" sprain* consists of pain on palpation above the level of the ankle joint at the distal tibiofibular joint. Often, swelling is not associated with the injury. Symptoms may be reproduced by either the compression test, in which the fibula is squeezed at midlevel against the tibia, or the external rotation test, in which the knee is flexed over the table as external rotation force is applied to the foot while the proximal tibia is stabilized. The *anterior impingement syndrome* consists of thickening and swelling in a bandlike fashion across the anterior ankle joint with tenderness elicited mainly along the anteromedial area. Restricted degrees of dorsiflexion often are associated. Pain is elicited when passively dorsiflexing the ankle joint and is relieved with plantar flexion. *Degenerative arthrosis* may consist of a ballotable ankle effusion in conjunction with painful crepitus while ranging the ankle joint.

Pain may be associated with a bandlike pattern along the interior ankle joint. Entrapment or damage to the *superficial peroneal nerve* may be associated with previous scars or with plantar flexion inversion injury. Occasionally, a Tinel's sign or percussion test will be positive overlying the nerve along the anterior lateral ankle joint line lateral to the extensor tendons. Finally, *osteochondral lesions of the talar dome* may elicit pain while the anterior lateral aspect of the talar dome is palpated with the foot held in plantar flexion.

Symptoms localized to the medial ankle joint and hindfoot consist of nerve entrapments and injury to the flexor tendon groups. *Tarsal tunnel syndrome* consists of entrapment of either the posterior tibial nerve or one of its branches, the medial and lateral plantar nerves under the flexor retinaculum (**Fig. 46-6**). A positive percussion test along the course of the neurovascular bundle may be associated with an injury to the nerve and dysesthesias in the distribution of the medial and lateral plantar nerves into the forefoot. Alternatively, the medial calcaneal nerve, which branches proximal to the tarsal tunnel, may be palpated along its course on the medial aspect of the heel. A *deltoid sprain* may often occur in conjunction with lateral ankle injuries and may be palpated inferior and anterior to the medial malleolus. Rarely do these sprains occur in isolation. *Tendonitis* and *tears of the tibialis posterior tendon* are common sources of medial ankle and proximal arch pain. Pain coursing the posterior tibial tendon along the posterior border of the medial malleolus and distally into the longitudinal arch is noted and may often be associated with swelling and thickening of the tendon. Attrition tears, which are

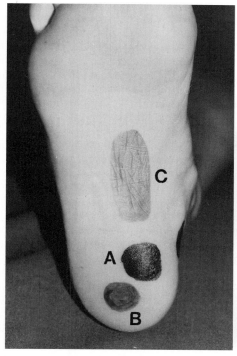
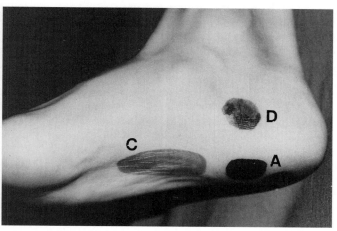

Figure 46-7 Common sites of plantar heel pain: *A*, medial calcaneal tubercle—origin of the plantar fascia as seen in heel pain syndrome; *B*, site for subcalcaneal bursitis and heel pad atrophy; *C*, central band of the plantar fascia; *D*, first branch of the lateral plantar nerve site of entrapment under the abductor hallucis muscle.

commonly seen in middle-aged females, are characterized by progressive loss of the longitudinal arch in association with medial ankle and arch pain. With weight bearing, a marked asymmetry with excessive hindfoot valgus is noted when viewed from behind. In addition, the medial longitudinal arch is depressed and the forefoot drifts into abduction; this creates the "too many toes" sign—visualization of a greater amount of the lateral foot area when viewed from behind. A heel rise test demonstrates the patient's inability to correct the hindfoot valgus, and often the patient will be unable to perform a single-stance heel rise on the affected limb. *Tendonitis* and *tears of the flexor hallucis longus tendon* are often seen in dancers and may be associated with a *posterior impingement syndrome.* Pain and inflammation are noted in the tendon along the posterior margin of the ankle proximal to the medial malleolus. The pain is aggravated by passive motion of the hallux when the ankle is brought from a dorsiflexed to a plantar-flexed position. When tears occur in the tendon, an associated fusiform thickening of the tendon creates a triggering effect, and stenosing tenosynovitis may result in complete loss of passive extension of the hallux while the ankle is in dorsiflexion.

Heel pain may have a variety of causes, including nerve entrapment, focal stress fracture, or inflammation of the plantar fascia (**Fig. 46-7**). Painful *heel pad syndrome* is localized to the central weight-bearing area of the heel and is painful on direct palpation of the heel pad. Atrophy of the heel pad or, alternatively, a subcal-

caneal bursitis is associated with the syndrome. *Calcaneal stress fractures* occur from repetitive high-impact loading. Diffuse swelling in association with tenderness elicited by compression of the medial and lateral aspects of the heel is suggestive of a stress fracture. *Plantar fasciitis or rupture* consists of tenderness along the central band of the plantar aponeurosis as it extends from the margin of the medial calcaneal tubercle to the hallux and lesser toes. Pain with passive dorsiflexion of the toes that puts the plantar fascia on stretch and tenderness on palpation of the plantar fascia are characteristic. In acute cases of plantar facial rupture, a palpable gap and localized swelling may be noted along the midarch level. Plantar fibromatosis unassociated with plantar fasciitis is a painful nodular thickening adherent to the plantar fascia, often in midsubstance. *Entrapment of the first branch of the lateral plantar nerve* (Baxter's nerve) is manifested as heel pain with associated tenderness on palpation above the abductor hallucis muscle medially.[1] Direct palpation may create a burning sensation on the plantar heel that may extend over to the lateral border of the heel. Finally, *heel pain syndrome,* or pain that is localized to the medial calcaneal tuberosity, is central medial on the plantar surface of the heel and is diagnosed through a process of exclusion once the aforementioned sources are evaluated and ruled out.

Midfoot Conditions

Conditions affecting the midfoot generally involve sprains of the various plantar ligaments of the tarsus or arthrosis of the joints caused by a variety of traumatic and inflammatory conditions. Selective palpation correlating with the bony anatomy is essential in isolating the specific joint(s) involved. The *accessory navicular* can be a painful symptomatic accessory bone along the medial aspect of the navicular tuberosity where part of the posterior tibial tendon inserts. Pain is usually elicited with resisted plantar flexion and inversion on palpation of this navicular. Sprains of the tarsometatarsal joint may or may not be associated with swelling through the midfoot. Pain is elicited with a pronation abduction force applied through the forefoot while the midfoot is stabilized. Any instability through these joints should be noted.

The most common afflictions involving the forefoot include disorders of the hallux and lesser toes and metatarsalgia. Disorders of the hallux include hallux valgus, hallux rigidus, and sesamoiditus and fractures. *Hallus valgus*, a lateral deviation of the great toe at the metatarsal phalangeal (MP) joint, may be multifactorial in etiology. Generally, the toe drifts laterally and pronates with subluxation in the dorsal plantar direction. This creates a painful prominence along the dorsal medial metatarsal phalangeal joint. Symptoms relate to mechanical pressure from shoe wear. Because of the altered position of the toe, painful overloading and hyperkeratotic development may exist under the medial base of the proximal phalanx. Similarly, a *transfer lesion* may occur with overloading of the second MP joint. Examination of the overall foot configuration, especially for a planovalgus foot, which may aggravate these symptoms and contribute to the faulty mechanics, should be noted. Trauma to the *dorsomedial cutaneous nerve* as it runs over a prominent medial exostosis may be manifested as a burning dysesthetic pain in the hallux with a positive percussion test overlying the dorsal medial bunion. *Sesamoiditis* secondary to inflammation or fracture is noted under the first metatarsal head and may be localized to either the medial or lateral sesamoid bones. *Hallux limitus and hallux rigidus* are degrees of involvement of arthrosis involving the MP joint. The pain initially is localized to the dorsum of the MP joint, and a palpable joint osteophyte overlying the metatarsal head may be noted. A more involved condition associated with hallux rigidus includes diffuse arthrosis manifested by diffuse joint swelling, thickening of the capsule, and painful crepitus. Motion through the MP joint will be restricted. When motion through the MP joint of the hallux is measured, it is recommended that the zero starting position be used as a reference (**Fig. 46-4**). The hallux is placed in the functional neutral position by aligning the great toe with the plantar surface of the foot. The plantar surface plane is based on a line connecting the calcaneal tuberosity to the head of the first metatarsal. Function is measured in the sagittal plane with plantar flexion and dorsal flexion, and in hallux deformities, mobility and passive correction in the coronal plane should be noted.

Disorders of the lesser toes include deformities of the toes, both fixed and flexible plantar callosities, and nerve entrapments. A *hammer toe* is characterized by a flexion contracture at the proximal interphalangeal (PIP) joint with an associated mild extension contracture at the MP joint, whereas a *claw toe* is typified by hyperextension of the MP joint and flexion contractures of both the PIP and distal interphalangeal (DIP) joints. *Mallet toe* deformities consist of isolated flexion contractures at the DIP joint. All lesser toe deformities may be categorized as either flexible or rigid with the joints being normally located, subluxed, or frankly dislocated. A *corn*, or hyperkeratotic thickening of the skin in response to mechanical pressure within shoe wear against the dorsum of the toe box, is commonly seen and can be painful. Determination of the flexibility in these deformities and the degree of extrinsic tightness is evaluated by pressing underneath the corresponding metatarsal head in a dorsal direction and observing whether the deformity can be corrected passively. A *soft corn*, or *clavus*, is typically seen in the fourth web space and is due to an abutment of the proximal phalanx of one toe against the metatarsal head of the other toe. Pain is recreated by compressing the two toes in the web space together. A synovitis may be noted in the MP joints as a diffuse swelling and thickening of the joint. Palpation by squeezing from a dorsal plantar direction will assess the effusion as well as recreate the pain. *Instability* of the MP joints with disruption or attenuation of the plantar plate may be best delineated by stabilizing the metatarsal shaft with one hand while grasping the base of the proximal phalanx with the other hand and attempting to translocate the toe in a dorsal and plantar direction. Involvement in multiple lesser toes with dislocation dorsally is seen in inflammatory arthropathies like rheumatoid arthritis.

Metatarsalgia is pain under the metatarsal heads that may develop from a variety of causes. In general, the thickness of the fat pad, which is often lost in inflammatory disorders such as rheumatoid arthritis, should be recorded as well as the development of hyperkeratotic lesions on the plantar skin. A *callus*, or localized thickening of the plantar skin in reaction to pressure over bony prominences, is painful with direct pressure on palpation and satellite lesions are not noted, in contrast. A *viral wart* may have satellite lesions, and maximum pain is recreated with side squeezing. The wart has a central core with punctuate hemorrhages unlike the corn where no punctuate bleeding exists, but a seed corn. An *interdigital or Morton's neuroma* occurs most frequently in the second and third web spaces. Applying pressure in the web space distal to the level of the metatarsal heads usually elicits tenderness and recreates the symptoms.

Percussion in the planar web space over the neuroma while the toes are extended may recreate the paresthesias extending into the digits. A click may be appreciated when the foot is squeezed from the medial lateral borders while the plantar web space is palpated distal to the intermetatarsal ligament (Mulder's click).

Fusiform swelling on both the plantar and dorsal metatarsal that is painful proximal to the metatarsal head may be a *stress fracture*. This may be caused by prolonged repetitive activities such as marching; those individuals with a long second ray relative to the first are at increased risk for overload and fracture.

SUMMARY

The step-off approach to clinical evaluation of the foot and ankle starts with a detailed history involving not only the patient's foot complaints but also a review of systems for any systemic condition. Once done, the examiner should evaluate the focus of the patient's symptoms in context and relationship to the remainder of the foot and ankle structures and the lower extremity as a whole. By performing a meticulous evaluation based on a solid understanding of the anatomy and soft tissue and bony landmarks of the foot and ankle, an accurate differential diagnosis and treatment plan can be generated.

References

1. Baxter D, Thigoen CM: Heel pain: operative results, *Foot Ankle* 5:16, 1984

2. Green WB, Heckman JD: *The clinical measurement of joint motion,* ed 1, Park Ridge, Ill., 1994, American Academy of Orthopaedic Surgeons; pp. 117-138.

3. Miller WE: General consideration in the examination of the foot and ankle, *Foot Ankle* 2(4):180-184, 1982.

4. Sammarco GJ, Diraimondo CV: Chronic peroneus brevis lesions, *Foot Ankle* 9:163-170, 1989.

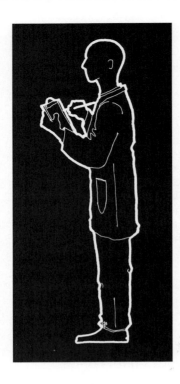

Chapter 47

Treatment and Indications for Surgical Treatment of Foot and Ankle Injuries

Per A.F.H. Renström
Ulf Eklund

CONTENTS

Injuries to the foot and ankle are common at work and in recreational activities. The foot is an anatomical masterpiece involving 29 bones, 19 muscles and tendons, and 115 ligaments. Most of these anatomical structures can be injured in one way or another, and it is therefore very important to secure a correct diagnosis if the treatment is to be a success. The ankle is the most commonly injured part of the body. This chapter includes a description of the different injuries that can occur in the foot and ankle during work and recreational activities. The focus has been to describe how these different injuries can be diagnosed and treated when surgery is indicated. An evaluation of when it is possible to return to work after surgery for the different injuries has been made.

Foot and ankle problems are common, especially in active people. In industrial life, not only are people walking a great deal on hard surfaces, but they are also climbing, jumping, and so forth, so the risk of foot and ankle injuries is increased. Many of these injuries are acute, and the treatment of acute injuries such as fractures and ligament and tendon ruptures is usually non-controversial. Many injuries, however, are overuse injuries, and they constitute a great clinical diagnostic and therapeutic problem. Treatment and indications for surgery are often controversial in these cases. In this chapter we try to shed some light on these injuries, give indications for surgery, and estimate the time to return to work after surgery.

ANKLE SPRAINS

In spite of the high frequency of ankle injuries, clinical diagnostic techniques and methods of treatment vary greatly, perhaps because the biomechanics of the ankle ligaments and their clinical evaluation are not fully known. The anterior talofibular ligament (ATFL), the calcaneofibular ligament (CFL), and the posterior talofibular ligament (PTFL) function as a unit. Although one may resist a specific motion, the primary stabilizing ligament is dependent on foot position. As the foot plantar-flexes, strain in the ATFL increases and strain in the CFL decreases. Although the ATFL is the weakest ligament, it is clinically the most significant ligament. It is involved in 85% of cases of common inversion ankle sprains and in 20% in combination with the CFL. Clinical ligamentous damage is primarily a function of tensile loading and is only secondarily affected by twisting and shear forces.

The most common mechanism of injury to the lateral ligaments of the ankle is plantar flexion and thereafter gradually increasing progression to inversion. The lateral joint capsule tears first, followed by rupture of the ATFL, which causes hemarthrosis and subcutaneous ecchymosis. With further inversion, the CFL ruptures, and the PTF and deltoid ligaments sustain varying degrees of injury: in 60% the ATFL tears alone, in 20% the ATFL tears in combination with the CFL, in 10% the PTFL tears, and in 3% the deltoid ligament tears.

Treatment of severe grade III lateral ankle ligament tears has generated much controversy, but a critical review of the literature shows that functional treatment provides the quickest recovery to full range of motion and return to work and physical activity without major residual problems.[5] Functional treatment should include a short period of protection by tape, bandage, or brace, followed by early weight bearing. This is recommended as the treatment of choice in most acute cases. Range-of-motion exercises and neuromuscular training should begin early. If residual problems persist after functional treatment, delayed surgical reconstruction or repair can be performed years after the injury with results comparable to those after primary repair.

Some authors have recommended operative repair of acute severe ankle sprains in young athletes. Indications for acute repair for athletes as listed by Leach and Schepsis[7] are (1) a history of momentary talocrural dislocation with complete ligamentous disruption, (2) a clinical anterior drawer sign, (3) 10 degrees more tilt on the affected side with stress inversion testing, (4) clinical or radiographic suspicion of tears in both the ATFL and CFL, and (5) osteochondral fracture. Most techniques described for repair of acute ligament injuries are similar. Ten percent to 20% of the cases, however, have residual problems. If a patient has continuous pain and swelling 3 to 4 months after an ankle ligament sprain, attention should be focused on intraarticular lesions or other differential diagnoses. It is very important to be aware of the many differential diagnostic possibilities.

Chronic Ankle Instability

Chronic ankle instability may be either mechanical or functional. Mechanical instability is characterized by ankle mobility beyond the physiological range of motion and is measurable by anterior drawer and talar tilt tests. Mechanical instability is present if anterior translation is more than 10 mm (or more than 3 mm greater than that of the uninjured ankle) or when talar tilt is more than 9 degrees (or 3 degrees greater than the uninjured ankle). Functional instability is a subjective feeling of giving way of the ankle during physical activity or walking on uneven ground. Chronic ankle instability of either type with pain, recurrent giving way, and positive stress testing is an indication for operative treatment.

Surgical Treatment

Chronic ankle instability, as demonstrated by pain, recurrent giving way, and positive stress tests, is a major indication for surgical treatment. A combination of mechanical and functional instability is the most frequently reported indication for surgery.

More than 50 procedures and modifications have been described for treating chronic ankle instability. These can be loosely grouped as nonanatomical reconstructions or anatomical repairs. The reported success rates for nearly all procedures are more than 80%.

Nonanatomic reconstructions use another structure or material to substitute for the injured ligaments. Structures commonly used for grafting are fascia lata and peroneus brevis tendon. Numerous modifications of these classic procedures have been described.

Anatomical reconstruction is based on the Broström report[3] in 1966 that direct suture repair of chronic ankle ligament injuries was possible, even many years after the initial injuries, and that the ends of the ligament could be found. Others reported that the elongated ligaments had healed encased in fibrous scar tissue. Several authors have reported successful imbrication or shortening and replantation of the ligaments to achieve good results with a technique (Peterson procedure) that includes shortening of the ligament, repair through bony tunnels, and imbrication with local tissue.[9] This anatomical technique repairs both the ATFL and CFL. Nonanatomical reconstructions, except for the Elmslie procedure and the Chrisman-Snook modification, repair only the ATFL. Repair of the CFL is important because insufficiency of this ligament may be a factor in the development of subtalar instability.

Anatomical repair of both the ATFL and CFL through bony tunnels produces good long-term results and is recommended as the initial procedure in most cases. If anatomical repair fails, a tenodesis procedure such as the Chrisman-Snook reconstruction is a good alternative. Nonanatomical reconstructions are also indicated in patients with moderate arthritis or lax joints.

Return to work. After surgery, it is possible to return to a desk job after 1 to 2 weeks depending on the pain. The patient will, however, depend on crutches for 2 to 3 weeks. Return to walking work will be possible after healing and rehabilitation, which most commonly is 3 to 4 months.

CHRONIC ANKLE PAIN

Persistent ankle pain has been attributed to many causes, including incomplete rehabilitation, chondral or osteochondral lesions of the talus, occult fractures, and impingement syndromes.

Osteochondral Lesions of the Talus

Osteochondral fracture, talar dome fracture, transchondral fracture, and osteochondritis dissecans are currently believed to be similar lesions. The etiology is traumatic, either as a single event or as multiple microtraumatic insults. Osteochondral lesions are staged in four levels: *Stage I* is a compression injury causing microscopic damage to an area of subchondral bone. Plain radiographs are negative. In *stage II*, a partially detached osteochondral fragment is detectable on careful examination of an adequate series of plain radiographs. In *stage III*, the osteochondral fragment is completely detached but remains in anatomical position, and in *stage IV*, the detached fragment is displaced elsewhere in the joint.

The patient usually has a history of a sprained ankle. Sometimes a "pop" was heard. With a recent injury, moderate or severe swelling of the joint can be seen. Tenderness is typically located just distal to the anterior tibiofibular syndesmosis or behind the medial malleolus, depending on the location of the lesion. Following an inversion injury, the symptoms of a concomitant anterolateral osteochondral lesion may be "mashed" in the signs of the ligament tear.

When an osteochondral lesion is suspected, a careful plain radiographic examination is needed with anteroposterior (AP), lateral, and oblique views of the ankle. Mortise views in plantar flexion should disclose a posteromedial lesion, and the corresponding view in dorsiflexion reveals an anterolateral lesion. If the patient is treated for a ligament injury alone (usually immediate functional rehabilitation), the symptoms persist—pain just distal to the anterior syndesmosis, recurrent swelling, and even catching or locking—and a renewed plain radiograph investigation is negative, further imaging of the ankle is necessary, including a bone scan, which is very sensitive although not specific. If the bone scan is not over the talus, further evaluation by plain tomography, computed tomography (CT), or magnetic resonance imaging (MRI) is sometimes needed to accurately determine the exact location and extent of the lesion.

Appropriate staging and early treatment of osteochondral lesions of the talus provide the best end results. Healing depends on capillary overgrowth from the body of the talus. Immobilization of the area seems to be necessary to prevent the frictional effects of an uneven joint surface and potential progress of the lesion into more advanced stages leading to nonunion. Lesions in stages I, II, and III without established nonunion signs (marked sclerosis, gross uneven joint surfaces, or osteoarthrosis) are treated with a non–weight-bearing lower leg cast for 6 weeks, followed by a weight-bearing cast until radiographic evidence of a healing. An interarticular injection of 10 ml lidocaine can be effective in stage I lesions. Delayed nonoperative treatment of stage III lesions often fails. These lesions, as well as stage IV lesions, are often treated surgically to prevent further deterioration of the joint. An experienced arthroscopic surgeon reaches many of these lesions arthroscopically (removal of the detached lesion and debridement of the lesion bed), but open approaches are occasionally needed. Reattachment of the osteochondral lesion might be considered in the acute phase. Proper access occasionally requires osteotomy of the medial or lateral malleolus. If an osteotomy is performed, it is essential that subsequent internal fixation is rigid to allow the important early motion rehabilitation. Postoperative weight bearing is delayed 2 to 6 weeks (a full 6 weeks if osteotomy of the medial malleolus was performed). Results are mixed. The prognosis following early nonoperative treatment in stages I, II, and III is good in 75% of patients; surgery in late stage III and in stage IV lesions yields a 40% to 80% rate of good results. Advanced lesions, where treatment has been delayed more than 1 year, generally have a poor outcome.[8]

Return to work. After arthroscopic curettage and drilling, return to work that involves walking is possible within 2 to 4 months after the surgery. In some cases, however, pain will be persistent and return to work may require a longer time. In 20% to 25% of cases, a second surgery with bone grafting may be necessary, but this will not really be apparent until 6 months after the first surgery.

Loose Bodies in the Ankle

Loose bodies in the ankle are typically seen on plain radiographs and are often related to intermittent pain, swelling, and clicking. They emanate either from a stage IV transchondral fracture of the talus, from osteophytes on the anterior distal rim of the tibia or the dorsal neck of the talus, or if multiple, from "synovial osteochondromatosis." Posteriorly located loose bodies must be differentiated from an extraarticular os trigonum. Chip fractures may appear as loose bodies as well. Pure chondral loose bodies from lesions in the tibial plafond or talar dome or from synovial chondromatosis cause the same symptoms. However, if plain radiographs are negative, more advanced measures are needed such as MRI or arthroscopy.

Arthroscopic removal of loose bodies by a skilled arthroscopic ankle surgeon is the treatment of choice. Far posteriorly located bodies and lesions should be approached by open means if the surgeon is not comfortable with the posterior arthroscopic portals.

Impingement Syndromes

Impingement synovitis of the lateral ankle following an inversion injury is not uncommon. Symptoms can totally mimic those of an anterolateral talar osteochondral lesion. Radiographic evaluation used for detecting osteochondral pathology should also reveal soft tissue abnormalities. In the absence of concomitant chronic ligamentous instability, treatment of impingement synovitis involves the surgical removal of impinging tissue by way of the arthroscope. When lateral ligamentous insufficiency is also present, open removal of impinging chronic synovitis tissue together with an appropriate stabilizing procedure is recommended. Postoperative results are generally excellent, provided that no chondral lesions are present.

Residual symptoms following an ankle inversion injury are quite common and are most often due to mechanical and/or functional instability of the joint. Occasionally, however, anterolateral ankle pain and a feeling of giving way persist in spite of normal stability and a well performed functional rehabilitation program. Examination reveals tenderness just anterior to the lateral malleolus, especially in dorsiflexion. Additionally, at times a snapping phenomenon from this region can be elicited when the foot is tested for inversion stability. In these instances, a *meniscoid lesion of the ankle* should be suspected. Radiographs are normal, as is bone scintigraphy, thereby excluding osteochondral lesions. A possible etiology is fibrosis that has developed in posttraumatic impingement synovitis following the inversion injury. Possibly, torn strands of the ATFL or distal parts of it are caught in the talofibular joint, with subsequent synovitis and ultimately fibrosis developing. An intraarticular injection of 10 ml lidocaine may limit the pain. This test and limited dorsiflexion will secure the diagnosis.

On exploration, which is readily done arthroscopically, the lesion has a hyalinized meniscoid appearance. Simple excision of the lesion and surrounding reactive synovitis leads to full recovery in the majority of patients.

Return to work. After an impingement syndrome that involves impingement synovitis or a meniscoid lesion that has been treated surgically, return to work can vary somewhat but should be possible within 1 to 3 months, depending on the type of work. Results and the prognosis are usually good.

Osteophytes at the anterior rim of the tibia—often called "soccer player's ankle"—is a condition with decreased dorsiflexion and pain over the anterior part of the ankle joint. Apart from soccer, the condition is seen also in sports such as American football and orienteering; however, it is only seen rarely in recreational athletes. Dorsiflexion is blocked because of the formation of osteophytes on the distal anterior rim of the tibia and sometimes on the corresponding area of the dorsum of the talar neck. The osteophytes probably result from repetitive traction microtrauma to the ankle joint capsule with subsequent bleeding and, ultimately, reactive osteophyte formation. The history, clinical examination, and plain radiographs reveal the condition.

Removal of the osteophytes, openly or arthroscopically, followed by rapid rehabilitation consistently yields good or excellent results, although ankle dorsiflexion is not always fully restored.

Sinus Tarsi Syndrome

Patients with a history of multiple lateral ankle sprains occasionally have residual pain and tenderness to palpation 2 cm anterior and distal to the tip of the lateral malleolus. This area, the sinus tarsi, is a funnel-shaped cavity bordered by the talar neck superiorly, the anterolateral calcaneus inferiorly and posteriorly, and the interosseous talocalcaneal ligament anteriorly. Recurrent subtalar sprains may cause microruptures in this broad, flat ligament leading to a chronic inflammatory reaction. The diagnosis is determined from the patient's history and localized tenderness slightly but significantly distal to the ATFL. Usually, subtalar motion is impaired and sometimes painful. Typically, ankle joint stability is not affected. Radiographs are negative, but temporary pain relief from a local anesthetic block into the sinus tarsi is highly diagnostic.

Initial treatment consists of rest and nonsteroidal antiinflammatory drugs (NSAIDs). Steroid injection into the sinus tarsi has proven helpful.[6] In the rehabilitation phase, peroneal remobilization is emphasized because a sinus tarsi syndrome may be related to functional instability of the ankle joint. In the rare cases where symptoms persist, surgical "decompression," that is, excision of the sinus tarsi contents, has been successful.

Return to work is often possible 1 to 2 months after surgery, but this can vary.

Arthrosis of the Ankle

The incidence of ankle arthrosis is low when compared with that of the hip and knee. It is most commonly seen following a fracture around the ankle, especially when fracture healing was allowed in a nonanatomic position. This leads to incongruency of the ankle mortise and, often, to rapid development of arthrosis. Other predisposing factors include severe ligamentous laxity and stage III and IV osteochondral lesions of the tibial plafond or the talar dome.

As yet, no curative treatment has been found for articular surface injury and/or degeneration. Symptomatic treatment aiming at unloading the surfaces and reducing the reactive inflammation is easy and often very helpful. Occasionally, especially with catching and locking sensations from detached osteophytes or pieces of cartilage, arthroscopic or open debridement and loose body removal are warranted. In severe cases, more extensive treatment must be considered. Ankle arthrodesis is an option often yielding pain relief. The functional disability can often be well compensated in young patients. In older patients, ankle arthroplasty may be an alternative.

TENDON INJURIES AROUND THE ANKLE

Traditionally, the term *tendinitis* has been used to describe most tendon overuse injuries. However, the tendon itself consists of dense connective tissue with little inherent vascularity and is not predisposed to inflammatory change. Instead, the term *tendinosis* is used to define structural (degenerative) tendon changes. The surrounding tendon sheath—peritenon—is usually highly vascularized and subject to inflammation, or *peritendinitis*, when overused. Tendon disease (excluding ruptures) can thus be described as tendinosis, peritendinitis, or a combination.

Achilles Tendon Overuse Injuries

Achilles tendon overuse injuries are common. A number of intrinsic and extrinsic factors predispose to these injuries: lower extremity malalignment (hyperpronation, increased femoral anteversion, cavus foot, etc.) and a tight Achilles tendon with poor flexibility. In recreational running athletes, poor shoes, hilly tracks, and training errors (such as sudden changes in mileage or speed and improper warm-up and cool-down) are related to heel cord overuse problems. Pain is the main symptom, and is typically located 2 to 6 cm above the Achilles tendon insertion at the dorsal aspect of the calcaneus. This region of the Achilles tendon complex is considered vulnerable and prone to overuse because of poor vascularity. Physical examination includes an evaluation of alignment and flexibility of the heel cord and inspection/palpation of the cord, the insertion, and the retrocalcaneal area. Four major differential diagnoses must be considered.

1. *Peritendinitis* is manifested as inflammation of the surrounding peritenon.
2. *Tendinosis,* or degenerative changes within the tendon itself, is characterized by gradual onset of pain, some stiffness, and diffuse tenderness and swelling of the tendon complex. With peritendinitis, crepitation is occasionally present. Acute condi-

tions usually heal with rest and correction of the underlying cause. Chronic conditions are difficult to treat successfully. Concentric and eccentric contraction exercises according to the slow-progression principle are used together with orthotics aimed at correcting malalignments.

3. *A partial rupture* typically has a sudden onset of pain. Clinical examination demonstrates localized swelling and distinct tenderness, which distinguishes this lesion from peritendinitis and tendinosis. The healing potential of partial Achilles tendon tears is poor, with more than 80% of patients having residual problems 5 years and 73% having problems 10 years after the injury.[1]

4. *Retrocalcaneal bursitis,* an inflammation of the bursa between the calcaneus and the anterior aspect of the Achilles tendon, is characterized by pain combined with tenderness and swelling anterior to the distal part of the heel cord.

   Treatment of Achilles tendon overuse injuries is primarily conservative (except for partial tears), the cornerstones being correction of malalignment, ice and NSAIDs, ankle range-of-motion exercises, and stretching/strengthening of the plantar flexors and dorsiflexors of the ankle. We strongly advise against the use of corticosteroid injections in the treatment of heel cord injuries. A 1-cm heel wedge can be useful in reducing symptoms in daily activities. It is important to avoid strenuous and repetitive heel cord loads for an extended period of time; the patient should be informed that healing of heel cord overuse injuries often requires treatment for 4 to 6 months. If conservative measures fail in spite of a 6-month period of adequate treatment, surgery may be indicated. Preoperatively, radiographic investigation will exclude calcifications, and MRI or ultrasonography will reveal the extent of structural changes within the tendon. This helps the surgeon plan the surgery and decide what procedure is appropriate.

   Surgery for peritendinitis includes incision/removal of the thickened, scarred peritenon. Surgery for a partial tear or tendinosis involves an incision longitudinally in the tendon and careful removal of pathologic tissue. Thereafter, the tendon should be carefully closed by adapting side to side. If retrocalcaneal bursitis is the diagnosis, the bursa should be removed and an osteotomy of the superior corner of the calcaneal tuberosity carried out. Postoperative care usually involves immobilization for 7 to 10 days and then mobilization-allowing plantar flexion of 0 to 20 degrees in a walking boot. With appropriate indications and carefully monitored postoperative rehabilitation for 4 to 6 months, surgery yields good results in 80% to 85% of patients.

   Return to Work. After surgery, return to work depends on the diagnosis and the type of work. The patient can return to desk work within the first week but should keep the leg elevated. If the patient has mobile work that includes lots of walking, the patient can return to limited activities after 1 month and walk in the walking boot. Return to full activity is usually possible 3 to 4 months after surgery.

5. *Complete Achilles tendon rupture* most commonly occurs in active people about 35 to 45 years of age. The most common situation is sports activity that involves a sudden change of motion. The typical history is a sudden pop and pain. Injured people often think that somebody has hit them from behind. An inability to plantar-flex the foot is typical, and Thompsen's test is diagnostic.

   The treatment for active people is most commonly surgery. Surgery allows early tension to be put on the tendon, which results in proper orientation of the collagen and thereby the possibility to regain full strength. Plantar flexion from 0 to 20 degrees is allowed after 1 week and this early motion makes it possible for an early return to work. The patient can walk in a walking boot after 2 to 3 weeks. Nonsurgical treatment is also possible for less active people. This involves at least 6 to 8 weeks of immobilization and a long rehabilitation. Return to desk work is possible at an early stage. The risk for rerupture is much higher with nonsurgical therapy and early motion is not possible.

Return to work. After a complete Achilles tendon tear, return to a desk job depends on crutch walking but is possible within 3 to 5 days regardless of treatment. The patient can often walk reasonably well after 1 month with a walking boot if surgery has been performed and can walk properly and go back to full activity 3 to 5 months after the surgery. Return to hard physical activity or work after conservative therapy is sometimes possible after 6 to 9 months.

Peroneal Tendon Injuries

The peroneus longus and brevis tendons run downward on the lateral aspect of the ankle and midfoot to their insertions on the plantar side of the first metatarsal, medial cuneiform, and navicular and on the proximal end of the fifth metatarsal, respectively. The tendons pass behind the lateral malleolus beneath the superior and inferior retinacula, by which the tendons are held in position.

Peroneal peritendinitis or *tendinosis* is typically elicited via stenosis under these retinacula. *A longitudinal tear* can occur by trauma or overuse. A common predisposing factor to peroneal tendon disease is distortion of the local anatomy caused by a fracture of the lateral malleolus or the calcaneus or by an ankle sprain. Pain, swelling, and joint tenderness are located posterior and inferior to the lateral malleolus. Pain may be increased on weight bearing, but forced plantar flexion and inversion and resisted eversion of the ankle are more painful. Physical examination must include an evaluation of tendon stability. Subtalar motion usually is decreased. Treatment is primarily conservative: active rest, ice, NSAIDs, and crutches as acute measures. Casting can possibly be helpful in some patients. Surgery with correction of the cause is sometimes necessary.

Recurrent subluxation or dislocation of the peroneal tendons is an important differential diagnosis. This kind of injury requires major trauma with internal rotation in combination with inversion. The patient can feel pain when this happens. This injury feels like the tendon is subluxing or dislocating over the lateral aspect of the lateral malleolus. When doing twisting activities, this can happen and is painful for the patient. Treatment of these injuries is often surgical, but some people prefer a short period of casting.

Surgery is indicated for subluxing or dislocating tendons in most cases if this injury tends to become chronic. When this condition is chronic, it is painful and the patient cannot carry out hard work without pain and fear of painfully dislocating or subluxing the tendon. Surgery includes deepening of the peroneal groove and imbrication of the retinacula. If the tendon also has a chronic pathologic condition, surgical incision and removal of the pathologic tissue can be valuable, although this kind of surgery is not very common.

Return to work. After surgery, return to a desk job is possible within the first 3 to 5 days. However, after surgery the rehabilitation time is 6 weeks in a walking boot and then 6 weeks of rehabilitation, so return to harder labor is possible after 3 months.

Flexor Hallucis Longus Tendon Overuse Problems

Overuse problems in the flexor hallucis longus tendon complex are common in ballet dancers because of frequent and forceful plantar flexion of the ankle and great toe (plié and point work). Repetitive push-off maneuvers also transmit substantial forces across the tendon and its sheath, with possible irritation, swelling, and nodulus formation following.

The result is pain and sometimes catching or even locking of the tendon—functional hallux rigidus. Symptoms are most often located behind the medial malleolus where the tendon passes through a narrow fibrous tunnel, thereby predisposing to impingement. Other tight areas for flexor hallucis longus tendon passage are under the base of the first metatarsal and between the great toe sesamoids.

Therapy consists of active rest, ice, NSAIDs, and crutches in the acute phase. A longitudinal arch support with firm soles is often helpful. Plié and point work in dancers, as well as forced toe-off exercises, must be avoided until the patient is symptom free. If symptoms persist, especially if they are stenotic, surgery is indicated. The fibrous tunnel is divided, and tenosynovectomy and tendon debridement are performed. Local swelling of the tendon proper, when present, is explored

and often reveals a partial rupture. Scar tissue excision and tendon reconstruction are performed. Postoperatively, the ankle is immobilized 2 to 10 days followed by a rehabilitation program.

Return to work. In jobs with hard labor, return to work is possible after 2 to 4 months.

Tibial Posterior Tendon Overuse Problems

Overuse tibial posterior tendon injuries are seen in young active persons such as runners. Hyperpronation is a strong predisposing factor because mechanical demands on the tendon along its course behind the medial malleolus to the insertion on the navicular bone are then significantly increased. Repetitive microtrauma leads to inflammation in the sheath and to partial tears and scar formation in the tendon itself. Complete ruptures are seen in the elderly population. Long-standing unidentified tibial posterior tendon ruptures result in a unilateral flatfoot and highly or totally impaired independent toe rise.

Clinical findings include tenderness and sometimes swelling along the course of the tendon behind the medial malleolus. Crepitus is frequently present. Passive pronation and resisted supination of the midfoot exacerbate the pain.

Treatment in the acute phase includes active rest, ice, NSAIDs, and a medially posted orthotic. In severe cases, a short leg non–weight-bearing cast for 2 weeks usually relieves the pain. Patients with flatfoot deformities need more advanced orthotic treatment following careful biomechanical evaluation. In chronic cases, surgical exploration is considered to address potential tenosynovitis, tendinosis, tendon tear, and stenosis along the tendon course.

Return to work depends on the resolution of pain. After surgery, 2 to 4 months is often needed for healing and rehabilitation before pain-free walking is possible.

SUBTALAR JOINT INJURIES

Subtalar Joint Dislocations

Subtalar joint dislocations are occasionally seen in athletes, but more commonly they are caused by a fall from a height or a traffic accident. Substantial torsional force is required to accomplish these dislocations because of the pronounced inherent bony and ligamentous (deltoid medially; calcaneofibular and talocalcaneal laterally) stability of the subtalar joints. The dislocation is classified according to the direction taken by the foot in relation to the talus: medial, lateral, posterior, or anterior. Medial dislocation is by far the most common subtalar dislocation reported, the injury mechanism being forced inversion. The condition is very painful to the hindfoot, and the deformity marked, with the midfoot and forefoot severely adducted. Prompt management is crucial because of compromise of neurovascular structures. Anteroposterior and lateral radiographs of the ankle and foot are taken without delay. Fractures of the malleoli, talus, fifth metatarsal, or navicular sometimes accompany these injuries. An attempt at closed reduction under intravenous sedation may be justified, but if not successful, immediate open reduction must follow. Once reduced, the subtalar and talonavicular joints are typically stable, and no internal fixation is needed. Postoperatively, immobilization in a short leg non–weight-bearing cast for 3 weeks is recommended, followed by gradual range-of-motion exercises and progressive weight bearing.

Provided that subtalar dislocations are treated promptly and reduction is successful, the prognosis is satisfactory in many patients. Severe soft-tissue problems and associated fractures tend to worsen the outcome. Late complications include impaired subtalar motion, arthrosis of the joints affected, and persistent swelling and pain. In selected patients, a triple arthrodesis is warranted.

FRACTURES

Fracture of the Talus

The talus holds a key position in the ankle joint—that of linking the leg and the foot. It articulates to the tibia and fibula, calcaneus, and navicular. More than 60% of the surface is covered with articular cartilage, which leaves only a limited area for nutritional blood supply. Talar blood supply is further compromised with trauma and/or surgery in this region.

Apart from the common minute avulsions from the lateral part of the talar neck following lateral ankle sprains, substantial trauma is required to fracture the talus. Most commonly, a talar neck fracture is sustained from a forceful passive dorsiflexion of the ankle joint, as occurs when landing on the feet after a fall from a height. In this situation, the anterior margin of the distal end of the tibia is thrust into the dorsal talar neck. The patient has significant swelling and pain. Radiographs give details as to the fracture pattern and possible subluxation or dislocations.

Displaced fractures require reduction and rigid fixation, followed by early non–weight-bearing range-of-motion exercises. For undisplaced fractures, 6 to 8 weeks' immobilization in a neutral-position short leg cast is recommended. Weight bearing is delayed until radiographic union is evident.

The prognosis after displaced, unreduced fractures is poor. Better results are achieved following anatomic reduction and stable screw fixation. However, even with apparently nondisplaced fractures, ankle joint arthrosis develops in one third of the patients at late follow-up.

Fractures of the Calcaneus

Like talar fractures, substantial force is required to create a fracture of the calcaneus. Landing on the heel after a fall or jump from a height is the most frequent injury mechanism. A calcaneal fracture is very painful and is usually associated with significant swelling. Plain radiographs give the diagnosis. However, further imaging using CT may give additional valuable information regarding the extent of the fracture and its effect on the subtalar joints. The risk of compartment syndrome in the intrinsic muscle compartments of the foot necessitates monitoring compartment pressures and performing a fasciotomy when indicated (pressure above 35 mm Hg) to prevent ischemic muscle injuries and clawing of the toes.

Treatment of calcaneal fractures is controversial. Because of the topographic complexity of the bone and the variable fracture patterns, it is difficult to obtain comparable groups when different treatments are evaluated. A full spectrum of treatment modalities ranging from no reduction/no surgery/no immobilization, by closed reduction/immobilization, to open reduction/internal fixation (ORIF) are used. However, at present, the trend seems to be increasing in favor of open treatment. The main indications are severely disrupted posterior subtalar facets, a significant upward displacement of the calcaneal tuberosity, or a valgus displacement of the tuberosity of the calcaneus with abutment against the lateral malleolus.

If a nonoperative approach is chosen, early motion is recommended while weight bearing is delayed 8 weeks. Operative treatment necessitates care by a surgeon with extensive hindfoot fracture experience.

The long-term prognosis after calcaneal fractures is guarded, regardless of treatment. Eighty percent to 90% of patients have residual symptoms. Typically, subtalar mobility is significantly inhibited. In many cases, a permanent custom-made heel orthotic is required to control pain and swelling.

Return to work. Depending on the location and extent of the injury, return to work varies. It is sometimes impossible to return to hard work because of persistent pain during walking.

STRESS FRACTURES

Stress Fractures of the Foot and Ankle

Stress fractures are the most common fractures of the foot and ankle in athletes and workers. Typical stress fracture locations are the distal fibula, tibia, calcaneus and navicular bone, and metatarsals. Bone is continuously adapting to new loading patterns. A stress or fatigue fracture is the failure point in a normal adaptive process. The periosteum gives early warning signs of overloading such as pain. If fatigue microdamage occurs too rapidly, new bone cannot develop fast enough, and the bone weakens. Gradually, a stress fracture develops.

The muscles play a major role in shock absorption. *Muscle fatigue* impairs shock absorption, which leads to altered stress distribution and increased compressive loads on the bone with a greater risk for stress fracture. Together with muscle fatigue, another important contributing factor in the development of a stress fracture is *biomechanical imbalance,* such as skeletal asymmetry and leg length discrepancy. A short leg is more susceptible to stress reaction and fracture. Some *anatomical abnormalities* predispose to stress reactions, however, on an unpredictable basis. For example, a rigid foot puts increased stress on the metatarsals. The second metatarsal is at risk in hard surface running with a tight heel cord, a long second metatarsal, or a flexible, nonsupportive great toe present. Other factors include exercises on hard surfaces, improperly supportive shoes, and injury to the opposite extremity. The patient protects the injured limb by placing more weight on the opposite limb.

A common clinical course is insidious onset of pain that is vague at first. With continued stress, pain increases and becomes more localized, with possible soft tissue swelling. Clinical examination reveals distinct tenderness over the lesion. The diagnosis is verified by scintigraphy. Plain radiographs typically become positive at 3 to 8 weeks. Treatment consists of activity modification to the limits of comfort. Nongravity exercises are initiated. Casting is recommended with multiple fractures, intolerable pain, or fragmentation. Healing of a properly treated stress fracture occurs in 4 to 15 weeks but could take 6 months. A useful clinical healing test is having the patient hop on the affected limb without pain. Screening for hormonal imbalance or endocrine dysfunction is indicated in multiple or recurrent stress fractures.

HINDFOOT STRESS FRACTURE

Calcaneal stress fractures are relatively uncommon. They have been reported in military recruits in vigorous physical training of more than 16 hours a day. Diffuse pain about the heel is aggravated by compression of the heel from a medial to lateral direction. Pain is *not* localized only to the plantar aspect of the heel. Weight bearing as tolerated with crutches, a shock-absorbing heel insert, NSAIDs, and at least 6 to 8 weeks are required for healing.

METATARSAL STRESS FRACTURES

Seventeen percent to 20% of stress fractures in the lower extremity are located in the metatarsals. The second ray is the most common site of a metatarsal stress fracture. Surgery for hallux valgus is related to stress fracture of the second metatarsal because of altered loading patterns. Hypermobility of a metatarsal can predispose to adjacent metatarsal stress fracture. Typical locations are: first metatarsal—medial base; second and third—distal diaphysis; fourth—middle or distal diaphysis; fifth—proximal (junction metaphysis/diaphysis). Typically, symptoms progress slowly in a "crescendo effect." It can take 1 to 2 months or more before stress fractures become visible on plain radiographs. A bone scan is the key to early radiographic confirmation of a stress fracture.

Metatarsal stress fractures are generally treated nonoperatively; in early nondisplaced fractures, activities are limited for 4 weeks. Running in 3 to 4 feet of water is beneficial, if the forefoot is protected from heavy repetitive loading.

However, stress fractures through the fifth metatarsal need special attention. Nonoperative treatment implies 6 to 8 weeks of non–weight-bearing casting. Less restricted non-operative treatments have shown high failure rates. An increasing number of investigators advocate internal fixation (screw) early because this markedly decreases healing time and return to strenuous activities.[4] Signs of chronicity of the fracture such as cortical thickening and intramedullary sclerosis strongly indicate that only open treatment will be successful. Surgical alternatives are curettage, bone grafting, and cerclage fixation of the fracture; drilling of the medullary canal followed by malleolar screw fixation without opening the fracture; or combinations of the two. Postoperative casting time varies from 2 to 8 weeks among authors. Return to strenuous activities requires clinical and radiographic evidence of healing in 8 to 12 weeks.

HALLUX SESAMOID STRESS FRACTURES

Hallux sesamoid stress fractures are rare, much rarer than sesamoiditis, a difficult differential diagnosis. Bipartition of the sesamoid is not uncommon, so radiographic diagnosis is also difficult. Furthermore, scintigraphy is positive in both stress fractures and sesamoiditis. Stress fractures, however, do not heal with immobilization or prolonged inactivity. If other causes of pain can be excluded, a sesamoid stress fracture is treated with excision, with a good prognosis thereafter. It should be noted that surgical access to the lateral sesamoid is difficult. The safe removal of the lateral sesamoid requires significant surgical experience in this area.

TARSAL NAVICULAR STRESS FRACTURE

Navicular stress fractures are uncommon in nonathletes. The condition is characterized by an insidious onset of vague arch pain, increased pain in the midfoot with motion, and limited dorsiflexion of the ankle. Activity increases the discomfort. Typically but not always, tenderness is localized over the navicular bone. Plain radiographs are most often normal, and a bone scan is required for diagnosis. Plain tomography or CT delineates the extent of the fracture. The fracture is typically sagittally oriented in the central third of the bone. This might be due to the relative avascularity of the central part of the navicular. Treatment of acutely displaced fractures calls for ORIF with screws. Nondisplaced fractures should be treated with a non–weight-bearing cast for 6 to 8 weeks to heal uneventfully. In patients not casted or given a weight-bearing cast, the complication rate is high with delayed union, nonunion, and recurrence of the fracture. Nonunion should be treated by bone grafting, with or without instrumentation. Postoperatively, the ankle and foot are immobilized in a non–weight-bearing cast until union has occurred, which may take 2 to 4 months.

Return to work. After surgery, return to work may be possible the same day if the work is a desk job. Return to work depends on the location and type of stress fracture. Non–weight bearing is sometimes necessary with hard labor for 1 to 2 months, so it can take 2 to 4 months before a patient returns to hard labor.

HEEL PAIN

Heel pain is a common and potentially disabling condition with many possible causes. Distinction of these is important because treatment and the expected outcome differ.

A thorough history of the patient's pain and a careful physical examination are mandatory tools in establishing a correct diagnosis. An evaluation of the patient's characterization of the pain, including onset, duration, nature, localization, and relation to physical activity, will help in establishing the diagnosis. Alignment of the lower part of the leg, ankle, and foot should be determined, as well as the range of motion of the ankle and subtalar joints and the status of the longitudinal and transverse arches of the foot. Skin abnormalities such as discoloration, wounds, bumps, and blisters and tender areas, including nerve branches (Tinel's sign) should be noted.

Plantar Fasciitis

True plantar fasciitis is an inflammation of a greater part of the plantar fascia with pain on passive dorsiflexion of the toes and tenderness over the proximal area of the plantar fascia. Therefore, symptoms predominate in the plantar aspect of the midfoot rather than the heel. Special orthotics designed to relieve the pressure on the plantar fascia should be used. If symptoms persist in spite of adequate rest and orthotic use (3 to 6 months), surgery such as proximal plantar fascia release should be considered.

Heel Pain Syndrome

Pain localized over the plantar fascia origin on the anteriomedial calcaneal tuberosity is termed *heel pain syndrome* or *plantar fasciitis*. Onset is insidious, proceeded by overuse. Pathogenesis is believed to be traction periostitis and microruptures at the plantar fascia origin. Symptoms include morning stiffness and pain that resolve during the day. However, pain increases following prolonged walking and can be intolerable with jumping and running. Palpation reveals pain in the very localized area just described, but the pain is typically not elicited with passive dorsiflexion of the toes, which causes traction on the plantar fascia. Plain radiographs are negative and may or may not show a calcaneal spur.

Primarily, conservative treatment consists of active rest, NSAIDs, and usually an orthotic device (shock-absorbing heel cup, custom-made nonrigid orthosis). Stretching exercises are advocated in the presence of a tight heel cord. Within a 3-month time frame, this treatment is usually successful, but up to 1 year may be required in some cases. In refractory cases, one corticosteroid injection may be considered; however, it is crucial that the cortisone be deposited *deep* to the plantar fascia to avoid plantar fat pad atrophy. In the few cases in which disabling symptoms persist, surgical treatment such as proximal plantar fascia release is indicated. The time needed for healing and rehabilitation is 2 to 5 months.

Heel Spurs

The relation between plantar heel pain and a heel spur on radiographs was considered to be very poor. Only half of the patients with heel pain have a spur, and of all people with a heel spur, only 10% to 15% have heel pain. Indeed, a heel spur, when present, is located *deep* to the plantar fascia origin in the non–weight-bearing substance of the flexor digitorum brevis muscle.

Plantar Fascia Rupture and Heel Spur Fracture

Plantar fascia rupture and heel spur fracture are characterized by pain in the same area as in heel pain syndrome, but the *onset is sudden*. Ruptures of the plantar fascia are not common, but they do occur. Complete ruptures are reported in the literature after cortisone injection in the plantar fascia.

In patients with acute trauma or persistent pain, a special x-ray projection (45 degrees medial oblique) that can reveal a fractured spur should be taken. Treatment is primarily conservative: active rest, NSAIDs, crutches, and very gradual, over a 6 to 10 week period, resumption of weight-bearing activities. If symptoms persist and nonunion is suspected, surgical removal of the detached fragment must be considered.

Fat Pad Atrophy

The plantar fat pad of the heel is a highly structured tissue designed to withstand repetitive impact loads. If the structure fails, as could happen following overuse, shock-absorbing capacity decreases. This could result in pain. On clinical examination the heel pad feels softer and thinner, with the underlying calcaneal tuberosity readily palpable. Maximum tenderness is located *centrally on the weight-bearing area* of the heel, as opposed to the anteromedial tenderness location in heel pain syndrome. Treatment is conservative with a cushioned heel cup and soft-soled shoes.

Fat Pad Inflammation

Inflammation of the fat pad produces symptoms similar to those of fat pad atrophy, except for no palpable thinning or softening of the heel pad. In this situation, the heel cup should be semirigid rather than cushioned. Prognosis is usually good, but symptoms may need 6 months to resolve completely.

Return to work. After a period of heel pain, return to work varies with the diagnosis. Most people can work during conservative treatment of heel pain, but walking should be restricted. After surgery for heel pain (which mostly involves release of the plantar fascia), the healing and rehabilitation time needed to return to walking is usually around 2 to 4 months. Sometimes tenderness remains, and the rehabilitation time can be extended.

NERVE INJURIES

Manifestations of peripheral nerve injuries include paresis/paralysis of extrinsic and intrinsic muscles, sensory defects, pain and contractures, and a risk for secondary changes such as pressure ulcers and neuropathic arthropathy.

In a neurological examination of the foot and ankle, careful assessment of *sensory, motor,* and *sympathetic* function is important. The examination includes an evaluation of gait, heel and toe walking, and the Trendelenburg sign. The presence of muscle paralysis, stiffness, contracture, spasticity, ataxia, pain, and fixed or functional present deformity should be registered. Foot contractures are first studied with flexed knees. Then the knees are straightened to evaluate the effect of the gastrocnemius on the deformity. Cavus, planus, varus, valgus, and equinus of the whole foot and forefoot are assessed together with flexibility of the arches, as well as claw toes and hammer toes. Skin moisture reflects sympathetic function. Peripheral nerve disease is often accompanied by sympathetic degeneration, with dry, thin skin resulting. The *Tinel's sign* is closely evaluated as regards *presence, intensity,* and *location.* Documentation with drawings and photographs of areas with nerve dysfunction is very helpful in the assessment and treatment of nerve disorders.

Causalgia is characterized by overactivity of the sympathetic nervous system because of irritative lesions of sympathetic nerve fibers. Burning pain and dry, hot skin are typical manifestations. A sympathetic nerve block often improves symptoms.

Charcot deformity is a joint deformity that can occur in conjunction with any neuropathy, with sensory deficit developing in a joint subjected to loading of the weight of the body. This is commonly seen in the midfoot joints in conjunction with diabetes mellitus.

Classification

Five degrees of nerve injury are traditionally distinguished, depending on the severity of the injury.

First degree: Conduction deficit, axon intact. Prognosis—good.
Second degree: Axon severed but intact endoneurium, wallerian degeneration. Regeneration follows the pattern of regrowth. Axon regeneration averages 1 to 2 mm/pday and is typical of a second-degree injury.
Third degree: Disorganization of internal structure of the funiculi, minor perineurium changes, irregular regeneration. In a third-degree

injury, regeneration is blocked by disorganization of the Schwann cell tubes. As soon as it is evident that recovery is slowed or absent (Tinel's sign along nerve route), exploration is considered. Distal tingling on percussion over a nerve marks the most distal point of regenerating sensory axons. This is very useful in mapping nerve regeneration.

Fourth degree: Axonal rupture, funicular and perineural disruption. The nerve trunk is intact, but nerve bundles are disorganized. Spontaneous functional recovery is rare.
Fifth degree: Loss of continuity of the nerve trunk. Fourth-degree and fifth-degree injuries may not be distinguishable unless an open injury has revealed the nerve status. Although motor nerve fibers are usually more susceptible to compression and are therefore the first to fail and the last to recover, this is not always true. Most compression neuropathies recover by the sixth month; when they do not, intraneural fibrosis and disorganization have occurred. Neurolysis, both external and internal, offers some hope of improvement. When severe third-degree and fourth-degree lesions are present with no further chance of recovery, resection of the lesions with autografting can improve the outlook in selected cases.

Entrapment Neuropathies

The pathogenesis of nerve entrapment is considered to be gradual constriction by anatomical structures about a nerve and chronic compression of a nerve against a nonyielding structure.

Nerve entrapments usually give mixed motor and sensory symptoms. Sensory deficits typically come relatively late. The relationship between nerve fiber size, motor/sensory containment, and vulnerability to compression is uncertain. Many believe that sensory fibers are more resistant to compression than motor fibers are, but others disagree. Entrapment of a sensory or mixed nerve results in tenderness over the entrapment point. If the compression has produced axonal interruption, a Tinel's sign may be elicited at the point of compression. Electromyographic (EMG) and nerve conduction studies can be helpful in identifying and localizing an entrapment lesion.

Valleix Phenomenon

Pain and hypersensitivity are sometimes seen proximal to a nerve compression. Blocking the nerve at the entrapment site relieves the proximal symptoms. It is postulated that compression can result in proximal nerve hyperirritability. External decompression leads to the relief of symptoms, provided that intraneural fibrosis is not established. Intraneural fibrosis is often present once motor denervation has occurred (atrophy, denervation signs on EMG). Hence surgery should not wait until late in the process. If, however, intraneural fibrosis has indeed developed, intraneural neurolysis under adequate magnification can yield some improvement in symptoms.

ENTRAPMENT OF THE COMMON PERONEAL NERVE

The common peroneal nerve transmits motor innervation to the peroneal muscles and to the extensors of the foot and ankle. The nerve is vulnerable to compression at the fibular head and neck. An intraneural or extraneural ganglion (with or without connection with the tibiofibular joint), an enlarged fabella, or a bone tumor in the proximal fibula can all cause compression at this level.

The peroneus longus muscle has two heads: a superficial head attaching to the head of the fibula and a deep head inserting at the fibular neck, below the nerve. Following subtalar motion of the foot, the nerve slides back and forth between the two muscle heads, potentially leading to compression of the nerve.

These injuries can be part of overuse syndromes. People who wear wooden shoes, walk on hard floors extensively, or make repeated flexion motions in their job, may be prone to this kind of injury.

Symptoms include pain and hypoesthesia in the lateral leg and ankle, a "weak ankle" feeling, and even footdrop. Objectively, there is a positive Tinel's at the compression site, together with sensory deficit and peroneal weakness. External decompression gives relief in most cases. Intraneural neurolysis is indicated when intraneural fibrosis is present. It should be noted that the peroneus longus muscle is a powerful plantar flexor of the first ray; it maintains the medial longitudinal arch of the foot along with being an important subtalar evertor. Weakness of this muscle leads to an altered distribution of the load on the foot when standing; more load must be borne by the second and third metatarsal heads, with potential metatarsalgia following.

The lateral cutaneous nerve of the calf and the sural communicating nerve, both sensory, emerge in the popliteal region from the common peroneal nerve. Compression at this level leads to pain on the lateral side of the lower leg, and/or dorsolateral foot. Local anesthesia blocks at the maximum point of tenderness usually relieve the pain permanently.

ENTRAPMENT OF THE SUPERFICIAL PERONEAL NERVE

From the division of the common peroneal nerve high in the lower leg, this strictly sensory nerve travels between the anterior intermuscular septum and the fascia of the lateral compartment and emerges through the fascia at the junction between the middle and distal third of the lower leg, as one or two nerves. It runs subcutaneously in front of the lateral malleolus to innervate the major part of the dorsum of the foot. The anatomy of the terminating branches varies greatly, and they are at risk in surgery around the first metatarsal head. Transverse skin incisions should be avoided on the dorsum of the foot.

The nerve can be trapped where it pierces the fascia. Recurrent ankle sprains, causing stretching of the nerve, predisposes to this condition. Pain is located over the lateral aspect of the calf and ankle and in the dorsolateral foot. Inversion and plantar flexion of the ankle can exacerbate the pain. Objectively, local tenderness and a positive Tinel's sign are present. Three milliliters to 5 ml of a local anesthetic relieves the symptoms, sometimes permanently. Cortisone may be tried as an additional nonoperative measure. However, occasionally pain recurs and requires surgical decompression.[10]

Peripheral branches on the dorsum of the foot may be compressed by tight shoes (skiboots), cicatrix, and tarsometatarsal joint osteophytes and produce symptoms. In these cases, preventive appropriate shoe correction is mandatory. Treatment with local anesthetics and sometimes a cortisone injection is usually successful.

ENTRAPMENT OF THE DEEP PERONEAL NERVE

The deep peroneal nerve runs together with the anterior tibial artery on the anterior aspect of the ankle, beneath the extensor retinaculum, and then between the extensor hallucis longus and the extensor digitorum longus tendons to the dorsum of the foot. A motor branch is sent laterally on the middorsum of the foot to the extensor digitorum brevis muscle. The nerve terminates with sensory innervation of the first dorsal web space. Compression between the fascia and adjacent skeleton (osteophytes from the medial tarsometatarsal joint) leads to pain over the dorsum of the foot with occasional radiation into the first web space. Local tenderness is present. The Tinel's sign is sometimes positive, and hypoesthesia in the first dorsal web space may be present. During treatment, tight shoes must be avoided, at least temporarily. Surgical removal of osteophytes may be necessary. Care must be taken to not injure the nerve during the procedure.[2]

ENTRAPMENT OF THE POSTERIOR TIBIAL NERVE AND BRANCHES

The posterior tibial nerve, a mixed motor and sensory nerve, runs together with the posterior tibial artery behind the flexor digitorum longus tendons in the distal third of the lower leg. It then courses behind and below the medial malleolus, covered by the flexor retinaculum. At this point, the posterior tibial nerve gives rise to the medial calcaneal nerve, a sensory branch that pierces the flexor retinaculum together with a small artery, runs directly under the posterior calcaneal tubercle, and innervates the skin of the heel pad. This nerve may be involved in heel pain syndrome. The tibialis posterior nerve divides beneath the flexor retinaculum to form the medial plantar nerve and the lateral plantar nerve. These nerves correspond to the median and ulnar nerves of the hand, respectively. The medial plantar nerve runs under the anterior part of the calcaneal tuberosity; gives motor branches to the abductor hallucis, flexor hallucis brevis, flexor digitorum brevis, and lumbrical muscles; and provides sensation to the medial part of the sole, including the medial 3½ digits. The lateral plantar nerve also runs down along the medioplantar aspect of the calcaneal tuberosity along its course to the lateral part of the plantar pedis and the lateral 1 ½ digits. Motor branches are sent to the adductor hallucis muscle, the interossei, and the small muscles on the lateral aspect of the foot.

Entrapment of the posterior tibial nerve at the level of the knee or lower leg is rare. However, entrapment of the nerve within the fibroosseous tunnel behind and distal to the medial malleolus is frequent and is referred to as *tarsal tunnel syndrome.* This syndrome is characterized by burning pain on the sole of the foot, often accentuated by ambulation but characteristically also annoying at night. Predisposing factors include chronic instability and/or edema, hyperpronation, and a posterior bony prominence of the talus. Motor deficits and intrinsic muscle paresis/paralysis typically come late. Tarsal tunnel syndrome is positively correlated with pregnancy, as is carpal tunnel syndrome, with which this condition has many similarities. Objectively, a positive Tinel's sign is usually present together with numbness of the sole and tenderness behind and below the medial malleolus. Delayed nerve conduction of the medial (greater than 6.1 ms) and lateral (greater than 6.7 ms) plantar nerves further supports the diagnosis.

The treatment of choice is surgical decompression. This involves dividing the flexor retinaculum and freeing the nerve proximally and distally. Internal neurolysis is indicated if the nerve is fibrotic. Occasionally an os trigonum, if causing the compression, is removed.

Jogger's Foot

Entrapment of the medial and lateral plantar nerves is occasionally seen as they pass under the abductor hallucis muscle. "Jogger's foot" is medial plantar apraxia: burning heel pain, aching arch, and loss of sensation on the sole of the foot behind the great toe. The entrapment site is typically at the point where the abductor hallucis crosses the navicular tubercle. Anesthetic blocks, steroids, and antivalgus orthotics are initial treatment modalities. Surgical decompression is sometimes indicated.

Morton's Neuroma

The plantar interdigital nerves are terminal branches of the medial and lateral plantar nerves. Morton's neuroma is currently believed by most investigators to be the reaction of a plantar interdigital nerve compression. The condition is characterized by metatarsal pain, often poorly localized but at times clearly radiating into the toes (usually the third and fourth but possibly any or all). Pain is aggravated by ambulation and by tight shoes. With dorsiflexion of the metatarsophalangeal (MTP) joints, the plantar interdigital nerves and vessels are angulated over the leading edge of the transverse metatarsal ligament at or just proximal to the bifurcation of the

nerve to two adjacent toes. Pseudotumor formation results from irritation to the nerve. The third-space plantar nerve is formed from both the medial and lateral plantar nerves, which possibly explains why this nerve is larger and more fixed than the other interdigital nerves and therefore more prone to compression. Other factors predisposing to this condition include cavus foot, high-heeled shoes, and weakness of the intrinsic and peroneal muscles.

Treatment consists of shoe correction, with the aim of diminishing pressure on the metatarsal heads and a reduction in MTP motion by using wider shoes. A metatarsal bar is often helpful. The bar should be placed posterior to, not at the level of, the metatarsal heads and preferably between the two soles of the shoe. The shoe should also have a wide toe box and a low heel. A metatarsal pad set just behind the point of tenderness may also be a successful alternative. Nonsteroidal anti-inflammatory drugs and local steroid injections are advocated by some investigators. Foot exercises meant to strengthen the intrinsic, the peroneus longus, and the tibial posterior are recommended. In refractory cases, surgical removal of the compressed part of the plantar interdigital nerve is warranted, usually through a dorsal longitudinal approach, or some prefer a transverse plantar incision near the MTP joint crease. Magnification is a strongly recommended technique. Surgery yields a 75% to 80% rate of good or excellent results. If secondary surgery is attempted, a longitudinal plantar approach is recommended by most authors to achieve the necessary, more extensive exposure.

Entrapment of the Sural Nerve

Entrapment of the sural nerve can occur anywhere along its course from the popliteal fossa to the toes. The sural nerve, purely sensory, arises from the tibial nerve 3 cm above the knee joint, runs deep to the deep fascia of the calf to the distal third of the lower leg where it becomes superficial, runs behind the lateral malleolus, and innervates the lateral aspect of the sole. The nerve is often sacrificed for grafting, with minor or no problems thereafter. Inadvertent traumatization, however, could cause annoying discomfort.

Conditions that may include local sural nerve compression include Achilles tendon peritendinitis, recurrent ankle sprains, lateral calcaneal or subtalar joint problems, and fractures of the base of the fifth metatarsal. Symptoms include shooting pain and paresthesias along the course of the nerve. Local tenderness and a positive Tinel's sign are characteristic. Occasionally numbness is noted.

Conservative treatment includes avoidance of external nerve compression. Nonsteroidal antiflammatory drugs and occasionally a local block can be tried. If these measures fail, surgical decompression is advised.

Entrapment of the Saphenous Nerve

Entrapment of the exclusively sensory saphenous nerve is rare. The saphenous nerve crosses over the tibia in a posteromedial to anterior direction 5 to 7 cm above the ankle joint and, together with the greater saphenous vein, runs anterior to the medial malleolus. It innervates the proximal, medial part of the dorsum of the foot.

Return to work. Depending on the nerve involved and the type of surgery performed, return to work varies. If decompression is carried out, the patient can return to work after a couple of weeks, even to work involving walking. Surgery that involves excision or extensive release may require longer recovery, and return to work is then possible in 2 to 4 months.

MIDFOOT INJURIES

Midtarsal Sprains

The midtarsal or transverse tarsal joint—often called Chopart's joint, that is, the talonavicular and calcaneocuboid joints—holds a key position in the medial and lateral longitudinal arches. The midtarsal joint also acts together with the subtalar joints in inversion and eversion. Midtarsal sprains are potentially disabling injuries, with healing times often much longer than anticipated. In general, substantial force is required to cause significant injury to these joints.

A comprehensive classification system has been developed that ranges from nondisplaced ligamentous injuries, through subluxations, to dislocations. Fractures of adjacent bones may or may not be present. Soft tissue engagement can be significant. In addition to plain radiographs, CT scans are most helpful in delineating the extent of severe injuries in this region. Undisplaced injuries are normally treated nonoperatively. Because of potential instability, 6 weeks in a non–weight-bearing cast is recommended, followed by 2 weeks in a walking cast. During rehabilitation, a shoe with a firm sole should be worn together with a longitudinal arch support. Displaced fractures, subluxations, and dislocations all need to be reduced. Occasionally, closed reduction is successful, but usually open means are required. Internal fixation is performed, followed by restricted weight-bearing casting for 3 to 6 weeks.

The prognosis after midtarsal injuries is highly dependent on whether reduction is achieved. Nonreduced injuries, as well as extensively comminuted fractures, often do poorly. A future arthrodesis will have to be considered in these cases.

Tarsometatarsal Injuries (Lisfranc's joint)

The second metatarsal base is the primary bony stabilizer of the tarsometatarsal articulation. It sits in a tight mortise between the distal parts of the first and third cuneiforms. The cuneiforms and the metatarsal bases are wedge shaped, being wider dorsally, and thereby contribute to the transverse arch of the metatarsals. Motion in the joints is restricted. Together they allow some pronation and supination of the forefoot. Severe trauma to Lisfranc's joint caused by direct or indirect forces on the midfoot can result in a varying pattern of fractures and dislocations. Indirect forces along the metatarsals may result in dislocation of the joint, with or without fractures through the plantar aspect of the metatarsal base. Soft tissue injuries are often extensive following fracture-dislocation of the Lisfranc joint complex. Tourniquet should be avoided when these injuries are treated because the soft tissues will be further compromised.

Injuries to the Lisfranc joint are notorious for missed initial diagnosis and inadequate treatment. The most constant, reliable radiographic sign is a slight widening between the bases of the first and second metatarsals, between the second and third metatarsals, or between either of the cuneiforms. Fractured fragments should be sought between the first and second metatarsal bases and between the medial and middle cuneiforms. Oblique views are necessary for adequate descriptions of radiographic findings.

The goal of treatment is a stable, anatomic reduction. Because of interposing soft tissues or fractured fragments, reduction is rarely successful by closed means. Open reduction/internal fixation is recommended; transfixion is accomplished with Steinmann pins or Kirschner wires (a standard Kirschner wire will not hold the first metatarsal rigidly enough) or by using appropriate screws as temporary (16 weeks) internal fixation. Postoperatively, partial weight bearing for 6 weeks is recommended, followed by a walking cast for 4 to 6 weeks thereafter.

Combinations with lower leg, calcaneal, or ankle fractures are common, and the risk of development of compartment syndrome is substantial. Intracompartmental pressure measurements are mandatory, and fasciotomy is performed without delay when indicated. The prognosis is good provided that the injury is closed and reduction/fixation is adequate. Degenerative arthritis may occur but is surprisingly benign if good primary reduction is achieved. However, open injuries, and inadequate reduction lead to unsatisfactory end results.

Metatarsophalangeal Sprains and Dislocations

Repetitive hyperextension loads on the first MTP joint predisposes to injury on the plantar aspect of the capsule around the joint. Alternatively, the dorsal aspect of the joint is sprained following a hyperflexion event. The clinical picture consists of local pain, tenderness, and swelling. In grade III injuries, stability is compromised. In these cases, osteochondral damage is occasionally seen.

Treatment of MTP sprains is nonoperative, but ice, compression, and elevation are used acutely. Initial immobilization is required with weight bearing as tolerated. Nonsteroidal antiinflammatory drugs are beneficial. Recovery time is often long, 10 weeks not being unusual. Injections of local anesthetics or steroids are potentially aggravating to the injury and should be avoided. An orthosis (steel or Orthoplast) limiting dorsiflexion of the first MTP joint is used during rehabilitation. Surgical capsule repair and removal of loose bodies are occasionally indicated. Strenuous activities such as running and jumping are resumed only after the patient is asymptomatic.

Forced hyperextension of the MTP joints beyond physiological limits may lead to rupture of the plantar plate either through the sesamoids as fractures or proximally. The latter is irreducible because of blocking from the plantar plate. Reduction is performed with a transverse plantar incision over the prominent metatarsal head. Great care must be taken not to sever the plantar digital nerves. The dislocation is reduced by grabbing the torn end of the plantar plate and manually relocating the phalanx to its normal position. Once reduced, the joint is usually stable. Postoperatively, a cast is worn for 4 weeks, with weight bearing as tolerated. Dislocations with sesamoid fractures are usually readily reducible by closed means.

Metatarsophalangeal joint dislocations of the lesser toes can typically be reduced by closed means. Once reduced, the joint is usually stable and crossover taping is sufficient.

Metatarsal Fractures

Soft tissue coverage of the dorsum of the foot is thin and vulnerable and has a suboptimal blood supply. Strong ligamentous connections are present between the metatarsal necks distally as well as strong bands between the bases, except between the first and second, where the soft tissue connection is located between the second base and medial cuneiform.

The injury mechanism is often a direct blow to the dorsum of the foot caused by a heavy object. It is a common industrial injury. Shoes with steel-reinforced toe boxes protect the toes but not the metatarsals. Direct force on the metatarsals usually results in transverse neck fractures of the second, third, and/or fourth metatarsals, whereas indirect force leads to spiral shaft fractures. The common plantar flexion–inversion trauma results in a fifth metatarsal base fracture. Following severe injuries to this region, compartment pressures in the foot should be carefully monitored and fasciotomy performed when indicated.

Treatment of nondisplaced fractures affecting the lesser metatarsals includes the use of a firm metatarsal pad, circumferential taping, and a firm boot with a crepe sole. Undisplaced fractures through the first metatarsal require a carefully molded non–weight-bearing short leg cast for 2 weeks, followed by progressive weight bearing as soon as tolerated.

In the treatment of displaced fractures, sagittal-plane displacement inevitably leads to altered weight distribution across the forefoot and should be avoided. Normally, the load on the first metatarsal head is twice that of any of the others (including the fifth). Moderate frontal-plane displacements are not as critical. Displaced first metatarsal fractures are best treated with ORIF. Chinese woven wire traps can be used to distract the hallux longitudinally and aid reduction. An elastic bandage around the ankle can be used for countertraction. It is crucial to regain length. Next, the metatarsal is

temporarily transversely transfixed to the second ray. If possible, rigid internal fixation is used; if not, multiple pins are used to secure the fractures. If the fracture is open and major soft tissue problems are present, wound care is possible only through the use of external fixation of the fracture.

With only one displaced metatarsal fracture, closed reduction is attempted. If successful, 6 weeks of non–weight-bearing casting follows. With multiple fractures, surgical fixation using either screws and plates or intramedullary retrograde pinning is recommended. Casting is unnecessary following stable internal fixation. With fractures through the metatarsal neck, closed reduction is virtually impossible. Fixation with Kirschner-wire is commonly used.

Return to work. Work that involves a lot of walking after midtarsal injuries may often require a long recovery time. These injuries are often either missed or contribute to secondary problems, and a treatment time of 3 to 6 months is frequently required. It is of greatest importance to secure a correct diagnosis early to provide optimal treatment and facilitate early return to work.

FOREFOOT PROBLEMS

Hallux Rigidus

Hallux rigidus is stiffness of the hallucal MTP articulation, usually secondary to arthrosis of the joint. The etiology can be (1) juvenile hallux rigidus secondary to osteochondritis dissecans of the first metatarsal head in some cases; (2) related to gout, especially in bilateral hallux rigidus in men; (3) posttraumatic arthrosis of the joint; and (4) most commonly, secondary to hallux valgus. Radiographs reveal a crown of osteophytes on the dorsal part of the metatarsal head, as well as around the proximal part of the proximal phalanx. Clinically, local pain and tenderness and a varying degree of range-of-motion restriction are evident.

Treatment is initially nonoperative; rest, ice, NSAIDs, and shoes with stiff, rocker-bottom soles. Steroid injections are often beneficial. The metatarsal rocker bar, in contrast to a true metatarsal bar, is curved rather than flat. It should *never* be put proximal to the MTP level because it would then only accentuate the bending of the sole at the MTP level. A combination with moderate heel elevation is often beneficial to rocker-bottom sole function.

Persistent pain when pushing off is a problem for many patients, who therefore ask for surgery. A number of surgical procedures are available to treat hallux rigidus: removal of osteochondrotic loose bodies, removal of osteophytes, wedge osteotomies, the Keller procedure, arthrodesis, and Silastic implants. However, for very demanding patients, arthrodesis is often preferred and is the treatment of choice today. The Keller procedure (extirpation of the base of the proximal phalanx) potentially results in a short, unstable great toe, which would impair push-off ability. Silastic implants are contraindicated because of synovitis and even implant breakage following strenuous loading.

Return to work. After surgery with arthrodesis, return to a desk job is often possible within 4 to 7 days. Return to work that involves walking requires 3 to 6 months' healing and rehabilitation.

Hallux Valgus

Patients with hallux valgus and bunions invariably have pronation deformities causing lateral pressure on the hallux. As the hallux is forced laterally, the medial portion of the first metatarsal head is uncovered and forms most of the dorsomedially directed bunion. The extensor hallucis longus tendon pull is displaced laterally, further accentuating the hallux valgus deformity. The incidence of hallux valgus is much greater in women than men, probably partly because of the use of high-heeled and pointed-toe shoes. Patients seek help because of recurrent pain/tenderness over the bunion or because of cosmetic problems and difficulties in finding appropriate shoes. Objectively, both the longitudinal and the transverse arches are insufficient. A very broad splayfoot is sometimes seen. The bursa over the bunion may be intensely inflamed: red, hot, swollen, and very tender. The great toe is angled laterally and may even be overriding or underriding the second and third toes. A hammer toe deformity of one or more of the lesser toes is often present.

Management of hallux valgus is nonsurgical in the majority of patients. Orthotics correcting arch insufficiency are most beneficial, and shoe modifications are in order. It is crucial to relieve pressure on the bunion. A ring-shaped pad around the bunion is sometimes helpful. Indications for surgery can vary and include a valgus angle of more than 15 degrees, toes lying on top of each other, recurrent painful bursitis, painful calluses, and an inability to wear shoes. A great number of surgical procedures address bunion and the angular deformity.

Return to work. After surgery, return to work depends on the technique used. After a simple bunionectomy it is possible to return to work within 4 to 6 weeks. If an osteotomy is carried out, return to walking work is not possible until a healing time of 3 to 5 months has elapsed.

Hammer Toes

Hammer toes are characterized by hyperflexion of the proximal interphalangeal (PIP) joints and are usually caused by curling of the middle toes from a tight sock or shoe. Painful corns on the dorsum of the PIP joints develop. If joint range of motion is unaffected, conservative treatment such as enough room in shoes, toe manipulation to maintain mobility, and strapping of the toe in extension is advocated.

If the toes are hyperflexed and restrict walking or if major callus formations are causing pain, surgery is indicated. Surgery includes excision of the distal end of the proximal phalanx and is often gratifying.

Return to work. With hammer toe surgery, return to work is often possible 1 month after surgery.

The Sesamoids

The sesamoids are two bones located on the plantar aspect of the hallucal MTP joint. The medial sesamoid is somewhat larger and bears more of the load, whereas the lateral sesamoid lies toward the first web space. From several ossification centers the sesamoids ossify in early childhood. However, partition is common, with 10% of the population having bipartite sesamoids (unilateral in 75% but bilateral in 25%). Fifteen percent of the population also has an interphalangeal sesamoid. The sesamoids have articular facets located superiorly, toward the metatarsal head. The facets are enclosed in the joint capsule, and the remainder of the sesamoids are embedded in the flexor hallucis brevis tendons. The flexor hallucis longus tendon passes between the sesamoids.

Injury mechanisms result from (1) a direct blow caused by a fall from a height, typically resulting in a comminuted fracture; and (2) forced hyperextension of the hallux leading to avulsion (transverse) fractures of the sesamoid. Such patients typically have a dislocated first MTP joint. Stress fractures are increasingly common, specifically in competitive athletes involved primarily in running or dancing. It is often very difficult to distinguish a stress fracture from a bipartite sesamoid. Radiographs (AP, lateral, and axial tangentials of the sesamoids, *not* the entire foot) may show smooth or irregular edges. A stress fracture is often undetectable on initial plain x-ray films. A bone scan shows increased uptake in stress fractures, but possibly also in sesamoiditis. Osteochondral lesions of the sesamoid have also been described, to further complicate the picture.

As opposed to sesamoid fractures resulting from a single traumatic event, sesamoid stress fractures seem to have a poor healing potential. The fracture will not heal despite 6 weeks of casting and months of activity restriction. Excision is recommended, with potentially good end results. Successful surgery, however, requires very careful technique to avoid the introduction of disabling complications such as neuromas, hallux valgus/varus, or cock-up deformity.

Metatarsalgia

Metatarsalgia, or pain in the MTP region, is a condition with many possible causes. Hallux rigidus, sesamoiditis, stress fractures, and Morton's neuralgia are discussed elsewhere in this chapter. A common predisposing factor to metatarsalgia is altered forefoot biomechanics, extrinsic or intrinsic, caused by the following:

- High-heeled shoes, which significantly alter the load from the hindfoot to the MTP region.
- An equinus foot, especially when caused by a tight heel cord and/or anterior impingement of the ankle, thereby preventing ankle dorsiflexion.

- A cavus foot, where support is maintained only by the metatarsal heads and the heel (and not also by the lateral longitudinal arch); this results in overload of the forefoot.
- Irregular distribution of load between the metatarsal heads. In the static standing position, all metatarsal heads bear load, the first metatarsal head bearing double the load of the others. In the dynamic take-off phase of walking and running, this relative first ray overload is even more evident. A disturbance of this load distribution between the metatarsals may be caused by an abnormally short or hypermobile first ray or by a long second metatarsal. With a hypermobile first metatarsal, a significant part of the load is transferred to the second and third rays.

Treatment is conservative in the majority of cases. Supporting orthotics that relieve the overload on the metatarsal heads are often beneficial. With a hypermobile first ray, a pad just proximal to the second and third metatarsal heads and/or underneath the first ray is tried. Stretching of a tight heel cord is essential. If significant discomfort persists in spite of adequate orthotics and flexibility treatment over a 6-month period, surgery must be considered. Here soft tissue as well as skeletal corrections may be indicated.

Capsulitis of the second MTP joint is related to hallux valgus, condition in which the hallux forces the second toe to sublux dorsally. Tenderness over the dorsal capsule and pain on passive dorsiflexion of the second MTP joint is diagnostic. Typically, no interdigital pain or tenderness is present. Strapping of the second toe in a reduced, plantar-flexed position is usually helpful. Rarely, an extensor tenotomy, with or without capsulotomy, is required.

SKIN CONDITIONS

Corns

Soft corns are interdigital clavi formed between toes as a result of pressure between adjacent phalangeal condyles. Hard corns represent accumulations of keratin layers of skin, typically on the dorsum of the toes, to prevent ulceration of the skin from chronic pressure that is usually extrinsic. The key to successful treatment is relief of extrinsic pressure. The corn should be softened and pared judiciously. Occasionally, surgical removal of intrinsic pressure is necessary, for example, with a prominent phalangeal condyle.

Calluses

Calluses are hyperkeratotic lesions similar to corns. They form on the plantar aspect of the foot following weight-bearing and shearing forces. Typical lesion areas are under the metatarsal heads and under the heel. Underlying structural deformities such as an insufficient transverse arch, forefoot varus or valgus, a plantar-

flexed first ray, or a long second ray are common. Local treatment of calluses equals that of corns; custom-made orthotics are generally needed. If these measures prove insufficient, a rare event, surgical correction of an underlying deformity must be considered.

The diagnosis of a cutaneous lesion is sometimes difficult. Scar formation, warts, inclusion cysts, and foreign body inclusions may all have the appearance of a corn or a callus. A careful history, clinical examination, and occasionally soft tissue radiographs are needed. If still in doubt, referral to a highly specialized institution without touching the lesion is indicated.

Warts (verrucae vulgares)

A wart is the result of a papillomavirus infection that is transferred between individuals in showers, saunas, and locker room floors. The incubation period is 1 to 6 months. The warts are typically located on the sole of the foot. They are round or oval and gray-white, have a crack or a dark spot in the center, and are often tender to pressure. They are commonly multiple.

Primary plantar wart treatment consists of weekly paring and application of keratolytics, including 50% trichloroacetic acid or 40% salicylic acid. Failure of this treatment to eradicate the wart may warrant the use of careful electrosurgery following infiltration of local anesthetic with epinephrine. We advise against excision of a wart by scalpel or curet because of the risk of scar formation from inadvertent penetration of the basilar layer of the skin. X-ray therapy may be considered when all else fails, provided that it is given by an experienced operator. Again, prevention is crucial, and the use of bathshoes in humid areas is strongly recommended.

Blisters

Blisters are caused by a shearing irritation of the skin, typically caused by the improper fitting of shoes and/or socks. The epidermal layers split, and the cavity formed is filled with a clear fluid. Treatment consists of prompt removal of extrinsic irritant and if needed, clean aspiration of the fluid. Deroofing of the blister should be avoided because the overlying skin is a good dressing and helps prevent secondary infection.

Fungal Infections (Tinea Pedis)

Occasionally referred to as "athlete's foot," fungal infections may develop in circumstances where foot hygiene is inadequate. The most common infecting organisms are *Trichophyton rubrum* and *Trichophyton mentagrophytes*. Both "dry" and "wet" varieties of tinea pedis exist. Predominant sites of infection are the web spaces. The dry form appears as gray-white scaling of the skin, whereas in the wet vesicular form, the web space skin has a macerated appearance. Diagnosis can be made by revealing hyphae and mycelia by light microscopic examination of scrapings from scaling and vesicle walls.

Treatment of the dry form of tinea pedis consists of local antifungal solutions, sometimes supplemented with oral griseofulvin. The wet form is best treated with potassium permanganate or silver nitrate. A secondary bacterial infection may necessitate erythromycin administration. Prevention such as good foot hygiene, including frequent change of socks, shoes allowing adequate aeration, and avoidance of barefoot walking in locker rooms, is essential.

NAILS

Ingrown Toenails

Ingrown toenails are common and potentially disabling. Posttraumatic nail deformation caused by injury of the nail matrix may elicit the problem. The shape of toenails is congenitally different. Some types are flatter, others are folded. Frequently, there is a conflict between the lateral and medial edges of a folded toenail, and the adjacent nail. The problem grows when external pressure is increased from a tight sock or a shoe with a narrow toe box. If the edge of the nail penetrates the skin, bacterial infection and voluminous granulation tissue will result. The condition, which is most painful, typically engages the lateral aspect of the great toe, but any toe could be affected.

Prevention is essential and includes good foot hygiene, properly fitting footwear, and appropriate nail trimming habits. Once a week the nails should be cut transversely because they may grow down into the nail fold if cut to a rounded outline. Once established, the acute-phase infection should be drained and the area soaked in an antiseptic solution followed by a dry cover. Surgery should be avoided in the acute phase because of the high risk of postoperative infection, including potential osteomyelitis. In chronic cases, the ingrown part of the nail, including the nail matrix of that part, should be surgically removed. Three weeks should be allowed for healing postoperatively.

Return to work. After surgery for ingrown toenails, return to work is possible in 3 to 6 weeks. These conditions are painful.

Subungual Hematomas (Black Nail, "Tennis Toe," "Soccer Toe")

Bleeding of the nail bed can be the result of a direct blow to the nail from being trodden on or from a too narrow toe box. The hematoma shines through the nail and renders it black or dark blue. The condition may be very painful in the acute stage. The hematoma is evacuated through a small hole through the nail made with a red-hot straightened paper clip. The procedure is most often painless and gives immediate relief. This procedure also preserves the nail, which would otherwise fall off after 2 to 3 weeks because of disruption of its blood supply.

Subungual Exostosis

As a result of repetitive direct blows, for instance, a basketball player's forefoot repeatedly being trodden on, reactive exostosis formation may develop on the dorsal aspect of the outer phalanx of the toe underlying the nail. Intense tenderness prompts treatment, typically nail removal and, occasionally, also removal of the exostosis.

Fissures

Fissures of the weight-bearing area of the sole can be very painful and most disabling. Fissures are mainly correlated with hyperkeratosis, but they are also seen in conjunction with psoriasis and fungal infection. Obesity and wearing of shoes without counters also contribute to the development of fissures. Hyperkeratosis-related fissures are treated with topically applied salicylic acid. Steroid ointments or creams might be added for a limited time. A concomitant fungal infection may need oral antifungal treatment such as griseofulvin, 2 doses of 125 to 250 mg.

References

1. Allenmark C: Partial Achilles tendon tears, *Clin Sports Med* 11(4):759-770, 1992.

2. Baxter DE, Thigpen CM: Heal pain, operative results, *Foot Ankle* 5(1) 16-25, 1984.

3. Bronstrom L: Sprained ankles. V. Treatment and prognosis in recent ligament ruptures, *Acta Chir Scand* 132:537-550, 1966.

4. DeLee JC, Evans JP, Julian J: Stress fracture of the fifth metatarsal, *Am J Sports Med* 11(5):349-353, 1983.

5. Kannus P, Renström P: Treatment for acute tears of the lateral ligaments of the ankle, *J Bone Joint Surg* 73A:305-312, 1991.

6. Komprda J: Le syndrome du sinus du tarse, *Ann Podol* 5:11-17, 1966.

7. Leach RE, Schepsis AA: Acute injury to ligaments of the ankle. In Evarts CM, editor: *Surgery of the musculoskeletal system,* Vol 4, New York, 1990, Churchill Livingstone International; pp 3887-3913.

8. Pettine K, Morrey B: Osteochondral fractures of the talus, *J Bone Joint Surg* 69B(1):89-92, 1987.

9. Renström P, Kannus P: Management of ankle sprains, *Oper Techn Sports Med* 2(1):58-70, 1994.

10. Styf J: Entrapment of the superficial peroneal nerve: diagnosis & results of decompression, *J Bone Joint Surg* 71B:131-135, 1989.

PART V

Legal

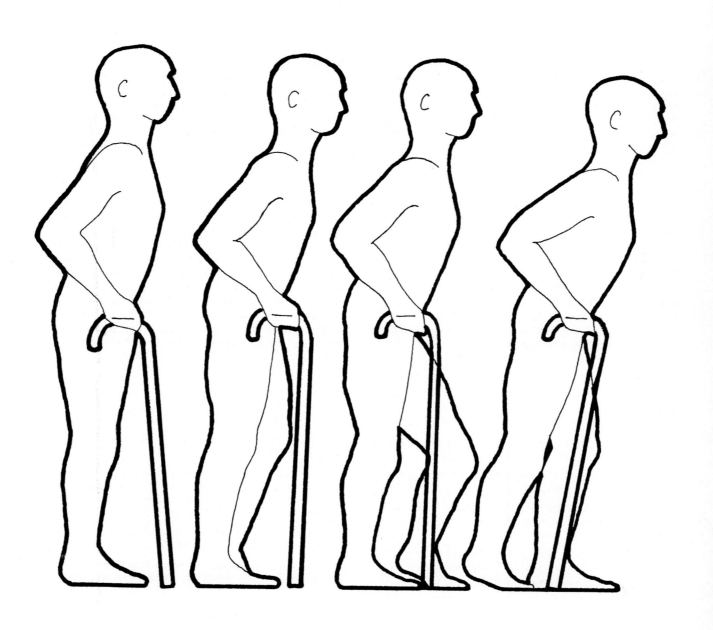

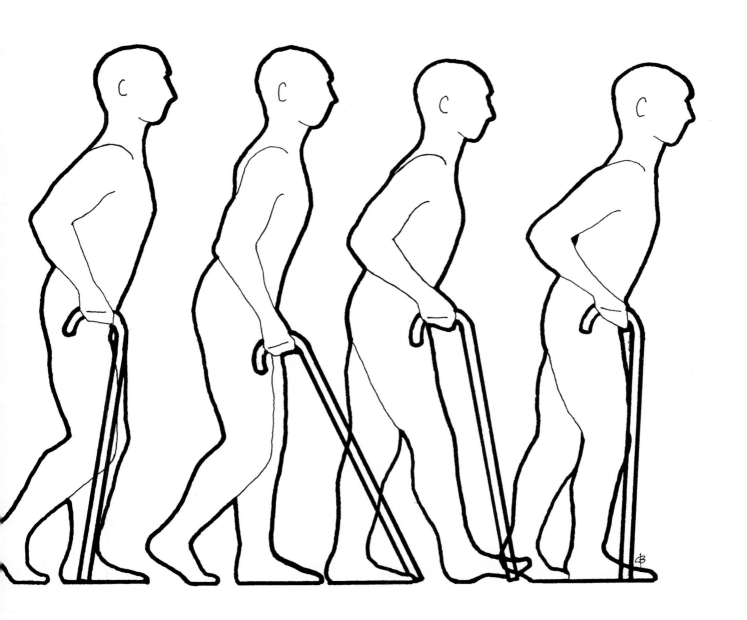

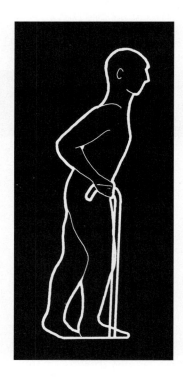

Chapter 48

The Worker's Compensation System

Judith Goodwin Greenwood
Edwin T. Wyman, Jr.

CONTENTS

OVERVIEW OF THE CURRENT U.S. SYSTEM

Interpretation of constitutional law in the United States in the early part of the twentieth century precluded any federal or national program for compensating workers with work-related injury and disability, even though such social programs had been and were being adopted in European countries. Therefore, it was left up to the individual states to adopt laws that statutorily instituted the principles of "no fault" and "limited liability" for compensating workers for on-the-job accidents and injuries. These laws established the famous quid pro quo: injured workers were barred from monetary recovery suits against their employers under tort law, whereas employers were required to pay limited wage replacement and medical benefits related to the injury. Under tort law, an injured worker had to bring a suit against the employer to obtain any monetary relief if the injury disabled the worker from performing job-related duties. If the employee won, the recovery could be substantial, including lost wages, medical care, and monetary awards for pain and suffering. The process was costly, however, and the majority of injured workers either could not afford the process or could not successfully prove negligence because employers had three strong defenses: the injured worker's contributory negligence, a co-worker's negligence, and the worker's acceptance of a risky job assignment

Worker's compensation laws prescribing some level of wage replacement and medical benefits under the aegis of state administrative agencies were intended to reduce the need for litigation, obviate the occasional and unpredictable large award against an employer, and at the same time, ensure certainty of fair monetary recovery for workers disabled from their jobs because of a job-related injury. By the middle part of the century, most state laws had expanded to include recognized work-related diseases. Exclusive remedy for economic loss because of work-related injury or disease was both the original and later intent of worker's compensation laws. Still, litigation, although appearing truncated by state laws and the administrative oversight of benefits, did not by any means disappear.

Although most benefits for temporary work disability and medical care today are provided without litigation, two issues remain that are frequently disputed: first, the issue of causality (whether in fact an injury or disease is work related); second, the issue of residual impairment and its effects on the worker's future earnings or even employability. Therefore, in worker's compensation jurisdictions in the United States, case law developed side by side with statutory law, sometimes dominating it. Worker's compensation laws, both statutory and case, cover over 56 major U.S. jurisdictions, including the 50 states and the District of Columbia, federal employees, longshore and harbor workers, and U.S. territories. In addition, railroad workers are covered by the Federal Employees Liability Act, and sailors on the high seas are covered by the Jones Act, both of which are basically tort law.

Because of its history, the United States has a complex system of legal redress for work-related injuries.[5] Both administrative and judicial interpretation of the issues must deal with whether an injury arose "out of and during the course of an employee's job" and, later, whether a particular work-related injury or disease may have resulted in some permanent impairment of an employee's functional capacity that results in economic losses related to job opportunity or performance. Challenges involving the necessity or appropriateness of medical treatment for the claimed injury or disease may be raised, and later, challenges may be made for any exacerbation of the original condition with regard to more disability, time lost from work, and need for medical care. Decisions in individual cases may vary according to jurisdictional laws and their interpretation.

The jurisdictional complexity of the U.S. system is compounded by the various ways that employers finance their coverage. Worker's compensation coverage can be secured in state jurisdictions in three ways: through private insurance carriers, through public state funds, and by employers who meet certain state bonding requirements to cover their own losses, commonly called "self-insurance." Not all are available in every state. Coverage through private insurance carriers is most common and is available in all but six states. These states (Nevada, North Dakota, Ohio, Washington, West Virginia, and Wyoming) have exclusive state funds that prohibit coverage through private carriers. The concept behind exclusive state funds addresses the social welfare notion behind worker's compensation in most European countries: state-mandated coverage for wage replacement and medical benefits provided through an arm of the state that "taxes" employers rather than through a private entity selling insurance premiums for profit. Otherwise, state funds operate similarly to private insurers.

Only Wyoming and North Dakota disallow employers from covering their own losses or "self-insuring." Self-insurance is not the logical opposite of an employer purchasing insurance through a private insurer or a state fund. When insurance is purchased by an employer, the basic premium is determined by spreading injury-related monetary losses, or risk, through a specified industrial class for a group of employers, for example, street and road construction. If an employee is injured on the job, the insurer takes care of any wage replacement and medical benefits, assigns the loss to an individual employer's account, and then tabulates that single employer's losses over a given time period as part of the losses for the given industrial class as a whole. Thus employers who voluntarily purchase coverage through an insurance premium have large claim expenses spread throughout their class. In contrast, an employer who self-insures is directly responsible for paying the wage replacement and medical benefits mandated by state law in every employee claim, including the occasional very large claim. In essence, self-insurers are betting that they will have less large-claim expense than that borne by employers insured as a group.

A large minority of states (over a third in 1993) have public or quasi-public state or mutual funds that compete with private carriers by offering insurance premiums based on loss experience and subject to rate regulation. Some of these competitive state funds have been in existence from the origin of the law. Others are relatively new. Recently, more states have established state mutual funds. Since 1988, five states—Rhode Island, Louisiana, Texas, New Mexico, and Maine—have enacted legislation creating state funds to cover the residential or assigned risk pool of employers unable to purchase insurance from private employers because of escalating premium rates. The major difference between these competitive state funds and private insurers is the absence of a profit motive for the state funds, which assumes that addressing social need is their primary goal.

Private insurance carriers can refuse coverage to employers whose estimated risk for work-related injuries and disease exceeds the maximum allowable premium rate permitted under state regulation for employers who voluntarily buy insurance. However, another mechanism must be available for employers who do not qualify for the voluntary market because worker's compensation coverage is commonly mandated by law. That mechanism is the assigned risk pool. In states where only private carriers provide coverage, the expenses incurred in the assigned risk pool are absorbed by all insurance carriers in the state. However, assigned risk pools have typically operated at a loss, too often resulting in higher premiums in the voluntary or open market where employers can choose their carriers. Presumably, competitive or mutual state funds that assume assigned-risk employers without a motive or need for profit can help lower premium costs overall and increase access to coverage. Still, if premium rates go up because benefit payments increase, even state fund rates must go up.

Whatever the coverage-financing mechanism, the system also includes administrative, fiscal regulatory, and adjudicatory bodies. In states with exclusively state funds, the administrative agency is perforce the same as the financing agency. In states with the other various combinations of coverage—private insurance, competitive state funds, and self-insurance—a specially designated administrative agency will enforce the state law through various rules and regulations and will serve as the first step in resolving disputed claim-related issues. In all jurisdictions where self-insurance is permitted, self-insured employers must abide by whatever legislation pertains to all regularly insured employers and the rules and regulations executed by the administrative agency.

Outside of states with exclusively state funds, a state's department of insurance commonly regulates the premium rates charged by state funds and private insur-

ance carriers, although a number of states have introduced open or competitive rating. In the large majority of states in which private insurance is the common vehicle for coverage, the carriers depend on a national rate-making body, the National Council of Compensation Insurance, to undertake the actuarial process of using employer loss experience in the aggregate to assess base rates for each of the many different classes of employers. The state insurance commissioner will then approve or disapprove the recommended rates. Currently, in many states, tight regulation and disapproval of recommended rates have brought about a clear and evident problem in how worker's compensation functions and how it is financed.

Adjudication of claims is generally similarly structured throughout state jurisdictions, irrespective of the manner of financing coverage. Basically, this three-step process begins with the initial administrative decision regarding "arising out of and in the course of employment." If this first decision is protested by the employer, the claim is reviewed by a specially appointed appeals body. The final appeal by either party in claim disputes is through a superior state court.

At any time during the life of an established claim, either party, the employer or employee, may dispute any administrative decision regarding any issue within the claim, including medical treatment, extent of disability, and any exacerbation of an original injury. The appeals body decides all protests to administrative decisions.

Despite the original no-fault intent of worker's compensation laws and the corollary concept of exclusive remedy through these laws, litigation abounds in many, if not most jurisdictions. In practice, worker's compensation claims can become entangled in causality and work-relatedness issues not only when disability and medical benefits are at stake but also when employer negligence issues appear to some observers to have eroded the exclusive-remedy concept.

THE MEDICAL NEXUS AND ITS REQUIREMENTS

Essential Communication and Reports

The worker's compensation system deals in large part with medical information; thus effective transmittal of that information is a major responsibility of the physician treating work-injured patients. In the treatment of a patient who is not injured at work, the physician, the patient, the patient's family, and the third-party payer are the only interested parties. Here, record keeping and reports are for the most part read only by physicians, so medical terminology and technical jargon are perfectly acceptable.

In a patient with a work injury, however, several other parties have a very active interest in the patient's treatment, recovery, and return to work. The interests of these parties are not the same, and the interest of any one may not be known to the others. In addition, the parties may not communicate well with each other, so misunderstandings are common. The parties include, in addition to the patient and the family, the patient's employer, often a union, attorneys for both the patient and the employer, the insurance company or state fund covering the worker's compensation claim, and the state administration of the worker's compensation law. Whereas the primary goal of the physician is returning the patient to full and painless function, the goals of the other parties may be different: returning the worker to employment and terminating benefits, simply terminating benefits because of questions regarding causation, or seeing that the worker maximizes disability and receives full benefits. Disputes may arise because of this disparity among the goals of the parties involved.

In every report, the physician should use lay language that can be easily understood by nonmedical personnel. Because of the diverse interests among parties, somewhere in every medical report related to the claim the treating physician should always answer the questions that the other parties in the system want answered, whether they are specifically asked or not:

- What is the present diagnosis?
- Is it work related? (Based on the patient's history.)
- Can the patient work?
- If the patient cannot work, when will the patient be able to work?
- What are the limitations of work?
- How long will any work limitations last?
- Is the condition at an end result?
- If so, is permanent impairment present?
- When can any permanent impairment be established and what is its specific level?

At each patient encounter, updated information should be given in regard to these questions and the information quickly dispersed to all other parties in the system. Not to do this simply confuses and delays administrative handling of the work-related injury claim. The use of standardized forms by the physician is often helpful in making sure this information is included.

Through medical reports at the initiation, during, and at the conclusion of treatment, the physician supplies the information that the worker's compensation administrators use to establish temporary wage replacement benefits and financial awards through lump sum and permanent disability settlements. The financial impact obviously greatly affects the patient's future behavior and productivity, so the physician needs to accept the responsibility to provide clear, concise, objective documentation.

The necessity for documentation begins at the first visit of the work-injured patient to a treating physician. This documentation (the "first report of injury") is the patient's entry key to the worker's compensation system. The worker's statement to the employer that this is a work injury is not enough. It must be documented by the physician even though the patient's history is the only evidence that it was a work injury. The patient/worker should be informed that this physician-signed documentation must reach the worker's compensation system administration because eligibility for treatment and benefits under this system will probably not be allowed without it. Besides the statement that the patient cited a work incident to be the cause of the reported symptoms, the other necessary information needed in this first report of injury is the diagnosis, abilities or limitations in work, and an estimate as to the duration of any inability to perform the regular job. Other information that is helpful, although not essential, includes a short outline of the patient's job history, both in the present job and previous jobs, as well as any other musculoskeletal problems in the past, especially if they were work related. A sample form developed by the Committee on Occupational Health of the American Academy of Orthopaedic Surgeons is presented in Appendix A as an example of a method to ensure that this information is obtained.[1]

At each treatment visit following the initial one, administrative and medical progress needs to be documented. The administrative section should include information about administrative and legal actions and any conflicts, as well as the need for activities such as vocational testing or case management assignment. Treatment options should be expressed so that a lay reader can understand them clearly, and it is probably well to repeat the information concerning causation, work ability, and the probable duration of time to the point of maximum medical improvement. The availability of limited or modified work activities for a specific duration of time may be very beneficial to an injured patient because the earlier the patient returns to work, the less adversarial and controversial administrative settlements become, the less confused the patient becomes, and the less cost for the system in both medical and indemnity payments. The treating physician, an insurance carrier's case manager, or both can work with employers to seek job modification for a limited time that would permit return to work until the claimant/patient reaches full physical function.

The final visit between the physician and patient after a work injury must address issues centered around the point of maximum medical improvement. This means that the patient has reached a medical end result, or a point at which either full recovery has occurred or further improvement is not expected in the foreseeable future. Some strictly palliative care may be necessary and should be specifically outlined as to type, frequency, and duration. It is also necessary to express any activity limitations in functional terms, particularly in regard to returning to regular employment. If any individual patient cannot return to the preinjury job, either with a modified work assignment or as before, a statement as to the need for vocational rehabilitation evaluation is needed. If full physical function has not been restored, a rating of permanent partial impairment (discussed later) by the treating physician is recommended and may negate the need for an independent medical examination. Interval and final visit forms from the American Academy of Orthopaedic Surgeons, which were developed along with the initial visit forms, are included in Appendix A.

The Use of Independent Medical Examinations

Independent medical examinations are often used to help the worker's compensation administrators resolve disputes regarding treatment efficacy as well as physical impairment. Thus examining physicians may be asked to act as independent examiners in a legal process that uses their expressed medical opinions to reconcile other medical opinions in a claim file. It is important that independent medical examinations be thorough and complete, that examiners be without bias or preconceived views, and that they clearly document the basis for the opinion given. Decisions may be difficult for physicians because they assume that they are being asked to be as accurate as when they are making patient treatment decisions. This feeling is enforced by attorneys asking physicians whether their decisions are "within reasonable medical probability." To the physician this means approximately 90%, which is actually the legal accuracy represented by the term "beyond a reasonable doubt." In actual fact, physicians are being asked in this system for accuracy levels that are better described by the term "more probable than not," which would translate to 51% probability or greater. Insistence by the physician for the highest accuracy level leads to indecisive medical reports full of disclaimers and exceptions. These are next to worthless to the administrative system in resolving a claim.

The independent medical examination report represents a summary of the medical events and recovery progress since the injury, as well as the administrative actions that have directly affected treatment. Much of the information in these reports is the same as that outlined under the treatment visit documentation. Because examiners have not had the advantage of seeing the injured worker over a period of time, they must pay special attention to inconsistencies. Physical examination tends to weigh objective findings more heavily than subjective findings. Objective physical findings are those that cannot be consciously controlled (e.g., deep tendon reflexes), whereas subjective findings can be consciously controlled (e.g., joint range of motion). The examination searches for inconsistencies in physical findings such as those described by Waddell.[7] The report should end with a description of further treatment needed if any, the establishment of a point of maximum medical improvement, a listing of the objective findings to support this conclusion, a description of functional activity limitations, any need for vocational rehabilitation or functional capacity testing, and a percentage of impaired function in physical ability if present. The American Academy of Orthopaedic Surgeons' outline for an independent medical examination is included in Appendix B.[2]

Dispute Resolution and the Physician— Preparing and Delivering Testimony

Because the worker's compensation system is medicolegal in nature, physicians treating or evaluating patients within it are often asked to provide testimony to assist in the resolution of litigation and disputes. Physicians usually abhor this because they feel that they are in a totally different world and are being attacked. Most physicians have little or no knowledge or experience in giving testimony until they are asked to be the medical expert in a legal setting governed by legal, not scientific rules.

If done correctly, the medical treatment records or the report of the independent medical examination should provide all the information needed for testimony whether by the physician's appearance at a worker's compensation board or court or the physician giving a deposition. Depositions are much more convenient for the physician because they are usually done in the office with or without video recording. Convenience and a familiar setting should not obliterate the fact that a deposition *is* a legal proceeding, however, for in actuality it is just as formal and authoritative as court testimony.

The medical records in any legal proceeding will be very familiar to the attorneys on both sides, the claimant's attorney and the employer's or insurance carrier's attorney, so the physician should also review these records to ensure familiarity. It may also be well for the physician to have a conference with the attorney who has requested the testimony to make the presentation more effective and allow the attorney to plan the direct testimony. It is most important for the physician to understand what is at issue in the litigation because it is often not what a medical viewpoint might dictate or assume. It is also necessary for the physician to know whether the testimony is to be presented to a judge or a jury. Juries will need to have a good bit more explanation of terms and concepts framed in lay language than will administrative law judges, who may have had considerable experience in hearing medical testimony.

At the time of court testimony, it is important that the physician be dressed neatly and conservatively and exhibit an attitude of confidence and helpfulness. If testimony is given before a jury, frequent eye contact with the jury will express the desire to transmit the information that they need for their decision making. Questions should be answered directly and simply. Care should be taken to give no more information than specifically requested because extraneous information may simply provoke more questions and confuse the essential message delivered to the jury.

Some specific points should be understood by the physician before the testimony. The term "authoritative" in legal terms means that it is accepted in its entirety as being true. Therefore, if the physician is asked whether a well-known text or paper is authoritative, an affirmative reply means that every concept and word of the text is accepted as true. It is better to say the work is one of several well-known and influential articles on the subject. A question about payment for the testimony being given may arise. The reply should be that payment is being made for the time involved in reviewing the records, examining the patient, writing a report, and giving testimony. The physician may be asked a long, convoluted, "hypothetical question" that usually summarizes the specific case but emphasizes only the points in favor of the particular party represented by the attorney outlining the question. The physician may feel manipulated and fear that the testimony will be slanted by answering such questions. However, if this is indeed the case, the other attorney will readdress the issue from another perspective in rebuttal and question the physician again, thus adding additional relevant information.

IMPAIRMENT AND DISABILITY

Impairment: A Medical Concept

Although physicians use the terms impairment and disability interchangeably, they are not the same, and the difference is important. Orthopaedic physicians are able to determine impairment, which means the anatomic or physiologic loss of function. It is expressed in terms such as abilities to stand, sit, bend, walk, reach, and climb. These abilities may be quantified in whatever way the physician feels comfortable and may be documented by specific "objective" measurements known under the general heading of physical functional capacity testing. This testing may be done by medical personnel other than the physician, including physical therapists, but the significance of these results remains to be determined by the physician. Disability, on the other hand, describes the limitations in specific work activities or activities of daily living resulting from impairment, coupled with other personal factors that affect a person's ability to function in a given job situation. Unless the physician has complete knowledge of the patient's job, as might be the case if practicing medicine at the patient's place of work, and has full knowledge of the patient as a person, disability determination will require information from other experts, including psychologists, psychiatrists, and vocational rehabilitation counselors. These experts can determine factors other than anatomic and physiologic impairments that may impair work performance, and vocational rehabilitation specialists can determine the availability of jobs that fit a worker's specific physical impairment and other functional factors.

Full function has been said to be a combination of a person's physical ability, needs, and will. In this regard, if full function is equated with the worker's employment or return to work potential, then the worker's ability to do a job depends on the functional limitations of the medical condition itself, the physical demands of the job, and the adaptability of the work station or job activities to the worker's physical limitations. The worker's needs involve such issues as living expenses, education and skill training, career advancement desires, seniority, and opportunities. The worker's will, or motivation, is influenced by factors such as family and social support systems, job satisfaction, and work ethic and sense of personal responsibility. By and large, the orthopaedic physician considers only issues related to the worker's physical function and reports findings to the worker's compensation administration. In most instances, decisions related to impaired function can be determined on these reported findings. However, for a small number of injured workers (fewer than 10%), factors related to need and motivation negatively interact to result in chronic pain syndrome. This is a subconscious psychological stress disorder that manifests itself by pain magnified far beyond that explained by physical findings. Chronic pain syndrome can severely delay a patient's recovery. In these cases, other experts, such as those already mentioned, must make determinations of a worker's actual disability beyond physical impairment and how such disability will affect any claim settlement or return to work.

Impairment rating systems have been developed to aid physicians in determining musculoskeletal physical function in a worker's postinjury recovery. Specific impairment rating systems may be state mandated or not. A majority of states either mandate or recommend use of the American Medical Association's (AMA) *Guides to the Evaluation of Permanent Impairment,* which is now in its fourth edition.[2] Some states such as Minnesota have developed their own systems.[6] Usually the impairment rating is expressed as a percentage, although at times it is requested that it be expressed in terms of length of time (in weeks or months) of total inability to work and partial inability to work. The ideal impairment rating system would be convenient, simple to apply, accurate, and relevant to the patient's function. It should also be fair, objective, cost-effective, and designed to give consistency in ratings between two physicians using the system. Unfortunately, none of the systems are ideal in this regard, although each edition of the AMA *Guides* seems to edge closer to these objectives and the fourth edition appears significantly improved in rating impairment.

Methods of impairment rating can be grouped under three general headings. *Diagnostic* methods simply assign a percentage of impaired function based on a diagnosis without any regard for individual variation. The advantage of this system is that it is consistent, simple, and cost-effective, but it may not be relevant or fair. *Anatomic* methods depend on physical findings, which in the musculoskeletal system usually mean range-of-motion determination. Although anatomic methods are also consistent, convenient, accurate, and timely, they are less relevant and objective. In theory, *functional* methods come closest to the ideal because it is physical function that is being rated. However, measurement techniques to quantify function are too new to guarantee relevancy, objectivity, and fairness, and the methods are neither simple nor cost-effective.

The current AMA *Guides* allow much more choice for diagnostic, functional, and anatomic evaluation, but it is too early to state whether this increased choice will decrease consistency and fairness levels. Clearly, no one "best way" has currently been found to reduce the multiple factors in human functional loss into a single number, so one can expect a continued search for better methods. For this reason, controversy will continue despite whatever methods are mandated by administrative entities, but impairment rating should edge continually closer to accurate measured values of functional loss. Even with an ideal impairment system, it will not be effective unless the physician using the given methods has an appropriate understanding of their purpose and knowledge concerning their use. Unfortunately, some physicians resist evaluating impairment and denigrate the process, which in the end only harms the worker.

Disability: A Multifactorial Concept

As indicated in the preceding section, full function as related to work disability can involve more than just physical ability in and of itself. Without consideration of the physical demands of the job and job activities, a secretary with an injured knee may have the same level of restricted physical function or impairment as a telephone company lineman. However, the secretary can be released to work relatively soon in the healing process given that accommodating transportation arrangements are available. The lineman, however, will require complete or nearly complete healing to return to work unless the telephone company has a good modified work assignment program. After healing is complete, their residual impairment (e.g., stiffness, muscle atrophy, or ligament looseness) may be very similar, but work-related disability may well be quite dissimilar if the lineman can no longer fully perform all required job functions but the secretary can.

The aforementioned example demonstrates the fine line between impairment and disability and the difficulty in evaluating either one or both. Physicians, in determining the time to return to work after time has been lost from work and then, if necessary, determining any residual impairment after maximum medical recovery is reached, may take known job-related and personal factors into account as well as restricted or limited physical function. The difficulty in determining maximum medical improvement or the amount of residual disability arises from the influence of the more subjective and more personal factors of disability introduced in the preceding section: will and motivation, job stress and dissatisfaction, family and medical support systems, economic needs and responsibilities, and level of education and transferable skills. A negative amalgam of these latter factors in combination with physical limitation

and required job activities can impede an individual's actual or perceived ability to perform work.

The Americans with Disabilities Act (ADA), which requires employers to hire or rehire disabled workers, does not directly address these subjective and personal factors. The ADA speaks directly to job modification and workplace accommodation. These factors may, in many cases, bridge the impairment-disability issue when physical impairment is a major contributing factor to work disability. In some cases, actions taken in compliance with the ADA may alleviate certain subjective factors such as job stress or dissatisfaction if the employer begins to show concern for employees and their jobs.

The crux, then, of problematic work-related disability is the amalgam of subjective and personal factors that impede the normal healing and job restoration process and that are not immediately or easily amenable to job modification, to workplace accommodation, or given a last alternative, to vocational job retraining.

Persons for whom most of the disability laws have been written and programs developed have been assumed to have some physical limitation or defect, usually visible, or some mental limitation, usually discernible, that impedes their expected productivity at work or their participation in the normal social milieu. Disability, however, has another dimension: it can serve as a fault line in personal development and human communication and relationships, particularly work-related disability. In the traditional context, all disability, including work-related disability, has been perceived as primarily a medical problem subject to medical treatment and evaluation. More recently, disability, particularly as related to the workplace, is perceived as an engineering problem related to the design or redesign of job tasks and work stations. What is beginning to unfold is the view that work-related disability may also be a psychosocial problem needing the restoration of personal development and basic human relationship commitments, beginning with the integrity of the employer-employee relationship. A major prospective study on factors influencing reported back injuries that included over 3000 Boeing company employees in Seattle showed job dissatisfaction to be the best predictor of all other factors studied, including physical factors such as lifting strength, aerobic capacity, spinal canal size, work history, and medical history factors.[3]

Whether medical treatment itself can resolve a work-related disability problem, whether after maximum medical improvement the reengineering of job tasks and/or work stations is also needed, or whether after some degree of medical resolution is achieved, addressing personal development and psychosocial problems is needed to restore an individual to some level of productivity, work or return to work has been a goal of disability policy following that of economic assistance during the time of recovery. However, if any party involved in the system has an economic incentive to maximize disability, the return-to-work goal will be compromised. Compounding that problem, disability has become an expanding concept as medical science provides more diagnostic categories for people to claim disabling conditions (e.g., ruptured disk, cumulative trauma disorder), as medical technology produces more diagnostic tests to show abnormalities that may or may not be actually disabling (e.g., magnetic resonance imaging), as the workplace requires more robotic and less diverse job activities, and as workers find themselves in dissatisfying jobs for whatever reasons. Still, that being said, physical or mental injury, illness, or limitation is presumed to be the primary cause of disability, and disability has been recognized as a legal status; thus physicians are perforce part of an adversarial medical-legal system with all of its incumbent problems.

WORKER'S COMPENSATION IN THE WIDER ARENA OF HEALTH CARE

A Retrospective View

When state worker's compensation laws were being enacted in the second decade of the century, there was also a strong movement led by the Progressive Party for national health care insurance. Providing medical coverage and wage protection to workers injured on the job was considered only a step in the direction of relieving poverty caused by illness. The AMA expressed interest in a model health insurance bill and, in 1916, appointed a committee to begin drafting such a bill. However, opposition from organized labor at the national level and by private insurance companies, along with World War I and U.S. opposition to anything German, including Germany's national health insurance program, quickly eroded any support for a national health plan. By 1920, it had become a nonissue.

Although national health insurance did become an issue again in the 1930s during President Franklin D. Roosevelt's first term, only the Social Security Act for old age pension insurance passed Congress in 1935. By the end of the decade, policy decisions had excluded both health care and worker's compensation from the new social insurance program, and worker's compensation became even more a world unto itself, divorced from the federal debates on disability and health care. President Harry S. Truman's proposal for a national health-care system in the mid-1940s did not gain needed support, in large part because voluntary nonprofit insurance plans pioneered by Blue Cross and Blue Shield were strong among the working middle class where the wage earner also had worker's compensation coverage. Later, federal intervention in the 1950s and 1960s did bring about coverage for disabled persons through the Social Security Act and then medical care coverage for the elderly and those in the population poor enough to qualify for medical aid.

Thus by 1970, over 50 years of national policy debate about disability and health care resulted in some wage support and medical care for workers injured on the job through state worker's compensation programs, then decades later support for others in the population too disabled to work for a year or more, and finally both Medicare and Medicaid.[5]

Although it had been frozen out of the national policy debates, worker's compensation did not remain untouched by the social energy unleashed during the 1960s. In 1972, the National Commission on State Workmen's Compensation Laws issued a report that set in motion a decade of state program reforms including wage replacement and medical benefit increases as well as other legislated and administrative reforms. Today, worker's compensation is being brought back into the mainstream of federal policy debate. The salient issues that are pulling worker's compensation back toward the center are physician reimbursement, managed care, and the proposed merger of the worker's compensation medical benefit into general healthcare plans.

Resource-Based Relative Value Scale

On January 1, 1992, the Health Care Financing Administration, which oversees the federal Medicare program, initiated a new method for paying physicians performing medical procedures that was based on resource input: the total time and work of the physician, as well as and practice costs, including malpractice liability. Called the Medical Fee Schedule, it was to be phased in over a 4-year period ending January 1, 1996.

Because the federal government has become such a dominant payer of healthcare providers, most other healthcare payers are following the lead of Medicare. Several state-level public payers, including worker's compensation programs, are either initiating or planning to initiate some version of a resource-based relative value scale (RBRVS). By the end of 1993, those states included Minnesota, Washington, Pennsylvania, Colorado, and West Virginia, with other states falling in behind. In at least two states—Washington and West Virginia—the impetus at the state level has been to move various public payers, such as public employees insurance, Medicaid, worker's compensation, and public health service, toward common reimbursement policies to better rationalize and simplify the basis and process of physician reimbursement.

One policy result inherent with the purpose of resource-based reimbursements is that primary care physicians who treat patients without performing procedures will be paid more equitably in comparison to specialists doing these procedures. Because the RBRVS has a "zero-sum" goal, procedural specialists will generally be reimbursed less than before, and thus many oppose it. Relative value units (RVUs) have been established and are being updated by the federal Health Care Financing Administration working in cooperation with the AMA. The RVUs are then multiplied by conversion factors that may be weighted for geographic location to account for differences in the cost of living and practice costs to arrive at the actual dollar reimbursement rates for given procedures. As states move to RBRVS systems of reimbursement, it is the conversion factor that is key for providers. Although the federally accepted RVUs remain in place, conversion factors can be made budget neutral and be developed independently from those of the Medicare Fee Schedule.

Constructing resource-based relative value medical fee schedules, although innovative, is not an overall structural change for most state worker's compensation programs because over two thirds of the states already had fee schedules of some sort in place by 1992. A greater change for worker's compensation has been the move toward managed care.

Managed Care as a Tool for Worker's Compensation

Managed care has emerged as the standard for group healthcare delivery during the past decade and is now being adopted by worker's compensation programs. To be adopted, however, it must be adapted to the special needs of worker's compensation. Because musculoskeletal injuries predominate in worker's compensation, a managed care organization must first ensure a provider mix heavily weighted with orthopaedic surgeons, neurosurgeons, outpatient treatment centers, physical therapists, and chiropractors, as opposed to the predominance of primary care physicians found in general health practice.

Further, managed care is a process, and managing medical care delivery in a worker's compensation claim is quite different from the process of managing an episode of care under group health insurance or within a general health maintenance organization (HMO). In worker's compensation, work-relatedness must be determined before treatment, and then treatment must be directed toward return to work. Managed care providers must understand the worker's compensation law within their jurisdiction and in bordering jurisdictions. They need to communicate treatment progress and outcomes to the insurer, to the employer, and also in many instances to the administrative agency in language free of medical jargon, as noted earlier in this chapter.

The need for directing treatment toward return to work cannot be overstated. To this end, state worker's compensation jurisdictions are moving away from a laissez faire approach to medical treatment and are adopting guidelines for providers to use in treating work-related injuries. Thus managed care in worker's compensation more and more will involve various review activities directed not only at controlling costs of care but also at ensuring quality of care and facilitating return to work. Because treatment is so highly discretionary in soft tissue injuries, which are the work-related injuries most commonly compensated, well-structured concurrent and retrospective managed care review using treatment guidelines can identify ineffective or inappropriate treatment patterns over time and help treating physicians redirect treatment to more productive outcomes. Some specifics of this, however, must await outcome data not presently available.

Retrospective review after treatment is usually done through medical bill review by relating procedures to diagnosis to determine appropriateness, frequency, and duration. Medical bills that fail these tests may then trigger manual review of the medical records. Whereas the first outcome of such a review may be to deny payment for services determined to be unnecessary or inappropriate, a second outcome can be to profile providers over time to identify those who most commonly are denied payment and the reasons for denial.

More productive to treatment itself is concurrent review. In group health, this commonly relates to inpatient hospital services and is performed by nurses. Although a review of inpatient hospital services is important for worker's compensation, outpatient services for musculoskeletal injuries are by far more prevalent than any other services. Therefore, specialized review programs now use computerized criteria or algorithms to monitor a patient's progress through a treatment regimen. Whether such outpatient services are monitored on a large scale by a computerized program or in a more traditional way by insurance company claim adjusters reviewing claims against specified treatment guidelines, an independent medical examination may be ordered to clarify the claimant's medical status.

Although the independent medical examination has already been discussed, it is well to review its purpose with regard to managed care. An independent medical examination *must* be objective because it becomes the basis for deciding whether the treatment is necessary for the work injury and whether the treatment regimen is progressing to achieve maximum medical stability. The decision maker acting on the information from the independent examination may be the insurance claims adjuster or, if any part of the claim has been disputed, an administrative commissioner or law judge. The report of a good independent examination clearly addresses the questions at hand regarding treatment and expected outcome and provides reasonable estimates of recovery and return to work. Often an independent medical examiner will need to address questions relating to preexisting conditions that may or may not affect recovery. Only treatment related to recovery from the work injury can legitimately be covered through worker's compensation.

As the study done at Boeing Aircraft shows, because nonmedical factors such as job dissatisfaction and poor performance appraisals by supervisors can be critical factors in achieving the return-to-work goal, case management is an essential activity in a significant number of claims. A case manager is the link between the treating physician and the employer and can arrange modified work assignments for job reentry or can help with workplace redesign. Regarding motivational issues, although case managers cannot cure past job dissatisfaction or amend a poor performance appraisal, they may find ways to help employers and employees better structure their role relationship.

Some insurance company claims adjusters may begin to function as case managers in some claims, but typically their caseload is too large to permit them to do anything more than monitor medical treatment and progress and make decisions about the extent of work disability. Case managers are most often specially trained nurses who can act as a worker's ombudsman in communicating with all other interested parties in the system. Employers themselves can often provide effective case managers who can personally interact on a face-to-face basis with claimants, their treating physicians, and their attorneys if a dispute arises. Otherwise, insurance companies and/or state worker's compensation administrative agencies may employ or contract with case managers. A case manager in state agency employment has the perceived advantage of neutrality, independent of any potentially contesting parties.

When injured employees are not able to return to their old job because of some residual impairment from injury, either with a modified assignment or to a modified work station, vocational rehabilitation becomes necessary. All worker's compensation jurisdictions provide vocational rehabilitation benefits, although some much more productively than others. Retraining for work first requires an accurate assessment of job availability in a particular geographic area. An assessment of a worker's skills and potential then follows. Retraining and schooling can be part of vocational rehabilitation, but these are usually significantly more expensive than job modification or workplace redesign.

Managed care is critical to the good overall management of worker's compensation claims, especially through a network of given providers who follow and are monitored by treatment guidelines designed to positively influence return to work, through continued effective case management that enables workers to return to work, and if needed, through vocational rehabilitation. However, managed care technologies in general have not been subject to careful examination because of their rapid diffusion, and this is particularly true in worker's compensation.

To date, only one worker's compensation HMO project in Florida has been evaluated,[4] and that evaluation was done after only 1 year in operation. After accounting for administrative fees in the HMO and adjusting for demographic and injury differences, the difference between the HMO and a control group's costs was 38.57%. Total medical costs were reduced almost 60% (with physician costs down 48%), and surgery rates were half those of the control group.[4] Still, true outcome measures in terms of reduced lost time and increased return to work take several years to assess. In theory, effective managed care in worker's compensation should not only control escalating medical costs but also have considerable effect on lost time claims by reducing recovery and return-to-work time for moderately severe injuries and by reducing disputes and litigation.

Worker's Compensation and a National Health Plan

In the fall of 1993, the White House released a proposed Health Security Act, the result of intensive deliberation the spring before by a national task force on healthcare reform. Title X of the Health Security Act required coordination of the medical portion of worker's compensation and automobile insurance within the proposed new delivery system. With coordination, insurers, both private carriers and state funds, would continue to maintain financial control of an entire worker's compensation claim, both medical and wage replacement benefits, but lose a certain amount of control over medical care delivery in a claim. Coordination is not without its problems, even though it is a logical and perhaps even necessary component of a national healthcare plan.

Although the very large employers (5000 employers or more) may set up their own health plans, the coordination approach proposed requires private insurance carriers, state funds, and self-insured employers to purchase medical coverage for worker's compensation claims from designated health plans within a geographic region. These health plans are paid on a capitation basis for general health care, but worker's compensation medical costs would be paid on a fee-for-service basis, thus providing an incentive for health plans and their providers to find many disabling conditions to be work related. Further, health plans are required to designate case managers with respect to worker's compensation services provided, but with no direct accountability to insurers or employers with regard to outcome. Thus conflict is possible between health plan case managers and case managers of employers, insurers, and even state agencies about the best course of treatment in terms of achieving early return to work. As discussed in the previous section, managed care must be specially organized and executed to facilitate this goal.

Another feature of the proposed coordinated health plan involves the use of specialized worker's compensation providers. Although well intended in terms of giving health plans a way out of setting up specialized services on their own and allowing injured workers a way of selecting providers outside their general healthcare plan, this provision could have unfortunate consequences as regards both cost and quality. It may be politically difficult for states to restrict the designation of specialized providers to channel workers to really qualified specialists, and these providers would presumably not be subject to either the case management provisions of the health plans or any utilization controls of employers and insurers. This clearly creates the possibility of injured workers doctor shopping, receiving unneeded services because of fee-for-services reimbursement, and having longer-duration disability.

The Health Security Act of 1993, as well as the other health-reform bills introduced to Congress, all concur on the need for treatment protocols overall. Title X of the act authorizes demonstration projects for the development of protocols to treat work-related conditions. Nationally accepted guidelines, if enforced by health plans and by states, would likely reduce unnecessary care and facilitate return to work. Guidelines for the treatment of low back conditions are especially critical because of the volume of back disability claims and the variation in both diagnosis and treatment patterns; the new guidelines from the Agency for Health Care Policy and Research are discussed in Chapter 22. Various states are also beginning to develop and adopt treatment guidelines or protocols by working with local medical specialists and borrowing work done by others. Well-documented demonstration projects are needed to test the efficacy of guidelines.

A Prospective View

As the twentieth century comes to a close, two of the social policy issues present at the beginning of the century are being revisited: the compensation of work-related injuries and national health care. Title X of the Health Security Act calls for the establishment of a Commission on Integration of Health Benefits that is mandated to study the integration of financial responsibility for all medical benefits into the health alliances discussed earlier. Political considerations play an important role in the resolution of these issues.

Full integration would mean that employers would no longer be responsible for that portion of the worker's compensation premium related to medical expenditures and designated health plans would receive payment directly from regional health alliances set up to purchase services. Although there is a provocative logic to a full integration of healthcare delivery, there is a persuasive counterlogic to such integration because of the unique nature of a worker's compensation claim.

Unlike general health care where one episode of care (e.g., an office visit or surgery) is an entire claim, in worker's compensation, a medical claim can last for years from the first treatment related to an occupational injury or illness to the point of maximum medical improvement. In computing premiums, actuarial calculations are based on injury and experience-based projections of total costs over time. Group health premiums, however, are calculated from one policy year to the next. Beyond the problem of how medical treatment over time would be financed by a health alliance that otherwise operated on a strictly annualized basis, unique legal issues of dispute resolution and provider testimony related to medical treatment and duration of disability arise because health alliances could offer different health plans from one year to the next to employers who would then offer them to their employees. Further, with the partial loss of direct employer premium rating based on the employer's previous medical expense experience, incentives for employer safety could be compromised.

More importantly and in corollary fashion, medical care benefits in worker's compensation are directly related to the payment of wage replacement or indemnity benefits. These too can extend over time. Disconnecting financial responsibility for the medical benefit from financial responsibility for the indemnity benefit could very likely increase indemnity benefits if health plans

and their providers do not understand the medical/indemnity benefit relationship and the impairment/disability issue with regard to return to work.

If worker's compensation medical care is fully integrated in health plans in the future, efforts could be undertaken to federalize disability benefits in some manner and eliminate the roles of state administration and private insurance carriers altogether. Organized labor would certainly be a major advocate of doing so inasmuch as it was the major proponent of a national worker's compensation program during the reform movement of the 1970s.

A national health and disability program in the United States would be truly evolutionary given the original constitutional challenges of due process to early worker's compensation laws, the nearly century-long resistance of organized medicine and private insurance to a national healthcare program, and the reluctance of Congress in midcentury to include nonoccupationally caused disability in the Social Security Act. As noted earlier, any disability compensated by the Social Security Administration has to be total in nature and prevent an individual from any gainful employment for 12 months or more. Worker's compensation programs, for all their variability in other respects, cover partial disability, a concept of some form of impaired earning capability because of the residual and permanent effects of an injury or illness.

How partial disability would or could be accommodated through a national program is at best unclear. The problems associated with measuring and compensating levels of partial disability have been the most resistant to any administrative or statutory resolution, and the ways in which states have sought to deal with permanent partial disability compensation (e.g., from impaired earning capacity to wage loss, from weekly benefits to lump sum settlements) have largely contributed to the variability among state worker's compensation programs.

There is some merit to the argument that the line between traumatic workplace injury and the gradual disability brought on by lifestyle and aging has blurred tremendously, thus introducing an illogic to compensating disability through different programs. And there is merit to the perspective that it is not the cause but the consequences of disability that should be the focus and concern of any administrative program. However, there is probably little if any merit to the idea that a national health and disability program would be any more cost-effective than state programs, especially given the recent experience of European countries with rising expenses in their social welfare programs. A national program would have no better ability, and perhaps less ability, to cope with the political pressures that accompany an ever-expanding concept of disability and the expansion of both medical and disability assistive technologies. The issues of maintaining state worker's compensation programs versus evolving to some national program or combination of programs need to be carefully studied and understood in light of our own century-long experience with state programs and what we can anticipate based on the experience of other countries that have some form of matured national social welfare. Is there some rational middle-ground approach that would be better than either of these two broad alternatives?

References

1. American Academy of Orthopaedic Surgeons, Committee on Occupational Health: *A physicians primer on worker's compensation,* Park Ridge, Ill, 1992, The Academy.

2. American Medical Association: *Guides to the evaluation of permanent impairment,* ed 4, Chicago, Ill, 1993, The Association.

3. Bigos SJ, Battie MC, Spengler DM, et al.: A prospective study of work perception and psychosocial factors affecting the report of back injury, *Spine* 16(1): 1-6, 1991.

4. Florida Department of Insurance: *Worker's compensation managed care pilot project: second interim report to the Florida Legislature,* Tallahassee, Fla, 1993, The Department.

5. Greenwood JG: A historical perspective on worker's compensation in the context of national health policy debate. In Greenwood JG, Taricco A, editors: *Worker's compensation health care cost containment,* Horsham, Pa., 1992, LRP Publications; pp. 1-26.

6. Minnesota Department of Labor and Industry: *Permanent partial disability rules,* Minnesota Rules Chapter 5223, Minneapolis, 1993, The Department.

7. Waddell G, et al: Chronic low back pain: psychological stress and illness behaviors, *Spine* 9:209, 1984.

Appendix A: AAOS Treatment Report Forms

INITIAL TREATMENT REPORT

General and History
Present job with brief description of physical effort—length of time in this occupation with this employer.

_____

_____

_____

Demographic History
Marital status, dependent children, educational level, past and current work history, race, alcohol and drug usage.

_____

_____

_____

Chief Complaint
The symptoms keeping the patient from his/her job.

_____

_____

_____

Present Illness
Describe history of chief complaint and outline casual connection to work (i.e., "the patient states that . . . "). Injury details should include those of medical significance only. Include medication history. Include pertinent laboratory and imaging studies and treatment.

_____

_____

_____

Past History
General health and systems review affecting complaint (GI, GU/GYN, and arthritis in the case of low back pain).

_____

_____

_____

Physical Examination
Medically significant findings related to present illness.

_____

_____

_____

Diagnosis
Specific diagnostic impression with short differential diagnosis if appropriate.

_____

_____

_____

Medical Treatment Issues
Planned treatment with basis for selection—note planned consultations (MD - PT - OT - etc.)

_____

_____

_____

Administrative Issues
Causation issue stated directly. Ability to work (full- or part-time, regular or adjusted job). Probable duration of inability for any work (temporary total disability) or usual work (temporary partial disability). Probable full recovery time (maximum medical improvement).

_____

_____

_____

Next Visit Date

INTERVAL TREATMENT REPORT

Interval Medical History

As with usual medical history, but including other treatments given, administrative and legal actions, and conflicts that are of medical importance (e.g., employer refuses to accept causation, lawyer medical referrals, worker not receiving wage benefits).

_____

_____

_____

Physical Examination

Changes for better or worse since last exam.

_____

_____

_____

Diagnosis

Any change from previous visit.

_____

_____

_____

Medical Progress Statement

Include treatment options and changes as well as a functional progress statement (walking and sitting tolerance, for instance).

_____

_____

_____

Administrative Progress Statement

Repeat causation statement and note ability to work (full- or part-time, regular or adjusted job). Estimate duration of no work (total temporary disability), limited work (temporary partial disability), and point of maximum medical improvement (MMI). Also note need for physical or vocational rehabilitation.

_____

_____

_____

Next Visit Date [   ]

FINAL TREATMENT REPORT

Remember that the reliability required of your decision is 51% ("more probable than not")

Interval Medical History
Including both medical and administrative developments as in the interval treatment reports.

_____

_____

_____

Physical Examination
Changes for better or worse since last examination.

_____

_____

_____

Diagnosis
This should remain unchanged from previous interval reports.

_____

_____

_____

Medical Progress Statement
There should be no significant further treatment changes or diagnostic testing advised. A statement should be made that the patient has reached a medical end result and that no significant change in physical findings or activity levels is expected in the foreseeable future. A need for vocational rehabilitation may be mentioned.

_____

_____

_____

Administrative Progress Statement
The point of maximum medical improvement (MMI) should be stated to have been reached with a date assigned that may be the date of the report. Long-term, (i.e., 20 years) future medical needs or decreased function may be mentioned here but should not affect the MMI. Ability to work (full- or part-time). Regular or another (or adjusted) job. Final determination of functional impairment expressed in percentage (AMA _Guides_ the most standard reference). Need for vocational evaluation.

_____

_____

_____

Appendix B: AAOS Independent Medical Evaluation Form

INDEPENDENT MEDICAL EVALUATION

Remember that the reliability required of your decision is 51% ("more probable than not")

Sources of History
Patient (comment on patient's ability as a historian) or records (list).

_____

_____

_____

Demographic History
Marital status, dependent children, educational level, past and current work history, race, alcohol and drug usage.

_____

_____

_____

General History
Educational level. Present job with brief description of physical effort required. Length of time at that occupation and with that employer. Prior work skill.

_____

_____

_____

Chief Complaint
The symptoms keeping the patient from his/her job.

_____

_____

_____

Present Illness
Start with initial episode of chief complaint. Include all work and nonwork episodes, treatment, and prior claims. Describe present complaint and claim status and recent treatment.

_____

_____

_____

Past Medical History

General health and systems review affecting chief complaint (GI, GU/GYN, and arthritis in the case of low back pain).

_____

_____

_____

Physical Examination

Describe objective and subjective findings. Note inconsistencies. Measure and describe scarring. Use check sheet.

_____

_____

_____

Pertinent Laboratory and Imaging Findings

Note dates of study. Note whether imaging source is actual films or reports.

_____

_____

_____

Diagnosis

Differential and specific impression. Remember to give basis of opinions (objective and subjective findings).

_____

_____

_____

Medical Treatment Issues

When was point of maximum medical improvement reached? Further necessary treatment? Likelihood of long-term progression.

_____

_____

_____

Administrative Issues

Causation, aggravation, or exacerbation stated. Ability to work (full- or part-time), regular or another (or adjusted) job. Describe functional impairments and need for or results of vocational evaluation or functional capacity testing.

_____

_____

_____

Impairment

Use AMA *Guides* or other methods to give percentage. Assign apportionment or second injury fund criteria if appropriate.

_____

_____

_____

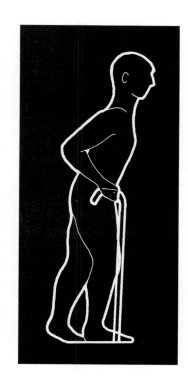

Chapter 49

Governmental Control

Nortin M. Hadler

CONTENTS

The industrial revolution took a great toll on workers, whose physical well-being was placed at risk by the conditions of labor. The mandate for change grew out of the workforce itself. All laborers lived in dread of loss of income. The English "Friendly Societies" and German "Krankenkassen" developed, usually in association with trades, and enabled artisans and more advantaged workers to purchase insurance that would provide some "sick pay," not medical treatment, should illness force them out of work. Workers often went into debt while attempting to pay medical bills, and medical practice was plagued by accounts receivable. Although all workers lived in dread of losing income as a consequence of illness, death was their greatest fear. As late as 1907, 7000 American workers were killed in just two industries—railroading and bituminous coal mining.[1]

"Common law" was fashioned by the ruling class to place the worker at an insurmountable disadvantage in gaining redress. The employer was exonerated by

> "that 'unholy trinity of defenses:' (1) *contributory negligence*—the worker could not recover if he himself had been negligent in any degree, regardless of the extent of the employer's negligence; (2) the *fellow-servant doctrine*—the employee could not recover if it could be shown that the injury had resulted from the negligence of a fellow worker; and (3) the *assumption of risk*—the injured man could not recover if injury was due to an inherent hazard of the job of which he had, or should have had, advance knowledge."[24]

Late in the nineteenth century it was estimated that 40% of all workplace accidents were no one's fault and that 30% were a result of contributory negligence. The "fellow servant" doctrine was articulated by Lord Abinger in England in 1837 and imported by Judge Shaw into Boston in 1842, where it was used to block redress for the remainder of workplace accidents.[19] Furthermore, this "unholy trinity of defenses" is only one facet of the casting off of feudal paternalism that characterized legislation of the mid-nineteenth century; all matter of poor relief was restricted in the belief that such programs impeded the circulation of labor and created disincentives to work.[23]

THE UNITED STATES

America did not roil with social reform at the turn of the century. That was not for lack of homeless people, almshouses, and the vestiges of the colonial Poor Laws. There even was unrest, but it was primarily agrarian and populist and not appeased by social insurance programs. The Socialist party was little political threat, and the union movement was far less developed than in Europe.[25] The movement for social reform was spearheaded by "social progressive" academicians such as the economists John Commons of the University of Wisconsin and Henry Seager of Columbia University, who founded the American Association for Labor Legislation (AALL) in 1906. The advocacy of the AALL was to reform capitalism, not abolish it.

The AALL was visible, but its impact was limited. Only worker's compensation insurance legislation survived the politics of the day, and not easily.[3] Congress would not abide a national program; bills were drawn up painstakingly, one state at a time. The worker could ill afford any insurance. Management stepped up if the program included "tort immunity" and the ability to pass on the cost to the consumer. By 1949, all states independently administered worker's compensation insurance programs. Today, the states are joined by the District of Columbia, the territories, federal employees, and railway workers; 58 independent jurisdictions administer insurance schemes, some of which are exclusively underwritten and managed by governmental agencies, some allow the employer to self-insure, and most are a marketplace for the private insurance industry. In accepting indemnification under worker's compensation, the American worker forfeits any other form of redress, including the right to sue the employer, except under very special circumstances.

A central tenet of all worker's compensation programs is the provision of medical care aimed at returning the injured worker back to the job. Neither the physicians of the time nor the hospitals were prepared for this challenge. In fact, Stevens' description[26] of the medical response to the compensable injury early in the century would pertain today.

> The average hospital organization, geared to undertake "careful and daring" surgery, was just not attuned to effective reconstruction (rehabilitation) work, including "unremitting after-care. . . ." Indeed, hospitals "never desired this sort of work particularly. . . ." The central core of treatment—the continuous care of an injured worker, both as inpatient and as long-term outpatient—was generally unavailable.

Worker's compensation claimants became the special purview of the trauma surgeon. In the beginning, the injuries that qualified were violent. However, the definition of "injury" became more expansive. Inguinal herniation could be considered an injury only if it were termed a "rupture." And back pain qualified once the concept of the "ruptured disk" gained general credence in the 1930s.[12,16] After World War II, most of the growth in compensation claims can be ascribed to expanding the definition of injury in this fashion. Worker's compensation in America underwrites extraordinary surgical zeal aimed at the ailing back and more recently the aching arm. The American worker—in fact, all Americans—have come to speak and think about musculoskeletal discomfort in an injury context. Seduced by the promise of dramatic diagnosis, unbridled interventions for cure, and the largess of wage replacement or more, the American worker has been urged on by surgeons, lawyers, and common sense to confront the contest of causation with escalating vigor. The proliferation of pain centers and rehabilitation facilities suggests that although someone may be benefiting from this trend, it is not necessarily the injured worker.

President Franklin Roosevelt's efforts to expand social welfare coverage to include the disabled American worker joined the struggle to define entitlements. Congress decided that "real" disease can be reliably identified by physicians through clinical techniques that quantify impairment. Social Security Disability Insurance (SSDI) came into being to ensure the American worker an adequate income if such could no longer be earned. The basis of an award was the magnitude of medically determinable disease—the amount of impairment[13]; workers had to be sufficiently impaired so that one could infer with confidence that they could not "maintain substantial gainful employment." A "handbook" was developed and listed examples of the magnitude of impairment that would be prerequisite. Once SSDI was in place, the previous strident objections of physicians to impairment rating schemes were superseded by acquiescence and remunerative participation. The American Medical Association was quick to leap onto the impairment bandwagon by publishing the *Guides to the Evaluation of Permanent Impairment*. All editions of this popular and profitable guide contain the disclaimer that impairment need not correlate with disability. If that disclaimer were heeded, the "Guides" would have limited utility. However, they are widely used, particularly in disability determination for worker's compensation insurance in some jurisdictions that require that they be followed. This occurs despite the overwhelming evidence that impairment, short of catastrophe, is a minor determinant of disability.[14]

Social Security Disability Insurance was developed to insure workers who become globally disabled by disease; the disabled who never or hardly ever worked still had to turn to the "welfare" systems of the states, each of which, in its fashion, carried on the tradition of the Poor Laws. Title XVI of the Social Security Act was passed into law in 1972 and by 1974 had imposed the rules and bureaucracy for administering SSDI on the state welfare programs. This Supplemental Security Income (SSI) program overwhelmed the agency and thereby led to a dramatic surge in cost of the federal disability insurance program. By 1977, nearly 3 million disabled Americans were receiving benefits, nearly three times the number in 1967.

In 1980, President Carter signed legislation requiring that the Social Security Administration commence periodic reviews of the validity of the disability claimed by all these recipients. The intent was to purge the rolls of the unworthy, of those who can work. PL 96-265, enacted a century after the birth of social reform, produced one of the bleakest chapters in the annals of the disabled. Many did not meet impairment criteria. These claimants ascribed their disability to symptoms, particularly the symptom of pain, and were infuriated by a process that discounted the veracity of their symptoms in favor of the dearth of impairment. Nonetheless, they were disallowed. This meant that a person who survived on a meager SSDI/SSI pension (monthly payments averaged nearly $600 for the disabled and $165 for a dependent spouse or child) had to find work or plead poverty. Even claimants who perceived themselves disabled and were turned down by SSDI/SSI could not find a niche in the labor force.[29] Until the process was halted by class action suits before the Federal Judiciary, Congress charged the Institute of Medicine with finding a solution. How can the symptoms of pain be validated and quantified so that pain will serve as a criterion for a disability award? A committee deliberated and produced a document that concluded, in essence, that more research was needed.[20] Neither this committee nor any other formal body is willing to replace impairment rating for disability determination; this is but one facet of the complicated task of healthcare reform currently under consideration in the United States.

Today, the United States has in place an unwieldy, inefficient, heavily bureaucratized system. Conspicuously missing is health insurance for the working-age population. In the absence of health insurance, these disability schemes may be the only recourse, short or long term, for anyone who cannot work, for anyone who will not work, and even for anyone who can work but is displaced or redundant.

JAPAN

The history of Japan is characterized by centuries of foreign interaction alternating with centuries of exclusion.[27] Social legislation remained sparse in Japan before the aftermath of World War II. The period of occupation under MacArthur saw the dismantling of imperial government and the creation of a constitutional democracy. It also witnessed the introduction, almost in pure form, of the Prussian template for workplace health and safety legislation; in 1947 the Diet enacted the Labor Standards Law and the Workmen's Accident Compensation Insurance Law. Modifications have been made in administration, but little in substance. Japan has a national Workers' Accident Compensation insurance scheme administered through the Ministry of Labor.[21] Employees of all but the smallest enterprises are provided with indemnification by virtue of premiums required of their employer. These premiums are established by experience rating on an industrywide basis. Other private sector workers can participate voluntarily. Aside from the fact that the program is national and not an "exclusive remedy," it is similar to the American worker's compensation insurance.[31]

In addition to worker's compensation, attention has been paid to occupational disease, setting of safety standards, recourse for marginal workers, and so forth.[22] In 1972, the Diet enacted the Industrial Safety and Health Law similar to the U.S. Occupational Safety and Health Act, with an emphasis on prevention. In 1975, the Ministry of Labor founded the University of Occupational and Environmental Health, a medical school whose graduates are bound to serve 9 years in the practice of occupational medicine. Furthermore, all Japanese workers and their families are indemnified for the direct and indirect costs of illness under the Health Insurance Act.[18,21] In addition to healthcare benefits, the insured is entitled to a substantial wage substitution if unable to return to work after 3 days. If employment is terminated (and it can be terminated even while on sick leave), the insurance coverage continues for 5 years. If the individual is still disabled, coverage reverts to the National Pension or Employees' Pension, less generous and more stigmatizing components of the national health and social security schemes.[28]

Medical intervention is at the discretion of the treating physician. Most care involves frequent, brief patient contacts, the provision of prescription pharmaceuticals, and even admission to private clinics. All this is readily underwritten for an employee with an incapacitating backache[8]; health insurance has covered over 24 million days of care for low back pain each year since 1970.[17] The risk of stigmatization for being ill and accepting care is minimal. The likelihood of surgical intervention is far less than in the United States, and the expectation of healing and return to work is facilitated by tradition and by the lack of a comparably appealing option. Worker's compensation is not the path of least resistance for a worker except in cases of a violent accident consequent to external force.

Comparisons with the United States are difficult because of the absence of a single insurer and the extraordinary variability of coverage from state to state and within each jurisdiction in the United States. Furthermore, these insurance schemes are social contracts that cannot be generalized from country to country. The fact that 25% of all indemnity claims under worker's compensation in the United States reflect disabling back "injuries"[32] must speak to these sociopolitical differences at least as much as differences in workplace safety and worker susceptibility to injury.

Japan has a labor force numbering over 40 million that has managed to be reconciled to the same worker's compensation paradigm that for most Western countries is a cause of some degree of contentiousness. Several explanations are possible: employment and job satisfaction are so high that worker's compensation is indeed a recourse of last resort in a flexible work environment and seldom a surrogate for job dissatisfaction. Return to work may be facilitated by the award system in Japan; there is so little to gain unless one remains under treatment, and the medical community does not foster such behavior. Because similar clinical care is available under health insurance if the condition is considered an illness rather than an injury and because temporary pensions of adequate magnitude are also forthcoming, the contest of causality is less pressing in Japan than elsewhere. Clearly, peer review is involved in a worker's decision to consider a regional backache an injury. Of course, these explanations and others one could imagine might be totally off base. Just because the Western world was able to impose its approach to workplace safety and health on Japan 45 years ago does not mean that the outcome can be appreciated from a Western perspective.

SWITZERLAND AND NEW ZEALAND

Switzerland and New Zealand decided that whether related to employment or not, injury deserved special consideration. In 1912, Switzerland established the Swiss National Accident Insurance Fund (SUVA), which remained a state-controlled monopoly until 1984 when private insurers were allowed into the market. The New Zealand Parliament passed the Accident Compensation Act creating the Accident Compensation Corporation (ACC) in 1972. Both SUVA and the ACC provide a national, no-fault insurance umbrella for all residents and citizens that covers medical expenses and lost wages consequent to an accidental injury, regardless of the setting in which the accident occurred. These programs—known as 24-hour coverage—draw on contributions from automobile licensing fees, wages, employer taxes, and the general fund. Both programs had been the target for reform and the subject of considerable criticism in the past because of escalating costliness, until the mid-1980s, when they were flourishing, seemed to be serving the common good, and were applauded for their cost-effectiveness.[5,9,11] The 24-hour coverage was achieved in very different ways under the two systems.

Adherence to a strict definition of "accidental cause" is required by SUVA for coverage. A SUVA physician determines causation, establishes wage replacement and any award for pain and suffering, and monitors each patient for a year if the injury is covered. Few backaches qualify under this definition, and backache patients may receive medical care but no pension or oversight. After 1 year of disability—covered or not—the wage earner's claim reverts to the Invaliden Verseherung, which is the agency that is responsible for further pensioning.

The issue of causation has been defused for the ACC in New Zealand. For example, a backache can qualify if the claimant can describe a precipitant that occurred within 3 months of the claim. If the incapacity precludes return to prior work, this status must be recertified monthly by the treating physician and is subject to review by the ACC. Limited lump sum awards for pain and suffering are provided. The ACC has open-ended responsibility for its awardees. This includes medical care and permanent total or partial awards. Sometimes these awards are debated within the agency, particularly if the impairment is minimal or questionable.

THE NETHERLANDS

The Dutch have taken the opposite tack from "24-hour coverage." For the Dutch, a social security system should provide benefits across the board that cover the entire adult working population with no further categorization. The Dutch program has discarded the issue of injury; all that matters is work incapacity. Furthermore, for the first year under the Sickness Benefits Act, the test is whether one can return to the former job. If not, 70% of the wages is replaced, medical care is provided, and the course of the injury is frequently monitored by agency physicians. If the patient is not well enough to return to the old job at 1 year, the case is turned over to another agency—the Gemeenschappelijke Medische Dienst (GMD)—for disability determination. If the patient is determined to be 80% incapacitated, a pension of 70% wage replacement continues. If the patient is 15% incapacitated, no pension will be rewarded. Some contentiousness arises in the middle areas, but the GMD decision usually prevails. The liberal approach of the Dutch, like that of most of the Scandinavian countries, is the product of their national conscience and continues regardless of the considerable cost and occasional opposition.

FRANCE

After World War II, France constructed a system that encompasses nearly all relevant clinical contingencies, the Sécurité Social. A national health insurance policy underwrites medical care from independent practitioners. The population is also served by local agencies, the Caisse, that provide administrative, allied health professional, and another tier of clinical support. A "corps" of physicians—the médicin conseil—based in the Caisse monitors the quality of care delivered by private physicians but underwritten by federal programs. These physicians review files, can suggest or question therapies, but cannot prescribe. For an employee, particularly of a large enterprise or one affiliated with a trade association, yet a third physician is involved, the médicin du travail. These are occupational physicians who are empowered to consider fitness to work and monitor worker health.

The major distinctiveness of the French paradigm relates to the ongoing nature of the clinical decision-making process regarding disability. The ability to return to work is a goal of health care from the outset. It falls upon the médicin conseil and the médicin du travail to ensure such. The Swiss serve the function with the kreisarzt, but only under SUVA for the injured worker. The French provide this level of care for the injured and the ill, although the benefits favor the injured.

CONCLUSION

Worker's compensation is supposed to ensure a safer workplace by "experience rating;" this means that companies or industries with a higher injury rate are charged a higher premium. The frequency of forceful injuries has remained constant while nonviolent "injuries" escalate. Furthermore, every advanced country has been compelled to enact legislation to inspect, regulate, and enforce standards for workplace health and safety in the past 20 years. This is compelling testimony to the ineffectiveness of worker's compensation. The workplace is only starting to come to grips with self-destructive behavior on the part of the workforce, and this initiative is from government regulators and, to a disappointingly small degree, from labor and management awareness. Finally, "caring" for the injured worker has produced even more outrageous behavior[7,15] on the part of the "providers" than what plagues society at large.[4,6]

Webster and Snook[30] have recently updated their analysis of the experience of the Liberty Mutual Insurance Company in indemnifying worker's compensation claims, particularly for backache. The analysis is a reproach to the worker's compensation concept. This insurer, and presumably others in the industry, finds itself forced to raise premiums to underwrite an escalating likelihood that American workers with back injuries will find themselves facing temporary total disability if not permanent partial disability. Furthermore, this fate has not been thwarted by underwriting the more and more costly ministrations of medical, chiropractic, osteopathic, and various other practitioners. Based on these descriptive statistics, Webster and Snook call for a concerted effort to identify responsible, remedial factors. It appears that the algorithm for recourse for low back pain that is promulgated by the worker's compensation system is dangerous.

Almost all the data presented by Webster and Snook[30] pertain to individuals with regional backache[15]: sufferers between the ages of 18 and 55 who would be otherwise well and who cannot ascribe their backache to a discrete traumatic precipitant. Such morbidity is ubiquitous, is always daunting, and always forces the patient to choose between three options[14]: most of us can cope most of the time. Some of us choose to be patients and seek the assistance of healthcare providers. Some of us seek care in the context of worker's compensation as claimants with a back injury. Choosing is a process that is easily perturbed by preconceived notions and the exigencies of life. For example, psychosocial challenges at the workplace outstrip psychometrics, ergonomic challenges, or the quality of the illness to explain why a worker with a backache chooses to be a claimant.[2] And once the choice to be a claimant is made, such variables as magnitude of the award, the paucity of wages, and litigation are readily demonstrable direct correlates of the likelihood of a claim eventuating in either temporary or permanent disability.[32] Furthermore, rather than a return to health, the fate of these claimants is a convoluted process of interventions and contests that all too often leaves them in a vortex of disability determination, mulling about America's pain, work hardening, and rehabilitation clinics trying to prove they hurt as much as they claim.[14] These and others are the pressures brought to bear on any worker's compensation claimant with a regional backache. No wonder that more and more they are rendered disabled in spite of more and more putatively palliative clinical or ergonomic interventions.

It follows that the enormously costly enterprise of worker's compensation insurance benefits so many who are involved in its execution far more than it benefits the unfortunate claimant with a regional backache.[10] It also follows that the remedy for the worker with a regional backache offered by worker's compensation has outlived its usefulness. Removing atraumatic "injuries" from compensability would decrease total claims only by some 25% (it would reduce cost by 75%, but again, that is a secondary consideration). The majority of the claims are a result of violent trauma, and although these claims are adjusted efficiently by worker's compensation

and at a predictable cost to industry, they also result in a predictable price paid by the workforce. Worker's compensation has proved itself to be a minor influence in rendering the workplace less hazardous in spite of experience rating.

Experiments in social policy may be difficult to enact, but once enacted they are even more difficult to alter, let alone retract. The Prussian paradigm—the first set of laws mandating compensation for work-related injury and illness, passed in Germany from 1884 to 1911—has dominated thinking for a century. Its administration employs legions (some 80,000 are employed by the Social Security Administration in the United States, for example). It is a lifeline for so many and a sacred entitlement for so many more.

Two principles are incontrovertible: Sensible health care should be ensured in all advanced countries. Sensible health care must make provision for sick leave. "Sensible" is meant to denote caring, compassionate recourse with all interventions based on established benefit/risk ratios. Likewise, safety in the workplace should be regulated to be "sensible," defined in a similar fashion, and employers held responsible in this regard. Neither sensible health care nor the provision of a sensibly safe workplace should be served by profit-driven enterprises. These issues must be considered in the debate over healthcare reform in the United States.

References

1. Berkowitz M, Burton JF: *Permanent disability benefits in workers' compensation,* Kalamazoo, Mich, 1987, WE Upjohn Institute; p 17.

2. Bigos SJ, Battié MC, Spengler DM, Fisher LD, Fordyce WE, Hansson TH, Nachemson AL, Wortley, MD: A prospective study of work perceptions and psychosocial factors affecting the report of back injury, *Spine* 17:177-182, 1991.

3. Bohlen FH: A problem in the drafting of workmen's compensation acts, *Harvard Law Rev* 25:328-348, 1912.

4. Burton JF: Workers' compensation costs, 1960-1992: the increases, the causes and the consequences, *John Burton's Workers' Compensation Monitor* 6:1-15, 1993.

5. Carron H, DeGood DE, Tait R: A comparison of low back pain patients in the United States and New Zealand: psychosocial and economic factors affecting severity of disability, *Pain* 21:77-89, 1985.

6. Greenwood J, Taricco A, editors: *Workers' compensation health care cost containment,* Horsham, Pa, 1992, LRP Publications: pp 1-374.

7. Hadler NM: Arm pain in the workplace. A small area analysis, *J Occup Med* 32:113-119, 1992.

8. Hadler NM: Backache and work incapacity in Japan, *J Occup Med* 36: 1110-1114, 1994.

9. Hadler NM: Disabling backache in France, Switzerland, and the Netherlands: contrasting sociopolitical constraints on clinical judgement, *J Occup Med* 31:823-831, 1989.

10. Hadler NM: Epilogue. In Greenwood J, Taricco A, editors: *Workers' compensation health care cost containment,* Horsham, Pa, 1992, LRP Publications; pp 339-344.

11. Hadler NM: Industrial rheumatology: the Australian and New Zealand experiences with arm pain and backache in the workplace, *Med J Austr* 144:191-195, 1986.

12. Hadler NM: Legal ramifications of the medical definition of back disease, *Ann Intern Med* 89:992-999, 1978.

13. Hadler NM: Medical ramifications of the federal regulation of the Social Security Disability Insurance program, *Ann Intern Med* 96:665-669, 1982.

14. Hadler NM: *Occupational musculoskeletal disorders,* New York, 1993, Raven Press; pp 227-262.

15. Hadler NM: Regional back pain, *N Engl J Med* 315:1090-1092, 1986.

16. Hadler NM: Regional musculoskeletal diseases of the low back: cumulative trauma versus single incident, *Clin Orthop* 221:33-41, 1987.

17. *Health and welfare statistics in Japan—1991,* Tokyo, 1991, Health and Welfare Statistics Association; p 90.

18. Inglehart JK: Japan's medical care system, *N Engl J Med* 319:807-812, 1988.

19. Larson A: *The law of workmen's compensation,* Section 4.30, New York, 1972, Matthew Bender; pp 25-32.

20. Osterweis M, Kleinman A, Mechanic D, editors: *Pain and disability,* Washington, 1987 National Academy Press, pp. 21-36.

21. *Outline of social insurance in Japan,* Tokyo, 1991, Japanese Government Social Insurance Agency.

22. Reich MR, Frumkin H: An overview of Japanese occupational health, *Am J Public Health* 78:809-815, 1988.

23. Rimlinger GV: *Welfare policy and industrialization in Europe, America and Russia, New York,* 1971, John Wiley & Sons.

24. Somers HM, Somers AR: *Workmen's compensation,* New York, 1954, John Wiley & Sons; p 18.

25. Starr P: *The social transformation of American medicine,* New York, 1982, Basic Books; pp 238-250.

26. Stevens R: *In sickness and in wealth,* New York, 1989, Basic Books; pp 84-89.

27. Sugimoto M, Swain DL: Science and culture in traditional Japan, New Haven, Conn, 1989, Yale University Press; pp 1-192.

28. Tsushima Y: *Annual report on health and welfare for 1989,* Tokyo, 1990, Ministry of Health & Welfare; p 112.

29. U.S. General Accounting Office Report to Congressional Requesters: *Social Security disability: denied applicants' health and financial status compared with beneficiaries',* GAO/HRD-90-2:1-78, Washington, DC, 1989, General Accounting Office.

30. Webster BS, Snook SH: The cost of 1989 Workers' Compensation low back claims, *Spine* 19:1111-1116, 1994.

31. Williams CA: How the Japanese workers' compensation system differs from ours, *NCCI Dig* 3:13-22, 1988.

32. Worrall JD, Appel D: The impact of workers' compensation benefits on low back claims. In Hadler NM, editor: *Clinical concepts in regional musculoskeletal illness,* Orlando, Fla, Grune & Stratton; pp 281-297.

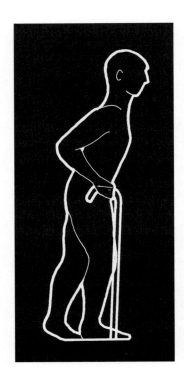

Chapter 50

The Physician's Role in Disability Evaluation

Scott Haldeman

CONTENTS

Most social systems throughout history have been forced to deal with the problems of a population containing individuals who have been injured, who are suffering from chronic disease, or who simply through aging have a reduced ability to perform the daily activities required for survival, both those associated with work and those at home. In nonindustrialized societies, the physical disabilities associated with aging are often perceived as being accompanied by increased wisdom and experience. Thus older members of society become the teachers and decision makers for the community. Those individuals with minor restrictions in ability are given tasks around the home in the preparation of tools or food and the care of children. Because of a lack of medical and health resources, the severely disabled inevitably succumb to infection or malnutrition and, occasionally in certain societies, some form of ritual suicide.

In modern industrialized nations, on the other hand, those individuals who are disabled have been given access to a wide variety of healthcare facilities and social resources in an attempt to reintegrate them into the community. To avoid abuse of these benefits, mechanisms have been developed to assess degrees of disability and assign responsibility for the cause of this disability. Rapid growth in the cost of these benefits has led to an increasing emphasis on the effects of chronic illness and injury on lifestyle and work capacity. Extensive legislation has been developed to set up rules for the provision of benefits to those unfortunate enough to have reduced capacity as a result of chronic illness or injury. Such legislation includes worker's compensation,[17] Social Security,[19] and the Americans with Disabilities Act (ADA). Furthermore, multiple private and industrial programs and insurance policies have been established to assist individuals who are ill, injured, or otherwise disabled.

In almost every determination of disability or ability, legislation or private contract requires the input of at least one and often several licensed healthcare practitioners. The basic assumption is that the most competent and best trained individual in society to determine the ability of other members of society to perform specific duties is the medical physician or, in certain areas, other healthcare practitioners such as osteopathic physicians or chiropractors. This decision has not been based on any well–thought out or scientifically investi-

gated competence but instead has fallen on the physician by default. Unfortunately, the skills necessary to perform this social function are not, as a rule, taught in medical school and until recently have not even been the subject of significant research. To some extent, therefore, physicians asked to perform this task have to do so based on personal opinion, great variability in experience, and usually poorly thought out legislation or social contracts.

ETHICS ASSOCIATED WITH DISABILITY EVALUATION

Physicians faced with the requirement that they determine the degree of impairment and the ability or inability of an individual to perform specific tasks must deal with a number of ethical dilemmas not commonly considered in clinical practice. Basic clinical practice is relatively simple in comparison to disability evaluation. Most physicians perceive their ethical duties to care for and relieve patient symptoms or illnesses by whatever means they can and without any consideration of the social position of their patients or the pressures exerted from outside authorities. The welfare of the patient is inherent in the Hippocratic oath. The contract for services is between the doctor and the patient.

One of two things happen when a physician is required to change roles and issue opinions on legal matters. If physicians are required to issue opinions that will have an impact on their own patients' ability to obtain compensation or work in a particular occupation, it is natural for physicians to be biased in favor of the patient's position in the matter. Failure to take a patient's position could seriously jeopardize the patient-doctor relationship and have an adverse impact on the ability to take care of the patient's healthcare needs. On the other hand, an inability to justify a particular position that may be strongly held by the patient can seriously jeopardize the physician's credibility within a worker's compensation or other healthcare delivery system. This can subject the doctor to deposition and increased paperwork to justify a position and can at times lead to ostracizing the physician or canceling a contract by worker's compensation, healthcare insurance, or the management agency.

If physicians are functioning as independent medical examiners, their ethics are subject to pressure from the referring source. Inevitably the patient has been referred to an independent medical examiner because of disagreement between the insurance carrier or agency and the patient or treating physician. Irrespective of the honesty of the independent medical examiner, insurance carriers tend to refer insured persons to physicians with a track record that tends to support their position. Further difficulty arises in that patients tend to be distrustful of the independent medical examiner and may attempt to justify their perceived position. This may lead to embellishment and other forms of exaggerated behavior to impress the assessing physician. Although the criteria of Waddell and associates[21] can be used to identify certain of these factors, the assessing physician may be tempted to be less sympathetic to such an individual irrespective of the underlying disability that may be camouflaged by this behavior.

Certain judicial systems have developed mechanisms to reduce the bias inherent in disability evaluation. One mechanism introduced in California is that of an Agreed Medical Examiner or rotating Qualified Medical Examiner. Under the Agreed Medical Examiner system, both the injured worker's counsel and the insurance carrier's counsel must agree in advance on a physician as an arbiter of the level of disability and other associated medical-legal questions. Under the Qualified Medical Examiner system, an unrepresented worker is given three names by the state in rotating order of registered examiners. Patients can then pick one of the three physicians as their evaluator. In other jurisdictions that have a permanent administrative judge, certain physicians develop a reputation for credibility in the community. The weight given to the opinion of such credible assessing physicians is much higher than that from either the treating physician or the biased independent medical examiner. Physicians fortunate enough to reach this level of credibility in a community, however, can find themselves overwhelmed by requests to do disability evaluations.

Hadler[10,11] has seriously questioned the ethics of any physician who performs disability evaluations. It is his opinion that the notion of impairment rating is fatally flawed and should be discarded completely. He believes that diminished working capacity as a result of musculoskeletal disorders, which is the most common cause of disputed disability, is overwhelmed by psychological and sociopolitical confounders and cannot be determined in the medical setting. The marked variation in medical opinion as to the nature and extent of disability given similar clinical findings tends to support this view. Further support comes from the work of Waddell,[20] Bigos,[3,4] Deyo[9] and their colleagues, in which it is demonstrated that the greatest predictors of disability from low back pain are psychosocial rather than pathophysiologic in nature.

A treating physician has a number of options in disability evaluation. In the private setting, the physician can simply refuse to perform the evaluation and under these circumstances force the administration body into an independent medical examination. This may, however, bring down the wrath of the patient who feels abandoned in the administrative part of medical care. Alternatively, in a managed care or group practice, another physician in the same group or an administrator can be designated to fill out the paperwork based on the patient's chart and further evaluation. The majority of doctors, however, find that they cannot escape the paperwork associated with disability evaluation.

MEDICAL OPINIONS REQUIRED DURING DISABILITY EVALUATION

The physician faced with a demand for a disability evaluation has to reach a number of conclusions and provide opinions on the topics explained on the next few pages. Not all disability schemes require that the physician address each issue. Furthermore, specific requirements or definitions inherent in the administrative procedure of a specific disability system might not be included in this outline.

Date of Permanent and Stationary Status

Regardless of whether one is a treating physician or an assessing physician, the point of maximum medical benefit or permanent and stationary status must be determined. This is the point where administrative rules concerning disability begin to take effect. It is virtually impossible for a permanent disability evaluation to be made before declaration of the point of maximum medical benefit.

The concept of maximum medical benefit, however, is not nearly as easy as it appears at first glance. Many diseases and injuries heal completely and leave the patient free of any disability. Under these circumstances, the point of maximum medical benefit can be determined without difficulty. In other conditions, a well-defined end point for recovery can be documented. For example, in the case of loss of a limb or an eye or even the healing of a fracture with residual deformity and limitation, it becomes evident at a specific point of time that further treatment will not be of any benefit and that the patient is unlikely to change in the future. Most legislation for disability and most contracts concerning disability have been established with the assumption that all diseases and injuries will eventually reach this point.

Certain injuries and illnesses, however, do not fall neatly into this administrative niche. Many degenerative or cancerous diseases progressively get worse and even become terminal over a number of years. At no point is this type of disease process stationary. On the other hand, diseases and illnesses such as multiple sclerosis have no known long-term treatment. Therefore it is possible to say that this person has reached a point of maximum medical benefit immediately following the diagnosis because future medical treatment may have an impact on progression of the disease process. In other individuals, an injury or illness may gradually heal over a number of months or years irrespective of the nature and extent of medical treatment. Such self-limiting disorders can again be said to have reached the point of maximum medical benefit early in the process but are neither permanent nor stationary in the classic sense of these words. Still other disorders become chronic, with periods of exacerbation and remission, and require continuous or intermittent treatment or monitoring of the patient. In these situations, medical care may be necessary for the rest of the patient's life and the disease may never reach a level of maximum medical benefit even though the patient's status may be both permanent and stationary.

Although no universal rule covers this point in time, it is reasonable to assume that the time of maximum medical benefit or permanent and stationary status is the point where the patient has shown no significant change in disability status for a number of weeks and it is unlikely that additional medical treatment in the future will cause improvement in medical status or level of disability.

Residual Subjective Complaints

Once it is determined that the patient has reached permanent and stationary status, most agencies request a statement regarding ongoing patient symptoms. The discussion of subjective complaints includes a list of the specific body parts or functions that are affected and the manner in which they affect the patient's functional ability. This can usually be obtained by simply asking the patient to list all symptoms and discuss how these symptoms affect specific daily functions or abilities. It is useful to note how patients perceive not only their disability but what their actual abilities are for specific functions.

Certain agencies such as the state of California worker's compensation system also demand some form of rating or judgmental statement on the part of the physician as to the severity and frequency of the subjective complaints. Such terms as 25% of the day, 50% of the day, 75% of the day, and 100% of the day may be categorized as occasional, intermittent, frequent, or constant. Similarly, subjective complaints may have to be rated as minimal, slight, moderate, or severe, depending on their own specific functions. In this setting, it may be necessary to subjectively state whether the patient is precluded from certain activities because of the nature and severity of the symptoms.

Residual Objective Findings

Inevitably, the physician is asked to list the abnormal physical findings noted on clinical examination as well as any and all abnormal laboratory findings. In certain disability evaluation systems such as Social Security, a simple listing of the objective findings is all that is necessary. In other systems, such as the American Medical Association (AMA) guidelines, it becomes necessary to not only list the objective findings but also classify their severity as degrees of loss of range of motion and degrees of loss of sensation, strength, or coordination.

Another decision that is often required in this setting is a statement as to whether the subjective complaints are consistent with and confirmed by the objective findings. Signs of nonorganic clinical patterns such as those developed by Waddell et al[21] for low back pain may be requested by name or by insinuation.

Diagnosis

Many disability evaluation systems begin with the diagnosis. The degree of disability is dependent on the diagnosis. The AMA guidelines, for example, give a specific impairment rating for specific diagnoses such as spondylolisthesis and disk herniation. The diagnosis usually does not define disability in the clinical setting. However, the diagnosis should be compatible with both the subjective complaints and the objective findings as noted from the clinical examination.

Work and Activity Restrictions

Perhaps the greatest amount of guesswork expected of the physician is the determination of work restriction.[7,8] This decision may also have the greatest impact on the patient. Work and activity restrictions not only focus on the patient's current occupation but, in many cases, have an impact on potential future employment or activities as well. Many disability insurance policies deal solely with the ability of individuals to do their usual and customary occupation. On the other hand, others require an assessment of the individual's ability to do any occupation. Detailed charts of restrictions based on the ability to lift, push, pull, climb, bend, stoop, crawl, and kneel and other similar activities are commonplace in disability evaluations.

One difficulty in this setting is to differentiate what a normal healthy person of similar age, sex, education, and body build would be capable of doing. This can often be inferred by National Institute for Occupational Safety and Health (NIOSH) or other standards.[18] It then becomes necessary to determine how a particular individual being evaluated differs from normal and how this affects the ability to do specific work. Nowhere in medical training or even in specialty training does this approach a science.

Work and Activity Ability

In the past, work ability has not been a major issue except when an insurance carrier asks for a list of what an individual is capable of doing to determine the restrictions to any reasonable occupation.

With the increasing interest in vocational rehabilitation following work-related injuries, it has now become important for a physician to determine whether a proposed occupation falls within the individual's work capacity. This must be considered an estimation on the part of the physician and tends to fall within the perceived or anticipated normal estimates that other physicians with similar training are likely to establish for an individual with a similar clinical picture. The utilization of strength testing equipment may be of value,[22] but as yet, no standardized manner for documenting disability has been associated with strength measurements.

This issue has gained even more importance with passage of the ADA in 1992. The emphasis and pressures on physicians doing an evaluation under this act may be the exact opposite of those that exist when they are asked to determine work restriction. It is not uncommon for an individual to claim to be able to do a particular occupation that other individuals seeking disability and having the same complaints would swear they were incapable of doing. This act is further complicated by the requirement that an employer make "reasonable accommodations" for qualified individuals with a disability. Often the physician is asked to decide what accommodations would be necessary for the individual to perform the essential functions of the job. The Equal Employment Opportunity Commission defines essential functions as "the fundamental job duties of the employment position." The ADA is discussed in greater detail in Chapters 51 and 52.

Ability to Perform the Usual and Customary Occupation

The physician is commonly asked to answer whether an individual can perform the usual and customary occupation with an absolute yes or no statement. This is usually based on a very superficial job review, job analysis, or a description by the patient as to what the required activities might be. The pressures here can be in opposite directions in different patients. Some patients seeking disability or retraining may swear that they cannot perform the activity, with very little or no objective basis for such a statement. On the other hand, other individuals who are scared of losing their job may swear that they are able to do all the activities of their normal occupation in the presence of extensive symptomatology, pathology, and obvious disability.

What is particularly distressing to a physician in this setting is that the checking of a single box on a form can have the result of causing individuals to lose their job, be disqualified from retraining to another occupation, or be denied Social Security or other benefits upon which they are dependent for daily survival.

Ability to Participate in Vocational Rehabilitation

Whether the worker can participate in vocational rehabilitation is often answered in the form of a check in a yes/no box and based on very minimal information. Sometimes it requires a simple statement that the patient cannot and is unlikely to do the usual and customary occupation in the future but, at a particular point in time, can begin to participate in retraining or the assessment of a potential future occupation. If the administrative system has trained vocational rehabilitation assessment personnel, the physician simply has to make a statement that it is safe to consider the vocational assessment process. It is only after patients have decided for which occupation they wish to retrain that the physician may have to make a final decision as to whether they can perform the duties of that particular occupation.

Causation

The issue of causation for a specific injury or illness can be the area of greatest legal dispute. It is in this setting where significant variation in medical opinion often occurs and where the physician is most likely to be subjected to cross-examination. The issue of fault can be of great financial consequence to the insurance carrier, agency, or individual who is perceived as causing the disability.

One reason for conflicting medical opinion is the legal concept of reasonable medical probability. In a court of law, a physician only has to determine that it is more probable than not that a disability is associated with a particular exposure or incident. This suggests a 51% chance that a direct cause of the disability can be identified.

The causation concept becomes even more complex when the compensation system has specific rules and regulations outlined. For example, the California Labor Code excludes from compensation those injuries caused by the employee's use of alcohol or illegal controlled substances, intentional self-inflicted injuries, suicide, or injuries resulting from an altercation in which the injured employee was the initial physical aggressor. On the other hand, the California legislature has defined certain conditions such as hernia, pneumoconiosis or tuberculosis, heart disease, and cancer as being work-related injuries when they affect firefighters, forestry officers, peace officers, and correctional employees. The law presumes that any disability associated with these complaints in this group of workers is due to their employment. It requires considerable evidence to the contrary to rebut this presumption.

Apportionment

Once a conclusion has been reached as to the cause or causes of disability in a particular patient, the physician is commonly asked to render an opinion as to whether all disability is due to a single injury or illness or whether multiple contributing factors are responsible for the level of disability. It is difficult in this situation to correlate medical opinion on the etiology of a disease process and the legal concept of causation and apportionment. Many disorders occur in the normal population for which no cause is known. Degenerative conditions of the musculoskeletal system occur in virtually the entire population as part of the aging process. In a certain percentage of these individuals, one could anticipate the development of symptoms and/or disability at some time in their future. If, however, the same individual has one or more injuries, it may become necessary to differentiate the level of disability that was likely to have occurred in the absence of the injury from that brought about by the injury itself. In other situations, the patient may have a preexisting level of disability that is simply increased by a specific injury and the level of increased disability has to be determined. In a third scenario, a patient may have been subjected to multiple injuries over a period of time and the physician is asked to apportion a level of disability to each of the multiple injuries.

A number of ways can be used to state apportionment. The arbitrary designation of a percentage of disability to each of a number of factors is clearly based on opinion and determined by the biases of the assessing physician. Another approach is to determine the ability of the patient to perform specific tasks at the time just before the injury in question and then attempt to subtract that level of disability from the total disability the patient is experiencing after an injury at the time of maximum medical benefit.

Ongoing and Future Medical Care Requirements

Insurance carriers are often required to keep reserves to pay for future medical treatment of individuals who have been injured. In personal injury litigation, argument is commonly made that the patient should be reimbursed for potential future medical costs that may be incurred as a result of a prior injury or disability. This poses its own unique difficulty to the assessing physician.

If the patient does not require surgical intervention at a particular time, for example, for a disk herniation or degenerative joint disease, it is always possible that surgery might be required in the future. It is, however, impossible to predict with any degree of security and particularly within "reasonable medical probability," which suggests a 51% level of security, that a patient will require surgery in the future. On the other hand, if one does not raise that issue and the patient does require surgery sometime in the future, the benefits may not be available.

The second question regarding future medical treatment that has not been resolved in most medical settings is that of palliative care. The use of treatment modalities that give some degree of relief of symptoms or simply support the patient through periods of exacerbation are extremely subjective. For example, no research has shown that physical modalities in a therapist's office result in any long-term or ongoing benefit to the patient. Nonetheless, many patients believe they do get some relief of symptoms for hours or days. Similar statements are commonly made regarding a variety of medications and even spinal manipulation. The question is raised whether some relief of symptoms and attempts to make the patient more comfortable reasonably justify the often high costs associated with such treatment.

It is probably more honest for a physician to state that a treatment is unlikely to give more than subjective temporary relief rather than state that the treatment is not medically necessary.

PRINCIPLES OF DISABILITY DETERMINATION

In an attempt to be fair and honest in the allocation of disability benefits, a number of medical organizations and governmental agencies have developed very specific disability or impairment rating systems. Each of these systems has been the subject of extensive debate and discussion, and clearly none have reached the goals of being truly objective and fair. Nonetheless, certain principles have developed.

Pathology

The physician is perhaps more competent in diagnosing pathology than in any other activity associated with disability determination. The diagnosis has therefore become inherent in the determination of disability. For example, the diagnosis of disk herniation or spondylolisthesis is considered important under AMA guidelines and must be listed if present.[2] In a similar vein, California guidelines have specific disability ratings for disorders such as posttraumatic head syndrome, which is considered a clinical diagnosis. The earlier method of evaluating permanent impairment put out by the American Academy of Orthopaedic Surgeons[1] relied heavily on diagnosis as the basis for determining disability.

Unfortunately, the relationship of disability to pathology is not as clear-cut as it would seem.[12] The documentation of extensive degenerative changes—such as stenosis and disk herniation in the back and neck in a large portion of the population who do not appear to be disabled—has raised serious doubt as to the value of a pathologic diagnosis as a guiding principle of disability determination. At the same time, large numbers of patients claim disability where no pathologic process can be documented on testing and examination.

Despite these difficulties, the presence or absence of pathology and the nature of the diagnosis are, in many instances, the only part of the evaluation in which evaluating physicians strongly agree.[1,5] This may be the reason why it is so attractive to administrative authorities. In Washington State, the worker's compensation system differentiates levels of disability in patients with back pain based on the clinical pattern associated with a disk herniation, for example, whether neurological deficit or symptoms in the lower extremities are present.

Range of Motion

One of the easiest measurements to make, especially in the extremities, is the range of motion of a particular joint. Most extremity joints have a well-defined normal range, and the use of goniometers permits an accurate measure of any loss of motion in a joint. The AMA guidelines have given specific impairment values to loss of range of motion of varying degrees for most joints.[2]

This has in fact become the mainstay for the AMA guidelines in the assessment of peripheral joint function.

Intraobserver reliability is reasonably good in the measurement of spinal range-of-motion measurements, particularly with the advent of the dual goniometer system.[14,15] One difficulty with spinal range-of-motion measurements, however, is that they require cooperation on the part of the patient to make an accurate measurement. A second problem is the lack of strong correlation between spinal range of motion and work capacity.

Neurological Loss of Function

In terms of the musculoskeletal system, neurological loss of function or impairment is usually based on an assessment of sensation, strength, and coordination. Although many purely neurological diseases and disorders exist, many musculoskeletal conditions directly affect neurologic function. This includes such disorders as spinal injuries with radiculopathy, myelopathy, or cauda equina syndrome, as well as peripheral entrapment neuropathies such as carpal tunnel syndrome and tarsal tunnel syndrome.

SENSATION

The most subjective of the neurological impairments following musculoskeletal injuries is a change in basic sensory function. This may include areas of anesthesia, dysesthesia, paresthesia, or hyperesthesia. It can also be described as a cold intolerance or as being associated with pain. In these settings, the physician is often asked to determine whether the area of sensory change is consistent with a specific nerve injury or dermatome or with a fairly nonspecific paresthesia or pain symptom. The anatomical distribution of the sensory change therefore becomes important.

A second component of the sensory change is whether it affects specific functions. The loss of fine-touch sensation in the hand following carpal tunnel syndrome may lead to an inability to use the hand for certain fine-motor activities. A similar loss of sensation in the foot, however, may result in no disability. In the case of causalgia or reflex sympathetic dystrophy, the pain and dysesthesia may be so severe as to critically limit the function of an extremity.

Sensory nerve conduction may be important in documenting the existence of a peripheral or entrapment neuropathy and confirming the presence of a subjective symptom. Although sensory nerve conduction can be described as normal, slightly abnormal, moderately abnormal, and severely abnormal or unobtainable, the exact correlation between the degree of abnormality and sensory changes has not been adequately documented. Somatosensory evoked responses may also document the presence of a lesion, particularly in the spinal cord. The localization of lesions, however, is not very accurate, and it is not possible at this point to extrapolate a level of impairment from the degree of abnormality in the somatosensory evoked responses.

MOTOR FUNCTION

The loss of motor function, particularly when associated with atrophy, is perhaps the most objective of the neurological findings that relate to disability. Partial or total loss of muscle function or strength can seriously affect the ability of an individual to perform specific tasks. In this setting, the physician is asked to document the nature and extent of the motor loss, as well as whether the distribution of motor loss fits with the documented diagnosis.

In the documentation of motor neurological deficits it may be necessary to perform electrodiagnostic studies. The diagnosis of many entrapment neuropathies may be fairly evident on clinical examination in certain patients. In other patients, however, the use of nerve conduction studies or needle electromyography may be necessary to confirm a diagnosis of carpal tunnel syndrome, tarsal tunnel syndrome, or even radiculopathy. Although electrodiagnostic testing can confirm the presence of a neurologic deficit, most tests have fairly poor sensitivity for the degree of loss. The AMA guidelines, however, require that motor loss be quantified. This has led to fairly crude quantitative descriptions from needle electromyography and motor nerve conduction studies as mild, moderate, or severe. The degree of severity, however, does not readily transfer to degree of weakness. It is still primarily the clinical examination that determines the degree and extent of weakness.

COORDINATION

Loss of coordination of the hand and/or lower extremities, particularly in such disorders as spinal cord injuries, must be differentiated from similar loss of function resulting from central nervous system disorders or even the loss of coordination resulting from a severe peripheral neuropathy or joint deformity. The ability to balance, move rapidly, and do fine coordinated movements with the hands or feet can seriously affect or have an impact on the ability of the individual to do certain activities.

Assessment of coordination is to a large extent dependent on the diagnosis. It is necessary to investigate vestibular, hearing, vision, and proprioceptive function, as well as the presence of peripheral neuropathies and myelopathies. In musculoskeletal disorders, the primary cause of incoordination, however, is loss of motor function or sensory function in an extremity as a result of bony deformity.

REFLEX FUNCTIONS

The loss of reflexes by themselves do not directly transmit into disability. The measurement of reflexes, however, is important in the confirmation of subjective complaints and in the determination of a diagnosis.

Electrodiagnostic studies may be important in determining the presence or absence of a reflex abnormality. This is particularly true in S1 radiculopathy in the lower extremities, which can be directly measured by means of the H-reflex. These tests, however, should not be used as a basis for impairment or disability but rather as confirmation of the diagnosis.

Pain and Other Subjective Complaints

The issue of impairment or disability secondary to pain and other subjective complaints can be considered the most controversial aspect of the disability evaluation.[16] Pain and many paresthesias cannot be readily measured either on the clinical examination or by specific tests. Pain is also influenced to a great extent by cultural and psychosocial factors. A recent paper by Jensen et al[13] showed a significant relationship between disability and patients' beliefs about their pain. If a patient believes that activity associated with increased pain should be avoided, the degree of perceived disability is likely to be much larger. The issue is so controversial that earlier editions of the AMA *Guidelines to the Evaluation of Permanent Impairment* gave virtually no impairment rating to pain in the absence of objective findings. Social Security similarly will not accept subjective symptoms that are not confirmed by clinical or laboratory findings.[6,19]

Despite the intense medical and administrative debate as to whether pain represents a disability or impairment, it remains the primary concern of many patients and a justification on their part for perceived disability. The fourth edition of the AMA guidelines has dedicated an entire chapter to the concept of impairment secondary to pain. Although these guides recommend that pain be rated as minimal, slight, moderate, and marked, as well as intermittent, occasional, frequent, and constant, they take care to not designate a specific percent impairment of the whole person as a result of pain and instead recommend that these descriptive terms be used.

California, on the other hand, has a long history of rating disability based solely on subjective complaints. To some extent, the AMA guidelines have followed the concepts drawn up by the California system. Under this system, minimal pain is annoying and slight pain is tolerable but does have an impact on certain specific activities. Moderate pain causes an extensive or marked decrease in an individual's ability to carry out specific tasks, and severe or marked pain precludes a specific activity. The terms occasional, intermittent, frequent, and constant have been given different values in the AMA and the California guidelines, but they have the net effect of dividing the amount of time in each day that individuals experience pain into 25%, 50%, 75%, or 100% quadrants.

Measurement of pain has been the subject of a significant amount of research, and a number of tools have been developed to give a clinician or researcher some means of comparing pain patterns between individuals. The Visual Analog Scale is the most common and the easiest to use of the tools that are available. This rating of pain in a scale by a patient varies from minimal or no pain to the most severe or incapacitating pain the patient has experienced. The disadvantage is its

assumption that pain is a unidimensional experience, and the assessment of pain is dependent on the patient's prior pain experience as a comparison. The McGill Pain Questionnaire presents another attempt at evaluation of the nature of a pain by dividing it into words that describe the qualities of the experience, that is, in terms of temporal, spatial, pressure, thermal, and other properties, and by describing the effect of pain in terms of the tension, fear, and autonomic changes with which it may be associated. It has been shown to be valid and reliable but has not developed into a tool that is widely used in disability evaluation.

ADMINISTRATIVE CONSIDERATIONS

The final decision whether an individual is eligible for benefits under a disability system is in all cases either legal or administrative in nature. Physicians performing disability evaluation must realize that they are simply providing information and an opinion on which administrative or legal decisions can be made. It is not unusual for a physician's perception of the amount of disability being offered to translate into either considerably more or less disability at the administrative level.

Each piece of legislation concerning disability and every administrative policy or contract has built into it very complex methods of taking a physician's medical report and translating that information into specific numbers that are used to distribute benefits. For example, the Social Security system and many disability policies are all-or-none decisions. An individual is either declared disabled or declared capable of returning back to the workplace. The AMA guidelines, on the other hand, ask for a specific percent impairment of the whole worker, and the physician is asked to derive these percentages by complex tables and measurements. The California worker's compensation system requires the physician to estimate the activities that an injured worker can or cannot perform, and this is transferred into a percentage of the workforce from which the patient is excluded.

This obvious difference between the physician's determination of disability and the final disability rating that the patient ultimately receives has led a number of individuals to differentiate impairment from disability. Under this concept, impairment is determined by a physician and disability by the legal or administrative system. The differentiation, however, is somewhat blurred, and physicians should be aware of the mechanisms by which their opinions will transfer into the disability rating.

Many administrative systems take into account the age and sex of injured workers, as well as their prior occupation, education, training, experience, and the availability of work that these individuals are capable of performing in the community. Many of these administrative decisions are made by professional government-appointed raters or claims adjusters hired by insurance carriers. Still other decisions are taken to either a worker's compensation court or an appeals court before a judge or administrative official. Inevitably, a further appeals process is available through superior court, particularly if it is claimed that certain jurisdictions are biased on the basis of race, sex, ethnic origin, or even sexual orientation. An appeal to the Superior Court can be made when a disability claim is perceived as being denied in an inconsistent or willful manner. The physician is simply the first step in the determination of disability benefits.

CONCLUSION

When physicians are asked to determine impairment or disability in a formal assessment, they must recognize that disability is in essence a social benefit or a private contract and that the final decision is being made by an administrative authority. The determination of eligibility for disability benefits is, however, based on the accuracy and consistency of the medical opinion. Inconsistent medical reporting, given the same facts, has been demonstrated within the California system and has resulted in marked discrepancies between the levels of disability given to individuals with similar injuries and physical findings. This has led to a perception of abuse and unfairness in the system, which in turn has led to multiple revisions of the Worker's Compensation Act.

The more objective the medical findings and the more consistent the medical opinion, the easier it is for an administrative system to provide a fair and equitable distribution of disability benefits. It must be recognized, however, that perceived abilities and disabilities of the injured person may not relate very well to objective medical observations and that medical opinion of the impact of subjective pain and other complaints may be no better than the opinion of other members of society.

In the final analysis, a physician who elects to give a disability evaluation must perform a complete and comprehensive examination, accurately describe the physical findings, and then express opinions in an objective and consistent manner. All efforts must be made to avoid undue influence on the medical opinion by outside sources, including the patient, attorneys, and administrative agencies. It is only through this objective medical analysis that the final distribution of disability benefits can be made in compliance with the appropriate law or contract.

References

1. American Academy of Orthopaedic Surgeons: *Manual for orthopedic surgeons in evaluating permanent impairment,* Chicago, 1966, The Academy.

2. American Medical Association: *Guides to the evaluation of permanent impairment,* ed 4, Chicago, 1993, The Association.

3. Bigos SJ, Battié MC, Spengler DM, et al.: A longitudinal study of work perceptions and psychosocial factors affecting the report of back injury, *Spine* 16:1-6, 1991.

4. Bigos SJ, Spengler DM, Martin NA, et al.: Back injuries in industry: a retrospective study. III. Employee-related factors, *Spine* 11:252-256, 1986.

5. Brand RA, Lehmann TR: Low-back impairment rating practices of orthopedic surgeons, *Spine* 8:75-78, 1983.

6. Carey TS, Hadler NM, Gillings D, et al.: Medical disability assessment of the back pain patient for the Social Security Administration: the weighting of presenting clinical features, *J Clin Epidemiol* 41:691-697, 1988.

7. Clark W, Haldeman S: The development of guideline factors for the evaluation of disability in neck and back injuries, *Spine* 18(13):1736-1745, 1993.

8. Clark WL, Haldeman S, Johnson P, et al: Back impairment and disability determination. Another attempt at objective, reliable rating, *Spine* 13:332-341, 1988.

9. Deyo RA, Diehl AK: Psychosocial predictors of disability in patients with low back pain, *J Rheumatol* 15:1557-1564, 1988.

10. Hadler NM: Backache and humanism. In Frymoyer J, editor: *The adult spine: principles and practice,* New York, 1991, Raven Press.

11. Hadler NM: Insurance against work incapacity from spinal disorders. In Frymoyer J, editor: *The adult spine: principles and practice,* New York, 1991, Raven Press.

12. Haldeman S, Shouka M, Robboy S: Computed tomography, electrodiagnostic and clinical findings in chronic workers' compensation patients with back and leg pain, *Spine* 13:345-350, 1988.

13. Jensen MP, Turner JA, Romano JM, Lawler BK: Relationship of pain-specific beliefs to chronic pain adjustment, *Pain* 57:301-309, 1994.

14. Keeley J, et al.: Quantification of lumbar function. Part 5: Reliability of range of motion measures in the sagittal plane and an in vivo torso rotation measurement technique, *Spine* 11:31-35, 1986.

15. Mayer TG, Tencer AF, Kristoferson S, et al.: Use of noninvasive techniques for quantification of spinal range of motion in normal subjects and chronic low back dysfunction patients, *Spine* 9:588-595, 1984.

16. Melzack R, Katz J: Pain measurement in persons with pain. In Wall PD, Melzack R, editors: *Textbook of pain,* ed 3, New York, 1994, Churchill Livingstone International.

17. Minnesota Medical Association: *Worker's compensation permanent partial disability schedule,* Minneapolis, 1984, The Association.

18. National Institute for Occupational Safety and Health: *A work practice guide for manual lifting,* Report 81-122, Cincinnati, 1981, US Department of Health and Human Services.

19. Social Security Administration: *Disability evaluation under Social Security: a handbook for physicians,* HEW Pub (SSA) 79-10089, Washington, DC, 1975, The Administration.

20. Waddell G, Main CJ, Morris EW, et al: Chronic low back pain, psychological distress and illness behaviour, *Spine* 9:209-213, 1984.

21. Waddell G, McCulloch JA, Kummel E, Venner RM: Nonorganic physical signs in low back pain, *Spine* 5:117-125.

22. Waikar AM, Schlegal RE, Lee KS: Strength tests for evaluation of low back injuries, *Trends Ergonom Hum Factors* 9:667-674, 1986.

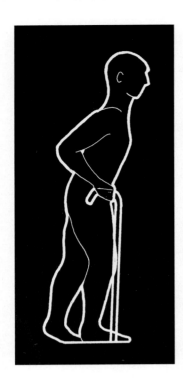

Chapter 51

The Americans with Disabilities Act

Dawn Leger
John D. Kemp

CONTENTS

In 1990, the Americans with Disabilities Act (ADA) was signed into law (PL 101-336). What is considered the most sweeping employment legislation since the 1960s went into effect in 1992. Based on years of local, state, and federal actions promoting education, vocational rehabilitation, and public access for people with disabilities, the ADA covers employment as well as access to public services and accommodations.

An estimated 49 million children and adults have disabilities in the United States, and by the year 2000, 20% of the U.S. population will have a disability.[5] The unemployment rate for disabled adults is 67%, and those who are employed are underpaid and underused. Congress found that individuals with disabilities have been discriminated against in a systematic manner, and this unfair discrimination restricts equal opportunity to participate and compete in society on an equal basis and costs the American taxpayer literally billions in necessary disability dependency payments.[7] The ADA will prohibit the exclusion of qualified disabled Americans from jobs and public services and will enforce laws against discrimination in the workplace. The removal of discriminatory practices from the workplace will reduce dependency and nonproductivity and encourage every American to pursue opportunities for education, employment, and participation in every aspect of modern life.

The highlights of the ADA and a discussion of its implications for employers is presented in this chapter. Additionally, we look at the role of the healthcare provider in interpreting the regulations for occupational health and safety. The law itself is being refined and clarified as various courts respond to challenges and litigation. Early indications are that the law has actually increased the productivity of business and saved money in retraining, insurance claims, and worker's compensation.[6]

DEFINITIONS

The ADA is geared to protect all "qualified individuals" from discrimination in employment at jobs that they can perform safely and in which they can benefit from "reasonable accommodation" when necessary. A qualified individual with a disability is anyone with a disability who has the skill, experience, education, and/or other job-related requirements for a particular position with or without reasonable accommodation. A "disability" is defined by the ADA as a physical or mental impairment that substantially limits one or more of the major life activities of an individual, or a record of same (ADA, Section 3). "Reasonable accommodation" may include making existing facilities readily

accessible to and usable by individuals with disabilities or restructuring the job, which might include modification of equipment, tools, or the work space. Employers may reasonably be expected to adjust work schedules, provide interpreters or modified training materials, or reassign workers to vacant positions for which they are equally qualified and compensated.

The ADA requires a good-faith effort on the part of employers to make reasonable accommodations, but because each job and each individual case are different, no blanket requirements of employers have been formulated. Employers do not have to make reasonable accommodations that would prove to be an "undue hardship" for the employer because of the cost, size, or disruption of the change or if it would affect operation of the business. This may become an issue in a small business. In these cases, other accommodations should be sought, as well as advice and assistance from employment specialists and vocational rehabilitation agencies, and possibly, employers may decide that they cannot hire such an individual with a disability. Funds to offset the cost may be obtained from government or private agencies, or the employee may desire to contribute to the modification in some way.

Employees with disabilities are the best resource for developing creative solutions to job modification. Other agencies may be able to assist employers in designing reasonable accommodations, and a growing market of assistive technology can be purchased or imitated for tool modification or accessibility. Ergonomists or human factors engineers are trained to design workplaces that fit the worker, regardless of ability or disability. Occupational therapists and vocational counselors are trained to assist individuals in their activities of daily life, including transportation, personal grooming, and purposeful work.

EMPLOYERS AND THE LAW

The equal opportunity and ADA regulations greatly restrict the type of information that employers can request from a job applicant. All the information collected during the application and interview process must be job related, that is, training, experience, and ability to perform job-related duties. A rebuttable presumption exists that a job description accurately reflects the real duties of a job. Employers cannot ask job applicants about the existence or nature of a disability. Employers must base hiring decisions on whether the individual is capable of performing the essential functions of the job, with or without reasonable accommodation. The employer cannot ask about a disability, but can ask whether applicants can perform the particular, essential job functions and may ask applicants to demonstrate how they would carry out the tasks as enumerated in a written job description. Employers have the obligation to inform all applicants and employees of the intention to provide reasonable accommodation for individuals with disabilities in both the application and employment stages.

Job Descriptions

Job descriptions, although always important, take on added significance under the new legislation. Interviewing and hiring for vacant positions must be based on written job descriptions that have been prepared in advance of advertisement and that categorically state the "essential job functions" for the position.[1] Traditional job descriptions are now inadequate for determining the physical and mental demands of a particular job and for finding the best person to fill the position according to these demands. Simply stating tasks—load boxes, transcribe tapes, assemble components—does not break down the physical demands of each task sufficiently. Employers need to know the exact weight, mass, and frequency of the boxes that need to be moved, the level of difficulty to hear tapes and transcribe the information quickly into a word processing system, and the dexterity required to assemble the specific components of the job.

Medical Screening

Employers may use medical screening of applicants for vacant positions only if it is job related and universally administered. An employer must ask every applicant—not only individuals with a disability—to undergo the same physical examination, and that examination must relate to the particular tasks in the job description. The employer should consider the physical requirements of the job and any public safety or environmental hazards associated with the work. Employers may deny employment to an applicant if the safety and health of the other workers might be affected by the presence of an individual with a disability, or denial may be based on other factors not related to the disability.

Job analysis systems have been developed over the past decade to assist employers in measuring the physical demands of particular jobs and the physical abilities of applicants or employees needed to carry out the job. These systems should objectively measure the physical requirements of each separate task component of a job, including cardiovascular, muscular, motor, vision, and hearing. They should also look at the conditions of the working environment, including noise, temperature, vibration, stress, and other environmental hazards that may be present.[4] These components are then linked to the medical screening to produce reliable tests to identify those applicants with the ability to perform the job with the least likelihood of causing injury to themselves or others.

Under the ADA, a determination of physical and mental requirements for each job is important and must be assessed on an individual basis and in an impartial and valid manner. Employers may seek professional assistance from ergonomists or physical/occupational therapists, special training for health and safety personnel, and new guidelines for occupational medical staff. These job analyses will also promote greater awareness of poor ergonomic design of jobs, work spaces, or tools. Ideally, this might lead to job redesign and a consequent reduction in work-related injury and disability claims, as well as a more productive work environment in compliance with the ADA and other job-related legislation.

Reasonable Accommodations

Of particular importance under the ADA is the distinction between essential and marginal job functions. Employees must be able to perform essential job functions with reasonable accommodations that employers are required to make, and marginal job functions are those that can be reassigned or modified.

When a worker already on the job is injured and disabled, these job descriptions will help the employer work with the disabled individual to assess the worker's ability to continue in the current position and to develop reasonable accommodations to facilitate that occurrence. Employers have a great deal to gain by retaining already trained individuals who become disabled, and society benefits from their continued employment. Reasonable accommodations are important techniques to adapt the workplace to the "new" capabilities of the employee.

Each case is different and must be evaluated individually by taking into consideration the specific abilities and functional limitations of a particular applicant or employee with a disability *and* the specific functional requirements of a particular job. Reasonable accommodations may include the following:

- Making facilities readily accessible and usable by an individual with a disability
- Restructuring a job by reallocating or redistributing marginal job functions (taking care to not cause an undue burden or hardship on other employees, which could in turn lead to resentment and a hostile working environment)
- Altering when or how an essential job function is performed
- Implementing part-time or modified work schedules
- Obtaining or modifying equipment or devices
- Modifying examinations, training materials, or policies
- Providing qualified readers and interpreters
- Reassigning the individual to a vacant position
- Permitting use of accrued paid leave or unpaid leave for necessary treatment
- Providing reserved parking for a person with a mobility impairment
- Allowing an employee to provide equipment or devices that an employer is not required to provide.[2]

Employers must make a good faith effort to make reasonable accommodations. If an employee poses a significant risk to the health and safety of others, the employer has a right to fire or refuse to hire that individual. Under this condition, employees with contagious diseases or infections that imperil the health or safety of their co-workers or the public may be dismissed. Employer rules such as prohibiting alcohol or illegal drugs in the workplace remain valid, and employers are required to conform to the Drug-Free Workplace Act. Rehabilitated drug users or alcoholics cannot be excluded from the workplace, and employers must demonstrate current drug or alcohol use before dismissal of an employee.

HEALTHCARE PROVIDERS AND THE LAW

Occupational medical staff, including physicians, nurses, and nurse practitioners, may participate in the evaluation of applicants and employees for placement in particular jobs. Medical screening guidelines are developed to provide physicians with information to make appropriate recommendations about the physical ability of the employee to perform the particular tasks outlined in the job description. Medical assessment may include testing of strength, manual dexterity, and lifting, as well as evaluation of visual, hearing, and other motor skills, based on the essential requirements of the job.

Under the ADA, an individual with a disability is a person who has a physical or mental impairment that substantially limits one or more major life activities, has a record of such an impairment, or is regarded as having such an impairment.[2] Occupational medical personnel are not involved in the determination of disability but, instead, the ability of the employee to carry out the essential functions of the job. If the employers choose to use a medical examination, it can only be given after a job offer has been made, it must be job related and necessary to the business, and all employees in the same job classification must undergo the same evaluation without discrimination, except when there is evidence of a job performance or safety problem. The scope of these examinations need not be identical, however, and a physician may conduct a more extensive examination if evidence of a physical or mental limitation that relates to the performance of the job is found. For example, all potential employees in a job category must be given a blood test, but if a person's initial test indicates a problem that may affect job performance, further tests may be given to that person only, in order to get necessary information.[2]

Under the ADA, a post-offer medical examination may be conducted to determine if an individual currently has the physical or mental qualifications necessary to perform the specific job and to determine that the person can perform the job without posing a direct threat to the health and safety of self or others.[2] Medical examinations may be conducted to ensure compliance with other federal safety laws, such as those for interstate truck drivers or pilots. The post-offer examination can include more than the ability to perform job functions, but any withdrawal of a job offer must be shown to be due to a health or safety issue or because no reasonable accommodation was available to enable the individual to perform the essential job functions. Job offers may not be withdrawn because of a perceived risk of injury to self or others, such as denial of employment because of the discovery of an asymptomatic curvature of the spine. If the medical examination reveals that the individual has had serious and multiple back injuries while performing similar work, it is reasonable to withdraw the job offer based on the significant risk that the individual would be further injured in the course of the job.[2]

The medical examination cannot be used to exclude individuals from jobs based on the speculation that they might incur injuries to themselves in the future, unless it is medically documented that the individual would pose a significant risk of substantial harm to self or others in the course of the job. If previous injury from similar tasks has been documented, and no reasonable accommodation can be made to reduce the risk of reinjury—such as the use of mechanical devices or restructuring of the job—the employer can withdraw the job offer. The physician is not responsible for making these decisions, however, and can only provide the best evaluation of the functional abilities of the individual in relation to the job functions and the health and safety requirements of the workplace. Although the physician may be provided with much specific detail about the job, the medical recommendations should focus on two concerns: whether the person is currently able to perform the specific job, with or without reasonable accommodation, and whether the person can perform the job without posing a direct threat to the health or safety of self or others.[2] Even though the physician may visit the job site and suggest specific reasonable accommodations, it is the responsibility of the employer to make the final decision based on the best available objective evidence. This may include consultations with health and safety personnel, as well as outside consultants such as rehabilitation counselors or therapists and organizations serving people with disabilities.

CONCLUSION

It is the responsibility of the employer to offer opportunities to all individuals, including individuals with disabilities, in a nondiscriminatory manner and to make reasonable accommodations to the known limitations of workers with disabilities that will allow them to perform their jobs without risk of injury to themselves or their co-workers. Medical and safety expertise facilitated by the presence of detailed job analyses and written job descriptions, can assist in the optimal, ergonomic placement of individuals in the workplace. Although the ADA does not require employers to undertake formal job analyses, the information collected is usually helpful to employers in identifying essential job functions and hiring individuals best qualified to carry out the job. Some job analyses are useful for setting wage rates and others may not link the essential job tasks to the specific tasks and functions that constitute a job. People with disabilities are often able to perform tasks by using other, often unexpected compensatory skills and abilities, sometimes with assistive devices or work site adjustments.

Employers must recognize that the major changes in federal law that result from passage of the ADA are intended to enable even more workers to enter the workforce in a nondiscriminatory manner. Everyone who interacts with business and industry—workers, managers, human resource officers, and occupational health physicians—should familiarize themselves with the new regulation to facilitate their smooth implementation. These are summarized briefly in the following list. If a question remains about a particular area, it is imperative to seek additional information to clarify the new regulations.

- The definition of "disability" is broad and includes individuals with human immunodeficiency virus infection or facial disfigurement, for example.
- The requirement for "reasonable accommodation" imposes a "de minimis" or minor obligation on employers to provide an accessible and usable work environment to qualified applicants and employees.
- Application and interview forms must be reviewed and changed to limit the type of health-related information that employers may now only obtain after a job offer has been made, and then only for purposes of medical coverage and job restructuring.
- Medical examinations are prohibited before the offer of employment, and examinations after an offer of employment must be requested of all employees in that job category. Employers must show reasonable cause for the withdrawal of a job offer, such as safety and health risks to other employees or the unreasonableness of accommodating a particular employee without any viable alternatives.
- Employers should clearly delineate the essential functions of a job in a written job description before interviewing for and filling a position, in order to hire individuals capable of performing those essential functions, with reasonable accommodation provided if necessary.
- Employment policies and practices should foster neither disparate treatment nor disparate impact, in which disabled employees experience a hostile or discriminatory working environment.
- Employees alleging intentional discrimination may seek punitive and compensatory damages from the courts and can request jury trials to hear the case.
- Employers may not discriminate against disabled employees in providing an equal work environment and benefits.[3]

Despite the predictions of unreasonable costs and demands on business, an ongoing survey by the Job Accommodation Network (JAN) shows that very few employees with disabilities request or need any accommodations, more than three fourths of the accommodations cost less than $1,000, and more than half cost less than $500.[6] The JAN, a resource service of the President's Committee on Employment of People with Disabilities, also found that almost half the surveyed firms making accommodations valued the benefits they receive at more than $10,000, both in increased productivity and money saved in recruitment, retraining, health insurance, and worker's compensation costs. Rather than being a cost burden, reasonable accommodations can lead to financial benefits to industry, particularly if the spirit of the ADA is applied proactively throughout the workplace. Often, reasonable accommodation is no more than work reorganization, and industrywide scrutiny of jobs and work environments can lead to a reduction in injuries and claims for work-related illness. This is especially true for the costly and difficult to diagnose and treat area of "low back pain."

An unexpected finding of the JAN survey was the discovery that "back impairment" is the disability most frequently cited in Equal Employment Opportunity Commission complaints since implementation of the ADA in 1992. More than 20% of the cases claiming violation of the ADA were back related, and only about 10% were from "traditional" disability claimants. This finding, disturbing to businesses because they fear that anyone with low back pain can sue if they are fired, is a positive move toward redirecting efforts in the treatment and prevention of back pain. According to Dr. Gerald Weisman, director of Rehabilitation Technology Services at the Vermont Rehabilitation Engineering Center in Burlington, these statistics show that back injuries are too often mishandled by business, mostly because people focused too much on curing back pain instead of curing the workplace.[6] The ADA, with its focus on task analysis and reasonable accommodation, will support a movement toward redesigning work in an ergonomic, creative way.

References

1. Carmean G: The Americans with Disabilities Act: tie medical screening to the job, *Human Resources Magazine,* Arlington, Va, July, 1992; p. 85.

2. Equal Employment Opportunity Commission: *Technical assistance manual on the employment provisions (Title I) of the ADA,* EEOC-M-1A, January 1992, EEOC; p I-5.

3. Fox JC: *Challenges and opportunities for occupational health professionals and human resource managers. The Americans with Disabilities Act of 1990: countdown to compromise: what to do now.* Paper presented at the American College of Occupational and Environmental Medicine Intensive Training Course, New York, Oct 30-31, 1992.

4. Grandjean E: *Fitting the task to the man: an ergonomic approach,* London, 1988, Taylor & Francis.

5. Job Accommodation Network: *The Americans with Disabilities Act of 1990,* PL 101-336, Morgantown, WVa, 1990, JAN.

6. Minton E: Accommodation between a rock and a hard place, *Occup Health Saf,* 63(8):60-64, 1994.

7. Public Law 101-336, 1990.

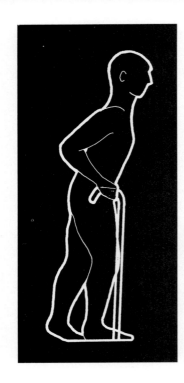

Chapter 52

Preemployment and Preplacement Evaluations and the Americans with Disabilities Act

Jay Himmelstein
Glenn Pransky
*David Fram**

CONTENTS

*David Fram is an ADA Policy Attorney in the Office of Legal Counsel, U.S. Equal Employment Opportunity Commission (EEOC). Before joining the EEOC, Mr Fram practiced law at the Washington, D.C., law firm of Hogan and Hartson after graduating from Cornell Law School. Mr. Fram contributed to this article in his private capacity. No official support or endorsement by the commission or any other agency of the U.S. government is intended or should be inferred.

Support for this project comes, in part, from NIOSH/CDC cooperative agreement No. U60/CCU106156.

Clinicians involved in primary care and orthopaedics are commonly confronted with situations in which employers attempt to control worker's compensation and other costs by using medical testing to identify the "most fit" or safest workers. Preemployment examinations (including preplacement/"postoffer" examinations, which are done after an employment offer has been extended but before work has begun) are but a subset of situations in which clinicians are asked to make determinations about a worker's employability. Broadly defined, *worker fitness and risk evaluations* include all evaluations that are administered by medical personnel to determine a worker's ability to perform specific job tasks and to determine risk in relation to anticipated workplace exposure. Although these examinations are usually done at the request of an employer in situations where jobs are thought to be especially physically demanding or hazardous, they are becoming increasingly common for nonhazardous jobs as well.

As illustrated by the following case examples, preplacement examinations used to determine employability can be complicated by a number of technical, ethical, and legal factors. Despite the prevalence of these examinations and the potential significance of the findings, a dearth of scientific literature is available to guide physicians on the proper collection, analysis, and use of the data requested. In these situations, clinicians must balance their ethical responsibilities as professionals in the context of liability, malpractice, and antidiscrimination law.

- A patient requests that his physician complete an employment form certifying that he can safely lift 100 lb. You know from the patient's medical history that he has had recurrent back pain. What should your response be to an employer who asks for such certification and what type of evaluation would be appropriate in this case?
- An individual is referred to you by a local employer for a preplacement evaluation for a forklift driver job. The individual has a history of having had successful low back surgery performed by one of your colleagues. The company is asking you whether it is "safe" for this former patient to do the forklift job, which requires driving a forklift in

the sitting position and involves occasional "heavy" lifting. How should you evaluate this patient and how should the results be reported to the employer?
- One of your private patients asks for an appointment for the purpose of filling out employment forms. He has been hired by a local warehouse company but does not know yet what his job will be. You are asked to certify his ability to do a job about which you have no information. What should you do?
- A local employer asks you to perform "preemployment" examinations on all new employees in the interest of controlling worker's compensation costs. The employer would like you to design a screening program that includes medical examination and strength testing so that only workers who are not at risk of back pain are cleared to work at heavy jobs in this factory. What should your response be?

Recent legislation has recognized that employment examinations have been a common cause of discrimination against people with disabilities. In passing the Americans with Disabilities Act (ADA) of 1990, Congress targeted a number of medical practices that were believed to be discriminatory, including (1) exclusions of individuals with disabilities based on risks that are uncertain or anticipated only years later, (2) exclusions of individuals with disabilities based on anticipated future health or worker's compensation costs, and (3) "blanket" exclusions of an entire group of people with similar disabilities if those exclusions are not "job related and consistent with business necessity."[6,8]

In this chapter we describe the key features and implications of the ADA as it applies to preplacement or postoffer examinations and develop an approach to decision making that concentrates on common misconceptions relating to these examinations. We also characterize the key elements of a model preplacement program. This review is intended to enable clinicians to implement preplacement examinations in a scientifically and legally sound manner.[4,5]

SCOPE AND CONTEXT OF THE AMERICANS WITH DISABILITIES ACT

The ADA has been described as the most sweeping antidiscrimination legislation in the United States since the Civil Rights Act of 1964. A previous federal statute, the Rehabilitation Act of 1973, prohibited discrimination against an otherwise qualified individual with a handicap on the basis of that handicap in any program or activity that received federal financial assistance, by certain federal government contractors, and by most federal government agencies. The ADA, on the other hand, is not tied to the receipt of federal funds and thus covers a much larger percentage of the American workforce.[10]

The ADA consists of five major sections or titles:

- Title I prohibits discrimination against "qualified individuals with disabilities" in job application procedures, compensation, promotion, discharge, job training, and other conditions of employment.
- Title II prohibits the exclusion of persons with disabilities from participation in benefits, services, and activities offered by government entities and requires that public transportation be accessible.
- Title III guarantees to persons with disabilities access to privately operated places of public accommodation (for example, restaurants, banks, retail and department stores, and other similar places).
- Title IV requires telephone companies to provide interstate and intrastate telecommunication relay services so that hearing- and speech-impaired individuals can communicate with individuals who do not have hearing or speech impairments.
- The miscellaneous provisions of Title V say, among other things, that state laws that offer greater or equal protection are not preempted by the ADA.

Americans with Disabilities Act Employment Provisions

Title I of the ADA prohibits employment discrimination against a "qualified individual with a disability" on account of that disability. An individual with a disability is defined in the ADA as someone who

1. Has a physical or mental impairment that substantially limits one or more major life activities
2. Has a record of such impairment
3. Is regarded as having such an impairment[11]

Individuals are "qualified" for a job if they meet the basic job prerequisites and if they can perform the "essential functions" of the job with or without "reasonable accommodation." The ADA requires employers to make reasonable accommodations for qualified individuals with disabilities unless these accommodations impose an "undue hardship." Reasonable accommodation means modifications or adjustments to the application process to enable someone with a disability to apply for a job, modifications or adjustments to the manner or circumstances in which a job is performed so that an individual with a disability can perform the job, and modifications or adjustments to enable an employee to enjoy equal benefits and privileges of employment.

Under the ADA, employers may not conduct *medical examinations* or make *disability-related inquiries* of applicants before they are extended a conditional offer of employment. These prohibitions help ensure that an applicant's nonmedical qualifications are considered before the medical condition is evaluated. Whether an examination is "medical" depends on the particular examination and revolves around a list of factors that are indicative of medical examinations. These include such factors as whether the examination is designed or

intended to reveal an individual's health or impairments, whether it is invasive, and whether it measures an individual's performance of a task or physiologic responses to performance. Whether inquiries are "disability related" depends on whether the inquiry is likely to elicit information about a disability.

After an individual is offered a job but before starting work, an employer may require such examinations and may make such inquiries if these are given to all entering employees in the job category. Although an employer may obtain medical/disability-related information at the post-offer stage, the ADA restricts employers' subsequent actions based on this information. An employer may withdraw a conditional job offer because of an individual's disability *only* if the employer can show one of the following:

1. The individual cannot perform the essential functions of the job despite reasonable accommodations.
2. The individual poses a "direct threat" to self or others in the position that cannot be reasonably accommodated.
3. Other federal laws or regulations—such as Federal Aviation Administration (FAA) or the Department of Transportation (DOT) regulations—require the employer to withdraw the job offer because of the individual's medical condition.

THE ROLE OF THE HEALTH PROFESSIONAL UNDER THE AMERICANS WITH DISABILITIES ACT

The ADA places requirements on employers that are aimed at providing equal employment opportunities for people with disabilities. The role of medical professionals in this process is primarily to provide guidance on whether an individual has a covered disability, whether the individual is qualified, and whether the individual poses a direct threat, and to provide recommendations regarding workplace accommodations. The U.S. Equal Employment Opportunity Commission[2] (EEOC) has issued a technical assistance manual to help employers and persons with disabilities learn about their obligations and rights under the employment provisions of the ADA. This manual provides numerous examples that illustrate the subjects discussed in the following sections and will be quite helpful to healthcare providers who are involved with patients who may have a covered disability.

Does the Individual Have a Covered Disability?

The health professional can assist the employer in determining whether an individual has a physical or mental impairment and whether the impairment substantially limits a major life activity such as seeing, hearing, speaking, breathing, learning, performing manual tasks, sitting, standing, lifting, reaching, and working. In the simplest case, this role can be fulfilled merely by providing information regarding an impairment that limits one or more major life activities. For example, a patient who has nerve damage that substantially interferes with walking would have an impairment that "substantially limits one or more major life activities" and would therefore have a covered disability. Likewise, a potential employee who has fully recovered from back surgery but is limited by an inability to lift objects weighing more than 5 lb from floor level would be considered to have a covered disability.

Interestingly, if individuals claim coverage under the ADA because they are substantially limited in the major life activity of "working," they must be unable to perform a class of jobs or a broad range of jobs. A person's inability to do one particular job generally would not make that person substantially limited in "working." For example, an individual whose back impairment prevented the performance of one specific job would not be covered under the ADA (unless, as described later, the employer regarded that individual as unable to perform a class of jobs or a broad range of jobs). On the other hand, if the individual's back impairment prevented the performance of any heavy-labor job, that person would be substantially limited in performing a class of jobs.

It is worth noting again that a physician's determination that someone has no actual disability does not completely resolve the matter. Individuals may have a covered disability if an employer simply "regards" them as having a disability. For example, an employer may regard potential employees who have successfully recovered from carpal tunnel surgery as high risk and thus unemployable in any position. This perception alone may, under certain circumstances, make the potential employee covered under the ADA.

Is the Individual Fit to Do the Job?

An employer may ask medical professionals to determine whether an individual is capable of performing a job. In general, this is a determination that is very difficult to make in the medical setting with any degree of certainty. The EEOC[2] has targeted medical disqualifications of employees with disabilities as a major area of concern because of the unnecessary discrimination in the hiring process that has resulted. For example, it is unlikely that certain medical conditions (such as mild scoliosis, previous back surgery, or asymptomatic spondylolisthesis), if present, would automatically result in an individual's inability to perform a job that involves some lifting. In fact, it would be hard to predict with any degree of certainty whether an individual with prior low back pain would or would not be able to perform certain tasks based on an examination in the doctor's office. Therefore it is most appropriate that questions of "fitness" be answered through approaches such as job simulation or job-specific testing rather than through guesswork based on physician examination.

Does the Individual Pose a Direct Threat?

An employer may require that an individual not pose a "direct threat" to the health or safety of self or others in performance of the job. However, the requirements to meet the direct-threat threshold as specified under the ADA are quite stringent. The risk must be significant (highly probable) and the potential harm must be substantial (severe); the risk factors must be based on objective medical data, not speculation or generalization from studies of large groups or similar persons; the risk must be constant, not temporary; and finally, the risk must be one that cannot be reduced below the direct threat level through reasonable accommodation.[1]

As described, the direct-threat standard is quite exacting and, in effect, makes it extremely risky for physicians to disqualify applicants based on future risk. Physicians performing preplacement examinations should become familiar with the limitations of these examinations' ability to determine fitness or risk, especially the limitations in predicting a future adverse outcome. A number of considerations are important here, including the possibility of compensatory changes (strength, ability, technique) over time, the ability of workers and employers to adjust the job demands, variability in the nature and manifestation of disease processes, regression to the mean of laboratory tests, and difficulty in using clinically derived normal ranges to define functionally significant abnormalities. The evaluating health professional should address these areas in advising the employer regarding the direct-threat standard.

What Accommodations Are Appropriate?

An important and positive role for medical personnel is the recommendation of reasonable accommodations that would allow a person to perform the essential functions of the job. This, of course, requires that the evaluating health provider have detailed information about the job requirements or personal knowledge of the job through visiting the workplace or by reviewing videotapes extensively reflecting the workplace and work performed (See Chapters 14 and 15). In the example of the patient with gait difficulties described earlier, it may be that the only accommodation needed is wheelchair access to a desk so that the patient can perform a data entry clerk job. In the case of the patient with prior back surgery, recommendations for accommodation may be more complex. For example, if "lifting" is not an essential function of the job, reassigning the lifting duties to another employee would be an appropriate accommodation. If "lifting" is an essential function, the clinician might suggest certain equipment to help the employee perform this function despite the physical limitations. In many cases, the physician may not be the ideal person to conceive such accommodations. It is important that clinicians recognize their limitations in this respect and request assistance in their decision-making process.

DESIGNING A MODEL PREPLACEMENT EVALUATION PROGRAM

Based on the requirements of the ADA, scientific principles, and ethical medical practice, several considerations are of paramount importance in designing an appropriate program for medical evaluations of fitness to work.[3]

A model program should begin with medical staff education about the ADA and the scientific limitations of preplacement examinations in predicting fitness or risk. Examiners should avoid participating in evaluations that occur before a conditional job offer, and both employers and examiners should have reasonable, realistic expectations about the benefits (if any) to be gained from conducting these evaluations. Each examiner should be familiar with the job for which the examination is being performed. This should include knowledge of job requirements, applicable medical standards, federal regulations, working conditions and hazards, emergency requirements, and available accommodations. Usually this information is best obtained through a work site visit. The examination should be designed with specific goals in mind—such as establishing a baseline for future medical surveillance, determining whether an individual can physically perform the job tasks required, determining what, if any, harm to the individual or others could result if the individual was placed in the job, identifying individuals with medical problems that could be exacerbated by work, or satisfying examination requirements of the U.S. Department of Transportation in relation to truck drivers.

Although not required by the ADA, examiners should also take the following steps to be in compliance with other legal and ethical precedents. Examiners should be aware that patient participation in preplacement medical examinations is not, in an ethical sense, entirely voluntary. Patients agree to participate because they want/need the job. Therefore, examiners must take great care in explaining the content and process of the examination. Patients should be informed of the rationale for each element of the examination, even though the examination does not have to be entirely work related. Examiners should explain what information will be released to the employer and what will remain confidential. Patients also need to understand the potential uses of the information generated by the examination, including the possibility that it could result in modification or, in rare instances, withdrawal of the job offer. Finally, patients should be informed that the medical evaluation is narrowly focused on work-related issues and in no way constitutes an overall assessment of their health status.

Examiners should be prepared to explain to both employers and patients the results of any test performed in relation to predictions of job fitness and risk; abnormal values should also be communicated to the patient, with advice for follow-up with a primary care provider.

Although this is not required by the ADA, specific communication forms can be used to ensure that only information that is essential for safe job placement be given to employers (for example, see Appendix A). If there are concerns about fitness or a direct threat to self or others, communication between the physician, employer, and patient should be an interactive, ongoing process to discuss abilities, limitations, and suggested accommodations. This is important, inasmuch as it is ultimately the employer's legal responsibility to make a decision regarding job qualification.

Additional information of a medical nature may be reported to qualified first-aid personnel if relevant (such as informing local first-aid providers at a plant site that a new employee has a seizure disorder). However, all medical information collected in the examination should be treated as confidential and kept in a medical file separate from personnel files. Although the ADA does not prohibit employers from obtaining this information, medical ethical considerations encourage healthcare providers to protect the confidentiality of medical information and release information to employers only as required under the ADA to make decisions on fitness or risk.[7]

A Note on the Use of "Objective" Tests and Devices

A typical physician office examination usually provides few objective data to aid in determining fitness or risk for a particular job. Similar "abnormal" findings are seen in job applicants, individuals who have had injuries performing certain tasks, and persons without *any* problems who are currently performing the same job activities. Numerous testing devices have been developed to provide more quantitative data on strength, range of motion, and nerve function. Measurements of maximum lifting, pushing, pulling, gripping, and pinching force, as well as range of motion measurements, can be obtained. For physical capacity measurements, these devices usually measure the force exerted by the subject against fixed object (isometric force) or a moving object with either a fixed (isotonic) or variable (isokinetic) resistance. Those devices used to measure back function may also record range of motion, usually as back flexion/extension. Other screening devices have been developed to measure median nerve motor or sensory function to target workers at risk for carpal tunnel syndrome. Frequently, these tests and devices are marketed to employers and medical professionals as "objective" and "legally defensible" under the ADA.

Very few data have been published on the reliability or validity of many of these measurements; independent studies have demonstrated test-retest reliability usually no greater than 0.5 to 0.8 in individuals with a history of back problems.[9] Validity is of even greater concern; the motions and tasks performed by subjects when using these machines usually differ significantly from work activities. In most heavy lifting jobs, for example, the work activities are usually much more complex and varied than the test activity. Although there may be some correlation between gross measures of strength, such as those derived from these devices, and risk of future low back injury in heavy lifting jobs, the predictive power for a given *individual* is low unless the tested individual demonstrates symptoms or an inability to perform a task in a similar position with a similar weight as that encountered on the job.

A reasonable alternative and a more valid, but less quantitative measure of work ability and risk can be obtained through work simulation. Many physical therapy practices have developed in-house work simulation capabilities. This process begins with work site assessment, where sample work materials are collected, work activities are videotaped, and weights and distances are measured. A work simulation is then developed during which prospective employees are observed while performing a variety of typical work tasks. These approaches may be most effective with heavy lifting jobs or jobs involving gross motor activities such as climbing, pushing, and pulling. However, employers concerned about risks of future cumulative trauma disorders should be aware that simulated work activities are unlikely to provoke short-term pain in upper extremity–intensive jobs in the work simulation setting. Minor muscle aches that develop in this setting are probably more consistent with early task adjustment, and no correlation with the development of future cumulative trauma disorders has been documented.

In summary, a variety of approaches are available to quantify a worker's maximal force capability in performing simple, stereotypic movements. Work simulation is less quantitative but has significant advantages with greater validity in determining actual work capability. All these approaches are limited in their ability to predict actual worker fitness or future risk; they cannot incorporate the effect of worker training, skills development, job changes or accommodations, and progression or regression of future medical problems. Nothing about these tests or devices changes the employer's responsibilities or liabilities under the ADA or the medical professional's obligation to scientific and ethical practice. Often, the most useful role for the ethical medical practitioner is to appropriately inform employers about the limitations of these approaches.

SUMMARY

It is clear that active participation in enhancing employment of people with disabilities requires an expanded base of information for practicing clinicians. Several caveats are worth emphasizing:

1. *The evaluation of workers must be individualized to a specific person and a specific set of job tasks.* Except for certain situations with requirements established

under federal laws, physicians and employers are prohibited from relying on nonspecific "physical standards" that exclude an individual on the basis of disability unless it has been demonstrated that those who fail to meet the standards because of a disability constitute a "direct threat" to themselves or others that cannot be reasonably accommodated or cannot perform essential job tasks with reasonable accommodations.

2. *A person's ability to do a job is often best determined by a job simulation or job trial.* Many of the best methods for determining fitness will therefore be nonmedical, and the role of the medical examination may be minimal in determining employability. Moreover, determining a person's future risk of injury or disease progression is especially complicated and filled with potential liability for the evaluating clinician and the employer. The physician should be careful to ensure that employers are aware of the very limited benefit of preplacement medical evaluations of worker fitness and risk.

3. *Healthcare providers are clinicians, not lawyers or personnel managers.* Although health professionals need to become conversant with their role under the law, it is not their duty to act as legal counsel to the employer or employee. Although providers should communicate with employers, they must remember that it is not their responsibility to make employment decisions. However, they should also recognize that in most cases, their advice will be given considerable weight in employment decisions. The physician's responsibility is to provide medical opinions and guidance regarding disability status, functional capability, and direct threat and, where appropriate, to recommend modifications and accommodations to mitigate risk or enhance capabilities. The responsibility for making employment decisions or deciding whether it is possible to make a reasonable accommodation for a person with a disability lies with the employer, who is expected to incorporate information from a variety of sources (including other health professionals and disability experts) in making employment decisions.

The ultimate impact of the ADA on the makeup of the American workplace will not be known for many years. However, it seems likely that if the ADA is successful in removing barriers for people with disabilities, physicians and other healthcare providers will play a key role in facilitating the integration of people with disabilities into the workplace. To accomplish this, clinicians need to shift from their traditional focus on diagnosing disability to recognizing and enhancing capability.

References

1. 29 C.F.R., Section 1630.2(r).

2. Equal Employment Opportunity Commission: *A technical assistance manual on the employment provisions (Title I) of the Americans with Disabilities Act*, Washington, DC, 1992, US Government Printing Office.

3. Goldsmith N: *Understanding the Americans with Disabilities Act: a compliance guide for health professionals and employers*, Beverly, Mass, 1993, OEM Press.

4. Himmelstein JS, Andersson GBJ: Low back pain: risk evaluation and pre-placement screening, *Occup Med*, 3:255-269, 1988.

5. Himmelstein JS, Pransky GS: The ADA and you: implications for the occupational health professional, *J Occup Med*, 34:(5): 501-502, 1992.

6. House of Representatives Rep No 485, pt 3, 101st Congress, 2nd session: *House Committee on the Judiciary,* Washington, DC, 1989, US Government Printing Office.

7. Rest K: Ethical issues in providing occupational health services, *J Ambul Care Manage*, 17(2):53-62, 1994.

8. Senate Rep No 116, 101st Congress 1st session: *Senate Committee on Labor and Human Resources,* Washington, DC, 1989, US Government Printing Office.

9. Troup J, Foreman T, Baxter C, Brown D: The perception of back pain and the role of psychological tests of lifting capacity, *Spine* 7:645-657.

10. 29 U.S.C. Sections 791, 793, 794.

11. 42 U.S.C. Section 12102.

APPENDIX A

SAMPLE: REPORT OF PRE-PLACEMENT MEDICAL EVALUATION

Entering Employee name _____ Date _____

Employer _____

Job title _____

Based upon my evaluation of this entering employee on this date:

_____ 1. There are no medical contraindications to performing the described job without accommodation.

_____ 2. There are no medical contraindications to performing this job, with the following recommended accommodations, or job training:

_____

_____

_____ 3. Without an accommodation, this employee may be at risk for substantial harm (as described below) in performing the job for which she/he was evaluated.

_____

_____

_____ 4. See attached statement of abilities.

_____ 5. Medical hold: waiting for additional data. Re-evaluate on _____.

_____ 6. Further testing is required to fully evaluate ability or risk.

Comments: _____

_____

If 2,3,4 or 6 above are checked, please call me at xxx-xxx-xxxx to discuss this further, including recommendations for other information which may aid in accommodations or clarification of risk.

Any attached information on medical conditions should be treated as confidential medical information, in accordance with the Americans with Disabilities Act, with distribution only as authorized under the law.

_____   _____   _____
Employee   MD   Date

Index

Note: Page numbers in *italics* indicate illustrations and legends; "t" following page numbers indicates tables.